Eighth Edition

Novak's

Gynecologic and Obstetric Pathology

With Clinical and Endocrine Relations

EDMUND R. NOVAK, A.B., M.D.

Associate Professor of Gynecology, The Johns Hopkins University
School of Medicine; Gynecologist, Johns Hopkins and Union Memorial
Hospitals, and Greater Baltimore Medical Center, Baltimore, Maryland

J. DONALD WOODRUFF, B.S., M.D.

Professor, Obstetrics and Gynecology,
Richard W. TeLinde Professor of Gynecologic Pathology,
Johns Hopkins Hospital, Baltimore, Maryland

902 illustrations—18 in color

1979

W. B. SAUNDERS COMPANY / Philadelphia / London / Toronto

W. B. Saunders Company: West Washington Square
                          Philadelphia, PA 19105

                          1 St. Anne's Road
                          Eastbourne, East Sussex BN21, 3UN, England

                          1 Goldthorne Avenue
                          Toronto, Ontario M8Z 5T9, Canada

Novak's Gynecologic and Obstetric Pathology
with Clinical and Endocrine Relations   ISBN   0-7216-6869-0

Last digit is the print number: 9   8   7   6   5   4   3   2   1

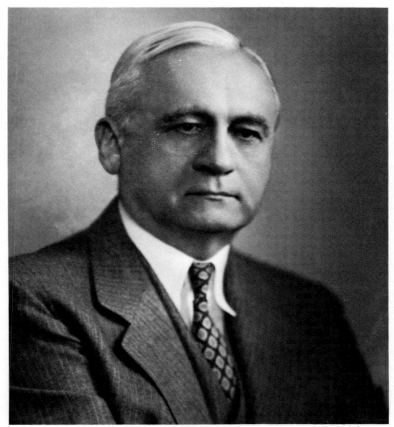

Udel Bros.

In Memoriam

EMIL NOVAK

February 3, 1957

To Our Families

CONTRIBUTORS

JOHN K. FROST, M.D. Professor of Pathology, Johns Hopkins University School of Medicine; Pathologist and Head, Department of Cytopathology, Johns Hopkins Hospital, Baltimore, Maryland
Cytopathology

CARL J. PAUERSTEIN, M.D. Professor of Obstetrics and Gynecology and Professor of Physiology, The University of Texas Health Science Center at San Antonio; Chief, Gynecologic Service, Bexar County Hospital District, San Antonio, Texas
Fertilization; Placental Abnormalities; Pathology of Abortion

PREFACE
TO
THE
EIGHTH
EDITION

The eighth edition of our textbook has appeared somewhat later than new editions usually appear, but the last revision was so well received and has continued to have such a wide sale that we have procrastinated. Actually in a pathologic text there are usually relatively few truly revolutional concepts and new thoughts in any decade, and this seems especially true in the 1970s. There has been considerable experimentation in various methods of population control, and we have attempted a more detailed explanation and illustration as to how these may modify pelvic pathology. Newer concepts of oncology have likewise been reevaluated. In an effort to save space, we have on occasion abbreviated the titles of certain references, but the references themselves seem up to date. Various older ones may be found in earlier editions.

We trust that this eighth edition of our textbook will receive the same warm reception, and will continue to have the same extensive sale, as our previous edition. We have tried to improve it in every way possible. At the same time we have tried to streamline it somewhat to avoid making it too bulky and cumbersome. We had occasion to note that the seventh edition was approximately twice the size of the fourth edition, which was published in 1956 by Novak and Novak.

Obviously any pathology textbook will be concerned with oncology, and every attempt has been made to update the book by covering the newest and most recent concepts without becoming too involved with the treatment of these diseases, which seems permissible in a primarily pathologic textbook. As mentioned in earlier editions, it is our feeling that the TNM method of classification of the extent of pelvic tumors is extremely cumbersome and impractical, and consequently we have not utilized it extensively in this text.

Since this pathologic textbook is widely read over the entire world and appears in many different languages, we have enlarged discussion of various tropical disorders that may afflict the female genital tract. This addition follows many suggestions by Middle and Far Eastern critics; although we have expanded our coverage, we still feel that these subjects belong primarily in various textbooks of tropical medicine, so coverage here is not extensive.

Adequate illustrative material is of extreme importance in any pathologic treatise, and we have continued to try to improve on these. In most instances black and white photographs seem satisfactory, but we have included a number of color plates, some of which are new in this textbook.

We should like to welcome Dr. Carl Pauerstein as a contributor to this text, and thank him for his outstanding chapters. We continue our appreciation to Dr. J. K. Frost for his well written chapter on cytopathology, which has received the highest approval in previous reviews of this textbook. Aside from these, we are the sole authors, and although each of us is responsible for certain chapters, there is frequent mutual discussion, so that the vast majority of the text represents a compendium of our ideas. This seems preferable to presenting isolated chapters by a variety of authors, who may discuss closely allied topics with a lack of consistency and coordination.

We wish to formally thank those who have been good enough to send material to our laboratory. In all cases we have attempted to give proper acknowledgment, but we may have inadvertently omitted credit in a few instances. On occasion we have utilized pictures that may not be of the highest technical quality, but this seems justifiable if it allows illustration of lesions only rarely encountered.

We are indebted to a number of individuals whose ideas or illustrations are incorporated. Thanks for invaluable help as always go to Miss Helen Clayton, as well as to Chester Reather and Raymond (Pete) Lund of our Photographic Department. We should also like to express our gratitude to the many nice people associated with the W. B. Saunders Company, who were so helpful and cognizant of the various difficulties associated with compiling this edition. Thanks again go to The Williams & Wilkins Company for permission to use various illustrations and figures, which we have done without specific notation.

We sincerely trust this edition of the text will represent continued improvement. We feel strongly that this is a legacy of Emil Novak and warrants our utmost dedicated efforts.

EDMUND R. NOVAK, M.D.

J. DONALD WOODRUFF, M.D.

CONTENTS

Mesothelial Reactions and the Mesothelioma..................................... 426

Unspecified Designations—Undifferentiated Carcinoma
(Primary Solid Carcinoma of Ovary)... 430

Extension and Metastasis of Ovarian Carcinoma........................... 430

Treatment and Salvage of Ovarian Cancer 433

Chapter 22

**OVARIAN NEOPLASIA: STROMOEPITHELIAL LESIONS
—PRIMARILY STROMAL (BRENNER TUMORS, FIBROTHE-
COMAS, SARCOMAS, ETC.)**.. 437

Brenner Tumors of the Ovary... 441

Tumors with Functioning Matrix 449

Chapter 23

**OVARIAN NEOPLASIA: PRIMARILY STROMAL LESIONS
(FIBROMA, FIBROTHECOMA INCLUDING THE MIXED
MESODERMAL TUMORS)**.. 451

Stromal Tumors 451

Fibroma (Fibrothecoma) 451

Other Solid Tumors 455

Ovarian Sarcomas 455

Lymphoma... 459

Chapter 24

OVARIAN NEOPLASIA: METASTATIC LESIONS 461

Tumors Arising in the Genital Canal... 461

Metastatic Lesions with an Extragenital Primary Tumor............... 464

The Krukenberg Tumor of the Ovary 471

Primary Krukenberg Tumors 473

Chapter 25

GERM CELL TUMORS.. 476

PART I. *DYSGERMINOMA OF THE OVARY*

Germ Cell Tumors... 476

Germ Cell Tumors and Precursory Conditions 476

Dysgerminoma (Germinoma)... 477

Gonadoblastoma 485

PART II. *OVARIAN TERATOMAS*

Chapter 26

GONADAL STROMAL TUMORS—FEMINIZING (GRANULOSA AND THECA CELL)

Chapter 27

Chapter 28

Chapter 29

PELVIC ENDOMETRIOSIS 561

Chapter 30

FERTILIZATION, IMPLANTATION, AND PLACENTATION 585

Carl J. Pauerstein

Chapter 34

GYNECOLOGIC AND OBSTETRIC CLINICAL CYTOPATHOLOGY

John K. Frost

Chapter 1

DISEASES OF THE VULVA

NORMAL HISTOLOGY OF VULVA

The external genitalia—specifically the labia majora and minora, the clitoris, and the vestibule with its associated glands—are of ectodermal origin (Fig. 1–1). The labia majora are longitudinal folds of fat whose lining epithelium is stratified squamous, with varying degrees of surface maturation and keratinization, and with an underlying layer of connective tissue corresponding to the dartos of the male scrotum. The labia majora are practically absent in the young child, their development—primarily the deposition of fat—being one of the secondary sex characteristics heralding puberty. The skin of the more prominent portions of the labia is pigmented. These folds are rich in hair follicles, sebaceous glands, and sudoriferous glands (Fig. 1–2). The latter include the unique apocrine glands found in special areas, e.g., the axilla, perianal region, and breast, and characterized by "decapitation" secretion, in contrast to the characteristic cellular loss of the sebaceous (holocrine) gland and the cytoplasmic secretory activity of the merocrine gland (Fig. 1–3). Because the onset of secretion occurs at puberty and the cyclic nature of the activity corresponds to that of the ovary, Way and Memmesheimer consider these apocrine glands to be "accessory sex glands." The knowledge of this cyclic activity is important in the diagnosis and treatment of certain vulvar diseases.

The mons pubis (mons veneris) is a cushion of fat covered by skin and its appendages, including the apocrine glands. The labia minora are firmer structures than the majora, and are composed primarily of vascular connective tissue. The surface stratified epithelium is characterized by a relative absence of both the granular layer of the epithelium and hair follicles. The numerous sebaceous glands secrete directly onto the skin through epithelial tunnels (Fig. 1–4). Apocrine glands, although present, are infrequent.

The clitoris, like its male homologue, is made up of vascular erectile tissue, differing from the penis in that it lacks the corpus spongiosum. From an embryologic standpoint the two vestibulovaginal bulbs, which are congeries of veins situated beneath the anterior portion of the labial structures, correspond in the female to a divided corpus cavernosum, i.e., they are made up of two corpora with an intricate network of nerves (Fig. 1–5).

The female urethra, opening externally at the meatus urinarius, is lined by transitional epithelium with the stratified epithelium of the vaginal mucosa present at or near the orifice. At the lower border of the meatus are the openings of the Skene's ducts (paraurethral ducts), tiny tortuous canals coursing just beneath the urethra for a distance of about 1.5 cm.; they are lined by squamous epithelium, and may be the seat of infection inaccessible to treatment by local applications. Studies have shown that the canal is almost completely surrounded by a labyrinth of paraurethral glands entering the distal urethra from its posterior aspect. Huffman considered these structures to be the homologues of the male prostate.

Occlusion of one or more of these glands produces cyst formation and the subsequent infection may result in the development of a suburethral abscess, an occasional cause of urinary retention in the female. In cases of recurrent urinary tract infection, the paraurethral canals should be suspected as a

Text continued on page 6

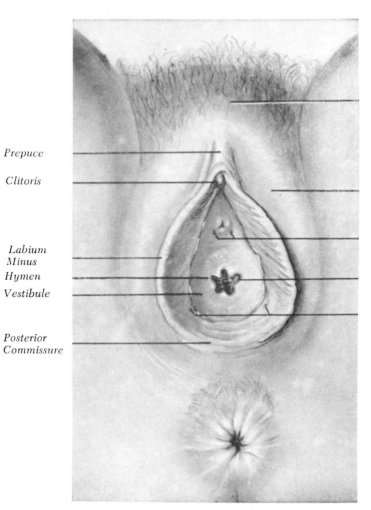

Mons Pubis

Prepuce

Clitoris

Labium Majus

Opening of Skene's Ducts

Labium Minus

Hymen

Vestibule

Vagina

Vulvovaginal (Bartholin's) Glands

Posterior Commissure

Figure 1–1. The Vulva.

Figure 1–2. Normal stratified epithelium of labium majus with hair follicles, sebaceous glands, and sweat glands.

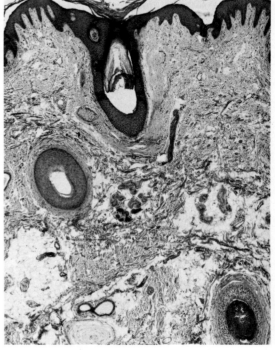

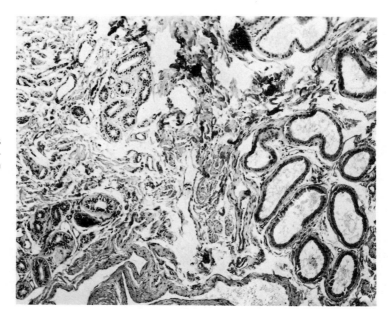

Figure 1–3. The larger apocrine glands on right, lined by cells with abundant pink-staining cytoplasm, may be compared with the smaller merocrine glands on left.

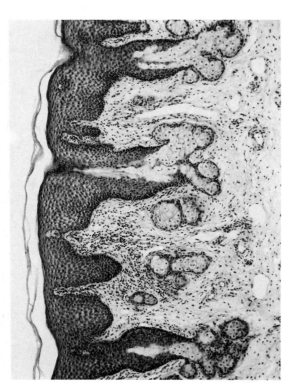

Figure 1–4. Section through labium minus showing sebaceous glands opening directly through stratified epithelium without hair follicles.

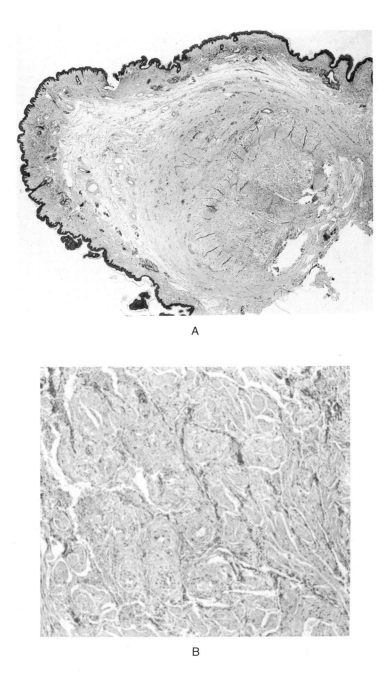

A

B

Figure 1–5. *A*, The clitoris, showing the two corpora cavernosa in right center with their striking vascular composition. *B*, Section through the erectile tissue of clitoris.

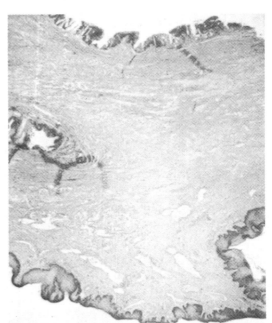

Figure 1–6. Section of hymen.

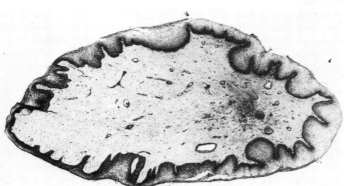

Figure 1–7. Section through a hymenal polyp removed from 2 day old child. Note the edematous stroma, somewhat suggestive of that seen in sarcoma botryoides.

Figure 1–8. High power of transitional epithelium in main duct of Bartholin's gland with the mucus-secreting acini.

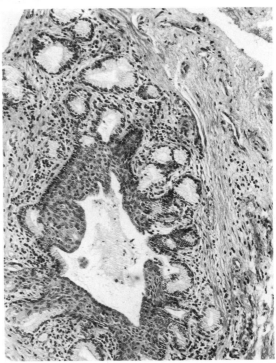

5

focus, especially in the absence of other pathologic lesions. Diverticula resulting from such processes may be demonstrated by positive pressure urethrography.

The hymen, partially closing the orifice of the vagina, consists of a double plate of stratified squamous epithelium (Fig. 1–6) between which is a well developed layer of firm, vascular, connective tissue. Residual tags of the hymen, carunculae hymenalis, are frequently noted at the introitus. "Hymenal polyps" have been reported in the first decade of life and must be differentiated from sarcoma botryoides (Fig. 1–7).

Finally, among these vulvar structures must be included Bartholin's glands (vulvovaginal glands), situated, one on each side, beneath the fascia in the depths of the perineum. The orifice of the gland occasionally may be seen at the introitus, approximately midway between the urethra and the fourchette. In chronic gonorrheal infections, which frequently involve this gland, the duct openings may be quite conspicuous and surrounded by an erythematous areola. These areolas initially were considered pathognomonic of gonococcal infection— the so-called gonorrheal macule of Sanger; however, many other organisms have been cultured from the purulent contents of the dilated duct.

The glands themselves are of racemose type, and their lobulation is of significance if surgical excision is indicated. Fortunately, such surgery is rarely necessary today, since marsupialization of the dilated duct usually affords adequate drainage and avoids more extensive dissection. Only if deep-seated infections recur or if the possibility of neoplasm exists is removal indicated.

The stratified epithelium at the orifice of the gland gives way to a transitional variety in the main duct. As the duct divides, the epithelium shows fewer and fewer layers, but the superficial layer of cells remains columnar or cuboidal. The acini themselves are lined by a mucus-secreting epithelium, with nuclei placed close to the basement membrane (Fig. 1–8).

It is important to appreciate that, as in the male, there are minor as well as major vestibular glands. The introitus, in many instances, is ringed with such small variants of the Bartholin's gland. These may be the seat of chronic or recurrent infections and irritation at the outlet.

IMFLAMMATORY DISEASE OF VULVA

Since the vulva is of ectodermal origin, the common inflammatory processes affecting it are similar to those found elsewhere on the skin. Probably the most frequent dermatitis is atopic or reactive resulting from an association of local moisture, retained by tight, "nonbreathing" clothing and local irritants (medications, colored or scented toilet paper, detergents, hygiene sprays, etc.). Often there is a history of recent use of antibiotics. In such cases the dermatitis is not the result of sensitivity to the antibiotic, but to a resultant candidiasis, both vaginal and vulvar. Thus it is important to study the vaginal flora, since the reaction to the discharge from the vaginitides may trigger the onset of acute vulvar inflammation.

During the acute phase of the dermatitis, there is erythema and edema, often associated with superficial traumatic excoriation due to pruritus. Specific patterns are usually noted in the more classic types. Acute lichen planus is diagnostically dramatic with its violaceous patches (Fig. 1–9), and intertrigo is seen as fissuring of the macerated skin in the intercrural or interlabial folds, most commonly in the obese patient. Biopsy in this phase shows the characteristic evidence of acute infection with superficial epithelial defects.

In the chronic dermatitides, classically the eczematoid, neurogenous, seborrheic and intertriginous types, the gross picture is altered by surface keratin, which produces a whitish or grayish white "leukoplakoid" discoloration (Fig. 1–10). Similarly, the microscopic pattern is characterized by hyperkeratosis, acanthosis, and chronic inflammatory infiltrate—features that have all been associated with "leukoplakia" (Fig. 1–11). The danger of basing a diagnosis on the microscopic pattern without thorough study of the gross lesion cannot be overemphasized. Furthermore, it must be *stated* and *restated* that the microscopic diagnosis of "leukoplakia" be eliminated because of the poor definition of the cellular criteria.

Pustular disease is not uncommon in the external genitalia. The hair follicle and its associated sebaceous gland form ideal bases for the entrapment of secretions due to occlusion of the shaft and subsequent focal infections. More significant in the develop-

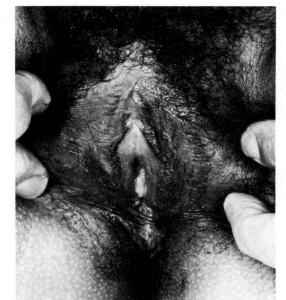

Figure 1–9. Lichen planus. The discolored areas to the left of clitoris and along the right inner labium majus represent the classic violaceous lesions of acute lichen planus.

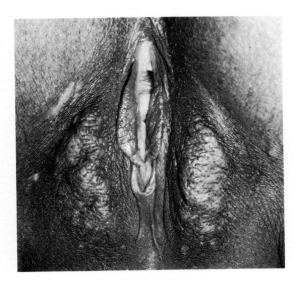

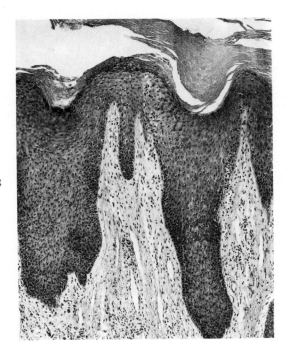

Figure 1–10. Chronic seborrheic dermatitis with marked edema and thickening and grayish white change in the skin.

Figure 1–11. Chronic dermatitis of the vulva showing marked hyperkeratosis and acanthosis.

ment of suppurative disease is the apocrine gland. As the result of its cyclic secretion and the frequency of local irritation, hidradenitis is not uncommon. The recurrent aspects of hidradenitis suppurativa (Fig. 1–12) indicate its association with this specialized gland and suggest a therapeutic approach to the problem—namely, modification of secretory activity by the use of oral contraceptives or cyclic estrogen. Antibiotics and local heat are often necessary in the acute phase and extensive "unroofing" incisions may be indicated for the more deep-seated, dissecting abscesses.

Fox-Fordyce disease is another manifestation of apocrine obstruction. Grossly the labia majora and mons are dotted with tiny, slightly elevated, firm, intensely pruritic papules. Microscopically there is a mild inflammatory infiltrate, particularly concentrated around the apocrine glands, with dilatation of the acini resulting from occlusion of the duct. Oral contraceptives and local antipruritic medications are usually effective therapeutic measures.

Crohn's disease, on rare occasions, may affect the vulva. In approximately 20 to 25 per

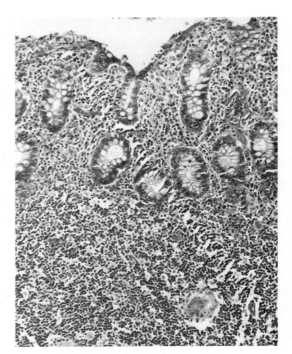

Figure 1–13. Crohn's disease of large bowel. Note giant cell.

cent of these cases, the regional enteritis is demonstrated on the perineum by the formation of rectoperineal or rectovaginal fistulae. The microscopic alterations are characterized by inflammatory infiltrate and occasionally the presence of granulomas (Fig. 1–13).

Behçet's disease is characterized by a triad of lesions (the triple symptom complex), consisting of recurrent aphthous ulcerations in the mouth, on the external genitalia, and in the eye. Any one or all three of these lesions may be present, but uveitis and similar infections in the eye are less frequent than the vulvar and oral ulcerations. In the chronic phase destruction of labia with fenestration may develop. The cause of the disease is unknown. Although thought to be an autoimmune disease, since there was evidence of an improvement with cortisone, more recently the theory of viral causation has been introduced (Figs. 1–14 and 1–15).

Histologically, in the chronic phase, the disease is characterized by an intense inflammatory infiltrate and vasculitis culminating in occlusion of many vessels in the subcutaneous tissues. These findings support the autoimmune theory (Fig. 1–16).

Clinically the lesions are frequently self-limiting and thus the effectiveness of various therapies is difficult to assess. Fatal cases are

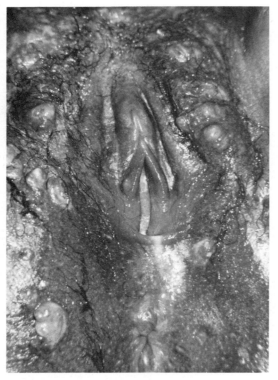

Figure 1–12. Suppurative hidradenitis. Note multiple draining pustules that intercommunicate.

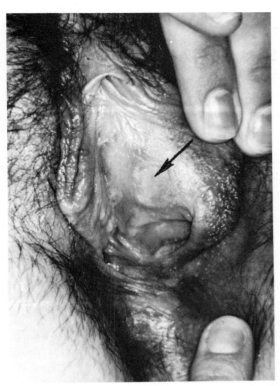

Figure 1–14. Healed ulceration at introitus in Behçet's disease. Note fenestration below the arrow.

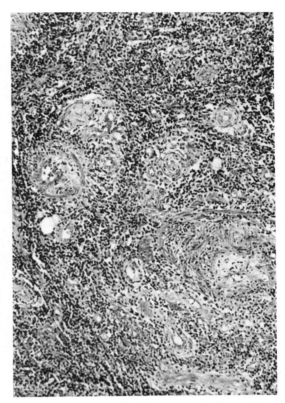

Figure 1–16. Inflammatory infiltration with vasculitis in Behçet's disease.

almost routinely associated with involvement of the central nervous system. More recently certain chemotherapeutic agents, particularly the alkylating variety, have reportedly been successful in controlling the progress of the neurologic lesions; however, more experience is necessary for proper assessment of the effects. Of interest is the reported cyclic nature of the exacerbations, and improvement with the use of oral contraceptives has been recorded. In spite of this, systemic cortisone is still the most widely used and effective therapy.

SYSTEMIC DISEASE OF VULVA

The vulva may reflect the presence of systemic disease. The presenting symptom in the diabetic patient is often vulvar pruritus. Grossly, the external genitalia are fiery red, reflecting the poor response of the diabetic to the commonly associated monilial infection (Fig. 1–17). Furthermore, chronic anemia is occasionally accompanied by vulvar ulceration, and a uremic frost may be appreciated as brownish-yellow patches on the external genitals in the terminal stages of kidney disease.

VIRAL DISEASE OF VULVA

Herpes simplex infection of the vulva is common; however, since initially it is rela-

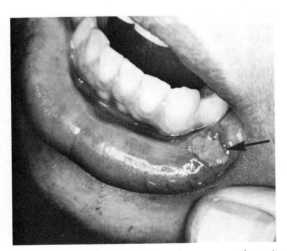

Figure 1–15. Ulceration of buccal mucous membrane in Behçet's disease.

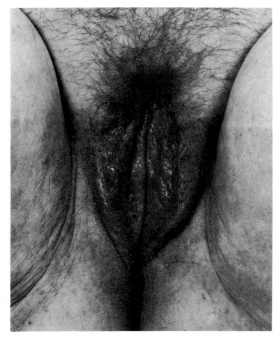

Figure 1–17. Diabetic vulvitis, showing the reddened, edematous external genitalia (darkened zone at outlet).

tively asymptomatic, the vesicular stage is rarely seen and the lesion usually has progressed to the symptomatic stage of superficial serpiginous ulceration by the time the physician is consulted (Fig. 1–18). Biopsy of the questionable lesion will be diagnostic with the finding of eosinophilic intranuclear inclusions (Fig. 1–19). Two aspects of herpetic infection of the vulva deserve special mention: (1) recently, herpes virus type II has been implicated as a potential etiologic agent in the development of cervical cancer, and in view of the relative frequency of multicentric foci of malignancy in the lower genital canal, the possibility of viral disease must be viewed more seriously; (2) vulvar herpes is undoubtedly only a local manifestation of infection existing throughout the lower canal. More careful study will often reveal lesions in the vagina and cervix. This association becomes of serious significance if the patient is pregnant and near term. If there is evidence of active infection within 2 to 4 weeks of predicted delivery, as demonstrated by the eosinophilic intranuclear inclusions in the vaginal smear, cesarean section should be entertained as the optimum method of delivery; although cultures are helpful, they rarely increase the accuracy of diagnosis over the careful cytologic study. Therapy in the acute stage includes the use

of local dyes, such as neutral red, and exposure of the area to strong light to take advantage of the "photosensitivity" of such viral lesions. The possibility that the use of such agents may be related to the later development of malignancy has limited its use in recent years; nevertheless, the studies of Friedrich and associates have not demonstrated abnormal activity in the epithelium of treated cases followed over a period of 30 to 60 months. However, in view of the controversy, therapy with such agents cannot be recommended. Local applications to eliminate secondary infections include ether, alcohol, Listerine, Betadine, and so forth. Fundamentally therapy is unnecessary if the lesions are relatively asymptomatic since agents have not been developed at present to prevent recurrences. As with other acute vulvar infections, inguinal lymphadenitis is common. During the acute phase, the vesicles are either intradermal or subepithelial. Biopsies demonstrate eosinophilic intranuclear inclusions, similar to those seen in the vaginal cytologic preparation. Latent or recurrent infections are common and are usually less symptomatic than the primary.

Herpes zoster infections are rare, associated with marked distress, and the lesions can often be traced along the course of the pudendal nerve over the adjacent buttock.

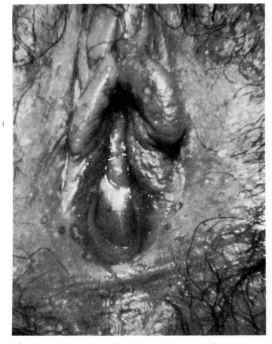

Figure 1–18. Superficial serpiginous ulcerations in perineum with edema and ulcerations of the labia minora.

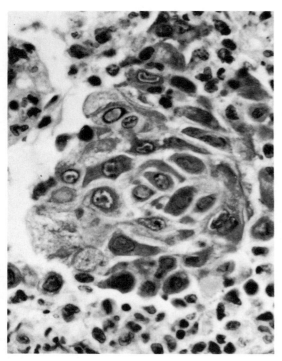

Figure 1–19. Intranuclear inclusions in a patient with herpes simplex II.

Recently molluscum contagiosum has been recognized more commonly in the external genitalia. Generally the lesions are asymptomatic, although rarely they are pruritic. The gross tumor is usually 5 to 8 mm. in diameter with an umbilicated center (Fig. 1–20). The latter contains the waxen kernel that may be evacuated by a tiny curette. Microscopically, the central area is seen to contain cells harboring the large inclusion bodies. The latter are classically eosinophilic at the base of the core and become more basophilic as they near the surface (Fig. 1–21).

Gonorrheal Inflammation

The adult vulvar mucosa, with its many layers of stratified squamous epithelium, is resistant to gonorrheal infection. The vulnerable structures in the external genitalia are the vulvovaginal glands, the urethra, and the associated Skene's ducts. On the other hand, gonorrheal vulvovaginitis is seen frequently in the young child because of the thinness of the vaginal mucous membrane, as will be discussed more fully in Chapter 2.

Bartholin Adenitis

Inflammation of the vulvovaginal glands is frequently due to gonorrheal infection; however, other organisms may be responsible, as noted in cultures from abscesses. In the acute stage of the disease, the gland is swollen, edematous, turgid, and painful, and the

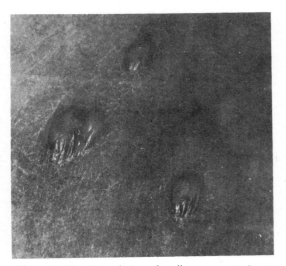

Figure 1–20. Gross lesion of molluscum contagiosum. Umbilicated center may be seen in the larger nodule.

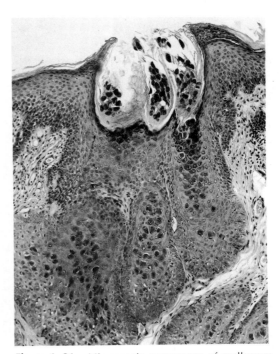

Figure 1–21. Microscopic appearance of molluscum. The umbilication is noted in center and dark inclusions are easily recognized.

overlying skin is reddened and very tender. Pressure over the gland may result in the expression of pus from the duct orifice; however, exquisite tenderness usually precludes such a procedure.

Microscopic examination in this stage shows the usual evidences of acute suppurative inflammation, with extensive infiltration of polymorphonuclear leukocytes, hyperemia, edema, epithelial degeneration, and perhaps desquamation.

The process terminates in one of two ways. In many cases, abscess formation supervenes, and the swelling and pain become more pronounced, with focal fluctuation. In such cases incision is indicated and the evacuation of the purulent contents of the gland results in immediate relief. Conversely, spontaneous rupture often occurs and the resultant small perforation furnishes inadequate drainage, so that the subsidence of the acute process is prolonged and recurrences are common unless the opening is enlarged.

In the less virulent infections, the process may subside without abscess formation, since drainage of the exudate may occur spontaneously through the natural channel. Resolution is occasionally incomplete, and chronic inflammation of the gland persists as it may after incision or spontaneous perforation of an abscess.

Chronic Bartholin adenitis presents clinically as an indurated nodularity of the gland, which is readily palpable deep in the perineum, lateral to the fourchette, but which remains asymptomatic for years. In other cases, exacerbations occur, with repetition of abscess formation, or with the development of cysts produced by occlusion of the ducts. If the main duct is thus blocked, the resulting cyst may be quite large (Fig. 1–22).

The lining of Bartholin's duct cysts varies greatly, from the classic transitional epithelium of the normal duct to a flattened, almost nonexistent layer, depending on the intracystic pressure and the destruction produced by the infectious process.

In the absence of a specific transitional epithelial lining, difficulty may be encountered in making positive histopathologic identification. In most instances, however, the mucus-secreting acini, similar in many aspects to those of the salivary gland, will be found in the chronically infected underlying tissue (Fig.1–23).

It must be appreciated that minor vestibular glands ring the introitus. Inflammatory

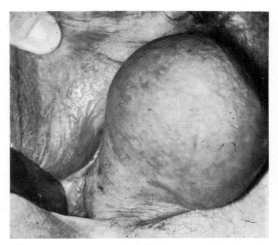

Figure 1–22. A large Bartholin duct cyst arising from the outlet.

reactions in such elements are common and biopsy may suggest atypical proliferation as a result of incorrect interpretation of transitional epithelium as a "loss of normal maturation and/or carcinoma in situ" (Fig. 1–24).

The gonorrheal form of vulvovaginitis in children is described in Chapter 2.

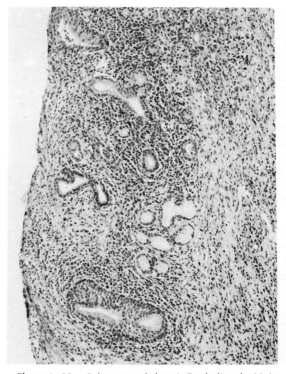

Figure 1–23. Subacute and chronic Bartholin adenitis in wall of a cyst. No surface epithelium is visible.

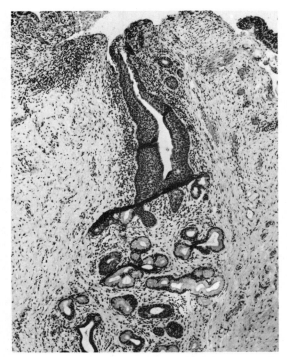

Figure 1–24. Excision of focal reddish lesion at outlet showing infiltrate in subcutaneous tissues with transitional epithelium in duct and mucus-secreting acini.

ULCERATIVE LESIONS OF VULVA

Simple Acute Ulcer (Aphthous)

This controversial lesion, first described by Lipschutz in 1895, involved either the epithelium of the vulva or the lower vagina. Of the three varieties described by Lipschutz, the first and second (gangrenous and venereal) are probably related to systemic disease, such as erythema multiforme, or regional enteritis (Crohn's disease). The third form is similar to multiple aphthous ulcers as seen in aphthous stomatitis. If vulvar and oral lesions occur simultaneously, Behçet's disease must be considered among the differential diagnoses.

It had been suggested that the common *Bacillus crassus* or *Lactobacillus*, found almost routinely in vaginal cultures, is the etiologic agent; however, there is no scientific validity for this thesis. Undoubtedly many such ulcerations are of viral origin, e.g., the herpetic or Behçet's lesions. Thus, the nebulous category of "Lipshutz ulcers" should be eliminated in favor of more specific diagnoses.

Chancroid (Ulcus Molle)

The ulceration of chancroid is typically ragged and irregular, especially in its later stages. It has an excavated appearance, with a granulating and often purulent surface, but with little or no surrounding induration. There is often associated edema of the vulvar structures. Pain is a more common clinical feature of chancroid than of the other ulcerative lesions of the vulva. Often the ulcer arises in the region of the clitoris or in the vestibule. When large, its outline is irregular and serpiginous because of the phagedenic tendencies of the lesion. The causative agent is the bacillus of Ducrey (*Haemophilus ducreyi*), which may be demonstrated by smears and cultures of the exudate. Associations with hemophilus vaginitis have not been described; however, some are undoubtedly existent.

Microscopically, the lesion presents few characteristics that distinguish it histopathologically from other chronic ulcerative lesions.

Granuloma Inguinale

The distribution of this venereal disease in the tropics is well known; currently it has become a rare entity in the United States, or at least is rarely diagnosed as such. Although both viral and protozoan agents have been proposed as the cause of the infection, recent investigations have suggested that the bacillus *Donovania granulomatis* (*Calymmatobacterium*) is the offender.

The disease begins usually on the labia minora or on the mons pubis as a small papular lesion, and tends to spread by superficial ulceration along the inguinal and pubic regions. The surface of the ulcerated area is covered with granulation tissue. The ulcerative process often involves the vulvar structures. Although generally it has been believed that there is no tendency to enlargement of the inguinal nodes, nevertheless, as with most acute inflammatory processes the local drainage tracts respond with enlargement and local discomfort.

The inclusions making up the Donovan bodies are recognized most readily in the large mononuclear cells as bilobed organisms appearing red with the Giemsa stain (Fig. 1–25). Although smears are adequate for most diagnoses of the acute infection, biopsy is necessary to eliminate the presence

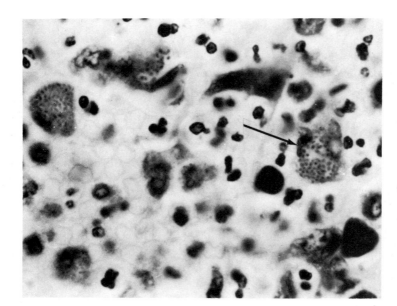

Figure 1–25. Donovan bodies—inclusions can be seen at arrow.

of malignancy in the chronic distorting lesions. In the later stages of the disease, the ulceration may be deep and extensive cicatrization may result. Cases of granuloma inguinale of the cervix, uterus, tubes, and ovaries, as well as some instances of extragenital infection, have been reported.

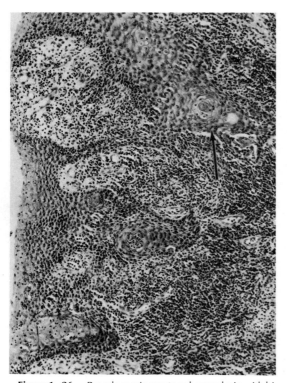

Figure 1–26. Pseudocarcinomatous hyperplasia with bizarre acanthosis, extreme inflammatory infiltrate, and abnormal maturation near rete tips (arrow).

Histologically, the disease is characterized by a transitory phase of subcutaneous infiltration with plasma cells, leukocytes, and large mononuclear cells, followed by the development of the typical granulation tissue. The so-called granuloma cells described by some authors, and characterized by a foamy, vacuolated cytoplasm, were regarded by von Haam as endothelial cells; however, most investigators feel that they are histiocytes with phagocytized degenerated cellular debris. Marked pseudocarcinomatous hyperplasia is recognized in the chronic stage, and differentiation from anaplastic alteration may be difficult. Of major importance is the abnormal maturation in the tips of the rete pegs. Intraepithelial pearl formation must be looked on with suspicion, and more adequate tissue specimen may show definite malignancy (Figs. 1–26 and 1–27). As in other distorting, nonhealing infectious processes, carcinoma may occasionally develop in these chronic lesions of granuloma inguinale.

Lymphogranuloma Venereum (LGV, Lymphogranuloma Inguinale, Lymphopathia Venereum)

The agent responsible for the lesions of lymphogranuloma inguinale was previously believed to be due to one of the large filterable viruses; however, recent studies have incriminated the chlamydia, members of the psittacosis granuloma species. Diagnosis is established largely on the basis of the skin

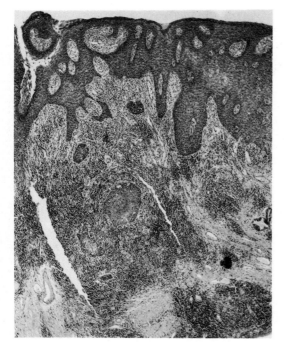

Figure 1–27. Area of invasive cancer adjacent to the pseudocarcinomatous change seen in Figure 1–26.

reaction to the Frei antigen. The complement fixation test has proved to be an effective diagnostic reaction and possibly more accurate and more available than the Frei antigen. Unfortunately, the tests remain positive indefinitely, so if the tests are performed in the acute phase of a process, other infectious processes must be ruled out.

The disease begins as small superficially ulcerated lesions of the external genitalia, followed by the development of pronounced inguinal adenitis. Further progress is characterized by extensive ulceration combined with marked lymphedema, often eventuating in focal or diffuse elephantiasis. The latter, associated with draining sinuses, is pathognomonic of lymphopathia venereum (Fig. 1–28) and confused only with extensive suppurative hidradenitis. In differential diagnosis it must be reemphasized that the latter rarely involves the labia minora except by minor degrees of edema. Occasionally, large indolent ulcers may destroy the vulvar structures and extend into the perineum and rectum. The term "esthiomene" was used to describe such ulcerative lesions. Whereas this designation formerly was loosely applied to all ulcerative processes of obscure etiology, it has now been eliminated since it was nonspecific. Combined lymphatic obstruction

and tissue damage may lead to either rectal and urethral strictures or destruction in these areas with resultant incontinence. Fenestration of the labia is not uncommon.

The microscopic picture is characterized by extensive infiltration with large mononuclear and plasma cells and an occasional eosinophil, dilatation of the lymphatic vessels with endothelial proliferation, and, in the later stages, marked fibrosis and scarring. In addition, microabscesses (probably originating with vascular occlusion) and giant cells with pseudotubercle formation are noted in the subacute phase (Fig. 1–29). Such abscesses are the seat of the classic draining sinuses. Pseudocarcinomatous hyperplasia with marked elongation and distortion of the rete pegs simulates malignant alterations. Conversely, carcinoma may develop in lymphogranulomatous lesions and be overlooked for years as a result of the similarity of the benign and malignant gross pictures. Salzstein and co-workers, Douglas, and others have recorded such experiences, and recognized the necessity for the liberal use of biopsy to establish the diagnosis in many of the chronic ulcerative conditions.

Extragenital manifestations of lymphogranuloma are well known. Extensive intes-

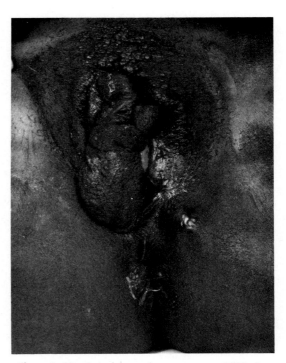

Figure 1–28. Lymphogranuloma venereum (LGV) showing lymphedema of right labium and draining sinuses in perineum on left.

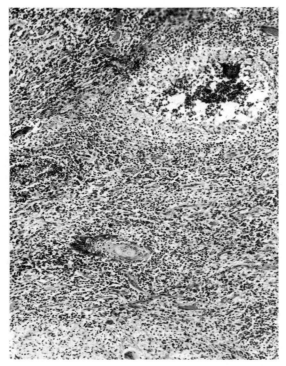

Figure 1–29. Focal abscess formation with giant cells in the adjacent area. The classic tubercle is absent.

tinal disease with cicatricial constrictions, particularly of the large bowel, have been reported and examples of meningitis have also been recorded.

Syphilitic Lesions of Vulva

Syphilis may affect the vulva in the form of primary, secondary, or tertiary lesions.

The primary lesion, or chancre, may pass without notice for it is much less conspicuous than similar lesions in the male and usually heals spontaneously in four to six weeks. It presents as a firm lesion with a "punched out" center, and there is less pronounced induration than is noted in males (Fig. 1–30). The primary lesion is more apt to be multiple in the female. The chancre is commonly located on the labia or at the introitus, and edema may be pronounced. Inguinal lymphadenitis is routinely present although not as striking as that associated with lymphogranuloma. Although the classic chancre is well known, it must be appreciated that primary syphilis may masquerade in many guises, and thus *all* ulcerated lesions must be studied thoroughly. Although the chancre is usually evanescent, a chronic variant is well known and may remain dormant for 4 to 6 months.

The characteristic secondary lesion in the vulva is the condyloma latum (Fig. 1–31). The lesion presents as a plateau-like excrescence, raised slightly above the surface. The surface has a grayish, necrotic, moist appearance, and is usually somewhat depressed at its center. Such lesions are commonly multiple, often confluent, involving not only the vulva but the adjacent perineum, perianal region, and the inner sides of the thighs. Histologically, the condyloma latum presents a granulomatous base, with superficial necrosis, as would be expected from the microscopic appearance. The spirochete is readily recoverable from both the primary and secondary lesions. The Warthin-Starry silver impregnation stain or fluorescent techniques may demonstrate the infecting agent. Serologic tests, as in other stages of the disease, are of basic diagnostic importance.

Tertiary lesions on the vulva are rarely seen, occurring either as gummatous tumors or ulcerations. Such syphilitic ulcers may extend widely and destroy the vulvar structures as well as the surrounding areas.

The histologic features of the tertiary syphilitic lesions are a marked granulomatous reaction, with a preponderance of lymphocytes, and prominent perivascular infiltration. Giant cells surrounded by epithelioid and mononuclear cells simulate tubercle formation.

Tuberculous ulceration of the vulva is

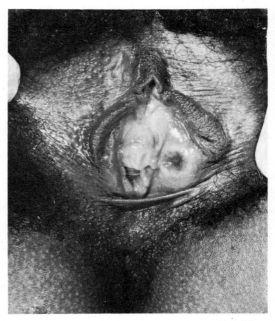

Figure 1–30. Chancre on inner surface of left labium minus.

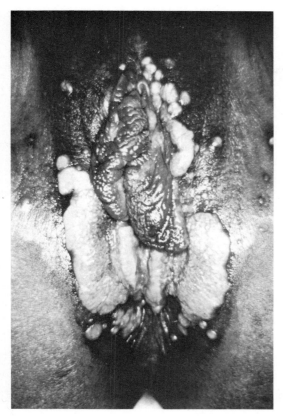

Figure 1–31. Condylomata lata.

appearance is that of an irregular, ragged ulcer of granulomatous or even caseous appearance.

The microscopic diagnosis is based upon the demonstration of the tubercles, characterized, as elsewhere, by the classic giant cells surrounded by epithelioid cells. Differentiation from syphilis in the tissue may be difficult; consequently, special techniques, e.g., acid-fast or fluorescent stain, should be used routinely to confirm the presence of the Koch-Weeks bacillus. Guinea pig inoculation with the infected material and the use of skin tests may assist in establishing the diagnosis.

Carcinomatous Ulcer

In its later stages carcinoma of the vulva produces extensive ulceration. Similarly, the very early but aggressive cancer may necrose as a result of its neoplastic potential. The lesion, however, can be readily diagnosed by the microscopic examination of biopsy specimens. The gross and microscopic characteristics are described in the section dealing with vulvar neoplasia.

Other Ulcerative Lesions

Vesicular lesions resulting in ulcerations occasionally appear on the vulva following smallpox vaccination. Factitious or self-induced ulcerations have been recognized in the psychologically disturbed patient (Fig. 1–32). The histopathology of such lesions is nonspecific.

very rare, but it may occur as a primary lesion due to exogenous infection and generally by direct inoculation from an infected sexual partner. The lesion begins as a nodule which later ulcerates, the usual seat being the labia or the vestibular region. The characteristic

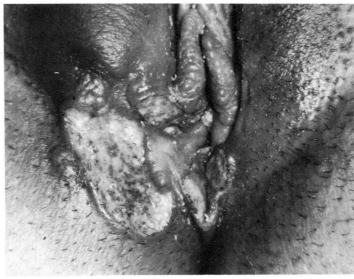

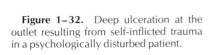

Figure 1–32. Deep ulceration at the outlet resulting from self-inflicted trauma in a psychologically disturbed patient.

HYPERPLASTIC AND "ATROPHIC" CHANGES

Schwimmer described leukoplakia of the tongue as a precancerous lesion in 1877, one of his 20 patients demonstrating concomitant patchy whitening of the vulva. Breisky, in 1885, recorded an atrophic, whitish, constricting change similar to "kraurosis." Bonney was impressed with the inflammatory origin of such lesions and recognized a relationship between the atrophic and hypertrophic stages. He suggested that the latter preceded the former and that the malignant potential was present only with the hypertrophic alterations. Taussig believed that the malignant potential was as great in one as the other; thus, definitive therapy was imperative in both varieties. The gross stages of the disease as described by Taussig are as follows: (1) erythema, edema, excoriation, and dryness; (2) thickening and flattening of whitened vulvar folds; and (3) cracking and superficial ulceration with parchment-like appearance to white or bluish white skin. The microscopic stages are: (1) minimal hyperkeratosis and acanthosis with inflammatory infiltrate, (2) hyperkeratosis and acanthosis with epithelial hypertrophy and round cell infiltration, and (3) hyperkeratosis, flattened rete pegs and a frayed basement layer with dermal collagen and inflammatory infiltrate.

Much of the confusion surrounding these lesions stems from the tremendous variety of conditions which have been labeled as leukoplakia. These may be classified as follows:

I Absence of pigment
   Leukoderma—congenital (Fig. 1–33)
   Vitiligo—acquired (result of scarring and trauma)

II Hyperkeratosis
   Infections
      Intertrigo, chronic dermatitis, etc., with lichenification
   Hyperkeratosis occurring on benign tumors—condyloma, papilloma, keratosis (Fig. 1–34), etc.
   Lichen sclerosus and allied conditions
   Hyperplasias, typical and atypical
   Carcinoma in situ
   Invasive carcinoma

The confusion that exists in differentiation of the gross patterns is reflected in the microscopic interpretation of such lesions. Too frequently the presence of mild hyperkera-

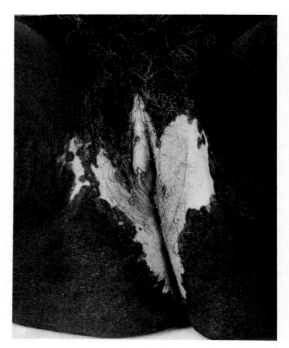

Figure 1–33. Leukoderma showing extensive whitish depigmentation of the vulva. No relationship to leukoplakia.

tosis, acanthosis, and inflammatory infiltrate has led to the diagnosis of leukoplakia when the lesion was in truth a chronic dermatitis with lichenification (Figs. 1–10 and 1–11). Furthermore, quite commonly the atrophic conditions are diagnosed as leukoplakia simply on the basis of the superficial white hyperkeratotic alteration. As a result of such interpretations of microscopic changes and the histopathologic diagnosis of "leukoplakia," the clinician felt the necessity for surgical elimination of the lesion in view of the malignant potentiality suggested by use of the term. The inevitable result was unnecessary surgery for many benign conditions and distortion of the outlet, with subsequent dyspareunia. Thus, it would seem important to modify the terminology in an attempt to convey to the clinician the degree of epithelial atypicality as connoted by the cervical diagnoses of mild, moderate, or marked basal cell hyperactivity and carcinoma in situ (CIN). Such an approach should suggest the proper course of further investigation and management of the specific case.

The cellular changes in vulvar anaplasia, however, are not as specific nor as characteristic as those described for their cervical counterparts. The degree of atypism cannot be based on the extent of epithelial penetration by the abnormal cells. The most suspi-

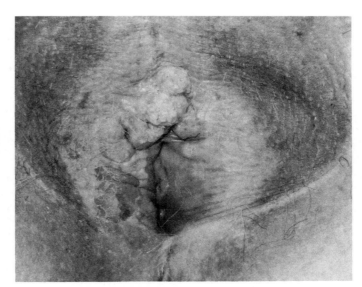

Figure 1–34. Extensive hyperkeratosis of prepuce with focal excoriations on left at outlet.

cious atypicalities are those noted at the rete tips in the form of rapid maturation characterized by an attempt at pearl formation (Fig. 1–35), or bizarre, anaplastic immature cells in these areas. The former change is recognized more commonly in premalignant conditions of the vulva, since squamous cell carcinoma is the most frequent variety of neoplasia. Nevertheless, in those lesions preceded by granulomatous disease, the transitional or more immature cell type of anaplasia is common.

In the effort to provide more information as to the malignant potential of the lesion, the term "hyperplasia," either typical or atypical, has been applied to the proliferating lesions. Such a term seems more meaningful to the clinician since it provides a point of reference, comparative with other atypical proliferations in the female genital canal, i.e., cervix and endometrium. Typical hyperplasia corresponds to the classic picture of chronic dermatitis with hyperkeratosis. The epithelium has proliferated to produce acanthosis, but there is no atypical maturation in the strata (Fig. 1–10) and thus the malignant potential is nil. The atypical hyperplasias are characterized by distortion and abnormal maturation of the epithelium. Mild to moderate degrees demonstrate individual cell maturation through the lower half of the epithelium with or without acanthosis (Fig. 1–36). Marked atypicality is characterized by "pearl" formation in the rete tips and/or extensive individual cell alterations (Fig. 1–37 A,B). In the former situation there is often collagenization of the underlying

stroma, while in the latter there is little, if any, change in the subcutaneous tissues. It has been recognized frequently that atypical hyperplasia and carcinoma in situ occur in multiple foci not only in the lower genital canal but also in the vulva, as noted in Figure 1–36; thus many biopsies are usually necessary in order to evaluate the differences in

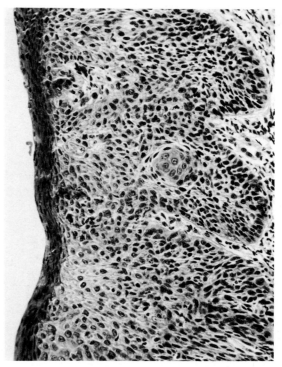

Figure 1–35. Atypical maturation. Note increased basal and parabasal cells and the attempt at intraepithelial pearl formation. There is moderate to marked atypical dystrophy.

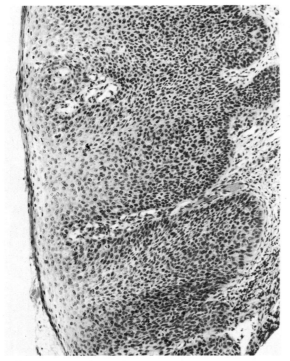

Figure 1–36. Atypical maturation with increase in the immature cells and lack of the normal layers of mature surface cells.

cellular aberration that may be appreciated from one section to the next. It should go without saying that the minor degrees of hyperplasia should be followed carefully and biopsy resorted to frequently if any suspicious gross alteration is noted. Toluidine blue has been helpful in localizing areas of increased nuclear activity; however, it must be appreciated that both false negative and false positive tests are not uncommon. Cytogenetics may prove to be an important adjunctive study to determine differential anaplastic activity, but more experience is needed to assess its validity.

The incidence of invasive disease developing in the setting of these hyperplastic epithelia is difficult to assess. Vulvar malignancy is not common; the hyperplastic and hyperkeratotic lesions, however, are frequent. Thus, it must be suspected that the incidence of cancer developing in such lesions is relatively low (2 to 3 per cent). Kaufmann and Gardner have reported on the follow-up of 120 cases of vulvar dystrophy. In only one patient did cancer develop, and atypical hyperplasia had been present in an earlier study. Nevertheless, it should be ap-

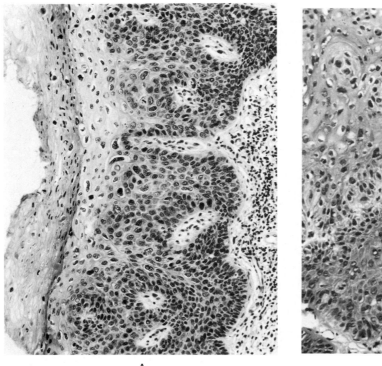
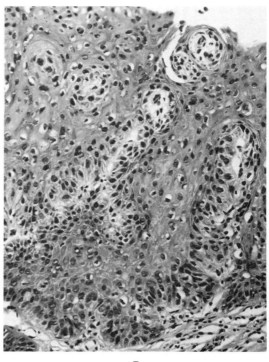

A   B

Figure 1–37. *A,* Marked atypicality of epithelium with individual cell anaplasia. *B,* Marked atypical hyperplastic dystrophy. Note lack of full-thickness alterations and abnormal maturation at rete tips (no basal layer).

preciated that the follow-up period varied from 6 months to several years, and all patients had been "treated." Consequently, this study does not necessarily record the natural "life history" of the dystrophy. The untreated case may progress, in due time, to cancer, as demonstrated in Figure 1–38. Thus, all patients with dystrophic alterations should be treated for the common symptom, e.g., pruritus, and biopsied if specific foci of atypicality develop—i.e., firm, cartilaginous areas or nonhealing superficial ulcerations.

Lichen Sclerosus

Lichen sclerosus may occur in various areas of the body and in any age group; however, it is more common and more extensive on the vulva. In the earliest phase, the lesion appears as a yellowish-blue papule. With coalescence of multiple lesions, an entire area becomes grayish, thin, and often parchment-like (Fig. 1–39). Generally, there are no early symptoms; however, the thinned tissue is easily and commonly irritated, and itching results, particularly in the postmenopausal state. Excoriation appears and hyperplasia may develop in certain areas. With the coexistence of atrophy and hyperplasia, malignancy may develop in the vulva in which apparently only a simple, thin atrophic le-

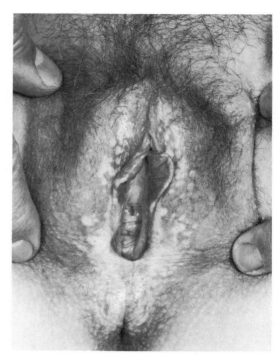

Figure 1–39. Lichen sclerosus —white punctate lesions on both sides with coalescence at the fourchette. (From Woodruff and Baens: Am. J. Obstet. Gynecol., 87:713, 1963.)

sion had existed previously (Figs. 1–40 and 1–41). This relationship in the postmenopausal patient may represent "incrimination by association" rather than a "cause and effect" situation. The incidence of so-called atrophic changes in vulvar epithelium in the late years is unknown but the unrealistic term "primary senile atrophy" may demonstrate the frequency.

Microscopically, lichen sclerosus is identified by hyperkeratosis, thinning of the epithelium, a subepithelial zone of collagen, and chronic inflammatory infiltrate beneath the collagen. Often the layer of keratin is thicker than the epithelium. The latter is markedly thinned and the basal layer is disturbed by the presence of atypical mature cells in the normally regular, spindle-celled zones. The homogeneous collagen area is often strikingly edematous if the process is acute or has been recently irritated. The underlying infiltrate is made up of lymphocytes with an occasional melanophore (pigment-laden macrophage), as is seen in many chronic lesions. Keratin plugging of the follicles is common but is not a differentiating feature between lichen sclerosus and kraurosis.

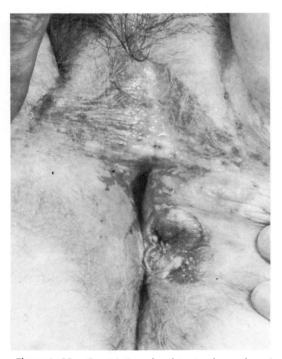

Figure 1–38. Constriction of outlet, atrophy, and carcinoma at fourchette on left side.

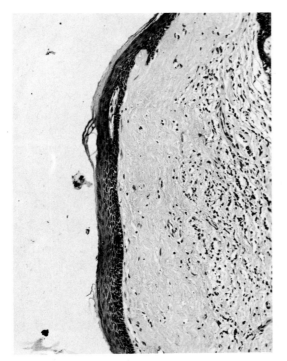

Figure 1–40. Thinned epithelium with dermal collagenization (see Fig. 1–41). (From Woodruff and Baens: Am. J. Obstet. Gynecol., 87:713, 1963.)

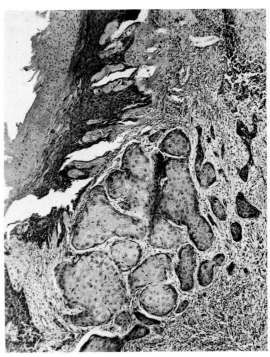

Figure 1–41. Invasive carcinoma adjacent to the area of lichen sclerosus seen in Figure 1–40. (From Woodruff and Baens: Am. J. Obstet. Gynecol., 87:713, 1963.)

The histologic changes in lichen sclerosus are similar to those described by Taussig for chronic atrophic vulvitis, later known as atrophic leukoplakia, kraurosis, and primary senile atrophy. The arguments for the use of one term in preference to the other are more than academic but are of clinical significance. Consequently if these alterations are histopathologically similar, it would be wise to use the histologic diagnosis of lichen sclerosus for all cases in which the cellular findings correspond to those noted above. The gross appearance should also be described without suggesting that the histology necessarily corresponds to the specific gross picture.

The connotation of any diagnosis is of obvious importance to the clinician. Historically leukoplakia has been associated with premalignant disease. Conversely, lichen sclerosus has been designated as a benign condition, almost never eventuating in cancer. This should not lull one into a false sense of security, since many cases can be cited to prove the fallacy of the latter statement. Possibly hypertrophy, which may

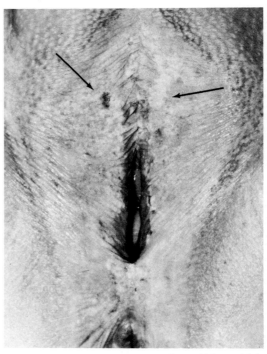

Figure 1–42. Constriction of outlet with loss of labia minora, superficial ulceration on right of clitoris, and hyperkeratotic plaque to left.

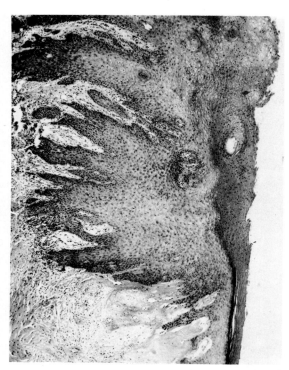

Figure 1–43. Mixed dystrophy with atypical hyperplastic alterations on the left, associated with thinning of the epithelium and underlying collagenization on the right. Surface parakeratosis on the left can be compared with the keratinization on the right (see Fig. 1–42).

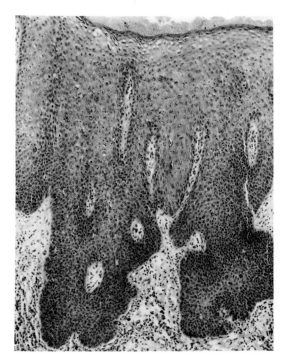

Figure 1–44. Atypical hyperplasia showing abnormal maturation in rete pegs. Compare with Figure 1–35 (intraepithelial pearl formation).

coexist with atrophy, is a necessary step in the transition from the benign to the malignant state (Figs. 1–35, 1–42, 1–43, and 1–44). Nevertheless, malignancy may eventuate with this atrophic pattern in 1 to 2 per cent of cases (Figs. 1–40 and 1–41).

Kraurosis

Kraurosis is a clinical term, not a histologic diagnosis, describing a shrinkage in the vulvar structures with loss of the normal architecture, decrease in or complete absence of the subcutaneous fat, and agglutination of the minor labia, reducing the normal appearance of the vulva to a flattened, smooth, grayish-white area, often superficially excoriated or fissured, especially at the fourchette. The outlet is constricted so that coitus is painful or impossible.

Microscopically, the picture is identical to that of lichen sclerosus. Although a diagnosis of kraurosis often is made on the basis of the microscopic findings, one cannot determine the degree of shrinkage of the vulvar structures by gazing through the microscope at a small fragment of tissue. Finally, despite many attempts, a definite microscopic dif-

ferentiation between kraurosis and lichen sclerosus has not been possible. Consequently, it would seem wise to reserve the use of the descriptive term "kraurosis" to the grossly shrunken constricted outlet and lichen sclerosus for the microscopic definition of the atrophic lesions.

The obvious explanation for these lesions is a withdrawal of the estrogenic hormones; however, such an etiology is not feasible in cases occurring in younger women in whom the estrogenic function of the ovaries is still active. One can only assume that for some unknown reason the vulvar tissues lose their responsiveness to the ovarian hormone. Obviously, since similar changes occur in apparently "nonsexual skin," other etiologies must be considered, such as local vascular alterations and trauma.

As noted above, the many terms, atrophic leukoplakia, primary senile atrophy, lichen sclerosus, and kraurosis, applied to the thin constricted white vulvar skin only serve to confuse the picture. Of major importance is not the name applied, but the correct evaluation of tissue changes. In this context of atrophy, malignancy rarely may develop as the result of disturbed metabolic activity.

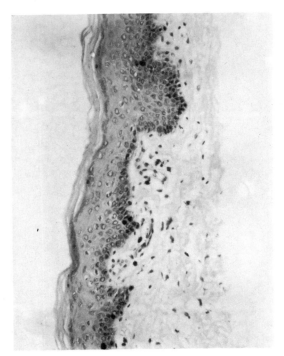

Figure 1–45. Autoradiogram of normal vulvar epithelium showing rare labeled cell. (From Woodruff et al.: Am. J. Obstet. Gynecol., 91:809, 1965.)

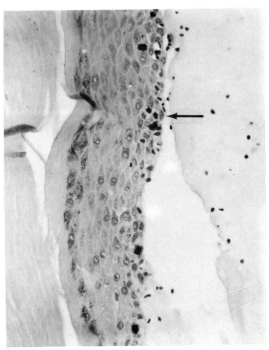

Figure 1–46. Autoradiogram of lichen sclerosus showing more labeled cells. (From Woodruff et al.: Am. J. Obstet. Gynecol., 91:809, 1965.)

Studies by Clark and co-workers, and by members of our staff, using acridine orange fluorescence and uptake of radioactive precursors for nucleic acid synthesis have demonstrated that such tissues are more active than normal epithelium (Figs. 1–45 to 1–47). This concept, however, was suggested by Taussig years ago in his description of the frayed basement membrane in the atrophic phase of leukoplakia or chronic atrophic vulvitis (Fig. 1–48). It is then of importance to control the common symptoms of pruritus in these cases and to use the biopsy freely when suspicious ulcerations or specific thickenings of the superficial tissues develop. *Vulvectomy* is necessary only when anaplastic alterations are recognized.

Elephantiasis Vulvae, Stasis Hypertrophy

The chief cause of such alterations is a blockage or stasis of lymphatic or vascular channels, or both. Probably the most common situation in which such stasis exists is that associated with pregnancy. Pathologically, the best illustration of this mechanism

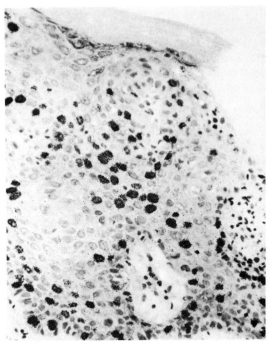

Figure 1–47. Autoradiogram of carcinoma in situ showing marked labeling. (From Woodruff et al.: Am. J. Obstet. Gynecol., 91:809, 1965.)

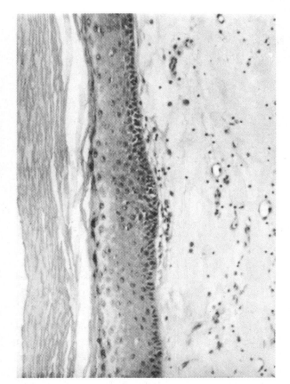

Figure 1–48. Microscopic pattern of lichen sclerosus with frayed basal layer.

may be seen in the cases of tropical elephantiasis, in which the parasitic worm *Filaria sanguinis-hominis* is responsible for the lymphatic block. Locally such stasis is a frequent concomitant of lymphogranuloma venereum. Other etiologies include chronic hidradenitis, Crohn's disease, extensive pelvic neoplasia, debilitating neurologic disease, and pregnancy (either nonspecific or related to the secretion in aberrant breast tissue on the vulva). In the patient with long-term lymphatic obstruction, the skin covering the lymphedematous, hypertrophic labia is greatly thickened, resembling elephant hide. The subcutaneous tissues are edematous and focally infiltrated with lymphocytes and plasma cells. Lymphatics are dilated and endothelial proliferation may be striking. Occasional giant cells may be recognized, although the classic tubercle with its epithelioid cells is missing.

BENIGN TUMORS OF VULVA

Cysts of Vulva

The most common member of this group is the Bartholin's duct cyst or vulvovaginal cyst. The characteristics have been fully described in a previous section under Bartholin adenitis.

Sebaceous cysts arise as a result of blockage of the ducts of the sebaceous glands so richly distributed over the vulva (Fig. 1–49), and are found frequently on the labia majora and minora. The contents are characteristically cheesy and, like sebaceous cysts elsewhere, they are very prone to infection and to abscess formation. Microscopically, the lining of the sebaceous cyst is characterized by the presence of irregular clumps of cells with small, dark nuclei and clear cytoplasm; thus, the term "cyst" may be supplanted by "sebaceous inclusions." Giant cells resulting from tissue reaction to the foreign sebaceous material are routinely found. Carcinoma arising in these cysts is rare, and when present has been reported to be of the basal cell variety.

Epithelial inclusion cysts are common and represent the residuum of the chronically obstructed sebaceous "duct." The desquamated superficial epithelium makes up the contents of such cysts and grossly may simulate sebaceous material. The microscopic appearance of such lesions is characterized by a stratified squamous epithelial lining, rep-

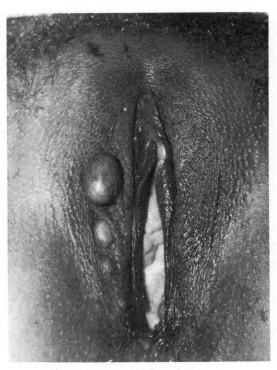

Figure 1–49. Multiple inclusion cysts.

resentative of the epithelium of the hair follicle, which has been included in the final process of the occlusion of the hair follicle shaft and its associated sebaceous gland (Fig. 1–50).

Mucinous Cysts

An occasional pedunculated, mucinous cyst develop lateral to the clitoris or in the inner aspect of the labium minus. Such lesions may represent aberrant mucinous epithelium, misplaced at time of the division of the cloaca by the urorectal fold. Another possible etiology involves the minor vestibular glands. These structures, like Bartholin's gland, have mucus-secreting acini and may reflect the same occlusive processes that affect the major glands.

Cyst of the Canal of Nuck

Finally, a cyst may arise from the peritoneal covering carried down with the round ligament to its insertion in the labium majus. Such cysts are lined by peritoneal epithelium. They correspond to the hydrocele in the male. Direct and persistent communication with the peritoneal reflection along the inguinal canal and its associated round ligament may result in the development of an indirect inguinal hernia presenting in the labium majus. Clinically, it is important to appreciate these relationships, since excision of the local dilatation, cyst, or sac will only

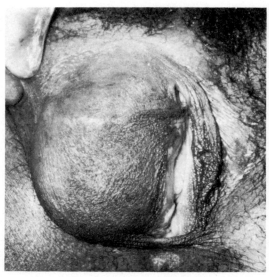

Figure 1–51. Large varicocele of right labium minus.

lead to recurrence, owing to the persistence of the communication with the peritoneal lining. Reactions in this peritoneal lining have led to the erroneous diagnosis of malignancy when the neoplasia represented only a mesothelial reaction.

Dilatation of the veins of the associated pampiniform plexus simulates the common varicocele of the scrotum (Fig. 1–51). Conversely, many of the varicose dilatations of the external genitalia relate to obstruction of branches of the pudendal vessels. The latter may be reflecting deeper pelvic disease. Most vulvar varices are unilateral.

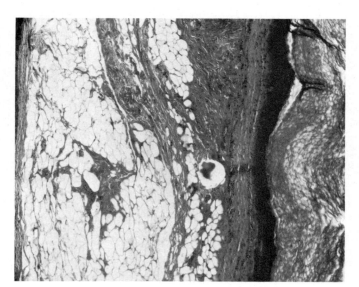

Figure 1–50. Stratified epithelial lining of inclusion cyst on left; adipose tissue is present in the center, with skin to far right.

Solid Benign Tumors

Among these must be included the verrucous lesions (condylomata acuminata), fibroma, fibromyoma, lipoma, angioma, hidradenoma, nevus, granular cell myoblastoma syringoma, and endometrioma. Isolated examples of other tumors, classified as lymphangioma and neurofibroma (von Recklinghausen's disease) have been reported.

Fibromas are uncommon and usually contain smooth muscle and fatty tissue; thus, most lesions should be diagnosed as fibromyoma or fibrolipoma. These tumors do not always arise from the vulvar tissues, but may merely present in the external genitalia. The sites of origin are occasionally the round ligament or the intrapelvic fibromuscular tissue. The tumors may attain an enormous size, a weight of 121 kg. (268 lb.) having been reached in the frequently quoted case of Buckner (1851). Those arising from the round ligament or deeper pelvic structures may present as firm, often nodular, diffuse masses. Those of vulvar origin tend to become pedunculated at an earlier stage (Fig. 1–52).

The microscopic features are characteris-

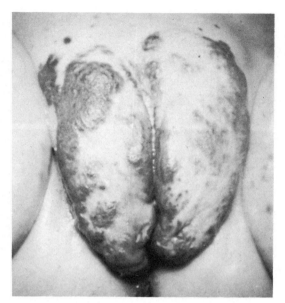

Figure 1–53. Congenital hemangioma of both labia in a 3 month child.

tic of those described in similar tumors at extrapelvic sites. In the larger tumors, extensive hyaline or cystic degeneration has been recognized. Leonard, from his study of vulvar tumors, found that as many as 22.5 per cent of the fibromas undergo sarcomatous change. Conversely, of the four sarcomas recorded in our laboratory, there was no history of a preceding tumor.

The hemangioma of the vulva may occur as a congenital lesion usually involving other sites in addition to the vulva (Fig. 1–53). It is important to recognize that such lesions regress spontaneously and rarely need active treatment. Although local therapy with liquid nitrogen and carbon dioxide snow has been promoted for such lesions, the vulvar tumors should be observed or treated surgically only in the event of excessive bleeding. Small, elevated hemorrhagic lesions commonly appear on the vulva in the postmenopausal patient. These are rarely hemangiomas, but rather represent multiple tiny varicosities. The microscopic picture of the true hemangioma is characteristic of such lesions elsewhere. The focal nests of dilated vessels show varying degrees of endothelial proliferation. The angiokeratoma (Figs. 1–54 and 1–55) is similar to other such lesions with surface hyperkeratosis. Of importance is the occasional misdiagnosis of hemangioma or hematoma in

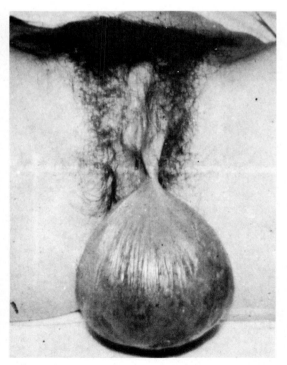

Figure 1–52. Large pedunculated fibroma of vulva. (Courtesy of Dr. Ed Foord.)

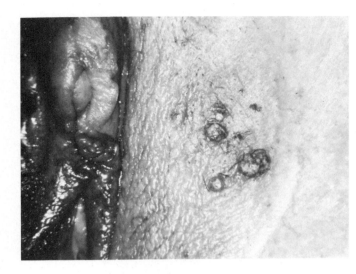

Figure 1–54. Angiokeratoma.

cases of malignant melanoma, particularly if the tumor originates in or around the clitoris.

Verrucous lesions of the vulva occur in one of two forms—the relatively rare true papilloma and the common condyloma acuminatum.

The squamous papilloma appears as a warty growth, arising usually from the labia majora, and having the treelike microscopic structure characterizing papilloma in gen-

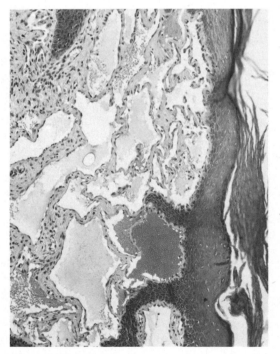

Figure 1–55. Angiokeratoma—keratin on surface. Subepithelial capillary dilatation with minimal endothelial prominence.

eral. These tumors generally grow slowly and occur most often in women beyond middle age. The common condyloma acuminatum has been classified in the past as a venereal wart. Although this relationship to venereal disease has been denied, it seems that there is more than a modicum of truth in the original designation since in a majority of cases the infecting agent has been transmitted by coitus.

Warts on the vulva, as elsewhere, are of viral origin. The common wart virus has been studied extensively, and although the virus of the acuminate wart and that of usual skin lesion appear similar with the electron microscope, they are, nevertheless, antigenically different; i.e., the antigen from the common wart does not cross react with that of the condyloma agent. Further investigation into the immunologic aspects of these viruses may provide a method of distinguishing patients who are prone to recurrences from those who have developed antibodies. It is hoped that such studies may also lead to a method of treating the patient with recurrences. This approach to the wart problem becomes more important since, particularly in young patients, carcinoma in situ often grossly simulates condylomata acuminata. The infectious origin of cervical neoplasia has been supported by many investigators, and the herpes hominis virus II has been implicated repeatedly. Possibly the condyloma virus may be playing the same role in the lower canal.

Since the virus is an obligatory biotroph and therefore necessarily associated with another agent, it is found most commonly in an area moistened by a variety of secretions and thus presenting an ideal atmosphere to support the growth of a variety of bacteria. Spontaneous regression is not uncommon, particularly if the lesions have appeared and grown rapidly during pregnancy. Nevertheless, if the vagina is markedly involved with condylomas, cesarean section should be entertained as the method of delivery because of the possibility of extensive lacerations and the difficulty in suturing such tissues. Furthermore, there are instances of laryngeal papillomas in the newborn which are thought to be related to infection with the wart virus in the mother.

Pathologically, the condyloma acuminatum is one of the verrucous lesions, and in this respect differs from the condyloma latum, which is a specific syphilitic lesion. By definition the lesion is a "pointed excrescence." The warts may be solitary (Fig. 1–56); however, most frequently they are multiple, involving the labia, the perineal and perianal regions, the upper inner thigh, and often the lower portion of the vagina (Fig. 1–57). Rarely they are noted in the upper vagina and on the cervix.

Microscopically, the condyloma acuminatum is a treelike growth with a heavy covering mantle of stratified squamous epithelium showing marked acanthosis and parakeratosis (Fig. 1–58). Papillomatosis may be present to a minor degree and occasionally hyperkeratosis is noted, particularly in the late stages of the lesion.

Microscopically, hyperkeratosis is charac-

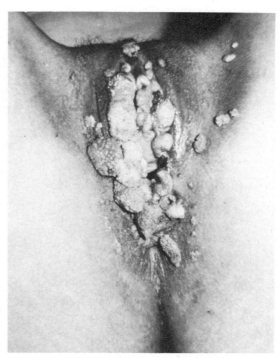

Figure 1–57. Extensive condylomatosis. Note that the small lesions are brownish while the larger and older ones are whitish.

terized by the presence of a well defined granular layer in the epithelium (stratum granulosum), superimposed on which is the layer of keratin, acidophilic material con-

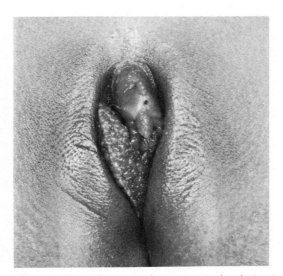

Figure 1–56. Solitary warty lesion at vaginal outlet in a 3 year old child.

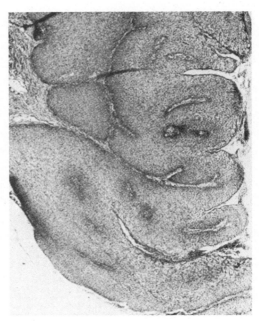

Figure 1–58. Benign papillomatous pattern of condyloma acuminatum.

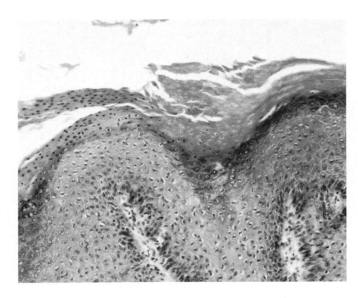

Figure 1–59. Hyperkeratosis (at right) and parakeratosis (at left) in condyloma acuminatum.

taining either no nuclei or the shadowy outlines of large, pale forms. Conversely, with parakeratosis (incomplete keratinization), there is an absence of the granular zone and the surface layers are composed of cell outlines containing small, dark nuclei (Fig. 1–59). The critical feature is the pre-eleidin or prekeratin, without which keratinization is obviously impossible. There is a sharp line of demarcation between the epithelium and the edematous vascularized underlying connective tissue. The latter always shows some degree of inflammatory infiltration, especially in the superficial layers. Occasionally, vacuolization may be seen in the nuclei displacing the chromatin, suggesting intranuclear inclusions (Fig. 1–60).

Malignant proliferation may occur in either the condyloma acuminatum or the true

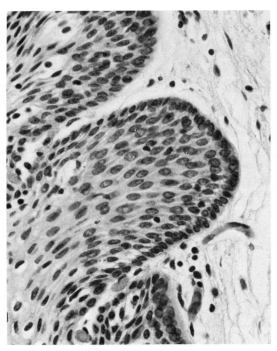

Figure 1–60. Vacuolization in the epithelial cells of condyloma acuminatum (?viral inclusions).

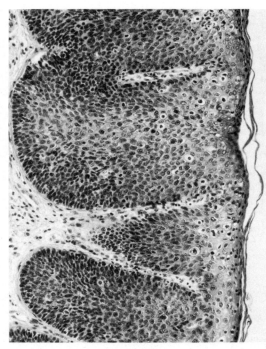

Figure 1–61. Condylomatous carcinoma in situ of the vulva—elongated rete pegs with classic atypical cells (corps ronds are abundant) and loss of normal maturation with surface parakeratosis.

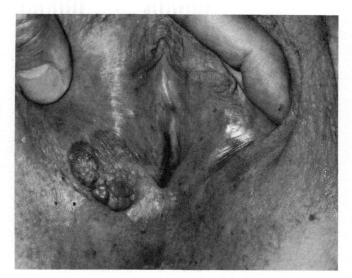

Figure 1–62. Condylomatous carcinoma in situ. Patient had other warts in vagina.

papilloma. The incidence is difficult to establish; however, with either lesion such anaplastic change is rare (Fig. 1–61). Nevertheless, it may be difficult to differentiate the gross appearance of the benign from the malignant lesion (Figs. 1–62 and 1–63). In neither of these illustrated cases was carcinoma diagnosed from the gross appearance, but in both instances the lesions had been present for 20 years or more.

Acrochordons (fibroepithelial polyps) are small polypoid fibrous tags which contain an edematous cord of connective tissue and a surface layer of stratified epithelium. They

may appear grossly white with superficial keratinization. Conversely, these are often dark as the result of melanosis and the accumulation of subcutaneous melanophores such as is commonly associated with any chronic irritation. Generally such lesions need no therapy unless they produce local irritation.

Seborrheic keratoses are common on the vulva, as on the skin elsewhere. Grossly the pigmented lesion may be confused with carcinoma in situ or melanoma (Fig. 1–64). The

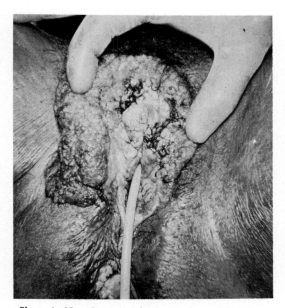

Figure 1–63. Carcinoma beginning in condylomata acuminata in 48 year old patient. First lesion had been removed at age of 18 years.

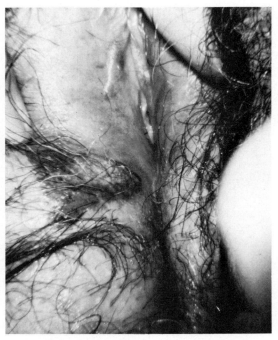

Figure 1–64. Pigmented seborrheic keratosis.

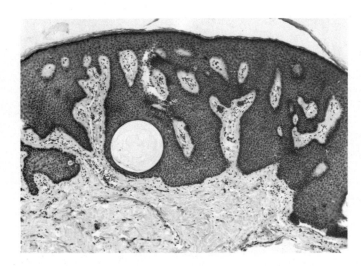

Figure 1–65. Seborrheic keratosis with its classic "horn cysts."

biopsy, which obviously should be done, confirms the histopathologic differential. The thickened epithelium with its keratin inclusions is pathognomonic of the seborrheic lesion (Fig. 1–65).

Hidradenoma of vulva (hidradenoma tubulare or adenoma hidradenoides) is a rare tumor of the vulva, but one that deserves special consideration since, although the lesion is benign, it has been mistaken for adenocarcinoma. It was first described by Pick in 1904. The histogenesis of this tumor is, on good evidence, believed to be from the vulvar apocrine glands, and in some cases a direct continuity of the tubules of the tumor with the sweat glands can be demonstrated.

Clinically, the hidradenoma presents as a sharply circumscribed, slightly elevated lesion, rarely much more than 1 cm. in diameter (Fig. 1–66). The skin overlying the nodule may be reddened or slightly ulcerated and granular, so that slight bleeding may at times be a clinical symptom. Most frequently, however, the lesions are asymptomatic and are usually found on routine examination of the genitalia. The location is most frequently on the labia majora or in the interlabial folds.

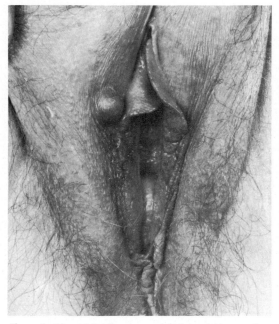

Figure 1–66. Hidradenoma on right inner labium majus.

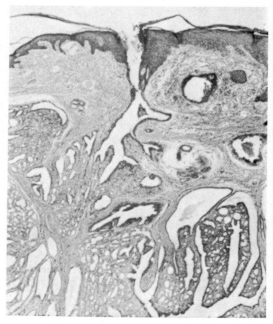

Figure 1–67. Hidradenoma of vulva.

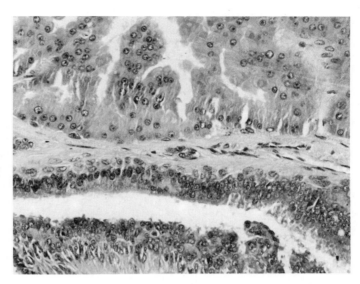

Figure 1–68. High power view of hidradenoma. Note the large, pale secretory cell in upper segment and the indifferent or myoepithelial cell beneath the cuboidal elements (lower middle).

The histologic appearance is quite characteristic. The pattern is papillary-adenomatous. The epithelial lining is characteristically a double layer of nonciliated columnar cells with clear cytoplasm and dark staining nuclei (Fig. 1–67). Large, pale cells with abundant acidophilic cytoplasm are seen as the very mature superficial cells that are the actively secreting elements of the acinus (Fig. 1–68). Underlying the superficial epithelial layers, especially in the smaller acini, are rounded or cuboidal cells simulating the reverse or indifferent cells of the cervix. Simple excision has effected permanent cures in nearly all reported cases, as noted by Woodworth and co-workers in a survey of 69 such lesions. Rare cases of hidradenocarcinoma have been recorded.

Beneath the epithelium is a layer of flattened myoepithelial cells (Fig. 1–68). Confusing microscopic patterns, suggestive of malignancy, are produced by proliferation of the stromal or myoepithelial elements; however, these "mixed tumors," nodular hidradenomas, and clear cell myoepitheliomas, despite their neoplastic appearance, pursue a benign course if wide local excision is performed (Fig. 1–69).

A lesion occurring in the duct of the apocrine system, the syringocystadenoma papilliferum, is characterized by papillary invaginations into the dilated ducts. Such lesions simulate and may be representative of aberrant breast tissue since the vulva lies along the nipple line. The gross appearance is suggestive only because of the nipple-like appearance of the slightly pigmented lesion.

Lactation may be recognized, as noted in a small tumor removed from the vulva at time of delivery (Fig. 1–70). A few cases of breast carcinoma have been reported as arising in the vulva or adjacent mons pubis.

The syringoma is a common skin lesion but is rarely diagnosed since most such

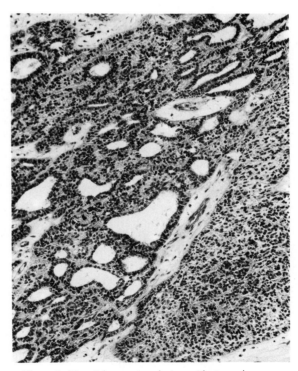

Figure 1–69. Adenomatous lesion with stromal component suggesting anaplastic change; nevertheless, such tumors behave in a benign, locally invasive lesion. Clear cell myoepithelioma is noted at lower right.

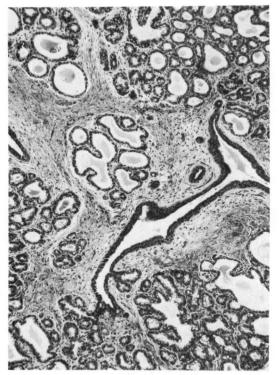

Figure 1–70. Lactating breast tissue from vulva. (From Woodruff and Seeds: Obstet. Gynecol., *20*:690, 1962.)

tumors are small and asymptomatic. They are usually multiple, tiny, elevated, nontender nodules. Histologically, the lesion is characterized by slightly dilated eccrine glands lined by thin stratified epithelium with terminal comma-like tails.

Sebaceous adenoma is similarly a rare entity on the vulva. Grossly it is multinodular and occupies the labia minora more commonly than the labia majora. The multiple sebaceous glands show a proliferation of the basal cell from which the well-differentiated gland arises. There is no cellular atypia.

Pigmented nevi are not uncommon on the vulva (Fig. 1–71). Although the vulva makes up only about 1 per cent of the entire surface of the body, nevertheless, approximately 3 to 5 per cent of malignant melanomas in the female arise in this area. The reasons for such statistics may be the variety of traumas to which the vulva is subjected and the frequency of "junction" activity in the vulvar nevus (Fig. 1–72). In the latter, the nests of nevus cells lie in the basal layer and the activity in "dropping off and invading" the underlying tissue is frequent. This per se is not tantamount to malignancy, but the activity, as demonstrated by the presence of in-

flammatory cells and free pigment, is ominous. Excision with wide margins is the treatment of choice.

The juvenile nevus, often designated as giant and spindle cell nevus, is benign but may be misinterpreted as malignant melanoma. The underlying vascularity with an intradermal component assists in differentiating this lesion from its malignant counterpart (Fig. 1–73). Biopsy of the pigmented lesion has not been recommended because of the possibility of dispersing cells if the tumor is malignant. However, there is no documented validity to this thesis, and in view of the many pigmented lesions on the vulva, biopsy is the only technique by which a positive diagnosis can be established.

Granular cell myoblastoma (Fig. 1–74) is a rare vulvar tumor found more commonly in other areas of the body, the most frequent being the tongue. Although the name suggests an origin from smooth muscle, the lesion undoubtedly arises from the nerve sheath and is more accurately described as schwannoma. The majority of the vulvar lesions have been found on the labia majora, and they are rarely more than 2 to 3 cm. in diameter. The surface is often superficially ulcerated. The characteristic cells are large, contain eosinophilic granules of various

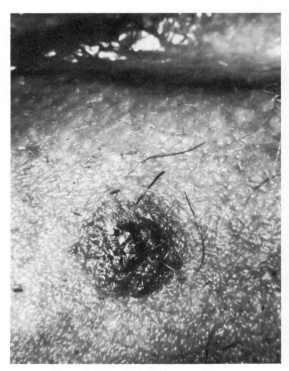

Figure 1–71. Grossly pigmented nevus.

Figure 1–72. Nevus showing marked junction activity at arrow.

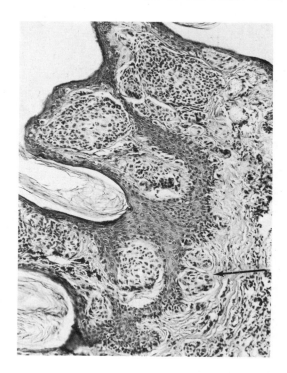

Figure 1–73. Juvenile nevus.

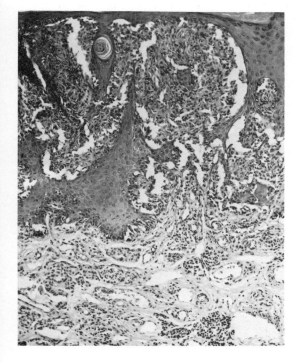

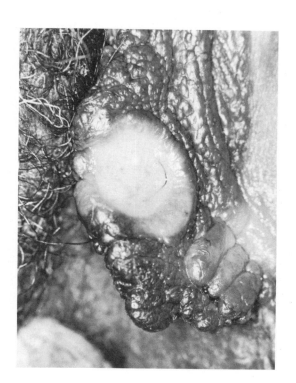

Figure 1–74. Granular cell myoblastoma.

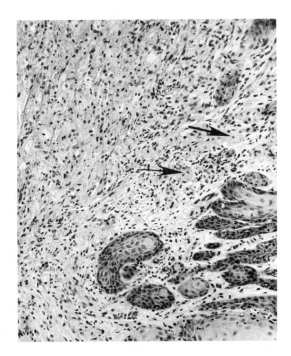

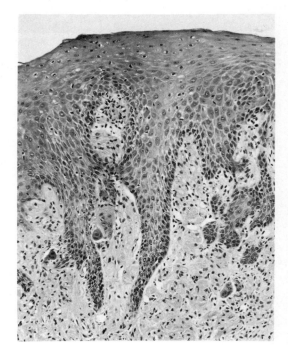

Figure 1–75. Granular cell myoblastoma. Pseudoepitheliomatous alterations are evident. Large cells with cytoplasmic eosinophilic granules are difficult to distinguish (at arrows).

Figure 1–76. Granular cell myoblastoma (schwannoma). The large pale cells containing prominent eosinophilic granules can be recognized in the stroma. The confusing pseudocarcinomatous hyperplasia suggests early invasive cancer.

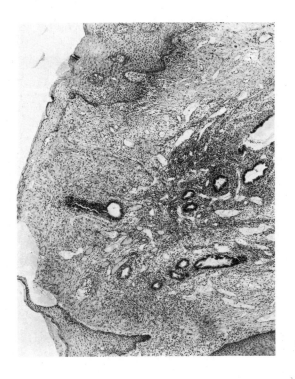

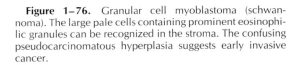

Figure 1–77. Endometriosis with extension to surface.

sizes, and have a slightly basophilic nucleus (Fig. 1–75). The routine pseudocarcinomatous hyperplastic changes in the overlying epithelium have been diagnosed as carcinoma in situ; however, they are benign (Fig. 1–76). Although local recurrences and occasional malignant changes have been reported, most cases of "metastases" are, in reality, instances of multiple primary tumors. The margins of the lesions are poorly identified and thus recurrences are not uncommon.

Endometriosis is an uncommon lesion in the vulvar area. It may occur in the Bartholin's gland region or in the incision resulting from surgery on the gland. The cyclic nature of the symptoms usually makes the diagnosis, and tissue excision confirms the presence of typical endometrial glands and stroma (Fig. 1–77). On other occasions it is found in the upper labium majus along the peritoneal investment of the round ligament.

MALIGNANT TUMORS OF VULVA

CARCINOMA IN SITU, INTRAEPITHELIAL CARCINOMA (FORMERLY BOWEN'S DISEASE, ERYTHROPLASIA OF QUEYRAT AND CARCINOMA SIMPLEX)

These lesions are grouped together in this discussion because they are basically all examples of preinvasive cancer. Recent reports suggest an increase in the incidence of such lesions, particularly in the third and fourth decades of life. Of interest is the association with multicentric anaplastic changes in the anogenital area. Numerous instances of in situ lesions occurring simultaneously on perineum, vulva, and cervix have been reported, and these associations suggest the possibility that an infectious agent may be the etiologic factor, particularly in the younger patient. This thesis is supported by the gross condylomatous appearance of some lesions.

Grossly carcinoma in situ presents a variety of pictures, varying from diffuse or localized white hypertrophic areas with or without a reddened background to atypically pigmented lesions. Toluidine blue may be a helpful diagnostic procedure to define the common multiple foci of neoplasia. How-

ever, false negative and false positive reactions are not uncommon, since the nuclear stain will be absorbed in excoriated but benign foci while neoplastic hyperkeratotic lesions remain unaffected (Figs. 1–78 and 1–79). The atypical pigmentation also is not well defined by such studies (Fig. 1–80). Microscopically, the changes may simulate the characteristic picture of Bowen's disease (Fig. 1–81). The epithelium is acanthotic, with alternating hyperkeratosis and parakeratosis. The former are characteristically white and the latter reddish. Although stratification is present, the abnormal cells are seen in all layers. Corps ronds, nuclear clumps and grains, and individual cell keratinization are evidences of the atypical type of maturation characteristic of Bowen's disease (Fig. 1–82). Such lesions have a very low invasive potential; nevertheless, they are a form of carcinoma in situ. Other conditions demonstrate changes more characteristic of the cervical lesion—namely, complete loss of the normal stratification, with absence of the superficial cells. A combination of these cellular alterations is not uncommon; thus, there are few instances of pure Bowen's disease. Finally, there may be no alteration in the superficial epithelium, the

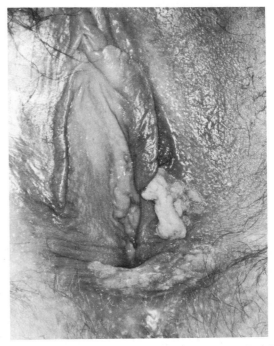

Figure 1–78. White lesion can be appreciated on the left vulva just above the fourchette. The irregular reddish area with white islands is poorly demonstrated at the fourchette.

A Flat and papillary vulvar condylomas in diabetic patient. B Pigmented seborrhoeic keratosis—differential diagnosis, including melanoma, carcinoma in situ, etc. C Carcinoma in situ associated with benign condylomata acuminata in vagina and cervix. D Granular cell myoblastoma treated as chronic chancre for 6 weeks. E Atypical hyperplastic dystrophy—developed invasive cancer in 18 months (see *F*). F Invasive cancer 18 months after excision of prepuce (see *E*) with atypical hyperplastic dystrophy—negative biopsy 9 months ago. G Large verrucous carcinoma—negative codes. H Classic ulcerative carcinoma with positive nodes.

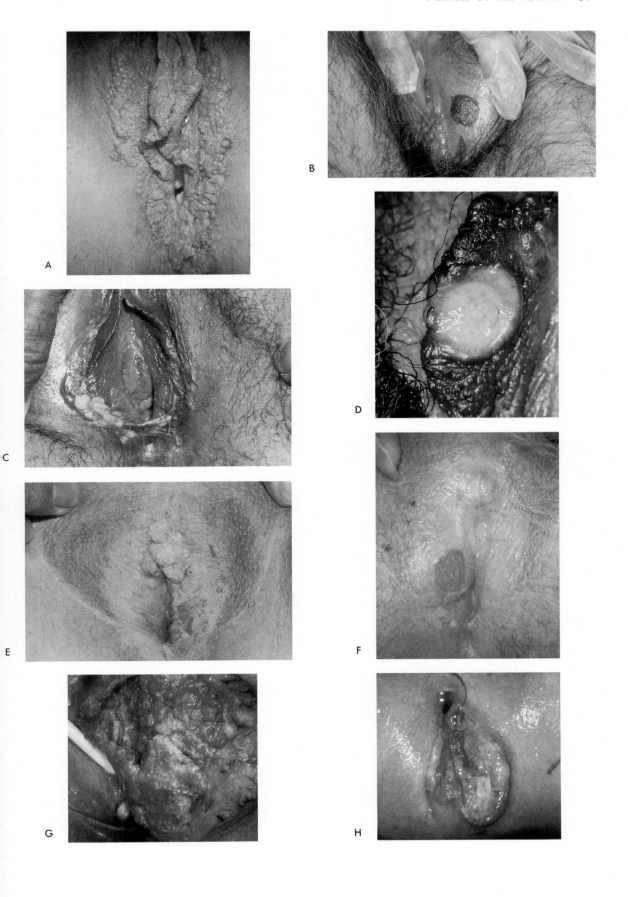

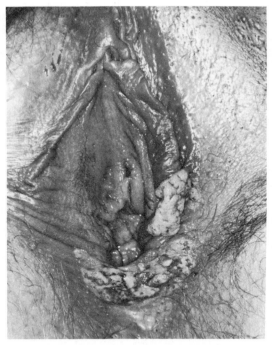

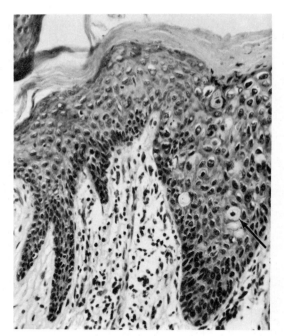

Figure 1–81. Carcinoma in situ on right (corps ronds at arrow) and normal epithelium on left.

Figure 1–79. Same lesion as seen in Figure 1–78 after toluidine blue staining. Note that the white lesion is poorly stained, while the reddish areas at fourchette are prominent.

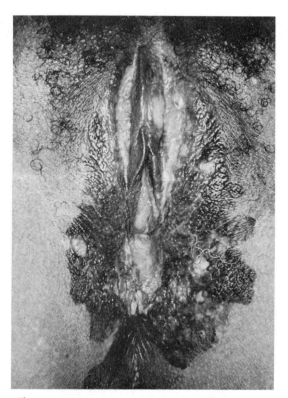

Figure 1–80. Carcinoma in situ of vulva with intense pigmentation.

only evidence of anaplasia being atypical maturation in the rete pegs with a tendency for these pearls to drop off into the underlying stroma. Multicentric origin of such lesions is well known and occasionally necessitates vulvectomy. Certainly in the young patient all such changes must be evaluated carefully, since reversible atypia has been reported. Finally, local chemotherapy may play a prominent role in the treatment of such lesions.

Paget's disease of the vulva is rare. Grossly, the picture simulates that seen on the nipple—a brick-red background with slightly raised edges and a variable number of white surface epithelial islands (Fig. 1–83). The breast lesion is characteristically associated with an underlying intraductal carcinoma, but in most cases of vulvar Paget's disease, the lesion is limited to the skin. The classic large cell with its abundant, finely granular cytoplasm and light, basophilic nucleus may be seen primarily in the parabasal layer of the epithelium (Fig. 1–84); however, individual elements are present throughout the various strata, as well as in the underlying appendages.

In approximately 25 per cent of the cases there is invasive disease. The latter is represented by an adenocarcinoma in the apo-

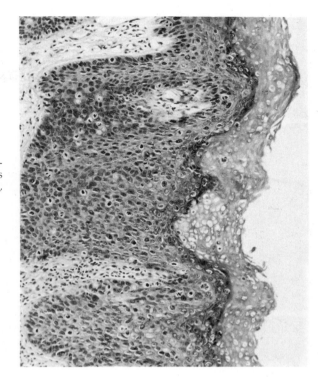

Figure 1–82. Carcinoma in situ showing hyperkeratosis and irregular acanthosis. Anaplastic cell alterations are characterized by individual cell keratinization (IK), chromatin clumping (CC), and corps ronds (CR).

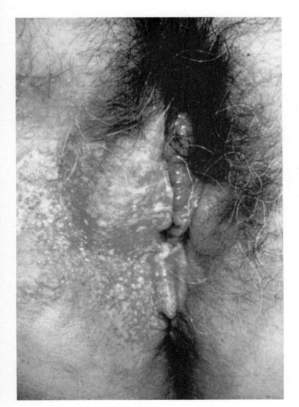

Figure 1–83. Paget's disease of the vulva. The white epithelial islands can be visualized with the red background (slate-colored in this photo).

crine system, or the individual cells may demonstrate malignant tendencies throughout the surface layers, with direct invasion into the underlying stroma. The metastases may reveal a squamous pattern with "pagetoid cells." The origin of the characteristic cell type remains somewhat controversial; many feel that it arises from the embryonal stratum germinativum as cells that are basically destined to be part of the apocrine system and may therefore be found in any of the appendages. Electron microscopic studies suggest that the classic cell is, in all respects, similar to the apocrine variety. In intraepithelial disease, the appendages are involved in 75 to 80 per cent of the cases.

There may be two varieties of Paget's disease. The most common lesion on the vulva seems to begin and remain as an intraepithelial disease. The characteristic sequence of excision and recurrence without metastasis over a period of many years suggests the persistent intraepithelial variety. Conversely, the neoplasm that begins in the underlying system, and invades early, often develops metastases before the surface epithelium is involved (Figs. 1–85 and 1–86). The latter affords little opportunity for curative surgery, and irradiation has not been a successful adjunctive therapy. Regrettably, recent

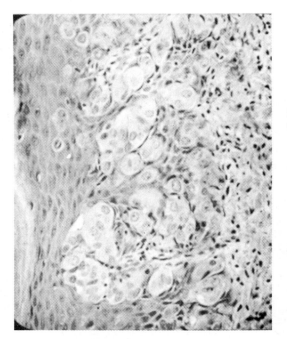

Figure 1–84. Paget's disease of the vulva, a rare lesion. Note typical Paget cells, identical with those seen in Paget's disease of the nipple.

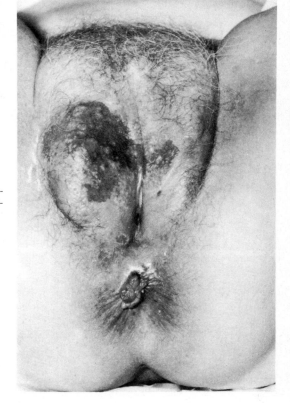

Figure 1–85. Malignant form of Paget's disease involving both labia majora. Patient had retroperitoneal and supraclavicular nodes involved at time of first visit.

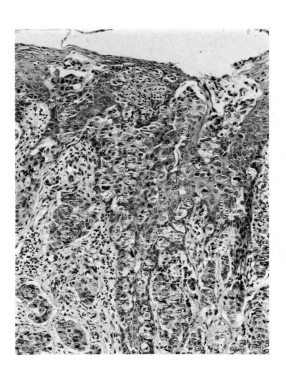

Figure 1–86. Microscopic appearance of lesion in Figure 1–85, showing extensive invasion of underlying tissues.

studies have been unable to demonstrate histologic differences between the invasive and the in situ lesions.

Malignancies of the vulva may be classified as follows:

I Epithelial
Squamous cell—mature, immature, and mixed
Basal cell
Verrucous carcinoma
Bartholin's gland carcinoma
II Melanoma
III Other
Fibroleiomyosarcoma
Lymphoma
Rhabdomyosarcoma

Carcinoma of the Vulva

Squamous cell carcinoma of the vulva is the most frequent of the vulvar malignancies. It ranks third in incidence among genital cancers, being exceeded only by uterine and ovarian carcinoma. Approximately 3 to 4 per cent of all primary malignancies of the genital canal arise in this area.

Classification

Most investigators have developed some special categorization of vulvar neoplasia. Most recently, the International Federation of Gynecology and Obstetrics (FIGO) proposed use of the TNM (tumor-node-metastases) nomenclature as follows:

FIGO Classification of Carcinoma of the Vulva

TNM Classification and Clinical Staging of Carcinoma of the Vulva (adopted in 1970, to be used from January 1, 1971.)

T—Primary Tumor
T1 Tumor confined to the vulva— 2 cm. or less in larger diameter
T2 Tumor confined to the vulva— more than 2 cm. in diameter
T3 Tumor of any size with adjacent spread to the urethra and/or vagina and/or perineum and/or the anus
T4 Tumor of any size infiltrating the bladder mucosa and/or the rectum mucosa, including the upper part of the urethral mucosa and/or fixed to the bone

N—Regional Lymph Nodes
N0 No nodes palpable
N1 Nodes palpable in either groin, not enlarged, mobile (not clinically suspicious of neoplasm)
N2 Nodes palpable in either one or both groins, enlarged, firm and mobile (clinically suspicious of neoplasm)
N3 Fixed or ulcerated nodes
M—Distant metastases
M0 No clinical metastases
M1a Palpable deep pelvic lymph nodes
M1b Other distant metastases

Clinical Stage Groups

Stage I			Stage II		
T1	N0	M0	T2	N0	M0
T1	N1	M0	T2	N1	M0
Stage III			*Stage IV*		
T3	N0	M0	T1	N3	M0
T3	N1	M0	T2	N3	M0
T3	N2	M0	T3	N3	M0
T1	N2	M0	T4	N0	M0
T2	N2	M0	T4	N1	M0
			T4	N2	M0
			T4	N3	M0

All other conditions containing M1a or M1b

Although this classification has merit, it is cumbersome and could be resolved into four stages that would cover adequately all the features of the FIGO proposal:

Stage I—Primary tumor of 2 cm. or less without palpable nodes or with nodes not clinically suspicious.

Stage II—Primary tumor larger than 2 cm. without palpable nodes or nodes not clinically suspicious.

Stage III—Tumor of any size with palpable nodes, suspicious or nonsuspicious, and with invasion into the urethra, vagina, perineum, or anal orifice; or tumor of any size with clinically suspicious nodes.

Stage IV—Tumor of any size with fixed or ulcerated nodes, with neoplastic infiltration of the bladder and/or rectal mucosas or fixed to the bony pelvis.

All metastatic disease is included in Stage IV. Furthermore, recent studies suggest that survival rates for Stage III and Stage IV M1a are similar, while there are essentially no survivors among the patients with Stage IV M1b lesions—i.e., those with distant metastases.

Primary carcinoma of the vulva is characteristically a disease of the seventh and eighth decades of life; however, the average age of patients in whom it is preceded by granulomatous disease is approximately 40 years—i.e., 20 years younger than the usually quoted age incidence. This cancer may arise from any area on the external genitalia, particularly in the postgranulomatous cases. The most common site for the classic lesion is the upper labia majora.

Several lesions have been mentioned in this chapter as possible precursors of vulvar carcinoma; chief among these are the atypical hyperplastic dystrophies characterized by thick, hard cartilaginous plaques often traversed by linear excoriations. Nevertheless, careful follow-up of the common typical dystrophies and lichen sclerosus has revealed that rarely do these lesions culminate in the development of invasive neoplasia. Douglas has reported that in the West Indies, 45 per cent of vulvar malignancies are preceded by granulomatous disease, and others record similar experiences. Charlewood and Shippel report four of 11 carcinomas beginning in condylomas. It would seem that some chronic irritative lesion is commonly the precursor of vulvar malignancy; consequently, such lesions warrant frequent biopsy if prompt healing does not take place (Fig. 1–87 A,B). Viral diseases must be considered seriously in view of the mutation changes in the nucleus associated with such infections. The initial lesion in vulvar carcinoma is apt to be an inconspicuous one, so that delay in seeking medical attention is the rule. A small nodular ulcerative lesion appears, gradually enlarges, and terminates in a papillomatous fungoid lesion (exophytic) (Fig. 1–88). The inguinal and femoral lymph nodes are the earliest extravulvar tissues involved. Extension into the adjacent vagina, rectum, and urethra is not uncommon in the more advanced lesions. Deeper involvement into the bladder or rectal sphincter may result in incontinence of urine or feces. Classification of vulvar malignancy is based on the size and extent of local invasion and metastases. The disease is not prone to cause widespread distant metastases, as noted by Lundwall, who found evidence of extrapelvic disease in only 14 or 186 autopsy cases. It is thus of major importance that the local lesions be excised widely if recurrences in the perineal area are to be

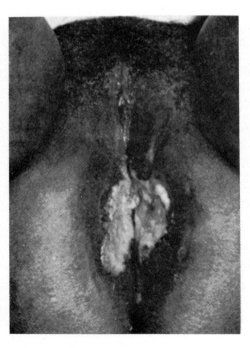

A

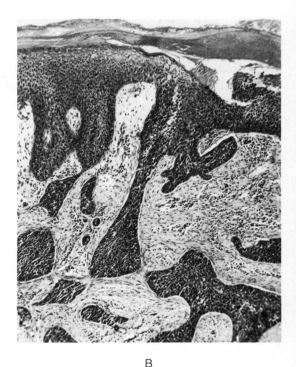

B

Figure 1–87. *A,* Lymphogranuloma with subsequent carcinoma involving most of vulva as well as posterior vaginal wall. (Patient alive and well after radical vulvectomy, Miles and Basset procedure.) Recurred as a carcinoma in situ in elephantiasis 9 years later. *B,* Invasive carcinoma associated with gross lesion of *A.*

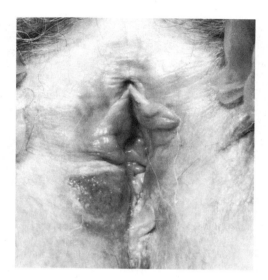

Figure 1–88.   Carcinoma of vulva.

avoided (Fig. 1–89). Furthermore, such recurrences should be widely excised since they may, in truth, represent re-occurrences of disease rather than demonstrations of incomplete excision.

Microscopically, the highly differentiated, keratinizing lesion constitutes approximately 75 per cent of all the epithelial lesions (Fig. 1–90*A*). Large nests and columns of such cells are seen to extend deeply into the stroma. The surface ulceration may be fictitious in that the granulomatous base is really covered by an atypical epithelium. At

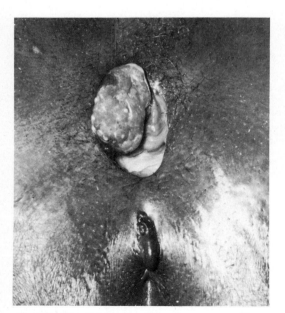

Figure 1–89.   Carcinoma of the vulva recurrent 18 years after radical vulvectomy.

the margin of the ulcer, the vulvar epithelium *often is quite normal.* Conversely, atypical hyperplasia, characterized by a central core of abnormally keratinized cells, or even carcinoma in situ may reside in the immediate vicinity. The connective tissue routinely shows chronic inflammatory infiltrate. More undifferentiated forms are not uncommonly associated with preexisting granulomatous disease (Fig. 1–90*B*); however, they may appear without any specific precursory disease. A recent report suggests that the cytogenetics of the mature and immature varieties are basically different, the former demonstrating a striking peri-triploid component and being associated with a higher incidence of nodal involvement. More studies are necessary to establish the importance of such findings.

In these lesions arising from the clitoris, Taussig emphasized a sarcoma-like pattern, the cells being of immature, embryonic type, with heavily staining nuclei and marked mitotic activity. This poorly differentiated or "epidermoid" tumor arises at any area and constitutes approximately 20 per cent of all primary carcinomas of the vulva. Although the tumor appears more aggressive histologically, in the author's opinion the survival has not been influenced by the degree of differentiation of the tumor. Therapy in most clinics consists of one-stage radical vulvectomy with lymphadenectomy. The latter is combined with extraperitoneal excision of the deep nodes if the superficial inguinal and femoral nodes are positive. Recently certain investigators are employing total pelvic irra-

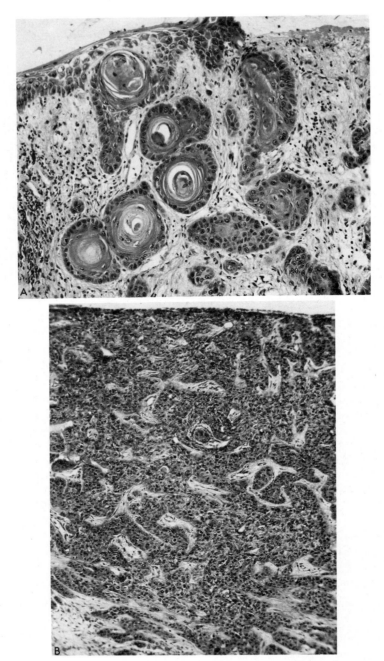

Figure 1–90. *A*, Invasive squamous cell cancer showing pearl formation. *B*, Epidermoid carcinoma of the vulva. Note difference in maturity of tumor cells. (From Saltzstein et al.: Obstet. Gynecol., 7:80, 1956. Courtesy P. B. Hoeber, Inc.)

diation in place of the deep lymphadenectomy in view of the minimal salvage rate if the pelvic nodes are positive; the results are yet to be evaluated. In stages I and II, 5 year survival figures approach 90 per cent, while with regional node involvement, a 35 to 40 per cent salvage can be expected (Fig. 1–91).

Verrucous carcinoma must be differen-

tiated from the classic invasive lesion. Such tumors are commonly large and exuberant (Fig. 1–92). Often regional nodes are palpable but negative for tumor. The histologic demonstration of true invasion is difficult to establish in view of the normal maturation of the invading cells (Fig. 1–93). This feature is in contrast to the pearl formation seen in the classic squamous cell lesion. Although this

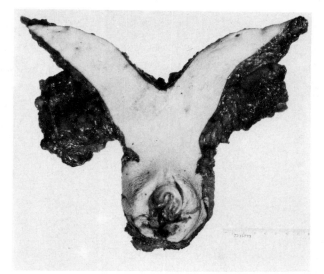

Figure 1–91. Resected vulva and adjacent nodal tissues.

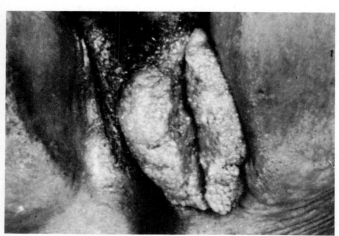

Figure 1–92. Verrucous carcinoma. Vulvo-inguinal nodes palpable and *negative*.

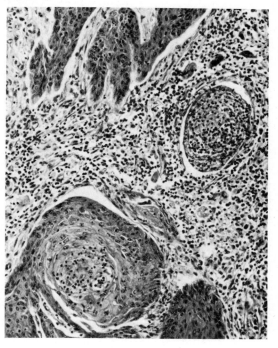

Figure 1–93. Verrucous carcinoma of the vulva. Nests of cells seem to be invading but the evidence of individual cell atypia and keratinization is absent or minimal.

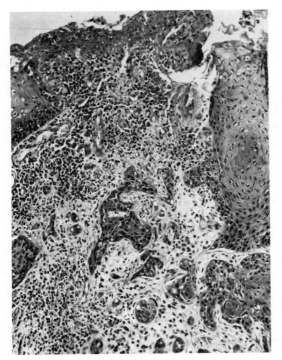

Figure 1–94. Microinvasive carcinoma of the vulva, less than 3 mm. invasion and less than 2 cm. in size, with positive inguinal nodes.

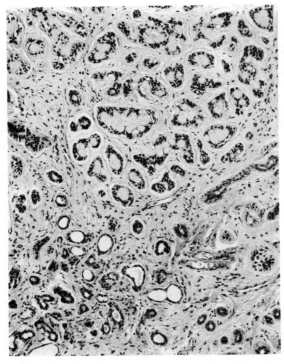

Figure 1–95. Adenoid-cystic "cribriform" type of adenocarcinoma of Bartholin's gland (simulates appendage tumor). (From Woodruff and Seeds: Obstet. Gynecol., 20:690, 1962.)

lesion is locally invasive and recurring, metastases, even to the regional nodes, rarely if ever develop. Consequently, wide local excision is the surgical procedure of choice.

In contrast to the large noninvasive verrucous lesion is the so-called microinvasive carcinoma. This dangerous designation has led to the use of simple vulvectomy for neoplasms with less than 3 mm. of invasion (Fig. 1–94). Unfortunately, there are several reports noting the development of widespread metastatic disease and death following such therapeutic programs. Consequently, any lesion, regardless of size, with true stromal invasion should be treated as other invasive tumors. As a matter of fact, these small invasive tumors may be much more aggressive than large lesions of 8 to 10 years' duration.

Microscopically, the tumor that originates at the orifice is of the squamous variety, since it arises from the stratified epithelium invaginating into the gland and is thus a classic carcinoma of the vulva rather than of Bartholin's gland. From the duct, lined by transitional epithelium, a very rare papillary type may develop. Finally, in the secreting area, the classic lesion is an adenocarcinoma quite similar to the adenoid cystic tumor of the salivary glands (Fig. 1–95 and 1–96). This cribriform carcinoma has a tendency to invade deeply into the adjacent tissue, to recur locally, and to metastasize late, often to the lung. Consequently, the treatment is extensive local excision, and removal of regional nodes is of questionable import. This adenoid-cystic tumor must be differentiated from the benign adenoma of Bartholin's gland (Fig. 1–97).

Basal Cell Carcinoma

In spite of the usually high degree of malignancy of vulvar cancer, occasional cases are seen in which the carcinoma appears, both microscopically and clinically, to be similar to the readily curable basal cell carcinoma noted elsewhere on the skin as "rodent ulcers." While locally malignant, these basal cell carcinomas rarely metastasize and appear to respond favorably to radiotherapy and wide local excision. Grossly, these lesions are ulcerative with slightly rolled, raised, and indurated edges (Fig. 1–98 A). Microscopically, the masses of small, dark,

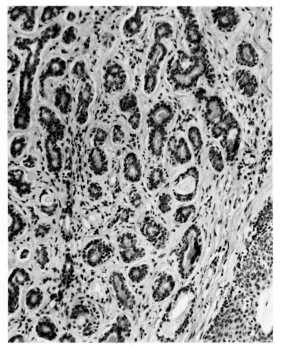

Figure 1–96. Adenoid-cystic tumor.

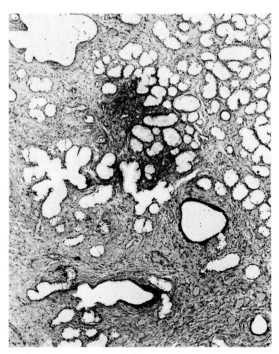

Figure 1–97. Benign adenoma of Bartholin's gland.

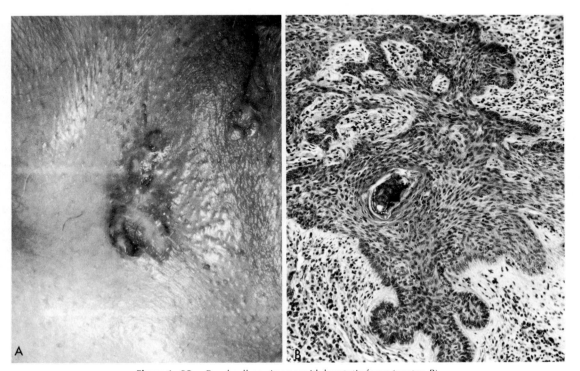

Figure 1–98. Basal cell carcinoma with keratotic focus (center, *B*).

basal cells with a monotonous pattern spread serpiginously into the underlying tissue but generally maintain continuity with the surface epithelium and as a result, as noted, metastasis is rare (Fig. 1–98 B) and is only to the regional nodes.

Rarely, the lesion may demonstrate both a basal and a squamous component (Fig. 1–99 A). Definition of prognosis depends on the relationship between the basal and the squamous elements. A well-identified basal cell carcinoma with keratotic foci behaves like the classic basal tumor and thus demands only wide local excision. Conversely, there are neoplasms composed of immature, anaplastic cells with focal maturation. Such tumors are aggressive and simulate cloacal cancer and demand more aggressive therapy. Extension of the tumor may reveal rather unique characteristics, as demonstrated by the invasion of the perineural spaces seen in Figure 1–99 B.

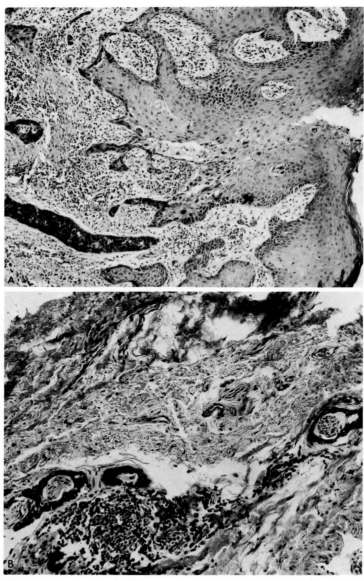

Figure 1–99. A, Infiltrative lesion demonstrating both the mature pearl-forming pattern and the small, dark, basal type. B, Extension of the basal element of the "basosquamous" cancer into the perineural space deep in the vulval tissues. (All the nodes were negative in this patient.)

OTHER MALIGNANT LESIONS OF THE VULVA

Malignant Melanoma

Although malignant lesions other than those of epithelial origin are rare, their presence must be recognized. Malignant melanoma composes approximately 2 to 3 per cent of vulvar neoplasms. These lesions may occur in any age group. Two basic gross patterns are recognized—the nodular and the spreading varieties. The former may be amelanotic. To identify the nature of the pigmented lesion, biopsy is necessary, since there are a large variety of such alterations that may occur on the vulva. The microscopic appearance commonly reveals "junction" activity, but rarely does an intradermal nevus become malignant. The malignant potential is determined by the level of involvement of the dermis. At level I only the interpapillary ridges are involved, basically an "in situ" lesion. In contrast, level V lesions extend beyond the reticular dermis into the adjacent fat. Survival corresponds to the level of involvement (Fig. 1–100 A,B), that is, approximately 100 per cent for level I and II lesions and 0 per cent for those with invasion of the fat. These true malignant melanomas must be differentiated from the "juvenile nevus." In the latter, although there is apparent involvement of the dermis, the deep cells do not invade from the junction area but are really intradermal. Early and radical surgical therapy as reported by Symmonds and others has resulted in excellent 5 year salvage. Unfortunately, radiation therapy has been unsuccessful in controlling extension of the disease. Recent reports suggest that chemotherapeutic agents, particularly DTIC, may be the adjunctive therapy of choice.

Fibrosarcoma

This is less frequent than melanoma, the incidence being about 2 per cent of all primary lesions in our series. The gross lesions were either hard and nodular or ulcerative. The common microscopic picture represents interlacing bundles of elongated cells with scant cytoplasm, demonstrating extreme nuclear pleomorphism and mitotic activity (Fig. 1–101). Leiomyo-, rhabdomyo-, neuro-, and fibrosarcomas have been reported by DiSaia, with generally poor survival. Treatment has been surgical, and adjunctive

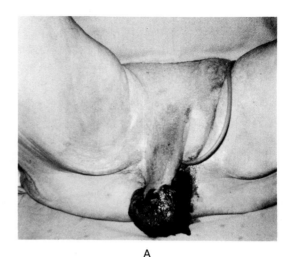

A

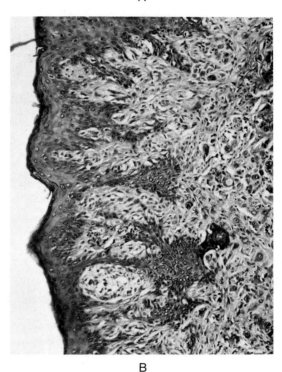

B

Figure 1–100. *A*, Large malignant melanoma simulating a hematoma. (Courtesy of Dr. E. Friedrich.) *B*, Malignant melanoma. Junction activity with invasion of underlying dermis (level II or deeper).

chemotherapy for extensive disease. The latter has not been dramatically successful, but it is better than irradiation.

Rhabdomyosarcoma

Rhabdomyosarcoma of the vulva generally occurs in the young, during the first two decades of life. A rapidly progressive lesion, the

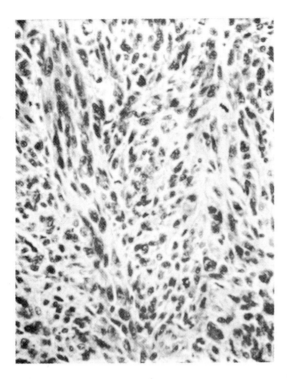

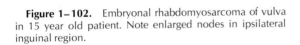

Figure 1–101. Sarcoma of clitoris.

Figure 1–102. Embryonal rhabdomyosarcoma of vulva in 15 year old patient. Note enlarged nodes in ipsilateral inguinal region.

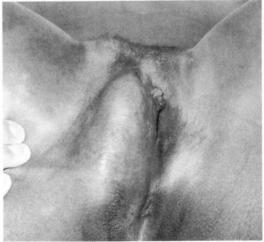

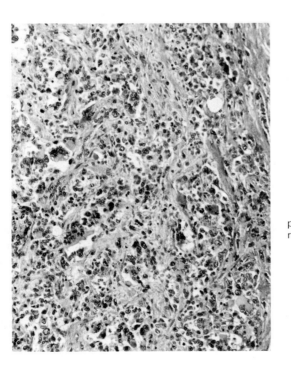

Figure 1–103. Bizarre cellular pattern in vulvar neoplasm of 15 year old patient (see Fig. 1–102). Embryonal rhabdomyosarcoma.

neoplasm extends into the regional and retroperitoneal nodes (Figs. 1–102 and 1–103). Prognosis, as for most such tumors, is poor, although chemotherapy and irradiation have offered a new and promising approach to treatment.

Tumors of Paraurethral Glands

These lesions arise at the vaginal outlet and will be discussed in Chapter 2.

Lymphoma

In this area, as in others, lymphoma is often a local manifestation of a systemic disease, although about 10 per cent of such lesions, as recorded by Gall and Mallory, seem to be localized and may be "cured" by radiation therapy and chemotherapy. Even more widespread disease has been controlled by such means.

Secondary Malignant Tumors

The vulva may be the seat of metastasis from cancer of the uterine body or cervix, or from the adjacent rectum (Figs. 1–104 and 1–105). Chorionepithelioma and hypernephroma also may metastasize to the vulva,

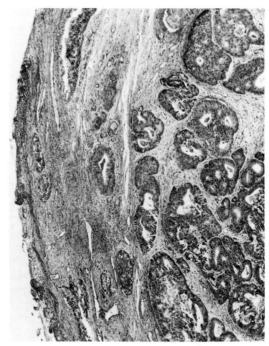

Figure 1–105. Metastatic carcinoma of endometrium to vulva.

though not nearly as frequently as to the vagina. Occasionally other primary tumors in distant organs may be associated with secondary malignancy in the vulva.

DISEASES OF THE URETHRA

Infections

Paraurethral Gland Infections

Skene's ducts are usually recognized at the posterior aspect of the external urethral meatus. They extend suburethrally for 1 to 2 cm. and are usually straight and tubular in structure. The orifice is lined by stratified epithelium and the main portion by transitional epithelium. The ducts are occasionally the seat of acute or chronic inflammatory disease. The orifice appears red, edematous, and everted, and a drop of purulent material can be expressed easily. Although the gonococcus has been recognized as a frequent cause of such infections, a variety of organisms, including *Trichomonas*, may be harbored in these structures. As a result of chronic infection, the orifice may be occluded, with the production of a cyst.

Similarly, the suburethral glands, well described by Huffman, are not uncommonly

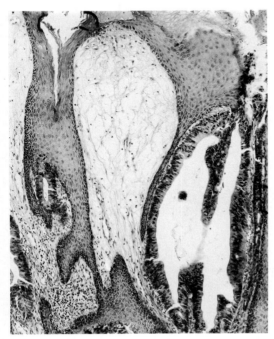

Figure 1–104. Adenocarcinoma of rectum metastatic to vulva. (From Woodruff and Seeds: Obstet. Gynecol., 20:690, 1962.)

chronically infected. As a result of such infections, patients complain of urethral burning and discomfort, often without excessive frequency. In the acute phase the symptoms are those of cystitis, and irritation of the region, as with coitus, may be the major factor in recurrent bladder infections. Cystic dilatations of the glands are well recognized as foci of infection, with pus exuding from the urethral orifice on evacuation of the suburethral sac. These suburethral diverticula are rarely congenital, and result almost routinely from the recurrent infections in the glands.

Microscopically, the usual infiltration into the adjacent submucosa and muscularis is seen. The epithelial lining may be absent, but when present is usually pseudostratified columnar (transitional) or, at the terminal portion, single-layered cuboidal, often mucus-secreting. The latter is similar to the epithelium seen in von Brunn's cell cysts, possibly related to remnants of the cloaca destined initially to become intestinal components.

Urethritis cystica is similar in every respect to its counterpart in the bladder. Small inclusions of transitional epithelium are surrounded by chronically infected submucosa. These may be seen grossly through the panendoscope; however, they more often are represented by a reddened, edematous mucosa from which float filamentous folds of mucous membrane. These are not true tumors but are related to the inflammatory process.

In the postmenopausal period, the epithelium at the urethral meatus takes part in the general atrophy of the adjacent vaginal mucosa. As a result,there is not infrequently a reddened eversion of the urethral tissue in this period. This change is misdiagnosed as caruncle or other tumor formation and treated radically. Most often this lesion is asymptomatic or produces slight traumatic bleeding (Fig. 1–106). Treatment with local estrogens is usually effective.

Benign Tumors

The caruncle is presumably the most common benign tumor occurring in the urethra. As noted previously, many such lesions are in reality prolapsed, chronically infected urethral mucosa, recognized most fre-

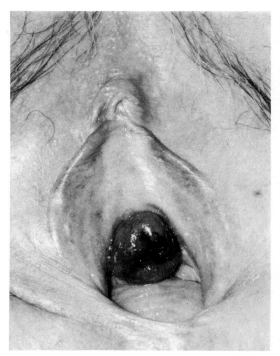

Figure 1–106. Prolapsed, infarcted urethral mucosa with uterine prolapse.

quently after the menopause, at which time the atrophy of the vaginal mucosa is reflected in the urethral orifice as well.

Characteristically, the caruncle is a reddened, tender, polypoid lesion, presenting usually from the posterior portion of the meatus. Tenderness is quite variable; most observers believe, however, that in many cases there are no presenting symptoms.

Microscopically, three forms have been described: papillomatous, angiomatous, and granulomatous. The latter two are quite difficult to distinguish by the usual hematoxylin and eosin stain, since granulation tissue simulates an angiomatous pattern very closely. There are innumerable small vessels surrounded by edematous, almost myxomatous stroma infiltrated with inflammatory cells (Fig. 1–107 A,B,C). The lining is frequently absent because of the inflammation, but if present may be transitional or stratified squamous epithelium. True papillomatous tumors are relatively uncommon.

Condylomata acuminata and squamous papillomas are seen most frequently on the vulva, but do occur in the vagina, in the cervix, and at the urethral meatus (Fig. 1–108). Rarely, the papilloma lined by transitional

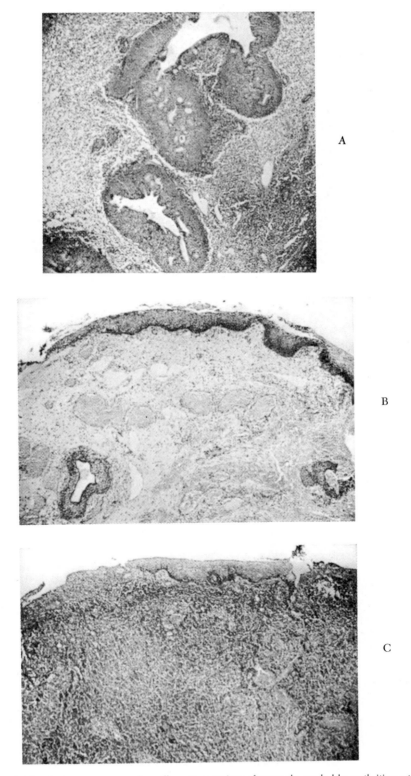

Figure 1–107. *A,* Histologic appearance of papillomatous variety of caruncle, probably urethritis cystica with infolded mucosa. *B,* Angiomatous variety of urethral caruncle, probably prolapsed mucosa with vascular distention. *C,* The granulomatous variety of caruncle, probably of inflammatory origin.

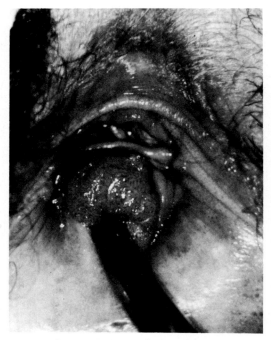

Figure 1–108. Urethral condyloma.

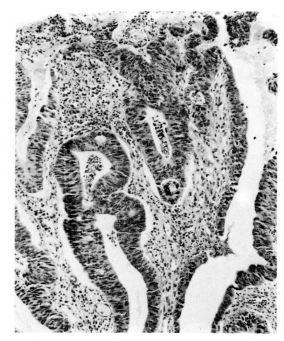

Figure 1–110. Adenocarcinoma primary in urethra.

epithelium, common in the bladder, may be seen in the internal urethra.

Malignant Tumors

Primary carcinoma of the urethra is rare. Of the two varieties—the vulvourethral and urethral—the former is more common. Most of these lesions are squamous carcinoma mi-croscopically and present as polypoid lesions. The urethral variety arises from the stratified epithelium and is therefore similar to papillary carcinoma of the bladder.

Occasionally, the rare mucus-secreting glands of the suburethral area are the site of an adenocarcinoma (Fig. 1–109). This tumor may present vaginally or intraurethrally (Fig. 1–110). The clear cell pattern in many

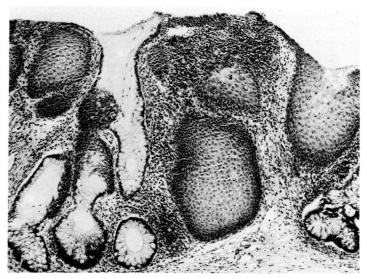

Figure 1–109. Mucus-secreting epithelium with goblet cells in urethra.

areas simulates the tumor of mesonephric origin occasionally arising in the lower genital tract.

Other Primary Malignant Tumors

Sarcoma, melanoma, and lymphoma have been reported to arise from the urethral area. These are so rare that only individual cases are reported, such as that of a malignant melanoma recorded by McBurney and Bale.

Secondary Malignant Tumors

Carcinoma of the bladder, vulva, vagina, and cervix involves the urethra by direct extension. Metastatic nodules secondary to fundal and ovarian carcinoma are occasionally recognized in the suburethral area. Choriocarcinoma may also involve the suburethral area secondarily.

REFERENCES

Alexander, L. J., and Shields, L. T.: Squamous cell cancer secondary to granuloma inguinale. A.M.A. Arch. Dermatol. Syph., 67:395, 1953.

Anderson, J. P.: Hidradenoma of vulva. A.M.A. Arch. Dermatol. Syph., 62:873, 1950.

Birch, H. W., and Sondag, D. R.: Granular-cell myoblastoma of the vulva. Obstet. Gynecol., 18:443, 1961.

Boehm, F., and Morris, J. McL.: Paget's disease and apocrine gland carcinoma of the vulva. Obstet. Gynecol., 38:185, 1971.

Bonney, V.: Leukoplakic vulvitis and conditions liable to be confused with it. Proc. Roy. Soc. Med., 31:1057, 1938.

Boschback, F. W.: Adenoid-cystic carcinoma of Bartholin gland. Geburtshilfe. Frauenheilkd. 29:473, 1969.

Brack, C. B., and Dickson, R. J.: Carcinoma of the female urethra. Am. J. Roentgenol., 79:472, 1958.

Brack, C. B., and Farber, G. J.: Carcinoma of the female urethra. J. Urol., 64:710, 1950.

Charlewood, G. P., and Shippel, S.: Vulval condylomata acuminata as a premalignant lesion in the Bantu. S. Afr. Med. J., 27:149, 1953.

Chiodi, N. E., Siegel, I. A., Guerin, P. F., and McCaughan, D.: Granular-cell myoblastoma of the vulva and lower respiratory tract. Obstet. Gynecol., 9:472, 1957.

Clark, D. G., Zumoff, B., Brunschwig, A., and Hellman, L.: Preferential uptake of phosphate by premalignant and malignant lesions of the vulva. Cancer, 13:775, 1960.

Cole, H. N.: Lymphogranuloma inguinale. J.A.M.A., 101:1069, 1933.

Collins, C. G., Kushner, J., Lewis, G. N., and LaPointe, R.: Noninvasive malignancy of the vulva. Obstet. Gynecol., 6:339, 1955.

Collins, C. G.: Invasive carcinoma of the vulva with lymph node metastases. Am. J. Obstet. Gynecol., 109:446, 1971.

Dawson, D. F., Duckworth, J. D., Bernhardt, H., and

Young, J. M.: Giant condyloma and verrucous carcinoma of the genital area. Arch. Pathol., 17:225, 1965.

DeSousa, L. M., and Lash, A. F.: Hemangiopericytoma of the vulva. Am. J. Obstet. Gynecol., 78:295, 1959.

DiPaola, G. R., Balina, L. M., Gomez-Rueda, N. M., et al.: Treatment of lichen sclerosus et atrophicus of the vulva with topical testosterone. Rev. Argent. Ginecol. Obstet., 2:224–230, 1971.

Di Saia, P. J., Rutledge, F., and Smith, J. P.: Sarcoma of the vulva. Obstet. Gynecol., 38:180, 1971.

Douglas, C. P.: Lymphogranuloma venereum and granuloma inguinale of the vulva. J. Obstet. Gynaecol. Br. Commonw., 69:871, 1962.

Fagan, G. E., and Hertig, A. J.: Carcinoma of the female urethra. Obstet. Gynecol., 6:1, 1955.

Friedrich, E. G., Julian, C. G., and Woodruff, J. D.: Acridine orange fluorescence in vulvar dysplasia. Am. J. Obstet. Gynecol., 90:1281, 1964.

Friedrich, E. G.: Reversible vulvar atypia. Obstet. Gynecol., 39:173, 1972.

Friedrich, E. G.: Vulvar Disease. Philadelphia, W. B. Saunders Company, 1976.

Greenblatt, R. B., Dienst, R. B., Pund, E. R., and Torpin, R.: Experimental and clinical granuloma inguinale. J.A.M.A., 113:1109, 1939.

Hart, W. R.: Paramesonephric mucinous cysts of the vulva. Am. J. Obstet. Gynecol., 107:1079, 1970.

Hart, W. R., Norris, H. J., and Helwig, E. B.: Relation of lichen sclerosus et atrophicus of the vulva to development of carcinoma. Obstet. Gynecol., 45:369–377, 1975.

Hassim, A. M.: Bilateral fibroadenoma in supernumerary breasts of the vulva. J. Obstet. Gynaecol. Br. Commonw., 76:275, 1969.

Hay, D. M., and Cole, F. M.: Post-granulomatous carcinoma of the vulva. Am. J. Obstet. Gynecol., 107:479, 1970.

Hester, L. J.: Granuloma venereum of cervix and vulva. Am. J. Obstet. Gynecol., 62:312, 1951.

Huber, C. P., Gardiner, S. H., and Michael, A.: Paget's disease of the vulva. Am. J. Obstet. Gynecol., 62:778, 1951.

Huffman, J. W.: Detailed anatomy of paraurethral ducts in adult human female. Am. J. Obstet. Gynecol., 55:86, 1948.

Japaze, H., Garcia-Bunuel, R., and Woodruff, J. D.: Primary vulvar neoplasia: A review of in situ and invasive carcinoma, 1935–1972. Obstet. Gynecol., 49:404, 1977.

Jeffcoate, T. N. A.: Chronic vulval dystrophies. J. Obstet. Gynecol., 95:61–74, 1966.

Jeffcoate, T. N.: Dermatology of the vulva. J. Obstet. Gynaecol. Br. Commonw. 69:888, 1962.

Katayama, K. P., Woodruff, J. D., Jones, H. W., Jr., and Preston, E.: Chromosomes of condyloma acuminatum, Paget's disease, in situ carcinoma, invasive squamous cell carcinoma and malignant melanoma of the human vulva. Obstet. Gynecol., 39:346, 1972.

Kaufman, R. H., Gardner, H. L., Brown, D., et al.: Vulvar dystrophies: an evaluation. Am. J. Obstet. Gynecol., 120:363–367, 1974.

Ketron, L. W., and Ellis, F. A.: Kraurosis vulvae (leukoplakia) and scleroderma circumscripta. Surg. Gynecol. Obstet., 61:635, 1935.

Langley, I. I., Hertig, A. T., and Smith, G. van S.: Relation of leucoplakic vulvitis to squamous carcinoma of vulva. Am. J. Obstet. Gynecol., 62:167, 1951.

Lipschütz, B.: Ulcus vulvae acutum. Jadassohns Handb. der Haut- und Geschlechtskrankheiten. Berlin, J. Springer, 1927.

McAdams, A. J., Jr., and Kistner, R.: The relationship of chronic vulvar disease, leukoplakia, and carcinoma in situ to carcinoma of the vulva. Cancer, *11*:740, 1958.

McBurney, R. P., and Bale, G. F.: Primary malignant melanoma of the female urethra. Surgery, *37*:973, 1955.

McDonald, J. R.: Apocrine sweat gland carcinoma of vulva. Am. J. Clin. Pathol., *11*:890, 1941.

Miller, N. F., Riley, G. M., and Stanley, M. G.: Leukoplakia vulvae. Am. J. Obstet. Gynecol., *64*:768, 1952.

Neilson, D. R., Jr., and Woodruff, J. D.: Electron microscopy in "in situ and invasive" vulvar Paget's disease. Am. J. Obstet. Gynecol., *113*:719, 1972.

Newman, B., and Gray, D. B.: Primary carcinoma of Bartholin's gland. Am. J. Surg., *92*:490, 1956.

Newman, W., and Cromer, J. K.: Multicentric origin of carcinomas of the female anogenital tract. Surg. Gynecol. Obstet., *108*:273, 1959.

Novak, E., and Stevenson, R. R.: Sweat gland tumors of vulva, benign (hidradenoma) and malignant (adenocarcinoma). Am. J. Obstet. Gynecol., *50*:641, 1945.

Nowak, R. J.: Basal cell carcinoma of the vulva. Obstet. Gynecol., *4*:392, 1954.

Palladino, V. S., Duffy, J. L., and Bures, G. J.: Basal cell carcinoma of the vulva. Cancer, *24*:460, 1969.

Pund, E. R., and Greenblatt, R. B.: Specific history of granuloma inguinale. A.M.A. Arch. Pathol., *23*:224, 1937.

Richart, R. M.: A clinical staining test for the in vivo delineation of dysplasia and carcinoma in situ. Am. J. Obstet. Gynecol., *86*:703, 1963.

Rutledge, F., Smith, J. P., and Franklin, E. W.: Epidemiology of carcinoma of the vulva. Am. J. Obstet. Gynecol., *106*:1117, 1970.

Sadler, W. P., and Dockerty, M. D.: Malignant myoblastoma vulvae. Am. J. Obstet. Gynecol., *61*:1047, 1951.

Salzstein, S. L., Woodruff, J. D., and Novak, E. R.: Postgranulomatous carcinoma of the vulva. Obstet. Gynecol., *7*:80, 1956.

Stone, M. J., and Abbey, F. A.: Sebaceous cyst: its importance as a precancerous lesion. Arch. Dermatol. Syph., *31*:512, 1935.

Symmonds, R. E., Pratt, J. H., and Dockerty, M. B.: Melanoma of the vulva. Obstet. Gynecol., *15*:543, 1960.

Taussig, F. J.: Diseases of Vulva. New York, D. Appleton-Century Co., 1921.

Taussig, F. J.: Leukoplakic vulvitis and cancer of the vulva. Am. J. Obstet. Gynecol., *18*:472, 1929.

Taussig, F. J.: Sarcoma of the vulva. Am. J. Obstet. Gynecol., *33*:1017, 1937.

Taussig, F. J.: Metastatic tumors of vagina and vulva. Surg. Clin. North Am., *18*:1309, 1938.

Walker, L. M., and Huffman, J. W.: Adenocarcinoma of female urethra. Rev. Quart. Bull., Northwestern University Med. School, *21*:115, 1947.

Wallace, H. S.: Vulvar leukoplakia. J. Obstet. Gynaecol. Br. Commonw., *69*:865, 1962.

Way, S. C., and Memmesheimer, A.: The sudoriparous gland. II. The apocrine glands. Arch. Dermatol. Syph., *38*:373, 1938.

Wharton, L. R., and Everett, H. S.: Primary malignant Bartholin gland tumors. Obstet. Gynecol. Surv., 6:1, 1951.

Wharton, L. R., and Kearns, W.: Diverticula of the female urethra. J. Urol., *63*:1063, 1950.

Woodruff, J. D.: Paget's disease of the vulva. Obstet. Gynecol., *5*:175, 1955.

Woodruff, J. D., Borkowf, H. I., Holzman, G. B., Arnold, E. A., and Knaack, J.: Metabolic activity in normal and abnormal vulvar epithelia. Am. J. Obstet. Gynecol., *91*:809, 1965.

Woodruff, J. D., and Brack, C. B.: Unusual malignancies of the vulva-urethral region. Obstet. Gynecol., *12*:677, 1958.

Woodruff, J. D., and Hildebrandt, E. E.: Carcinoma in situ of the vulva. Obstet. Gynecol., *12*:414, 1958.

Woodruff, J. D., Julian, C. G., Puray, T., et al.: The contemporary challenge of carcinoma in situ of the vulva. Am. J. Obstet. Gynecol., *115*:677, 1973.

Woodworth, H., Jr., Dockerty, M. B., Wilson, R. B., and Pratt, J. H.: Papillary hidradenoma of the vulva. Am. J. Obstet. Gynecol., *190*:501, 1971.

Yackel, D. B., Symmonds, R. E., and Kempers, R. D.: Melanoma of the vulva. Obstet. Gynecol., *35*:625, 1970.

Zelle, K.: Treatment of vulvar dystrophies with topical testosterone propionate. Am. J. Obstet. Gynecol. *109*:570–572, 1971.

Chapter 2

DISEASES OF THE VAGINA

EMBRYOLOGY

The origin of the vaginal epithelium continues to be a controversial subject. The existing concept proposes that the upper one half to two thirds develops from the paramesonephric system while the distal one third derives from the urogenital sinus. Alterations in the transitional area seen in the diethylstilbestrol (DES)-exposed individual seemed to substantiate this thesis in that apparently the paramesonephric epithelium extends into the vagina, resulting in a transitional zone nearer to the introitus (vaginal cervix). Recent studies of Forsberg suggest the involvement of the mesonephric (wolffian) ducts in the formation of the vaginal plate—the intermediate zone between the paramesonephric duct (müllerian tubercles) and the urogenital sinus (Fig. 2–1). Elucidation of the latter thesis awaits further study but would explain some of the vagaries in the response of the vaginal epithelium to hormones and the existence of the transverse vaginal septum.

NORMAL HISTOLOGY OF VAGINA

Histologically the vaginal wall consists of three layers, an outer fibrous, a middle muscular, and an inner epithelial. The fibrous coat is derived from the pelvic fascia, while the muscular coat consists of an inner circular and an outer longitudinal layer (Fig. 2–2). The epithelium and underlying lamina propria are of major interest to the clinician and pathologist. Alterations in the maturation of the epithelium reflect the hormonal status of the individual, as well as the presence of local modifying factors, such as prolapse or

vaginitis, and the influence of certain medications, e.g. steroids, amphetamines, and digitalis. Glands are not recognized in the normal vagina; however, mesonephric remnants have been described in the fornices and the studies of Sanberg have demonstrated the frequency with which paramesonephric "glands" may be found in routine study of the vaginal tract.

VAGINAL HISTOLOGIC CYCLE

For many years there has been discussion as to whether the human vagina undergoes a cycle of histologic changes corresponding to the cyclic changes that undoubtedly occur in many laboratory animals. Although the majority opinion suggests that cyclic changes do occur, a number of excellent investigators fail to find evidence of such alterations.

Diercks, in 1927, described three layers in the epithelium—the basalis, the functionalis, and between them, an intraepithelial cornified layer. As in the case of the endometrium, he suggested that the functioning layers were desquamated and the epithelium then regenerated from the basal layer. These observations were confirmed in monkeys by Davis and Hartman. More recently, electron microscopic studies have demonstrated the usual lamina densa and lamina lucida with cyclic functional activities probably related to transfer of substances through the "basement membrane."

There are definite demonstrable alterations in this epithelium at various stages of life. During the prepubertal and postmenopausal years, the vaginal epithelium is thin, the mature superficial cells are absent, and the smear shows only parabasal and interme-

59

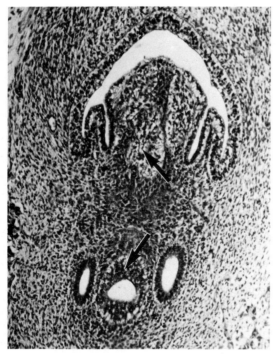

Figure 2–1. Section through the region of the developing vagina at 10 weeks of embryonic life. Upper opening is the urogenital sinus. The upper arrow shows the paramesonephric tubercle before development of uterovaginal canal. To either side of tubercle are the mesonephric ducts entering the sinus. Lower arrow points to paramesonephric duct with mesonephric ducts laterally.

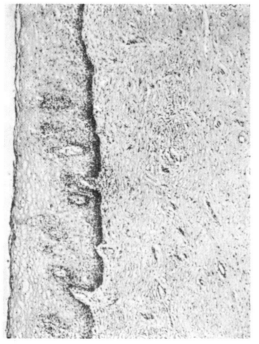

Figure 2–2. Histologic appearance of normal vaginal wall.

diate cells. In such a setting infections are common. Conversely, in the menstrual years, the superficial cells are prominent and reflect the estrogenic status of the patient. Indeed, this method of assessing estrogen function in the postmenopausal female has been utilized by Randall and others. The progesterone effect can also be detected cytologically in similar fashion (see section on cytopathology).

It seems highly unlikely that the vaginal mucosa responds as fully or precisely as does the endometrium; however, the ovarian hormones do not produce their effects only on tissues of paramesonephric origin. Most students agree with Meyer that the vaginal epithelium is derived not from the müllerian ducts but as an upward growth of the urogenital sinus. It must be recognized, however, that the upper portion of the vagina is of müllerian origin, and that stratified epithelium is present at müllerian tubercles prior to union of the urogenital sinus and the paramesonephric system (Fig. 2–3). Certain congenital structures found in this area suggest a malfunction between two systems of different origins that eventually fuse. The position of fusion is most dramatically demonstrated by the occasional presence of a transverse septum at about midvagina, with a cavity superiorly at the cervix and a short invagination at the outlet. A diagnosis of congenital absence of the vagina is usually made in most of these cases, when in truth the abnormality is an incomplete fusion of the two systems. Anastomosis of the two systems usually can be accomplished in most instances without use of a skin graft.

The complete absence of the vagina as seen in the Rokitansky-Custer syndrome is due to the failure in development of the terminal portions of the paramesonephric ducts. The tubes and ovaries are commonly quite normal, and a small fibrous band at the junction of the tubes represents the rudimentary fundus. In such cases, formation of the vagina by means of a skin graft, as proposed by McIndoe, has been effective. The common association of renal anomalies, which include agenesis and pelvic kidney, must be appreciated. When a vagina is constructed by making use of such a procedure, the transplanted skin often will assume certain characteristics of the vagina, including response to estrogen, after a period of several years.

The studies of Forsberg introduce a new

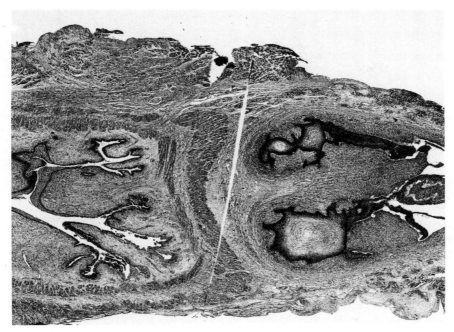

Figure 2–3. Section through the developing uterovaginal canal in 20 week old embryo. Transverse septum can be centrally located. To the left is the urogenital sinus; to the right, mullerian tubercles. (From Woodruff and Williams: Am. J. Obstet. Gynecol., *85:* 724, 1963.)

factor into the embryologic equation. His description of a "vaginal plate" possibly arising in midvagina by fusion of the mesonephric ducts may assist in explaining the point of

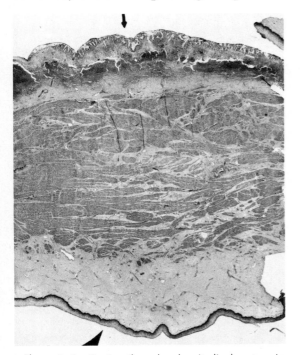

Figure 2–4. Section through a longitudinal septum in vagina with one blind canal. The closed vagina lined by mucus-secreting epithelium (small arrow); the normal vagina is lined by stratified squamous epithelium (large arrow).

junction between the epithelia of the uterovaginal canal and the variable responses to hormones. The lack of such a plate presents a better explanation for the transverse septum and also for the embryologic problems found in the child whose mother received DES in the early phases of her pregnancy. The importance of environment in this embryologic equation is well demonstrated in the congenital defect represented by the longitudinal septum in the patient with a double system. If the septum is complete and both vaginae open externally, the epithelium is normally stratified. Conversely, if one canal is blind, even though the cervical and endometrial epithelia are normal, the blind vagina is lined by mucus-secreting elements, as noted in the patient exposed to DES (Fig. 2–4).

INFLAMMATORY LESIONS

Because of its histology, the adult vaginal mucosa is relatively resistant to the gonococcus; however, other infections are quite common, often the result of bacterial, protozoan, and fungal agents, such as *Trichomonas vaginalis*, *Monilia*, and *Haemophilus vaginalis*. There has been a dramatic change in comparative incidences of these common invaders, probably due to the introduction

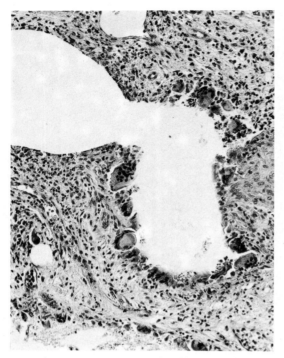

Figure 2–5. Cystic space lined by giant cells.

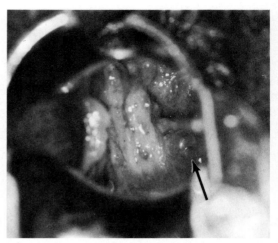

Figure 2–6. Vaginitis emphysematosa (cysts of various sizes) in a case of heart failure.

of metronidazole so that at present the fungus and *Haemophilus* infections are more prevalent than the *Trichomonas* type. In the prepubertal and postmenopausal patients, a variety of the common cocci and bacilli may be cultured from the vaginal canal. Treatment with antibiotics should *not* be predicated on such cultures unless the upper tract is involved.

Herpetic infection of the vagina is present in nearly all of these patients with vulvar lesions, and commonly goes unrecognized due to the absence of symptoms and lack of careful inspection. On occasion the vaginal lesion may become large and excavated, suggesting malignancy. Biopsy and cytology are necessary to confirm the diagnosis and rule out neoplasia.

Vaginitis emphysematosa is an unusual infection of the vagina and the adjacent cervix. The lesion is characterized by numerous small cysts lined by a syncytium of foreign body giant cells. The cervicovaginal tissue is diffusely infiltrated with inflammatory cells (Fig. 2–5). No specific bacteria have been recovered from the cysts, but the gas has been analyzed as carbon dioxide. The lesions are

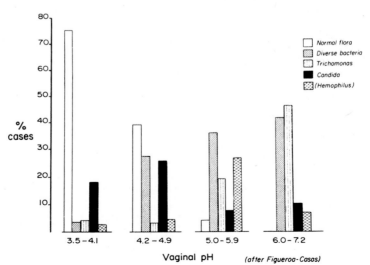

Chart I. Vaginal pH and infection with various microorganisms. (From Baggish and Woodruff: Obstet. Gynecol. Surv., 22:69, 1967.)

noted especially with pregnancy or in heart failure and are asymptomatic (Fig. 2–6). *Trichomonas* is commonly associated with such alterations.

The pH plays a major role in protecting the vagina from the various potentially infecting agents. Chart I documents the data demonstrating this relationship. It is obvious that the presence of *Lactobacillus* plays a major role in assisting the vagina to resist the invasion by many of the infecting agents. Nevertheless, reducing the pH from 6 to a more realistic 3.5 to 4 is more easily said than done. Most acidifying agents, such as vinegar douches and acid-gel, exert only temporary effect.

Cytologic preparations are of major import and, with determination of the pH, should be performed on all patients complaining of discharge, irritation, or odor. Therapies for the specific infections have been well outlined in clinical texts but consist mainly of Flagyl for *Trichomonas* infestations; Mycostatin, Monistat, or Lotrimin for the monilial lesions (including Mycolog for the associated vulvar disease), and triple sulfa cream or Terramycin suppositories for *Haemophilus* infections. It is imperative to appreciate the frequency with which such infections are transmitted by coitus, and thus both patient and consort should be treated simultaneously, particularly if there are recurrences. Recently Flagyl has been used successfully as a treatment for *Haemophilus* vaginitis.

Gonorrheal Vulvovaginitis of Children

Whereas the many-layered vaginal mucosa of adults is resistant to invasion by the gonococcus, the thinner, less vascular prepubertal epithelium is susceptible. Gonococcal vaginitis in children may be a very persistent infection, with recurrent bouts of purulent discharge and vulvar irritation. Histologic examination reveals the classic thin, stratified epithelium with subepithelial inflammatory infiltrate and bacteriologic study confirms the diagnosis.

Although recurrences are common during childhood, spontaneous cure of the local infection occurs at the menarche. Upper tract disease may develop at this time if the vaginal infection has not been controlled. This sequence of events suggested the use of estrogen in the therapy of gonococcal vaginitis, and many reports have recorded the effectiveness of such treatment.

Such nonspecific vaginitis is also common in the prepubertal years, again because of the thin, easily irritated mucosa. It is important, with persistent or recurrent infections, to rule out foreign bodies or tumors by the use of the vaginoscope. In the absence of such pathology, the problem usually responds to local estrogenic hormone therapy, although many prefer to use systemic antibiotics.

Postmenopausal Vaginitis

Similar to the prepubertal situation, the vaginal epithelium of the postmenopausal woman is characteristically thin, and thus prone to local infection (Fig. 2–7). The vaginitis thus produced is of clinical importance because the bleeding that results from local trauma suggests more serious disease. Careful inspection of the vaginal mucosa often reveals the vaginal source of the bleeding; however, it is important in such cases to investigate the entire genital canal and the adjacent rectal and urinary structures.

Aside from the bleeding, postmenopausal vaginitis may cause troublesome discharge with a sensation of vaginal burning and itching, and dyspareunia. Treatment by estrogenic therapy produces proliferation of the epithelium and effectively eliminates the ir-

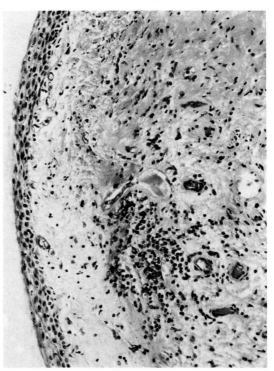

Figure 2–7. Thinned epithelium in postmenopausal vaginitis with underlying inflammatory infiltrate.

ritation, although recurrences are common unless therapy is continued. Local application usually produces a more rapid effect than systemic medications. It should be appreciated that some absorption takes place and reactions in the breast and endometrium are not uncommon. Thus, continuous daily therapy is contraindicated and unnecessary. One application every 10 days is usually sufficient to maintain a well-supported vaginal mucosa.

Histologic examination of the postmenopausal vagina reveals a thin epithelium without evidence of surface maturation. The subepithelial connective tissue usually shows a nonspecific infiltration with plasma cells and lymphocytes, although polymorphonuclear leukocytes and superficial ulcerations are not uncommon. It should be appreciated that vaginal cytologic preparations taken during the postmenopausal period may be misleading due to the pressure of the immature parabasal cells. Consequently, careful examination and repeat cytology after the use of local estrogen are important if previous studies have been inconclusive (see Chapter 35).

ULCERATIVE LESIONS

Syphilitic lesions of the vagina are rarely seen. Chancre usually appears at the introitus or on the vulva, although condylomata lata and mucous patches may involve the distal vagina. Tertiary syphilitic ulcerations, chancroid, granuloma inguinale, lymphogranuloma venereum, herpes, and tuberculosis (Fig. 2–8 A) may produce extensive destructive lesions on the vulva, vagina, and cervix. The gross appearance gives the clinical impression of malignant disease, and it is of obvious importance to establish the correct diagnosis by biopsy prior to instituting therapy.

Decubitus ulceration is characteristically associated with complete prolapse of the uterus and inversion of the vagina (Fig. 2–8 B), with hyperkeratosis developing over the exposed part. Keratin is protective and thus results from the traumas to which the vaginal epithelium is exposed.

After total hysterectomy, granulation tissue is commonly seen at the apex of the vault (Fig. 2–9 A). Such lesions are to be differentiated from anaplastic change and from the prolapsed fimbriated end of the tube (Fig.

2–9 B). The latter is more commonly seen after vaginal procedures and often can be differentiated from granulation tissue or carcinoma by biopsy of the exposed tissues. Little pain is associated with the excision of the granulation tissue; however, if the tube is traumatized, pain—often referred to the flank—usually results. Biopsy, of course provides the ultimate answer.

Ulceration of the vaginal vault is seen at times as a result of the pressure and irritation of foreign bodies, especially improperly fitted pessaries. A rare form of ulcerative lesion may occur in the lateral fornices of the vagina, in association with adenomatous changes in the wolffian or mesonephric duct vestiges located in this portion of the vagina. Similar surface irritations may be associated with adenosis and its malignant counterparts. Biopsy of such lesions, which may be clinically suggestive of cancer, will show the acinous or tubular elements characteristic of benign or malignant mesonephric or paramesonephric epithelia.

Finally, factitious ulcerations occur in the patient with psychiatric problems, particularly a woman who wishes to avoid coitus.

BENIGN TUMORS

Vaginal Cysts

These constitute the most common type of benign vaginal tumor, though rarely are they of the genuinely neoplastic or proliferative type. The most common varieties are Gartner's duct (wolffian duct) cysts and inclusion cysts.

Gartner's Duct Cysts. These are not rare. It will be recalled that the vestigial wolffian duct courses in the mesosalpinx, extends downward along the lateral margin of the uterus (occasionally being included in the uterine musculature itself) and into the anterolateral wall of the vagina, often to its outer third. The importance of these structures in the formation of the vaginal plate has been stressed by Forsberg. As a result of cystic distention of imperfectly obliterated regions of the duct, a cyst may arise in various portions along its course. In the vaginal segment, therefore, Gartner's duct cysts are found in the anterolateral portion of the wall. Such cysts may be segmented or multiple, in the former case resembling a tiny string of

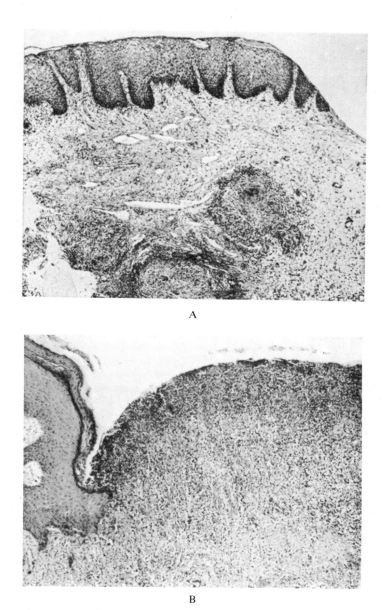

Figure 2–8. *A*, Tuberculous ulcer in vagina. *B*, Ulceration of vagina associated with prolapse (decubitus ulcer).

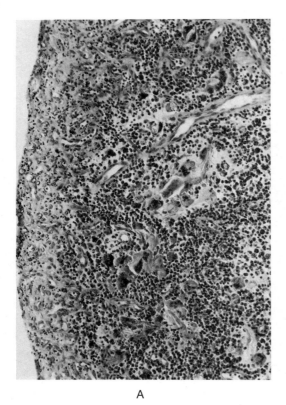

A

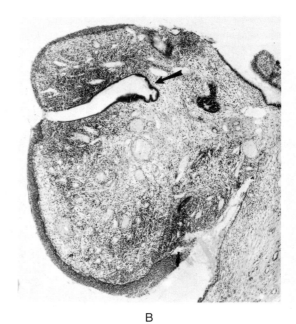

B

Figure 2–9. *A,* Granulation tissue showing extreme infection, old blood pigment, and foreign body giant cells. *B,* Prolapsed tube into vagina. Stratified epithelium is present on surface with tubal type at arrow.

sausages. While the Gartner's duct cysts are usually small, they may become large enough to project into the introitus and simulate a cystocele (Fig. 2–10).

Microscopically, the wall of such cysts is lined by an epithelium, often exhibiting

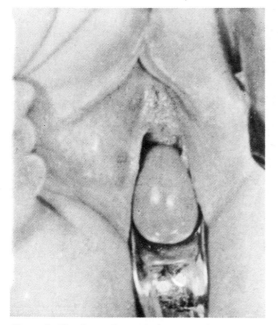

Figure 2–10. Large Gartner's duct cyst of anterior vaginal wall, clinically simulating a large cystocele.

marked variation in cell type. Usually there is a single layer of cuboidal or cylindrical cells, some containing secretory vacuoles, faintly positive for mucopolysaccharide, and a few possessing cilia (Fig. 2–11). A flattened layer of stratified metaplastic epithelium may be appreciated in certain foci. When the cyst is large, the epithelial layer may be so flattened by pressure atrophy as to be almost unrecognizable.

Vaginal Inclusion Cysts Although of little import clinically, these are numerically more frequent than the Gartner's duct variety. They are classically small—rarely larger than 2 to 3 cm. in diameter. Characteristically they are found in the posterior or lateral wall of the vagina, near the introitus. They are not infrequent at the apex of the vagina after inclusion of the vaginal epithelium in the performance of a hysterectomy.

The cause of these cysts is the inclusion of small islands of stratified vaginal epithelium beneath the surface. The desquamation and degeneration of the lining stratified epithelium results in the accumulation of cheesy yellowish contents within the cyst. Inclusion of vaginal mucosa beneath the surface occurs in one of two ways. In the perineal lacerations incurred at childbirth, tags of mucosa may be buried beneath the surface during the healing process, or in the repair of

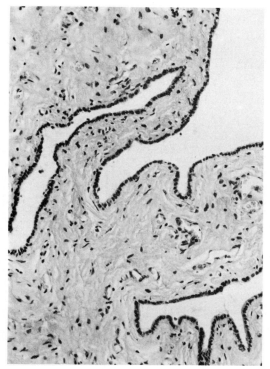

Figure 2–11. Typical lining of Gartner's duct cyst—low, flat cuboidal epithelium.

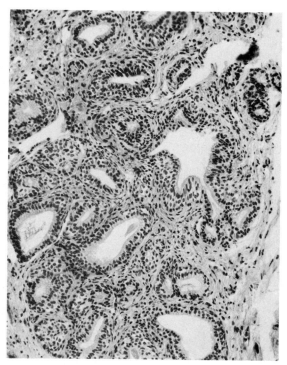

Figure 2–12. Glands lined by mucinous and transitional epithelium, and minor vestibular glands, found at the introitus.

such lacerations. The gynecologist may unwittingly cause such cysts by incomplete denudation of the mucosa in perineorrhaphy, or in the process of Bartholin's gland excision.

Other Cysts. Mucinous cysts at the outlet are rare and probably represent remnants of the incomplete separation of the rectum and urogenital sinus by the urorectal fold. As a result, mucus-secreting epithelial elements may reside in or near the introitus, with cystic dilatations. As noted in the discussion of the Bartholin's gland (Chapter 1), the major vestibular gland is a common site of cyst formation; conversely, minor vestibular glands are less well known but probably would be found frequently if routine sections were made through tissues at the introitus (Fig. 2–12).

Endometriosis and Adenomyoma

Endometriosis may occur anywhere in the vagina; however, the common site is the posterior fornix, where it is seen as a perforation of endometriosis from the cul-de-sac (Fig. 2–13). Other lesions may appear as reddened, superficial ulcerations that resist the usual douches, creams, and local applica-

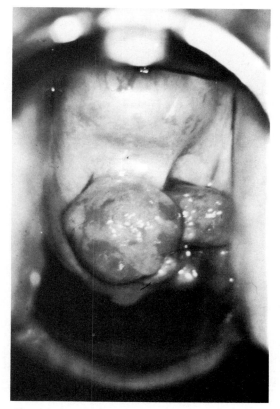

Figure 2–13. Endometriosis perforating through the cul-de-sac. The cervix can be seen anteriorly.

tions. On occasion the endometriosis may develop as a tumor or adenomyoma presenting in the posterior fornix. Biopsy will confirm the diagnosis (Fig. 2–14).

Rare cases of adenocarcinoma arising in endometriosis of the vagina have been reported. Lash and co-workers recorded a total of eight cases collected from the literature. The criteria suggested by Sampson, as noted by others, seem too rigid, but certainly both benign endometriosis and its malignant counterpart should be demonstrable in order for such relationships to be accepted.

Adenosis

The finding of glandular structures in the vagina is uncommon. As noted previously, mesonephric remnants and ectopic endocervical glands have been recognized. Lesions arising from these mucus-secreting, endocervical-type glands often present as roughened, pebbly elevations in the middle third of the vagina (Figs. 2–15 and 2–16). Excessive mucus discharge may be the presenting symptom, but the majority of cases are asymptomatic. Sandberg has demonstrated the frequency with which such structures may be recognized if routine sections are

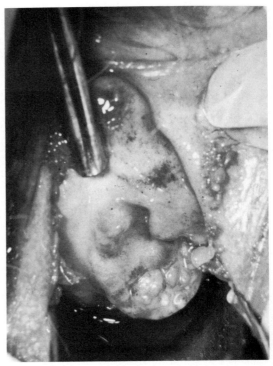

Figure 2–15. Irregular, pebbly elevations on the posterior wall of the vagina, simulating small nabothian cysts of the cervix.

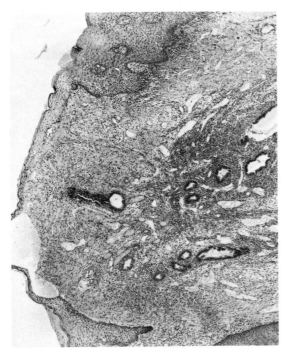

Figure 2–14. Endometriosis of the vagina. Note the thinning of the vaginal epithelium over the center of the endometrial tissue.

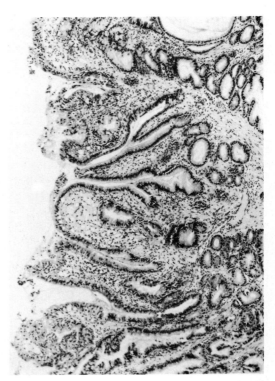

Figure 2–16. Adenosis. Adenomatous, pedunculated lesion in anterior vault. Mucus-secreting acini suggest endocervical origin.

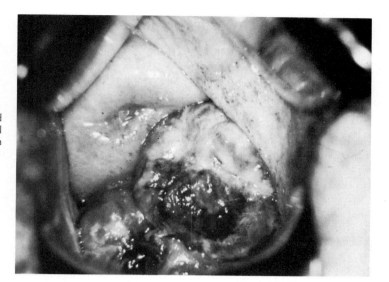

Figure 2–17. Tumor occupying and probably arising in the posterior vaginal fornix. External cervical os can be seen above and to the left of the tumor.

taken through the area. Obviously, malignancy may arise from these structures and should simulate that seen in the endocervix, i.e., either adenocarcinoma or the adeno-epidermoid variety (Figs. 2–17 to 2–19). Plaut and Dreyfuss recorded two cases and suggested that these glands may be the origin of adenocarcinoma.

Attention in the last decade has been

directed at the frequency with which adenosis may be found in the vagina of the young female whose mother received DES during pregnancy. As many as 90 per cent of such children have had adenosis demonstrable by colposcopy if the medication was received during the first 8 weeks of pregnancy. Conversely, fewer than 10 per cent demonstrated such alterations if DES was adminis-

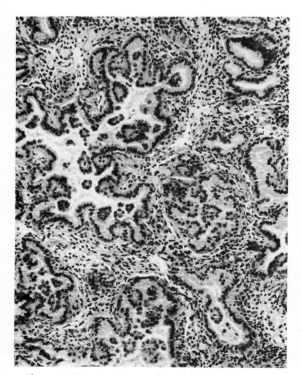

Figure 2–18. Mucinous adenoid lesion of the vagina (same lesion as in Figure 2–17; the malignant transformation is noted in Figure 2–19).

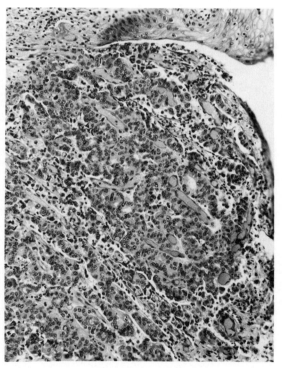

Figure 2–19. Adenocarcinoma arising as a malignant transformation of the adenomatous lesion seen in Figure 2–17.

tered only after the sixteenth week. The association of these changes with neoplasia will be considered later in this chapter.

SOLID BENIGN TUMORS

The acuminate wart, so common on the vulva, is a frequent invader of the vagina. The clinical and histopathologic features are similar to those recounted in Chapter 1.

Other such tumors are relatively rare, and they may be of any one of several pathologic types—e.g., leiomyoma, fibromyoma, neurofibroma, and polyps. The leiomyoma and fibromyoma may arise de novo from the musculature of the vagina or migrate extraperitoneally as subserous uterine tumors having become "divorced" from the fundus. The latter occupy any position, though usually occurring laterally or posterolaterally. Major problems develop in the surgical dissection since the ureter and major vessels are in close proximity.

The true vaginal polyp is uncommon although mucosal tags resulting from lacerations are frequent. The true polyp is composed of a loose, edematous stroma and thus simulates sarcoma botryoides, as noted by Norris and Taylor (Fig. 2–20). Nevertheless,

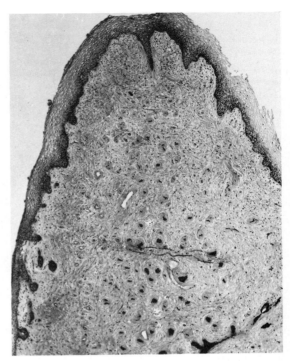

Figure 2–21. The loose texture of a vaginal polyp is evident here.

these lesions in the adult are routinely benign, need only excision to establish the correct diagnosis, but may recur if the base is not destroyed. Careful histopathologic evaluation demonstrates that the edematous stroma and occasional bizarre fibroblast are not evidences of malignancy (Fig. 2–21).

MALIGNANT TUMORS

Primary malignancies of the vagina are rare, and include carcinoma, sarcoma, and melanoma. Secondary malignancy is much more common, since cervical cancer extends first to the vagina.

Carcinoma

Carcinoma in situ of the vagina has been described frequently and under a variety of circumstances. Following both surgical (Graham and Meigs) and radiation (Koss and co-workers) therapy for cervical cancer, intraepithelial anaplasia has been recognized in the adjacent vagina. Multicentric foci in cervix, vagina, and vulva have been reported by numerous investigators. Commonly, cursory examination does not reveal a specific

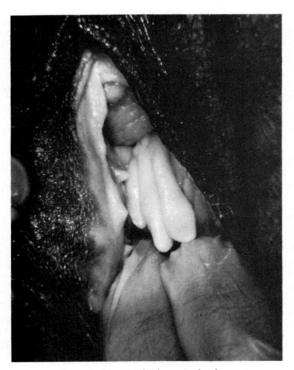

Figure 2–20. Multiple vaginal polyps.

gross lesion; however, whitish hyperkeratotic and erythroplastic foci, simulating those lesions described on the vulva, may be recognized in the vagina (Fig. 2–22). Histologically this lesion resembles, in all respects, carcinoma in situ of the cervix (Fig. 2–23), often demonstrating the classic full-thickness alterations of the epithelium or variations from mild to marked atypia or dysplasia. Rarely the lesion is keratinizing. The patients are almost routinely asymptomatic and thus the diagnosis is made by study of the vaginal cytologic preparation. Consequently it is important to obtain cells from both the proximal and the distal vagina, particularly in the patient who has had cervical neoplasia.

Invasive carcinoma of the vagina may be primary or secondary. The primary variety is rare, constituting about 0.5 per cent of all primary genital canal malignancies. The etiologic factors may relate to a variety of irritative agents. Circumstantial evidence supporting an infectious origin of cervical malignancy has been cited repeatedly and the vaginal lesion may be caused by similar agents. The invasive neoplasm arising in later years has been associated with prolapse by some investigators, but this etiology is not

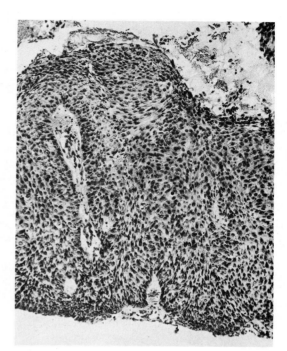

Figure 2–23. Carcinoma in situ of vagina 18 months after hysterectomy for carcinoma in situ of cervix.

generally accepted. Although it may occur at almost any age, the highest incidences are in the sixth and seventh decades of life.

The most common locations are the anterior or posterior walls of the vagina, especially in its upper half (Fig. 2–24 A,B). As the lesion enlarges, there is increasing induration and ulceration, and subsequent involvement of the rectovaginal septum and rectum, or, if anterior, the vesicovaginal septum and bladder. In the late stages, fistulas, extending into either of these organs, may be produced. Lymphatic extension of the disease is along the same route as that of cervical cancer, involving especially the iliac, hypogastric, and retroperitoneal glands if the lesion arises in the upper two thirds of the vagina. When the neoplasm is situated in the lower portion of the vagina, the inguinal glands are the first areas of extra-genital involvement, as in vulvar cancer.

The International Federation of Gynecology and Obstetrics has classified vaginal carcinoma as follows:

Preinvasive Carcinoma of the Vagina
    Stage 0   Carcinoma in situ, intraepithelial carcinoma
Invasive Carcinoma of the Vagina
    Stage I   The carcinoma is limited to the vaginal wall

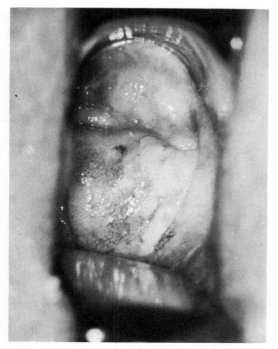

Figure 2–22. Carcinoma in situ of the vagina showing thick white leukoplakic changes. Atypical vascularization can be recognized grossly.

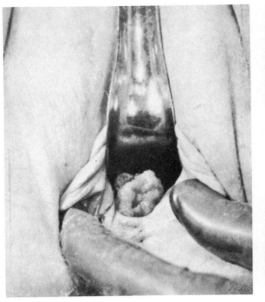 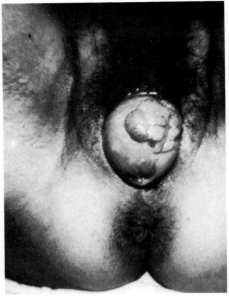

A   B

Figure 2–24. Carcinoma of the vagina. *A,* Posterior wall. *B,* Large nodular tumor of the anterior wall.

Stage II The carcinoma has involved the subvaginal tissue but has not extended onto the pelvic wall

Stage III The carcinoma has extended onto the pelvic wall

Stage IV The carcinoma has extended beyond the true pelvis or has involved the mucosa of the bladder or rectum; however, bullous edema does not permit one to classify a case as Stage IV.

Cases should be classified as carcinoma of the vagina when the primary site is in the vagina; the neoplasm involving the cervix is classified as carcinoma of the cervix; that which has extended to the vulva as carcinoma of the vulva; and that limited to the urethra as carcinoma of the urethra. These designations are important because treatment is dependent on the lymphatic drainage of the individual lesion.

Microscopically, primary vaginal carcinoma is, with rare exceptions, of the epidermoid type with various degrees of maturation (Fig. 2–25); however, the squamous, pearl-forming variety is more common in the vagina than in the cervix (Fig. 2–26).

Adenocarcinoma is rare. Benign and malignant adenomatous tumors arising in the cervix and vagina, lined by cells varying from the irregular hobnail epithelium to a clear, secretory cell, simulated the clear cell adenocarcinoma of the kidney and were thought to be of mesonephric origin. Al-

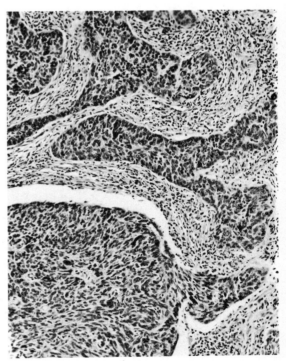

Figure 2–25. Epidermoid carcinoma of the vagina.

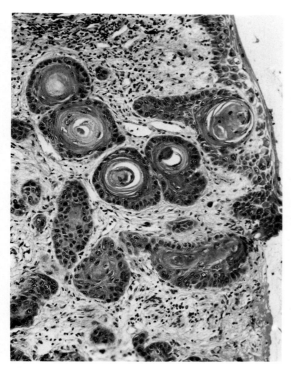

Figure 2–26. Mature, pearl-forming carcinoma of the vagina.

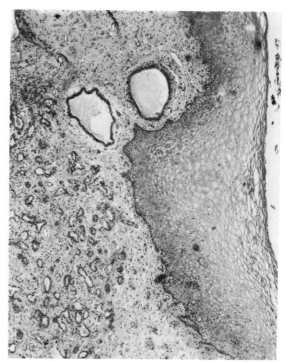

Figure 2–27. Normal stratified epithelium of the vagina. The adenoid structures beneath it appear quite benign and generally resemble those seen in mesonephric duct. Tubal type epithelium is present.

though such lesions undoubtedly occur, recent information suggests that the majority are of paramesonephric rather than mesonephric origin.

In the past decade Herbst and others have described a specific variety of adenocarcinomas arising in young women whose mothers received stilbestrol during pregnancy. The risk factor at present appears to be between 1 in 1000 to 1 in 4000. Thus, although adenosis is common in such exposed patients, the possibility of the development of malignancy is uncommon. The classic cell types found in adenosis are those seen in the endocervix and endosalpinx (Fig. 2–27). These tumors classically are found in the pericervical areas although occasionally they involve the middle and outer segments of the anterior or posterior walls of the vagina in the second and early third decades of life. At present, approximately 350 to 400 cases have occurred, primarily during the second and third decades of life, the youngest patient being 7 years and the oldest 29 years of age.

The microscopic picture is that of the clear cell tumor with papillary projections simulating the lesion classified previously as mesonephroma (Figs. 2–28 and 2–29 A,B).

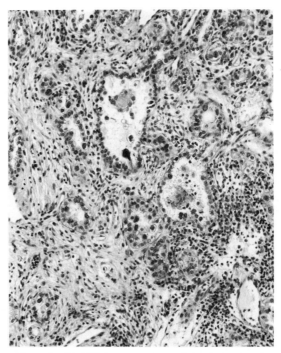

Figure 2–28. High power view of the lesion just beneath that seen in Figure 2–27. Both hobnail and clear cell patterns can be recognized.

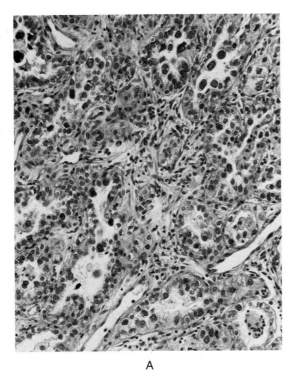

A

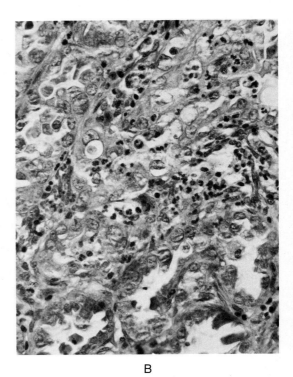

B

Figure 2–29. *A,* High power view showing the classic cellular changes in the mesonephroid carcinoma. *B,* High power view of mesonephroid carcinoma of the vagina.

As noted, such neoplasms undoubtedly arise from paramesonephric elements described as adenosis on electron microscopic studies.

The stimulation of embryonic tissue, with development of a neoplasm many years later at menarche, the time at which ovarian hormone production is initiated, represents a unique process. Nevertheless, the great majority of such lesions arise at the age of 14 years or later, suggesting that the thesis is valid.

An added problem has been the finding of epidermoid atypia or dysplasia in adenosis, suggesting that in situ neoplasia, similar to that seen at the cervical tranformation zone, may occur. Undoubtedly such will develop if the stimulating agents are present; however, the incidence should be no greater than that developing at the classic area. Nevertheless, careful follow-up should identify the precursory changes as demonstrated by routine cytologic studies in cervical neoplasia.

Malignant Melanoma

Melanosis is not an uncommon finding in the vagina. The basal layer of the epithelium demonstrates marked concentration of melanin and acanthosis (Fig. 2–30). Such changes demonstrate the ability of stratified squamous epithelium to reveal its relationship to the neural crest elements. Malignant melanoma of the vagina is undoubtedly a rare lesion, but a sufficient number of cases have been reported to accept their authenticity (Fig. 2–31). The prognosis has been poor primarily because the tumors have extended to level III or beyond prior to diagnosis (Fig. 2–32).

Sarcoma (Fibro- or Leiomyo-)

Such lesions are very rare and commonly develop as a solitary mass in the anterior or lateral vaginal walls. The focal nature suggests that most arise as secondary malignancies from a pre-existing benign fibroma or leiomyoma. The majority of those found in patients under the age of 50 years are low grade but tend to recur locally. Even those that appear benign histologically, if they attain a size of more than 8 to 10 cm., follow this pattern of the low grade malignant tumor. It is wise to alert the clinician to the clinical course of these lesions, since surgery is the primary and secondary method of therapy. Adjunctive radiation or chemotherapy has proved to be of little or no value.

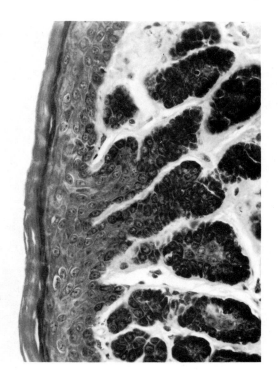

Figure 2–30. Melanosis of the vagina.

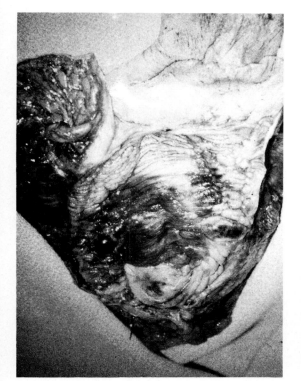

Figure 2–31. Malignant melanoma of the vagina treated by radical surgery.

Figure 2–32. Malignant melanoma—level II involvement.

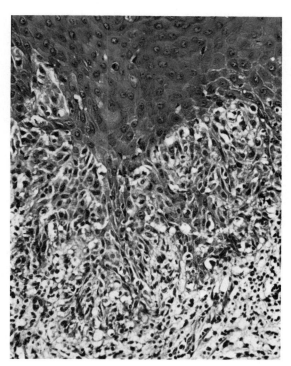

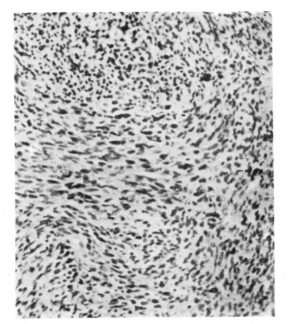

Figure 2–33. Sarcoma of vagina.

Conversely, such malignancies arising in the patient over the age of 50 years tend to follow a much more aggressive course and similarly appear more malignant histopathologically, the usual cellular criteria of malignancy being found in focal areas (Fig. 2–33). Since degeneration in the larger lesion is common, it is of obvious importance to differentiate such changes from true neoplasia. As with the low grade lesions, local recurrence is common; however, metastases may develop in distant organs. Extensive, and even exenterative, surgery is the treatment of choice, although this may be inadvisable or impossible in this age group. Triple chemotherapy has been reportedly effective in temporarily controlling the lesions and must be considered in these patients.

The lesion formerly known as "round cell sarcoma" may, in truth, represent an endometrial stromal lesion (stromatosis) either as an extension of a uterine tumor or arising de novo in the pelvic peritoneum with subsequent involvement of the vagina. Differential diagnosis may be difficult but every effort should be made to evaluate the tumor accurately since hormonal treatment for the stromal tumor should be given primary consideration.

Even rarer than the above neoplasms are the lymphomas. Examples of histocytic lymphoma have been reported and although they are rarely primary in this area, nevertheless accurate diagnosis is imperative if appropriate therapy is to be instituted.

Sarcoma Botryoides

This unusual lesion, found in the vagina during the first decade and usually in the

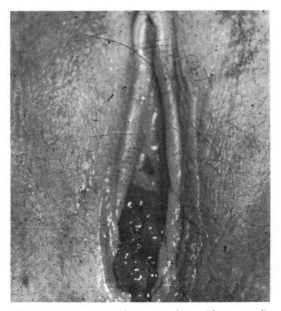

Figure 2–34. Fungoid sarcoma botryoides protruding from infant vagina.

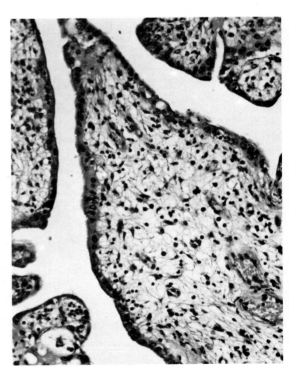

Figure 2–35. Sarcoma botryoides. Loose stoma suggests benignity. Differentiation from benign polyps is difficult.

first five years of life, was described by Spiegelberg in 1879 as "sarcoma colli uteri hydropicum papillare." The tumor arises from the upper vagina and the adjacent cervix. Thus, it may be said that the point of origin is the growing tip of the müllerian (paramesonephric) duct, with its very active stroma. Two cases in the newborn have been reported by Ober and associates.

Grossly, the disease is characterized by a mass of edematous grayish red polyps, filling and frequently extruding from the vagina (Fig. 2–34). A bloody discharge is the usual presenting complaint. Extension to the uterus, parametrium, and regional nodes is common, and distant metastases are late developments. Few five-year salvages have been recorded in the report by Daniel and others. These authors, in stressing a vaginal origin, comment on the frequency of multicentric foci in the subepithelial layer; the groups of fusiform tumor cells elevate the overlying epithelium to produce the papillary appearance.

Rarely does such a malignant tumor appear histologically so innocuous. Because of extensive edema, the first appearance suggests acellularity, and an erroneous diagnosis of benign vaginal polyp is often forthcoming (Fig. 2–35). Individual details of the cells in the more concentrated areas must be

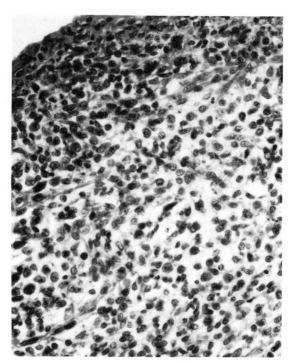

Figure 2–37. Stromal aspect of sarcoma botryoides (similar to endometrial stromal sarcoma).

studied carefully to establish the malignant nature (Fig. 2–36). Such a study will also frequently reveal the presence of rhabdomyoblasts. In fact, many of these tumors have been included in the group of rhabdomyoblastomas in children. Nevertheless the lesion is basically a paramesonephric stromal sarcoma with the occasional dedifferentiation of the stromal cell to one of the elements seen in many endometrial lesions (the mixed mesodermal tumors) (Fig. 2–37).

The pathologic report indicating a benign lesion unfortunately results in delay in diagnosis and treatment. Such delay is the paramount reason for poor salvage. The mere presence of a polypoid vaginal mass in a young infant should be almost pathognomonic of this disease; nevertheless, proof of the nature of the disease must be established pathologically. There are benign polypoid tumors in the vagina of the young child that simulate the botryoid sarcoma except for the definitive presence of a cambium layer. Even with the electron microscope absolute differentiation is difficult. Nevertheless the benign polypoid lesion clinically has a solitary stalk and can be treated by local excision (Fig. 2–38).

Although sarcoma botryoides has much in common with mixed mesodermal tumors,

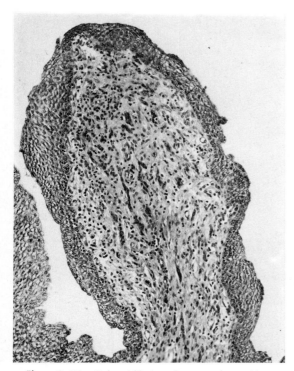

Figure 2–36. Polypoid lesion of sarcoma botryoides.

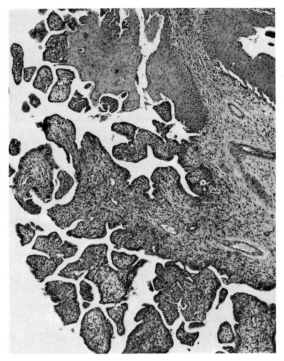

Figure 2–38. Benign polypoid vaginal lesion removed from 5 year old child (living and well after 4 years).

cartilage, bone, and abnormal epithelial elements are rarely present. Rhabdomyoblasts, as mentioned, are recognized occasionally if search is diligent. Daniel points out that sarcoma botryoides has been reported in the urinary bladder, bile ducts, and the region of the eustachian tube.

Radical surgery offers the best salvage. At present exenteration procedures are uti-

lized, distasteful as they may be in the young female. However, the proximity and deep extension of the vaginal lesion to bladder or bowel may demand such surgery. Of the handful of survivors, a few have received adjuvant radiotherapy, although radiotherapy as the only treatment is rarely more than palliative (Fig. 2–39). Triple chemotherapy offers promise; however, too few cases have been treated to evaluate the long-term results.

Endodermal Sinus Tumor

These unusual tumors, classic of that described in the ovary by Teilum, may arise de novo in the vagina. Most commonly appearing during the first decade of life, the lesion grossly simulates the sarcoma botryoides as a polypoid tumor filling the vagina and protruding beyond the outlet. Of germ cell origin (the lowest point of the base of the embryonic mesentery), these neoplasms grow rapidly and are routinely fatal unless the proper diagnosis is established and triple chemotherapy instituted. The histopathology is identical to that seen in its ovarian counterpart and must be differentiated from the mesonephroid lesion and sarcoma botryoides (Fig. 2–40).

Tumors of Paravestibular Glands

A few tumors developing at the vaginal outlet have been described as tumors of paravestibular glands, but the basic histopathologic features do not justify this desig-

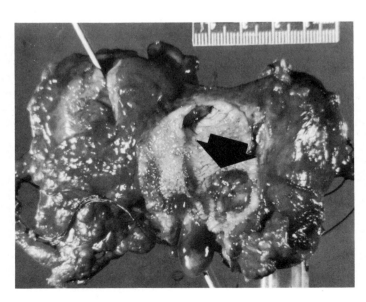

Figure 2–39. Exenteration specimen from a child of 22 months with sarcoma botryoides. The opened vagina can be seen in right center with the polypoid lesion near the outlet (at arrow). The entire vagina and cervix were involved.

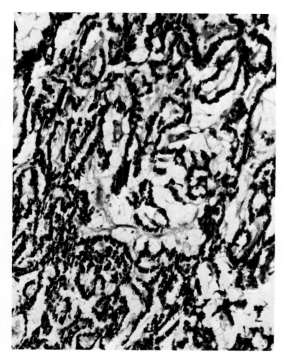

Figure 2–40. Endodermal sinus tumor of vagina in 2½ year old child (died 3 months after radical surgery).

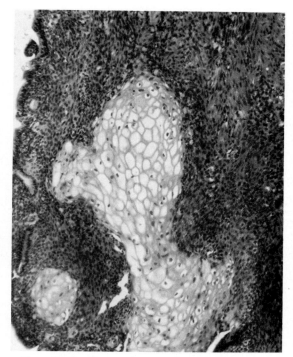

Figure 2–41. Tumor of paravestibular glands. Note proliferating stromal component.

nation. They generally occur in the third and fourth decades of life, and wide local excision has resulted in long-term survival. The epithelial elements are proliferative but not neoplastic. In contrast, the stroma seems more aggressive, suggesting that the para-mesonephric tissues may, on occasion, extend to the vaginal outlet and involve the vestibular glands but act like a stromal neoplasm (Fig. 2–41).

Metastatic Carcinoma

Whereas primary vaginal malignancies are rarities, secondary neoplasia is common. Cervical cancer extends into the vagina early in the course of the disease. Prior to the use of radium in the pre- or postoperative treatment of endometrial carcinoma, secondary deposits, either in the "cuff" or in subepithelial lymphatics, developed in 10 to 20 per cent of the cases if any myometrial invasion of the primary tumor was discovered. By direct extension, intra-abdominal neoplasia involves the posterior fornix while rectal and bladder malignancies may invade the contiguous areas of the vagina (Fig. 2–42). As noted above, uterine trophoblastic neoplasia may appear first as a nodule in the upper vault.

True metastatic disease from the kidney, upper intestinal tract, or other foreign sites is rare, although in most instances endometrial cancer seems to invade the vagina through vascular channels rather than by implantation.

Trophoblastic Disease

Choriocarcinoma of the vagina is a common site for the development of secondary lesions in the patient with primary uterine trophoblastic neoplasms. In a few cases the occurrence of the vaginal metastasis has furnished the first clue to the existence of chorionepithelioma. The vaginal growth appears as a dark blue hemorrhagic nodule. It is apt to be friable and to bleed on slight touch. The microscopic characteristics are described elsewhere (see Chapter 33).

The presence of villous and trophoblastic tissue in the vaginal vault, however, is not a justification for assuming that the intrauterine lesion is a malignant chorionepithelioma, since it may also occur with the so-called invasive or malignant moles. These are characterized by a local invasion of the contiguous vaginal vault or parametrium, with very little tendency to distant metas-

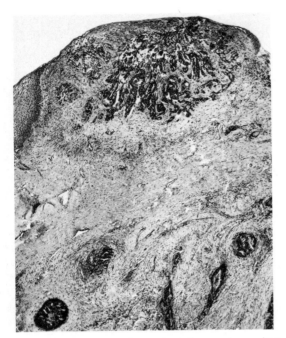

Figure 2–42. Metastatic ovarian adenocarcinoma into vaginal vault.

tases, such as is seen with chorionepithelioma. Adequate chemotherapy and careful follow-up will lead to approximately 100 per cent survival, thus explaining at least some cases reported as cures of chorionepithelioma even after incomplete removal (see Chapter 34).

REFERENCES

Ariel, I. M.: Malignant melanoma of the vagina. Report of a successfully treated case. Obstet. Gynecol., 17:222, 1961.

Ariel, I. M.: Five-year cure of a primary malignant melanoma of the vagina by local radioactive isotope therapy. Am. J. Obstet. Gynecol., 82:405, 1961.

Arronet, G. H., Latour, J. P. A., and Tremblay, P. C.: Primary carcinoma of the vagina. Am. J. Obstet. Gynecol., 79:453, 1960.

Ayre, J. E.: Cyclic ovarian changes in artificial vagina. Am. J. Obstet. Gynecol., 48:690, 1944.

Batsakis, J. G., and Dito, W. R.: Primary malignant melanoma of vagina. Obstet. Gynecol., 20:109, 1962.

Bivens, M. D.: Primary carcinoma of the vagina (a report of 46 cases). Am. J. Obstet. Gynecol., 65:390, 1953.

Boutselis, J. G., Ullery, J. C., and Bair, J.: Vaginal metastases following treatment of endometrial carcinoma. Obstet. Gynecol., 21:622, 1963.

Brenner, P., Sedlis, A., and Cooperman, H.: Complete imperforate transverse vaginal septum. Obstet. Gynecol., 25:135, 1965.

Burt, E. P., Roark, S. P., and Couri, P. J.: Vaginitis emphysematosa. Obstet. Gynecol., 4:335, 1954.

Burt, R. L., Prichard, R. W., and Kim, B. S.: Fibroepithelial polyp of the vagina. Obstet. Gynecol., 47:525, 1976.

Daniel, W. W., Koss, L. G., and Brunschwig, A.: Sarcoma botryoides of the vagina. Cancer, 12:74, 1959.

Diercks, K.: Der normale mensuelle Zyklus der menschlichen Vaginalschleimhaut. Arch. f. Gynäk., 130:46,1927.

Duckett, H. C., Davis, C. D., and McCall, J. B.: Sarcoma botryoides. Obstet. Gynecol., 9:517, 1957.

Fenn, M. E., and Abell, M. R.: Melanomas of vulva and vagina. Obstet. Gynecol., 4:902, 1973.

Fluhmann, C. F.: Simple round ulcers of vagina. Am. J. Obstet. Gynecol., 18:832, 1929.

Forsberg, J. G.: Cervicovaginal epithelium: its origin and development. Am. J. Obstet. Gynecol., 115:1025, 1973.

Forsberg, J. G.: Estrogen, vaginal cancer and vaginal development. Am. J. Obstet. Gynecol., 113:83, 1972.

Freund, D. R., Kegel, E. E., and Dugger, J. H.: Primary malignant melanoma of the vagina. Am. J. Obstet. Gynecol., 78:290, 1959.

Gardner, H. L., Dampeer, T. K., and Dukes, C. D.: Prevalence of vaginitis: study in incidence. Am. J. Obstet. Gynecol., 73:1080, 1957.

Gardner, H. L., and Kaufman, R. H.: Benign Diseases of Vulva and Vagina. St. Louis, C. V. Mosby Co., 1969.

Geist, S. H.: Cyclical changes in vaginal mucous membrane. Surg. Gynecol. Obstet., 51:848, 1930.

Graham, J. B., and Meigs, J. V.: Residual carcinoma in vaginal cuff after radical hysterectomy with bilateral pelvic lymph node dissection. Am. J. Obstet. Gynecol., 64:402, 1952.

Greenwalt, P., Barlow, J. J., Nasca, P. C., and Burnett, W. S.: Vaginal cancer after maternal treatment with synthetic estrogens. N. Engl. J. Med., 285:392, 1971.

Herbst, A. L., and Scully, R. E.: Adenocarcinoma of the vagina in adolescence. Cancer, 25:745, 1970.

Herbst, A. L., Green, T. H., Jr., and Ulfelder, H.: Primary carcinoma of the vagina: an analysis of 68 cases. Am. J. Obstet. Gynecol., 106:210, 1970.

Hummer, W. K., Mussey, E., Decker, D. G., and Dockerty, M. B.: Carcinoma in situ of the vagina. Am. J. Obstet. Gynecol., 108:1109, 1970.

Koss, L. G., Melamed, M. R., and Daniel, W. W.: In situ epidermoid carcinoma of the cervix and vagina following radiotherapy for cervical cancer. Cancer, 14:353, 1961.

Lang, W. R.: Premenarchal vaginitis. Obstet. Gynecol., 13:723, 1959.

Lash, S. R., and Rubenstone, A. I.: Adenocarcinoma of the rectovaginal septum probably arising from endometriosis. Am. J. Obstet. Gynecol., 78:299, 1959.

Laufe, L. E., and Bernstein, E. D.: Primary malignant melanoma of the vagina. Obstet. Gynecol., 37:148, 1971.

Livingstone, R.: Primary carcinoma of the vagina. Springfield, Ill., Charles C Thomas, 1950.

Marcus, S. L.: Primary carcinoma of the vagina. Obstet. Gynecol., 60:673, 1960.

Marcus, S. L.: Multiple squamous cell carcinoma involving the cervix, vagina and vulva: the theory of multicentric origin. Am. J. Obstet. Gynecol., 80:802, 1960.

Meyer, R.: Zur Frage der Entwicklung der menschlichen Vagina. 1-4. Arch. Gynäk., 158:639, 1934; 163:205, 1936; 164:207, 1937; 165:504, 1938; 166:306, 1938.

Norris, H. J., and Taylor, H. B.: Melanomas of the vagina. Am. J. Clin. Pathol., 46:420, 1966.

Norris, H. J., and Taylor, H. B.: Polyps of the vagina—a benign lesion resembling sarcoma botryoides. Cancer, 19:227, 1966.

Novak, E., Woodruff, J. D., and Novak, E. R.: Probable mesonephric origin of certain genital tumors. Am. J. Obstet. Gynecol., 68:1954.

Ober, W. B., Smith, J. A., and Rovilland, F.: Congenital sarcoma botryoides: report of 2 cases. Cancer, 11:620, 1958.

Plaut, A., and Dreyfuss, M. L.: Adenosis and its relation to primary adenocarcinoma. Surg. Gynecol. Obstet., 71:756, 1940.

Randall, C. L., Birtsch, P. K., and Harkins, J. L.: Ovarian function after the menopause. Am. J. Obstet. Gynecol., 74:719, 1957.

Ruffolo, E. H., Foxworthy, D., and Fletchner, J. C.: Vaginal adenocarcinoma arising in vaginal adenosis. Am. J. Obstet. Gynecol., 110:167, 1971.

Sandberg, E. C., Danielson, R. W., Cauwet, R. W., and Bonar, B. E.: Adenosis vaginae. Am. J. Obstet. Gynecol., 93:209, 1965.

Sandberg, E. C.: The incidence and distribution of occult vaginal adenosis. Am. J. Obstet. Gynecol., 101:322, 1968.

Schiller, W.: Mesonephroma ovarii. Am. J. Cancer, 35:1, 1939.

Silverberg, S. G., and DiGiorgi, L. S.: Clear cell carcinoma of the vagina (a clinical, pathologic and electron microscopic study). Cancer, 29:1680, 1972.

Singh, B. P.: Primary carcinoma of vagina. Cancer, 4:1073, 1951.

Smith, F. R.: Primary carcinoma of the vagina. Am. J. Obstet. Gynecol., 69:525, 1955.

Stafl, A., and Mattingly, R.: Vaginal adenosis: A precancerous lesion. Am. J. Obstet. Gynecol., 120:666, 1974.

Stieve, H.: Über angebliche zyklische Veränderungen des Scheidenepithels. Zbl. f. Gynäk., 55:194, 1931.

Stieve, H.: Das Schwangerschaftswachstum und die Gerburtserweiterung der menschlichen Scheide. Ztschr. f. mikros. anat. Forsch., 3:307, 1925.

Studdiford, W. E.: Vaginal lesions of adenomatous origin. Am. J. Obstet. Gynecol., 73:641, 1957.

Taussig, F. J.: Metastatic tumors of vagina and vulva. Surg. Clin. North Am., 18:1309, 1938.

Tobon, H., and A. I. Murphy: Benign blue nevus of the vagina. Cancer, 40:3174, 1977.

Tracy, S. E.: Sarcoma of vagina. Am. J. Obstet. Gynecol., 19:278, 1930.

Traut, H. F., Block, P. W., and Kuder, A.: Cyclical changes in the human vaginal mucosa. Surg. Gynecol. Obstet., 63:7, 1936.

Veridiano, N. P., Weiner, F. A., and Tancer, M. L.: Squamous cell carcinoma of the vagina associated with vaginal adenosis. Obstet. Gynecol., 47:689, 1976.

Whelton, J., and Kottmeier, H. L.: Primary carcinoma of the vagina: a study of a Radiumhemmet series of 145 cases. Acta Obstet. Gynecol. Scand., 41:22, 1962.

Whitacre, F. F., and Wang, Y. Y.: Biological changes in squamous epithelium transplanted to pelvic connective tissue. Surg. Gynecol. Obstet., 79:192, 1944.

Zondek, B., and Friedmann, M.: Are there cyclical changes in the human vaginal mucosa? J.A.M.A., 106:1051, 1939.

Chapter 3

HISTOLOGY OF THE CERVIX

Introduction

The cervix uteri is differentiated into two segments—namely, the portio or exocervix, that area covered by stratified epithelium, and the endocervix, lined by high columnar mucus-secreting elements. The exocervix derives from the invading epithelium of the urogenital sinus, or possibly the vaginal plate epithelium of the united mesonephric ducts. The endocervix is of paramesonephric origin. Embryologically, there is definable secretory activity in the endocervical glands during late embryonic life. Functionally and grossly, the cervical segment of the uterus is larger than the fundal portion during the embryonic and early developmental years. In addition to the epithelial elements there is a very active stromal component, particularly beneath the stratified squamous epithelium of the müllerian tubercles (Fig. 3–1). Interestingly this stratified epithelium is pres-

ent before the dissolution of the transverse septum in the formation of the uterovaginal canal.

The cyclic histologic response to the ovarian hormones is very striking in the endometrium, while in the cervix there is still doubt as to its nature. As a matter of fact, with the exception of a few studies, which are rather contradictory, there is little well-documented information on this subject. It would seem incredible, however, in view of the müllerian origin of this portion of the uterus, that there should not be some cyclic response, since such can be demonstrated in its secretory activity (cervical mucus). Furthermore, during pregnancy the cervix responds to hormonal influence by specific histologic changes, namely an often impressive decidual reaction that has been misinterpreted as malignant in character.

Neoplastic variations demonstrate dramat-

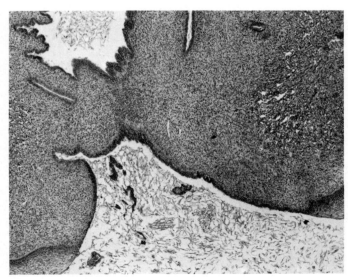

Figure 3–1. Stroma and glands at 16 to 20 weeks of embryonic life. Note active stroma of paramesonephric system, the adjacent squamous epithelium of the vaginal plate, and the glands of endocervix with uterine cavity above.

ically the embryologic differentials. Endocervical adenocarcinoma simulates that seen in the endometrium and ovary. Conversely, the lesions arising at the squamocolumnar junction are lower genital canal neoplasms. The importance of such differentials in embryology and the nature of the neoplastic stimuli are features of basic interest and demand the concern of clinicians and pathologists.

HISTOLOGY

Histologically, the cervix differs from the corpus primarily in the character of its epithelium.

As noted previously, there are two clearly defined types of cervical epithelia. The pars vaginalis, protruding into the vagina, is lined by stratified epithelium similar to that of the vagina. Since the area adjacent to the squamocolumnar junction is originally lined by everted high columnar epithelium and later converted to a metaplastic stratified variety, the dermal papillae, composed of the stroma between the clefts, are more prominent in this area than in the vagina. The epithelium normally does not demonstrate cornification, although if the cervix is prolapsed, it may become keratinized and skinlike. The stratified epithelium extends approximately to the external os, but there are individual variations, the line of demarcation being frequently distal or proximal to the anatomic os. It must be recognized that this transformation zone changes during life and often cannot be visualized in the postmenopausal patient. Ostergard has noted the differences in position of the squamocolumnar junction related to age, gravidity, and parity. This critical zone is found in the endocervical canal beyond the age of 60 years in 100 per cent of the cases. Thus, if most cervical malignancies arise at this squamocolumnar junction, endocervical specimens are of major importance in the evaluation of the cytology, particularly in the postmenopausal patient (Fig. 3–2).

The junction between the epithelium and the underlying stroma is usually referred to as the basement membrane or basal lamina; the mucopolysaccharide layer (which can be demonstrated by special stains) is irregularly present and often cannot be clearly defined beneath the gland epithelium. Furthermore, since invading tumor cells often produce their own mucopolysaccharide, the basal lamina represents an unrealistic and indefinable barrier. Finally, the structure recognized by the electron microscope does not correspond to the previously known basement membrane. Thus, the light microscope does not offer a specific method by which a "breakthrough" of malignant cells into the underlying connective tissue can be determined.

The epithelium of the endocervix differs from that of the portio, and the transition between the two may be abrupt or gradual (Fig. 3–3). Fluhmann clearly demonstrated that there is a gradual or prosoplastic transition between these epithelia in more than 90 per cent of cervices (Fig. 3–4). The cylindrical picket-fence type of cells lining the endocervix are much taller than the cells of the endometrial epithelium and normally exhibit no cilia. The nuclei, as compared with those of the corpus, are more deeply stained, and are placed basally, whereas those of the endometrium are vesicular and vary in position, depending on the stage of the cycle. The cytoplasm of the two epithelia also differs— that of the endometrial cell is usually acidophilic while that of the endocervix, because of its richness in mucin, shows either a clear neutral or a slightly basophilic reaction.

So-called "glands" of the cervix, although initially thought to be of the compound racemose type, have been described accurately by Fluhmann as an intricate system of tunnels and clefts that give an illusory impression of glands (Fig. 3–5). Intense scru-

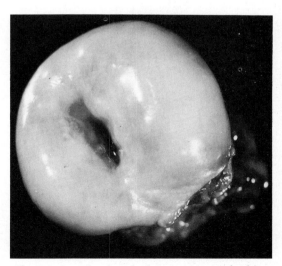

Figure 3–2. The squamocolumnar junction can be visualized just inside the anatomic external os.

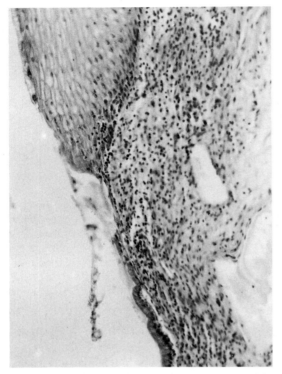

Figure 3–3. Abrupt transition between the high, columnar epithelium of the endocervix and the stratified epithelium of the portio.

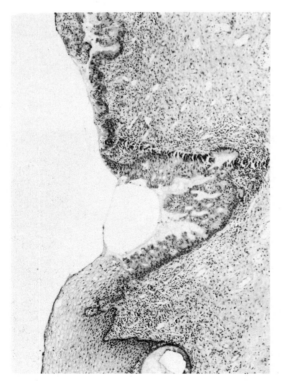

Figure 3–4. Prosoplastic transition at squamocolumnar junction—the common picture.

tiny of serial sections of both normal and pregnant uteri leaves little doubt of the validity of Fluhmann's thesis. Such "glands" may be recognized on the portio and adjacent vagina (adenosis vaginae) (Figs. 3–6 and 3–7).

At higher levels of the endocervix, variations in the cellular elements of the glands can be recognized frequently. In one and the same gland, transitions from the classic mucus-secreting cell to tubal or endometrial types produce the illusion of atypical alterations (Fig. 3–8). These changes simply demonstrate the totipotency of the paramesonephric epithelium.

Cervical Mucus Arborization

Zondek and Rozin have reported on the often observed tendency for dried cervical mucus to crystallize in specific palm leaf fashion, termed "arborization." By studying the viscosity of the cervical mucus, it is possible to determine whether ovulation has occurred. Although such a study is valuable and simple to perform, few clinicians depend solely upon this method to detect ovulation, especially since more accurate information can be obtained by basal body temperature and endometrial biopsy. Nevertheless, students of infertility place great stress on the viscosity of the cervical mucus (spinnbarkeit) at ovulation, with special emphasis on its receptivity to or rejection of the sperm. Furthermore, the studies of Mishell, Davajan, and Israel demonstrate the importance of the cervical architecture in the movement of sperm through the canal and the import of the "compartments" on fertility.

The stroma of the cervix is histologically unlike that of the endometrium, since it consists primarily of connective tissue; however, the ability of this stroma to respond to ovarian stimuli is demonstrated by the frequency with which it responds with a decidual reaction during pregnancy. As the internal os is approached, there is an increasing admixture of smooth muscle approximating the subepithelial zone. Cystic remnants of the mesonephric duct are frequent findings in the deeper stroma of the endocervix (Fig. 3–9). These elements, noted in 7 to 10 per cent of all serially sectioned cervices, may demonstrate the ability of mesonephric epithelia to respond to hormonal stimuli—e.g., during pregnancy tubal differentiation

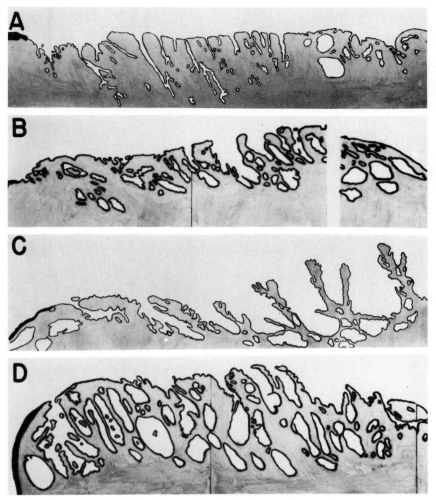

Figure 3–5. Appearance of the endocervix in various physiologic conditions. *A*, nonpregnant; *B*, pregnancy at 13 weeks; *C*, pregnancy at 35 weeks; *D*, pregnancy at term. (Courtesy of Dr. C. Frederic Fluhmann.)

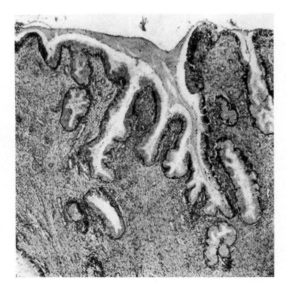

Figure 3–6. Microscopic appearance of cervix with characteristic picket-fence epithelium and spindle-celled fibrous stroma. The glandlike appearance is evident.

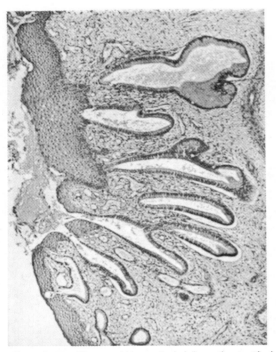

Figure 3–7. Characteristic cervical clefts on the stratified squamous epithelium of the pars vaginalis.

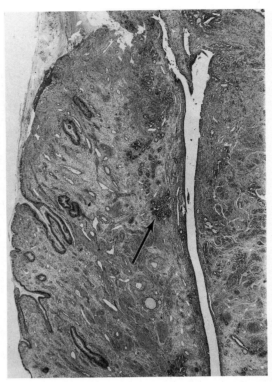

Figure 3–9. The mesonephric duct, deep in the substance of the cervix, with the nests of tubules along its course (at arrow).

may be appreciated in these deep-seated epithelial elements. Adenomatous patterns are occasionally seen in the mesonephric remnants and simulate a well-differentiated carcinoma (Fig. 3–10 A). Careful inspection reveals the epithelium to be low cuboidal with only rare secretory elements and the absence of abnormal nuclear activity (Fig. 3–10 A,B).

Stromal reaction around such elements occasionally simulates that seen in the paramesonephric derivatives (Fig. 3–11).

Contrasts with Endometrium

To summarize, therefore, the chief histologic differences between the endocervix

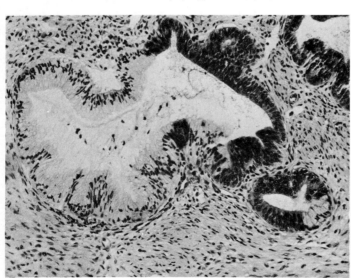

Figure 3–8. Benign alterations in cell type, commonly seen in the endocervical glands; both tubal and endometrial cells can be visualized in these clefts.

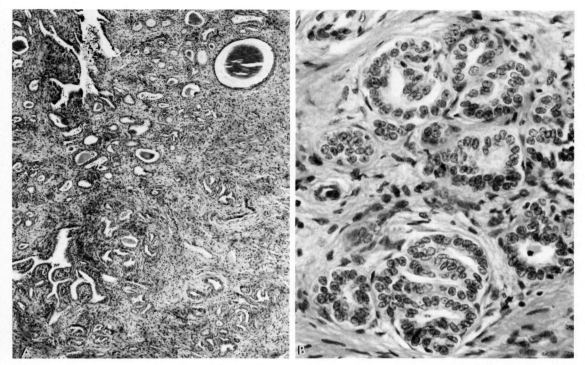

Figure 3–10. *A*, Mesonephric adenoma deep within cervical stroma. *B*, Low cuboidal epithelium lining mesonephric elements. Note absence of abnormal nuclear activity.

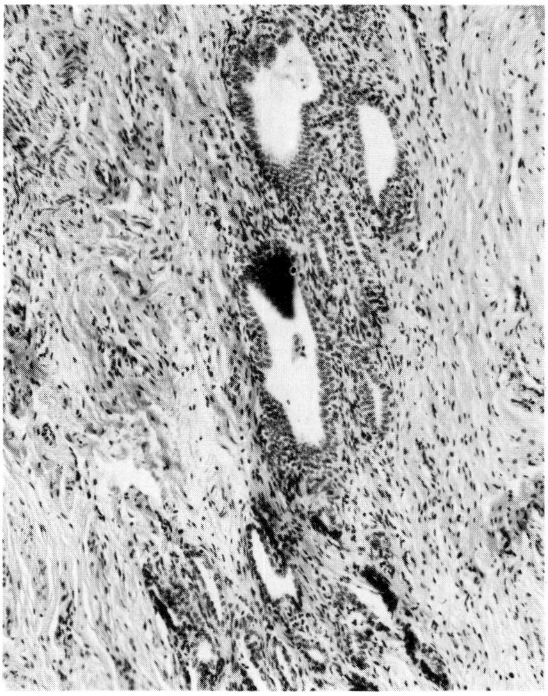

Figure 3–11. Stromal reaction around mesonephric remnants simulates that seen in association with paramesonephric elements.

and the endometrium are (1) the epithelium of the cervix is of the tall picket-fence type with basally placed nuclei containing uniformly dispersed chromatin, while that of the endometrium is cuboidal or columnar, with more centrally placed vesicular nuclei, depending on the phase in the cycle, and prominent nucleoli; (2) the cervical tunnels and clefts make up an intricate pattern since there is no cyclic loss of the majority of the cytoplasm as occurs in the endometrium; (3) the cervical stroma is composed of connective tissue with an indefinable subepithelial layer and variable amounts of smooth muscle. Smooth muscle is nonexistent in the portio but increases as the internal os is approached. The stroma of the endometrium consists of round or spindle cells that routinely demonstrate cyclic variations culminating in a decidual reaction during the premenstrual period.

These differences are emphasized because they constitute the basis for the proper identification of tissues in the pathologic examination of uterine curettings. The curette brings away fragments of endometrium as well as endocervix, and only a familiarity with the normal histologic features will enable one to identify the source of the tissue.

As in other parts of the genital tract, rare segmental anomalies of the cervical epithelium of the portio may be encountered, such as the presence of sebaceous glands (Fig. 3–12) and melanin in the basal layer. In view of these findings, it is not surprising that certain cervical lesions (Fordyce's disease, adenoid basal carcinoma, and melanoma) may simulate those seen primarily on the skin (see Chapter 5).

Possible Cyclic Changes in Cervical Mucosa

As already mentioned, it seems difficult to believe that the endocervix, especially in view of its müllerian (paramesonephric) origin, would not exhibit some cyclic histologic changes, as do the endometrium and the tube. Nevertheless, the few studies relative to such variations leave the question still confused. The extensive investigations of Sjövall led him to conclude that the cervical columnar epithelium, under the influence of estrogen, increases in height until after ovulation, and then becomes lower and increasingly secretory under the influence of progesterone.

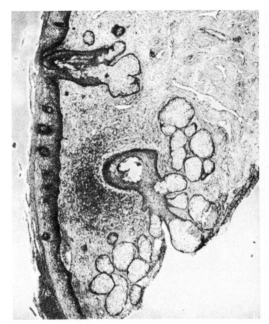

Figure 3–12. Sebaceous glands on vaginal surface of cervix—an uncommon occurrence.

On the other hand, Wollner's somewhat less impressive studies, based on biopsy specimens obtained usually at 2 week intervals and in a small series of women, resulted in his conclusions that the maximal development of the endocervix is reached premenstrually, when complete denudation of the surface took place followed by rapid regeneration. There appears to have been no acceptance of Wollner's views. Topkins' and Duperroy's investigations suggested that a specific histologic cycle in the cervix cannot be defined at this time, and this conclusion coincides with our own observations.

Cervical Changes in Pregnancy

Fluhmann and others have documented the histologic changes that occur in the cervix during pregnancy. As noted previously, the cervix is composed of three elements: a stroma, a "glandular" epithelium of the endocervix, and a stratified squamous epithelium of the ectocervix. Each of these is affected by pregnancy. There is marked increase in vascularity and edema of the stroma, and leukocytic infiltration is present in over 50 per cent of cervices. Decidual reaction of stromal cells was documented in 10.4 per cent (Epperson et al.) of the studied cases, but in hysterectomy specimens such alterations are much more common. Frequently this change occurs in small patches, but often large fields of typical decidual cells are observed (Fig. 3–13). The large pale cells may seem to be attached to the surface epithelium and have been misinterpreted as atypically maturing and superficially invading squamous elements. The absence of nuclear activity and the associated clinical and histologic findings establish the correct diagnosis (Fig. 3–14). The change is limited to the stromal elements, so that it would be illogical to assume that the decidua is merely a pregnancy response to a preexisting cervical endometriosis. The cervical stromal elements of paramesonephric (müllerian) origin demonstrate this characteristic response to the hormones of pregnancy, as may the submesothelial elements in the ovary and pelvic peritoneum. Decidual reaction has been demonstrated in the cervix of the newborn, again demonstrating the ability of this tissue to respond to hormonal stimuli.

The glands of the endocervix are influenced in four ways by pregnancy. It is true that each of these changes can be seen in the nonpregnant state, but they are much more striking in the parturient woman.

1. As described by Fluhmann, there is a marked increase in the actual number of glands. The individual glands are increased

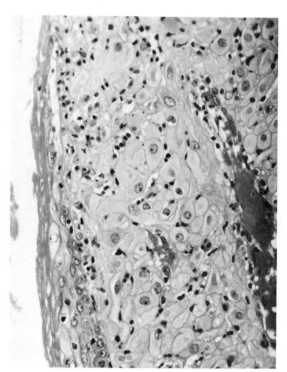

Figure 3–14. Decidual reaction beneath stratified cervical epithelium. The decidual cells seem to be a part of the epithelium and may be misconstrued as evidences of abnormal maturation.

in size and tortuosity, so that at the end of pregnancy the mucosa forms a spongy mass which makes up as much as one half the entire bulk of the cervix. Histologic examination shows a lacy adenomatous pattern. The glands are filled with mucus because of the secretory overactivity of the glandular epithelium (Fig. 3–15). For the sake of clarity, this change has been termed glandular hyperplasia.

2. There is a tendency for the glandular epithelium to "pile up" into two or three layers, with the formation of actual epithelial projections into the lumina of the glands. This has been termed glandular epithelial hyperplasia (Fig. 3–16).

3. When the epithelium shows a tendency to proliferate, new glands are formed within the lumen of the original glands. These new glands are lined with columnar or flattened epithelium. The change can become so marked that those not familiar with it may be tempted to think of adenocarcinoma. This phenomenon has been termed adenomatous hyperplasia.

4. Finally, the common types of metaplasia—both squamous and mucoid—are rec-

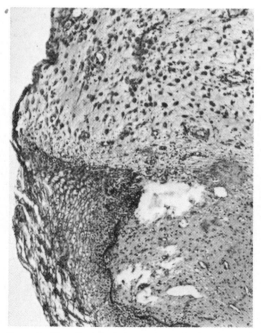

Figure 3–13. Decidual change in cervix (fourth month of pregnancy).

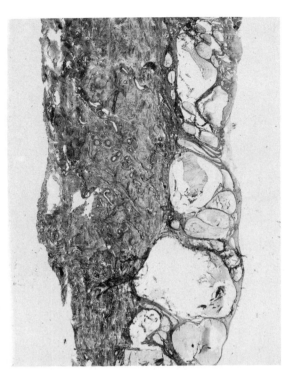

Figure 3–15. Marked dilatation of glands, producing an adenomatous appearance during pregnancy.

ognized frequently. Although these are noted in the nonpregnant state, the dramatic reactions, particularly the adenomatous changes seen with gestation, may cause concern.

Although changes in the stratified squamous epithelium of the ectocervix are not striking, there may be an apparent increase in the actual thickness of the stratified squamous epithelium and an associated hyperactivity of the basal and parabasal layers, to the extent that they compose more than half of the thickness of the epithelium. In an effort to cover the exposed glandular epithelium of the endocervix, the stratified squamous epithelium seems to proliferate. Frequently, this "healing" effort is accomplished only by basal cells, which appear overactive, with hyperchromatic nuclei. Overactivity of this basal layer in pregnancy is associated with changes in cervical cytology, and in many instances dyskaryosis with an increased number of parabasal cells and abnormal forms is found. The interpretation of these atypicalities is explained more fully in Chapter 34.

In a small percentage of cases the hyperactivity of the basal layer is marked and ap-

pears to completely replace the usual mosaic pattern of the stratified squamous epithelium. These basal cells show loss of nuclear polarity, increased mitotic activity, and varying degrees of cellular abnormalities suggesting a diagnosis of carcinoma in situ. Nevertheless, Epperson and his co-workers and Nesbitt have reviewed and followed these cases, and pointed out that they regress following the termination of pregnancy.

Conversely, it must be noted that carcinoma in situ *does* exist during pregnancy. The cellular changes may be more difficult to evaluate, but as Greene and Peckham have recognized, the criteria for establishing the unequivocal diagnosis of carcinoma in situ remain the same in the pregnant as in the nonpregnant state. The individual cell anaplasia must be definite and must extend through the full thickness of the epithelium, either on the surface or in the clefts. Basal cell hyperactivity should be studied very critically and conservatively because of the extensive reserve cell hyperplasia of pregnancy (Fig. 3–17). If the suspected lesion is true preinvasive cancer, expectant therapy with colposcopy and cytologic studies will not jeopardize the patient or her pregnancy, and should lead to proper therapy. With the

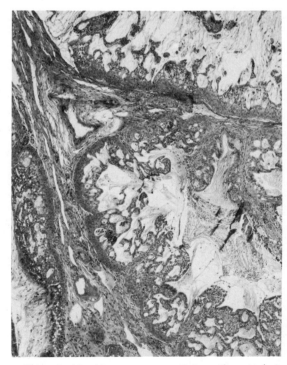

Figure 3–16. Hypersecretory activity with metaplasia classically seen during pregnancy.

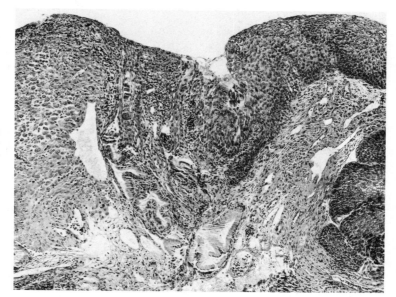

Figure 3–17. Decidual reaction on the left. Atypism is recognized in the epithelium on the right at the squamocolumnar junction. (Carcinoma in situ was diagnosed in later studies.)

marked eversion that occurs in pregnancy, colposcopic studies are particularly valuable since the extent of the lesion can be defined more accurately. Conization may be necessary occasionally; however, in our experience this procedure during pregnancy has not led to full evaluation of the situation, since in approximately 75 per cent of the cases residual tumor has been found in the follow-up studies, be they cytologic, colposcopic, or histologic. The management of these pre-invasive lesions in obstetric patients is reviewed by Johnson and associates.

In summary, different patterns must be recognized as pregnancy changes and not true anaplasia:

1. Increased adenomatous proliferation, which may be so marked as to mimic adenocarcinoma.

2. Reserve or indifferent cell metaplasia (suggesting basal cell hyperactivity).

3. Decidual reaction with a mosaic pattern suggesting squamous cells in the stroma.

In addition to a stromal decidual reaction, there are changes in the cervical vasculature. The intense cuffing of the small arteries (Fig. 3–18) is similar to that seen beneath the implantation site in the fundus. It has been suggested that this cuffing may represent the residuum of a marked perivascular decidual reaction. The exact etiology is unknown but in the myometrium it may remain for months or possibly years.

Thus, the cervix demonstrates a variety of pathophysiologic responses to pregnancy, all of which are of importance in differentiating the pathologic from the physiologic.

Finally, the Arias-Stella reaction may be noted in the endocervical glands (Fig. 3–19). The bizarre hyperchromatic cells, as in the

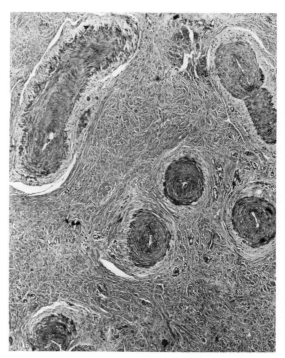

Figure 3–18. Perivascular cuffing in cervix during pregnancy.

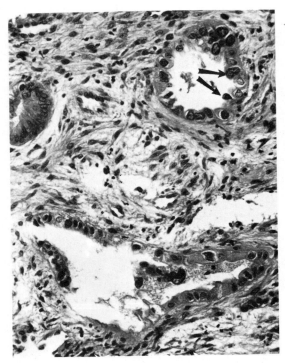

Figure 3–19. Arias-Stella reaction in endocervical curettage. Note hyperchromatic nuclei at arrows.

endometrium, are suggestive of malignancy. Furthermore, the superficial atypical nuclei are similar to those appreciated in the endocervical atypism associated with adenocarcinoma in situ. Careful study of the adjacent epithelium and correlation with the clinical picture will assist in establishing the correct diagnosis.

REFERENCES

Bergman, P.: Spermigration and cyclic changes in cervical mucus. Fertil. Steril., 4:183, 1953.

Bowles, H. E., and Tilden, L. L.: Decidual reactions of the cervix. Western J. Surg., 59:168, 1951.

Carrow, L. A., and Greene, R. R.: Epithelia of pregnant cervix. Am. J. Obstet. Gynecol., 61:237, 1951.

Danforth, D. N.: The squamous epithelium and the squamocolumnar junction of the cervix during pregnancy. Am. J. Obstet. Gynecol., 60:5, 1950.

DeAlvarez, R. R., Figge, D. C., Brown, D. V., and May, K. J.: Biologic behavior of human uterine cancer. Am. J. Obstet. Gynecol., 75:945, 1958.

Duperroy, C.: Morphological study of the endocervical mucosa in relation to the menstrual cycle and to leucorrhea. Gynaecologia, 131:73, 1951.

Epperson, J. W. W., Hellman, L. M., Busby, T., and Galvin, G. E.: Morphologic changes in cervix during pregnancy, including intraepithelial carcinoma. Am. J. Obstet. Gynecol., 61:50, 1951.

Fluhmann, C. F.: Nature and development of glands of cervix uteri. Am. J. Obstet. Gynecol., 74:753, 1957.

Fluhmann, C. F.: The glandular structures of the cervix uteri during pregnancy. Am. J. Obstet. Gynecol., 78:990, 1959.

Fluhmann, C. F.: The squamo-columnar transitional zone of the cervix uteri. Obstet. Gynecol., 14:133, 1959.

Fluhmann, C. F.: The developmental anatomy of the cervix uteri. Obstet. Gynecol., 15:62, 1960.

Fluhmann, C. F., and Dickmann, Z.: Glandular structures of the cervix. Obstet. Gynecol., 11:543, 1958.

Greene, R. R., and Peckham, B. M.: Squamous papillomas of the cervix. Am. J. Obstet. Gynecol., 67:883, 1954.

Greene, R. R., et al.: Preinvasive carcinoma of cervix during pregnancy. Surg. Gynecol. Obstet., 96:71, 1954.

Hamilton, C. E.: Ovulatory cycle in cervix of monkey. Anat. Rec., 94:466, 1946.

Huffman, J. W.: Mesonephric remains in cervix. Am. J. Obstet. Gynecol., 56:23, 1948.

Johnson, L. D., Hertig, A. T., Hinman, C. H., and Easterday, C. L.: Pre-invasive cervical lesions in obstetric patients. Obstet. Gynecol., 16:113, 1960.

Lapan, B.: Deciduosis of cervix and vagina simulating carcinoma. Am. J. Obstet. Gynecol., 58:743, 1949.

Linhartova, A.: Unusual lesions of the uterine cervix. Int. J. Obstet. Gynecol., 10:34, 1972.

Murphy, E. J., and Herbut, P. A.: Uterine cervix during pregnancy. Am. J. Obstet. Gynecol., 59:384, 1950.

Nesbitt, R. E. L.: Basal cell hyperactivity of cervix with postpartum follow-up. Obstet. Gynecol., 6:239, 1955.

Ostergard, D. R.: Effect of age, gravidity and parity on the locale of the cervical squamo-columnar junction. Am. J. Obstet. Gynecol., 129:59, 1977.

Saga, M., and Davajan, V.: Mechanism of crystallization of purified human midcycle cervical mucus. Am. J. Obstet. Gynecol., 129:154, 1977.

Sjövall, A.: Studies of cervical mucosa during menstrual cycle, childhood, senility and some hormonal disorders. Acta Obstet. Gynecol. Scand. (Suppl. 4), 18:3, 1938.

Stander, H. J.: Williams Obstetrics. 7th ed. New York, D. Appleton-Century Co., 1936.

Topkins, P.: Histologic appearance of endocervix during menstrual cycle. Am. J. Obstet. Gynecol., 58:654, 1949.

Urdan, B. E., et al.: Crystallization of cervical mucus. Obstet. Gynecol., 5:3, 1955.

Wollner, A.: Menstrual cycle in human cervical mucosa and the clinical significance. Am. J. Surg., 57:331, 1942.

Zondek, B., and Cooper, K.: Cervical mucus in pregnancy. Obstet. Gynecol., 4:484, 1954.

Zondek, B., and Rozin, S.: Cervical mucus arborization. Obstet. Gynecol., 3:463, 1954.

Chapter 4

BENIGN LESIONS OF THE CERVIX (CERVICITIS, THE METAPLASIAS, AND BENIGN TUMORS)

CERVICITIS

Introduction

Bacterial cervicitis may be the result of infection by the gonococcus, various pyogenic organisms, bacteroides, or a variety of other aerobic or anaerobic organisms. The initial attack is upon the "gland-bearing" areas, since the normal, intact stratified epithelium is usually resistant to the insults of such agents. Nevertheless, since the transitional zone commonly includes the endocervical areas that have been re-covered by metaplastic and later stratified epithelium, the infected occluded glands produce a diffuse inflammatory junction, generally referred to as chronic cervicitis.

Acute cervicitis may exist without systemic response, as is recognized in many biopsy specimens. The cervix under such conditions is grossly erythematous with edema of the everted endocervical mucosa. Bacteriologic study of the associated mucopurulent discharge may reveal the presence of gram-negative intracellular diplococci. The histologic examination is characterized by dilatation of the blood vessels and infiltration of the subepithelial and periglandular tissues with polymorphonuclear leukocytes and plasma cells.

Chronic Cervicitis

Chronic infection of the cervix is the most frequently encountered of all pathologic conditions, both in the clinic and in the laboratory, and is a common cause of leukorrhea. Actually the more correct term would be "chronic endocervicitis" since the glandular portions are the commonly affected elements, while, in contrast, the stratified epithelium of the portio protects its underlying tissues to a major degree. On examination one may find a grossly normal cervix except for lacerations or endocervical eversion (Fig. 4–1). A purulent discharge may exude from an otherwise innocuous-appearing cervical os.

More characteristically, the intracervical infection is associated with erythema of the lacerated, everted endocervix, the so-called eversion or ectropion (Fig. 4–2). The normally endocervical mucosa thus becomes hyperemic and edematous, often grossly suggestive of malignancy. Retention or Nabothian cysts (Fig. 4–3) of the cervical glands may be revealed by speculum examination, appearing as pearly gray vesicles or even whitish if the contents are purulent. If the cysts are deep-seated, they may cause only a surface irregularity on palpation. When punctured, such cysts yield an exudate that is either clear and mucoid, mucopurulent, or purulent (Fig. 4–4).

In other cases, even when no laceration is present, the cervical os may be surrounded by a circle of reddish, granular tissue, appearing as the so-called cervical erosion, the mechanism of which will be discussed later.

Microscopically, chronic cervicitis is characterized by an extensive subepithelial inflammatory infiltrate of plasma cells, with

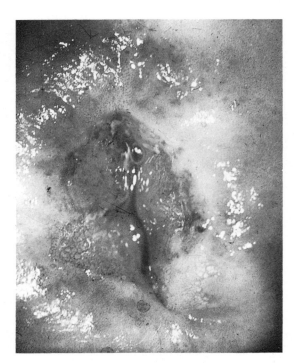

Figure 4–1. Marked eversion in old laceration with transformation zone exposed.

Figure 4–2. Erosion and ectropion of cervix.

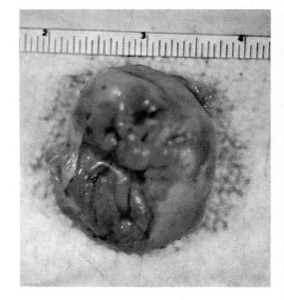

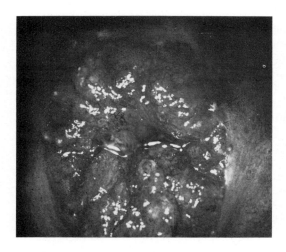

Figure 4–3. Marked chronic infection with cyst formation. The transformation zone is far out on the portio.

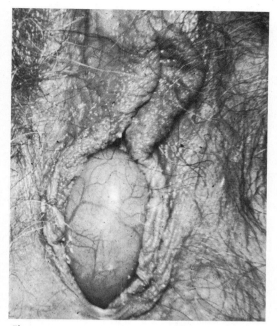

Figure 4–4. Large cervical retention cyst presenting at vaginal outlet.

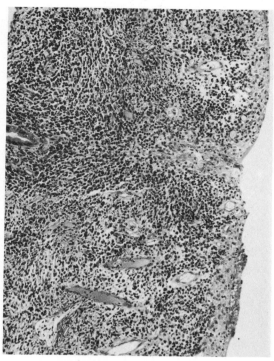

Figure 4–6. Marked chronic cervicitis. This section from the squamocolumnar region shows distortion of the surface epithelium and atypical maturation of the metaplastic elements. The underlying stroma is densely infiltrated with plasma cells, and vascularity gives the impression of granulation tissue. Epithelium of the gland is distorted.

scattered polymorphonuclear leukocytes and large mononuclear cells. The epithelium may be quite normal (Fig. 4–5), flattened to appear cuboidal or squamoid, or desquamated as a result of the intense reac-

tion (Fig. 4–6). Some pathologists have attempted to distinguish between the gonorrheal and the nongonorrheal forms, stressing especially the deep periglandular infiltration of the former, but this is not a reliable criterion.

In milder forms the inflammatory infiltrate may involve chiefly the superficial subepithelial connective tissue layer, but often diffuse or somewhat circumscribed collections of chronic inflammatory cells may be seen far beneath the surface. A less frequent finding is a marked hyperplasia of the glands, with the resultant adenoid appearance of the infected tunnels. Adenomatous hyperplasia, on the other hand, usually is associated with little evidence of infection. The aggregation of cystic clefts is ominous in pattern, but the individual flattened epithelial cells are benign. The process may be the result of the occlusions of many channels by a noninflammatory, nonneoplastic process (Figs. 4–7 and 4–8); however, the characteristics of the lining cells are suggestive of the flattened, irregular mesothelium seen in the

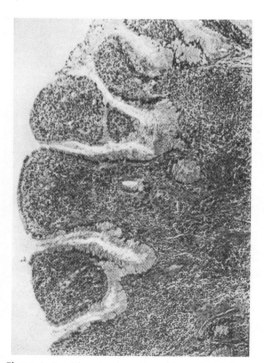

Figure 4–5. Chronic cervicitis, with marked inflammatory infiltrate in the underlying tissue.

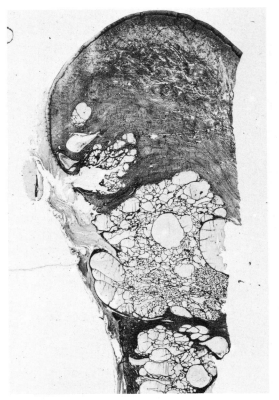

Figure 4–7. Lacy pattern characteristic of adenomatous hyperplasia.

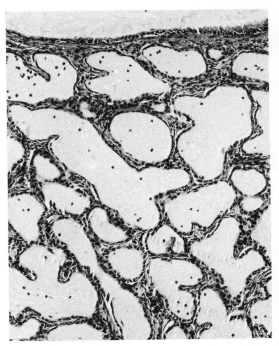

Figure 4–8. High power view of adenomatous change in endocervix. Epithelium is flattened, possibly of mesothelial origin.

adenomatoid tumor. The essential absence of secretory activity and infection supports this thesis.

GRANULOMATOUS DISEASE

Tuberculous Cervicitis

This is an uncommon infection, but may be seen as a late secondary manifestation of upper tract disease, most frequently salpingitis. In rare cases it appears to be primary in the cervix, introduced by a male partner with tuberculous epididymitis or other genitourinary disease. It produces in the cervix an ulcerative and at times hypertrophic lesion which grossly simulates carcinoma. The distinction between the two is made only by microscopic examination.

Microscopically, the lesion is characterized by chronic infiltration—primarily of lymphocytes associated with the classic tubercle, made up of a central giant cell and surrounding epithelioid cells (Fig. 4–9). Caseation may be noted in the acute phase of the infection (Sered et al.) with superficial

ulceration and pseudoepitheliomatous hyperplasia at the periphery. Except in this acute caseous stage, cultures, stains, and guinea pig inoculation may be negative, and microscopically the only acceptable diagnosis is granulomatous cervicitis.

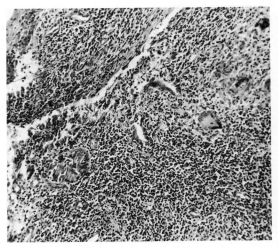

Figure 4–9. Squamous epithelium upper left; extensive lymphocytic cell infiltration below with typical granulomatous change, including giant cells and surrounding epithelioid reaction.

Other Granulomatous Infections

Although more frequent on the vulva, syphilis, granuloma inguinale, and lymphogranuloma venereum may involve the cervix and grossly resemble cancer. Other more definitive findings suggestive of the various specific diseases are similar to those stated in Chapter 1. Special stains, cultures, and antigen-antibody reactions are of assistance in establishing the final diagnosis. Furthermore, the geographic locale is of prime importance in the study of granulomatous disease. Schistosomiasis, so rare in our culture, is not uncommon in South Africa, and the telltale features may be recognized in both microscopic and cytopathologic preparations (Fig. 4–10).

Recently, with the increased use of intrauterine devices, associated infectious processes of the fungus variety have been found.

Cultures have been taken from the devices and are often positive for actinomyces. Rarely is major surgery necessary for such problems, but the offending agents may be found in several sites, including the cervix (Fig. 4–11).

VIRAL DISEASES

Condylomata acuminata have been described frequently in all areas of the lower genital canal and are of viral origin. Their classic warty appearance is well known; however, undoubtedly the smaller lesions go unrecognized, both grossly and microscopically (see Fig. 4–32). In view of the recent interest in a viral etiology for cervical cancer, such diseases take on added significance.

Similarly, the vesicular lesions of herpes

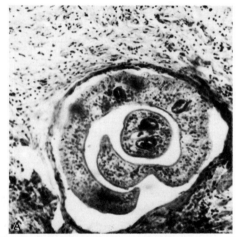

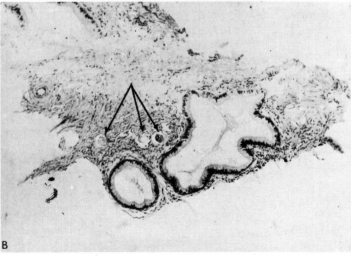

Figure 4–10. *A*, Bilharzial worms, the female embraced by the male, in a venous channel of the cervix. *B*, Bilharzial ova in cervical curettings. (Courtesy of Dr. M. F. Fathalla, Dept. Obstet. Gynecol., Mabarrah Hospital, Assiut, Egypt, U.A.R.)

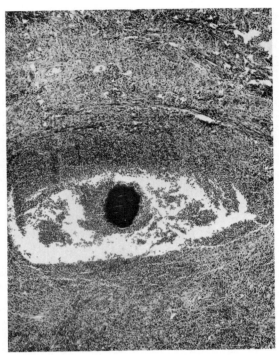

Figure 4–11. Actinomyces in the body of cervix. Patient had extensive pelvic inflammatory disease associated with intrauterine device.

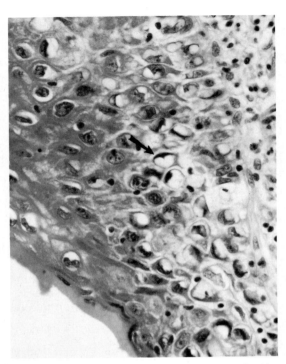

Figure 4–12. Condylomatous change in cervical epithelium. Note inclusions(?) at arrow.

simplex are routinely present on the cervix and vagina if the vulva is affected, but often go unnoticed since they produce few symptoms at the former sites. The characteristic intranuclear inclusions (see Chapter 1) are described frequently in cytologic spreads. Biopsies of the cervix in such cases may show either intraepithelial or subepithelial blebs, which may contain the classic inclusions. Other cellular alterations suggestive of viral disease are degenerative multinucleation and vacuolization of the nuclei (Fig. 4–12). These are sometimes difficult to distinguish from neoplastic processes and it must be appreciated that, if cancer and viral disease are related, there is no reason to doubt that the benign and in situ neoplastic alterations would be combined in many instances. Consequently, careful evaluation of these atypical changes is mandatory if overtreatment of benign lesions, particularly in the young girl, is to be avoided.

CERVICAL EROSION

There has been much discussion as to the mechanism involved in the production of the cervical erosion. It should be distinguished from ectropion, or eversion, which is usually the result of laceration, with a "turning out" of the edematous, vascular endocervix. The term "ectopy" has been applied to the foci of endocervical tissue, isolated on the portio, usually as the result of incomplete healing of an ectropion.

Erosion literally indicates an actual denudation of the epithelium as seen in the prolapsed cervix. Runge and Veit believed that the superficial layers of the stratified squamous epithelium are destroyed, leaving only the basal columnar or cuboidal cells and resulting from the erosive effects of pH changes in the vagina and the consequent increase in the pathogenicity of the vaginal flora. The congenital (Fischel) and the acquired erosions are characterized by diffuse patches of endocervical epithelium protruding from the canal beyond the squamocolumnar junction, and thus, in reality, constituting eversion of the endocervix.

Epidermidalization or Squamous Metaplasia

The presence of a stratified or epidermoid epithelium in the tunnels or clefts of the endocervix has been explained by three mechanisms: (1) direct invasion into the cleft by stratified squamous epithelium from the surface; (2) a metaplasia of the columnar epithelium into a less well differentiated epidermoid variety; or (3) a squamous metaplasia produced by proliferation of the reserve or indifferent cell. The last is the most well accepted theory at the present.

Epidermidalization. In the healing process of an erosion, the surface stratified squamous epithelium seems to invade the tunnels along the basal lamina directly, a process termed epidermidalization (or epidermoidization). The entire gland lumen may be filled, and the cylindrical epithelium may, as it were, be "choked to death" (Fig. 4–13). Nevertheless, small central, gland-like, mucin-filled cavities often remain as the residua of the preexisting, tall, columnar epithelium.

This pattern demonstrates the usual process of maturation of the basal or undifferentiated cells, following the stages of maturity noted normally in the epithelium of the portio, rather than the uniform, monotonous cell type recognized in squamous metaplasia. Consequently, since the developmental process in both metaplasia and epidermidalization is the same, the latter term is of historic interest only.

Metaplasia. Although the theory of metaplasia has been well accepted by most observers, there are differences of opinion as to the cell from which the metaplastic epithelium arises. The possibility of the mature, tall, columnar, mucus-secreting cell reverting to the round or ovoid metaplastic cell seems relatively inconceivable. The reserve or indifferent cell hyperplasia is considered by most authorities to be the logical explanation for the partial or complete obliteration of the tunnels by the metaplastic or epidermoid cell. These cells initially are uniform in type, rather than stratified, and the multilayered pattern may suggest an anaplastic change, such as is seen in basal cell hyperactivity. Careful study of the individual elements will demonstrate the uniformity of the cell and the benign nature of this alteration.

In the latter stages of metaplasia, maturity of the cells takes place and a characteristic stratified pattern results. The evidences of the preexisting endocervical gland–like arrangement are noted in the undulating basal layer, with tiny vascular canals near the surface and underlying normal clefts. The residua of the initial mucus-secreting epithelium often remain as tiny basophilic-staining central cores (Fig. 4–14). Further, it must be recognized that this reserve or

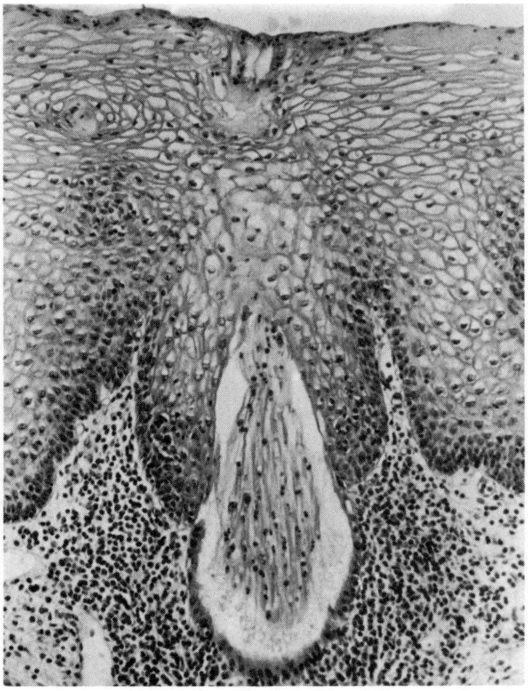

Figure 4–13. Epidermidalization of the endocervical cleft with mature stratified squamous epithelium. Extensive inflammatory infiltrate is noted in the underlying stroma.

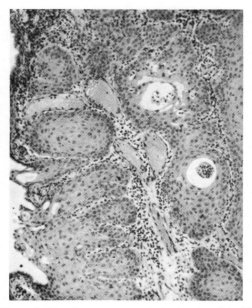

Figure 4–14. Squamous metaplasia showing clefts filled with the uniform type of cells. Residua of the mucus-secreting cells may be seen in right central area.

indifferent cell undoubtedly has the ability to produce either the common epidermoid variety or a mucopolysaccharide-containing cell (Fig. 4–15). The latter may never mature to the typical tall, pale, columnar variety, but special stains demonstrate the evidences of secretory activity.

The importance of these metaplastic changes cannot be overemphasized. As noted previously, Fluhmann and others have recognized the frequency of this pattern at the transitional zone of the cervix. It is the rule, rather than the exception, that the epithelial change from the stratified squamous to the high columnar cell is a gradual rather than abrupt alteration (Chapter 3). This intermediate epithelium simulates a metaplastic type; however, it is more commonly designated "prosoplasia." Furthermore, this zone is not stationary, but fluctuates throughout life. Certainly, the position of this transition varies from high in the canal during the late postmenopausal years, to a situation well out on the portio during pregnancy, in women with acute infections, and often in those using oral contraceptives.

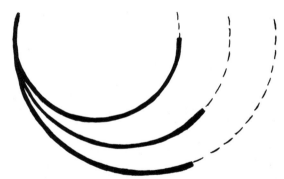

Figure 4–16. Diagrammatic representation of the changes in position of the squamocolumnar junction related to mechanical variations in the bulk of the cervix. (Broken line, endocervix; solid line, stratified squamous epithelium.)

These alterations may well be caused by the variations in the actual bulk of the structure (Fig. 4–16) (see also Chapter 3).

Of major importance to the pathologist are the confusing pictures that may develop from these patterns. Superficial evaluation may lead to the erroneous diagnosis of adenocarcinoma, adenoacanthoma, adenosquamous cancer, or the common epidermoid malignancy. Conversely, it must be recognized that all of these anaplasias may arise in the cervix; therefore, the investigator would be wise to study the individual cells carefully for evidences of anaplastic alteration. Such atypicalities suggest that the common epidermoid carcinomas arise, in truth, as malignant metaplasias, both changes developing in the same transformation zone. Even more suggestive is the adenoepidermoid neoplasia which originates in the tunnels or clefts, commonly without association to the surface.

Differentiating from Cancer

Differentiation of the benign from the malignant invasion of the endocervical tunnels and clefts may be difficult. Of fundamental importance are the surface changes, since it is here that the best possibility exists for study of the well-oriented full thickness of the epithelium. Nevertheless, it must be reemphasized that the tunnels may be the site of the most striking cellular changes. Tangential sections produce atypical pictures, suggestive of pearl formation (Fig. 4–17). Similarly, sectioning through an involved gland, without knowledge of the position of the present or preexisting lumen,

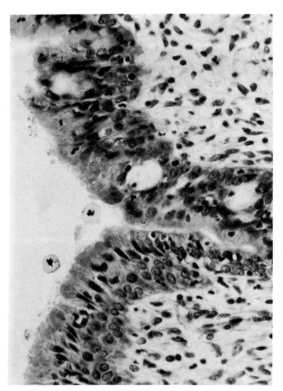

Figure 4–15. High power view of metaplasia showing mucus-secreting epithelium on surface (below) and acinous pattern (above).

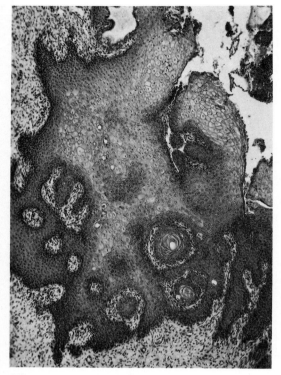

Figure 4–17. Tangential cut showing normally maturing surface epithelium with pseudo–pearl formation in lower central area, which simulates condylomata.

plasia is difficult, if not impossible, and repeat studies are imperative after attempt at treatment with local antibacterial and tissue reparative agents.

Pseudo-epitheliomatous or Pseudocarcinomatous Hyperplasia. The problems inherent in such conditions have been discussed in Chapter 1. Suffice it to say here that the elongation and distortion of the rete pegs produce patterns suggestive of anaplasia, especially when tangential cuts separate the epithelial tips from the surface, resulting in a picture of invasive disease. Careful study of cell detail in such situations is made more difficult if the patient has had a conization, in which case stratified epithelium, benign or neoplastic, may be buried beneath the surface (Fig. 4–19), and serial sections to establish connection of tips with the surface will usually result in the correct evaluation. Nevertheless, abnormal maturation and attempted keratinization at the basal layer with or without inflammatory reaction should increase the index of suspicion and demand more thorough study.

Atypical Metaplasia. The general characteristics of squamous and mucoid cell meta-

may give the false impression of full-thickness involvement of the epithelium by the malignant cells. Determining the degree of individual cell anaplasia in a satisfactorily oriented epithelium is imperative if accurate assessment of the lesion is to be made.

Many of the most difficult problems in the differentiation of the benign from the malignant epithelium arise in the inflammatory diseases. Five basic processes in this area deserve special mention.

True Ulceration (Erosion). In ulcerative disease, exclusive of malignancy, the initial tissue response is protective, as evidenced by the appearance of both polymorphonuclear leukocytes and lymphocytes for the purpose of debridement and development of antibodies to the irritative process. As healing begins, the active epithelial cells initiating the reparative process are not stratified and mitoses are more frequent. Unless this process is recognized, a diagnosis of basal cell hyperactivity or hyperplasia may be entertained. As regeneration continues, more bizarre cells appear in the superficial layers and these are commonly termed dysplastic (Fig. 4–18). Differentiation from true ana-

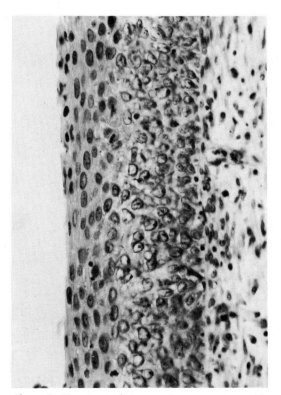

Figure 4–18. Atypicalities seen in regenerating epithelium. Atypical metaplasia.

plasia have been discussed. With squamous metaplasia, the cells are usually uniform, with abundant eosinophilic cytoplasm and pale blue nuclei and occasionally a "coffee-bean" configuration. Maturity may occur later, but it too is generally regular. On occasion, however, particularly when the inflammatory reaction is severe, cellular atypicalities appear, as seen in the regenerating epithelium. The cytoplasm may be clear or vacuolated, and the nuclei quite dark and irregular; however, mitoses are uncommon.

Adenomatous appearance may develop with tiny pseudo-acini lined by two to three layers of metaplastic cells. Such patterns simulate adenocarcinoma (Fig. 4–19). These formations are due to the proliferating metaplastic cells which enclose the remaining mucus-secreting cells, the centers being mucous blebs rather than keratin. Individual cellular atypism again is the absent feature that differentiates these changes from true anaplasia.

Microcystic mucoid metaplasia (microglandular metaplasia) associated with the use of oral contraceptives and prolonged estrogen therapy produces an adenoid pattern that may be confused with malignancy. The characteristics include a compression of the stroma, an increased secretory activity of the cell, and displacement of the classic basal nucleus to the middle or luminal edge of the cell. This position of the nucleus is classic of that seen in the earliest endocervical atypia and adenocarcinoma in situ and thus adds to the difficulty in interpretation. There is mucoid infiltration into the stroma, and this myxoid change enhances the ominous adenomatous pattern. These alterations are focal in nature and frequently do not disappear with the discontinuation of medication. Similar, although not as dramatic, alterations are noted in endocervical polypi of the postmenopausal woman who is receiving estrogen therapy (Figs. 4–20, 4–21, and 4–22).

On rare occasions, an Arias-Stella reaction may be noted in the endocervical tissues, particularly when a polypoid fragment is pedunculated into the canal. This is a further demonstration of the ability of the endocervix to respond to hormonal stimuli in a fashion similar to that of the endometrium even if not as dramatic (see Chapter 3, Fig. 3–19).

Stromal Reactions. The cervical stroma, as noted previously, can respond to hormone stimuli and the reactions occasionally may be confused with large mature squamous cells. The proliferative, swollen endothelial cell, so commonly seen with severe infections, may well be confused with invading epithelial elements, particularly when the cells blend into the stroma. Fibroblastic reaction, particularly that seen early in the reparative process when the youngest and most active cells are prominent, further confuses the picture. Nevertheless, although they are often large and distorted, these cells show no nuclear anaplasia.

The inflammatory infiltrate is both a blessing and a liability. Although the lumina of the clefts frequently are lost by metaplastic and anaplastic proliferations, the regular arrangement of the routinely associated infiltrate is common to both types of change. The characteristic processes demonstrated by the surrounding stromal concentration and its infiltrate stands in sharp contrast to true stromal invasion, which is patternless. The relationship between the malignant epithelial element and the inflammatory cell is not distinctive. On the other hand, at times the cellularity is quite suggestive of the lymphoid follicle, with histiocytosis and the occasional mitotic figure. The predominance of plasma cells in the surrounding tissue and the appearance of germinal centers of lym-

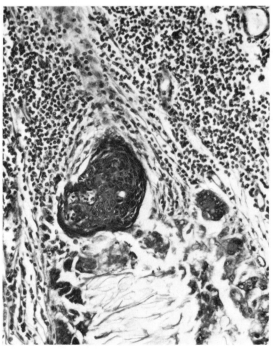

Figure 4–19. Nests of squamous epithelium buried beneath the surface following conization.

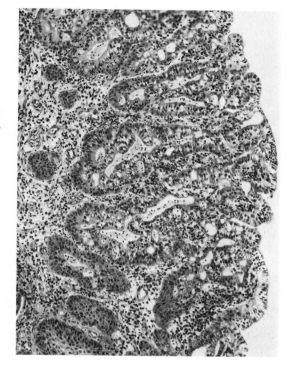

Figure 4–20. Low power view of the microcystic mucoid metaplasia associated with oral contraceptive. Squamous metaplasia may be recognized at the inner tips of the glands.

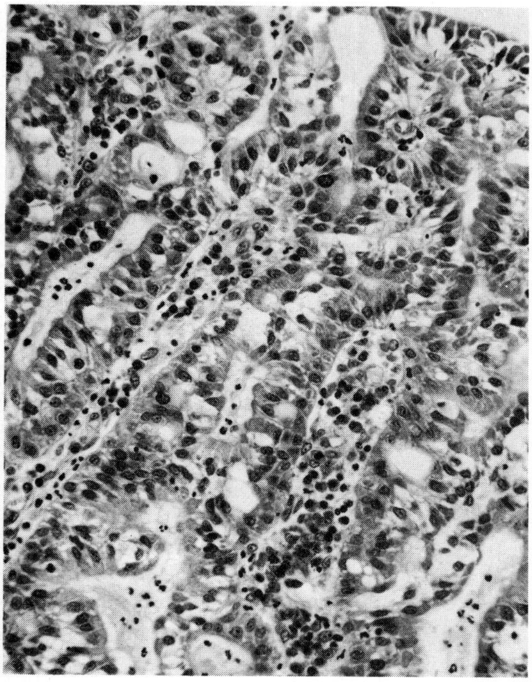

Figure 4–21. High power view of Figure 4–20, showing the basic features of microcystic mucoid metaplasia. (Note that the mucus is in various positions in the cells.)

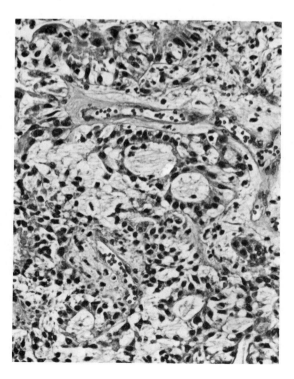

Figure 4–22. Microcystic or microglandular metaplasia of cervix associated commonly with use of oral contraceptives. Note mucoid infiltration into stroma.

phoid hyperplasia serve to establish the diagnosis of an inflammatory as opposed to microinvasive carcinoma or a lymphomatous infiltrate (Fig. 4–23).

Finally, the importance of the reaction is not definite. On one side this may be the evidence of the destructive nature of the invasive process and a breakdown of local resistance. Conversely, it may suggest the presence of antibodies that attempt to protect the host. Both may be true and may differ from case to case.

Hyperkeratosis and Parakeratosis. These changes are not routinely present on the surface of the stratified epithelium of the cervix. Often there are one or more layers of flattened superficial cells which simulate parakeratosis; however, this change is a normal process of maturation in the transition between metaplasia and the more classic stratification of the portio epithelium. Under pathologic conditions, both may be present. In prolapse, hyperkeratosis is common, and the so-called leukoplakia (white patches) microscopically shows surface keratin with its usual underlying granular zone (Fig. 4–24). Similarly, parakeratosis and acanthosis are the hallmarks of condylomata acuminata.

The possibility that viral agents may be etiologic factors in the genesis of cervical

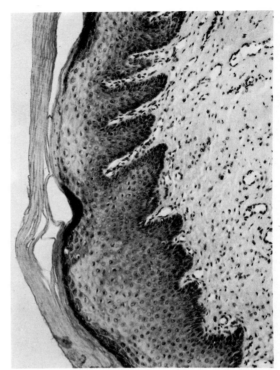

Figure 4–24. Hyperkeratosis on surface with prolapse of uterus—granular layer is prominent in the epithelium.

neoplasia has been suggested by numerous studies; thus, as noted previously, the condyloma acuminatum may take on additional significance in the area of the lower genital canal (Fig. 4–12). In spite of these benign states, the presence of either hyper- or parakeratosis should increase the pathologist's index of suspicion and demand further study. Confusing malignancies, specifically the very mature cancer, are uncommon in the cervix, but may be associated with such atypical patterns.

CERVICAL POLYP

Gross Pathology

The cervical polyp is a localized proliferation of the cervical mucosa presenting as a bright red, vascular, fragile growth, which is usually pedunculated but occasionally is sessile. Polyps may be single or multiple, often presenting as a cluster of small growths lying at the cervical os. They are generally small, sometimes not over a few millimeters in diameter, but may reach a diameter of several centimeters. The pedicle is usually

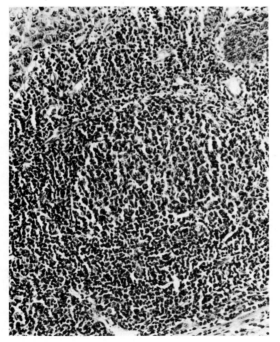

Figure 4–23. Inflammatory infiltrate with hyperplastic lymphoid center—mitoses are common in such centers.

quite small, so that the polyp can be removed easily by twisting the pedicle close to its attachment, or by use of a biopsy clamp or a sharp curette. It is not uncommon to recognize small cervical polyps in sections of uterine curettings.

In most instances the polyp springs from the endocervix, even though it protrudes well beyond the os. Much less frequently the origin is the squamous epithelium of the pars vaginalis, at or near the external os. In cases in which the polyp develops from the vaginal surface of the cervix, the growth may be of rather firm consistency and of the same grayish-pink color as the cervix itself. However, the characteristic cervical polyp, arising as it does from the endocervix, is red, the larger growths being strawberry-like in appearance (Fig. 4–25). Finally, on rare occasions, the endometrial polyp may extend through the cervical canal and into the vagina. It is obvious that only the microscopic characteristics will determine the exact origin of the lesion (Fig. 4–26). Proliferation of the stroma may produce ominous patterns suggestive of stromal sarcoma or mixed tumors. The latter, of course, may develop in the cervix and are often polypoid. Nevertheless, atypical and confusing cellular altera-

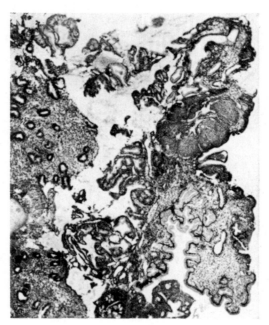

Figure 4–26. Uterine curettings, including cervical tissue in lower right, with tag of benign cervical squamous metaplasia in upper right.

tions may simulate malignancy but, as noted by Norris in the study of vaginal polyps, they pursue a benign course.

The vascularity associated with the frequency of infection and ulceration explains the bleeding which is produced by these small tumors, and which is so similar to the contact bleeding of early carcinoma.

Microscopic Characteristics

The covering epithelium varies according to the point of origin of the polyp, being usually identical with the normal endocervical mucosa (Figs. 4–27 and 4–28). Although chronic endocervicitis often exists, and is considered by many to be the etiologic factor, this seems unlikely in view of the frequency of infection. Some polyps are lined partly by the gland-bearing endocervical mucosa and partly by stratified squamous epithelium. Marked lobulation is characteristic of the endocervical type, the pattern being definitely treelike. Lesions arising on the portio are often not true polyps but rather condylomas, papillomas, or simply tags of tissue resulting from old lacerations.

The stroma is a loose-textured, often edematous, fibrous tissue. Variable degrees of inflammatory infiltrate are recognized in

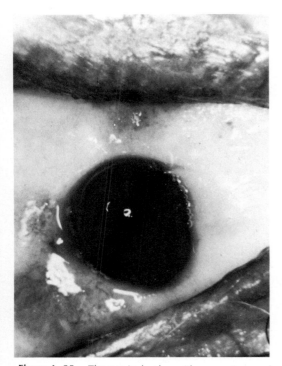

Figure 4–25. The cervical polyp with congestion as obvious cause of bleeding.

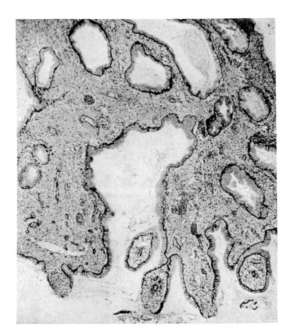

Figure 4–27. Typical benign cervical polyp.

the vascular stalk, and congestion with infarction of the tip produces ulceration and a granulation tissue reaction. The stroma during pregnancy may show extensive decidual change, especially if the lesion arises high in the canal, and the glands may even demonstrate an Arias-Stella reaction, as noted above.

A frequent histologic feature is the occurrence of squamous metaplasia or epidermidalization, described previously. When this is marked, a picture may be produced which might lead to the suspicion of cancer. In other cases the lacy, labyrinthine pattern produced by mucoid and squamous metaplasia of the gland epithelium may even lead to the erroneous diagnosis of adenocarcinoma (Figs. 4–20 to 4–22).

Malignant Changes

In a small percentage of cases epidermoid cancer may arise in a cervical polyp. In some instances, as in Figure 4–29, the malignant change is found only in the polyp and not in the adjoining portions of the normal cervix.

Adenocarcinoma may likewise arise in cervical polyps (Fig. 4–30). On the other hand, it must be remembered that adenocarcinoma may, in certain forms, begin as a small polypoid excrescence. In deciding whether one is dealing with a polypoid carcinoma or a polyp that has undergone secondary malignant change, the examination of the base or pedicle of the polyp is of importance. If this shows no sign of neoplasia, and if the malignant changes are seen in only a localized area or segment of an otherwise benign polyp, the secondary nature of the carcinoma

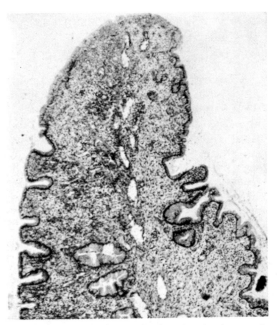

Figure 4–28. Tip of cervical polyp, showing the vascular injection and ulceration which so often cause bleeding.

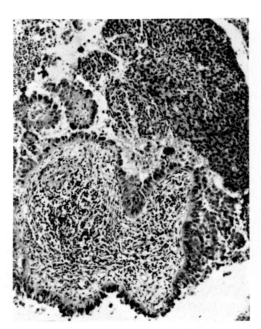

Figure 4–29. Epidermoid carcinoma developing in cervical polyp. Upper right shows carcinoma with endocervical polyp evident in lower portion.

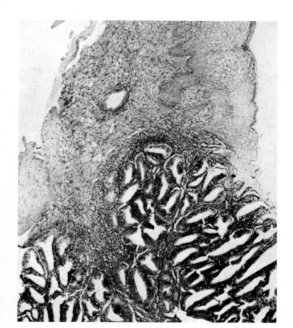

Figure 4–30. Adenocarcinoma developing in cervical polyp. Note the stratified epithelium covering the polyp.

can be assumed. On the other hand, if the polyp is solidly carcinomatous, with evidences of carcinoma also in the adjoining cervical tissue, one may conclude that the carcinoma is a primary one that has assumed the polypoid architecture. Mixed mesodermal tumors may present as polyps, and although they more commonly arise in the fundus of the uterus, they may develop from the endocervix. The edematous stroma may appear quite innocuous and may be the predominant component of the neoplasm. Careful microscopic evaluation is imperative in order not to under- or overestimate the stromal elements.

Clinical Significance

Most polyps produce no symptoms, and are found incidentally on speculum examination; nevertheless, bleeding is a common symptom. As a rule, this bleeding is scanty and intermenstrual. Especially characteristic is the contact bleeding, produced by coitus, by the examining finger, or perhaps by the edge of the speculum. Even light rubbing with a cotton-tipped applicator may start a trickle of blood because of the fragility and the vascularity of the growths.

It will be seen later that the chief symptom of cervical polyps—i.e., the intermenstrual staining or bleeding—is the same as in the far more serious condition of early carcinoma of the cervix. It is obvious, therefore, that this symptom demands thorough cytologic and histopathologic study to rule out more serious disease.

OTHER BENIGN LESIONS

Endometriosis

This is occasionally seen in the cervix with adenomyosis of the uterus or pelvic endometriosis. Nevertheless, since the endocervix is part of the paramesonephric system, it would not be surprising to find heteropia of this totipotential epithelium into an endometrioid variety. Endometriosis is probably more common than reported on the mucosal surface, since inflammatory reactions and associated alterations in the epithelium make endometriosis a diagnosis difficult to establish (Fig. 4–31). Grossly, a bluish nodule may be present; however, more commonly the diagnosis is made on histopathologic study of biopsy, conization, or hysterectomy specimens.

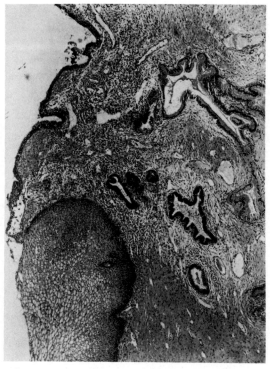

Figure 4–31. Endometriosis, showing typical endocervical glands and similarly typical endometrial glands and stroma at external os, adjacent to squamous epithelium.

Condyloma Acuminatum

The cervical acuminate wart is less common than the similar lesion of the vulva or vagina. As with the vulvar condylomas, pregnancy is likely to cause a marked stimulation of growth. In the series reported by Woodruff and Peterson, malignancy was rare, but degrees of cellular atypism were difficult to evaluate. The warty pattern, the uniformity and mosaic arrangement of the cells in spite of the enormous thickening of the epithelial layer, and the sharp dividing line between the latter and the stroma should make the distinction in most cases. The viral etiology of such lesions, and the resultant potential association with the development of neoplasia, makes these proliferations worthy of more intensive study. Furthermore, the vascular pattern (as described in Chapter 1) may confuse the colposcopist and lead to an erroneous diagnosis of neoplasia (Fig. 4–32).

Leiomyoma

The common leiomyoma of the fundus is found occasionally in the cervix; however, the majority of these arise in the region of the isthmus or fundus, since smooth muscle is rare in the distal segment. Because of the small caliber of the cervical canal, the latter may be partially occluded by such lesions (Fig. 4–33). Abell has described a polypoid fibromatous lesion, or papillary adenofibroma, of the uterine cervix.

Nevoid Lesions

Primary nevoid lesions of the cervix are rare, but a variety of such lesions have been described in the literature.

Mesonephric Tubules or Adenomas

Although the vestigial mesonephric (Gartner's) duct is usually situated just lateral to the cervical duct, its remains are occasionally seen in the form of tubules deep in the cervical substance, and these at times present an adenomatous appearance. Meyer has stated that, if routine serial sections were made, such remnants would be found in 10 per cent or more of all cervices. Greene and co-workers have discussed the difficulty in differentiating these remnants from the tips of the endocervical glands. Mesonephric tubules seem to demonstrate a basal lamina of PAS-positive material, although this structure is rarely present beneath the endocervical epithelium. These findings are not definitive since the basal lamina is not distinctive. In rare cases, the typical metamesonephroma containing clear cell and "Schiller hobnail" patterns, may arise from these vestigial structures.

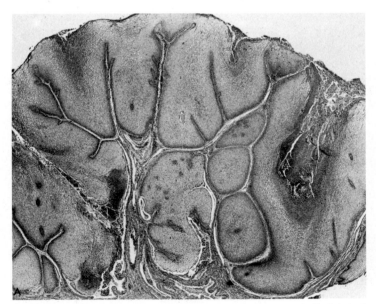
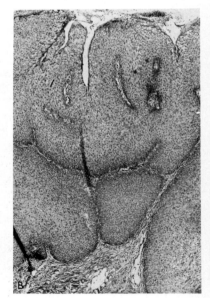

Figure 4–32. *A,* Benign condyloma of cervix in pregnancy. *B,* Slightly higher power, depicting well-differentiated pattern of cells.

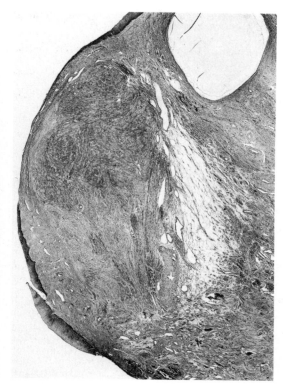

Figure 4–33. Leiomyoma lying directly beneath squamous epithelium of portio.

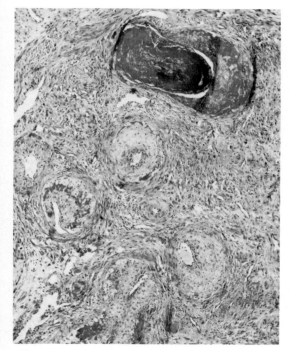

Figure 4–34. Cervical pregnancy. There is extensive perivascular thickening of intima and muscularis with intravascular coagulation.

CERVICAL PREGNANCY

This rare entity causes confusion and consternation both clinically and histopathologically. The common alterations of pregnancy were described in Chapter 3. With true cervical implantation, the vascular changes may simulate those seen with intrauterine gestation but are more dramatic, often with evidences of intravascular coagulation (Fig. 4–34). The latter is most commonly a systemic as well as a local problem but may result in serious hemorrhage. The presence of invading trophoblast establishes the diagnosis (Fig. 4–35).

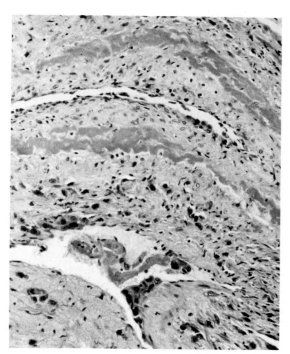

Figure 4–35. Cervical pregnancy with trophoblastic infiltration of vascular channels and thickening of vessel wall.

REFERENCES

Abell, M. P.: Papillary adenofibroma of the endocervix. Am. J. Obstet. Gynecol., *110*:990, 1971.

Adams, J. Q., and Packer, H.: Granuloma inguinale of the cervix. Southern Med. J., *48*:27, 1955.

Bishop, E. L.: Tuberculosis of cervix; with report of case. Am. J. Obstet. Gynecol., *19*:822, 1930.

Burd, L. I., and Esterly, J. R.: Vesicular lesions of the uterine cervix. Am. J. Obstet. Gynecol., *110*:887, 1971.

Crossen, R. J.: A case of gumma of cervix. Am. J. Obstet. Gynecol., *19*:708, 1930.

Danforth, W. C.: Tuberculosis of cervix. Ann. Surg., *106*:407, 1937.

Fluhmann, C. F.: Squamous metaplasia of the cervix uteri and endometrium. Am. J. Obstet. Gynecol., *68*:1447, 1954.

Geiger, C. J.: Benign and malignant polyps of cervix uteri. Am. J. Obstet. Gynecol., *32*:465, 1936.

Greene, R. R., and Peckham, B. M.: Squamous papillomas of the cervix. Am. J. Obstet. Gynecol., *67*:883, 1954.

Hoffmeister, F. J., and Gorthy, R. L.: Benign lesions of cervix. Obstet. Gynecol., *5*:504, 1955.

Jiji, V.: Blue nevus of the endocervix. Arch. Pathol., *92*:203, 1971.

Kistner, R. W., and Hertig, A. T.: Papillomas of the uterine cervix. Obstet. Gynecol., *6*:147, 1955.

Marsh, M. R.: Papilloma of the cervix. Am. J. Obstet. Gynecol., *64*:281, 1952.

Meyer, R.: Die Epithelentwicklung der Cervix und Portio Vaginalis Uteri und die Pseudoerosio congenita. Arch. f. Gynäk., *91*:579, 1920.

Meyer, R.: Die Erosion und Pseudoerosion der Erwachsenen. Arch. f. Gynäk., *91*:658, 1910.

Meyer, R., and Kaufmann, C.: Über den Wert der Stückchendiagnose. Zbl. f. Gynäk., *50*:20, 1926.

Motyloff, L.: Epidermoid heteroplasia (heterologous epidermoid differentiation) of basal cells of endometrium versus squamous-cell metaplasia. Am. J. Obstet. Gynecol., *60*:1240, 1950.

Novak, E.: Pathologic diagnosis of early cervical and corporeal cancer with special reference to the differentiation from pseudomalignant inflammatory conditions. Am. J. Obstet. Gynecol., *18*:449, 1929.

Novak, E. R., and Galvin, G. A.: Mistakes in interpretation of intraepithelial carcinoma. Am. J. Obstet. Gynecol., *62*:1079, 1951.

Novak, E., Woodruff, J. D., and Novak, E. R.: Probable mesonephric origin of certain female genital tumors. Am. J. Obstet. Gynecol., *68*:1222, 1954.

Parmley, T. H., Sherrer, C. W., and Woodruff, J. D.: Adenomatous hyperplasia of the endocervix. Obstet. Gynecol., *49*:1, 1977.

Raftery, A., and Payne, W. S.: Condylomata acuminata of cervix. Obstet. Gynecol., *4*:581, 1954.

Rainey, R.: Association of lymphogranuloma inguinale and cancer. Surgery, *35*:221, 1954.

Ruge, C.: Epithelialveränderungen und beginnender Krebs am weiblichen Genitalapparat. Arch. f. Gynäk., *109*:102, 1918.

Schneppenheimer, P., Hamperl, H., Kaufmann, C., and Ober, K. G.: Beziehungen des Schleimepithels zum Plattenepithel an der Cervix Uteri. Arch. f. Gynäk., *190*:303, 1958.

Schröder, R.: Die Anatomie der chronischen Cervix Gonnorhoë. Zbl. f. Gynäk., *55*:3429, 1931.

Sered, H., Falls, F. H., and Zummo, F. H.: Recent trends in management of tuberculosis of the cervix. J. Int. Coll. Surg., *20*:409, 1953.

Stein, A.: Carcinomatous degeneration of a cervical polyp without uterine involvement. Am. J. Surg., *10*:136, 1930.

Stevenson, C. S.: Cervical tuberculosis with report of so-called primary case. Am. J. Obstet. Gynecol., *36*:1017, 1938.

Wilbanks, G. D., Campbell, J. A., and Kaufmann, L. A.: Cellular changes of normal human cervical epithelium infected in vitro with herpesvirus hominis, type two (herpes simplex). Acta Cytol., *14*:538, 1970.

Woodruff, J. D., and Peterson, W. F.: Condylomata acuminata of the cervix. Am. J. Obstet. Gynecol., *75*:1354, 1958.

Youssef, A. F., Fayad, M. M., and Shafeek, M. A. E. D.: Bilharziasis of the cervix uteri. J. Obstet. Gynaecol. Br. Commonw. *77*:847, 1970.

Chapter 5

CERVICAL NEOPLASIA

Introduction

Primarily as the result of widespread use of vaginal cytology and the concerted effort to educate the population, there has been a dramatic decrease in the incidence of invasive cervical cancer. Nevertheless, neoplastic precursors (CIN) of invasive disease continue to increase. As noted in the preceding chapters, many problems arise in attempting to differentiate microscopically the common benign cellular aberrations from their malignant counterparts. In addition to the complicated benign patterns, various degrees of anaplastic change, from mild atypism to carcinoma in situ (CIN), must be evaluated carefully to insure that optimum therapy may be instituted. In view of the wide variety of cellular patterns and the frequency of both benign and malignant cervical disease, these alterations present major challenges to the pathologist.

EPIDEMIOLOGY

Incidence

It has been estimated that 2 of every 100 untreated women will develop cervical cancer by the age of 40. Many of the cytologic screening programs indicate that this is probably a reasonably accurate figure. Davis has reported an incidence of cervical neoplasia of 11.8 per 1000 women in a geographically controlled study with two screenings at 2 year intervals of almost 5000 women in the 30 to 45 age group. Obviously such figures will vary in different social and ethnic groups, with a low incidence in Jewish and certain Moslem women and a high incidence in Puerto Rican and Negro populations.

The American Cancer Society estimates that cancer of the cervix accounts for approximately 6000 to 7000 deaths a year in the United States. Whereas the mortality from breast and cervical cancer was equal 50 years ago, at present breast cancer causes four to five times and ovarian cancer one and a half times as many deaths as cervical malignancy. This is a tribute to improved detection of cervical carcinoma in its precursory and early developmental stages and the ease with which this can be accomplished. Realistically, with total screening, invasive cervical cancer could be eliminated.

Pathogenesis

Many of the studies relative to the etiologic agents in cervical malignancy support the thesis that multiple traumas play a major role. Wynder and associates; Christopherson; and others stress the importance of socioeconomic factors, such as early sexual activity, mixed sexual partners, and poor penile hygiene. Rewell states that in India, where marriage at the age of 14 and 15 years is common, cervical cancer occurs about 10 years earlier than the usually quoted age in the United States. Conversely, Gagnon was unable to discover a single case of cervical malignancy in a study of death certificates of 13,000 nuns. Coppleson and co-workers in Australia suggest a direct association, based on the finding of sperm heads within the cytoplasm of undifferentiated cervical epithelial cells. Recognizing the role played by viruses in the induction of neoplastic disease, many have proposed that they may be the carcinogenic agents. Davis and Aurelian; Kaufman; and others have reported strong circumstantial evidence to support this thesis by showing that patients with cervical neo-

111

plasia demonstrate the presence of positive titers to type II herpesvirus antigen. Recently, a specific antigen has been identified to emphasize and document the relationships. Although more thorough documentation of such statistics is necessary, it must be admitted that, at present, the evidence is very strong in favor of the theory that infection plays a major role in the production of cervical neoplasia.

PRECURSORS

The term "precancerous" has been used for many years in different senses by different writers and with differing degrees of enthusiasm. One group has applied the designation rather generally to lesions believed to predispose to cancer, embracing especially chronic irritative and inflammatory conditions, even though these in themselves are frankly benign. The other definition of the term precancerous refers to lesions that exhibit cellular activity unusual in benign conditions yet lack certain characteristics of actual cancer. When used in this sense, the term conveys the impression that the atypical cervical epithelium in question represents a histologic stepping stone between the benign and the malignant.

Precursory Aberrations

A variety of terms have been used to describe the cellular alterations which have been found to precede or to be associated with cervical anaplasia. Dysplasia, basal cell hyperactivity or hyperplasia, anaplasia, dyskaryosis, dyskeratosis, precancerous metaplasia, and atypia or atypical epithelium are a few of the more common appellations. Regardless of the term used, it is important that the clinician receiving the report be fully cognizant of the degree of abnormality and aware of its potentiality. *Atypism* (atypical hyperplasia or dysplasia) is the term used in our laboratory, and the degrees of change vary from mild, moderate, or marked to carcinoma in situ. Richart has introduced the terms CIN and CIS for in situ neoplasia and in situ carcinoma; these terms cover the broad spectrum of cervical neoplasia from its mildest forms to the classic in situ malignancy and are at present well accepted in most circles, both clinically and pathologically.

Of major importance is recognition of the potentiality for progression or regression of these cellular aberrations. They may proceed to invasive cancer or may at any point be reversible, undoubtedly as the result of local tissue or systemic defense mechanisms, as noted by Galvin. Conversely, Richart suggests that CIN represents a progressive spectrum of histologic abnormalities that will, in the majority of cases, progress inexorably to carcinoma in situ. Again it must be noted that much of the difference of opinion as to the final stage of CIN depends on the interpretation of the pathologist. Richart's mild dysplasia or CIN I might well be another observer's moderate to marked atypicality. Thus, it may be said that the degrees of CIN are truly "in the eye of the beholder."

Gross Pathology

There is no typical gross picture associated with these cellular atypisms nor with carcinoma in situ. Most of the changes are found in the chronically infected and lacerated cervix. When eversion is present, the commonly involved squamocolumnar junction or transitional zone is readily visible. Nevertheless, in the postmenopausal years this critical area is usually not visible to the naked eye. In such instances, the endocervical specimen, for either histologic or cytologic study, is of major import and obviously difficult to obtain.

Microscopic Patterns

The cellular changes associated with atypia are basically related to loss of normal maturation of the epithelium. There may be a tendency for the basal and parabasal cells to proliferate abnormally with the concurrent lack of the usual layers of differentiated surface cells. This is the pattern seen in *basal cell hyperactivity* or *hyperplasia*. Conversely, increased maturation is demonstrated by the appearance of the superficial type of cell with atypical changes, such as attempted keratinization with marked *acidophilia* of the cytoplasm and *bizarre nuclear figures* in the deeper layers of the epithelium. The depth of penetration of these abnormal cells is described by the modifying terms—mild, moderate, or marked.

In *mild atypism*, the neoplastic cells extend one quarter to one third of the way from

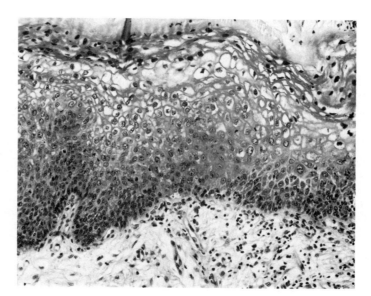

Figure 5–1. Minimal atypical proliferation of basal cell with koilocytosis.

the basal layer to the surface (Fig. 5–1). Great difficulties are encountered in differentiating these mild abnormalities from the epithelial reactions to infection, especially since both marked inflammatory changes and neoplasia commonly occur at the same squamocolumnar junction (Fig. 5–2 A,B). For example, Figge and co-workers followed 46 women in whom atypical epithelial hyperplasia was diagnosed. However, in 7 years the lesion progressed in only four cases and in none to carcinoma in situ. Coppleson and Reid studied the "native and regenerate epithelium" colposcopically, and described a juxtanuclear vacuole in the parabasal cell of the native epithelium.

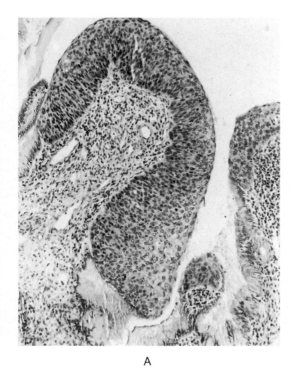

A

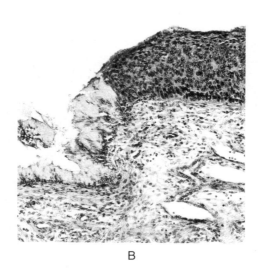

B

Figure 5–2. *A,* Abnormal surface epithelium showing atypical cells in lower one half but stratification in upper one half. Atypism near squamocolumnar junction with gland involvement. *B,* Carcinoma in situ at squamocolumnar junction. The classic point of origin for epidermoid carcinoma of the cervix.

However, these cells were more common in the superficial layers of the regenerate type. Differentiation between the inflammatory and neoplastic aberrations in the epithelium is difficult. The presence of marked subepithelial infiltrate obviously suggests an inflammatory rather than a neoplastic response. Nevertheless, if cervical malignancy is infectious in origin, all cellular proliferations should be followed carefully and looked upon with suspicion.

In *moderate atypism*, the cellular aberrations extend through one half to two thirds of the thickness of the epithelial layer. These atypical cells may demonstrate too rapid maturation, as seen in Figure 5–3 (*A,B*), or penetration of parabasal and basal type cells well into the upper layers; however, it is readily apparent that "pure" varieties of change are rare, as pure cell types of cancer are rare. Characteristically, the atypism includes the small cell nonkeratinizing, the

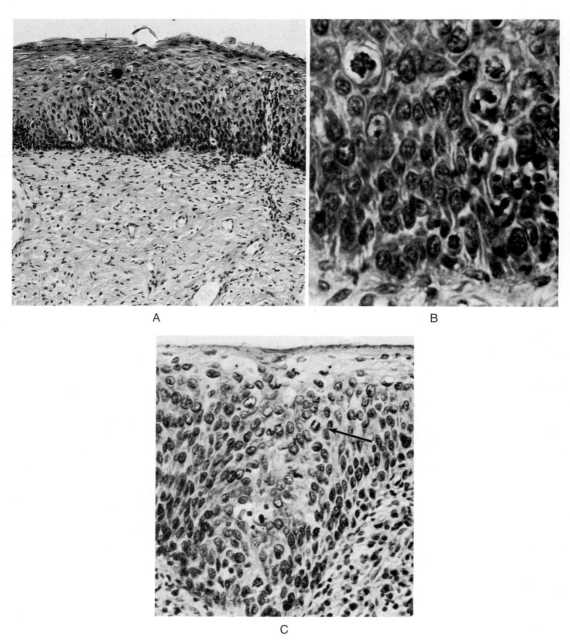

A   B

C

Figure 5–3. *A,* Moderate atypism. *B,* High power view of central area in *A.* Cell disarray is evident. CIN II. *C,* Moderate atypism with atypical maturation and basal cell hyperplasia through one half of epithelial layer (at arrow).

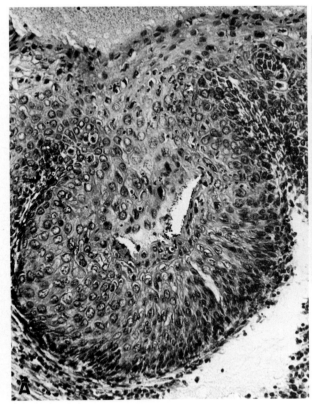

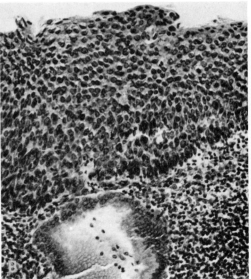

Figure 5–4. Variations in cellular atypia in the same case. *A,* Mature. *B,* "Small cell." (From Lambert, B., and Woodruff J. D.: Spinal cell atypia of the cervix. Cancer, *16*:1141, 1963.)

large cell nonkeratinizing, and the large cell keratinizing varieties (Fig. 5–4). In addition to the individual cellular anaplasia, the loss of polarity and the general disarray of the growth patterns are prominent (Figs. 5–5 and 5–6). It must be recognized that on rare occasions diagnosis of the degree of atypism and actually of early invasive cancer must be established on this disarray, loss of polarity, and individual cell changes in the basal layer, as noted in the spray carcinoma of Schiller. In such cases intraepithelial pearl formation in the rete tips may be the outstanding feature of anaplasia (Figs. 5–7 and 5–8).

It has been recognized by Galvin, and

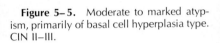

Figure 5–5. Moderate to marked atypism, primarily of basal cell hyperplasia type. CIN II–III.

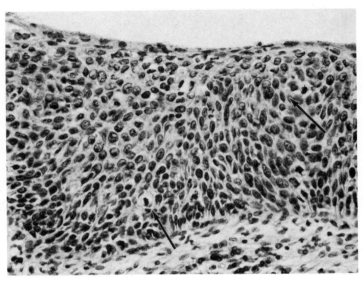

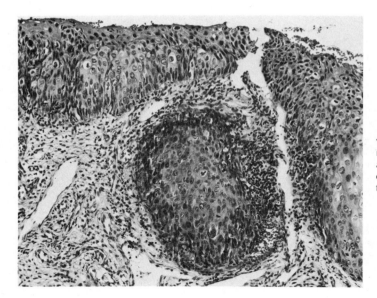

Figure 5–6. Carcinoma in situ showing various cell types. Large pale cells are prominent in the epithelium on far left. Similar cells are intermingled with the less mature atypical elements in the central plug and the upper central surface layer.

Lambert and Woodruff, that approximately 20 to 25 per cent of the cases diagnosed as moderate degree of atypism will progress to or, on further study, will be found to be associated with carcinoma in situ.

In *marked atypism,* the anaplastic cells penetrate through 75 to 90 per cent of the epithelium. As with invasive cancer, the ab-

normal cells do not follow a specific pattern. Areas in which the basal and parabasal cells extend into the superficial zone are adjacent to those in which the atypism is characterized by early and bizarre maturation, i.e., individual cell keratinization, multiple nuclei and nucleoli in large, pale cells, and variable chromatin patterns (Figs. 5–5, 5–6, 5–7, and 5–8). Careful study of the basal layers is of major importance in these cases. Loss of polarity and disarray of the cells in the deeper

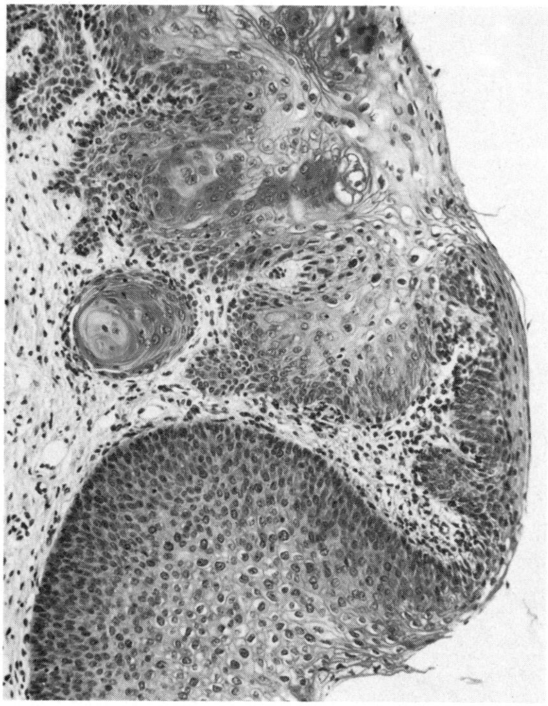

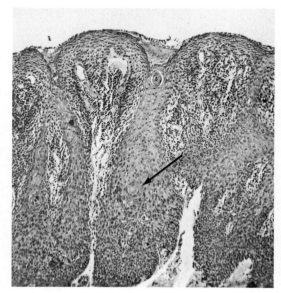

Figure 5–7. Mild to moderate atypical epithelium (basal cell hyperplasia) below, with mature, pearl-forming microinvasive cancer in center. Differences in cell types are striking in this tumor.

Figure 5–8. Intraepithelial pearl formation without loss of surface layers, but with invasive cancer. (From Woodruff, J. D. and Mattingly, R. F.: Epithelial changes preceding spinal cell carcinoma of the cervix. Am. J. Obstet. Gynecol. 77:977, 1959.)

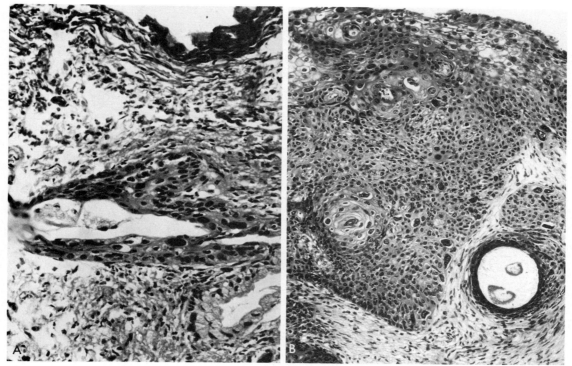

Figure 5–9. *A,* Atypical epithelium in endocervical gland (biopsy specimen). *B,* In situ carcinoma of cervix with microinvasion(?)—"cutdown" of biopsy specimen in *A.*

zone may be associated with early stromal invasion or microinvasion even though complete loss of stratification is not present (Fig. 5–9 *A,B*). It must be remembered that in some cases of invasive cancer the surface epithelium demonstrates less than the full-thickness alterations noted with the classic carcinoma in situ. The latter is particularly true in the so-called Schiller spray carcinoma, as stated previously (Fig. 5–10 *A,B*). Furthermore, it is important to realize that the available study material may not contain the most marked changes. This is evidenced strikingly by the approximate 65 per cent of these cases of marked atypism which, on follow-up, demonstrate carcinoma in situ. Undoubtedly, in some of the latter cases, the disease was present at the time of initial study.

Richart and others have suggested that true cellular neoplasia is one phase of a progressive process leading eventually to in situ cancer. By using nontraumatic means of follow-up, Richart eliminates the possibility of altering the natural course of the disease or, as may happen on occasion, of even eliminating it completely by repeated biopsy. Cytogenetic analyses have also demon-strated that many of the moderate or marked atypias demonstrate the same chromosomal aberrations as those seen with in situ cancer. Further studies are necessary to confirm these important approaches to the investigation of cervical neoplasia.

IRRITATIVE REACTIONS SIMULATING NEOPLASIA

Of the lesions of the cervix that are at times grossly and microscopically confusing but frankly benign, by far the most important group is that represented by the chronic inflammatory and irritative lesions. Even in the most intense forms of chronic cervicitis there is usually not the slightest pathologic evidence of malignancy, although clinically there may be great justification for suspicion. One frequently sees cervices that are badly eroded, irregularly hypertrophied, and apparently indurated, with granular mucosa that bleeds readily on slight touch and in which, therefore, the clinician would be very remiss if he did not at least suspect the possibility of a malignant condition. And yet in such cases one often finds, in spite of ex-

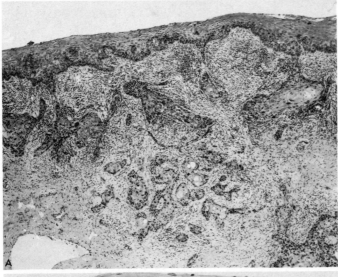

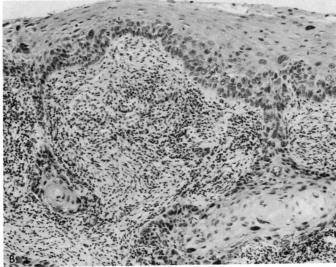

Figure 5–10. *A,* Invasive spray carcinoma of the mature type, with normal surface layers. *B,* High power view of *A* showing essentially normal surface epithelium with deeply invasive carcinoma.

tensive inflammatory changes, not the slightest suspicion of histologic malignancy if a biopsy is done, as it should be. On the other hand, in lesions that clinically are far less conspicuous, one may find definite evidence of cancer.

There is a difference of opinion among gynecologists as to the importance of chronic irritative lesions as precursors of cervical malignancy; nevertheless, the predisposing role of chronic irritation in the causation of cancer seems to be generally accepted in many other locations. It is undoubtedly true that heredity plays an important role in the predisposition to develop malignancy; however, the local irritants, particularly those of infectious nature, must be the major offenders.

Wilbanks and co-workers have grown cells from cervical in situ neoplasia in tissue culture. Their observations suggest that the in situ carcinoma behaves like invasive cancer; however, the growth pattern of the dysplasias is difficult to assess in view of the differences of opinion as to the degree of abnormality. The attempts to determine the cellular atypicalities produced by the introduction of herpesvirus into the tissue cultures of normal epithelial cells have not produced the proliferations suggested by clinical studies, but abnormalities in nuclei were observed.

Although trichomonal infections may lead to atypical cytologic and biopsy findings, Koss and Wolinska believe that these bear no true resemblance and no causative relation to true intraepithelial cancer. Kaminetzky and Swerdlow and others have stressed the atypical changes that may develop with the use of podophyllin; however, again these have not progressed to actual malignancy.

In many inflammatory lesions and polyps, one may observe marked evidence of so-called *epidermidalization* or *squamous cell metaplasia*. This condition, which is fully described in Chapter 4, is of special importance because it may so readily be mistaken for cancer, with which it actually has no more direct relation than other chronic irritative and inflammatory lesions. This error in diagnosis has been a very frequent one, and is still not uncommon, in spite of the much wider familiarity of pathologists with these special varieties of cellular microscopic pictures.

Special Varieties of Cellular Aberration

Koilocytotic Atypia. Koilo, meaning hollow or concave, has been applied to the atypism characterized by vacuolization of the cytoplasm in the upper layers of the epithelium. Various nuclear disturbances may be associated with this change and the seriousness is dependent on these disturbances rather than on the vacuolization. For example, although the patterns are similar, the nuclear abnormalities are obviously less striking in Figure 5–11 than in Figure 5–12. Interestingly, the surface cells in this variety

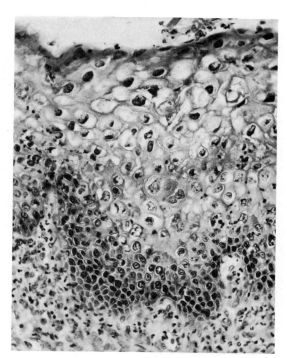

Figure 5–12. Atypia showing cellular abnormalities throughout all layers.

of change contain little *glycogen*. It seems quite possible that these changes are related to viral infection, and that the cellular aberrations are not neoplastic but rather viral in origin.

Hyperkeratosis and Parakeratosis. Neither of these changes is normally seen on the surface of the cervical epithelium, so that the presence of either should increase the pathologist's index of suspicion. Both indicate basically some metabolic disturbance; however, the individual cellular changes, as previously noted, must be evaluated to determine the degree of atypism. Marked aberrations associated with these atypicalities of maturation and metabolism are demonstrated in Figure 5–13 (*A,B*). Such alterations may well indicate the presence of a viral disease, specifically the acuminate wart. Nevertheless, as noted in Chapter 4, keratin may be present in the prolapsed cervix without any evidence of cellular atypia.

Other atypicalities of maturation are noted in Figure 5–14. Here, the thin atypical epithelium of the postmenopausal cervix may be confusing, both histopathologically and cytopathologically. The small dark cells on the surface suggest atypia; however, these alterations are usually related to an atrophy or poor hormone support for the tissues.

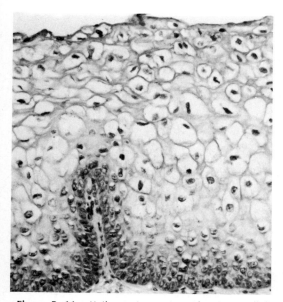

Figure 5–11. Koilocytotic atypia with minor cellular changes (almost no glycogen in surface layers).

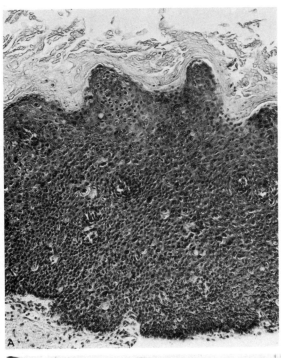

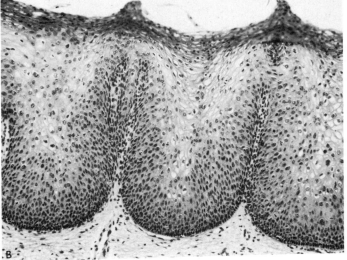

Figure 5–13. *A*, Hyperkeratosis with slight papillomatosis and Bowenoid type of marked atypism. *B*, Parakeratosis with slight papillomatosis and mild atypia of the epithelium (condylomatous).

Many of these atypicalities can be eliminated by the use of intravaginal estrogen.

Atypia in Squamous Metaplasia. Of importance is the recognition that major degrees of anaplasia may be demonstrated in the stratified epithelium of the tunnels while the surface changes are less marked (Fig. 5–15). Because of the frequency of tangential cutting in the underlying tortuous clefts, it is more difficult to orient the surface layers; nevertheless, the most marked atypicalities may be in these areas, and numerous serial sections must be made to aid in the correct evaluation of the invaginated epithelium (Fig. 5–16).

CARCINOMA IN SITU

(INTRAEPITHELIAL CARCINOMA, PREINVASIVE CARCINOMA)

Carcinoma in situ may be defined as a lesion in which the entire thickness of the squamous epithelial layer is replaced by cells microscopically indistinguishable from those of frank invasive cancer, with com-

Figure 5–14. Thin, atypical epithelium of the postmenopausal cervix. Cytopathologic study was reported as inconclusive. Follow-up was negative.

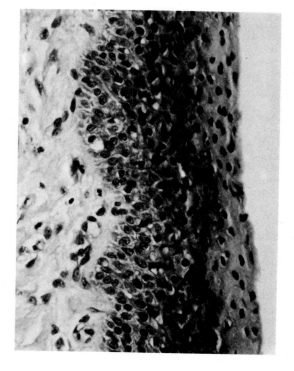

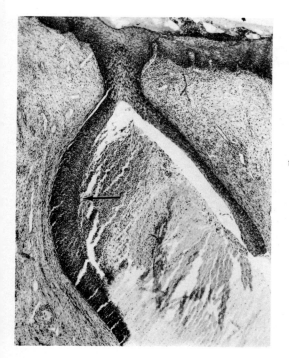

Figure 5–15. Atypia in epidermidalization. Surface epithelium appears essentially intact.

Figure 5–16. Carcinoma in situ with gland involvement. Surface changes are less dramatic.

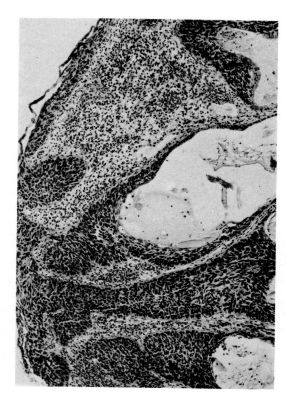

plete loss of stratification, but with no evidence of stromal invasion. Similar lesions in other organs have long been known to general pathologists. The cervical lesions were described by Schauenstein in 1907. Cullen, in the 1900 edition of *Cancer of the Uterus*, described a typical picture of premalignant cervical cancer with gland involvement adjacent to invasive disease. Rubin in 1910, and Schottländer and Kermauner in 1912 also called attention to the zone of preinvasive carcinoma often found adjoining an invasive lesion. The latter observation would suggest that frank invasive cancer is preceded by a stage in which the malignant changes are limited to the surface epithelium, with later penetration of the basement membrane and lymphatic permeation.

The chief credit for emphasizing the importance of carcinoma in situ as a forerunner of the invasive lesions belongs to Schiller (1927). The fact that he flatly called such lesions *Beginnendes Karzinom* created much controversy. The concept meant that it was no longer necessary to insist upon either clinical or histologic invasiveness as essential to the microscopic diagnosis of cancer; thus, an opinion could be substantiated on the basis of morphologic criteria alone. Initial acceptance of this thesis was delayed when follow-up of these cases revealed that only a minor percentage of the patients subsequently developed invasive lesions. For example, in only two of the 17 intraepithelial carcinomas followed by Stevenson and Scipiades did malignancy appear, even after many years, and similar observations have been made by others.

Nevertheless, in the succeeding years, evidence has mounted to substantiate the validity of such an entity as carcinoma in situ. Of major importance to both clinician and pathologist is the long latent period that usually exists between the diagnosis of intraepithelial disease and the final demonstration of true invasive cancer. This latent period is reflected in the fact that patients with carcinoma in situ are on an average 10 years younger than those with invasive cancer, as recorded by Galvin and co-workers. McKay and associates report similar statistics, with the mean of 48 years for patients with invasive cancer, 38 years for those with carcinoma in situ, and 34.9 years for those demonstrating atypical epithelial hyperplasia. Recent statistics based on more current

cytologic and colposcopic studies indicate that these average ages have been reduced by at least 5 years.

Nevertheless these reports indicate that cancer of the cervix may be a disease of extremely long duration, extending over perhaps as much as 15 or 20 years, if one includes both the preinvasive and the invasive stages of the disease. Many gynecologists have in the past expressed doubt as to whether one could properly designate as real cancer the preinvasive lesion, which should be readily curable by simple excision, and yet today no one can doubt that it is clearly related to cancer, representing at least a precursory stage. That most cervical cancers begin in preinvasive fashion seems possible; that carcinoma in situ as we know it today is not inevitably followed by invasive cancer may or may not be a valid statement. Too few studies have followed the progression of the disease without interfering with the natural history by repeated biopsies or minor forms of therapy. Invasive cancer may well have other forms of genesis, as suggested by the so-called spray carcinoma reported by Schiller, and described previously (Fig. 5–9). Furthermore these lesions may have a shorter life history as demonstrated by the 60 year old woman who, after careful yearly cytologic study, suddenly appears with invasive cervical cancer. Such experiences could be explained on a persistently reported false negative rate for routine cytologic studies of ± 20 per cent; on poor sampling procedure, particularly in the postmenopausal patient with an endocervical transformation zone; or on a lesion arising in the canal, in which instance cells may be shed late in the life history of the disease.

A few reports indicate that at least some cases of carcinoma in situ may regress and completely disappear, either spontaneously or following such minor procedures as biopsy (Wespi, Younge et al., Diddle et al.). Epperson and associates reported five cases recognized during pregnancy in which follow-up biopsies made post partum revealed complete disappearance of the lesion. Similar observations have been made by other investigators. In spite of the occasional histopathologic difficulty in evaluating proliferative epithelial changes associated with pregnancy and infection, the degree of cervical neoplasia can be evaluated accurately in most instances by careful study. Richart is of the opinion that true CIN will not regress but progress if the process is not interrupted by such procedures as biopsy.

The occurrence of multiple squamous cell cancers involving cervix, vagina, and vulva has been noted repeatedly. These multicentric foci of malignancy undoubtedly represent an area response to a carcinogenic agent rather than metastatic disease. The moral is that every clinician who treats an early lesion of one organ should be mindful of the possibility of neoplasia being present or developing in an adjacent area.

To assess the course of this disease more accurately, the ideal approach would be that of diagnosis followed by careful surveillance *without* definitive therapy (conization, cauterization, amputation, hysterectomy, or radiation). The studies conducted by Richart and others, as noted, indicate a progression of the neoplastic process, slow or rapid, if uninterrupted. Kottmeier's reappraisal of his microscopic sections has led him to believe that invasive cancer develops in about 25 per cent of women followed for 5 years after a diagnosis of intraepithelial cancer. Peterson reported a group of 127 women who were observed following a biopsy diagnosis of carcinoma in situ. Within 5 years, 22 per cent had developed invasive cancer. In a reevaluation of these cases, Peterson accepted only those cases in which the initial diagnosis had been confirmed by one additional biopsy. In this reconfirmed group, 50 per cent developed invasive disease in 10 years and four ended in death.

Difficulties in Diagnosis

There are several difficulties in the diagnosis of carcinoma in situ. First, this diagnosis cannot be made on the basis of a single biopsy, which often fails to reveal the full extent of the neoplastic process that may be present in an immediately adjoining area. Repeated and multiple biopsies must, therefore, be made, with the employment, in many cases, of other diagnostic procedures supplemented by cytopathology. Usually there is no urgency in reaching the final diagnosis on which treatment is to be based, and it is better for the patient to have a thorough study than for the clinician to institute treatment on the basis of inconclusive appraisal of the lesion.

There is marked disparity in reports as to the finding of invasion by further study of lesions originally considered to be intraepithelial by biopsy. Galvin and TeLinde recognized *invasion* in 76 per cent of their original group; however, this referred to gland *involvement* rather than true stromal invasion. In series by Dilts and co-workers and by Silbar and Woodruff, stromal invasion was noted in the conization specimen in 1.5 per cent and 5.9 per cent of cases in which the biopsy revealed only in situ change. Others have quoted greater degrees of error; however, with better evaluation of the biopsy material, recognition of the absence of the all-important transitional zone as evidence of an inadequate study (Fig. 5–17 A,B), and more use of additional specialized techniques in the individual case, missed invasion on biopsy material should be reduced to essentially zero. In a series of 196 consecutive cases in which the cytopathology, the colposcopy, and the directed biopsy all indicated that no more than microinvasive disease was present, no evidence of invasive cancer was found in specimens removed by conization and subsequent hysterectomy.

MICROINVASIVE CARCINOMA

A lesion is properly considered invasive if there is a "breakthrough" of the so-called basal lamina, with cancer cells spreading into the stromal tissue. In interpreting this feature, one must be cognizant of the false impressions often given by tangential section. Furthermore, the basement membrane as seen by the light microscope is an indefinite mucopolysaccharide layer beneath the epithelium and its presence is not regular or specific even in nonmalignant situations. In addition, it has been suggested that invading tumor cells lay down their own surrounding "membrane." Nevertheless, *microinvasion* is quite definite in some instances (Figs. 5–18, 5–19A,B). A common feature of the earliest invasive cell is its tendency toward an abundant eosinophilic cytoplasm, a finding that Genadry and co-workers have interpreted as evidence of the presence of actin and myosin. The latter proteins are associated with movement of the cell and thus possibly invasion. In flagrant invasive disease, obviously all types of cells are recognized in the underlying stroma (Figs. 5–20 A,B and

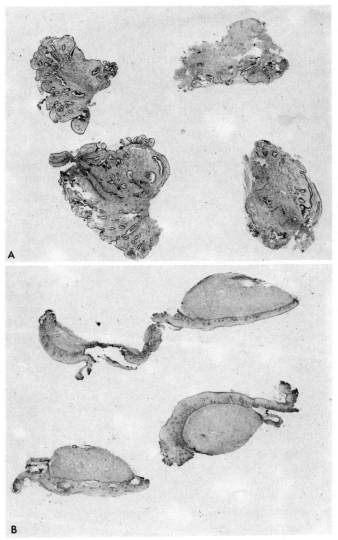

Figure 5–17. Inadequate biopsy—no squamocolumnar junction is present; stratified epithelium only.

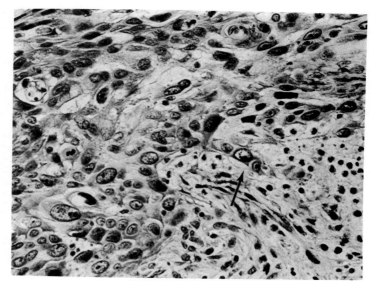

Figure 5–18. Microinvasion—note cellular atypism, particularly abnormal maturity.

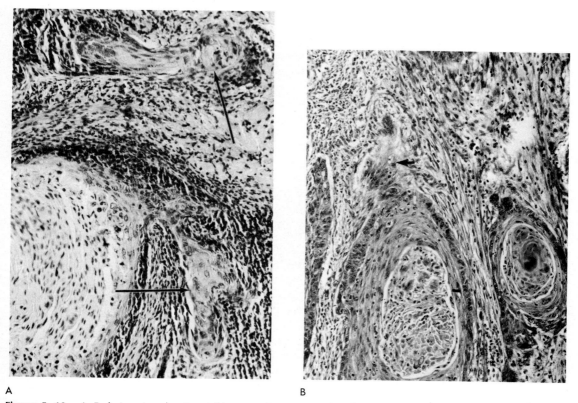

A

B

Figures 5–19. *A,* Early invasion showing striking maturity at penetrating tips (arrows). *B,* Early stromal invasion with foci of atypical cells (arrow).

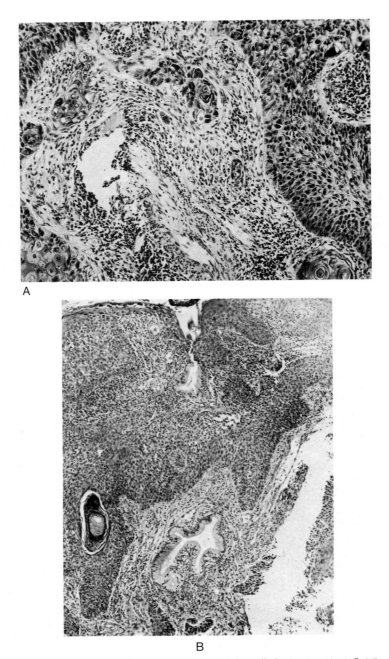

Figure 5– 20. *A,* Invasive cancer with lymphatic invasion (?) (might be called microinvasion). *B,* Microinvasive carcinoma. Multiple cell types with pearl formation are present on left, immature pattern on right. Invasive nests of cells are seen in low center. Note tissue space with malignant cells suggestive of lymphatic invasion.

5–21); however, if a tendency to normal maturation is present, gland involvement should be suspected and further sections obtained in an attempt to demonstrate residual glands (Fig. 5–22). Furthermore, the orderly arrangement of cells with an eosinophilic band at the periphery is tangible evidence of the preexistence of a gland. More decisive is the finding of nests of cancer cells in the lymphatics beneath the epithelium (Fig. 5–23). Such apparent "cancer emboli" must be evaluated accurately. Norris and others feel that it is almost impossible to differentiate tumor in tissue spaces immediately beneath the epithelium and adjacent to glands from lymphatic invasion. Nevertheless reported

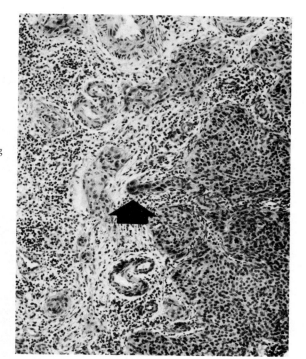

Figure 5–21. Microinvasive cancer at arrow showing breakthrough with invasive disease in the underlying tissue.

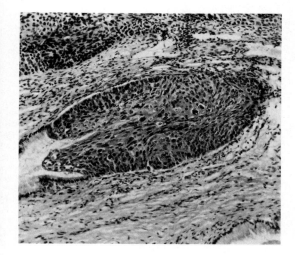

Figure 5–22. Gland lumen filled by atypical cancer cells but there is no breakthrough of gland or adjacent stroma. (Courtesy of Dr. G. A. Galvin.)

Figure 5–23. Invasive cancer with vascular invasion.

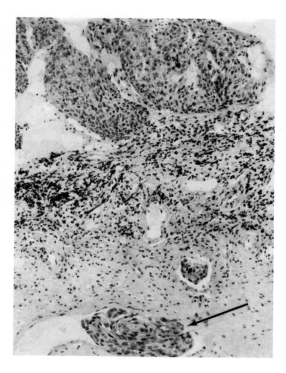

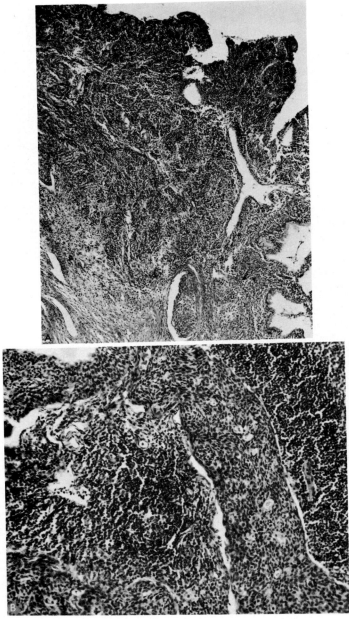

Figure 5–24. *A.* Microinvasive carcinoma of the cervix (2 mm. below basal layer of epithelium; glands can be seen to right) with vascular invasion in low center (see Figs. 5–20 and 5–21). *B,* Hypogastric lymph node with metastatic cancer from same tumor as in *A.*

cases of carcinoma in situ with lymph node involvement demonstrate the possibility of lymphatic penetration with minimal stromal invasion.

Involvement of the endocervical glands by intraepithelial carcinoma does not imply invasion and is still compatible with an in situ status. Care must be exercised in distinguishing glandular involvement from benign squamous metaplasia, but in the latter condition the individual cells are well differentiated and obviously benign, quite in contrast to the anaplastic cells of in situ cancer (Figs. 5–15 and 5–16). Nevertheless, distinction between marked glandular involvement and early stromal invasion cannot always be absolute. This is particularly true if the invading cells are poorly differentiated, i.e., of the small cell variety.

In spite of the obvious danger that even early stromal invasion may be associated with lymph node involvement, the current tendency is to treat microinvasive disease as carcinoma in situ. Latour suggests the term "preclinical" for intraepithelial and early invasive lesions, meanwhile indicating that their behavior is similar. Many cases of FIGO Clinical Stage IA fall into the latter category. For both, total hysterectomy with conservation of ovarian tissue in the young is the preferred treatment. At present, attempt is being made in some areas to define depth of stromal involvement as an index of actual invasion. Our current program is based on the usual limits of the normal tunnel epithelium (5 mm. or less) beneath the basal layer. Consequently, regardless of whether the pattern seems to suggest gland involvement, penetration of more than 5 mm. is considered to be invasive cancer. More recent studies would suggest that 1 mm. or less of stromal invasion is associated with no lymph node involvement. Similarly, invasion of 1 to 3 mm. will rarely demonstrate such extension. The 3 to 5 mm. depth of stromal invasion appears to carry approximately a 3 per cent incidence of positive pelvic nodes (Fig. 5–24 A,B).

GROSS CHARACTERISTICS OF EPIDERMOID CANCER

The Earliest Stages

The earliest stages of invasive cervical cancers are generally not recognized grossly,

and the finding of such a lesion represents a tribute to the zealous use of cytology and histopathology (Fig. 5–25).

The grossly suspicious lesions may appear in various forms. Most characteristically one finds at the margin of the external os a hardened, rather granular area which bleeds on the touch of the examining finger or the edge of the speculum, or on gentle rubbing with a cotton applicator. In many cases the cervix is the seat of an old laceration with eversion, and the cancer may appear as a slightly vegetative or finely papillary area of firm consistency, or as a definite small ulcer with a granular vascular surface and an indurated base. Any such lesion should be viewed with suspicion, and a biopsy made directly from the questionable area often shows undoubted cancer. Even with early invasive tumors, lymph node extension occurs in approximately 15 to 20 per cent of cases, as noted by Claiborne and associates. With increasing disease, nodal involvement obviously increases. Indeed, it is our inability to control lymphatic spread that is responsible for the high mortality of cancer.

The Moderately Advanced Stage

The later appearance of the growth varies considerably, chiefly depending on whether it assumes the *everting (exophytic)* form or the *inverting (endophytic)* form. In the former, the cancer becomes more and more papillary and cauliflower-like in appearance, often infiltrating the adjacent vaginal mucosa. The surface vegetations are fragile and perishable, so that they bleed freely, and necrosis and ulceration soon appear. In the inverting variety, however, the chief direction of growth seems to be into the cervical tissues. The cervix, therefore, becomes large, nodular, and often quite stony in consistency, with infiltration of the surrounding vaginal wall, as already mentioned. The degree of surface ulceration varies greatly.

The epidermoid carcinoma characteristically arises from the margin of the external os at the transformation zone or squamocolumnar junction. However, it may occasionally spring from the squamous epithelium covering the portio vaginalis at some distance from the os, and in others it may arise entirely within the cervical canal (Fig. 5–26). In the latter instances, the clinical onset is apt to be more insidious, as bleeding may occur late because of the protected situation.

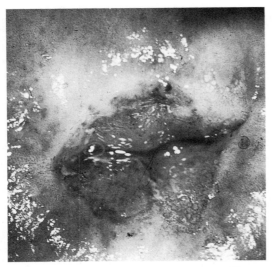

Figure 5–25. Early invasive cancer—no specific gross lesion.

Moreover, it is apt to be overlooked on speculum examination, as the cervix may appear quite normal. In later stages, the polypoid nature of the lesion is recognized by its protrusion through the os. In cases of this type, the diagnosis is made more readily by curettage of the canal than by biopsy.

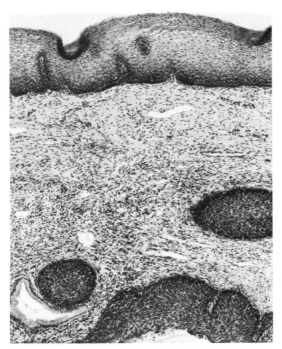

Figure 5–26. Normal surface epithelium with carcinoma in situ in tunnels.

The Advanced Stage

The late stages of the disease are characterized by widespread destruction and infiltration. The vagina may be almost filled with a huge cauliflower-like mass, the base of which may involve only a part of or almost all of the cervix. Or the cervix, in the inverting variety, may have been so completely destroyed that it presents only as a foul, excavated cavity lined by ragged necrotic cancer tissue. The adjoining vaginal wall is boardlike and infiltrated, as are the broad ligaments. The advance of the disease along the vesicovaginal and rectovaginal septa may produce fistulas into the bladder and rectum, while the parametrial involvement may block the ureters and hasten the uremia which most often is the immediate cause of the patient's death. Lymph node involvement, as might be expected, increases with advancing disease. Roughly interpolating the varied statistics gathered by Claiborne and co-workers, it would seem fair to state that nodal involvement occurs in 15 to 20 per cent of Stage I lesions and in 25 to 35 per cent of Stage II cases. In patients studied by autopsy, Solto and associates found extrapelvic metastasis in 85 per cent of 93 patients with gross cervical cancer.

CLINICAL CLASSIFICATION OF CERVICAL CANCER

It is obvious that for comparative study of the results of treatment there must be some standard to indicate the clinical stage of the disease. Various systems of classification have been devised (League of Nations, Schmitz, American College of Surgeons). The most widely employed had been that established by the League of Nations in 1937. Stage I of this classification has been a target of criticism, since it included all cases in which the cancerous lesion was limited to the cervix, whether it was only a few millimeters in size or whether most of the cervix was involved. Also included was the noninvasive, intraepithelial carcinoma in which the curability rate should be about 100 per cent.

The International Congress of Obstetrics and Gynecology at its meeting in New York in May, 1950, segregated carcinoma in situ into a special group (Stage 0). This International Classification, revised in 1971 by the International Federation of Gynecology and Obstetrics (FIGO), has been widely endorsed and adopted by clinicians, pathologists, and investigators.

Stage-grouping in Cancer of the Cervix International Classification

Preinvasive Carcinoma
  Stage 0 Carcinoma in situ, intraepithelial carcinoma. Cases of Stage 0 should not be included in any therapeutic statistics.
Invasive Carcinoma
  Stage I Carcinoma strictly confined to the cervix (extension to the corpus should be disregarded).
    Stage Ia—The cancer cannot be diagnosed by clinical examination.
      (1) Early stromal invasion, and (2) occult cancer.
    Stage Ib—All other cases of Stage I.
  Stage II The carcinoma extends beyond the cervix but has not extended on to the pelvic wall. The carcinoma involves the vagina but not the lower third.
    Stage IIa—No obvious parametrial involvement.
    Stage IIb—Obvious parametrial involvement.
  Stage III The carcinoma has extended on to the pelvic wall. On rectal examination there is no cancerfree space between the tumor and the pelvic wall. The tumor involves the lower third of the vagina.
    Stage IIIa—No extension on to the pelvic wall.
    Stage IIIb—Extension on to the pelvic wall.
  Stage IV The carcinoma has extended beyond the true pelvis or has involved the mucosa of the bladder or rectum.

Bullous edema as such does not permit allotment of a case to Stage IV.

The TNM classification has been proposed by the joint commission. It is cumbersome and confusing, as demonstrated by Tarlowska. In the classification of 6193 cases of cervical carcinoma, there were 10 categories into which *not a single case* was found to fit! Consequently, at present, the TNM classification is essentially worthless.

DIAGNOSIS OF CERVICAL CANCER

Obviously, a thorough history with special emphasis on menstrual irregularities, intermenstrual staining, or postmenopausal bleeding is of major import in the study of any pelvic disease; however, it is just as apparent that the patient with early cervical neoplasia is usually asymptomatic. The first suspicion of such lesions is the unsuspected report of atypical cells in the routine vaginal cytologic study. Further investigation of the patient with abnormal vaginal cytology is a major issue in our discipline.

It is imperative to appreciate that even with the best available laboratory staff and facilities there will be an unavoidable percentage of false positive and false negative results. Cytology may be quite unsatisfactory in the malignancy associated with extensive infection and necrosis or in the patient with severe but benign vaginitis, especially the trichomonal or postmenopausal types. Furthermore, the specimen may be poorly taken and false negative results obtained, as in the series reported by Silbar and Woodruff. Ruth Graham has further demonstrated the variations in cytologic diagnosis of 25 spreads read by eight different cytopathologists. Although false negative rates of 20 to 30 per cent have been reported with one cytopathologic study, it has also been demonstrated that this defect will be reduced to 9 per cent if the second preparation is negative, and to less than 1 per cent if there is a third study.

In spite of these inconsistencies, this technique is still the best screening method available today, and routine vaginal cytology should be obtained on all married females and all who have had coitus regardless of age. In the final analysis, it is the histopathologic report on which most treatment is based. Suspicious or positive smears should be followed by repeat cytology and cervical biopsy. If there is a gross lesion, biopsy should be taken immediately, since invasive disease may be determined with the one study, and since cytology is less accurate in these exuberant or ulcerative neoplasms (Fig. 5–27).

It is important to emphasize that, in the very early lesion, evidence of cancer may be lacking in one section but present in another. At least three sections, at intervals of several micrometers, should be made from each

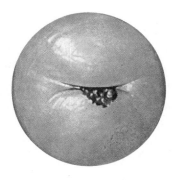

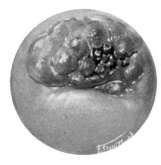

Figure 5–27. Clinical appearance of epidermoid carcinoma of cervix in early (above) and moderately advanced (below) stages.

block of biopsy material. Many times one is inclined to the diagnosis of intraepithelial carcinoma, only to find in other sections undeniable evidence of invasive carcinoma. It must be reemphasized that *the site of predilection for epidermoid cancer is the region of the squamocolumnar epithelial junction.* The studies of Foote and Stewart, mapping the sites of early carcinoma in situ, indicate that biopsy bites at the squamocolumnar junction at four equidistant points would reveal the lesion in all but a small proportion of cases. Nevertheless, it is also important to recognize that the anterior and posterior lips are the sites of origin of 60 to 75 per cent of cervical neoplasms, and thus biopsies should be concentrated in these areas rather than in the "3 and 9 o'clock" zones. Finally, biopsies which do not include the squamocolumnar junction should be so reported since, in spite of the size of the tissue fragments, cancer may be missed if the critical area is not included (Fig. 5–28 A,B).

In the presence of *suspicious lesions in pregnant women,* there should be no hesitation in resorting to biopsy, as it carries with it very little risk of disturbing the pregnancy or causing undue bleeding. There is need of much caution, however, in the interpretation of the biopsy sections, since squamous metaplastic changes, at times resembling intraepithelial carcinoma, may be found in a small proportion of pregnant women, with later spontaneous regression, as has been discussed in Chapter 3. There is often a clearer indication for repeat biopsies on the cervices of pregnant women than for the nonpregnant because of the variety of proliferative patterns, the common severe inflammatory infiltrate, the edema, the frequent, confusing decidual reaction, and microcystic metaplasia.

Conization

Conization has become the prime method for confirmation of the inconclusive smear and biopsy. Nevertheless, too frequently this procedure has been carried out after cytologic study only, and without use of the biopsy. Merrill reports that only 23 per cent of conization specimens from a group of community hospitals revealed any evidence of neoplastic alteration. Thus 77 per cent of the procedures were unnecessary for either diagnosis or treatment. Although, admittedly, this type of investigation is necessary in many instances, it is important to remember that, if invasive disease is discovered by biopsy, the more traumatic conization is unnecessary; indeed, it is *contraindicated,* since the most effective program for irradiation must be modified in the "coned" cervix. Furthermore, an additional anesthetic is eliminated if accurate diagnosis can be made by simple biopsy. Although the complications of conization are few, there seems little need for this procedure in the study of the majority of patients with abnormal vaginal cytology. Certain complications in future pregnancy, i.e., early fetal loss or dystocia due to cervical incompetence or stenosis, may be avoided if conization is eliminated. Finally, by the development of more accurate methods of investigation, such as colposcopy and colpomicroscopy, the limits of the lesion may be visualized, and directed biopsies may determine the degree of cellular anaplasia without the use of more traumatic procedures.

Thus our goal should be the elimination of unnecessary diagnostic procedures which add to the possibility of complications but do not add to the accuracy of the study. Our

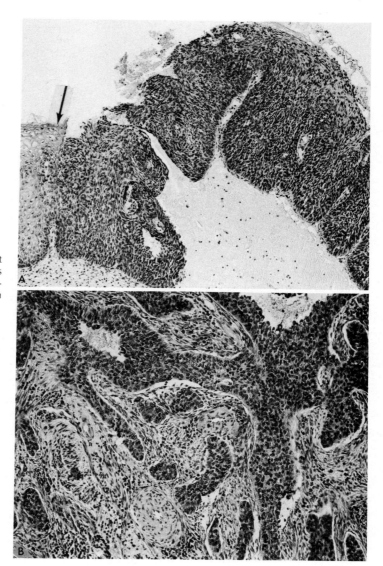

Figure 5–28. *A,* Carcinoma in situ at squamocolumnar junction—arrow shows dramatic transition from normal to anaplastic epithelium. *B,* Invasive carcinoma from *A*—missed by biopsy.

findings in 196 consecutive cases of in situ cervical cancer have demonstrated that, if cytologic, colposcopic, and directed biopsy histopathology indicated that no invasive disease is present, treatment may be instituted without the use of conization, unless such a procedure is to be employed as therapy in the young patient who desires to preserve her childbearing potential.

In spite of the accuracy of these simple diagnostic studies, there are instances in which "cold" conization is necessary. When there is wide divergence in the results of the diagnostic studies, e.g., negative colposcopy and positive cytology, or in cases where the extent of the lesion cannot be determined by the colposcopist, more extensive procedures

such as conization are imperative. The type of conization is less important than the tissue preparation and evaluation. It must be emphasized that the bulk of the cervical stroma is unimportant. Conversely, the necessity of inclusion of the area of the squamocolumnar junction with adequate margins on the portio and into the canal cannot be stressed too strongly. The removed tissue should be marked at the most anterior position (12 o'clock) and opened at this point. The tissue may then be flattened on a porous surface (e.g., cork) with the epithelial side exposed and floated face-down in the fixative. The entire specimen is then cut into four quadrants and each fixed separately, again sliced into three or four fragments, each through the squamocolumnar junction area, and finally three to four sections made from each quadrant. A total of 36 to 64 fragments, each demonstrating the transitional zone, are available for study. The cryostat has been used in several laboratories to eliminate the necessity for two surgical procedures, and to reduce hospital stay and postoperative complications. A report can be rendered to the surgeon in 25 minutes in our laboratory, where adequate trained personnel are available, and the permanent sections have confirmed the frozen section diagnosis.

Cervical conization has been proposed generally as adequate therapy for carcinoma in situ. Recurrence rates of 2 to 6 per cent have been reported by various investigators (Kolstad and Klem, Krieger and McCormack, and others). Such therapy is of obvious importance in the young patient desirous of maintaining fertility. The adequacy of the cone specimen is of major significance. If the margins are not clear, i.e., if atypia extends to the margin, the incidence of recurrence (basically residual disease) will be high. Nevertheless this recurrence rate is not as great as the incidence of residual disease in the postconization specimen, as noted by Silbar and others. It must be suspected that tissue reaction at the surgical margins probably eliminates minor amounts of such residual disease. Recently cryosurgery has been championed as a therapeutic approach to carcinoma in situ. It must be appreciated that the cases should be evaluated very carefully since the tissues will not be available for study with such procedures. Thus, colposcopy must be able to delineate the full extent of the disease, the directed biopsy must show no more than in situ cancer, and cytology must correlate with the above studies. The incidence of invasive cancer following all destructive procedures is small but sometimes masked by the healing process so that detection is delayed. Consequently, in the patient who has had her family, the most definitive therapy is total hysterectomy. A vaginal cuff should be included with the specimen only if the lesion extends out onto the portio, as demonstrated by careful gross study of the area, use of the Schiller reagent, and colposcopic evaluation. However, the great majority of in situ cancers extend into the cervical canal, and thus excision of a segment of vagina, which may result in a shortened vaginal canal, is unnecessary in most in-stances. Even with such therapy, about 1 per cent of the patients will demonstrate atypism in the vagina in the follow-up period; thus, continued cytologic study is necessary.

Schiller Tinctorial Test

This test is based on the fact, pointed out by Lahm, that the normal vaginal mucosa, as well as the stratified squamous epithelium of the pars vaginalis, is rich in glycogen. Cancerous epithelium, however, is glycolytic, and this fact has been utilized by Schiller in the iodine test which he devised. This consists of painting the cervix thoroughly with Gram's solution, consisting of 1 part of iodine and 2 parts of potassium iodide to 300 parts of water. This solution gives better results than Lugol's solution, which has often been used for the test.

Schiller advises that the solution be poured into the vagina and liberally mopped over the cervix, with care being taken to avoid traumatism to the mucous membrane, as this may lessen its tinctorial response. Henriksen suggests as a modification that the solution be sprayed freely over the cervix with an atomizer. Excessive mucous secretion should first be gently removed and, after a half minute or so to allow the stain to take hold, the excess solution should be sponged out (Figs. 5–29 and 5–30).

Normally, the squamous epithelium of the cervix takes a homogeneous deep mahogany-brown stain, while cancerous areas remain unstained, so that they stand out in sharp contrast. Unfortunately, the matter is not quite so simple and decisive, for other lesions which are not malignant may remain unstained, while trauma to the mucosa may also interfere with the reaction. The cylindrical epithelium of the cervical canal normally takes a rather light brownish-pink stain, and this must be taken into consideration in the cervices in which eversion or erosion is present. In ulcerated carcinoma, a dirty brownish stain may be present in the ulcerated area, though a whitish zone may be noted surrounding this, corresponding to the advancing margin of growth. We would point out, however, that certain cases of proved cancer have shown a negative Schiller stain, as noted by Friedell and coworkers. The main value of the Schiller test is to point out specific areas of abnormal glycogen metabolism for further study.

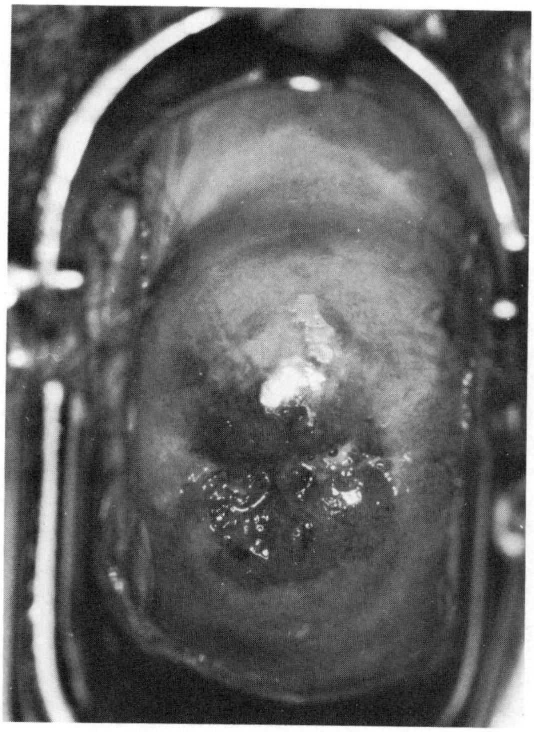

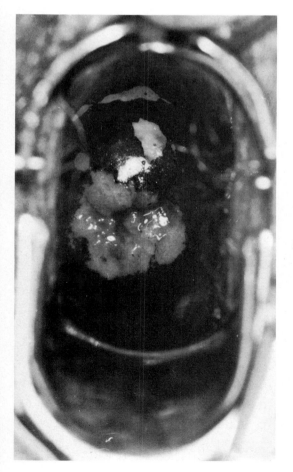

Figure 5–29. Eversion with patch of whitish change (carcinoma in situ) on anterior lip.

Figure 5–30. Schiller test on same cervix as in Figure 5–30, outlining the nonglycogen–containing areas.

Toluidine Blue

Richart has reported on the use of 1 per cent aqueous solution of toluidine blue to delineate areas of cervical dysplasia and carcinoma in situ. The preparation of the area with acetic acid to dissolve the mucus and the post-dye washing with a similar agent have resulted in the delineation of the abnormal cellular zones by a royal blue color. The dye is a nuclear stain, and the author believes that it affords a better pattern than that produced by the Schiller reagent. In the past two decades both of these tinctorial tests have been superseded, at least in part, by the use of colposcopy.

Histochemical Studies

A variety of enzymatic histochemical studies have been used in the attempt to produce a specific reaction that might differentiate benign from malignant epithelia. Although initially β-glucuronidase and later 6-phosphogluconic acid dehydrogenase appeared as specific enzymes to label the anaplastic cell, neither has fulfilled expectations. Consequently, at present, no specific enzyme reactions are of sufficient value to be useful aids in the diagnosis of cervical cancer.

Colposcopy and Colpomicroscopy

Kolstad, Stafl, and others have demonstrated the characteristic patterns present in the diseased cervix and have been able to differentiate the benign from the anaplastic changes. The mosaic pattern of the endocervical glands can be readily delineated from the smooth surface of the portio and the "punctation" with hairpin capillaries of carcinoma in situ (Fig. 5–31). Benign patterns of metaplasia and endocervical fold agglutination can be distinguished from the anaplastic changes (Fig. 5–32). The vascular changes associated with in situ and early invasive disease are shown in Figures 5–33 and 5–34. If the endocervix can be visualized, the limits of the lesion can often be discerned, and directed biopsies will determine the histologic extent of the anaplasia (Fig. 5–31). Further application of such specialized techniques has, to a major degree, obviated the necessity for conization in many questionable instances in which minor degrees of dysplasia were suggested by cytopathology. The absence of positive findings in the well-defined transformation zone has allowed the physician to follow the patient without having to perform a traumatizing conization.

Types of Cervical Cancer

There are two basic pathologic types of cervical cancer. The most common or *epidermoid variety* arises predominantly at the squamocolumnar junction or transformation zone, although an occasional pure *squamous* lesion appears on the portio, and an adeno-

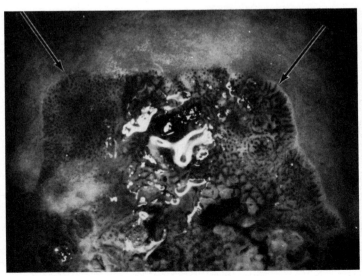

Figure 5–31. Colposcopic pattern of carcinoma in situ with "punctation" and "hairpin" capillaries at arrow on right, and mosaic pattern in center. (Courtesy of Dr. A. Stafl.)

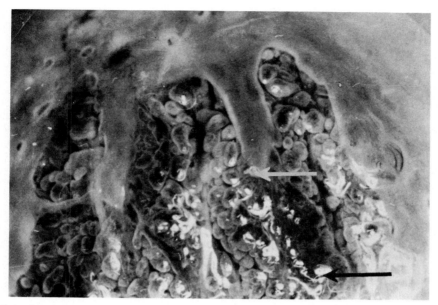

Figure 5-32. Colposcopic picture with tongues of metaplasia at upper arrow and agglutination of endocervical folds (ectopy) between arrows. (Courtesy of Dr. A. Stafl.)

epidermoid type develops primarily in the glands. The latter is histologically more epidermoid than adenoid. In contrast to the epidermoid and squamous tumors is the *true adenocarcinoma*, which arises in the gland-like area of the endocervix, i.e., in the tunnels or clefts. Martzloff noted that 94.5 per cent of cervical malignancy was of the epidermoid type and most authors agreed with

this ratio of one adenocarcinoma to 20 epidermoid carcinomas.

HISTOLOGIC GRADING OF EPIDERMOID CANCER

It has been proposed that the more immature the cell type, the more actively growing

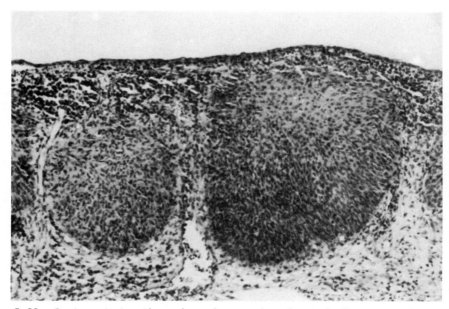

Figure 5-33. Carcinoma in situ with vessels seen between plugs of atypical cells. (Courtesy of Dr. A. Stafl.)

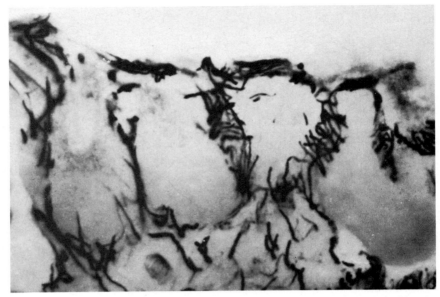

Figure 5–34. Vascular pattern in same specimen as in Figure 5–33. (Vessels outlined with alkaline phosphatase.) (Courtesy of Dr. A. Stafl.)

and malignant will be the tumor, and this general principle is embodied in the various histologic classifications of cervical cancer. The German subdivision into three grades—*ripe*, *unripe*, and *intermediate*—is based on this general principle. Martzloff in 1923 also depended on the cell maturity in his classification into the *spinal cell*, the *transitional cell*, and the *basal cell* varieties. Similarly, Broders differentiated cervical neoplasia, as well as any other variety, on the ability or

lack of ability of the epithelial cell to mature (Figs. 5–35 and 5–36). It is important to emphasize the extreme rarity of pure tumor forms. Most anaplasias are composed of all three cell types, with one type usually predominant.

Significance of Histologic Cell Gradation

In spite of the enthusiasm of these investigators for histologic classification of the cer-

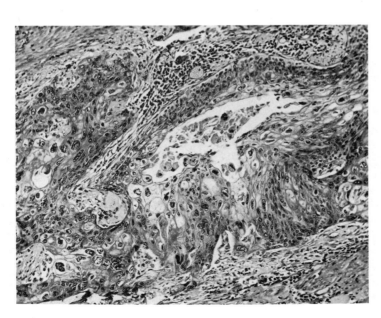

Figure 5–35. Invasive cancer showing mature pattern with attempt at pearl formation.

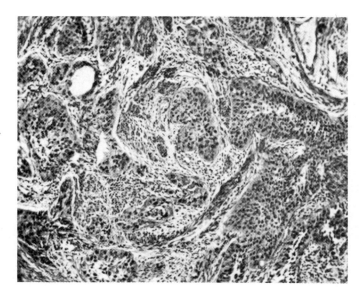

Figure 5–36. Strands and sheets of highly malignant cells in typical invasive cancer.

vical neoplasm, it is important to recognize that there are few pure cell types. Too frequently, the cells in one area demonstrate a striking tendency to mature; in other areas, the predominant cell type is more characteristic of the intermediate or even the small cell type. Furthermore, the initial purpose for such histologic classifications, namely the development of a method by which the most effective therapy (surgery or irradiation) could be selected, has not been justified by the statistical analyses. Prognostically, the clinical stage of the disease and the tumor mass have proved to be more important than the predominant cell type, as noted by Van Nagell and co-workers and by Burghardt. The original enthusiasm for cell type classifications as a guide to treatment has been dampened, though more studies are necessary to document or negate the validity of these current theses.

The term "glassy-cell carcinoma" has been used to describe a specific histologic variant of the classic squamous cell or epidermoid lesion. The characteristic cell in these neoplasms is large, with abundant glassy cytoplasm and a relatively uniform hyperchromatic nucleus (Fig. 5–37). In the author's opinion such lesions often show other, more routine cell types in nearby areas. Furthermore, the tumors made up largely of this cell variant do not demonstrate any unique biologic features. Nevertheless, few cases consisting primarily of glassy-cells have been observed in our lab-

oratory, and thus no positive statement can be made relative to specific behavior.

Clinical Studies to Evaluate Course of Disease

Recently the local reaction to the application of DNCB (dinitrochlorobenzene) has

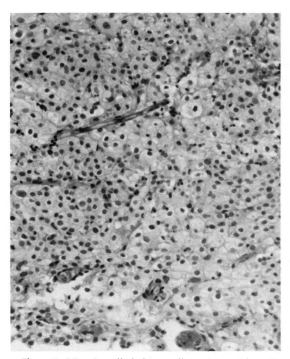

Figure 5–37. So-called glassy-cell carcinoma of cervix. In other areas foci of keratinization were present.

proved to be of great prognostic significance. Morton has noted, in a small series of cervical cancers, that a positive reaction is associated with an excellent cure rate, while the converse is also true. Possibly more experience in this area will lead to better immunologic techniques, not only for purposes of prognostication but possibly also for the development of methods to improve the patient's resistance to the onslaughts of the neoplasm.

The studies of infiltrates in the area adjacent to the invasive disease have been interpreted as demonstrations of both tissue destruction by the tumor and immunologic response to the malignancy (T or B cells). A specific decision has not been reached as to the prognostic significance of this infiltrate. Current techniques offer an opportunity for further studies to evaluate the importance of such infiltrates.

ADENOCARCINOMA OF CERVIX

Introduction

Adenocarcinoma of the cervix makes up about 5 per cent of primary cervical cancer. The average age for patients with adenocarcinoma is approximately the same as that for the epidermoid variety; however, one case has been reported in a 7 month old infant.

Gross Characteristics

Adenocarcinoma may arise either within the cervical canal or in the region of the external os. The former site, however, is the more characteristic, just as the latter is with epidermoid cancer. When adenocarcinoma develops within the cervical canal, it presents as a hardened, slightly papillary area which later undergoes ulcerative and necrotic changes. In such cases the cervix may appear entirely normal externally, but when the canal is dilated and curetted, masses of cancerous tissue are often brought away by the instrument, so that only a shell of cervical tissue (the barrel lesion) may be left. On the other hand, adenocarcinoma may present as a papillary or ulcerative lesion at the external os and the adjoining cervical area, so that in most cases one cannot be sure of the type until microscopic examination is made. When adenocarcinoma is found, it may be difficult to be certain whether it represents a primary cervical malignancy or a downward extension from the more common endometrial lesion. Differential curettage of the canal and cavity may sometimes be helpful; i.e., if a large amount of fungoid material is obtained from the cavity and little from the canal, an endometrial origin is suggested. Sometimes, however, the primary source cannot be ascertained, and the microscopic appearance may not be particularly helpful. Acanthosis is rare in primary cervical adenocarcinoma (as compared to the endometrium) but may sometimes occur, as noted by Fricke and associates.

The difference in the secretory activity of the endocervical cell versus that of the endometrial cell has been believed to be of major importance in differentiating the benign from the malignant adenomatous uterine lesions. Although such features are helpful, nevertheless, mucous secretion has been demonstrated both in the normal endometrial gland and in the endometrial adenocarcinoma. Furthermore, with the more undifferentiated tumor, less secretory activity can be demonstrated histologically and the site of origin of the lesion is undetermined. As noted later, if both endocervix and endometrium are involved, the FIGO classification designates such lesion as Clinical Stage II.

Microscopic Characteristics

To appreciate the abnormal gland pattern on which the microscopic diagnosis is based, one must remember that in the normal cervix the glands are quite uniform, are distributed discretely throughout the stroma, and are lined by a single layer of uniform, high, columnar, secreting cells of the characteristic picket-fence type. In adenocarcinoma, on the other hand, the glands are increased in number, and are lined by epithelium which shows varying degrees of neoplastic departure from the normal prototype.

The *in situ adenocarcinoma* is characterized by a loss of polarity and hyperchromatism of the nuclei. The large, irregular, basophilic nuclei occupy various positions in the cytoplasm and often appear to project from the luminal surface (Fig. 5–38 A,B), as described by Abell and Gosling. Inflammatory infiltrate confuses the issue by causing disturbances in the height of the cells, variations in the position of the nucleus, and the false appearance of hyperchromatism; nevertheless, mitotic activity is absent. Other

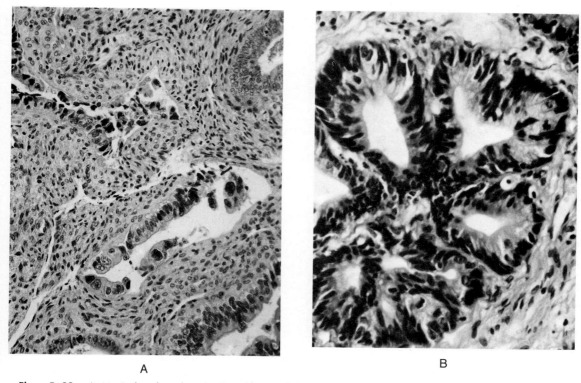

A   B

Figure 5–38. *A,* Atypical nuclear alteration in endocervical glands associated with adenocarcinoma in situ. *B,* Adenocarcinoma in situ. Note hyperchromatic nuclei near luminal edge of cell.

confusing pathophysiologic alterations, such as the Arias-Stella reaction and microcystic mucoid metaplasia, have been described in Chapters 3 and 4.

Transitions may not be easily recognized between this in situ stage and the well-differentiated adenocarcinoma (Figs. 5–39 and 5–40). In the mature variety the epithelial cell maintains its ability to secrete mucin, but its anaplastic quality is demonstrated by the irregular and bizarre arrangement of the closely packed glandular elements (Fig.

Figure 5–39. Mature, mucus-secreting adenocarcinoma of cervix in lower left.

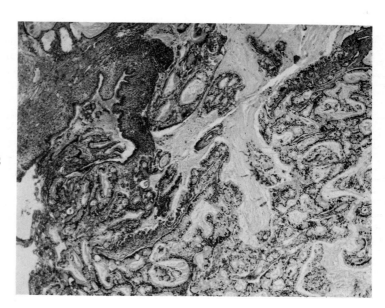

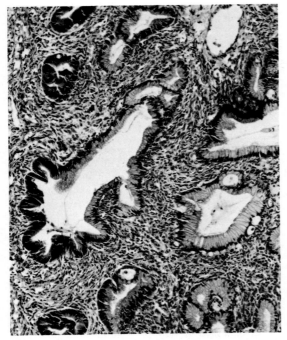

Figure 5–40. Adenocarcinoma in situ. Note transitions in normal glands. Metaplasia of tubal or endometrioid types must be ruled out by finding secretory and ciliated elements.

5–41 *A,B*). This rare lesion has been classified as gelatinous or mucoid adenocarcinoma and makes up approximately 3 to 5 per cent of all adenomatous malignancies of the cervix. It must be differentiated from the microcystic mucoid metaplasia associated with oral contraceptives (see Chapter 4). In the more classic type, the pattern simulates that seen in the endometrium, with an increase in the size of the nuclei, a concomitant reduction in cytoplasm, and a marked epithelial proliferation essentially eliminating the intervening stroma. The cytoplasm becomes eosinophilic, and little mucin can be demonstrated by special stains (Figs. 5–42 and 5–43). Again, grading of the lesion is similar to that of the corresponding endometrial cancer; i.e., the histologic grade increases as the proliferation of the lining cells eliminates the glandular pattern, until, in Grade IV, it may be almost impossible to define such elements, although the epithelial nature of the neoplasm is still recognizable. In rare instances a stromal component may be present, as in the mixed mesodermal tumor of the fundus. As noted in the most recent FIGO classification, if both endocervix and endometrium are involved, the neoplasm arbi-

trarily falls into the category of a fundal lesion with cervical extension.

A rare variety of adenocarcinoma arises from mesonephric vestiges deep in the substance of the cervix or in the lateral vaginal vault. Although there are undoubted cases of neoplasia developing in such remnants, the majority of these tumors develop in patients whose mothers received estrogenic agents during pregnancy. This mesonephroid or clear cell carcinoma occurring in the young adult has been described in Chapter 2. It must be appreciated that at least one third of these lesions involve the cervix (Fig. 5–44). Finally, a rare case of mesonephric papilloma of the cervix has been described in the literature. These occur in the young child and pursue a benign course. Their association with the mesonephric system has not been documented, and thus such papillomas must not be confused with the mesonephroid tumors.

ADENOSQUAMOUS AND ADENOEPIDERMOID CARCINOMA

Squamous metaplasia, as noted in Chapter 4, is a common alteration in the tunnels, apparently arising from the indifferent or reserve subcolumnar cell. Such a change occurring in adenocarcinoma results in the development of adenoacanthoma. It must be recognized, and will be discussed later, that the metaplastic epithelium in such a context is benign. The malignant component is the adenomatous element; therefore, this lesion is basically an adenocarcinoma in which squamous metaplasia has developed. If, as rarely occurs, the acanthomatous areas become anaplastic, a true squamous carcinoma results.

Conversely, if the indifferent or reserve cells demonstrate malignant alterations, the resulting anaplasia is epidermoid. Fundamentally, this is representative of the characteristic carcinoma arising at the squamocolumnar junction, with the normal columnar epithelium of the endocervix being replaced by the underlying malignant elements. If such a change occurs diffusely in the tunnels or clefts without concurrent alterations in the surface epithelium, an adenoepidermoid tumor results. Although maturity may take place in such a metaplastic epithelium, with the subsequent production of a true strati-

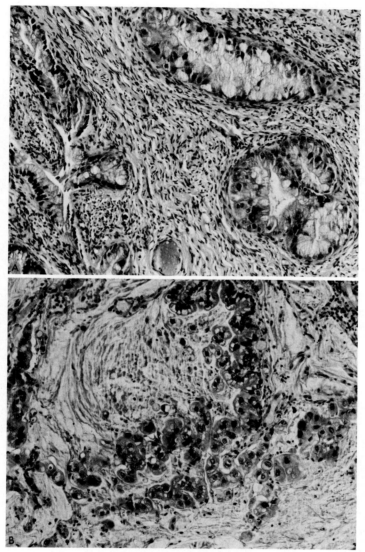

Figure 5–41. *A,* Individual nuclear aberrations in gland epithelium characterized by hyperchromatic nuclei in atypical positions in the tall picket-fence type cell. *B,* The well-differentiated mucus-secreting carcinoma recognized 18 months after the initial biopsy shown in *A.*

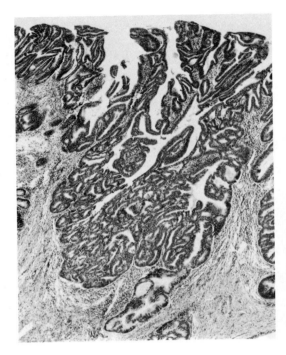

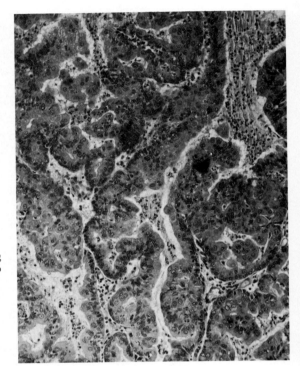

Figure 5–42. Adenocarcinoma invading from surface with few mucus-secreting glands in lower middle.

Figure 5–43. Adenocarcinoma of the cervix showing transition from the well-differentiated portion in lower left to the less well-differentiated area on right.

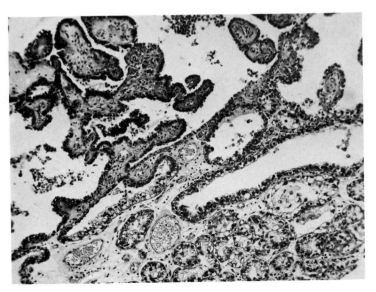

Figure 5–44. Mesonephroid carcinoma of cervix with clear cell pattern in lower right and papillary pattern in upper left.

fied or squamous lesion, this is a more unusual development in the experience of the author.

The adenoepidermoid lesion is characterized by a multilayered anaplastic tumor on the surface of which is a single layer of malignant cells. Thus, the adenoid pattern is maintained, although in many areas the overproduction of the indifferent cell has wiped out the last vestiges of the glandlike pattern (Figs. 5–45 A,B and 5–46). Abell has commented on the frequency with which this type of lesion is found in pregnancy, further evidence of the importance of the indifferent cell activity in the development of the tumor. The malignant potential of the adenoepidermoid as compared with epidermoid carcinoma is debatable, although certain studies would suggest that the prognosis is poorer in the former. Nevertheless, it seems likely that, stage for stage, the survival rates are comparable, since the adenoepidermoid lesion is rarely discovered in the early stages due to the area of the cervix in which it arises. Furthermore, many of the barrel lesions are of this adenoepidermoid variety. Obviously more clinical and pathologic evaluation of these lesions is necessary to deter-

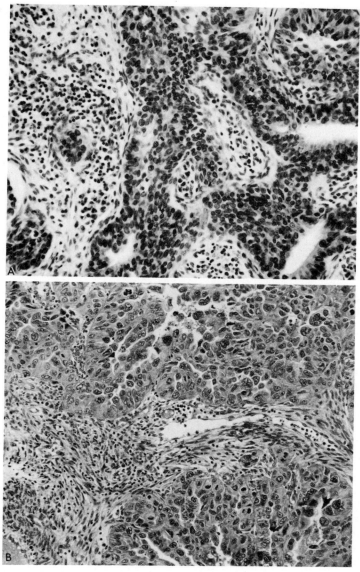

Figure 5–45. *A,* Adenoepidermoid carcinoma showing glandlike pattern on right but almost solid area in middle. *B,* Adenoepidermoid carcinoma showing almost solid epidermoid elements with gland epithelium almost eliminated.

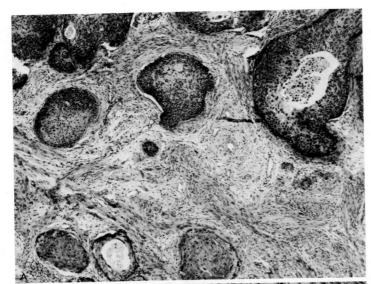

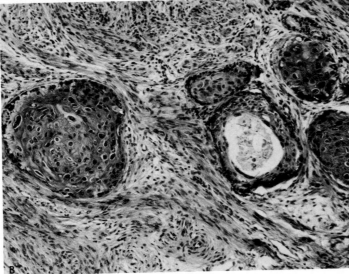

Figure 5–46. *A,* Adenosquamous cancer. The remains of glands can be seen in several areas and the maturation of the epithelium is evident. The lesion was fairly high, in the endocervix only, at the time of hysterectomy for pyometra. There were no atypicalities found in the tissue studies from the endocervix, endometrium, or portio, and no cytologic atypicalities were demonstrated. *B,* High power of *A.*

mine more accurately the prognostic significance of these unusual tumors. At present, approximately 8 per cent of all primary cervical malignancies fall into the category of adenoepidermoid carcinoma in our laboratory.

Adenosquamous carcinoma represents a lesion in which maturation of the metaplastic element in the glandular area of the cervix is predominant. These alterations must be quite rare; in our experience they develop high in the endocervix and may be recognized late in the developmental stages of the disease. Furthermore, since the tumor primarily involves the stroma, there may be no surface changes, thus denying the possibility of early cytologic diagnosis. The tumor

seen in Figure 5–46 (A,B) was found in a 66 year old patient with a pyometra.

EXTENSION AND METASTASIS OF CERVICAL CANCER

In view of the direct continuity of the squamous epithelium of the portio, the vagina is the most common site of secondary involvement with cervical cancer. Again, in the more advanced stages, the malignant process often extends upward along the surface into the corpus uteri. An interesting though rather rare form of epidermoid cancer is that in which the upward extension remains superficial, like the sugar coating of a cake, spoken of by the Germans as the "Zuckerguss" carcinoma. Parametrial extension is also common, though it is difficult to differentiate direct extension from lymphatic permeation.

It is the lymphatic route of dissemination of cervical cancer that is chiefly responsible for the difficult and often insoluble problems of therapy presented by this disease. The route of lymphatic extension is primarily via the hypogastric, iliac, and obturator nodes. Since staging is performed before therapy is begun, many Stage I lesions are found, by surgical staging, to have already metastasized to the regional nodes. It is now generally accepted that 12 to 15 per cent of Stage I cervical cancers will demonstrate regional node involvement. Furthermore, in approximately 50 per cent of these cases with iliac and hypogastric node metastasis, there will be para-aortic node involvement. It would thus seem that the 85 to 90 per cent 5 year survival for Stage I cervical cancer is due directly to the unrecognized 12 to 15 per cent of such lesions that are, in reality, Stage IV lesions. Finally, it has been recognized that this 50 per cent relationship of pelvic node to para-aortic node involvement holds true for each stage of the disease. Unfortunately, therapy for such metastases has been relatively unsatisfactory to date. The parametrium is involved in a large proportion of even relatively early cases, and practically all of the advanced group.

Evidences of lymphatic extension are often encountered even in very early cancers, in which the cervical lesion is small. Several authors have reported instances of so-called cervical in situ cancer in which subsequent laparotomy revealed positive lymph nodes. One must infer that at some point, undisclosed by microscopic sections, there had been lymphatic spread (Fig. 5–24 A,B). Thorough study of the suspicious lesion and better identification of micro-invasion have greatly reduced this incidence of unexpected pelvic lymph node invasion. Nevertheless it must be appreciated that the ±10 per cent mortality rate in Stage I cervical cancer is related primarily to unrecognized extracervical disease at time of first evaluation. Some clinics have resorted recently to pretreatment surgical staging in order to more accurately define the stage of the disease and thus institute more appropriate and "patient-designed" therapy. (Fig. 5–24 A,B). Involvement of

the perineural spaces (Fig. 5–57) has previously been thought to be evidence of lymphatic invasion. Such invasion may be appreciated relatively early and appears to be less ominous prognostically than true invasion of the vascular channels.

Metastasis to distant organs is not uncommon, as demonstrated by the studies of both Henriksen and Brunschwig and Daniel, in which approximately 40 per cent of patients dying of cervical cancer had extrapelvic tumor. Nevertheless, a majority of deaths are due to local extension with resultant urinary insufficiency, intestinal obstruction, and cachexia.

Kelly and co-authors have found a high incidence of tumor in postsurgical patients studied by autopsy, although the immediate cause of death was not necessarily the spread of cancer but rather surgical complications. They concur, with other impressions, on the futility of lymphadenectomy, since they found residual tumor in all 29 cases in which radical surgery revealed positive nodes. Both the lymphatics and the bloodstream may participate in dissemination of the disease. Metastasis to the ovaries, tubes, and uterine ligaments may occur by way of the lymphatics, although the bloodstream route must generally be invoked to explain the occasional metastases which occur to the skin, brain, liver, pancreas, spine, long bones, and other distant sites.

EFFECTS OF RADIOTHERAPY ON CERVICAL CARCINOMA

In view of the frequency of radium therapy for cervical carcinoma, it is important for the pathologist to be familiar with the effects of such treatment upon the histologic appearance of the normal epithelium and stroma as well as on the anaplastic cell, especially since follow-up biopsies are frequently done to determine the presence or absence of active cancer. The gross changes produced by radium have been well described by various authors, who suggest the following sequence: hyperemia appearing about one week after the application of radium; slough formation three weeks later; separation of the slough one month later; contraction due to the formation of fibrous tissue after still another month; and a final stage of marked contraction.

The cellular changes produced by radium also have been described by a number of authors. The initial effect appears to be an inhibition of nuclear division, soon followed by degenerative changes in both the cytoplasm and nuclei, and a tendency to clumping of nuclear material. The cells often show a vacuolated or clear cytoplasm. In other cells, the nuclei become hyperchromatic but with fuzzy borders, and the bland cytoplasm is increased (Fig. 5–47). With these changes there is marked chronic inflammatory infiltration of the stroma, with later increasing fibrosis. Often endothelial proliferation produces cells which simulate abnormal epithelium.

Despite our knowledge of morphologic changes in postirradiated cancer, the pathologist is often faced with the problem as to whether tumor cells are still viable. It is our belief that on occasion this distinction is frankly impossible and, therefore, prognosis based on sequential biopsy during and after treatment is commonly inaccurate. This is in contrast to certain European workers who believe that microscopic evaluation of cell changes during therapy is an accurate index of the radiosensitivity of the tumor and hence the outcome. Our own studies would suggest that there are so many variables present as to nullify the importance of such tissue studies. Among these variables are: (a) the probability that biopsy is not representative of the tumor as a whole, (b) inability to identify accurately the clinical stage of the disease and lymph node involvement, (c)

lack of uniform response to irradiation, and (d) above all, the difficulty in determining the viability of postirradiated tumor cells.

This last is perhaps the greatest problem for the pathologist. Application of any criteria for irradiated tissue is frequently difficult, for the immediate postirradiation changes of edema, nuclear clumping, pyknosis, etc., can be distinguished from malignant tendencies only with uncertainty. Late irradiation changes toward hyperkeratinization and fibrosis can also be a problem, and we have seen patients with a supposedly persistent or recurrent lesion live for years without treatment (Fig. 5–48), or show no disease if radical surgery is performed. Experience would suggest, however, that an unequivocally positive biopsy more than three months after irradiation suggests a resistant lesion. A positive biopsy, however, may persist at least four to six weeks posttherapy with no dire implication, for apparently in some tumors there is a certain time lag before the full irradiation effect is felt. Biopsies, although inconclusive, are definitely worthwhile during and after therapy.

Several investigators have attempted to correlate the responsiveness of the neoplasm to irradiation with the reaction of normal cells to this agent. At present, these studies have not been helpful in determining the ideal therapy.

Although Diddle and his co-workers found tumor cells in the blood of patients with epidermoid cancer, most workers agree

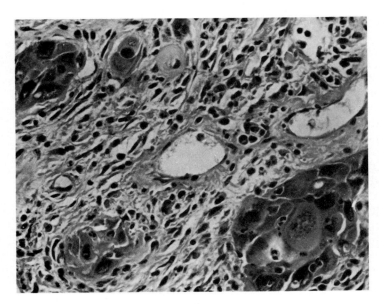

Figure 5–47. Postirradiation epidermoid carcinoma—cells show bland and irregular nuclei.

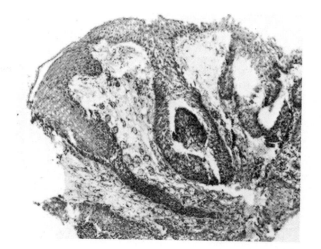

Figure 5–48. Biopsy four months after irradiation interpreted as probable recurrent or resistant tumor, but patient is alive without further treatment (6 year salvage).

that they are of little prognostic significance. It becomes apparent that the presence of circulating tumor cells is not serious unless emboli adhere to the vessel wall, penetrate, and invade the adjacent tissue. Therefore, it would seem that operative trauma with subsequent showering of tumor cells into the bloodstream is not necessarily an ominous event.

RECURRENT CANCER

Although a few clinics are utilizing surgery with or without preoperative irradiation as the primary therapy of early invasive cancer, irradiation alone is the most widely accepted mode of treatment. Radical surgery generally has been reserved for radioresistant or recurrent cases; however, a protocol for the selection of certain Stages Ib and IIa cases for primary surgical therapy has been presented by many students. Generally the group studied is made up of young patients who are good surgical risks. The elimination of gonadal function and the late effects of irradiation on the vaginal and bowel mucosas are thus avoided. Frequently loss of blood supply and fibrosis results in a rigid vagina that is unresponsive to hormone therapy, and severe dyspareunia is a common complication of irradiation.

When invasive disease is recognized in the local area following any type of treatment, prognosis is poor; however, 5 year survival rates of 25 per cent and more have resulted from exenterative procedures if extrapelvic disease is not present. Recurrence in the deep pelvis and lymphatic system is more difficult to evaluate, and may be mistaken for merely an irradiation reaction. Brack and co-workers found that increasing pelvic induration, sciatic radiation of pelvic pain, and pedal edema should increase the physician's index of suspicion that recurrence is present in spite of the absence of tissue confirmation.

Great care must likewise be taken to guard against the advent of another malignant growth, for it is well known that multiple primary lesions are not uncommon.

When cancer recurs in the cervix after treatment (and this has been reported up to 17 years following therapy), it may show the same histology as the original lesion. However, the evaluation of anaplastic change in the residual cervix and in the adjacent vagina offers one of the more perplexing problems to the pathologist. Such changes may indicate deeper, underlying invasive tumor. Conversely, as Koss and co-workers, and Julian and Woodruff, have noted, the malignant alterations are often in reality intraepithelial and may be related to the radiation therapy (Fig. 5–49). Careful study is imperative since simple hysterectomy with vaginal cuff should be sufficient therapy for these lesions. Furthermore, exenteration procedures in face of the extensive radiation damage are followed, in a high percentage of cases, by serious complications and a high mortality rate. Nevertheless, with a team surgical approach to these extensive procedures, mortality and morbidity have been reduced, and a ± 20 per cent 5 year salvage can be expected in the well selected cases.

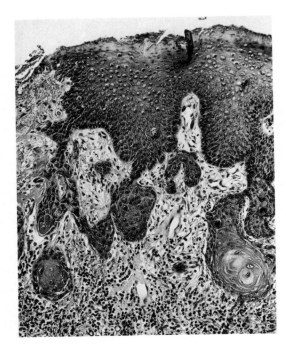

Figure 5–49. Atypical picture diagnosed as carcinoma 6 years postirradiation for invasive cervical cancer. (No further tumor found in hysterectomy specimen.)

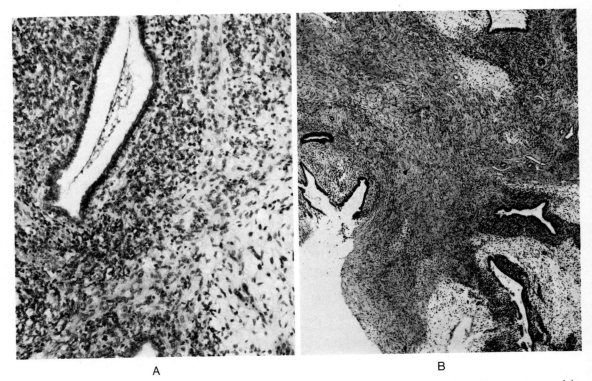

A   B

Figure 5–50. *A,* Low power view of stromal sarcoma of cervix. Note the benign glands with proliferating stroma of the paramesonephric system. *B,* Stromal sarcoma of cervix (known erroneously as adenosarcoma). There is no glandular neoplasia.

No evidence of carcinoma of the cervix 5 years after treatment is considered a 5 year salvage. Arneson has indicated that there are few recurrences after this period, so that 5 years seems a valid criterion for cure. Nevertheless, it must be understood there are a few late recurrences. Five year survival rates, stage for stage, have changed little in the past 25 years. In general they are:

FIGO	Stage I	88–92 per cent
	Stage II	60–65 per cent
	Stage III	30–35 per cent
	Stage IV	12–15 per cent

OTHER MALIGNANCIES

Sarcoma

Primary leiomyosarcoma and leiomyosarcoma arising in a preexisting benign myoma are rare in the cervix. The patterns are similar to those of the more common neoplasms of the fundus and will be described in succeeding chapters.

Mixed Mesodermal Tumors

Stromal Sarcomas. These lesions may be included under the heading of "mixed mesodermal" tumors since they arise from the paramesonephric stroma of the endocervix but may be found beneath the stratified epithelium of the portio. They generally occur in the third and fourth decades of life and are classically asymptomatic in the early stages.

On occasion the glands are atypical but not neoplastic. The lesion may be quite superficial, as noted by Abell and Ramirez and simple hysterectomy may result in long-term cures (Fig. 5–50 *A,B*). It should be appreciated that bizarre stromal cells such as those described in the vaginal polyp by Norris, may be seen in the cervical stroma and do not represent true neoplasms. Conversely the aggressive stromal sarcoma (Fig. 5–51) reacts like the similar lesion of the fundus and may rapidly invade the body of the cervix with fatal outcome.

Sarcoma botryoides has been described in Chapter 2 since it commonly fills a major portion of the vagina in the infant. Nevertheless, it must be recognized that it arises from the terminal portion of the müllerian duct (the tubercle); thus, the cervix is routinely and extensively involved. The pattern is identical to that described in Chapter 2.

In the adult, a mixed mesodermal tumor, similar to that found in the fundus in later years, may arise in the cervical canal, demonstrating all of the gross and microscopic features of the fundal lesion. It is usually polypoid. Striated muscle cells, cartilage, and other metaplastic mesodermal elements may be recognized in addition to atypical and anaplastic changes in epithelium and stroma (Fig. 5–52). Too few cases have been documented to form a basis for prognostication; however, the outcome undoubtedly would be similar to that of most of the fundal lesions, if not worse.

Melanosis, as noted in Chapter 3, has been

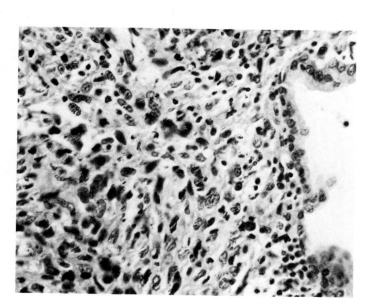

Figure 5–51. Stromal sarcoma. Note normal surface epithelium to far right.

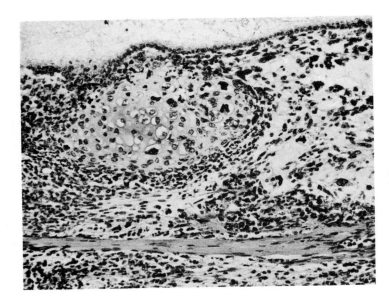

Figure 5–52. Mixed mesodermal tumor of cervix—cartilage seen in mid-upper portion.

noted on the cervix as well as the vagina; thus, primary malignant melanoma may develop de novo in these areas. Furthermore, recent cases of blue nevus have been recorded. These are benign; however, the blue color may also be indicative of the malignant melanoma and the latter, as in other areas of the body, pursues an aggressive and usually fatal course.

Adenoid-Basal Carcinoma

This unusual variety of carcinoma has been reported by Tchertkoff as "cylindroma." This term at present should be eliminated. Microscopically, it resembles the basal cell tumor of the skin (Figs. 5–53 and 5–54). The cells are small with regular dark nuclei. The invading nests do not destroy the

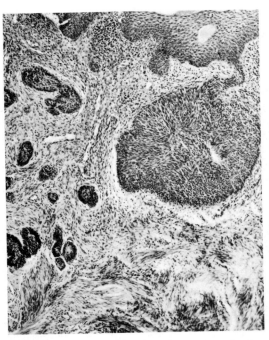

Figure 5–53. Adenoid-basal carcinoma extending from basal layer of lining epithelium.

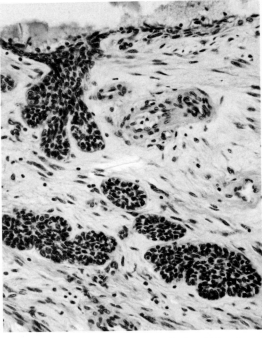

Figure 5–54. High power view of adenoid-basal carcinoma showing the uniformity of cells.

cervical stroma and, in general, this tumor seems to be locally invasive but amenable to excision by hysterectomy. Differential staining often reveals a small central core of PAS-positive, diastase-negative material. These lesions arise commonly on the portio of the cervix and are routinely associated with the more common histologic variety of epidermoid carcinoma in situ. The patients are usually in the late sixth or seventh decade of life—20 or more years older than the classic individual with cervical cancer. More cases need to be studied to determine the true life history of this unusual lesion.

This lesion must not be confused with the adenoid-cystic tumor which behaves like the adenoid-cystic tumor of the salivary gland (Fig. 5–55), which is locally aggressive and metastasizes late.

METASTATIC MALIGNANCY

The cervix is a common site for the extension of endometrial and vaginal cancer. As the result of the frequency of such occurrences, the most recent FIGO classification proposes that all adenocarcinomas involving both cervix and endometrium be classified

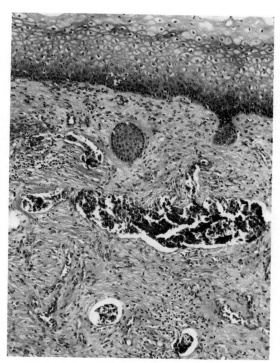

Figure 5–56. Metastatic carcinoma from endometrium into cervical stroma.

as primary fundal lesions, while, conversely, all epidermoid neoplasias found in both areas are to be classified as primary cervical cancer. Whereas extension to the cervix from adjacent disease is common, metastatic disease of extrapelvic origin is rare. Metastasis from endometrial malignancy may be seen in the subepithelial lymphatics of the cervix, suggesting the method by which the fundal lesion arrives in the vagina (Fig. 5–56). Local extension of the cervical tumor in the perineural spaces (Fig. 5–57) and in the lymph nodes (Fig. 5–58) is representative of common modes of spread of the disease.

Multiple Sites of Malignancy

The lower genital canal, i.e., the ectocervix, vagina, vulva, and perianal area, offers an ideal opportunity to study the regional effect of a carcinogenic agent. Reference has been made to this subject in Chapters 1 and 2. Suffice it to say that all lesions, in situ or invasive, deserve thorough and prolonged follow-up. The treatment of the initial lesion does not necessarily remove the carcinogenic agent!

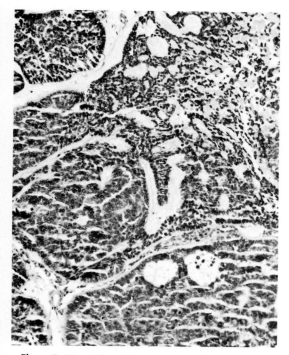

Figure 5–55. Adenoid-cystic carcinoma of cervix in an 83 year old patient. Compare with Figure 5–54.

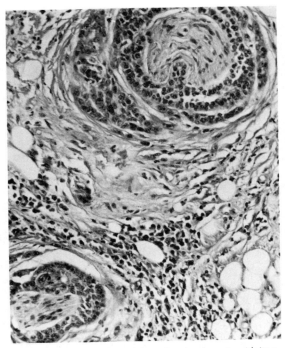

Figure 5–57. Epidermoid carcinoma of cervix with invasion of perineural spaces.

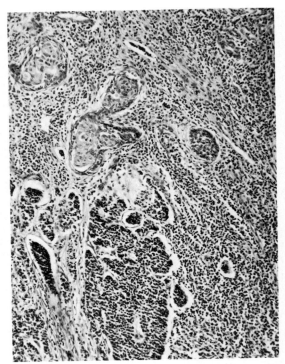

Figure 5–58. Metastatic carcinoma in iliac node. Note mature and immature patterns in adjacent areas.

REFERENCES

Abell, M. R., and Gosling, J. R.: Intraepithelial and infiltrative carcinoma of vulva: Bowen's type. Cancer, *14*:318, 1961.

Abell, M. R., and Ramerez, J. A.: Sarcomas and carcinosarcomas of the uterine cervix. Cancer, *31*:1176, 1973.

Allen, E., and Gardner, W. U.: Cancer of the cervix in hybrid mice following long-continued administration of estrogen. Cancer Res., *1*:359, 1941.

Aurelian, L., Strand, B. C., and Smith, M. F.: Immunodiagnostic potential of a virus-coded tumor associated antigen (AG-4) in cervical cancer. Cancer, *39*:1834, 1977.

Averette, H. E., Nasser, N., Yankow, S. L., and Little, W. A.: Cervical conization in pregnancy. Am. J. Obstet. Gynecol., *106*:543, 1970.

Baggish, M. S., and Woodruff, J. D.: Adenoid-basal carcinoma of the cervix. Obstet. Gynecol., *28*:213, 1966.

Baggish, M. S., and Woodruff, J. D.: Adenoid basal lesions of the cervix. Obstet. Gynecol., *37*:807, 1971.

Baker, H. W., Brack, C. B., and Dickson, R. J.: Adenocarcinoma of the cervix uteri. Obstet. Gynecol., *4*:664, 1954.

Barron, B. A., and Richart, R. M.: An epidemiologic study of cervical neoplastic disease. Based on a self-selected sample of 7,000 women in Barbados, West Indies. Cancer, *27*:978, 1971.

Bergsjø, P.: Cervical adenocarcinoma. Acta Obstet. Gynecol. Scand., *42*:85, 1963.

Boyes, D. A., Hardie, M., and Agnew, A. M.: Carcinoma of the cervix in an infant. Am. J. Obstet. Gynecol., *72*:1353, 1956.

Brack, C. B., Townsend, L., and Burns, B. C.: Prognostic factors in radioresistant cervical cancer. Obstet. Gynecol., *16*:1, 1960.

Broders, A. C.: Grading of carcinoma. Minn. Med., *8*:726, 1925.

Brunschwig, A., and Daniel, W.: Surgical treatment of cancer of the cervix uteri. Am. J. Obstet. Gynecol., *75*:875, 1958.

Burghardt, E., and Holzer, E.: Diagnosis and treatment of microinvasive carcinoma of the cervix uteri. Obstet. Gynecol., *49*:641, 1977.

Bushnell, L. F.: Prevention of complications of cervical conization. Obstet. Gynecol., *22*:190, 1963.

Carrow, L. A., and Greene, R. R.: Epithelia of pregnant cervix. Am. J. Obstet. Gynecol., *61*:237, 1951.

Claiborne, H. A., Thornton, W. N., and Wilson, L. A.: Pelvic lymphadenectomy for carcinoma of the uterine cervix. Am. J. Obstet. Gynecol., *80*:672, 1960.

Creadick, R. N.: Carcinoma of cervical stump. Am. J. Obstet. Gynecol., *75*:565, 1958.

Davis, H. J., and Jones, H. W., Jr.: Population screening for cancer of the cervix with irrigation smears. Am. J. Obstet. Gynecol., *96*:605, 1966.

Davis, H. J., Aurelian, L., and Royston, I.: Antibody to genital herpes simplex virus: association with cervical atypia and carcinoma in situ. J. Natl. Cancer Inst., *45*:455, 1970.

Diddle, A. W., Sholes, D. M., Jr., Hollingsworth, J., and Kinlaw, S.: Cervical carcinoma: cancer cells in the circulating blood. Am. J. Obstet. Gynecol., *78*:582, 1959.

Dilts, P. V., Elesh, R. H., and Greene, R. R.: Reevaluation of four quadrant punch biopsies of the cervix. Am. J. Obstet. Gynecol., *90*:961, 1964.

Epperson, J. W. W., Hellman, L. M., and Galvin, G. E.: Morphologic changes in cervix during pregnancy, including intraepithelial carcinoma. Am. J. Obstet. Gynecol., 61:50, 1951.

Fayemi, A. O., Ali, M., and Evalyane, V. B.: Müllerian adenosarcoma of the uterine cervix. Am. J. Obstet. Gynecol., 130:734, 1978.

Figge, D. C., de Alvarez, R. R., Brown, D. V., and Fullington, W. R.: Long-range studies of the biologic behavior of the human uterine cervix. Am. J. Obstet. Gynecol., 84:638, 1962.

Foote, F. W., and Stewart, F. W.: Anatomical distribution of intra-epithelial epidermoid carcinomas of cervix. Cancer, 1:431, 1948.

Fricke, R. E., Soule, E. H., and Craig, R. M.: Adenoacanthoma of the uterine cervix. J. Am. Geriat. Soc., 4:113, 1956.

Friedell, G. H., Hertig, A. J., and Younge, P. S.: Carcinoma in Situ of the Uterine Cervix. Springfield, Ill., Charles C Thomas, 1960.

Gagnon, F.: Etiology and prevention of cancer of the cervix of the uterus. Am. J. Obstet. Gynecol., 60:516, 1950.

Galvin, G. A., Jones, H. W., and TeLinde, R. W.: Basal cell hyperactivity in cervical biopsies. Am. J. Obstet. Gynecol., 70:808, 1955.

Genadry, R., Olson, J., Parmley, T., and Woodruff, J. D.: The morphology of the earliest invasive cell in low genital tract epidermoid neoplasia. Obstet. Gynecol., 51:718, 1978.

Glucksman, A.: Role of tumor bed in the treatment of squamous-cell cancers by irradiation. J. Obstet. Gynaecol. Brit. Emp., 57:322, 1950.

Graham, J. B., Graham, R. M., and Liu, W.: Prognosis in cancer of the cervix (the sensitization response). Surg. Gynecol. Obstet., 99:555, 1954.

Greene, R. R., and Peckham, B. M.: Preinvasive cancer of the cervix and pregnancy. Am. J. Obstet. Gynecol., 75:551, 1958.

Greene, R. R., et al.: Preinvasive carcinoma of the cervix during pregnancy. Surg. Gynecol. Obstet., 96:71, 1953.

Gusberg, S. B., and Guttman, R.: Pelvic lymph node dissection following radiotherapy. Am. J. Obstet. Gynecol., 76:629, 1958.

Hart, W. R., and Norris, H. J.: Mesonephric adenocarcinomas of the cervix. Cancer, 29:106, 1972.

Heins, H. C., Jr., Dennis, E. J., and Pratt-Thomas, H. R.: Possible role of smegma in carcinoma of the cervix. Am. J. Obstet. Gynecol., 76:726, 1958.

Henriksen, E.: The lymphatic spread of carcinoma of the cervix and body of the uterus. Am. J. Obstet. Gynecol., 58:924, 1949.

Jimerson, G. K., and Merrill, J. A.: Cancer and dysplasia of the post-hysterectomy vaginal cuff. Gynecol. Oncol., 4:328, 1976.

Jones, H. E.: Cervical epithelial changes over a thirteen-year period terminating in epidermoid carcinoma. Am. J. Obstet. Gynecol., 60:1369, 1950.

Jones, H. W., Jr., Goldberg, B., Davis, H. J., and Burns, B. C., Jr.: Cellular changes in vaginal and buccal smears after radiation: index of radiocurability of carcinoma of cervix. Am. J. Obstet. Gynecol., 78:1083, 1959.

Jones, H. W., Jr., Katayama, K. P., Stafl, A., and Davis, H. J.: Chromosomes of cervical atypia, carcinoma in situ and epidermoid carcinoma of the cervix. Obstet. Gynecol., 30:790, 1967.

Julian, C., and Woodruff, J. D.: Multiple anaplasias in the lower genital canal. Am. J. Obstet. Gynecol., 95:681, 1966.

Kaminetzky, H. A., and Swerdlow, M.: Podophyllin and the mouse cervix: assessment of carcinogenic potential. Am. J. Obstet. Gynecol., 93:486, 1965.

Kelly, J. W. M., Parsons, L., Friedell, G. H., and Sommers, S. C.: A pathologic study in 55 autopsies after radical surgery for cancer of the cervix. Surg. Gynecol. Obstet., 110:423, 1960.

Kistner, R. W., Gonback, A. C., and Smith, S. V.: Cervical carcinoma in pregnancy. Obstet. Gynecol., 9:554, 1957.

Kjorstad, K.: Carcinoma of the cervix in the young patient. Obstet. Gynecol., 50:28, 1977.

Kolstad, P.: Carcinoma of cervix, stage Ia. Am. J. Obstet. Gynecol., 104:1015, 1969.

Kolstad, P., and Klem, V.: Long-term follow-up of 1121 cases of carcinoma in situ. Obstet. Gynecol., 48:125, 1976.

Kolstad, P., and Stafl, A.: Atlas of Colposcopy. Baltimore, University Park Press, 1972.

Koss, J., and Wolinska, J.: Trichomonas vaginalis cervicitis and its relationship to cervical cancer: a histocytological study. Cancer, 12:1171, 1959.

Koss, L. G., and Durfee, G. R.: Cytologic and pathologic study of koilocytotic atypia. Ann. N.Y. Acad. Sci., 63:1245, 1956.

Krieger, J. S., and McCormack, L. J.: Conservative treatment for intraepithelial cancer. Am. J. Obstet. Gynecol., 76:312, 1958.

Lambert, B., and Woodruff, J. D.: Spinal cell atypia of the cervix—a clinico-pathological study. Cancer, 16:1141, 1963.

Marcus, S. L.: Multiple squamous cell carcinomas involving the cervix, vagina, and vulva: the theory of multicentric origin. Am. J. Obstet. Gynecol., 80:802, 1960.

Martzloff, K. H.: Cancer of cervix uteri. A pathological and clinical study, with particular reference to the relative malignancy of the neoplastic process as indicated by the predominant type of cancer cell. Bull. Johns Hopkins Hosp., 34:141, 184, 1923.

Martzloff, K. H.: Epidermoid carcinoma of the cervix uteri. Am. J. Obstet. Gynecol., 16:578, 1928.

Martzloff, K. H.: Recognition of early manifestations of cervical carcinoma. J.A.M.A., 111:1921, 1938.

Martzloff, K. H.: Cancer of the cervix. Some fundamental considerations. West. J. Surg., 53:255, 1945.

McKay, D. G., Hertig, A. T., and Younge, P. A.: Carcinoma in situ. J. Int. Coll. Surg., 21:212, 1954.

Melnick, J. L., and Rawls, W. E.: Herpesvirus in induction of cervical carcinoma. Hosp. Pract. 4:37, 1969.

Meyer, R.: Basis of histologic diagnosis of cervical carcinoma, and similar lesions. Surg. Gynecol. Obstet., 73:14, 1941.

Meyer, R.: Histological diagnosis of early cervical carcinoma. Surg. Gynecol. Obstet., 73:129, 1941.

Mikuta, J. J., and Celebre, J. A.: Adenocarcinoma of the cervix. Obstet. Gynecol., 33:753, 1969.

Morris, J. McL., and Meigs, J. V.: Carcinoma of cervix. Statistical evaluation of 1938 cases and results of treatment. Surg. Gynecol. Obstet., 90:135, 1950.

Mussey, E., Soule, E. H., and Welch, J. S.: Microinvasive carcinoma of the cervix. Am. J. Obstet. Gynecol., 104:738, 1969.

Nesbitt, R. E. L.: Basal cell hyperactivity in the pregnant cervix. Obstet. Gynecol., 6:239, 1955.

Nesbitt, R. E. L., Jr., and Stein, A. A.: Histochemical evaluation of carcinoma in situ of cervix uteri. Surg. Gynecol. Obstet., 107:161, 1958.

Norris, H. J., and Taylor, H. B.: Polyps of the vagina—a

benign lesion resembling sarcoma botryoides. Cancer, 19:227, 1966.

Novak, E. R.: Radioresistant cervical cancer. Obstet. Gynecol., 4:251, 1954.

Novak, E. R., and Galvin, G. A.: Mistakes in interpretation of intraepithelial carcinoma. Am. J. Obstet. Gynecol., 62:1079, 1952.

Novak, E. R., and Villa Santa, U.: Factors influencing the ratio of uterine cancer in a community. J.A.M.A., 174:1395, 1960.

Parker, R. T., Cuyler, W. K., Kaufmann, L. A., Canter, B., Thomas, W. L., Craedick, R. N., Turner, V. H., Peete, C. H., and Chenny, W. B.: Intraepithelial (Stage 0) cancer of the cervix. Am. J. Obstet. Gynecol., 80:693, 1960.

Peightal, T. C., Brandes, W. W., Crawford, D. B., Jr., and Dakin, E. S.: Conservative treatment of carcinoma in situ at the cervix. Am. J. Obstet. Gynecol., 69:547, 1955.

Pemberton, F. A., and Smith, G. V.: Early diagnosis and prevention of carcinoma of cervix. Am. J. Obstet. Gynecol., 17:265, 1929.

Petersen, O.: Spontaneous course of cervical precancerous conditions. Am. J. Obstet. Gynecol., 72:1063, 1956.

Peyton, F. W., and Rosen, N. A.: Cervical cauterization and carcinoma of cervix. Am. J. Obstet. Gynecol., 86:111, 1963.

Plate, W. P.: Carcinoma of mesonephric duct (in adults and children). Gynaecologia, 130:203, 1950.

Prystowsky, H., and Brack, C. B.: Carcinoma of the cervix in pregnancy. Obstet. Gynecol., 7:522, 1955.

Rainey, R.: Association of lymphogranuloma inguinale and cancer. Surgery, 35:221, 1954.

Rewell, R. E.: Ethnological factors in the etiology of cancer of the uterine cervix. J. Obstet. Gynaecol. Brit. Emp., 64:821, 1957.

Richart, R. M.: A clinical staining test for the in vivo delineation of dysplasia and carcinoma in situ. Am. J. Obstet. Gynecol., 86:703, 1963.

Richart, R. M.: Natural history of cervical intraepithelial neoplasia. Clin. Obstet. Gynecol., 10:748, 1967.

Rutledge, F. N., and Fletcher, G. H.: Lymphadenectomy after supervoltage irradiation. Am. J. Obstet. Gynecol., 76:321, 1958.

Schauenstein, W.: Histologische Untersuchungen über atypisches Plattenepithel an der Portio und an der Innenfläche der Cervix. Arch. Gynäk., 85:576, 1908.

Schiller, W.: Early diagnosis of carcinoma of cervix. Surg. Gynecol. Obstet., 56:210, 1933.

Schiller, W.: Untersuchungen zur Entstehung der Geschwülste. 1. Teil. Collumcarcinomen des Uterus. Virchow's Arch., 263:279, 1927.

Schottländer, W., and Kermauner, F.: Zur Kenntnis des Uteruskarzinons. Berlin, S. Karger, 1912.

Schulman, H., and Cavanagh, D.: Intraepithelial carcinoma of cervix. The predictability of residual carcinoma in the uterus from the microscopic study of the margins of the cone biopsy specimen. Cancer, 14:795, 1961.

Selzer, I., and Nelson, H. M.: Benign papilloma (polypoid tumor) of the cervix uteri in children. Am. J. Obstet. Gynecol. 84:165, 1962.

Silbar, E. L., and Woodruff, J. D.: Evaluation of biopsy, cone and hysterectomy in intraepithelial carcinoma of the cervix. Obstet. Gynecol., 27:89, 1966.

Solto, L. S. J., Graham, J. B., and Pickner, J. W.: Postmortem findings in cancer of the cervix. Am. J. Obstet. Gynecol., 80:791, 1960.

Stafl, A., Dohnal, V., and Linhartova, A.: Über kolposkopische, histologische und Gefassbefunde an der krankhaft veranderten portio. Geburtshilfe Frauenheilkd., 5:437, 1963.

Stevenson, C. S., and Scipiades, E., Jr.: Noninvasive potential "carcinoma" of cervix. Surg. Gynecol. Obstet., 66:822, 1938.

Stoll, P.: Carcinoma of Gartner duct in 15 year old girl (cervix). Geburtshilfe Frauenheilkd., 10:219, 1950.

Tarlowska, L., et al.: Comparison of the FIGO and TNM staging systems for uterine cervix cancer based on classification of 1693 cases. Gynecol. Oncol., 4:270, 1976.

Tchertkoff, V., and Sedlis, A.: Cylindroma of the cervix. Am. J. Obstet. Gynecol., 84:749, 1962.

TeLinde, R. W., and Galvin, G.: Minimum histological changes in biopsies to justify diagnosis of cervical cancer. Am. J. Obstet. Gynecol., 48:774, 1944.

TeLinde, R. W., Galvin, G. A., and Jones, H. W.: Therapy of carcinoma in situ: implications from study of its life history. Am. J. Obstet. Gynecol., 74:792, 1957.

Towne, J. E.: Carcinoma of cervix in nulliparous and celibate women. Am. J. Obstet. Gynecol., 69:606, 1955.

Tremblay, P. C., Latour, J. P., and Dodds, J. R.: Adenocarcinoma of the cervix uteri. Obstet. Gynecol., 15:299, 1960.

Van Nagell, J. R., Donaldson, F. S., Parker, J. C., VanDyke, A. H., and Wood, E. G.: Prognostic significance of cell type and lesion size in patients with cervical cancer treated by radical surgery. Gynecol. Oncol., 5:143, 1977.

Wall, J. A., Mastrovito, R., and Earl, D. M.: Team approach in cervical neoplasia. Am. J. Obstet. Gynecol., 75:606, 1958.

Waters, E. G.: Carcinoma of the cervix in a seven months old infant. Am. J. Obstet. Gynecol., 39:1055, 1940.

Weiner, I., Burke, L., and Goldberger, M. A.: Carcinoma of cervix in Jewish women. Am. J. Obstet. Gynecol., 61:418, 1951.

Wentz, W. B., and Reagen, J. W.: Survival in cervical cancer with respect to cell type. Cancer, 12:384, 1959.

Wespi, H.: Early Carcinoma of Uterine Cervix. New York, Grune and Stratton, 1949.

Wheeless, C. R., Jr., Graham, R., and Graham, J. B.: Adenoepidermoid carcinoma of the cervix. Obstet. Gynecol., 35:928, 1970.

Wilbanks, G. D.: Tissue culture in early cervical neoplasia. Obstet. Gynecol. Surv., 24:804, 1969.

Woodruff, J. D., and Mattingly, R. F.: Epithelial changes preceding spinal cell carcinoma of the cervix uteri. Am. J. Obstet. Gynecol., 77:977, 1959.

Woodruff, J. D., and Williams, T. J., Jr.: Multiple sites of anaplasia in the lower genital canal. Am. J. Obstet. Gynecol., 84:724, 1963.

Wynder, E. L., Cornfield, J., Schroff, P. O., and Doraiswami, K. R.: Environmental factors in carcinoma of the cervix. Am. J. Obstet. Gynecol., 68:1016, 1954.

Wynder, E. L., Mantel, N., and Lickliden, S. G.: Statistical considerations on circumcision and cervical cancer. Am. J. Obstet. Gynecol., 79:1026, 1960.

Younge, P. A.: Cancer of the uterine cervix (a preventable disease). Obstet. Gynecol., 10:496, 1957.

Younge, P. A., Hertig, A. T., and Armstrong, D.: A study of 135 cases of carcinoma in situ of cervix at free hospital for women. Am. J. Obstet. Gynecol., 58:867, 1949.

Chapter 6

ENDOCRINOLOGY OF THE ENDOMETRIUM AND OVARY

One should not attempt to evaluate the histology of the endometrium without correlating the interrelated functions of the ovary, the pituitary, and the hypothalamus. Although the exact function of the hypothalamus is not understood, it is generally accepted that there is a single releasing factor for each anterior pituitary hormone except prolactin. Yen states that only the LH releasing factor is valid. The existence of a separate FSH factor has not been established. Both positive and negative feedback mechanisms are operational, and the recent study by Van de Wiele elaborates on neurohormonal functions.

Figure 6–1A portrays diagrammatically the important pituitary-ovarian-endometrial relationships, and the reader should keep this in mind while reading the following text. Illustrated in Figure 6–1B is the action of the hypothalamic LH releasing hormone (LRH), which modulates pituitary function directly, by virtue of varied feedback mechanisms. The term Gr-RH, as utilized by some (Homburg et al.) seems more cumbersome than LRH.

The gynecologist designates the first day of menstrual bleeding as day 1 of the cycle. As desquamation of the functional zone (upper two thirds) of the endometrium is occurring, there begins secretion of the first of the important pituitary substances, the follicle-stimulating hormone (FSH), which leads to production of the two important ovarian hormones, estrogen and progesterone.

OVARIAN HORMONES

ESTROGEN

FSH has a very definite effect on the ovary, which responds by maturation of a number of the primordial follicles. As this occurs there is increasing secretion of *estrogenic substances*. It is generally accepted that the theca cell is responsible for the production of estrogen, although Falck, using intraocular transplant in animals, has indicated that the proximity of granulosa cells is necessary. Such observations have been confirmed by histochemical studies. The chief forms of estrogen found in the human body are estradiol, estrone, and estriol, although there are many other variants. It is believed that FSH requires small amounts of the *luteinizing hormone (LH)* to effect estrogen production from the follicular theca cell. At the same time, estrogen tends to facilitate production of LH with suppression of FSH just prior to ovulation.

The primary effect of estrogens is to stimulate the growth of the genital tissues, and this is evidenced by the marked increase in the height of the endometrium during the proliferative or nonsecretory phase of the cycle. A similar effect is exerted on the tubal and vaginal epithelia as well as on various extragenital tissues such as breast and bone. In addition to the natural C_{18} estrogens, of which there are many commercial varieties that need not be mentioned by name, there

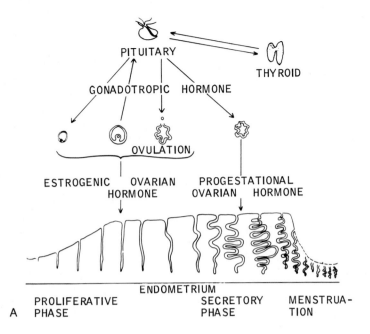

Hypothalamic-pituitary-
ovarian axis

Figure 6–1. *A*, Pituitary-ovarian-endometrial relationships. *B*, Hypothalamic relationships to events in *A*. (*B*, from M. Taymor: J. Reprod. Endocrinol. Courtesy of MedCom, Inc.)

are a number of other synthetic substances that are potently estrogenic, although chemically they are unrelated to the C_{18} steroids. Chief among these is diethylstilbestrol, which is in wide usage because it is quite inexpensive.

Somewhere at midcycle (in the normally menstruating woman generally between day 9 and day 18) ovulation occurs. The precise mechanism is still uncertain, but various pituitary gonadotropins are certainly instrumental in its production. A luteinizing hormone, LH, is probably influenced by estrogen produced by the developing follicles. It would seem that gonadotropic FSH and LH are produced, with ovulation occurring when there is an optimal ratio between these two trophic substances. As noted earlier, the hypothalamus is of extreme importance in the production of ovulation by virtue of certain neural *releasing factors* which govern FSH and LH production; these in turn are motivated by ovarian function and by reciprocal feedback mechanisms. In any case, there are many uncertainties in the ovulatory process.

PROGESTERONE

Whatever the mechanism, ovulation takes place, and the ovum is extruded from the surface of the ovary. Normally this occurs only from a single follicle, and the other developing follicles slowly become atrophic as they undergo the process called *atresia folliculi*. From the site in the follicle at which the egg was extruded there begins formation of the corpus luteum, which is the source of the second of the ovarian hormones, *progesterone.*

Progesterone is produced mainly by the granulosa cells, which have undergone lutein changes. Indeed, it has been suggested that progesterone formation occurs even prior to ovulation, at which stage of the cycle the granulosa cells do not have a discrete blood supply. Consequently, any progesterone produced would be passed through the theca interna zone, where it is converted into estrogen. Following ovulation, however, the vascular system of the theca interna invades the luteinized granulosa cells, carrying into the blood the progesterone that has now been biosynthesized to estrogen. However, estrogen is still produced by the other follicles as well as by portions of the corpus luteum.

Progesterone is a C_{21} steroid, and represents an initial step in the degradation of cholesterol. Other organs, such as the adrenal cortex and the placenta, also share in the production of progesterone. Progesterone is excreted in the urine in the form of pregnanediol, and assay of this is sometimes of clinical importance if one appreciates the fact that only a small portion (less than 25 per cent) of progesterone is excreted in such fashion.

While estrogen should be thought of as a growth hormone, progesterone is predominantly a secretory hormone, and following ovulation, the endometrium presents a secretory or progestational phase. Increasing amounts of glycogen and glycoprotein are liberated from the cells lining the epithelial glands into the gland lumina, and this glycogen may be detected by suitable stains. The characteristic changes of the progestational phase of the cycle, as noted in Chapter 7, result from the sustained stimulus of the ovarian steroids. As their blood level increases, there is a subsequent reciprocal inhibition of the gonadotropins, and this "feedback mechanism" leads to increasing involution of the corpus luteum, a decrease in the ovarian hormones, and ultimate withdrawal bleeding. In the event of pregnancy it is, of course, progesterone that is responsible for the characteristic decidual reaction which is merely an exaggerated progestational effect.

There is a difference of opinion regarding the effect of progesterone on the myometrium. Although many believe that progesterone is the normal inhibitor of the characteristic contractility of the uterine musculature, as indicated by Reynolds, there are an increasing number of investigators who have produced evidence that progesterone has no such inhibiting effect. It is, however, an inhibitor of ovulation, which does not occur as long as there is a normally functioning corpus luteum. In the rabbit it is absolutely essential to the maintenance of pregnancy in its early stage, but in the human it is certainly not indispensable, although it is undoubtedly of considerable importance from this standpoint. The recent study by Csapo and Pulkinnen would seem to substantiate this.

ANDROGENS

It is also well established that certain androgenic substances are produced by the normal female gonad. Rough estimation of these is sometimes possible by determination of the 17-ketosteroids found in the urine. It is important to emphasize that the most potently virilizing androgen, testosterone, is not a 17-ketosteroid, although it is partially excreted as such. Thus, in many cases of clinical virilism, the level of 17-ketosteroids may be quite normal if the androgen concerned is testosterone, whereas no virilism may be apparent with extremely high levels of 17-ketosteroid (when weak metabolites are present). Androgens are also produced by the adrenal cortex, but an increased level of 17-ketosteroids, if produced by adrenal cortical activity, is generally suppressed by use of dexamethasone, except in cases of an adrenal tumor.

While increased androgen production is more common in such abnormal conditions as the Stein-Leventhal syndrome and arrhenoblastoma, normal adult ovaries do produce a certain amount of androgenic substances. An excellent review by Jeffcoate summarizes rather extensively the biochemical and endocrinologic background of the bisexual potentialities of the ovary, and this has been reaffirmed by numerous other histochemical and biochemical studies.

HISTOCHEMICAL STUDY OF THE ENDOMETRIUM

It is becoming increasingly apparent to all gynecologic pathologists that study of hematoxylin-eosin preparations is often insufficient for adequate distinction and evaluation of tissues. Consideration of their various biochemical properties with differential stains capable of detecting certain histochemical characteristics is often necessary.

Appropriate techniques have led to the determination of a great many important metabolites of the endometrium at various stages of the menstrual cycle. Since these sequential changes involve glands, stroma, lining epithelium, and blood vessels in differential fashion, it would seem unwise to attempt a complete discussion of the many phases of histochemistry. Instead, the interested reader is referred to the studies of McKay and coauthors, Atkinson and Gusberg, and Boutselis and associates. The striking color plates of the last authors illustrate more vividly than words the precise results of their studies.

It is impossible to become involved in all of the ramifications of histochemistry and biochemical study of cell metabolism in this text. It is one of the most constantly changing facets of our specialty, and we have attempted to mention only a few of the many articles pertaining to it. Unfortunately, it would appear that there has been relatively little advancement in histochemical techniques in the last five years; it is to be hoped that this represents merely a temporary lull in what seemed an eminently promising area.

On the other hand, electron microscopy is becoming of increasing importance, and Ferenczy has contributed a number of studies of the endometrium. It seems unjustified to go into details about this highly specialized procedure.

HISTOCHEMICAL STUDY OF THE OVARY

Since it is desirable to consider ovarian stimulus and endometrial response together, it seems appropriate to consider certain histochemical features of the ovary here, although the histology of the ovary will be fully covered in Chapter 17. McKay and coworkers have performed extensive histochemical studies on the ovary at all stages of the cycle, and their preliminary work has provided a firm background for much of the recent application of biosynthetic properties. Their contributions have been concerned primarily with the close association of alkaline phosphatase and steroid activity, at the same time indicating certain histochemical similarities and differences between various steroid producing cells. Their observations seemed to indicate certain enzyme deficiencies as a probable cause of abnormal steroid function.

Their visionary work has been enlarged on by many biochemists who have pointed out certain biosynthetic pathways to the formation of the various ovarian hormones. Unquestionably the most popularly accepted scheme is that proposed by Smith and Ryan (Fig. 6–2). From cholesterol (derived from acetate) there are two alternate pathways (via pregnenolone or progesterone) by which testosterone may be produced. There is very possibly an equilibrium between this and the estrogenic hormones which may vary in certain physiologic and neoplastic disorders. Kase and Carter have suggested that in many instances the progesterone route is bypassed, with production of the end products via pregnenolone.

A comparison of normal ovaries and testes with abnormal gonads permits a semiquantitative estimate of the enzymatic reaction of certain component cells. Many previous authors have used these methods in studying

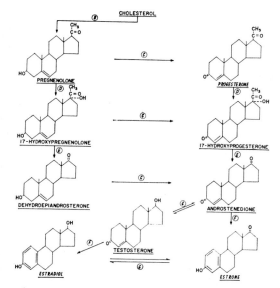

Figure 6–2. (Pathways of steroid biosynthesis in the ovary: *A*, Formation of sterol (cholesterol) from acetate; *B*, cleavage of cholesterol side chain—converts C_{27} to C_{21} compound; *C*, 3 β-ol dehydrogenase and Δ4,5-isomerase reaction; *D*, 17 α-hydroxylation; *E*, cleavage of side chain—converts C_{21} to C_{19}; *F*, aromatizing reaction; *G*, 17 β-ol dehydrogenase (reversible). (Courtesy of O. W. Smith and K. J. Ryan: Am. J. Obstet. Gynec., *84*:141, 1962.)

estrogenic ovarian tumors, and the usual techniques utilized have been reviewed by Woodruff and co-workers. Similar observations have been made on various *virilizing* neoplasms such as a Brenner tumor (Ullery et al.), a Krukenberg tumor (Ober), and others reported by Scully and Cohen. (These are more fully discussed with references in Chapter 28, but it seems that the ovarian stromal cell can be converted into either a theca-like (estrogenic) or Leydig-like (androgenic) cell by adjacent tumor. Scully and Cohen have published a very comprehensive summation of the behavior of certain ovarian stromal cells which are enzymatically active and are referred to as "enzymatically active stromal cells" (EASC). These are closely related if not identical to the luteinized thecal stromal cell. Deane and associates have also provided excellent references to histochemical study of cellular biosynthesis; Dorfman points out the probability that many other uncertain biosynthetic pathways to steroid formation probably exist.

By utilizing various substrates and by determining the reaction exhibited by normal cells of the testis and ovary, it would appear that this knowledge might be utilized to determine enzyme activity necessary to steroi-

dogenesis in certain equivocal cells in ovarian tumors or dysfunctions. Leventhal and Scommegna have contributed an excellent publication on histochemical techniques in evaluating possible steroidal function in a variety of tumors and abnormal conditions. As noted earlier, however, there have been disappointingly few new advances in the last 10 years.

Summary of Menstrual Endocrines

To summarize, the estrogenic hormone produced by the growing follicles brings about a steadily advancing proliferative phase in the endometrium. With the rupture of a follicle, the newly formed corpus luteum, through its secretion of both estrogen and progesterone, produces a still greater endometrial development, distinguished especially by increasing evidence of the secretory response evoked by the progesterone. The corpus luteum begins to retrogress, according to the results of many investigations, on about the twenty-second or twenty-third day of the cycle. The resulting withdrawal of the ovarian hormones is, as a matter of fact, believed to be the cause of the menstrual bleeding.

The mechanism whereby this is brought about is not yet entirely clear, though there is little doubt that the immediate factor is to be sought in the effect of these hormone changes upon the vascular apparatus of the endometrium. The studies of Markee and others have thrown much light upon this problem, indicating that the endometrial degeneration and desquamation of the bleeding phase are due to ischemia resulting from intense and prolonged vasoconstriction of the spiral arterioles of the endometrium.

Blood Supply of the Endometrium

This is furnished by two sets of arterioles: the *straight,* and the *spiral or coiled* (see Fig. 7–5). The former serve a merely nutritional function, but the latter, passing upward from the basalis well into the functionalis, play an important part in the physiologic and histologic cycle of the endometrium.

Through the study of endometrium that had been transplanted to the anterior chamber of the eye in monkeys, Markee has shown that the spiral arterioles undergo a periodic vasoconstriction and vasodilatation, producing the so-called "blushing-blanching" phenomenon, the pulsations alternating at intervals of 60 to 80 seconds.

As the cycle advances, the spiral arterioles lengthen more rapidly than the endometrium increases in thickness, so that the vessels accommodate themselves to the endometrium by increased coiling, which in the premenstrual period becomes so marked as to slow down the blood flow and bring about a stasis. It is the latter that Markee believes is responsible for the endometrial necrosis and the degenerative blood vessel changes that lead to hemorrhage by progressive ischemia and increased diapedesis. The possible contributing role of arteriovenous anastomoses is still a matter of dispute.

Shortly before the onset of menstrual bleeding, the vasodilatation gives way to an intense vasoconstriction, which some investigators believe is due to a toxic protein product which they call a euglobulin, although others describe a toxic factor designated as necrosin (Markee) or menotoxin. It should be added that the existence of such an agent must be regarded as rather nebulous, and some authors have flatly denied that it represents any specific entity. However, prostaglandin is important in inducing constriction, as noted below. The innervation of the endometrium is the subject of an extensive review by Dallenbeck and Vonderlin.

Depolymerization

Israel and co-workers believe that estrogen influences endometrial localization of certain hydrolytic enzymes which accumulate and ultimately lead to cell destruction and menstruation. Certain endometrial enzymes are enclosed in *lysosomes*—specific subcellular particles—and are inactive if the cell membrane is intact, but if released can destroy the cell. Estrogen is also responsible for deposition of glycogen and many acid mucopolysaccharides (AMPS).

The appearance of progesterone or a decrease in estrogen leads to synthesis of *prostaglandin,* which increases vasoconstriction and causes increased endometrial breakdown. There is a gradually increasing permeability of the lyosomal membrane, leading to release of the destructive hydrolases into the tissues, and this leads to endometrial breakdown and bleeding. This process of *depolymerization* is enormously complex, and any interested reader would do well to refer to the article of Israel and co-workers, who also attempt to explain the mechanism of dysfunctional uterine bleeding on this basis.

THE HORMONES OF PREGNANCY

It was pointed out many years ago by Zondek and Ascheim that even in early pregnancy the urine contains large amounts of a substance that has physiologic effects that in many ways parallel those of the pituitary hormones. The usual designation is human chorionic gonadotropic hormone (HCG). Detection of this is responsible for the many early immunologic tests for pregnancy that are now used; at the same time, quantitative measurement of this particular hormone is of extreme importance in the early detection of the hydatidiform mole and choriocarcinoma. It is now generally accepted that the cytotrophoblast (Langhans' cells) is the predecessor of the syncytiotrophoblast and produces HCG, although it may also be stored in the syncytium. Only a living, functioning trophoblast can produce HCG.

Like the pituitary sex hormones, the chorionic gonadotropins may be of dual nature, with both follicle-ripening and luteinizing components. It should be added, however, that some investigators at one time believed that the different effects of both the pituitary and the chorionic gonadotropic hormones represented only different manifestations of the activity of a single principle. Indeed, Goss and Lewis point out that purified preparations of LH and HCG are partially related antigens, but it was technically extremely difficult to obtain pure preparations of the respective gonadotropins. The main function of HCG is to maintain the corpus luteum through the first two or three months of pregnancy, by which time the placenta is "self-sufficient"; after this the level of HCG drops gradually.

That the trophoblast produces the gonadotropic hormone which finds its way into the urine is well established, and it has been possible to demonstrate the formation of this substance by trophoblast growth in tissue culture (Gey et al.). It is upon the presence of this trophoblastic or chorionic principle in the urine of pregnant women, even in the early weeks of gestation, that the validity of the various biologic tests of pregnancy depends. However, after about 60 days the level declines, so that a valid result should not be expected after 100 days. Aside from being useful in the diagnosis of pregnancy, these titers are of extreme importance in following women with trophoblastic disease (TRD). Immunoassays specific for the beta subunit (which eliminates any LH contaminant) is more precise and more accurate for lower levels. Finally, it has long been known that the placenta is the chief source of the large amounts of estrogenic hormone found throughout pregnancy. Even if the ovaries are removed in the early stages of pregnancy, the estrogenic hormone is still present in undiminished amount.

In the early stages of pregnancy, progesterone plays an important role in maintaining the nidation of the egg, and in some animals, especially the rabbit, this role is an absolutely indispensable one. In the human this does not seem to be true, as a considerable number of cases have been reported in which bilateral removal of the ovaries in early pregnancy has not been followed by abortion, though often it is.

It seems likely that there are certain estrogen receptors in the human endometrium, most apparent where there is a low level of endogenous estrogen. Henderson and Schalch indicate that these receptors are not demonstrable during pregnancy since all binding sites are occupied. However, progesterone receptions seem necessary for egg implantation (Baulieu).

THE ANOVULATORY CYCLE IN WOMEN

The fact that menstrual periods that are normal in character, amount, and rhythm may at times occur without the accompaniment of ovulation is now established beyond the shadow of a doubt. Frequently, however, there are disorders in duration, interval, and amount of bleeding. This was pointed out by Corner, who suggested that the anovulatory type of cycle seen so often in monkeys might perhaps be at times encountered also in the human female.

Opposed as this was to the then existing theory of menstruation, according to which ovulation is an absolutely essential part of the menstrual cycle, the correctness of Corner's view has now been fully established. This is not the place to review all the evidence now available. Suffice it to say, however, that the widely used diagnostic procedure of endometrial biopsy, when employed at the very onset of menstrual flow, has in many instances revealed an endometrium that shows not the slightest evidence of the secretory changes commonly accepted as the criterion of corpus luteum activity, and therefore of ovulation.

It would be unsafe to hazard any estimate as to the frequency of the anovulatory type of cycle in women. Certainly it is the unusual mechanism, the majority of menstrual cycles being of the ovulatory type. As a matter of fact, the problem has been studied chiefly in the relatively small group of women in whom a search is being made for the cause of existing sterility, and even in this group widely differing figures as to the incidence of the anovulatory cycle have been reported. Even in fertile women, however, and in those in whom sterility is not a consideration, as in young girls or perimenopausal women, there is evidence that the anovulatory mechanism is not rare. The recent widespread usage of basal temperature charts would suggest that certain women on occasion fail to ovulate although their general pattern is ovulatory. This seems well attested to by the occurrence of a flat temperature chart in normally menstruating groups of young student nurses, schoolgirls, and other control patients.

The menstrual phenomena with the anovulatory cycle are due to the functional activity of the follicle alone, instead of the sequential action of follicle and corpus luteum that characterizes the common biphasic type of cycle. The follicles advance to maturity or perhaps somewhat beyond, and then, instead of rupturing and extruding the ovum, they undergo degeneration, with cessation or sharp diminution of estrogen production.

It is this abrupt hormone deprivation that brings about bleeding after a considerable number of days, so that the rhythm of the flow, as well as its amount, may be quite like that of the ovulating woman. Such a cycle may therefore well be called, as it sometimes is, an incomplete one. Like dysfunctional bleeding (DFB), it is basically a disorder of ovulation, and must be of pituitary origin, though little is known about the immediate cause.

The endometrium in such cases, as might be expected, shows only various degrees of proliferative activity, with no evidence of secretory changes. Sometimes it resembles the preovulatory interval picture of the ovula-

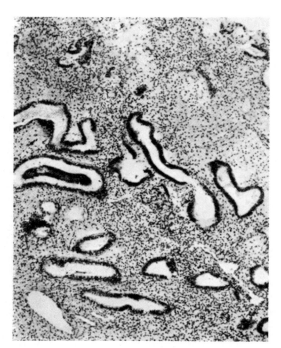

Figure 6–3. Anovulatory type of endometrium, obtained just before menstrual onset. Compare with usual premenstrual pattern.

tory cycle (Fig. 6–3). In other cases the growth effect of the estrogenic hormone has been carried farther, so that the premenstrual endometrium may show a well marked hyperplasia of the Swiss-cheese pattern, such as is seen so often in cases of DFB. The latter, therefore, represents only a pathologic exaggeration of the phenomena of the anovulatory cycle. The clinical severity of the bleeding rather than the histologic study would differentiate between the normal and the abnormal. In the same way, certain cases of functional menorrhagia may show a secretory endometrium, with only a quantitative abnormality of the factors concerned in the normal ovulatory type of cycle (Taw).

Some specialists regard the anovulatory cycle as pathologic because it represents the infrequent type; they argue that the periodic bleeding in such cases is not menstruation but pseudomenstruation. Those who hold this view urge that menstruation presupposes ovulation, corpus luteum formation, and predecidual changes in the endometrium. Such a limitation of the definition does not seem very sound.

The term menstruation is of very ancient vintage, the word "menstruous" being used a number of times even in the Bible, many centuries before anyone knew of ovulation or of hormones. The time-honored definition of menstruation is that it is a periodic physiologic bleeding from the uterine mucous membrane, and this would seem to apply regardless of the exact mechanism in the individual case. Childbirth is childbirth regardless of whether the mechanism is of the common vertex type, or, for example, by the much less common breech or face presentation.

INDUCTION OF OVULATION

Until recently there was no satisfactory agent for inducing ovulation. All previous endocrine methods of treating anovulatory bleeding consisted of providing hormonal hemostasis for the control of bleeding without incurring ovulation. Today, however, there are several agents which appear to be effective in instigating ovulation.

Clomiphene citrate (Clomid) is a synthetic nonsteroid analogue of chlorotrianisene (Tace), which is a long-acting estrogen. A variety of authors have utilized this in bleeding or sterility problems characterized by such forms of anovulation as the Stein-Leventhal syndrome and related disorders. There is still uncertainty as to the exact mechanism whereby clomiphene is effective. Its action appears to be at the hypothalamic-pituitary level, and most students think that it is antiestrogenic, although certain authors, such as Pildes, Marcus, and others, imply that in smaller dosage the effect is estrogenic. In any case, it seems to be quite effective in inducing ovulation by opposing estrogen and permitting gonadotropin stimulation of the ovary. Ovarian overstimulation with as many as 14 corpora lutea and massive ascites has been reported by Scommegna and Lash, and many of the publicized cases of multiple pregnancies have followed clomiphene therapy.

The endometrium will often show the same type of glandular-stromal disparity seen with birth control pills. The stroma is frequently a week or so more advanced than the glands, as with progesterone stimulation (Fig. 6–4). The recommended dosage of 50 mg. for 5 to 10 days is by no means standardized, but ovulation seems to occur frequently 7 to 10 days after inception of therapy. Clomiphene in larger, more prolonged dosage may be of importance in treating certain atypical endometrial hyperplasias, and

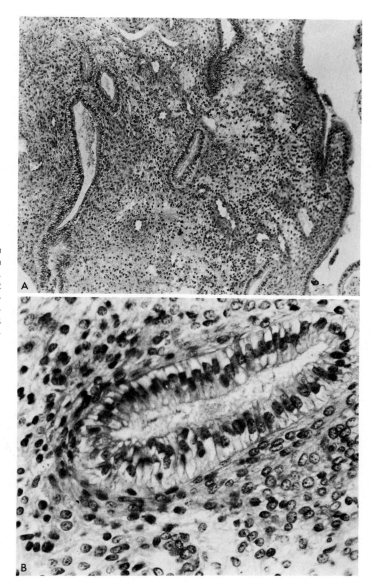

Figure 6–4. *A,* Postovulatory pattern with pronounced decidua-like changes in stroma following clomiphene therapy. *B,* High power of gland showing prominent vacuoles, but little tufting and budding. Clomiphene-induced changes seem less advanced in glands than in stroma. There is sometimes marked stratification of the surface epithelium.

even early adenocarcinomas, in the young woman.

Gonadotropins have in recent years been sufficiently purified so that they too have seemed to be useful in inaugurating ovulation, especially when there is an intrinsic pituitary defect. Most clinicians would of course prefer the less expensive clomiphene, but various combinations of pituitary and chorionic gonadotropins have been utilized by Gemzell and by Buxton and Hermann, as well as by various British authors. A substantial number of pregnancies have been reported. Human menopausal urine has been utilized to obtain the predominantly FSH fraction marketed under the name of Pergonal; the LH is more expensive and difficult to obtain, but sequential treatment with this following Pergonal administration is necessary to produce ovulation. Dosage is not standardized, and there is no place in this text for full discussion.

With *both ovulatory agents* it must be emphasized that superovulation and multiple pregnancies are common. Lutein cystic enlargement of the ovaries with occasional rupture represents a very real possible complication. The role of LRF as a therapeutic agent is uncertain at this time, but it will probably prove helpful in selected cases of amenorrhea.

Although it may seem that therapeutic

suggestions have no place in a pathology treatise, such details as these are almost indispensable for proper pathologic evaluation of a case. Charles has aptly commented on the iatrogenic patterns produced in the endometrium by various endogenous and exogenous agents. For example, if large theca-lutein cysts of the ovaries appear in the pathology laboratory, a much better interpretation will be forthcoming if the pathologist is cognizant of previous therapy.

PROGESTOGEN THERAPY

The up-to-date gynecologic pathologist must be familiar with the appearance of the endometrium as it is modified by therapeutic use of certain synthetic progestogens which have been widely utilized in the treatment of various functional and anatomic diseases of women. In the past, some occasionally exerted certain rather distressing virilizing effects. When used in the treatment of habitual or threatened abortion, the fetus was sufficiently virilized as to mimic true intersexuality, but this sequel rarely occurs today. Additional indications for the drugs, however, are such entities as dysfunctional uterine bleeding, primary dysmenorrhea, and, above all, inhibition of ovulation, for they are widely utilized as a contraceptive agent ("the pill"). They are also utilized in more sustained, long-range, and larger dose therapy for treatment in such diseases as endometriosis, and tend to incur very specific effects on the endometrium, although short-term cyclic therapy produces patterns not dissimilar to a normal progestational type of pattern.

A large number of combination steroids are available which may be given on a 20, 21, or 28 (21 active pills and 7 placebos) basis. A low estrogen content minimizes the possibility of thromboembolic complications. Use of sequential estrogen and progesterone has come into certain disfavor because of various complications in experimental animals; whether these are applicable to humans is questionable, although Silverberg and others have reported a number of "post-pill" (generally sequential) adenocarcinomas. Certain sequential pills have been taken off the market. Craig has discussed very adequately the pathology associated with birth control methods.

Prolonged large dosage of most progesto-gens tends to produce a profound decidual reaction on the part of the stroma, and indeed the main purpose of this drug in the treatment of endometriosis is to produce pseudopregnancy. Although there is an extensive decidua-like response of the stromal elements, there is, at the same time, a marked decrease in the glandular components up to a point of almost complete glandular exhaustion with nearly total disappearance of the endometrial glandular components (Fig. 6–5). This is a virtually constant finding in progestogen therapy for endometriosis. These steroids have also proved useful in actual treatment of recurrent endometrial carcinoma (see Chapter 9), and cause reversion of certain atypical endometria that closely mimic endometrial adenocarcinoma. The pathologist should certainly have knowledge of any prolonged steroid therapy before being called upon to make a diagnosis of any endometrium.

Even the relatively small dosage of progesterone utilized in the contraceptive pills seems to enhance the development of the stroma and retard the glands, producing a type of glandular-stromal disparity, although this is not so marked as with large dosage progesterone therapy for endometriosis. Indeed, we are classifying endometria having decidua-like stroma and exhausted or retarded glands as compatible with contraceptive pills; where there has been long-standing use of these steroids, the endometrium will show generalized atrophy.

Incidentally, the term "progestogen" is considered more appropriate than progestin, progesten, or gestogen by no less an authority than Dr. Willard Allen, who was instrumental in much of the early work in isolating progesterone as a specific endocrine agent. He has kindly consented to publication of his ideas.

POSTMENOPAUSAL OVARIAN FUNCTION

That there is evidence of postmenopausal estrogen production long after the cessation of menses is strongly indicated by a number of studies which note cytopathologic evidence of estrogen stimulation in the vaginal mucosa of aging women. McLennan and McLennan suggested that 40 per cent of postmenopausal women show moderate estrogenic activity for protracted periods of

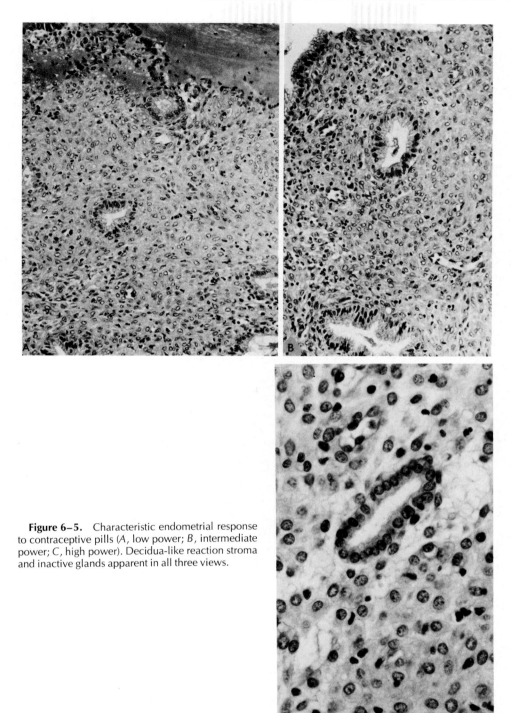

Figure 6–5. Characteristic endometrial response to contraceptive pills (*A*, low power; *B*, intermediate power; *C*, high power). Decidua-like reaction stroma and inactive glands apparent in all three views.

time as long as they live. The major source of this is probably the adrenal gland, and the androstenedione produced may be converted to other hormones. On occasion, however, the aging ovary may show evidence of endocrine activity.

By histochemical studies of the postmenopausal ovary, it has been found possible to demonstrate enzymatic activity suggestive of steroid function more than 25 years after the cessation of menstruation. The aging gonad, of course, harbors no follicles or cor-

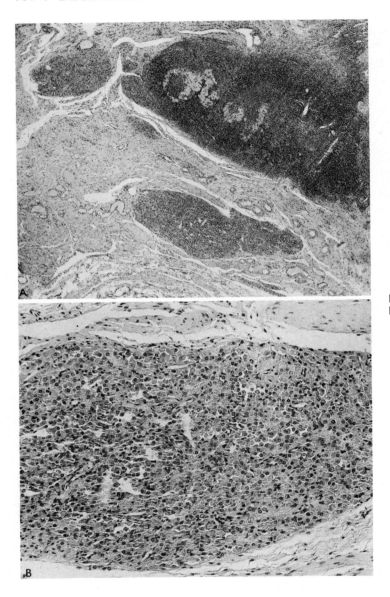

Figure 6–6. *A*, Characteristic cells in hilus near cortex. *B*, High power view of hilus cells.

pora lutea; the enzymatically active cells seem to be *hilus cells* (Fig. 6–6) and the *theca-like cells* of the ovarian stroma (Fig. 6–7).

The *hilus cells* behave histochemically like the androgen-producing interstitial cells of the testis, although the clinical effect is more apt to be associated with such conditions as endometrial hyperplasia (a presumed estrogen effect) and adenocarcinoma. The *stromal cell* also exhibits enzymatic activity suggesting steroid function of some type, although there is considerable difference from the true theca interna cell of the younger woman's ovarian follicle.

Enzymatic activity is found more commonly in ovaries removed because of such clinical abnormalities as hyperplasia or adenocarcinoma of the endometrium, but is not rare in the ostensibly normal woman whose ovaries are removed (for control study) at the time of vaginal hysterectomy because of prolapse with no evidence of an associated endocrinopathy. Correlation of the cytopathologic maturation index, the clinical status, and the histochemical activity has led us to deduce that the postmenopausal ovary may produce a mixture of estrogens and androgens, which might neutralize one another so that no overt endocrine effect is

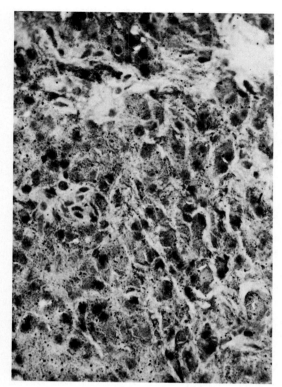

Figure 6–7. Fat stain of postmenopausal ovarian stroma showing high lipid content.

produced. This "neutral gender" does not, however, signify an ovary devoid of endocrine capabilities.

As Riley has indicated, there is a marked increase in HCG in the climacteric woman, and this may serve as the stimulus to increased hilar and stromal steroidogenesis. An admixture of androgens and estrogens would not appear to represent an unusual sequel in the normal ovary, and would serve as a ready explanation for the vagarious behavior and appearance of certain ovarian dysfunctions and tumors. For fuller details, the articles by Novak and associates and by Yen are recommended. As noted earlier, fresh ovarian tissue is frozen, after which cryostat sections are incubated with various substrates and an indicator dye. Enzyme activity may be demonstrated (rather than the steroid itself), but the presence of enzymatic histochemical activity in certain ovarian cells strongly suggests steroidal activity. Although absolute distinction between estrogen- and androgen-producing cells is not possible at present, there is additional biochemical evidence by Mattingly and Huang and by Plotz and co-workers that the

postmenopausal ovary manufactures androgen, which is converted to estrogen at other sites.

REFERENCES

Atkinson, W. B., and Gusberg, S. B.: Histochemical studies on abnormal growth of human endometrium; alkaline phosphatase in hyperplasia and adenocarcinoma. Cancer, 1:248, 1948.

Baulieu, E. E.: Steroid receptors and hormone receptivity. J.A.M.A., 234:404, 1975.

Boutselis, J. G., DeNeef, J. C., Ullery, J. C., and George, O. T.: Histochemical and cytologic observations in the normal human endometrium. Obstet. Gynecol., 21:423, 1963.

Buxton, C. L., and Hermann, W.: Induction of ovulation in the human with human gonadotropins. Am. J. Obstet. Gynecol., 81:584, 1961.

Charles, D.: Iatrogenic endometrial patterns. J. Clin. Pathol., 17:205, 1964.

Corner, G. W.: Fate of the corpus luteum in rhesus monkey. Contr. Embryol., 192; 87, 1941.

Craig, J. M.: The pathology of birth control. Arch. Pathol., 99:233, 1975.

Csapo, A. I., and Pulkinnen, M.: Indispensability of the human corpus luteum. Obstet. Gynecol. Surv., 33:69, 1978.

Czernobilsky, B., et al.: Effect of intrauterine device on histology of endometrium. Obstet. Gynecol., 45:64, 1975.

Dallenbeck, F. D., and Vonderlin, D.: Innervation of the endometrium. Arch. Gynäk., 215:365, 1973.

Deane, H. W., Lobel, B. L., and Romney, S. L.: Enzymic histochemistry of normal human ovaries of the menstrual cycle, pregnancy, and the early puerperium. Am. J. Obstet. Gynecol., 83:281, 1962.

Dorfman, R. I.: Steroid hormones in gynecology. Obstet. Gynecol. Surv., 18:65, 1963.

Falck, B.: Site of production of estrogen in rat ovary as studied in micro-transplants. Acta Physiol. Scand. (Suppl. 163), 47:1, 1959.

Ferenczy, A.: Cytodynamics of human endometrial regeneration. I. Scanning electron microscopy. II. Transmission electron microscopy and histochemistry. III. Experimental endometrial regeneration. Am. J. Obstet. Gynecol., 124:64, 1976; 124:528, 1976; 128:536, 1977.

Gemzell, C. A.: The induction of ovulation in the human by human pituitary gonadotropin. In Control of Ovulation. C. A. Villee (Ed.). New York, Pergamon Press, 1961.

Gemzell, C., and Roos, P.: Pregnancies following treatment with human gonadotrophins. Am. J. Obstet. Gynecol., 94:490, 1966.

Gey, G. O., Seegar, G. E., and Hellman, L. M.: Production of gonadotrophic substance (prolan) by placental cells in tissue culture. Science, 88:306, 1938.

Goss, D. A., and Lewis, J., Jr.: Immunologic differentiation of luteinizing hormone and human chorionic gonadotropin in compounds of high purity. Endocrinology, 74:83, 1964.

Greenblatt, R. B., et al.: Steroid production in postmenopausal woman. Obstet. Gynecol., 47:383, 1975.

Hall, J. E.: Alkaline phosphatase in human endometrium. Am. J. Obstet. Gynecol., 60:212, 1950.

Henderson, S. R., and Schalch, D. S.: Estrogen receptors in the human uterus. Am. J. Obstet. Gynecol., *112*:762, 1972.

Homburg, R., et al.: The hypothalamus as regulator of reproductive function. Obstet. Gynecol. Surv., *31*:485, 1976.

Israel, R., Mishell, D. R., and Labudovich, M.: Mechanisms of normal and dysfunctional uterine bleeding. Clin. Obstet. Gynecol., *13*:386, 1970.

James, V. H. T.: The excretion of individual 17-ketosteroids by normal females. J. Endocrinol., *22*:195, 1961.

Jeffcoate, T. N. A.: The androgenic ovary, with special reference to the Stein-Leventhal syndrome. Am. J. Obstet. Gynecol., *88*:143, 1964.

Kantor, H. I., and Kamholz, J. H.: Cyclic endometrial changes without menstruation. Fertil. Steril., *6*:353, 1955.

Kase, N., and Conrad, S. H.: Steroid synthesis in abnormal ovaries. Am. J. Obstet. Gynecol., *90*:1251, 1964.

Kistner, R. W.: Induction of ovulation with clomiphene citrate (clomid). Obstet. Gynecol. Surv., *20*:873, 1965.

Leventhal, M. L., and Scommegna, A.: Multiglandular aspects of the Stein-Leventhal syndrome. Am. J. Obstet. Gynecol., *87*:445, 1963.

Marcus, S. L.: Biologic effects of clomiphene citrate in the castrated rhesus monkey. Am. J. Obstet. Gynecol., *93*:990, 1965.

Markee, J. E.: Morphological basis for menstrual bleeding. Anat. Rec., *94*:481, 1946.

Mattingly, R. F., and Huang, W. N.: Steroidogenesis of the menopausal and postmenopausal gonad. Am. J. Obstet. Gynecol., *103*:679, 1969.

McKay, D. G., Hertig, A. T., Bardawil, W. A., and Velardo, J. T.: Histochemical observations on endometrium; normal endometrium. Obstet. Gynecol., 8:22, 1956. Histochemical observations on endometrium; abnormal endometrium. Obstet. Gynecol., 8:140, 1956.

McLennan, M. T., and McLennan, C. E.: Estrogenic status of menstruating and menopausal women assessed by cervico-vaginal smears. Obstet. Gynecol., 37:325, 1971.

Meyer, R.: Anovulatory cycle and menstruation. Am. J. Obstet. Gynecol., *51*:39, 1946.

Novak, E. R.: The endometrium. Clin. Obstet. Gynecol., *17*:31, 1974.

Novak, E. R., Goldberg, B., Jones, G. S., and O'Toole, R. V.: Enzyme histochemistry of the postmenopausal ovary associated with normal and abnormal endometrium. Am. J. Obstet. Gynecol., *93*:669, 1965.

Pildes, R. B.: Induction of ovulation with clomiphene. Am. J. Obstet. Gynecol., *91*:466, 1965.

Plotz, E. J., et al.: Enzymatic activities related to steroidogenesis in postmenopausal ovaries of patients with and without endometrial carcinoma. Am. J. Obstet. Gynecol., *99*:182, 1967.

Reynolds, S. R. M.: Physiology of the Uterus. New York, Paul B. Hoeber, 1939.

Riley, G. M.: Endocrinology of the climacteric. Clin. Obstet. Gynecol., *7*:432, 1964.

Scommegna, A., and Lash, S. R.: Ovarian overstimulation, massive ascites, and singleton pregnancy after clomiphene. J.A.M.A., *207*:753, 1969.

Scully, R. E., and Cohen, R. B.: Oxidative-enzyme activity in normal and pathological human ovaries. Obstet. Gynecol., *24*:667, 1964.

Song, J., Mark, M. S., and Lawler, M. P.: Endometrial changes in women receiving oral contraceptives. Am. J. Obstet. Gynecol., *107*:717, 1970.

Stewart, H. L.: Hormone secretion by human placenta grown in eyes of rabbits. Am. J. Obstet. Gynecol., *61*:990, 1951.

Sturgis, S. H.: Arias-Stella phenomena. Am. J. Obstet. Gynecol., *116*:589, 1973.

Taw, R. L.: Secretory endometrium in menstrual disorders. Am. J. Obstet. Gynecol., *122*:490, 1975.

Van de Wiele, R. L.: Neurohormonal control of gonadotropic secretion. Am. J. Obstet. Gynecol., *124*:832, 1976.

Wallach, E. E.: Physiology of menstruation. Clin. Obstet. Gynecol., *13*:366, 1970.

Wiley, C. A., and Esterly, J. R.: Human corpus luteum. Am. J. Obstet. Gynecol., *125*:514, 76.

Woodruff, J. D., Williams, T. J., and Goldberg, B.: Hormone activity of the common ovarian neoplasm. Am. J. Obstet. Gynecol., *87*:679, 1963.

Yen, S. S. C.: Hypothalamic pituitary discharge. Reprod. Endocr. (MedCom), 1973, p. 15.

Yen, S. S. C.: The biology of menopause. J. Repr. Med., *18*:287, 1977.

Chapter 7

HISTOLOGY OF THE ENDOMETRIUM

The endometrium is the uterine mucous membrane above the level of the internal os; below this point the mucosa is termed the endocervical epithelium. This sharp distinction is predicated on the remarkable ability of the endometrium to respond in cyclic fashion to the ovarian hormones, with resultant monthly menstruation. One must not assume that the vaginal, cervical, and tubal epithelia necessarily show no response to the gonadal influence, but certainly there is not the complete and well-defined response that is apparent within the fundus. Indeed the cyclic response is so specific that there are those who feel it is possible to date an endometrium to the day by appraisal of curettings. We do not agree, for apparently there is considerable variation in endometrial response among women at a comparable stage of the cycle, as well as in the same patient in different months. Likewise, there is a considerable disparity in the response of glands and stroma to a progesterone influence, one or the other on occasion showing a markedly exaggerated or decreased response. Nevertheless it should be possible to evaluate an endometrium within 24 hours, and this is our policy, which may have value in certain cases of infertility characterized by an inadequate luteal phase.

The endometrium is a specialized form of connective tissue characterized by a remarkable lability and sensitivity to the ovarian secretions and an amazing regenerative capacity for restoration after menstrual slough. At one time it was considered to be a type of spread-out lymph gland, and frequently there are focal areas of lymphocytes or lymphoid tissue scattered about (Fig. 7-1).

The endometrium consists of a number of

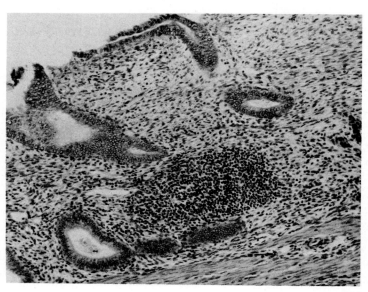

Figure 7–1. Many lymphoid follicles are often present in the endometrium at all stages of the cycle. Postmenstrual phase; note surface endometrium regenerating from the basal glandular epithelium (at right).

component parts, all responsive to the endocrine influence; a knowledge of each of these is paramount to an ability to assess in accurate fashion the appropriate stage of the menstrual cycle. Most informative is the appearance of the *endometrial glands* with their lining epithelium. In the immediately postmenstrual phase these glands are rather straight and tubular, but as the cycle progresses, there is increasing convolution and tortuosity, especially when the progesterone influence is felt. Initially the lining epithelium is tall columnar, with a basal nucleus, but with beginning progesterone secretion the nucleus migrates toward the gland lumen, producing a clear zone below it. This so-called subnuclear vacuole (Fig. 7-2) is taken as the first evidence of ovulation; subsequently the gland lumen may contain increasing amounts of glycogen and mucin, which are detectable by special stains. With this secretory effect, the epithelial cells become less distinct and exhibit a rather frayed and ragged appearance.

Much less helpful is the appearance of the *epithelium lining the endometrial surface,* although there is a gradual increase in its height from a cuboidal to a tall columnar appearance at ovulation, with subsequent re-

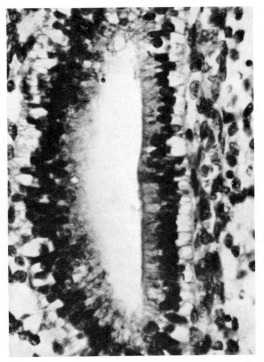

Figure 7–2. The subnuclear vacuoles, the first histologic evidence of secretory activity.

gression. Mucoid or squamous metaplasia (epidermidalization) may occur, and ciliated cells may be present.

The *stroma* throughout the interval phase is composed of cells with little cytoplasm that feature a disproportionately large dark spindle or round nucleus. In the preovulatory phase the stromal area is rather dense and compact, but in the premenstrual area there is increasing edema and vascularity with actual hypertrophy of the cells. They become enlarged, polyhedral, and pale-staining, so that a true decidual reaction is suggested, beginning around the stromal arterioles. This, of course, is an extreme response to progesterone, and it may occur in the absence of pregnancy. Obviously chorionic villi, of fetal origin, are pathognomonic of intrauterine pregnancy; a decidual reaction is only suggestive, and may occur merely as an exaggeration of the normal progesterone response. Indeed, it is impossible to distinguish an advanced progestational endometrium from an early pregnancy, except for the presence of trophoblast.

Thus, correlation of the component parts of the endometrium provides a good approximation of the stage of the cycle. Although it is unlikely that completely pathognomonic changes in the endometrium occur on any respective day of the cycle, Figures 7-4 to 7-19 seem to summarize the course of events during the usual month. The date indicated refers to the observed calendar status of the endometrium, and the histologic pattern may closely conform to this. However, we repeat our opinion that it is rarely possible to pinpoint the day, although we believe a close approximation (within 48 hours either way) can be made.

MENSTRUATION

If fertilization has not taken place, transformation of the predecidual endometrium to actual decidua does not occur. Instead there is regression and impaired function of the corpus luteum beginning four or five days before menstruation. There is a resultant decrease in the circulating hormones, and when there is a sufficiently low level of these, bleeding occurs. It is important to emphasize that bleeding does not occur when the hormonal level is high, but only when it decreases, and this "withdrawal bleeding" mechanism is utilized repeatedly in the handling of various functional endocrine problems.

The endometrium may be divided into a superficial *functional* zone consisting of an upper *compact* zone below which is the so-called *spongy* area (Fig. 7–3). Only this functional zone is responsive to a biphasic hormonal stimulus, and it alone participates in menstruation. The *nonfunctioning* basal layer is composed of young undifferentiated endometrium that has not achieved the capacity for full response to progesterone, although separate electron microscopic studies by Flowers and Wilborn and Nogales-Ortiz and co-workers suggest some response.

Even in the premenstrual phase of the cycle, it shows only an estrogen effect, and it is not desquamated in toto at menstruation. Indeed, it is from these basal buds as well as from the stroma (Baggish et al.) that the endometrium grows and regenerates itself after menstrual bleeding. In fact, regeneration of the surface endometrium begins before menstruation has completely ceased as a result of growth of this basal tissue (Fig. 7–4).

In any case, the teleologic interpretation would be that every menstrual cycle is dedicated to getting the endometrium into the best possible condition to maintain a fertil-

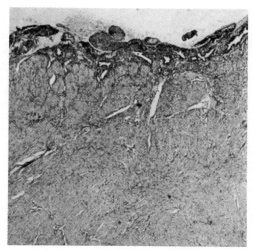

Figure 7–4. Endometrium on fourth day of bleeding, showing the surface being restored from the stumps of the glands.

ized egg in the event that pregnancy occurs. The mucous surface is thick, vascular, and contains abundant glycogen as a source of nutrition for any implanted conceptus. If, however, pregnancy does not take place, menstruation occurs, and the whole process is repeated the next month. The foregoing then represents merely a succinct sketch of the most important details of endometrial behavior. These will be discussed more fully after consideration of the vascular behavior which is the direct initiating cause of menstrual bleeding.

Vascular Behavior

Reference has been made to the important role played by the so-called *spiral* or *coiled* arterioles in the mechanism of menstruation, particularly in desquamation and bleeding (Fig. 7–5). The fragmentary character of the desquamation is readily explained by the almost terminal nature of these spiral vessels, which exhibit intense and prolonged vasoconstriction, shortly before the onset of the period, with resulting ischemia in the endometrial segments supplied. The role of prostaglandin was noted in Chapter 6. The deterioration of the blood vessel walls also explains their frequent rupture, and this, with probably also increased diapedesis, is responsible for the menstrual hemorrhage that occurs when the vasoconstriction is followed, as it is, by a long phase of vasodilatation. Menstruation may thus be looked upon as a summation of innumerable tiny menstrual hemorrhages in the endometrium

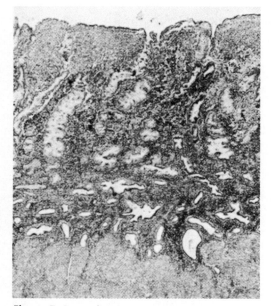

Figure 7–3. Endometrium at twenty-second day of cycle, showing contrast between the pale-staining secretory epithelium of the upper or functional layers of the endometrium and the nonsecretory epithelium of the glands in the basal layer.

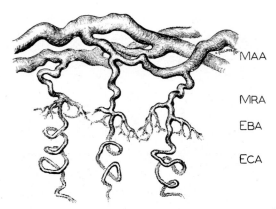

Figure 7–5. Stereographic representation of myometrial and endometrial groups of arteries in the macaque monkey. Above are shown parts of myometrial arcuate arteries (*MAA*) from which proceed myometrial radial arteries (*MRA*) towards the endometrium, in which two types of arteries are found: the larger endometrial coiled arteries (*ECA*) and the smaller endometrial basal arteries (*EBA*). (From H. Okkels and E. T. Engle: Acta Path. Microbiol. Scand., *15*:150, 1938.)

supplied by individual spiral arterioles. A study by Fanger and Barker, utilizing special staining techniques, confirms the varied vascular patterns in different phases of the cycle.

HISTOLOGIC PHASES OF MENSTRUAL CYCLE

In the common type of menstrual cycle, the occurrence of ovulation at approximately the middle of the intermenstrual interval serves to divide the cycle into a preovulation and a postovulation phase. Physiologically, these are distinguished by the fact that before ovulation only *estrogen* is produced by the ovary, and only a proliferative effect is therefore exerted upon the endometrium. During the postovulation phase, however, the corpus luteum secretes not only the estrogenic hormone but also *progesterone*, which brings about the characteristic secretory phase in the endometrium. On the basis of these differences, therefore, the entire cycle may be divided into a *proliferative*, a *secretory*, and a *bleeding* phase.

Although this differentiation of the chief phases is a sound one, it is too broad to be of great value for the more sharply descriptive purposes of laboratory classification, and we believe that the classification of phases as originally suggested by R. Meyer is still the most serviceable one, viz.:

1. Postmenstrual Phase. This corresponds roughly to the few days immediately following the cessation of a menstrual period. During this phase the endometrium is grossly quite thin, measuring usually only 1 or 2 mm. in thickness. The surface epithelium is low and cuboidal, the glands are straight, with little or no tendency to convolution, and their epithelium is like that of the surface, with no suggestion of secretory activity. During the latter part of this phase, mitoses begin to be seen in the epithelial cells. The stroma is dense, compact, and nonvascular in appearance (Figs. 7–6 and 7–7).

The immediate postmenstrual phase is sometimes called the *rest phase*, but it is questionable whether in the normally menstruating woman the endometrium is ever completely at rest. In women with abnormally long cycles, however, there may be virtual quiescence for a good many days, and this may be properly called a rest period.

2. The Interval Phase. This stage, beginning approximately one week after menstruation and extending to about one week before the next period, is therefore about two weeks in duration (Figs. 7–8 and 7–9). The growth activity already evident toward the end of the postmenstrual phase becomes more and more pronounced, so that the surface epithelium usually becomes taller and definitely columnar, while the glands become more and more hypertrophic, with gradual widening of the lumina and steadily increasing convolution. The gland epithe-

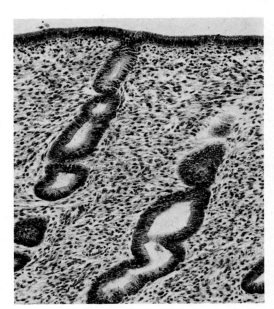

Figure 7–6. Postmenstrual endometrium (sixth day of cycle).

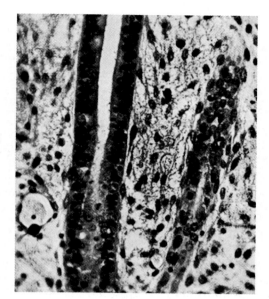

Figure 7–7. Numerous mitoses in both epithelium and stroma during the postmenstrual phase. They are also frequent in the early interval phase.

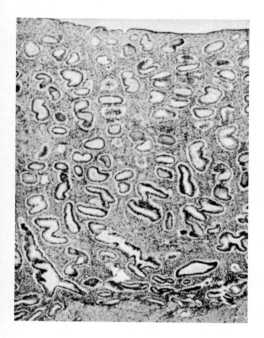

Figure 7–8. Endometrium at about midinterval period (fifteenth day), showing increasing size and moderate tortuosity of the glands.

Figure 7–9. Early secretory pattern (sixteenth day) with obvious subnuclear vacuoles, although there are only moderate changes in tortuosity of the glands.

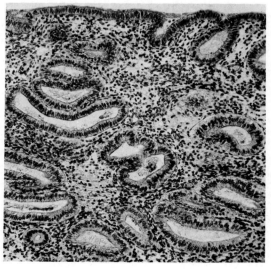

lium in the earlier, preovulation phase of the interval (early interval phase) shows no trace of secretory activity, but later one finds the nuclei pushed toward the lumina of the glands as a result of the formation of the so-called *subnuclear vacuoles*, already mentioned. These are commonly interpreted as representing the earliest evidence of ovulation in the human female. As a result of continued glycogen secretion into the gland lumen, the nucleus subsequently slips back to its original basal position.

Later in the interval (late interval phase) the secretory activity of the epithelium becomes increasingly marked, so that there is seldom any doubt as to this point on histologic examination alone (Fig. 7–10). When any doubt exists, demonstration of glycogen by differential staining usually clears up the uncertainty. In the late stages of the interval, the glycogen granules are found not only in the epithelium, but at times even in the lumina of the glands. The stroma in this stage is more abundant and somewhat more hyperemic than in the preceding phase.

The following chart notes the criteria utilized in our laboratory in dating the secretory endometrium; this is of considerable importance in studying certain sterility problems. Although the daily changes are enumerated, we always date the endometrium by using a 48-hour span (e.g., day 18–19 or day 24–25), and believe our accuracy to be 95 per cent provided the endometrium has not been modified by contraceptive pills. There is no purpose to be served in dating the proliferative endometrium.

Endometrial Dating

16th day
  Subnuclear vacuoles
  Pseudostratification
  Mitoses in glands and stroma

17th day
  More or less orderly row of nuclei
  Cytoplasm above nuclei and subnuclear vacuoles below
  Gland and stromal mitoses
  Extremely minimal secretion

18th day
  Vacuoles above and below nuclei
  Improved linear arrangement of nuclei
  Gland mitoses rare
  Stromal mitoses rare
  Bubbles of secretion seen at luminal border

19th day
  A few vacuoles remain in cell, but mainly active evacuation with intraluminal secretion
  No gland or stromal mitoses
  May look like day 16 but no pseudostratification

20th day
  Peak secretion with ragged luminal border
  Vacuoles are rare

21st day
  Abrupt onset of stromal edema
  Gland secretion prominent
  "Naked" stromal nuclei begin to appear

22nd day
  Peak edema
  Marked appearance of "naked" stromal nuclei
  Active secretion, but subsiding
  Rare stromal mitoses

23rd day
  Prominent spiral arterioles
  Periarteriolar cuffing with enlargement of stromal cell nuclei and cytoplasm (earliest predecidual change)
  Stromal mitoses

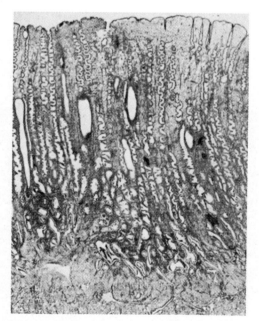

Figure 7–10. Endometrium at twentieth day, showing rather marked tortuosity of glands. The gland epithelium at this stage is definitely secretory.

24th day
Definite predecidual cells around arterioles with early subepithelial changes
Greater stromal mitoses
Ragged cell borders, i.e., secretorily exhausted

25th day
Definite subcapsular predecidua
Inspissated secretion noted to begin
Early stromal infiltration with lymphocytes and occasional polymorphonuclear leukocytes

26th day
Generalized decidual reaction
Polymorphonuclear leukocytic invasion
Inspissated secretion

27th day
Solid sheet of decidua
Marked leukocytic infiltrate
Inspissated secretion with variable intracellular secretory activity

28th day
Focal necrosis and hemorrhage
Peak leukocytic infiltration
Cells may show secretory exhaustion or may show active secretion
(Variable)

Menstruating
Stromal clumping
Glandular break-up and hemorrhage
Variable leukocytic infiltration
Edema
After 24 hours, metaplastic alterations on surface

3. Premenstrual (Progestational or Secretory) Phase. It may seem unfortunate that so many terms are applied more or less synonymously to the phase represented by the week or so prior to menstruation, when the maximum of secretory activity is noted in the endometrium. As a matter of fact, the terms are all self-explanatory, and descriptive from the standpoint of chronology, teleology, and histologic pattern, so that the objection is not as serious as it might appear at first thought.

In this phase (Figs. 7–11 to 7–13) the mucosa is thick, soft, and velvety, measuring from 3 to 8 mm. in thickness. It is usually of rather pale, edematous appearance. The surface epithelium remains quite tall and nonsecretory. The glands exhibit a steadily increasing tortuosity, the necks being often rather straight and nontortuous, but the mid-

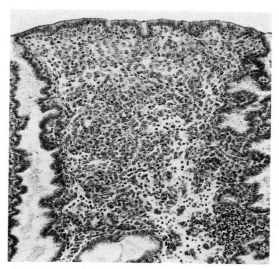

Figure 7–11. Premenstrual endometrium (twenty-fifth day). Glandular as well as stromal changes are apparent. Note the "saw-tooth" pattern incurred by budding of glands and beginning infiltration by pseudo-inflammatory cells.

dle sections presenting marked scalloping and often a "saw-tooth" appearance on longitudinal section. On the other hand, the very tips of the glands, immediately adjacent to and often dipping into the interstices of the muscle layer, commonly show little or no tortuosity. The basal layer varies much in thickness, sometimes being well marked, in other areas almost absent.

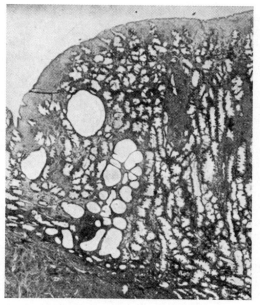

Figure 7–12. Marked premenstrual reaction on the twenty-seventh day, showing secretory activity and gland hypertrophy with convolution.

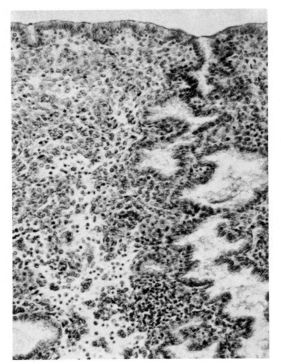

Figure 7–13. Endometrium from patient just before menstruation (twenty-eighth day), showing marked infiltration with leukocytes and wandering cells. Note decidua-like appearance of the stroma.

Corresponding to this stratum difference in gland outline, the gland epithelium likewise shows differences in secretory response at the different levels. In the middle spongy layer, corresponding to the greatest tortuosity of the glands, the epithelium is low and pale-staining, with a frayed-looking lumen edge suggesting a melting down of the cytoplasm. The nuclei have receded toward the basement membrane. The spiral twisting of the glands produces on section small tuftlike eminences of epithelium with an appearance of stratification. On the other hand, the epithelium of the basal layer often shows no secretory response at all, presumably because the immature epithelium near the growing tips of the glands, while responding to the estrogenic growth hormone, is not capable of responding to progesterone.

The stroma is most abundant in the superficial layer, between the necks of the glands. Here the cells show varying degrees of hypertrophy. Whereas in the earlier stages of the cycle there is almost no cytoplasm surrounding the nucleus, in the premenstrual phase a definite and sometimes rather broad cytoplasmic zone is often evident, giving a

decidua-like appearance to the cells. In the middle zone, the stroma is much less abundant, forming narrow septa between the glands, while in the basal layers the decidua-like change is apt to be absent. A conspicuous feature of this phase is the prominence of the basal and spiral arterioles, especially the latter, which frequently appear as small tufts of vessels in the deeper and middle layers of the endometrium (Fig. 7–14).

The described differences in the histologic response at different levels of the endometrium have led very naturally to a division into three strata, viz.: *compacta, spongiosa,* and *basalis.* While these are usually well differentiable in the pregravid phase, they are more sharply marked off in the decidua of early pregnancy, as will be discussed later.

The progestational picture described is a progressive one until shortly before the onset of menstruation, when the catabolic changes produced by the retrogression of the

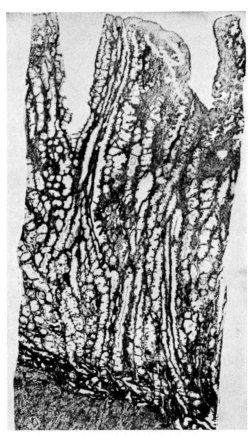

Figure 7–14. Typical premenstrual endometrium, showing by contrast the darker staining basalis near the muscle. The basalis takes no part in the functional cycle of menstruation, but is important in the reparative process.

corpus luteum begin to be expressed histologically. A rather massive infiltration of leukocytes occurs, chiefly polynuclear, but with many mononuclear cells (Fig. 7–13). The superficial layers take on a granular appearance, with poor staining and imperfect cell differentiation. These degenerative changes are indicative of the impending death of the superficial layers. It is important to recognize the normality of the immediately premenstrual pseudo-inflammatory infiltration, as otherwise this phase might be readily mistaken for a genuine endometritis. The presence of numerous plasma cells might suggest an infectious process.

Figure 7–15 summarizes the changes occurring in the cycle.

4. Bleeding Phase. That the endometrial surface is actually desquamated at menstruation is now universally accepted, though there was much difference of opinion on this point until the work of Schröder in 1915, followed later by that of Novak and TeLinde (1924) and others. It is only by a systematic chronologic study of endometria removed on the various days of the cycle that the progress of these retrogressive changes can be demonstrated and traced. Even before desquamation begins, its imminence is indicated by the degenerative changes in the upper layers, as suggested by the poor staining and granular appearance of both the epithelial and stromal elements.

Even with the onset of actual bleeding, tissue loss may be rather slight, with perhaps only a small patch of the superficial layer being cast off here and there. The blood vessels are widened and congested. This fact, together with the thinness of their walls—most of them being small venules or capillaries—makes it easy to understand why both rhexis and diapedesis are probably factors in the bleeding. Small punctate hematomas are often noted, lifting the superficial layers, and thus promoting further tissue loss, so that usually on the second day of bleeding most of the surface has been lost (Figs. 7–16 to 7–21).

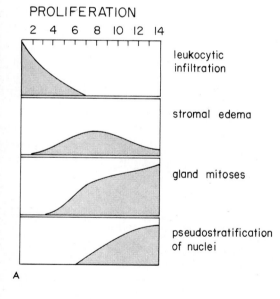

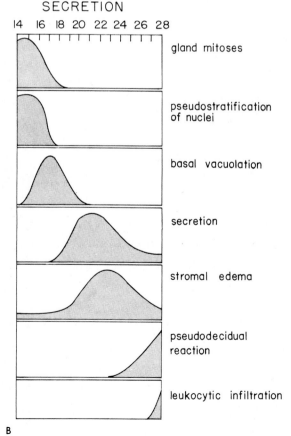

Figure 7–15. _A_, Diagrammatic description of proliferative phase. _B_, Secretory phase. (Courtesy of Dr. E. Friedrich, Milwaukee, Wisconsin.)

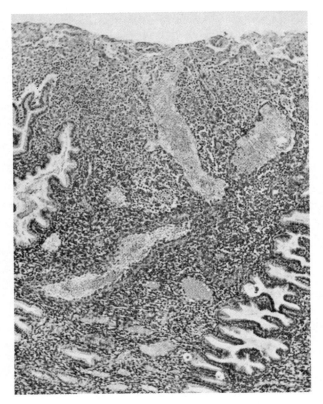

Figure 7–16. Endometrium on first day of menstruation. Note the dilated blood vessels, some of which are opening directly on the surface. There is marked infiltration of the upper layers, and small particles of the surface are being cast off. There are considerable individual differences in the degree of tissue loss on the first day.

Figure 7–17. More extensive crumbling of surface at another portion of same endometrium shown in Figure 7–16.

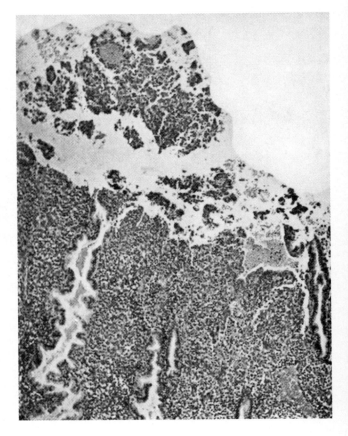

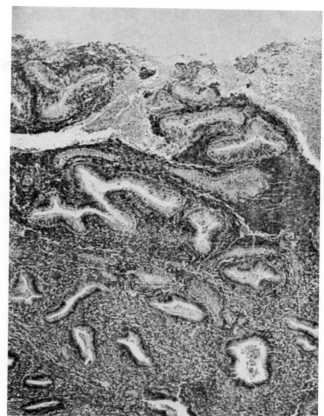

Figure 7–18. Endometrium on second day of menstruation.

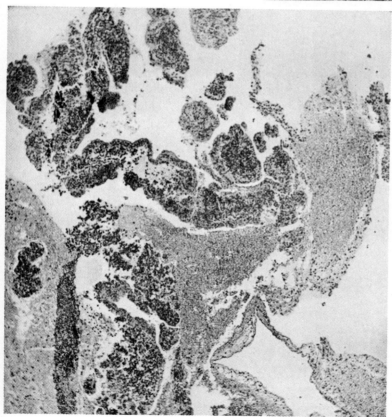

Figure 7–19. Blood clot, containing cast-off particles of endometrial tissue, from cavity of the uterus whose endometrium is shown in Figure 7–18.

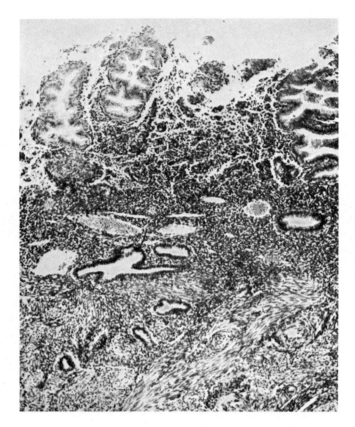

Figure 7–20. Another endometrium on second day of menstruation, showing loss of compacta and most of spongiosa.

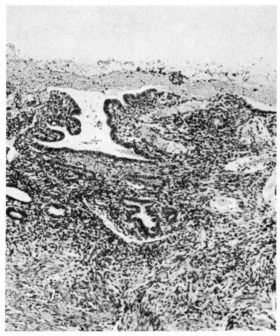

Figure 7–21. Endometrium on third day of menstruation, showing epithelialization of surface by outgrowth of epithelium from stumps of glands.

The tissue loss proceeds in a fragmentary or molecular fashion, with particles crumbling away here and there. In rare instances, however, the endometrium may be shed in the form of a more or less complete cast, constituting one variety of uterine cast, and often associated clinically with the so-called *membranous dysmenorrhea.*

By the third day, the desquamation has commonly reached its limit, though the latter differs markedly in degree in different cases. The compacta and a variable thickness of spongiosa are usually lost, and it is from the proliferative, nonsecretory epithelium of the surviving stumps of the glands and stroma that the new surface epithelium is to be restored. Indeed, one often sees evidence of this epithelial regeneration even while desquamation is still going on, with fragments of degenerated epithelium still lying on the surface. McLennan and Rydell have indicated wide variation in the normal process of menstrual shedding and regeneration; at the same time, grossly normal and abnormal (myomatous) uteri reveal a similar menstrual pattern.

5. Regeneration. The epithelium is restored with amazing rapidity, so that if one examines a uterus removed immediately after the cessation of menstruation, the surface is found to be already completely epithelialized. Mitoses are rarely seen at this stage, so that it seems possible that direct rather than indirect reproduction of cells may be concerned. Others have suggested that there may be a metaplastic transformation of stromal into epithelial cells, a view which is plausible because both the uterine epithelium and stroma have a common mesodermal origin. Electron microscopic studies by Ferenczy seem to indicate that regeneration occurs only from the remaining basal glands and surface endometrium without involvement of the stroma. Complete resurfacing seemingly is completed by day 5 and is independent of hormonal stimulus, although this is necessary for subsequent growth.

McLennan has indicated that *following curettage,* regeneration of the endometrium proceeds more slowly, and there is a dormant period of from two to three days unless curettage was performed early in the menstrual period. There is, incidentally, a striking absence of an inflammatory reaction of the postcurettage endometrium if subsequent hysterectomy is performed. Reyniak and co-workers have performed endometrial biopsies on postabortal patients and have found ovulation as early as day 9, with at least one third showing evidence of ovulation prior to their first menstruation.

Deviations from Normal Histologic Cycle

In general, the histologic response to the ovarian hormones is a fairly uniform one, though the degree of change is not always the same at all portions of the uterus. As a rule, too, the division between the functional layers (compacta and spongiosa) and nonfunctional (basalis) is fairly sharp, but in many areas the basalis may be so thin as to be scarcely perceptible.

Moreover, one may find in the functional layers areas of endometrium which, like the basalis, are immature, so that they do not respond to progesterone (Fig. 7–22). During the premenstrual stage such areas stand out in sharp contrast to the surrounding secretory endometrium. Histologically they may resemble the normal basalis, but often they present the more marked proliferative pattern of hyperplasia. These islands of local-

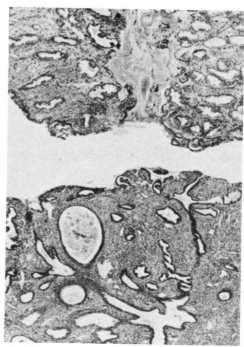

Figure 7–22. Uterine curettings, showing in same field area an immature or unripe endometrium (bottom) and a premenstrual or secretory stage (top). The name of "mixed endometrium" is often applied to such cases. (Courtesy of Dr. Herbert L. Traut.)

ized hyperplasia or *unripe endometrium* were described by Novak and Matzloff in 1924, and they have been noted by various other authors. They may form large scattered areas or they may form long columns extending through the whole thickness of the endometrium, and perhaps even rising as polyps above the surface. Such polyps are characterized by a noncyclic hyperplastic pattern (see Chapter 10).

An occasional finding in cases of functional uterine bleeding is that of so-called *delayed and irregular shedding of the endometrium.* Although this condition has been recognized for many years, attention has been called to it by McLennan and more recently by Taw, whose studies suggest that approximately 25 per cent of such women come to hysterectomy. It is characterized by the abnormal persistence of islands of the progestational functional layers of the endometrium which normally are shed and rather rapidly autolyzed. It is evident, therefore, that the lesion cannot be recognized histologically at the beginning of a bleeding phase, but only after the bleeding has persisted for a few days, usually about four or five. An abnormal persistence of progesterone effect is believed to be the important factor in bringing about this abnormal prolongation of the desquamation phase.

THE ENDOMETRIUM OF PREGNANCY

In the event of pregnancy the hypertrophic and secretory changes of the pregravid phase become even more marked, so that there is an imperceptible transition between the premenstrual picture in the nonpregnant woman and the very early *decidua* of the woman in whom the ovum has been fertilized. In fact, it is not always easy to make the distinction in the laboratory unless embryonic elements, such as villi, are present in the section. The *glands* of the decidua present marked saw-tooth convolution and scalloping, and the *epithelium* is low, pale-staining, and actively secretory. At a later stage the tortuosity of the glands is much less and the epithelium becomes very flat, so that there may be difficulty in distinguishing the glands from lymphatics or venules.

In our experience, a full-fledged Arias-Stella reaction (ASR) (Fig. 7–23A), as noted in Chapter 28, is found in less than 25 per cent of the cases of uterine or extrauterine gestation, although the knowledge of a definite pregnancy tends to influence even an unbiased pathologist to make this diagnosis. Unquestionably, there are borderline degrees of tufting and budding of the glandular epithelium, with slight cellular atypia—hyperchromatism, mitotic activity, or other alterations. Such changes should be marked before a positive diagnosis is made. Paradoxically, this response to trophoblastic tissue may be found following clomiphene or progestogen therapy. Novak points out the extreme difficulty in distinguishing minor degrees of ASR and the futility of utilizing this as a method of differential diagnosis between ectopic pregnancy and hydrosalpinx. He further notes that Sturgis had described these changes many years before Arias-Stella.

Other studies, such as Silverberg's, note an ASR in 75 per cent of all endometria in conjunction with abortion. It is at least as common with therapeutic as with spontaneous abortion, and this suggests an exaggerated response to elevated hormones rather than an involutional sequel to fetal death.

The *stromal cells* become large and polygonal, with a wide zone of cytoplasm sur-

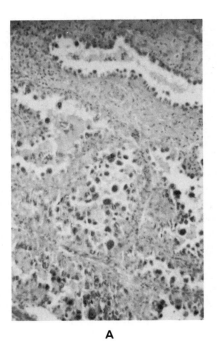

A

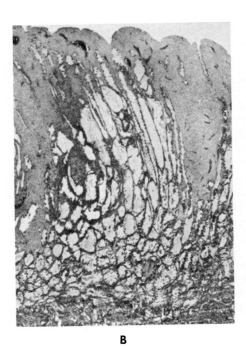

B

Figure 7–23. *A*, Arias-Stella reaction. Note hyperchromatic atypical cells lining glands. *B*, Decidua of early pregnancy, showing the superficial compact zone in contrast with the spongy middle portion. The basalis is not well shown in the field.

rounding the nucleus. They now constitute the characteristic *decidual cells,* and are arranged in mosaic or tilelike fashion. They occur in large fields in the superficial compact layer of the endometrium in which the gland elements are sparsest (Fig. 7–23*B*).

In the middle or spongy zone, on the other hand, the hypertrophy and convolution of the glands are most pronounced, with delicate interglandular septa, so that an intricate lacy pattern is produced. Finally, the basalis stands out in even sharper contrast with the upper layers of the endometrium than is seen in the nonpregnant woman, the tips of the glands being lined by a nonsecretory type of epithelium quite different from that in the upper reaches of the gland.

Ectopic Decidua

Undoubted decidual reaction has been described in many portions of the abdomen far removed from the endometrium, viz., the anterior or posterior peritoneal surface of the uterus, the anterior surface of the rectum, the floor of the cul-de-sac, the omentum, the ovary, the appendix, the cervix, the vagina, the peritoneum of the small intestine, and certain pathologic structures (such as adenomyosis of the uterus, parovarian cyst, bands of adhesions).

Not much of a definite nature can be said as to the general significance of this decidual reaction. As to its occurrence in many locations in the pelvis, one point is worthy of mention. In general, the locations at which decidual islands have been observed are quite similar to those in which endometrial islands—the endometrial implants described by Sampson—have been found to occur. However, the possibility of metaplasia of the coelomic epithelium, perhaps due to the stimulation of the pregnancy hormones, also deserves consideration. Parmley and co-workers believe that this is of etiologic importance in leiomyomatosis peritonealis disseminata. In the decidual islands, glands are usually absent, the reaction apparently involving patches of mesenchymal cells which, like the stroma of the endometrium, exhibit a sensitivity to the pregnancy hormones. As will be noted later, a decidual reaction on the surface of the ovary or tube may occur in a proved absence of any type of pregnancy so that decidua must not be regarded as pathognomonic of gestation (Fig. 7–24).

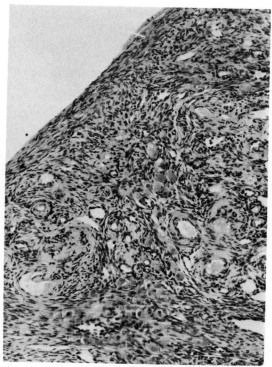

Figure 7–24. Probable decidual cells in subcortical stroma.

Postmenopausal and Senile Changes in the Endometrium

With the usual partial withdrawal of estrogen at the menopause, the endometrium, like the other genital tract tissues, may undergo atrophic changes. It becomes thin, the surface and gland epithelia appear low cuboidal in type, and the glands become very sparse (Fig. 7–25). At times they are cystic, possibly because of blockage by the contracting stroma, which becomes increasingly fibrotic with the years. However, the occasional presence of numerous large cystic glands is probably explainable by a different mechanism, as will be discussed. The thin senile endometrium is quite prone to infection, so that senile endometritis is relatively common. Bleeding may occur, most likely because of blockage of the venules by overdistended glands rather than because of focal arteriosclerosis (Meyer et al.).

The character of the hormonal transition from the menstruating to the postmenopausal epochs exhibits wide variation in different women. For example, the terminal menstrual cycles are sometimes ovulatory, but very often anovulatory, and in the latter

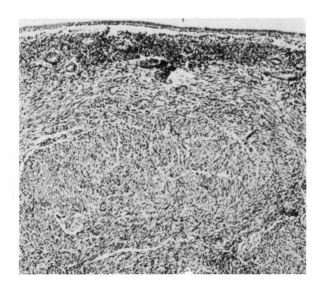

Figure 7–25. Senile endometrium.

group the endometrium often shows a hyperplastic pattern. These variations in terminal menstrual life appear to have an influence on the postmenopausal histology of the endometrium. The best illustration of this is seen in the frequent finding, long after the cessation of menstrual function, of a typical Swiss-cheese pattern of the glands, exactly like that seen with hyperplasia of the endometrium found in so many women toward the end of menstrual life. Sometimes the glands are lined by a tall columnar epithelium and there is a proliferative hyperplasia. This pattern is highly suggestive of active estrogen support, even in the nonbleeding postmenopausal patient. There is considerable evidence (see Chapter 8) that estrogen secretion may be present in certain climacteric females.

With the onset of the menopause, however, the growth stimulus is often removed. The stromal cells retrogress and may ultimately become fibrotic in appearance, and the epithelial cells no longer exhibit mitotic evidence of active growth. Many of the glands remain large and cystic, and this might explain the cystic glands that are common in the senile endometrium. Such cystic glands have in the past been assumed to be the result of cicatricial blockage of these ducts, but this view is not supported by histologic studies. On the other hand, the study of large numbers of hyperplastic endometria encountered in women from the active menarche to all ages beyond this epoch reveals all phases of transition between active hyperplasia, retrogressive hyperplasia, and se-

nile endometria with cystic glands (Fig. 7–26). If this general concept is correct, one would probably be justified in assuming that the terminal cycles of menstrual life had been anovulatory, provided one finds the hyperplasia signs still present on the retrogressive endometrium of the woman long after the menopause.

However, it must be remembered that the endometrium of the postmenopausal woman is subject to the influence of postmenopausal estrogen stimulation, now a well established possibility. This postmenopausal estrogen presumably originates from androstenedione, of ovarian or adrenal origin, which is converted to estrogen by various undefined organs. Thus, we not infrequently find typical hyperplasia, identical with that seen so often in the reproductive epoch, in women far beyond the menopausal age, even as old as 80 years.

After the menopause, as before, the endometrium appears to vary in the degree of its sensitivity or its refractoriness to the estrogenic stimulus and these variations are often seen in different parts of the same endometrium. Just as in the reproductive epoch one may find large areas of unripe or immature endometrium in an otherwise fully functioning mucosa, so one may find in a senile retrogressive endometrium localized areas of typical active hyperplasia. Not infrequently these localized areas are polypoid, just as one often finds polyps of hyperplastic pattern in a progestational endometrium during reproductive life.

Still another possibility after the meno-

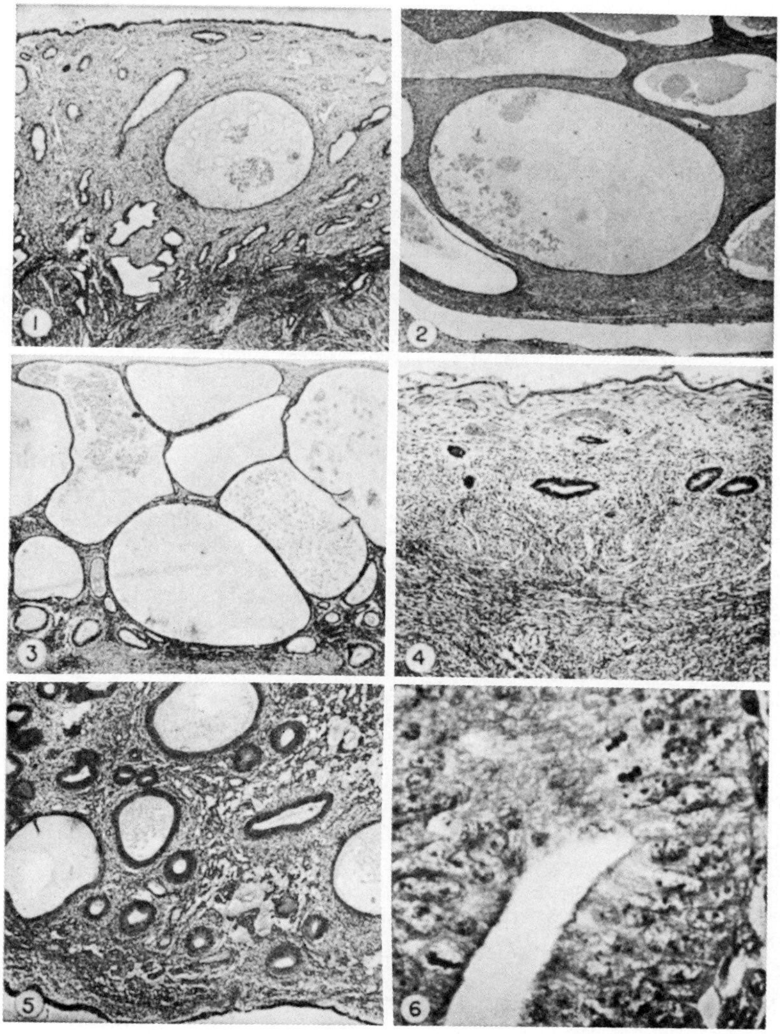

Figure 7–26. *1*, Retrogressed hyperplasia, with persisting cystic glands, 7 years after menopause, in a patient 49 years old. Note fibrous stroma. *2*, Retrogressed hyperplasia 10 years after menopause, in a patient 51 years old. Note flat atrophic epithelium and fibrous stroma. *3*, Extreme cystic enlargement of gland, representing persistence of hyperplasia pattern (retrogressive) in 57 year old patient 3 years after menopause. *4*, Typical atrophic senile endometrium 9 years after menopause, in a woman of 58 years. *5*, Active Swiss-cheese hyperplasia 30 years after menopause in a patient 80 years old. See high power of mitoses in 6. *6*, Mitoses in gland epithelium from another area of same patient as in *5*.

pause is the finding of a secretory endometrium, though this is very rare. Such an endometrium is ordinarily considered to be evidence of a preceding ovulation, so that it might be looked upon as paradoxic to encounter it after cessation of the menstrual function. True progestational endometrium has always been regarded as uncommon in the aging patient. For example, in the 137 endometria studied by Novak and Richardson, no case was included unless at least one year had elapsed since bleeding; in none of these was a secretory endometrium observed. However, in a more recent study we have found ovulation not infrequent in the woman over 50 years of age, and sometimes as long as several years after the last menstrual period. Pregnancy is rare, presumably owing to a faulty corpus luteum in the female past 50 years old. Theoretically these women could have become "postmenopausally pregnant," for most consider a year without bleeding as suggestive of this process. Psychogenic amenorrhea may occasionally suppress periods in the woman past 50 years of age, and may be presumed to represent a menopause, unless FSH determination is carried out.

In any case, it should be mentioned that certain forms of atypical hyperplasia are characterized by a tall pale-staining epithelial lining cell with varying degrees of intraluminal budding and tufting. Even the trained pathologist may have difficulty in distinguishing these from a genuine secretory endometrium of the menstrual era, although the hyperplastic epithelium is generally considerably taller than the secretory type and there are no predecidual changes in the stromal cells. We have seen repeated

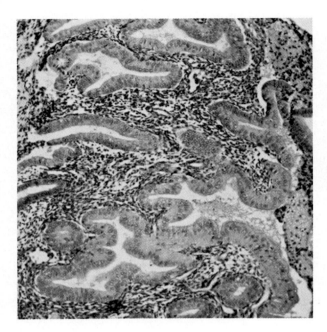

Figure 7–27. Tall, pale-staining epithelial lining glands with intraluminal tufting not unlike that seen in a progestational endometrium. The stroma is extremely compact with no evidence of progesterone stimulation.

cases in which women many years post menopause were supposed to have progestational endometria, but more discriminating study showed only a proliferative hyperplasia as in Figure 7–27. Indeed, in some respects, early adenocarcinoma has the histochemical appearance of progestational endometrium, and this is difficult to reconcile with the possibility that estrogen is the usual stimulus to endometrial adenocarcinoma.

Summarizing these observations on the postmenopausal endometrium, the following variations may be noted:

(1) A thin, atrophic mucosa, so commonly called the senile endometrium. This is numerically the most frequent finding in women beyond the menopause.

(2) A mucosa of varying thickness, but often not very thin, showing the Swiss-cheese pattern of hyperplasia but obviously of inactive, retrogressive type. Many of the glands are cystic and distended, others are small and atrophic.

(3) Active hyperplasia, either diffuse or, more frequently, in scattered patches, large or small, and not infrequently polypoid. Various combinations of these patterns, conditioned by different degrees of sensitivity or refractoriness, are seen in different parts of the same endometrium.

Thus, the postmenopausal ovary can no longer be presumed to be an inert, function-less gonad, but is seemingly capable of some type of steroidogenesis (Chapter 6).

REFERENCES

Baggish, M. S., Pauerstein, C. J., and Woodruff, J. D.: Role of stroma in the regeneration of the endometrial epithelium. Am. J. Obstet. Gynecol., 98:459, 1967.

Bartelmez, G. W.: Human uterine mucous membrane during menstruation. Am. J. Obstet. Gynecol., 21:623, 1931.

Bartelmez, G. W.: Menstruation (endometrial changes). J.A.M.A., 116:702, 1941.

Bartelmez, G. W.: Phases of menstrual cycle and their interpretation in terms of pregnancy, Am. J. Obstet. Gynecol., 79:931, 1957.

Bartelmez, G. W., Corner, G. W., and Hartman, G. C.: Phases of menstrual cycle in macaque monkey. Anat. Rec., 94:512, 1946.

Boutselis, J. G., DeNeef, J. C., Ullery, J. C., and George, O. T.: Histochemical and cytologic observations in the normal human endometrium. Obstet. Gynecol., 21:423, 1963.

Corner, G. W.: Relation between menstruation and ovulation in monkey. J.A.M.A., 89:1838, 1927.

Daron, G. H.: Arterial pattern of the tunica mucosa of the uterus in macacus rhesus. Am. J. Anat., 58:349, 1936.

Fanger, H., and Barker, B. S.: Capillaries and arterioles in normal endometrium. Obstet. Gynecol., 17:543, 1961.

Ferenczy, A.: Cytodynamics of human endometrial regeneration. I. Scanning electron microscopy. II. Transmission electron microscopy and histochemistry. III. Experimental endometrial regeneration. Am. J. Obstet. Gynecol., 124:64, 1976; 124:582, 1976; 128:536, 1977.

Fleming, S., Tweedale, D. N., and Roddick, J. W.: Ciliated endometrial cells. Am. J. Obstet. Gynecol., *102*:186, 1968.

Flowers, C. E., Jr., and Wilborn, W. W.: New observations on menstruation, Obstet. Gynecol., *51*:16, 1978.

Irwin, J. B.: Lymphoid apparatus of the endometrium with report of primary lymphoma. Am. J. Obstet. Gynecol., *72*:915, 1956.

Macht, D. I.: Further historical and experimental studies on menstrual toxin. Am. J. Med. Sci., *206*:281, 1943.

Markee, J. E.: Morphological basis for menstrual bleeding. Anat. Rec., *94*:481, 1946.

Markee, J. E.: Rhythmic vascular uterine changes. Am. J. Physiol., *100*:32, 1932.

McBride, J. H.: Normal postmenopausal endometrium. J. Obstet. Gynaecol. Brit. Commonw., *61*:691, 1954.

McLennan, C. E.: Current concepts of prolonged or irregular menstrual shedding. Am. J. Obstet. Gynecol., *64*:988, 1952.

McLennan, C. E.: Endometrial regeneration following curettage. Am. J. Obstet. Gynecol., *104*:185, 1969.

McLennan, C. E., and Rydell, A. H.: Extent of endometrial shedding during normal menstruation. Obstet. Gynecol., *26*:605, 1965.

Meyer, W. C., Malkasian, S. D., Dockerty, M. B., and Decker, D. G.: Postmenopausal bleeding from atrophic endometrium. Obstet. Gynecol., *38*:731, 1971.

Nadji, P., et al.: Endometrial dating and progesterone levels. Obstet. Gynecol., *45*:193, 1975.

Nogales-Ortiz, F., et al.: The normal menstrual cycle. Obstet. Gynecol., *51*:259, 1978.

Novak, E. R.,: Ovulation over fifty. Obstet. Gynecol., *36*:903, 1970.

Novak, E. R.: The endometrium. Clin. Obstet. Gynecol., *17*:31, 1974.

Novak, E., and Martzloff, K. H.: Hyperplasia of the endometrium—A clinical and pathological study. Am. J. Obstet. Gynecol., *8*:385, 1924.

Novak, E., and Richardson, E. H., Jr.: Proliferative changes in the senile endometrium. Am. J. Obstet. Gynecol., *42*:564, 1941.

Novak, E., and TeLinde, R. W.: The endometrium of the menstruating uterus. J.A.M.A., *83*:900, 1924.

Noyes, R. W., and Haman, J. O.: Accuracy of endometrial dating. Fertil. Steril., *4*:504, 1954.

Noyes, R. W., Hertig, A. T., and Rock, J.: Dating the endometrial biopsy. Fertil. Steril., *1*:3, 1950.

Parmley, T. H., et al.: Leiomyomatosis peritonealis disseminata (LPD). Obstet. Gynecol., *46*:511, 1975.

Payan, H., Daino, J., and Kish, M.: Lymphoid follicles in endometrium. Obstet. Gynecol., *23*:570, 1964.

Reyniak, J. L., et al.: Post-abortal endometrial regeneration. Obstet. Gynecol., *4*:203, 1975.

Schröder, R.: Anatomische Studien zur normalen und pathologischen Physiologie des Menstruationszyklus. Arch. Gynäk., *104*:27, 1915.

Schueler, E. F.: Ciliated epithelium of the human uterine mucosa. Obstet. Gynecol., *31*:215, 1968.

Silverberg, S. G.: Arias-Stella phenomenon in spontaneous and therapeutic abortion. Am. J. Obstet. Gynecol., *112*:777, 1972.

Speert, H.: The endometrium in old age. Surg. Gynecol. Obstet., *89*:551, 1949.

Sturgis, S. H.: Arias-Stella phenomenon. Am. J. Obstet. Gynecol., *116*:589, 1973.

Taki, I., Lijima, H., Doi, T., Uetseki, Y., and Moni, M.: Histochemistry of hydrolytic and oxidative enzymes in the human and experimentally induced adenocarcinoma of the endometrium. Am. J. Obstet. Gynecol., *94*:86, 1966.

Taw, R. L.: Secretory endometrium in menstrual disorders. Am. J. Obstet. Gynecol., *122*:490, 1975.

Wienke, E. C., Jr., Cavazos, F., Hall, D. G., and Lucas, F. V.: Ultrastructure of the human endometrial stroma cell during the menstrual cycle. Am. J. Obstet. Gynecol., *102*:65, 1968.

Chapter 8

HYPERPLASIA OF THE ENDOMETRIUM

Concepts of endometrial hyperplasia have undergone considerable change in recent years, regarding not only its histology but also its significance. No intelligent discussion of the subject is possible without some knowledge of the pathologic physiology of so-called dysfunctional uterine bleeding (DFB), the clinical syndrome with which this endometrial lesion is so often associated. DFB may be defined as bleeding without a causative uterine lesion (such as tumor, infection, or complication of pregnancy), although frequently there may be associated follicle cysts of the ovary. It should be understood that DFB and hyperplasia are not synonymous, the former being a clinical and the latter a pathologic term. Indeed, bleeding may occur with other endometrial patterns such as "irregular shedding" of a secretory endometrium, as emphasized by McLennan.

DFB, then, may occur with any type of endometrium, but most commonly with anovulation and resultant hyperplasia. Anovulation is most common at the two extremes of menstrual life, when ovarian function is just beginning (menarche) or when it is starting to taper off (menopause). It may, however, occur at any age and be associated with fairly regular menses or abnormal bleeding of any type; it has been noted that women who generally ovulate may occasionally have an anovulatory period.

Pathologic Physiology of Functional Uterine Bleeding

There are many cogs in the menstrual machine, and functional derangements of more than one type may result in abnormal bleeding, even with grossly normal pelvic organs. The most common of these is due to a *failure of ovulation*, with an abnormal persistence of a graafian follicle, or perhaps a group of follicles. As a consequence, the endometrium is subjected to an abnormally prolonged and excessive action of the estrogenic hormone. Since under such conditions the corpus luteum is not formed, the endometrium shows no evidence of the secretory and other predecidual characteristics evoked only by progesterone.

Under the influence of the relatively excessive unopposed estrogenic stimulus, there is an abnormal growth response in the endometrium, the degree of this being apparently dependent not only upon the amount and duration of the estrogenic stimulus, but also upon the degree of receptivity of the individual endometrium. Bleeding does not take place from an endometrium that is receiving steady supporting doses of estrogen, but occurs when a sharp drop or withdrawal of the hormone takes place. Such drops are believed to be due to the reciprocal relationship between the hypothalamic-pituitary axis and the ovaries.

At the menopause there is often ovarian failure, decreased estrogen, and a reciprocal rise in pituitary FSH, which leads to the characteristic vasomotor symptoms of menopause. With anovulatory bleeding, one finds exactly the opposite situation. Excessive amounts of the ovarian hormone cause inhibition of the pituitary, with a resultant decrease in FSH and diminished stimulation of the ovarian theca cells. This is followed by a drop in blood estrogen and consequent withdrawal bleeding. Benedict and co-workers and Sobrino and Kase have indicated that prolonged anovulation may lead to occasional adrenal hypersecretion and certain virilizing symptoms, as may occur with the closely related Stein-Leventhal syndrome.

Although there can be little doubt that the quantitative interrelationship between the ovaries and the hypophysis-hypothalamus is the underlying cause of the bleeding, there is no parallelism between the amount of bleeding and the degree of endometrial histologic response. We know very little about the local mechanism of the bleeding, but it would seem that an endometrium that shows comparatively little or no hyperplastic change may at times be associated with profuse bleeding, while in other cases a striking hyperplasia may exhibit less bleeding, or perhaps none at all. The most constant feature of DFB seems to be an absence of secretory changes, as would be expected of anovulation, and the absence of corpora lutea and progesterone. It should be added, however, that there are other types of functional bleeding that can occur from practically any type of endometrium. Bleeding, of course, occurs only when there is a decreased level of estrogen; consequently a sustained hormonal stimulus may result in prolonged nonbleeding phases. This clinical observation seems usual although it does not necessarily agree with the laboratory findings of Brown and co-workers, who find no correlation between bleeding tendencies and the urinary estrogen level.

Significance of the Term Hyperplasia. Bearing these facts in mind, one can understand the confusion that has arisen with regard to the use of the designation *endometrial hyperplasia*, some limiting it to the full-blown growth picture not infrequently seen; others include the milder degrees of growth effect, perhaps not distinguishable from those seen in the first half of the normal cycle, but characterized by an estrogen-induced type of bleeding. Perhaps it would be better to speak of the entire group as proliferative or nonsecretory, reserving the term hyperplasia for those cases in which genuine hyperplastic changes are observed, being always mindful of the stage of the cycle at which curettage was performed.

However, premenstrual pathologic evidence of hyperplasia or a nonsecretory endometrium represents merely varying degrees of the same basic difficulty: failure to ovulate. A diagnosis of hyperplasia would be much more frequent if women presented themselves for curettage before bleeding had persisted too long. It seems possible that continued bleeding may lead to desquamation of most of the surface epithelium, the most responsive zone, so that later curettage may show only a nonsecretory type of pattern.

Hysteroscopy or hysterograms for the diagnosis of hyperplasia do not seem feasible or even remotely comparable to the value of curettage. X-ray interpretation of the uterine cavity after injection of Lipiodol is not easy and it is doubtful that a pattern pathognomonic of anovulatory bleeding is recognizable, although on occasion the presence of unsuspected submucous myomas or endometrial polyps might be detected.

GENUINE HYPERPLASIA OF THE ENDOMETRIUM

Gross Characteristics

The gross characteristics of hyperplasia present much variation, even with the same histologic pattern. In the most pronounced cases the endometrium is enormously overgrown and polypoid, so that curettage in such cases yields great quantities of polypoid tissue (Figs. 8–1 and 8–2). It is this condition which was for so many years misnamed polypoid endometritis. Real endometritis is rarely polypoid, and with hyperplasia, evidence of inflammation is usually absent. When large quantities of such polypoid material are revealed in perimenopausal women, the surgeon inexperienced in pathology may well jump to the conclusion there is adenocarcinoma of the body.

The distinction is usually easy if one remembers that with a corresponding amount of tissue in cancer, friability and necrosis would undoubtedly be conspicuous whereas the polyps of hyperplasia are firm and intact, with a smooth nonulcerated mucosa. In a proportion of cases the endometrium shows no polypoid overgrowth, though it may be much thicker than normal. In still others it may be normal. On superficial examination the mucosa may seem smooth and intact, though careful inspection often reveals tiny areas of tissue loss, the significance of which will be discussed later.

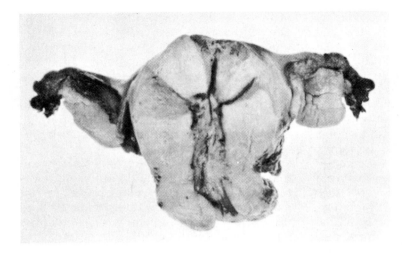

Figure 8–1. Gross appearance of marked hyperplasia of the endometrium. However, in most cases hyperplasia is associated with little or no thickening of the endometrium and is not polypoid.

Microscopic Appearance

Microscopically, the pattern of frank *hyperplasia* is very distinctive, so that the diagnosis is readily made after a glance through the microscope. By hyperplasia is meant an increase in the number of tissue elements, both epithelial and stromal. The surface epithelium is taller than normal, whereas that of the glands is likewise tall, with heavily stained nuclei which frequently show many mitoses. Similar activity may likewise be seen in the stroma (Fig. 8–3) which is compact-looking and abundant, with no sugges-

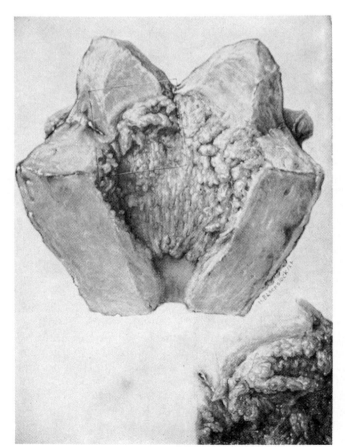

Figure 8–2. Gross appearance of marked polypoid hyperplasia. Note the sharp limitation of the condition to the endometrium proper and the non-involvement of the cervix. It is easy to see how curettage in such cases might lead to the suspicion of malignancy.

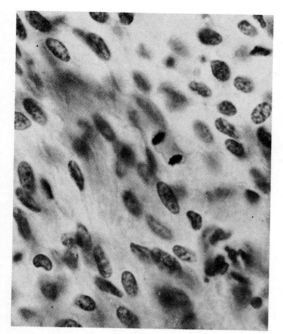

Figure 8–3. Mitotic figures in stroma of hyperplastic endometrium, which are less numerous in the epithelium.

tion of progesterone stimulation nor any evidence of inflammatory infiltration unless secondary infection has occurred.

Most distinctive, from a diagnostic standpoint, is the gland pattern. Whereas, in any phase of the normal cycle, there is a rather striking uniformity in the size and configuration of the glands, in hyperplasia the glands show marked disparity. Some are large and cystic, although others in the immediate vicinity may be very small. There is thus produced the so-called *Swiss-cheese pattern*, like the large and small holes of Swiss cheese (Figs. 8–4 and 8–5). This term, suggested in 1924, has been widely adopted in the literature. The large glands are usually lined by only a single layer of epithelium, but the smaller ones may show stratification or pseudostratification. Similar changes may occur with ectopic endometrium (Fig. 8–6).

Localized Areas of Necrobiosis. In examining sections of hyperplasia, one often encounters areas in which the endometrium shows marked degenerative change, with much round cell infiltration and with numerous thromboses of the blood vessels (Fig. 8–7). These areas are commonly rather sharply marked off from the surrounding endometrium, much like infarcts, and there is not the generalized inflammation seen with a true endometritis. They represent, as a matter of fact, the infarct-like areas of necrobiosis which Schröder especially has stressed as the source of bleeding in cases of hyperplasia. It is difficult to believe that they can explain the frequently massive hemorrhage which one not infrequently observes from an endometrium which is essentially intact. Sippe stresses the role of dilated endometrial sinusoids, which act in a similar manner to angiomas.

It seems more likely that these localized areas of necrobiosis are in some way produced by abnormalities in the behavior of the "coiled or spiral" arterioles of the functioning endometrium, which, according to

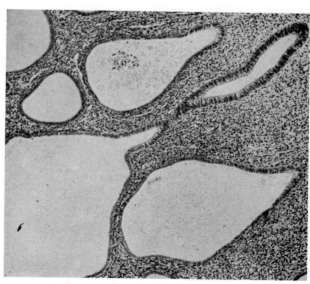

Figure 8–4. Characteristic Swiss-cheese pattern in marked hyperplasia of the endometrium.

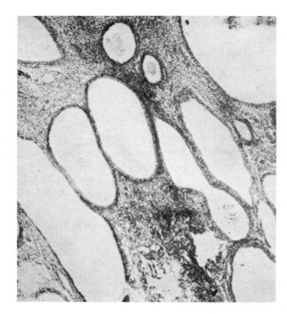

Figure 8–5. Swiss-cheese pattern in hyperplasia associated with profuse menorrhagia of 8 month's duration in a patient of 43 years.

Figure 8–6. Typical hyperplasia in an endometrial island of adenomyosis of the uterus, a common finding.

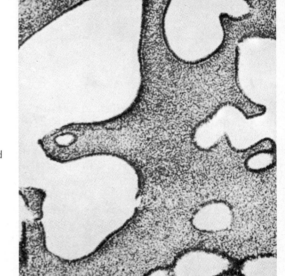

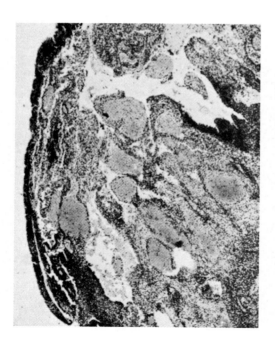

Figure 8–7. Necrobiotic area, with thrombosis, in a patient with hyperplasia of the endometrium.

the studies of Markee and co-workers, and other authors, play such a fundamental role in the mechanism of normal menstrual bleeding. Underlying the role of this vascular apparatus must be that of the ovarian hormones, and it is logical to believe that abnormalities in the latter would bring about an impaired vascular mechanism and thereby functional bleeding. It is useless to speculate about the details of this mechanism until more is learned about the nature of the vascular participation in the cycle and also the nature of its control by the endocrine hormones.

PROLIFERATIVE PICTURES IN ENDOMETRIUM ASSOCIATED WITH FUNCTIONAL BLEEDING

The typical hyperplasia of the endometrium as described is a frankly benign lesion, both clinically and histologically. As seen in women *during reproductive life*, there is no evidence to indicate that it predisposes to carcinoma, as has been implied by Chamlian and Taylor. It is worth emphasizing, too, that the hyperplasia in itself is not a cause of bleeding, representing as it does simply an exaggerated proliferative or growth effect upon the endometrium. The hormone abnormality responsible for this may likewise, though not invariably, be responsible for bleeding, as has already been stressed. This is well illustrated by a case of massive endometrial hyperplasia described by Tacchi (Fig. 8–8). The 57 year old woman consumed 2 mg. of stilbestrol in tablets almost daily for 7 years, and "from time to time she stopped taking them, but as vaginal bleeding began, she commenced taking them again" and bleeding would cease.

In other words, the growth response does not necessarily go hand in hand with the

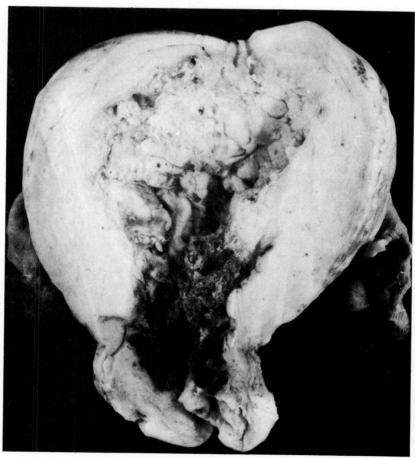

Figure 8–8. Marked polypoid hyperplasia (histologically benign) following prolonged estrogen therapy. (Courtesy of D. Tacchi: J. Obstet. Gynecol. Brit. Emp., 65:817, 1958.)

bleeding propensities, so that certain cases of DFB in which the underlying cause is a failure of ovulation may reveal hyperplasia of mild or severe grade, or one may find an endometrium showing only very moderate proliferative activity, similar to that found in the interval or even the postmenstrual phases of the normal cycle (Fig. 8–9). The common characteristic of the endometrium in all cases of this group is an absence of the changes produced by progesterone, for the latter hormone is lacking in such instances.

Occasional Finding of Tubal Type of Epithelium in Hyperplasia

An interesting finding in some cases of hyperplasia of the endometrium is that the epithelium may exhibit metaplastic changes of one sort or another. Normally the uterine epithelium is nonciliated, but a search for cilia by fresh technique will at times reveal sparse distribution of cilia, and this is common in cases of hyperplasia. When such tissues are fixed and stained, one not infrequently finds scattered areas in which the epithelium is of a typically tubal variety, with often all three types of tubal epithelium represented, viz., the ciliated or nonsecretory, the nonciliated or secretory, and the so-called peg cells.

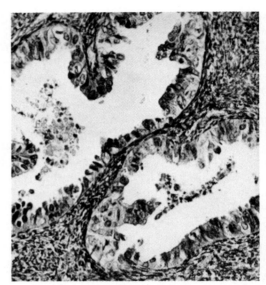

Figure 8–10. Tubal type of endometrial epithelium seen at times in certain areas of hyperplasia.

Occasionally, as in Figure 8–10, the epithelium of the glands may exhibit what is apparently a definite metaplastic change, so that it resembles quite perfectly the endosalpinx; acanthosis is a frequent concomitant. This is a reflection of the multipotential differentiating capacity of the coelomic epithelium.

PROLIFERATIVE AND PSEUDOMALIGNANT TYPES

In the milder degrees of departure from the typical benign Swiss-cheese pattern so common in hyperplasia, one may find only an *unusual degree of epithelial proliferative activity,* evidenced by increased pseudostratification or actual stratification, most frequently in the smaller glands (Fig. 8–11). The epithelial nuclei may be larger and may take a much heavier stain than normal, although the glands themselves may be closely placed, so that the questionable area stands out quite sharply from its surroundings. In other instances, it is the *paler staining* of the questionable area which, as in many cases of actual cancer, sets it out in relief to the surrounding tissue (Fig. 8–11*B*). Mitotic activity, so characteristic of hyperplasia in general, is of little value in the differential diagnosis between this condition and adenocarcinoma.

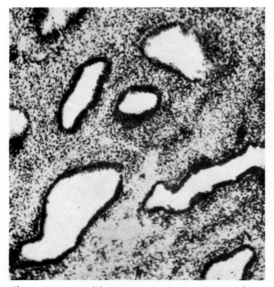

Figure 8–9. Proliferative (nonsecretory) but not hyperplastic endometrium in a patient with functional bleeding.

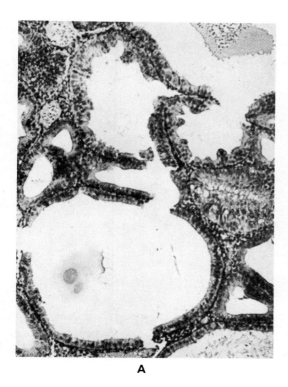

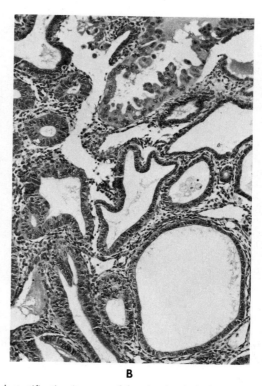

Figure 8–11. *A*, Markedly proliferative hyperplasia, with pseudostratification in some of the glands, producing pictures which may be confused with adenocarcinoma. *B*, Contrast typical hyperplasia (below) with beginning atypia (top). Note stratification and early papillae with paler epithelial cells (top right).

In other cases there is such extreme proliferation of the glands as to literally obliterate any intervening stroma ("back to back crowding") as seen in Figure 8–12. The epithelium is markedly convoluted, with intraluminal tufting and budding. The cells, instead of being one cell layer in thickness, may show some piling up and exhibit evidence of unusual mitotic activity (Fig. 8–13). It is easy to see how such a picture, coupled with such epithelial overactivity as has been described in the preceding paragraph, might make one suspect adenocarcinoma or a secretory (progesterone-induced) endometrium even in an older woman, although there are not the characteristic predecidual changes in the stromal cells (Fig. 8–14). As a matter of fact, even expert pathologists will disagree in the interpretation of certain cases. Most laboratories grade these atypical hyperplasias as mild, moderate, and marked.

Since these perplexing problems most frequently arise in the diagnosis of tissue obtained by diagnostic curettage, their vital bearing upon the patients' welfare is obvi-

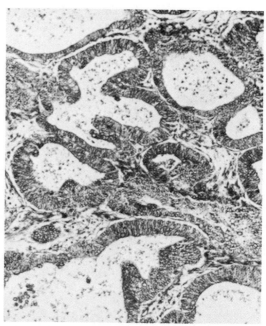

Figure 8–12. Atypical gland picture in hyperplasia, often mistaken for carcinoma. This patient, age 50, has remained well for many years following simple curettage.

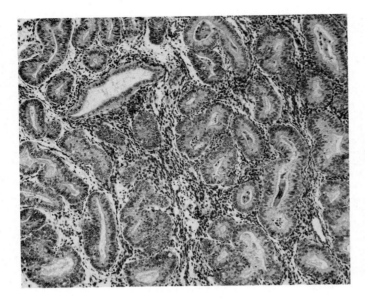

Figure 8–13. Markedly atypical hyperplasia. Beginning stratification and tufting of the lining epithelium with adenomatous crowding, although with still abundant stroma.

ous. No wonder, therefore, that in the occasional case the decision will be that of an eminent foreign gynecologist (Halban) who, on examining such an equivocal section in our laboratory, gave as his verdict, "Nicht Karzinom, aber besser heraus" ("Not carcinoma, but better out").

The simple fact is that in a very small proportion of cases it is impossible for any pathologist to distinguish between highly atypical but benign hyperplasia and genuine adenocarcinoma, so that the safe clinical practice is to treat such cases as probable adenocarcinoma. This subject is further discussed in Chapter 9.

In certain cases during the reproductive epoch we have encountered such evidence of proliferative activity as to raise the question of possible malignancy. Occasionally, in a young woman whose endometrium is frankly suspicious, we might perform a repeat curettage three to four months later. *Progesterone* or *clomiphene* therapy has been suggested by some, the rationale being that if the endometrium can be converted, it is not a malignant process. This procedure may be worthwhile in an occasional case, provided there is careful analysis of subsequent curettings so that a small polypoid malignancy is not overlooked.

Syncytium-like Epithelial Changes

Aside from such cancer-like areas as have been described, we have been interested in a rather curious epithelial reaction noted in a few cases. This is illustrated in Figure 8–15. This epithelial change, which is seen only in scattered areas, is characterized by stratification and acanthosis, with often a syncytial merging of the cells of either the surface or gland epithelium. The cells become large and often develop vacuoles which may become so large that compression of surrounding cells may produce a pseudoglandular picture. The syncytial suggestion is accen-

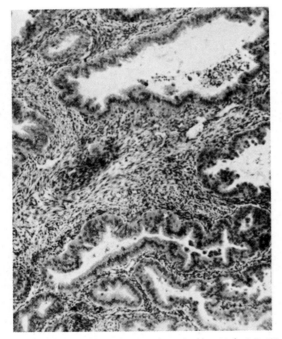

Figure 8–14. Postmenopausal atypical hyperplasia in 57 year old woman. Note resemblance in progestational endometrium. Seven years later frank adenocarcinoma evolved (see also Fig. 7–27).

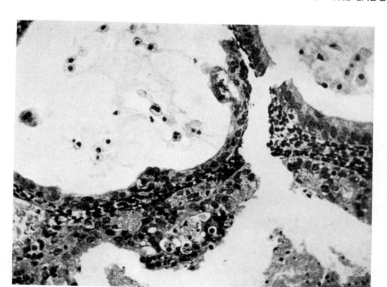

A

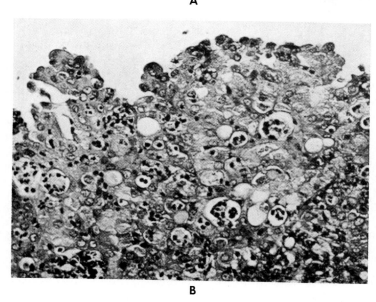

B

Figure 8–15. *A*, Synctium-like epithelial proliferation in hyperplasia, a rather rare finding. *B*, Higher power view of process shown in *A*.

tuated by the fact that the basement membrane is blurred, and appears at times to be completely lost. An interesting feature is the infiltration with many eosinophilic leukocytes; mitosis may likewise be noted.

Squamous Metaplasia or Epidermidization

Another interesting epithelial change at times encountered is the so-called *squamous metaplasia* (Fig. 8–16). This is a relatively frequent finding described by a number of authors (Novak and others). It involves primarily the glands, often filling the lumen, although surface epidermidization is not infrequent. The squamous cells are well differentiated and often spinal; although the novice pathologist may be concerned by their presence, in no way do they indicate a malignant tendency. The prognosis depends entirely on the glandular component, for if this is benign, so then is the whole process irrespective of the associated acanthosis. If the adenomatous element is malignant, the lesion is then defined as an *adenoacanthoma*, a variant of adenocarcinoma that will be discussed later.

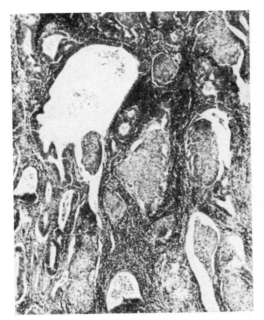

Figure 8–16. Squamous or acanthomatous plaques seen at times in benign hyperplasia of Swiss-cheese pattern.

The source of these squamous cells is speculative, but Meyer has favored an origin from so-called reserve cells which are presumed to lie between the epithelium of the glands and the stroma in the endometrium. These cells have never been demonstrated, and their existence seems rather nebulous. On the other hand, it would seem that there may be a direct transition from lining epithelium or stroma to squamous cells (Fig. 8–17 and 8–18), for on occasion we have seen all

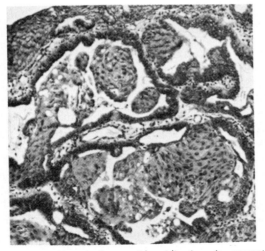

Figure 8–17. Surface epidermidization is present. Note transition forms between epithelium of glands into mature, well-differentiated squamous cells.

intermediate forms. As to what mediates the process, a number of conditions are associated with acanthosis, such as adenocarcinoma, senile endometrium, chronic or tuberculous endometritis, pyometra, submucous myoma, radiation, endometrial polyps, or uterine inversion. Acanthosis is also seen rather frequently today in conjunction with the intrauterine contraceptive device (IUD), as noted by Ober and coworkers. In experimental animals acanthosis can be produced by such agents as estrogen, infection, trauma, vitamin A deficiency, and various dyes, and certainly the first two of these stimuli must be regarded as possible stimulants in women.

In addition to squamous metaplasia, *mucoid* changes may be noted in the lining endometrium or endometrial glands. These may be confirmed by appropriate stains.

Pseudomalignant Hyperplastic Changes in Polyps

A special word seems necessary regarding the striking pseudomalignant proliferative changes that are found not infrequently in the polyps so often seen in cases of hyperplasia. This applies more particularly to the multiple polyposis of marked hyperplasia rather than to the single polyps of the stationary hyperplasia pattern which may be found even when the endometrium as a whole is of the normal functioning type. The latter represents one type of so-called focal hyperplasia, corresponding to the localized areas of hyperplasia or "unripe endometrium" which may be found at various levels in the endometrium proper. Such hyperplastic polyps, if atypical, may be a precursor to endometrial cancer, especially in the menopausal era (Fig. 8–18). Indeed, if such changes were seen in the endometrium proper, this diagnosis would no doubt be made by many pathologists, and yet their significance in polyps is much less. Interpretation may be difficult, for the polyp removed at curettage is often so macerated that it cannot be recognized as such.

Actual carcinomatous changes can of course occur in uterine polyps, but they are relatively rare. Of the cases that have been reported, some at least are polypoid carcinoma, for adenocarcinoma occasionally begins in just this polypoid form. It is especially this type in which, in a considerable number of reported cases, complete removal has apparently been accomplished by the

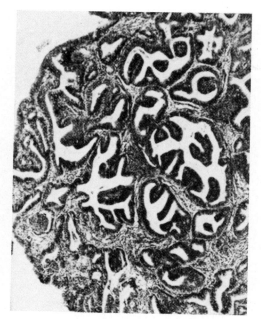

Figure 8–18. Adenomatous crowding of glands in a case of clinically benign but atypical hyperplasia in a polyp.

curette, the microscopic examination of the uterus after removal showing no evidence of cancer. The examination of the pedicle is of great importance in deciding whether one is dealing with a polypoid cancer or a benign polyp which has undergone malignant change. The latter assumption is justified if there is no trace of cancer in the pedicle.

Stromal Hyperplasia

In an occasional instance it is the stromal elements that react most prominently and in extreme forms apparently tend to the development of *actual sarcoma* of endometrial origin. A striking instance of this kind occurred in a patient of 28 years, who had had two curettements for persistent uterine bleeding, the scrapings showing typical hyperplasia. The endometrium in the last curetting showed marked stromal activity, with an unusual number of mitoses and at least some nuclear hyperchromatosis. One year later she died in another city, and autopsy tissue which was received in our laboratory showed extensive sarcoma of the endometrium. However, extensive stromal hyperplasia may occur without malignant connotation (Fig. 8–20).

Postmenopausal Hyperplasia

Today it is well recognized that one may find a perfectly typical and actively growing hyperplasia in women often far beyond the menopause, even when there is no history of

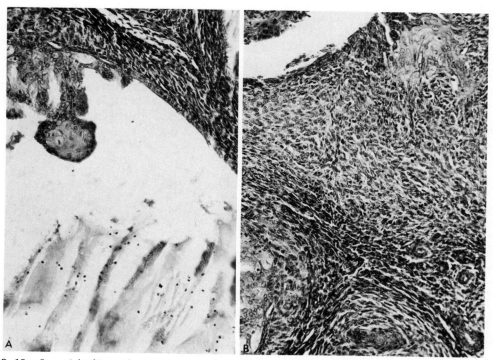

Figure 8–19. Syncytial tufting with squamous metaplasia, suggesting origin from lining epithelium (*A*) and possibly stroma (*B*) at upper right.

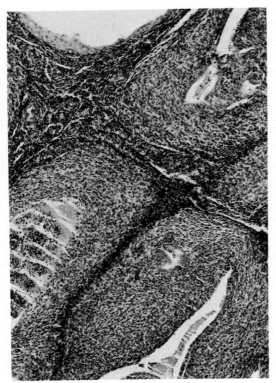

Figure 8–20. Marked proliferation of stroma in endometrial hyperplasia.

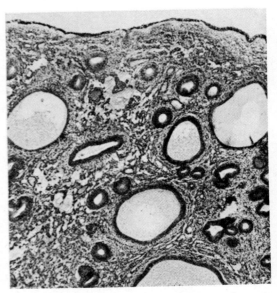

Figure 8–21. Postmenopausal Swiss-cheese hyperplasia, 30 years after menopause, in a patient of 80 years.

estrogen therapy. The general view had always been that hyperplasia is a disease of reproductive life, though it may be observed for at least a short time after the actual cessation of menstrual function, in conformity with the not infrequent existence of hyperestrinism during the earlier phases of the menopause.

In past years it was believed that hyperplasia could rarely persist for more than a year or two after the cessation of menstruation, but today the concept of postmenopausal steroid function by the adrenal, ovary, or other site is generally accepted. Novak and Yui found a considerable number in which typical hyperplasia was present in women from one to 40 years after the last menstrual period (Fig. 8–21). Fuller discussion of hyperplasia after the menopause and its possible premalignant role will be found in Chapter 9.

Although it is undoubtedly true that active hyperplasia, whether in localized or in diffuse forms, may be found in the endometrium long after the menopause, it should be emphasized that in a large proportion of cases postmenopausal hyperplasia is of an obviously retrogressive character. In other words, the Swiss-cheese pattern characterizing the endometrium of many women at the menopause, because of the fact that the terminal cycles are of the anovulatory type, is likely to persist for perhaps a good many years, even in the absence of any further estrogenic stimulation. In such retrogressive cases, even though the Swiss-cheese pattern persists, the stroma is likely to be more or less fibrotic, whereas the gland epithelium is low and inactive, with none of the mitoses so commonly seen in active hyperplasia. These postmenopausal changes have already been fully discussed in Chapter 7. Obviously the finding of postmenopausal hyperplasia mandates close inquiry about usage of exogenous estrogen.

REFERENCES

Benedict, P. H., et al.: Ovarian and adrenal morphology in cases of hirsutism or virilism and Stein-Leventhal syndrome. Fertil. Steril., 13:380, 1962.

Brown, J. B., Kellan, R., and Matthew, G. D.: Preliminary observations on urinary oestrogen excretion in certain gynecological disorders. J. Obstet. Gynaecol. Brit. Commonw., 66:177, 1959.

Campbell, P. E., and Barter, R. A.: Significance of atypical endometrial hyperplasia. J. Obstet. Gynaecol. Brit. Commonw., 68:668, 1961.

Chamlian, D. L., and Taylor, H. B.: Endometrial hyperplasia in young women. Obstet. Gynecol., 36:659, 1970.

McBride, J. M.: Premenopausal cystic hyperplasia and

endometrial carcinoma. J. Obstet. Gynaecol. Brit. Commonw., 66:288, 1959.

McLennan, C. E.: The major types of dysfunctional uterine bleeding. Clin. Obstet. Gynecol., 2:218, 1959.

Meyer, R.: Über seltenere gutartige and zweifelhafte Epithelveränderungen der Uterusschleimhaut im Vergleich mit den ihnen ähnlichen Karzinomformen. Arch. Gynäk., 115:394, 1922.

Munnell, E. W.: The management of dysfunctional uterine bleeding. Bull. Sloane Hosp., 7:21, 1961.

Novak, E., and Rutledge, F.: Atypical endometrial hyperplasia simulating adenocarcinoma. Am. J. Obstet. Gynecol., 55:46, 1948.

Novak, E., and Yui, E.: Relation of hyperplasia to adenocarcinoma of uterus. Am. J. Obstet. Gynecol., 32:674, 1936.

Novak, E. R.: Postmenopausal endometrial hyperplasia. Am. J. Obstet. Gynecol., 71:1312, 1956.

Ober, W. B., Sobrero, A. J., Kurman, R., and Sold, S.: Endometrial morphology and polyethylene IUD; a study of 200 endometrial biopsies. Obstet. Gynecol., 32:782, 1968.

Ostergaard, E.: Adenomatous hyperplasia following estrogen therapy. Acta Obstet. Gynecol. Scand. (Suppl.), 29:97, 1974.

Payne, F. L.: Endometrial hyperplasia. Am. J. Obstet. Gynecol., 34:762, 1957.

Schröder, R.: Endometrial hyperplasia in relation to genital function. Am. J. Obstet. Gynecol., 68:294, 1954.

Shearman, R. P.: Progress in the investigation and treatment of anovulation. Am. J. Obstet. Gynecol., 103:444, 1968.

Silverberg, S. G.: Current concepts in endometrial cancer and endometrial hyperplasia. Contemporary Obstet. Gynecol., 9:123, 1977.

Sippe, G.: Endometrial hyperplasia and uterine bleeding. J. Obstet. Gynaecol. Brit. Commonw., 69:1015, 1962.

Sluder, H. M., and Lock, F. R.: Uterine bleeding. South. Med. J., 44:820, 1957.

Sobrino, L. G., and Kase, N.: Endocrinological aspects of dysfunctional uterine bleeding. Clin. Obstet. Gynecol., 13:400, 1970.

Tacchi, D.: A case of massive endometrial hyperplasia associated with prolonged stilbestrol administration. J. Obstet. Gynaecol. Brit. Emp., 65:817, 1958.

Taylor, H. C.: Endometrial hyperplasia and carcinoma of body of uterus. Am. J. Obstet. Gynecol., 23:309, 1932.

Chapter 9

CARCINOMA OF THE ENDOMETRIUM

Introduction

Whereas clinical carcinoma of the cervix was believed to occur six to eight times more frequently than adenocarcinoma of the endometrium in previous years, today it would seem that the incidence is nearly equal if in situ cervical cancer is not considered. The basic cause for the relatively increased frequency of endometrial adenocarcinoma is that today's woman is living to an age at which she is more likely to develop this malignancy of the older female. Another primary reason is the widespread routine use of the cytopathologic smear so that cervical atypias are detected and treated in their incipiency. Indeed, the clinician in private practice today sees very few cases of invasive cervical cancer, for the current vogue of routine checkup, including smear, rarely allows the genesis of invasive cervical malignancies.

Novak and Villa Santa have summarized current concepts of carcinogenesis and indicate that the ratio between cervical and endometrial cancer is dependent on the type of patient admitted to any clinic. Patients from poor socioeconomic groups, with early and frequent intercourse, a resultant high number of pregnancies, and poor obstetric care, might be expected to have a disproportionate frequency of cervical cancer. Marnett and co-workers point out that in Connecticut the incidence of endometrial cancer has almost doubled in the last decade or so (figures from the Connecticut Tumor Registry).

Today's American woman has an average life span of more than 70 years, and it is probable that more women develop endometrial cancer, which is a disease of the older woman; this is unquestionably *the prime cause* of increased fundal cancer. In addition, the presumed increase in cases of endometrial adenocarcinoma is in part due to misinterpretation of so-called adenocarcinoma in situ. Recent studies by Smith and co-workers, Ziel and Finkle, and many others would seem to implicate estrogen therapy as a causal factor in the development of endometrial adenocarcinoma. In separate publications they point out that women using estrogen have four to five times greater risk of developing endometrial cancer, and the risk increases proportionately with the degree of exposure. In California the incidence of this malignancy has increased 50 per cent in the years 1969 to 1974 despite the fact that more liberal hysterectomy in younger patients would seem to have eliminated the possibility in many cases. Certain gynecologists who are endocrinologically oriented dispute the estrogen-adenocarcinoma relationship, primarily on the basis of the difficulty in distinguishing adenocarcinoma from a markedly atypical hyperplasia, possibly reversible. It would seem to us that a significant endometrial atypia warrants hysterectomy, so this seems no more than an academic point. However, the American College stresses that the estrogen-adenocarcinoma relation is not certain but urges cautious use of hormones.

Endometrial adenocarcinoma is characteristically a disease of postmenopausal women, with fewer than one fourth of all cases occurring in the menstrual era. The average age is 57 years, a full decade later than in women with cervical cancer. There is no

204

question that cancer involving the fundus is a much more favorable disease to treat than the cervical variety, and 5 year salvage approximates 75 per cent, or about twice that of the usual figures quoted for epidermoid cervical cancer of all stages.

Gross Characteristics

Diffuse Adenocarcinoma. In this form a large area of the endometrial surface, or perhaps the whole interior of the uterus, is involved. The cancerous area is thickened and irregularly polypoid with surface ulceration and necrosis in the later stages. Even in comparatively early cases, the surface involvement may be quite extensive and diffuse. Unlike the ordinary benign polyp, or the multiple polyps which may fill the uterus in some cases of benign polypoid hyperplasia, the polypoid outgrowths of cancer are of bulkier appearance, friable in consistency, with often superficial necrosis, in contrast with benign polyps, which are covered by a smooth mucosa.

Although polypoid hyperplasia may involve the entire endometrium, it ends in a sharp line corresponding to the internal os, for the cervix is never involved in the abnormal functional response represented by hyperplasia. Carcinoma, on the other hand, is no respecter of physiologic lines of demarcation, so that in extensive adenocarcinoma of the corpus the disease may extend well down into the cervical canal.

Not only does the disease extend along the surface, but it also pushes into the underlying musculature (Fig. 9–1). It is surprising how much surface involvement there may be with no involvement of the muscle wall. In other cases, one finds beneath the surface broad irregular zones in which the firm trabeculated appearance characteristic of the uterine musculature is replaced by an amorphous friable mass of cancer tissue.

Finally, in advanced disease, the involvement may extend to the peritoneum. In such cases the uterus may be grossly enlarged and on its surface one may see nodules, singly or in clusters, representing areas of lymphatic metastasis. These may arise long before the gross disease reaches the serosal surface.

Circumscribed Adenocarcinoma. There are many cases of adenocarcinoma in which the gross lesion seems definitely circumscribed, involving only a small area of the endometrial surface. In this type must be included a group in which the carcinoma begins in the form of a *localized polypoid* growth in any portion of the uterine cavity (Fig. 9–2 A). This does not imply that it arose in a benign polyp, for malignant change in a polyp is actually extremely uncommon. In such instances, the surface area may remain comparatively small, although the malignant process penetrates deeply into the musculature (Fig. 9–2 B).

The *polypoid form* is especially interesting because it represents the group in which diagnostic curettage has, in many reported cases, apparently removed all gross trace of

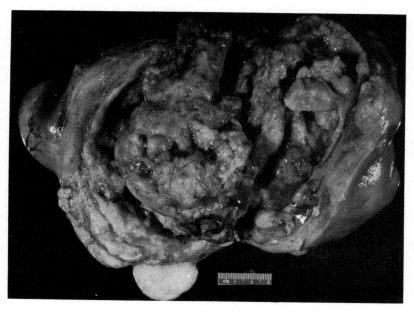

Figure 9–1. Uterine cavity filled by extensive diffuse adenocarcinoma with beginning myometrial extension. (Previous amputation of cervix).

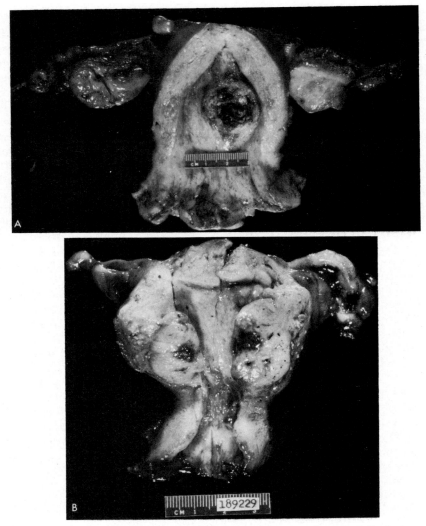

Figure 9–2. *A*, Circumscribed lesion of posterior uterine wall with no invasion of muscle. *B*, Beginning myometrial spread of localized endometrial cancer.

the lesion, so that examination of the uterus after hysterectomy shows no evidence of the disease. The absence of gross disease in such cases does not mean that the patient would be cured by simple curettage, although the prognosis after complete operation is very favorable.

From a practical laboratory standpoint, in cases in which the curettings show cancer and the macroscopic and microscopic examination of the removed uterus does not, the first suspicion should be of a possible mix-up in sections, and this should be eliminated. Even when this is done, however, a certain number of instances are observed in which contradictory findings occur, and these are explained by the fact that the curette has apparently brought away all demonstrable evidence of the uterine lesion. This can be readily appreciated when one sees such small polypoid lesions as that shown in Figure 9–3.

It is quite possible that localized and polypoid carcinomas represent merely early stages of a process that later becomes diffuse, but the fact remains that certain adenocarcinomas have a tendency to spread diffusely over the surface, whereas others tend to remain rather localized even when quite infiltrative.

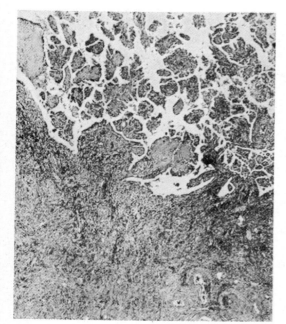

Figure 9–3. Section of small papillary adenocarcinoma of uterus.

Microscopic Characteristics

The microscopic picture of adenocarcinoma is characterized by a marked departure from the normal pattern, as regards both the disorderly atypia of the glands and the abnormal hyperactive histologic characteristics of the lining epithelial cells (Fig. 9-4).

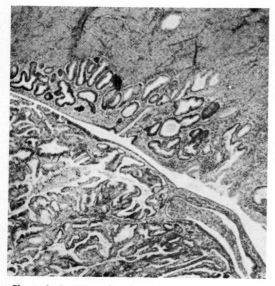

Figure 9–4. Normal endometrium above as contrasted with adenocarcinoma (Grade II) below.

In general, there are two chief features in the microscopic study of adenocarcinoma: (1) the pattern or architecture of the growth, and (2) the individual cell changes.

Pattern or Architecture. This gives at once the impression of a disorderly departure from the normal. Ordinarily the glands are distributed discretely throughout the stroma, and they are more or less uniform in appearance. In the postmenopausal endometrium, moreover, they are characteristically narrow and atrophic.

In adenocarcinoma, on the other hand, the glands present all degrees of departure from normal. They are increased in number, and show all sorts of irregular and often bizarre convolutions. Sometimes the gland atypia is comparatively slight: the glands are closely placed and moderately atypical, with an epithelium which in some places seems normal, although in others the cells are closely packed, polyhedral, with dark-staining nuclei, and a number of mitoses.

On the other hand, one frequently finds a far more atypical gland pattern, and in addition the gland epithelium is stratified, with beginning tufting and papillae, and marked anaplastic changes in the epithelial cells—nonuniformity in size and shape of cells and nuclei, mitoses, hyperchromatosis, etc. In advanced forms the glands may be solidly filled with dedifferentiated cells, so that in many areas the resemblance to solid epidermoid cancer may be perfect (Fig. 9–5).

Invasion of the stroma by epithelial cells is commonly seen in the highly malignant types but is often lacking in the forms in which the gland pattern is more moderately atypical. Even though invasiveness is looked upon as the most decisive feature of cancer, the mere absence of stromal invasion by the epithelium should not influence the diagnosis since vascular or lymphatic involvement may occur. In many instances the stroma is completely obliterated because of the massive hyperplasia of the glandular elements ("back to back crowding") (Fig. 9–6).

In many adenocarcinomas, especially when not too advanced, one finds a characteristic papillary or treelike pattern, as shown in Figure 9–3, although a papillary pattern is more suggestive of an ovarian origin. Psammoma bodies may be found on certain occasions (Factor). Finger-like processes are seen, consisting of a central delicate stem of connective tissue contain-

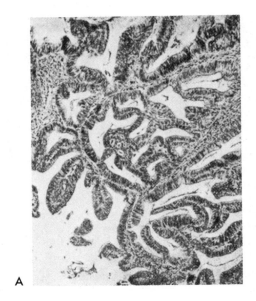
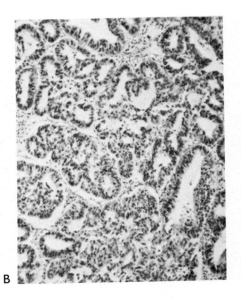

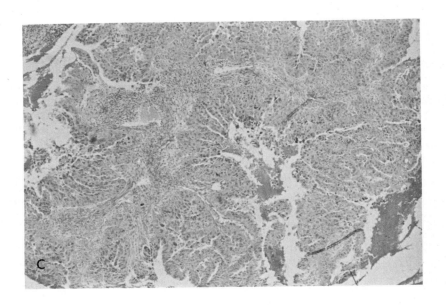

Figure 9–5. *A,* Grade I adenocarcinoma; *B,* Grade II lesion; *C,* Grade III lesion. (See FIGO classification, page 214.)

ing frequent blood vessels, and covered with a treelike growth of epithelium showing the malignant characteristics described, with often many acinus-like gland spaces. No such pictures are found in the normal endometrium or in benign polyps.

Cell Changes. In many adenocarcinomas a large proportion of the cells may retain essentially normal characteristics, but in others almost all the cells show a high degree of dedifferentiation, being polyhedral or rounded, closely packed, with heavily stained nuclei, and many mitotic figures, both typical and atypical. The stromal cells of a malignant growth play no essential part in the disease process, but usually show marked reactive inflammatory infiltration with round cells and leukocytes.

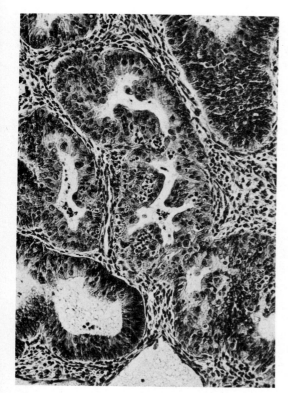

Figure 9–6. Markedly adenomatous atypical hyperplasia of borderline type. Beginning loss of stroma due to "back to back crowding."

With certain exceptions, as noted by Katayama and Jones, endometrial carcinoma is characterized by diploidy rather than the tetraploidy found in most cervical cancer. Stanley and Kirkland confirm this observation, and possibly this may account for the more innocuous course of the usual endometrial lesion.

Diagnosis

A decisive pathologic diagnosis can be made only by microscopic examination of the endometrium, so that diagnostic curettage is the most important procedure in all cases of abnormal bleeding, especially in the postmenopausal variety. While Doran and Thompson have pointed out that any type of operative manipulation may increase the percentage of suspiciously malignant cells in the peripheral blood, there is no certainty that clinical metastases are incurred. Seemingly, the pathologic diagnosis as determined by curettage offsets any questionable adverse effects. Endometrial washing such

as the jet-irrigation technique (Gravlee), aspiration, or brushing seem uncomplicated and accurate, but a thorough curettage is warranted even when other studies are negative. We have not found hysterography (Schwartz et al.) or hysteroscopy (Sugimoto) to be particularly helpful.

Bleeding, even from adenocarcinoma, is often scanty and intermittent with long nonbleeding phases. This should be emphasized to the climacteric female who may inquire why curettage is necessary when bleeding has ceased. When postmenopausal bleeding has occurred, *curettage is mandatory* despite a negative smear, for cytopathologic studies of the endometrium do not enjoy the high degree of accuracy, as with the cervix. A shift to the right of the maturation index is often noted despite an inconclusive smear, and this suggestion of increased postmenopausal estrogen activity should alert the clinician, assuming that the patient is receiving no hormone therapy.

Secondary Ulceration

As with other carcinomas, necrosis is a common feature, especially of the more advanced stages, so that in these the uterine cavity is covered with a ragged, ulcerated, fungoid mass. Even in the earlier stages, ulcerative and necrotic changes often take place, and it is easy to understand, therefore, the production of the slight spotting or bleeding that may mark the early stages. In the advanced forms, with extensive ulceration, bleeding may be profuse and constant. Pyometra may occur, but it is less common than in cervical malignancy.

Differential Microscopic Diagnosis

Although the microscopic diagnosis of adenocarcinoma is often simple enough, there is at least one endometrial lesion that may offer great difficulty in this respect. We refer to the *atypical, proliferative,* or *adenomatous* varieties of hyperplasia, which have been described in the preceding chapter. When the atypical changes are of mild degree, the differentiation is simple enough. When the lesion is an extensive adenomatous one, with marked epithelial proliferation, the simulation of low grade carcinoma is so perfect that pathologists differ in their diagnostic interpretation.

As a matter of fact, *there is a small group in*

which no pathologist can be absolutely sure. In any form of hyperplasia mitoses are present, often in large numbers, so that they are not helpful in the microscopic differentiation. In the lower grade adenocarcinomas there is little dedifferentiation of the epithelial cells, while in either the benign or malignant lesion the epithelial layer may be stratified (Fig. 9–7). Again, a large proportion of adenocarcinomas show little invasion of the myometrium. As a matter of fact, there is usually far more invasion of the muscle in the entirely benign adenomyosis than is seen in many adenocarcinomas.

The clinically malignant nature of the latter, as indicated by its extension to lymph glands, is proof that its cells do actually break through basement membrane and in certain cases this penetration, as well as its extension to the muscularis, is easily demonstrable (Fig. 9–8). It thus appears that there is a whole series of gradations, a species of histologic stepping stones, between atypical hyperplasia and adenocarcinoma, and there is no specific criterion as to the point at which the lesion assumes actually malignant characteristics. Certainly these *atypical hyperplasias* should be regarded as a precursory, if not the earliest, stage of malignancy, and the safe clinical plan is to treat them surgically.

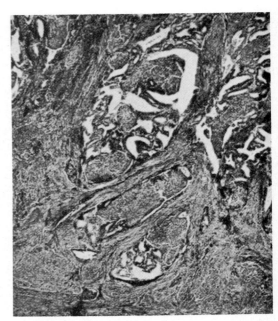

Figure 9–8. Adenocarcinoma invading uterine musculature.

Adenocarcinoma In Situ

We dislike this term, which has no specific criteria. In situ *cervical* cancer shows full-thickness replacement of the surface epithelium by abnormal, generally basal cells; what constitutes an *endometrial* in situ lesion is often simply a whim of the individual pathologist. Thus, many referred cases in which this diagnosis is made represent merely a benign cystic or mildly proliferative hyperplasia. Occasionally a normal premenstrual pattern may be present.

If the latter sounds ridiculous, let us state that it may be difficult to distinguish between a secretory pattern and proliferative hyperplasia. In each case there is tufting and infolding into the gland lumen. The cells in each instance are tall and pale, and even with hyperplasia there may appear evidence of secretory activity. The appearance of the stroma is decisive, for with hyperplasia, it is dense and compact; with progesterone stimulation, it is edematous, more vascular, and pseudodecidual.

Although cognizant of what the term adenocarcinoma in situ implies when used by expert pathologists like Hertig, we must reject usage of the term until some standardization is accomplished. Too liberal interpretation seems to invite an unnecessary index of

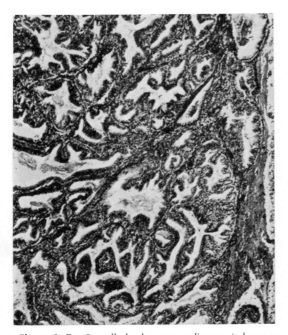

Figure 9–7. So-called adenoma malignum (adenocarcinoma Grade I).

suspicion and, as mentioned earlier, serves as a factor in the increasing incidence of presumed endometrial cancer. Likewise, very early lesions, seemingly compatible with an in situ status, can occasionally metastasize, although this is excessively uncommon (Figs. 9–9 and 9–10).

Histologic Grading of Adenocarcinoma of Uterine Body

It is useful to classify adenocarcinoma into various histologic types or grades. Aside from its prognostic significance, it at once conveys at least a rough idea of the microscopic appearance of the tumor.

The FIGO Cancer Committee has recently recommended three grades:

1. Highly differentiated adenomatous carcinomas;

2. Differentiated adenocarcinomas with partly solid areas;

3. Predominantly solid or undifferentiated carcinomas.

It would also seem that *myometrial invasion* as evident in the removed uterus is of primary importance in formulating a prognosis. Even well-differentiated tumors can on occasion penetrate deeply and extend into lymphatics, with recurrence and death.

On other occasions somewhat anaplastic lesions may be rather superficial and compatible with a prolonged life. *As a rule, however, the degree of differentiation parallels myometrial extension.*

Clinical Classification of Endometrial Carcinoma

The International Federation of Gynecology and Obstetrics in its Annual Report on the Results of Treatment in Carcinoma of the Uterus and Vagina (15th volume) has recommended that *carcinoma of the endometrial corpus* be staged as follows:

Stage 0 Histologic findings suggestive of malignancy, but not proved.

Stage 1 The carcinoma is confined to the corpus.

    1a Uterine cavity 8 cm. or less.

    1b Uterine cavity greater than 8 cm.

Stage 2 The carcinoma has involved the corpus and the cervix.

Stage 3 The carcinoma has extended outside the uterus, but not outside the true pelvis.

Stage 4 The carcinoma has extended outside the true pelvis or has obviously involved the mucosa of the bladder or rectum.

Stage I cases should be further qualified as

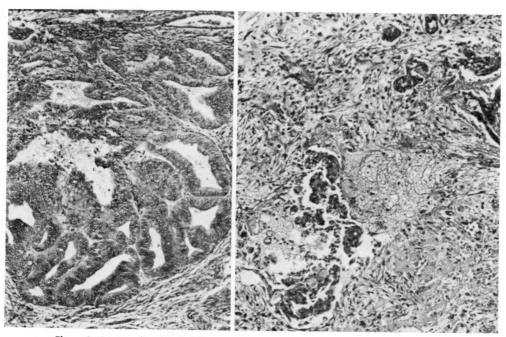

Figure 9–9. Localized well-differentiated adenocarcinoma (none present elsewhere).
Figure 9–10. Metastasis of adenocarcinoma (Fig. 9–9) to ovarian hilus.

A Early polypoid lesion with granulosal–thecal cell tumor. *B* Advanced disease with extensive myometrial involvement. *C* Adenoacanthoma (benign squamous component). *D* Adenoepidermoid tumor (malignant squamous component). *E* Beginning atypical endometrial hyperplasia (lower left). *F* Significant atypia (reverted following progesterone therapy, with subsequent pregnancy).

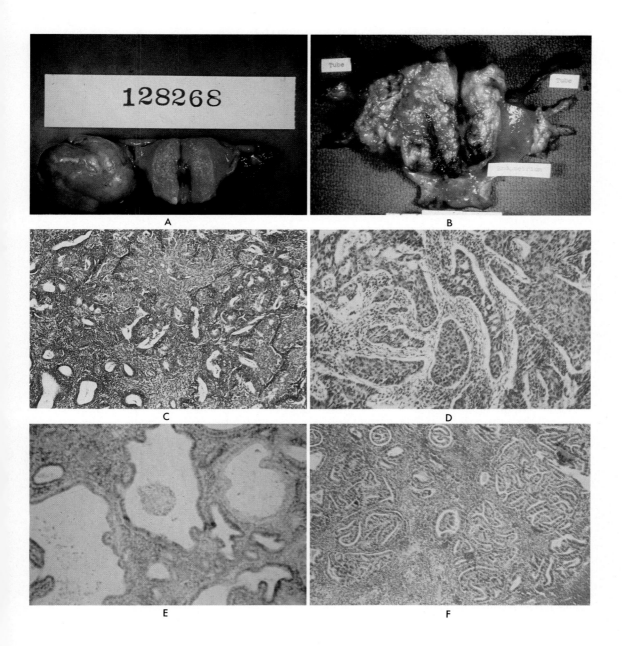

to whether they are (1) highly differentiated adenomatous, (2) differentiated but with partly solid areas, (3) predominately solid or undifferentiated.

This is a logical if not ideal method of classification. In subdividing Stage I into Ia and Ib, the size of the uterus hardly seems valid, for such concomitant diseases as myoma or adenomyosis are not rare, and one may find a large uterus with only minor degrees of cancer.

Carcinoma corporis et endocervicis is the suggested terminology when the presence of tumor in both locales makes it impossible to assign a primary site. Fractional curettage of first the endocervix and then the corpus, with tumor in both, may indicate the likely primary source, and histologic niceties may suggest an endometrial origin (if there is acanthosis) or an endocervical origin (if mucus-forming). Treatment of carcinoma of corpus and cervix is less satisfactory and standardized. In noting an approximate 15 to 20 per cent incidence of these Stage II lesions, Rutledge advocates radical hysterectomy *only* in those women who have some contraindication to the more usual irradiation followed by conservative hysterectomy.

When microscopically indistinguishable cancer involves ovary and endometrium, the term *carcinoma uteri et ovarii* has been proposed. This combination of endometrial and gonadal tumors occurs with some frequency, and on occasion it is impossible to ascertain which is the primary, or if there are two lesions (multicentric origin).

The American Joint Committee for Cancer Staging has advocated qualification of any tumor by such terms as T (primary tumor), N (lymph node involvement), and M (metastases); all of these are qualified numerically according to the extent. Although recognizing the need for standardization, we dislike having such a cumbersome classification applied to uterine malignancy.

Adenoacanthoma of Uterus

In Chapter 8, mention was made of the fact that squamous metaplasia of either the surface or the gland epithelium may occasionally be noted. The same type of change may be noted in adenocarcinoma, and often in exaggerated degree, giving rise to the so-called adenoacanthoma (Fig. 9–11). This change has most often been seen in adenocarcinomas of the lesser degrees of malignancy,

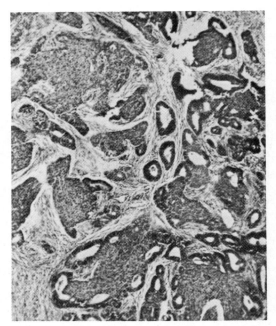

Figure 9–11. Adenoacanthoma of uterus, showing large metaplastic plaques resembling squamous epithelium.

and this no doubt explains why the adenoacanthomatous group has yielded relatively favorable results, although many (Badib et al., and others) feel that there is no particular difference in the salvage of adenocarcinoma and that of adenoacanthoma of comparable stage and grade. Acanthosis may occur in poorly differentiated tumors on occasion.

A remarkable histologic picture is produced when this metaplastic change is extensive. Between the gland lumina, and often pushing into them, are broad solid fields of cells that may resemble sheets or nests of squamous epithelium. Where they infringe on the glands, they may obliterate the epithelium of the latter, so that masses of the metaplastic epithelium may seem to be growing within the gland lumina themselves. Surface epidermidalization may also occur.

The earlier view as to the origin of this interesting histologic change was that it arose from certain indifferent cells beneath the normal columnar uterine epithelium, these cells possessing a differentiating potency, which under certain conditions might lead to the formation of a squamous type of epithelium (Fig. 9–12). More recent observations have suggested a direct metaplastic transformation from glandular epithelium into squamous cells, for at times all seem-

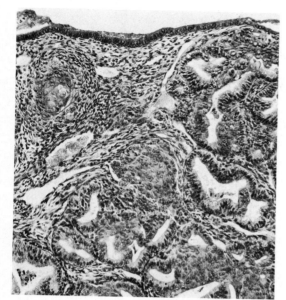

Figure 9–12. Well-differentiated adenoacanthoma of very low grade malignancy.

ingly transitional forms can be recognized. In spite of the rather forbidding appearance of the pronounced cases of adenoacanthoma, the squamous cells are mature and well differentiated although malignant change may occur. Generally speaking, therefore, it is upon the behavior of the epithelial and glandular elements that one must base one's evaluation of the malignancy of the adenoacanthoma.

A publication by Novak and Nalley has dealt with a small series of 16 adenoacanthomas. They found that squamous metapla-

sia occurred primarily in the early well-differentiated type of endometrial adenocarcinoma and was rarely, if ever, associated with myometrial or other extension. Indeed, the finding of acanthosis almost guarantees a good result. This of course does not include the very rare case in which true cervical epidermoid and endometrial adenocarcinoma coexist.

Adenoepidermoid (Squamous) Lesions

On occasion one may find a combined epidermoid and adenocarcinomatous malignancy involving the endometrium when the cervix is normal. We prefer to refer to this as an *adenoepidermoid* tumor, and this carries a much worse prognosis than an adenoacanthoma, from which however, it may have arisen (Fig. 9–13). These lesions, as well as the more differentiated *adenosquamous* tumors, are becoming more frequent for uncertain reasons, and there is a distressing 30 per cent 5 year salvage. They are relatively radioresistant, with a tendency to extensive infiltration and metastasis. At times histologic differentiation from the much more innocuous *adenoacanthoma* is difficult, as noted by Julian and co-workers.

Studies such as those by Charles and by Liggins and Way, indicating a 25 to 35 per cent extrauterine extension of adenoacanthoma, seemingly include cases of adenosquamous lesions, for the epidermoid component is prompt to invade or metastasize. In the usual adenoacanthoma, however, invasion or extension is rare with the usual

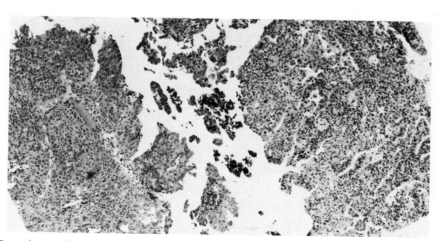

Figure 9–13. Adenoepidermoid cancer of endometrium showing epidermoid component (left) and adenocarcinoma (right).

well-differentiated tumor; in the one that is poorly differentiated (although there is an associated benign squamous metaplasia) the prognosis parallels that of the histologic grade of the adenomatous component (Fig. 9–13).

Mesonephric Pattern

Certain instances of endometrial adenocarcinoma portray a lipoid or a clear cell pattern as well as a tubular pattern lined by a flat cuboidal "peg-like" epithelium identical to that found in Schiller's mesonephroma. Kurman and Scully record 21 such cases, many of which showed both a clear cell and a tubular pattern, with psammoma bodies in a few (Figs. 9–14 to 9–16).

Obviously, the endometrium is not the usual site at which vestigial remnants of the mesonephric ducts would be expected. Perhaps these may on occasion occur in an aberrant location, yet may it not be likely that ordinary adenocarcinoma arising from a mesothelial surface can exhibit metaplastic changes that lead to the histologic picture of mesonephroma? On the other hand, mesonephroma has been suspected by some (Scully and Barlow) to arise from müllerian (paramesonephric) elements. Diverse origins seem possible.

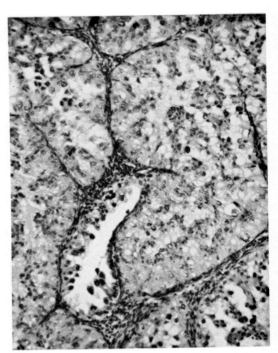

Figure 9–15. Mesonephroid pattern; note Schiller appearance in central portion. (Courtesy of Dr. McGillivray, University of Alberta.)

Adenocarcinoma Developing in Endometrial Polyps

Although carcinoma may begin as a localized polypoid lesion, as already described, it should be remembered that a previously benign endometrial polyp may undergo adenocarcinomatous degeneration (Fig. 9–17). It may be difficult to distinguish between the primarily and secondarily malignant polyps. The study of the base of the polyp is most apt to be decisive. If the base shows no cancer in a polyp that otherwise reveals the definite cancer, it may be concluded that the malignancy is secondary. If, on the other hand, the entire polyp, including the base, shows adenocarcinoma (not infrequently extending into the surrounding endometrium), it would seem certain that the lesion is primary.

Malignant degeneration of endometrial polyps is rare. In the consideration of possible malignant degeneration of endometrial polyps, mistakes are easily made because many polyps show a markedly adenomatous and proliferative pattern, which can readily be mistaken for adenocarcinoma. If such interpretative errors could be eliminated from

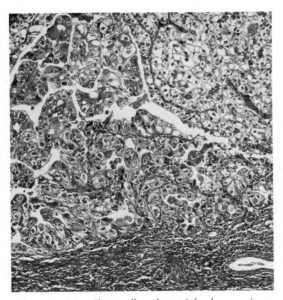

Figure 9–14. Clear cell endometrial adenocarcinoma with positive fat stain and no evidence of ovarian tumor. On occasion the pattern of Schiller's mesonephroma is found. (Courtesy of Dr. Umberto Villa Santa, Baltimore.)

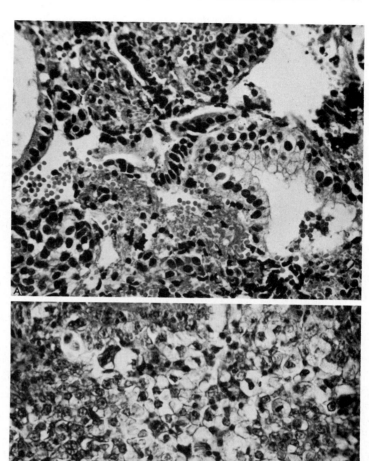

Figure 9–16. *A,* Clear cell pattern. *B,* Higher magnification of *A.*

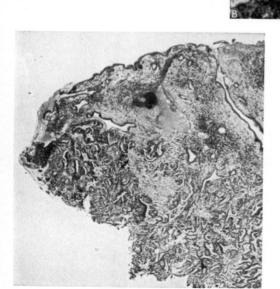

Figure 9–17. Endometrial polyp showing adenocarcinomatous change (below).

the statistics, the incidence of secondary cancer in polyps would be considerably less.

Although endometrial polyps rarely undergo malignant degeneration, it is not uncommon to find associated malignancy, especially around and after the menopause. Peterson and Novak found polyps to be associated with malignancy in over 15 per cent of all postmenopausal cases, the majority being adenocarcinoma of the adjacent endometrium. It would seem that the finding of an endometrial polyp, though benign, should suggest careful observation of the postmenopausal woman.

Relation of Uterine Myoma to Corporeal Adenocarcinoma

Myoma is such a common tumor that it would be strange if it were not often coexistent with carcinoma, and it is difficult to see how subserous or intramural growths could exert any irritative effect upon the mucosa. On the other hand, it is easier to believe that submucous tumors, with associated ulcerative and inflammatory changes, might theoretically predispose to cancer in some cases. Although no one now accepts the old view that myoma plays an important predisposing role, there are still many who speculate on the relationship of such estrogen-dependent lesions as myoma and adenomyosis.

The frequent association of abnormal bleeding should not lead one to the assumption that when myoma and bleeding coexist they are necessarily related as cause and effect, for an adenocarcinoma may possibly be concealed within the myomatous uterus (Fig. 9–18). Diagnostic curettage should be done routinely in any patient with a seemingly myomatous uterus, since an unsuspected cancer may be present despite a negative cytopathologic report. In most cases, the uterus should be opened immediately after hysterectomy and before closure of the abdomen, so that a more complete procedure can be carried out if unexpected carcinoma is revealed.

Secondary Adenocarcinoma

This occurs most often as a result of metastasis from carcinoma of the ovary (Fig. 9–19), but may be secondary to malignancy of more distant organs, such as the stomach or breast. Simultaneous multicentric malignancy of

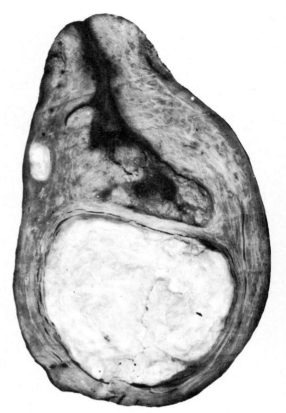

Figure 9–18. Large subserous myoma coexisting with adenocarcinoma of the endometrium; obviously myomectomy without previous curettage would have been unfortunate. (Courtesy of Prof. Robert Keller, Edinburgh.)

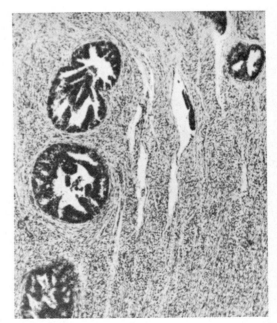

Figure 9–19. Secondary adenocarcinoma in uterine muscle, primary lesion being in ovary.

areas of common mesothelial origin, such as ovary, endometrium, tube, and endocervix, may occur, and should not be construed as metastatic phenomena (Woodruff and Julian).

Extension and Metastasis of Adenocarcinoma of Uterine Body

The dissemination of carcinoma of the body is chiefly through the lymphatics, though direct extension is also of importance. In advanced cases the disease may extend well into the cervical canal, so that gross examination may make it difficult to be sure whether the disease has originated in the cervix or in the uterine body.

The *lymphatics* that drain the body of the uterus, like those of the tube and ovary, empty chiefly into the lumbar group of glands situated near the lower end of the aorta. If the cancer site is low in the uterine body, the upper hypogastric glands, near the bifurcation of the iliacs, may be involved quite early, and they are almost always involved in the very late stages. Carcinoma arising near the uterine cornu may find its way along the round ligament lymphatics to the inguinal glands. However, radical surgery is not the usual treatment, since nodal involvement is relatively uncommon (approximately 10 per cent in Stage I).

The *ovaries* are the seat of metastases in some cases, though the incidence of this occurrence is considerably less than one might expect from the richness of the lymphatic intercommunications between the two organs. In only 7 of 147 cases (less than 5 per cent) of uterine adenocarcinoma did we find ovarian metastasis in our laboratory, although Gusberg and Yannopoulos note nearly 12 per cent.

The *tubes* may likewise be involved, probably by a mechanism similar to that described in connection with the ovary. The lymphatic connections of the tube with the uterus are even more direct than those of the ovary. It is of interest to note that metastasis to the tube is often submucous and interstitial, with an intact mucous membrane, speaking again for the importance of the lymphatic route rather than implantation. On the other hand, the whole lumen of the tube may be filled by extensive adenocarcinoma (Fig. 9–20).

The *peritoneum* of the pelvic and abdominal cavities is involved in many advanced cases, with nodules appearing over the parietal peritoneum, or in the visceral peritoneum covering almost any abdominal organs, including also the omentum. The *cervix* is likewise involved in certain advanced cases, as already noted, as may also be the *bladder* or *rectum.* Involvement of *distant organs,* such as the liver or lungs, may occur, but is relatively rare. Postoperative pelvic recurrence is the most common problem.

In general, however, endometrial cancer is frequently a "surface rider." It is much less prone to local or lymphatic extension than is cervical malignancy.

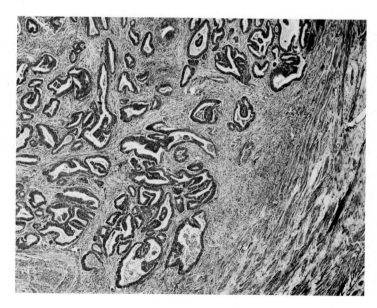

Figure 9–20. An unusually well-differentiated lesion has extended to fill the tubal lumen although muscularis is uninvolved.

Relationship of Endometrial Hyperplasia to Adenocarcinoma

It is generally accepted that endometrial hyperplasia as found in the menstrual era is an innocuous process, frequently transient, and in no way related to malignant trends, although it may sometimes represent a difficult clinical problem. Various earlier students have carried out separate studies which concur in this impression, but they also point out the increased significance of hyperplasia in the postmenopausal years, especially if it be of a proliferative variety. Other more recent authors, such as Gusberg, stress the role of adenomatous hyperplasia as a possibly precancerous lesion, and this is our own belief. His classification of *mild* (intense microcystic change), *moderate* (epithelial infolding and protrusion into the glandular lumen), and *severe* (back to back glandular crowding and a pale epithelial dysplasia) seems appropriate.

A much larger series of publications have concerned women with definite adenocarcinoma in which earlier endometrial curettement or biopsy had shown endometrial hyperplasia, often recurrent and frequently proliferative. Many authors have reported this sequel, and Hertig has designated some of these atypical hyperplastic patterns as adenocarcinoma in situ. Although not in complete agreement with this term, we are in accord with the possible, if not inevitable, tendencies of these adenomatous endometria toward cancer.

Observation of cases of hyperplasia around and after the menopause has convinced us that patients with hyperplasia show exactly the same features that are frequently, if not always, associated with women developing cancer. A late menopause, obesity, hypertension, diabetes, a poor fertility index, a history of previous curettages indicating anovulation are common denominators of (post) menopausal hyperplasia and adenocarcinoma. For fuller details the reader is referred to an earlier publication by Novak. From this observation one must form the very definite impression that hyperplasia (postmenopausal) and adenocarcinoma are variants of the same basic process, with fundal cancer evolving if there is a sufficiently prolonged or potent stimulus. If this stimulus is withdrawn, malignancy need not develop; if it is continued, adenocarcinoma frequently evolves. As to what this stimulus is, it is difficult to deny that it may be some type of estrogenic steroid.

Estrogen as a factor in the production of endometrial cancer has frequently been under suspicion, but has usually been absolved because endometrial cancer had not been produced experimentally in animals by this steroid. One must realize that most animals so treated develop an aseptic pyometra which might serve to nullify this development, but many workers have produced extreme degrees of endometrial proliferation (Fig. 9–21). Interestingly enough, cervical cancer has been produced in mice by estrogen as reported by Gardner and co-workers.

Meissner and associates produced endometrial adenocarcinoma in a certain strain of rabbit (Fig. 9–22). Once the neoplasm was produced, it went on to metastasize and kill the animal; obviously the lesion was not merely of pseudocarcinomatous nature. Meriam and co-workers have induced adenocarcinoma in one horn of the bicornuate rabbit uterus by inserting a string saturated with methylcholanthrene. Malignancy evolved following initial phases of cystic hyperplasia through proliferative forms to the genesis of true cancer.

It is accepted that unopposed estrogen is the normal stimulus to endometrial hyperplasia, and that there may be proliferative atypical forms of hyperplasia to the degree that they are indistinguishable from genuine fundal cancer. It has been noted that exogenous estrogens may be associated with the development of endometrial adenocarcinoma.

However, it would be syllogistic to assume that since (a) exogenous estrogen leads to endometrial hyperplasia, and (b) endometrial hyperplasia may be so proliferative as to exactly mimic corpus cancer (Fig. 9–23), therefore (c) endogenous estrogen causes cancer. Nevertheless, estrogen deserves certain consideration from many approaches as a possible cancerocidal agent, although other factors are most certainly involved. Knab has published an extensive resume of the problem.

Charles and co-workers have found normal urinary estrogen levels in eight patients with endometrial adenocarcinoma despite high cornification in the maturation index, and they suggest that the vaginal smear is not a reliable index of estrogenic activity in patients with endometrial cancer. One must be

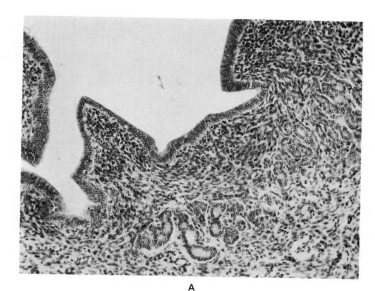

A

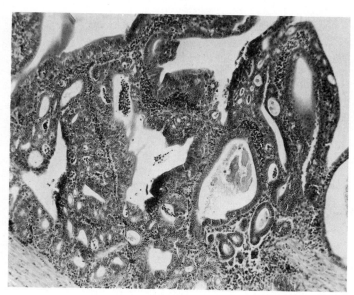

B

Figure 9–21. *A*, Control uterus of hamster. *B*, Proliferative hyperplasia following estrogen therapy for 280 days.

mindful of the technical difficulties in various bioassays as well as the possibility of convertibility of the closely related steroids so that detection in the urine may be impossible by current methods of assay.

In any case certain genetically inclined individuals may require only a small stimulus to trigger carcinogenic development; in others less inclined, no amount of stimulation would initiate the chain reaction. Many different observations suggest that estrogen may serve a role in the development of endometrial adenocarcinoma; no one of these is conclusive, but in conjunction with one another they must be regarded as suggestive. Briefly these may be summarized as follows.

Late Menopause

Repeated observations have noted the late and protracted menopause of women who subsequently develop fundal cancer. Since anovulation in this era is frequent, the opportunity for unopposed estrogen stimulation is present for prolonged periods of time, and it seems likely that this may persist, even in the absence of bleeding.

Previous Curettage

Adenocarcinoma patients have a high incidence of antecedent bleeding around the menopausal era, and curettings show a significant occurrence of hyperplasia or anovu-

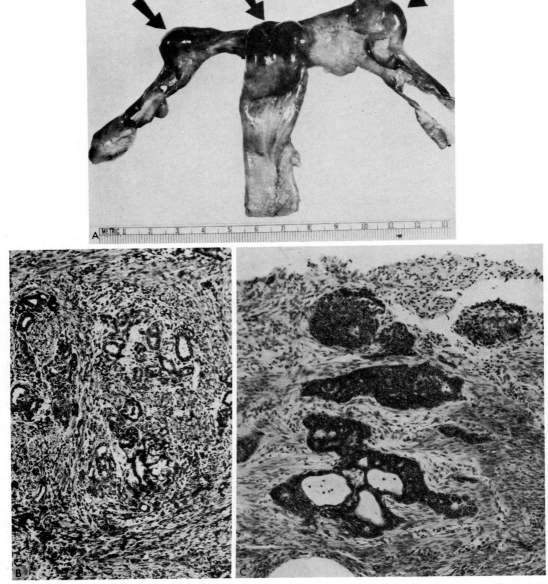

Figure 9–22. *A*, Adenocarcinoma of uterus developing in rabbit following sustained estrogen therapy. *B*, Myometrial extension. *C*, Distant metastasis. (Courtesy of Dr. Sheldon Sommers, Boston.)

latory bleeding (Fig. 9–24). The fact that prolonged nonbleeding phases thereafter may precede the appearance of endometrial cancer by no means implies that estrogen production is not continued, for proliferative endometria are frequent in the postmenopausal era, even without vaginal bleeding. Various cytologic studies by Randall would suggest frequent estrogen activity in the postmenopausal woman, and this has been confirmed by McLennan and McLennan.

Castration

Bilateral oophorectomy or adnexectomy, a frequent surgical procedure until about 1940, was practically never followed by the advent of corpus cancer. The development had always been deemed sufficiently rare to warrant isolated case reports. Articles by Hofmeister and Vondrak and by Cianfrani, reporting cases of postcastration adenocarcinoma, represent contradictory series; however, the technical difficulties in removing

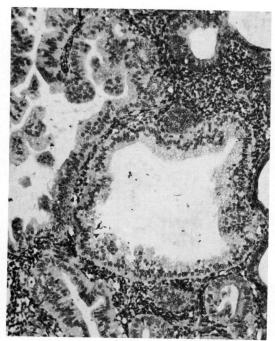

Figure 9–23. Postmenopausal endometrium following prolonged estrogen therapy. Cessation of therapy led to no further bleeding, and later curettage showed no endometrium. Note the tall, pale epithelium with marked intraluminal tufting and budding.

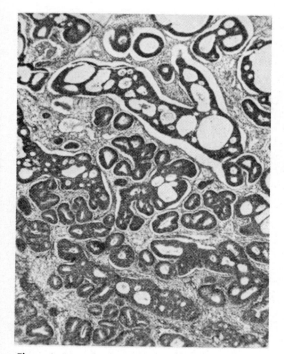

Figure 9–24. Third curettage in 56 year old woman in whom earlier sections had shown only hyperplasia. Hysterectomy was refused, but two years later Grade II adenocarcinoma was noted.

all ovarian tissue in cases of inflammatory disease or endometriosis might well explain this discrepancy. The frequent confusion of diagnosing early microscopic stages of the disease may also be a factor. Brown and coworkers report the concurrence of ovarian agenesis, but obviously there are extraovarian sources of estrogen.

Anovulation with the Stein-Leventhal Syndrome

As this interesting lesion is discussed more fully in Chapter 20, suffice it to say here that this type of ovarian dysfunction is associated with uninterrupted anovulation with resultant unopposed estrogen. It might be pertinent to note that Jackson and Dockerty have found up to 40 per cent concurrence of this type of ovarian pathology and endometrial adenocarcinoma, although Stein himself states he has never noted this sequence. A report by Andrews and Andrews reviews the literature. We have seen several instances of it (Fig. 9–25).

It should be added that Kaufman and coworkers have been able to cause a reversal of atypical hyperplasia (up to a certain point) by wedge resection of the ovary with resultant ovulation, corpus luteum formation, and progesterone secretion. However, when a certain degree of endometrial atypia has occurred, the process appears irreversible, with evolvement of undoubted adenocarcinoma. Kistner has achieved similar results in converting atypical hyperplasia by utilizing progestogens, and Wall and co-workers have suggested clomiphene to obtain the same results.

McDonald and his associates compared 72 endometrial cancer patients with polycystic (SL) ovaries or feminizing ovarian tumors to patients with only endometrial disease. The former have a better prognosis, as do women whose tumors follow estrogen therapy. This conforms to our own impressions.

Feminizing Ovarian Tumors

Certain estrogen-producing tumors of the ovary have been noted as coexisting with endometrial cancer in a much higher ratio than the laws of chance would permit. These granulosa and theca cell tumors (feminizing gonadal stromal) are associated with fundal adenocarcinoma in 15 to 25 per cent of all cases (see Chapter 26). This so-called *spon-*

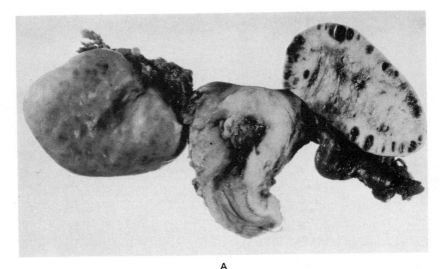

A

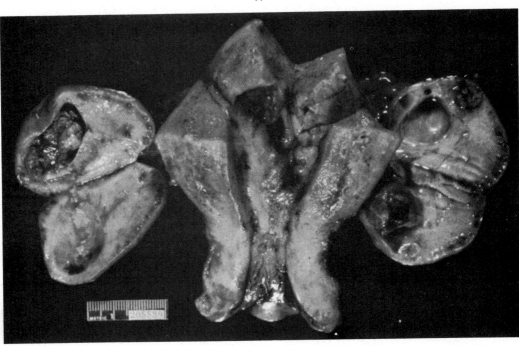

B

Figure 9–25. *A*, Adenocarcinoma in 15 year old girl with large polycystic ovaries. (Courtesy of Dr. Robert Greenblatt, Augusta, Ga.) *B*, Polypoid endometrial adenocarcinoma with Stein-Leventhal ovaries and incidental bilateral dermoids. (Incidental tumors occur in approximately one fifth of such ovaries.) (From Novak, E. R., et al. [Eds.]: Novak's Textbook of Gynecology. 8th Ed. Baltimore, Williams & Wilkins Co., 1970.)

taneous biological experiment would seem to afford a very real and valid basis for our concepts of estrogen as a potent stimulus to neoplastic development.

Estrogen Therapy

An increasing number of cases have been reported with a history of prolonged estrogen therapy and the later development of uterine cancer. Gusberg has reported 23 cases in 20 years at a single clinic. The role of estrogen therapy in the genesis of adenocarcinoma has been discussed earlier and should cause discriminating gynecologists to discourage protracted estrogen therapy. Of particular interest in some of these cases is the presence of all intermediate patterns from simple cystic through more proliferative adenomatous hyperplasia to the pro-

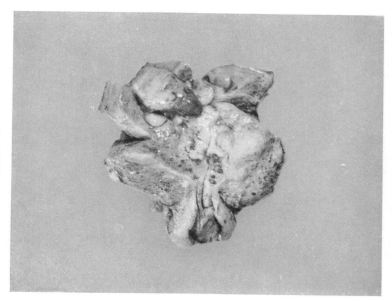

Figure 9–26. Estrogen therapy for 11 years. Note the thick myometrium with endometrial proliferation and the polypoid adenocarcinoma at left cornu.

duction of frank unquestioned corpus cancer (Figs. 9–26 and 9–27). We have recently seen a patient with gonadal dysgenesis and histologically proved streak ovaries after a 7 year regimen of estrogen (four weeks on and one week off); Cutler and associates record six cases.

Association of Hyperplasia and Adenocarcinoma

This has been observed repeatedly by interested pathologists since the initial articles by Taylor (1932) and Novak and Yui (1936). Simple cystic or proliferative hyperplasia (or both) may be found in conjunction with frank cancer, and all gradations may occur, just as all degrees of atypical hyperplasia may precede the development of endometrial adenocarcinoma (Figs. 9–28 and 9–29).

Postmenopausal Hyperplasia

As noted previously, postmenopausal hyperplasia and corpus cancer have so many features in common as to suggest that they are merely different degrees of a similar endocrine or metabolic process with the malignant end process occurring if there is a sufficiently prolonged and potent stimulus. Recurrent bleeding due to repeated and *increasingly atypical hyperplasia does not deserve procrastination* but warrants hysterectomy to forestall the possibility of developing cancer. A single episode of post-

menopausal hyperplasia may be treated expectantly, but continuation suggests a sustained stimulation which may culminate in adenocarcinoma unless the end-organ is removed.

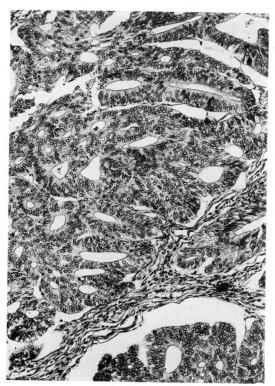

Figure 9–27. Microscopic pattern of Figure 9–26. Early adenocarcinoma in polyp; other areas show all gradations of hyperplasia.

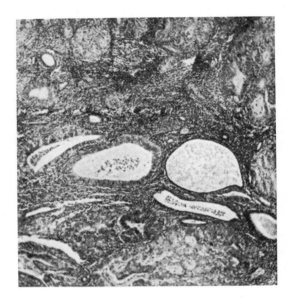

Figure 9–28. In the center is an area of benign hyperplasia (postmenopausal), while surrounding it is definite adenocarcinoma.

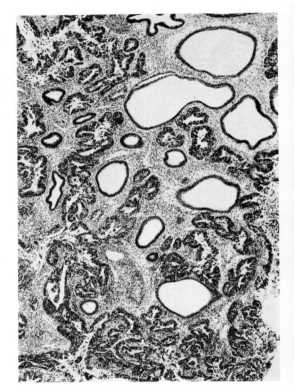

Figure 9–29. Associated hyperplasia and adenocarcinoma.

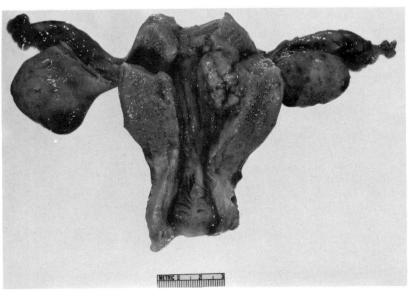

Figure 9–30. Adenoacanthoma arising in conjunction with a fresh corpus luteum of right ovary and generally secretory endometrium.

There are certain dissenters to the so-called "estrogen therapy." Much of the disbelief stems from the earlier work of Jones and Brewer, who reported a group of young menstruating women whose endometrium showed cancer in conjunction with a progestational endometrium and a fresh corpus luteum (Fig. 9–30). There is no question that this occurs, but as the exception to the usual picture of postmenopausal adenocarcinoma.

It is by no means rare to find patches of endometrium that are not in accord with the stage of the cycle, and are probably composed of refractory basalis tissue (Fig. 9–31). Schroeder enlarges on this advent in a discussion of the genesis of polyps. These localized foci or polyps may show only a hyperplastic pattern despite a generally premenstrual pattern. In other words, these unripe islands are incapable of progesterone response, and even in the face of a biphasic cycle they respond only to estrogen (Fig. 9–32). This constant stimulus, unopposed in these refractory foci, might easily be expected to result in varying degrees of proliferative architecture. This would seem to serve as an explanation to the dissenters to the theory that estrogen is a factor in the development of fundal cancer.

In recent years we have witnessed several

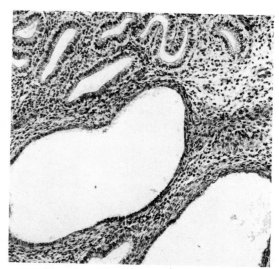

Figure 9–32. Section from compacta: note secretory changes associated with hyperplastic glands.

cases in which women had been on contraceptive pills for years. Ultimately bleeding occurred, and curettage revealed focal areas of adenocarcinoma despite a generally secretory endometrium, as in Figs. 9–33 and 9–34. It would seem logical to presume that these patients had localized areas of endometrium of the immature type, reactive only to the estrogen component, with the ultimate development of endometrial adenocarcinoma. Silverberg has collected over 20 cases, mostly occurring after use of sequential pills. Lyon and Kelley and associates note additional cases.

The source of estrogen in the postmenopausal woman has evoked considerable speculation, though it is accepted that the adrenal gland is capable of estrogenic activity. In his excellent study on estrogens in the postmenopausal patient (56 cases), Procopé has emphasized the role of both the adrenal gland and the ovary. Certainly the postmenopausal ovary should not be discounted as a potential source of steroidogenesis, as indicated by histochemical studies performed by Novak and co-workers (Chapter 6). There have been several different papers by Woll and colleagues, Hertig and associates, Novak and Mohler, and others, noting a frequent association of hyperplasia of the ovarian stromal cells and adenocarcinoma of the endometrium. These hyperplastic ovarian stromal cells may be arranged in clumps or whorls but may be diffuse. The resem-

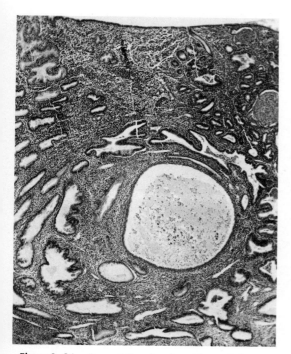

Figure 9–31. Progestational endometrium at left; nonsecretory pattern with acanthosis at right.

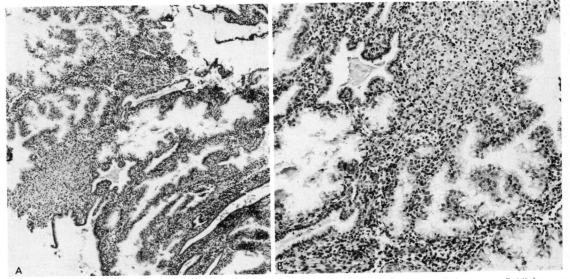

Figure 9–33. *A*, A generally secretory endometrium in a 31 year old para 2 on contraceptive pills for 4 years. *B*, High power view of *A*. Hypersecretory glandular pattern with decidua-like changes in stroma.

blance to theca cells is very real, but whether they may, like the normal theca cell, actively liberate estrogen is still uncertain, although they take up fat avidly. However, this ovarian stromal hyperplasia or diffuse thecosis has been found to be nearly three times more common in conjunction with endometrial cancer than in control series. It is likewise disproportionately common with breast cancer.

Finally, it must be emphasized that the role of estrogen in the development of endometrial cancer is still speculative. Further

work is necessary before there should be any final acceptance of this tenet, but the possibility of its carcinogenic role, especially in the genetically predisposed patient, warrants full consideration. More recent study indicates that the major hormone produced in the postmenopausal era is androstenedione, which may be converted to estrogen (estrone in the woman with endometrial adenocarcinoma).

In conclusion, then, although there are few who insist categorically that estrogen is *the* cause of endometrial cancer, most stu-

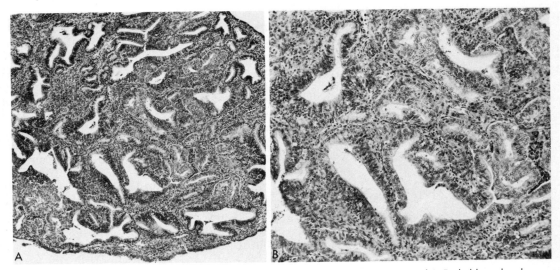

Figure 9–34. *A*, Small foci of hyperactive refractory endometrium. *B*, High power view of *A*. Probably early adenocarcinoma arising from areas nonresponsive to progesterone and thereby reactive only to the estrogen component of "the pill."

dents admit that adenocarcinoma arises in an estrogen-conditioned endometrium or in the abnormal foci that do not participate in a response to progesterone. For many editions of this text, we have been outspoken in indicating belief that estrogen may be the ultimate stimulus when the woman is constitutionally predisposed to develop a malignancy; when this predisposition is not present, perhaps the most potent carcinogen might not provoke the disease.

In reviewing cases of endometrial cancer with antecedent hormone therapy, it is important to note that the steroid has generally been administered in uninterrupted sustained fashion over the course of years. Large dosage estrogen over shorter periods of time (as administered to certain patients with breast cancer) seems less likely to be followed by endometrial disease. Although not condemning the use of estrogens for the symptomatic postmenopausal patient, we urge a discriminating method of administration when the uterus is present in a patient with a familial history of cancer. The repeated assertions by Greenblatt that estrogen is a rather innocuous drug which should be administered frequently are totally unacceptable—even if concomitant progesterone is utilized, there is no guarantee that cancer may not ensue (Fig. 9–34).

Epidermoid Carcinoma of Endometrium

This is a rare lesion, usually occurring in older women in whom there has been a previous metaplasia of the columnar epithelium into squamous epithelium (Fig. 9–35). The occurrence of patches of squamous epithelium is not rare in the senile endometrium, and in extreme cases the entire endometrium is replaced by stratified squamous epithelium (the so-called *ichthyosis uteri*) from which an epidermoid cancer can arise. The occurrence of squamous metaplasia has been noted with long-standing pelvic inflammatory disease, following radium application, vitamin A deficiency, continued use of IUD, etc., and there would seem to been noted with long-standing pelvic inflammatory disease, following radium aprence is exceedingly rare, and most of the reported cases of combined adenocarcinoma and epidermoid carcinoma are misinterpretations, the squamous component being of benign nature.

TREATMENT OF ENDOMETRIAL ADENOCARCINOMA

A complete discussion of treatment hardly is warranted in a pathology text; on the other hand some understanding is paramount for full comprehension of our approach to the disease. Three basic modes of therapy exist, and there is no complete agreement among leading gynecologists as to just what the routine treatment should be. Fortunately approximately 75 per cent of endometrial cancer presents as Stage I or less. An excellent review of the treatment of endometrial carcinoma (Jones, 1975) is strongly recommended.

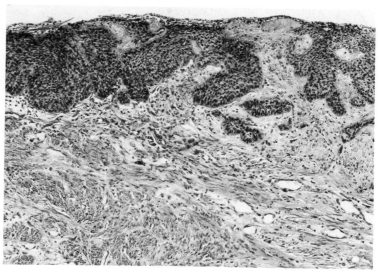

Figure 9–35. Epidermoid cancer of endometrium. Cervix and endocervix are normal.

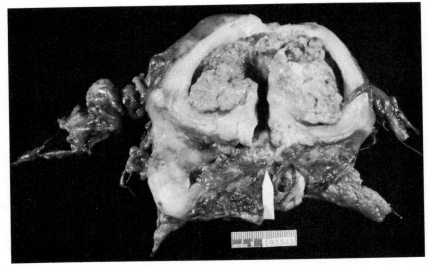

Figure 9–36. Carcinoma of endometrium following irradiation for cervical cancer 5 years previously. Cervix (arrow) is completely sloughed. The carcinogenic effect of irradiation must be considered.

Irradiation Therapy (33 Per Cent Salvage)*

Most are agreed that, as the only treatment, irradiation should be reserved for those patients who are considered to be poor medical risks because they are incapable of tolerating more definitive surgery. Fortunately this is a rare occurrence in this day of improved anesthesia, and in addition the possible carcinogenic role of irradiation, while difficult to accept with 100 per cent assurance, is likewise difficult to deny. Endometrial adenocarcinoma may follow small dosage irradiation, as occurs with an irradiation menopause or "scatter" following treatment of cervical disease (Fig. 9–36).

Surgery Alone (50 Per Cent Salvage)*

There are few who deny that surgery is the most important part of any therapeutic program for fundal cancer, although the majority opinion is that it alone is not sufficient for any but the most superficial and well localized forms of the disease. Others indicate that superior salvage can be achieved without irradiation, and this is usually standard treatment in many European centers. Indeed, it is generally believed that irradiation is unnecessary and does not improve the salvage in Stage 1 tumors (85 per cent survival).

Irradiation and Surgery (75 Per Cent Salvage)*

This represents the so-called preferential or optimal approach to the disease, and most gynecologists believe this should be the usual method of treatment. Although this text does not propose to enlarge on specific therapy, there seems little doubt that the best results of all cases accrue with combined therapy, whether irradiation consists of x-ray or radium, followed some weeks later by surgery. How important the postirradiation delay before surgery really is seems speculative; in Johnson's study, patients having hysterectomy immediately postirradiation had no more complications than patients with a 6 to 8 week interim period, and salvage was comparable. It is curious that the uterus, subsequently removed, often shows that there is viable-appearing tumor in the specimen. We can only postulate that irradiation does something to the tumor cells, despite their apparent viability, to render them incapable of subsequent implantation or metastasis. Shah and Green, Frick and coworkers, and Graham have indicated that it makes little difference as to whether the irradiation is administered pre- or postoperatively; either will decrease recurrence in the vaginal vault and other sites.

Today there is increasing dependence on postoperative (rather than preoperative) irradiation in the form of vaginal sources and/or full pelvic cobalt therapy. This has certain advantages in that (1) the total extent of the disease is apparent, (2) there is not the risk of radiation complications that may occur with certain distorted myomatous uteri, (3) better

---

* All figures approximate from aggregate studies.

results are achieved in cases in which there is an associated adnexal mass, and (4) hospital expenses may be minimized by avoiding a separate admission for insertion of radium.

Where there is cervical extension with endometrial cancer, our policy is to irradiate the cervix (as with epidermoid cancer), and after 6 weeks to perform simple hysterectomy. Occasionally radical surgery is utilized but, irrespective of the type of therapy, salvage is impaired by nearly 50 per cent.

Hormone and Chemotherapy

That endometrial adenocarcinoma may be an estrogen-dependent tumor seems probable, and since estrogen and progesterone sometimes appear antagonistic, there have been an increasing number of studies advocating the use of *progesterone* in treating certain cases of endometrial neoplasm. Although the results are perhaps not as spectacular as those obtained with methotrexate therapy for trophoblastic lesions, they represent a valuable contribution in the increasingly successful attempts at treating cancer in a systemic fashion. Richardson has indicated that progesterone may be bound to a *receptor* protein in the cytoplasm, and that this complex then enters the nucleus where it binds to an *acceptor* protein. The hormone-receptor complex is then activated, and after transport to the nucleus it will interact with the DNA to stimulate messenger RNA synthesis (Fig. 9–37). The mRNA then returns to the cytoplasm, where it plays an important role in the synthesis of specific new proteins. It is similarly recognized that various end-organ targets of estrogen contain these estrogen receptors, and thus it might be possible to predict which endometrial or breast carcinoma might respond to changes in the hormonal milieu. Young and co-workers indicate that evaluation of progesterone

binding will indicate which lesion will be affected.

It would appear that certain steroids, notably androstenedione, are produced by the postmenopausal ovary or adrenal, or both, and may be converted into estrogen by an as yet uncertain mechanism. In any case, increased conversion of androgen to estrogen has been noted with endometrial carcinoma by Siiteri and co-workers, and it may be manufactured or stored in body fat. Rubin and associates note a decreased estriol-estrone relationship in women with fundal adenocarcinoma, and speculate that estriol may exert a guarding effect, whereas increased estrone seems more apt to be associated with adenocarcinoma. In any event in the usual postmenopausal female there is no longer the anti-estrogenic effect of progesterone normally found only in the younger ovulating female.

Progesterone. *Therapy of Advanced and Often Recurrent Treated Tumor.* Kelley and Baker, Kennedy, Mussey and Malkasian, and Varga and Henriksen have been enthusiastic about prolonged remission (up to 2 years) in approximately one third of the patients treated. Most responsive were those women who had prolonged symptoms prior to initial surgery and irradiation therapy and a sustained interval before recurrence, i.e., a slow-growing tumor (Figs. 9–38 and 9–39). Treatment consisted of no less than 750 to 1500 mg. of intramuscular progesterone (Delalutin) per week, and patients have been maintained on such therapy for as long as 18 months. Our own experience would suggest that endocrine therapy is less effective in treating local recurrence than metastatic disease; we have seen several satisfactory results in treating biopsy-proved pulmonary recurrences (Fig. 9–40), as well as certain disappointing results when there was pelvic disease. Smith and co-workers indicate that

Figure 9–37. Sequence of the steroid hormone complex. The steroid hormone estrogen or progesterone (*1*) enters the cell. The cytoplasm contains a protein that binds specifically to the particular steroid (*2*). This protein is thought to be a receptor specifically involved in hormone action. The steroid receptor (*3*) enters the nucleus, which contains a protein (*4*), associated with the chromatin, which acts as an acceptor that specifically binds the steroid-receptor complex (*5*). The whole unit acts as a key that turns on the cell, possibly by activating a portion of the genome (*6*). DNA is transcribed into RNA, and RNA is translated into protein. (Courtesy of Dr. G. Richardson. Reprinted, by permission, from New England Journal of Medicine, *286*:645, 1972.)

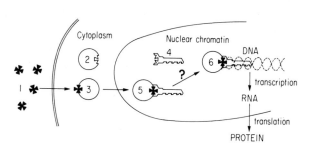

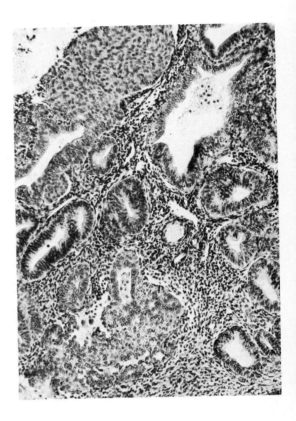

Figure 9–38. Low grade adenoacanthoma found in young patient.

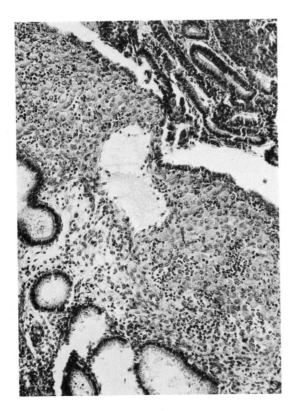

Figure 9–39. Carcinomatous endometrium removed (for study) one month after progesterone therapy. Note beginning drug effect (below) with residual tumor (above).

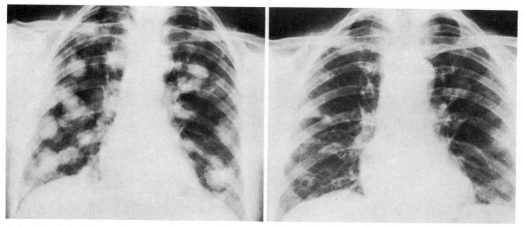

Figure 9–40. (*left*). Recurrent adenocarcinoma one year following irradiation and surgery with biopsy-proved metastasis. (*right*). X-ray 8 months later after large dose progesterone. Patient now has complete 6 year remission. (Courtesy of Dr. P. A. Nilsen, Oslo, Norway.)

the younger patient with a well-differentiated tumor seems most responsive; low dosage oral progesterone (Megace) may be continued indefinitely, and this is our own policy.

Treatment of Markedly Adenomatous Hyperplasia. Kistner and Wall and associates have been successful in causing reversion of a markedly atypical endometrial pattern and possibly adenocarcinoma after large dosage of progesterone for many months. Curettage after prolonged progesterone therapy generally reveals almost total absence of the glands (glandular exhaustion) and a marked decidual reaction of the stroma, identical to that shown in Figure 28–17. At present, it is impossible to state dogmatically how long treatment should be continued and what should be expected following cessation of the progesterone. Probably a 3 to 6 month trial period of progesterone may be utilized, followed by curettage, but if the endometrial atypicality persists, hysterectomy seems indicated. It must be understood that even the well-differential endometrium in a youthful patient cannot always be converted (Fig. 9–41).

Clomiphene. The use of clomiphene in such conditions as anovulatory bleeding and the Stein-Leventhal syndrome has been dis-

cussed in other chapters of this text. Wall and co-workers have extended this mode of therapy to include certain postmenopausal patients whose endometrium showed an atypical hyperplasia or even a frank adenocarcinoma (and their photomicrographs are convincing). In 2 of 10 patients with adenocarcinoma treated by clomiphene there was a gradual regression of the malignancy, with conversion into initially a secretory and then an atrophic pattern. This type of therapy should be reserved for the young anovulatory patient anxious for pregnancy.

Pregnancy

Kistner has indicated that the optimal therapy for endometrial hyperplasia is pregnancy. O'Neill has reported a case (and reviewed the literature) of a 17 year old patient with an apparently authentic endometrial adenocarcinoma who was treated by progestogens and who shortly afterward conceived; she has remained well. At least six cases are recorded by Karlen and associates. Obviously pregnancy is a form of "treatment" applicable to only a very few women who are afflicted with malignant endometrial patterns.

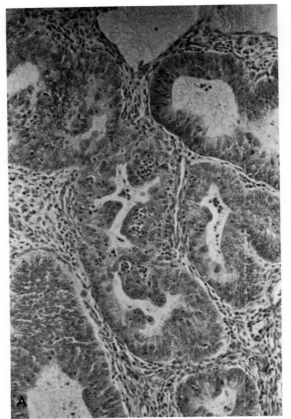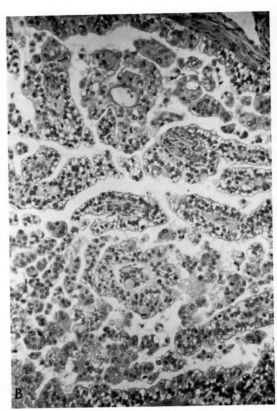

Figure 9–41. *A*, Extremely atypical endometrium in 26 year old para 0. *B*, Papillary adenocarcinoma has developed despite 6 months' progesterone therapy. (Courtesy of Dr. Julian Meyer, Roanoke, Va.)

SALVAGE

There is no question that endometrial adenocarcinoma is an infinitely more favorable disease than cervical cancer insofar as prognosis is concerned. Yet it is unrealistic to be too optimistic, as noted in the recent discussion by Henriksen on the spread of this disease, although admittedly this was based on autopsy findings. Boronow's review emphasizes that endometrial cancer is not "a benign disease." Familiarity with a large number of reports and studies of fundal cancer of varied degrees treated by different modes of therapy prompts the following *approximates:*

1. When the disease is confined to the endometrium, the salvage should exceed 90 per cent irrespective of treatment.

2. When there is superficial myometrial involvement, salvage should exceed 80 per cent with a slightly better result when there is preferential or optimal (irradiation plus surgical) treatment.

3. When massive myometrial or cervical extension occurs, salvage drops to 50 per cent, irrespective of the type of therapy, but a combination of irradiation and surgery is somewhat preferable.

4. When there is extrauterine spread of the disease one must expect a marked decrease in curability (25 per cent or less), but irradiation and/or progesterone may lead to an increased remission.

5. All of these generalizations apply to a moderately well differentiated tumor; when there is increased undifferentiation or involvement of the cervix, there is decreasing salvage.

REFERENCES

American College of Obstetricians and Gynecologists, Technical Bulletins, 43:1, 1976.

Anderson, D. G.: Management of advanced endometrial adenocarcinoma with methoxyprogesterone acetate (Provera). Am. J. Obstet. Gynecol., 92:87, 1965.

Andrews, W. C., and Andrews, M. C.: Stein-Leventhal syndrome with associated adenocarcinoma of the endometrium. Am. J. Obstet. Gynecol., 80:632, 1960.

Arneson, A. N.: Long term follow-up observations in corporeal cancer. Am. J. Roentgenol., 91:3, 1964.

Badib, A. O., Kurohara, S. S., Vongtama, V. Y., et al.: Biologic behavior of adenoacanthoma of endometrium. Am. J. Obstet. Gynecol., 106:205, 1970.

Bailar, J. C.: Multiple tumors with uterine cancer. Cancer, 16:842, 1963.

Beck, R. P., and Latour, J. P. A.: Necropsy reports on 36 cases of endometrial cancer. Am. J. Obstet. Gynecol., 85:307, 1963.

Benjamin, F., and Deutsch, S.: Plasma estrogens and hormones in endometrial carcinoma. Am. J. Obstet. Gynecol., 126:638, 1976.

Beutler, H. K., Dockerty, M. B., and Randall, L. M.: Precancerous lesions of the endometrium. Am. J. Obstet. Gynecol., 86:433, 1963.

Boronow, R. C.: Endometrial cancer. Obstet. Gynecol., 47:630, 1976.

Brown, J. M., Dockerty, M. B., Symmonds, R. E., and Bonner, E. A.: Vaginal recurrence of endometrial carcinoma. Am. J. Obstet. Gynecol., 100:544, 1968.

Calanog, A., et al. Testosterone metabolism in endometrial carcinoma. Am. J. Obstet. Gynecol., 124:60, 1975.

Charles, D.: Endometrial adenoacanthoma. Cancer, 18:737, 1965.

Charles, D., Bell, E. T., Loraine, J. A., and Harkness, R. A.: Endometrial carcinoma-endocrinological and clinical studies. Am. J. Obstet. Gynecol., 91:1050, 1965.

Chen, G. Y., et al.: Cellular hypersensitivity with adenomatous hyperplasia and adenocarcinoma of the endometrium. Am. J. Obstet. Gynecol., 121:370, 1976.

Cianfrani, T.: Endometrial cancer after bilateral oophorectomy. Am. J. Obstet. Gynecol., 69:64, 1955.

Cohen, C. J., and Deppe, G.: Endometrial carcinoma and oral contraceptives. Obstet. Gynecol., 49:390, 1977.

Cutler, B. S., Forbes, A. P., Ingersoll, F. M., and Scully, R. E.: Endometrial carcinoma after stilbestrol therapy in gonadal dysgenesis. N. Engl. J. Med., 287:628, 1972.

Di Saia, P. J., et al.: Carcinoembryonic antigen in patients with gynecologic malignancies. Am. J. Obstet. Gynecol., 121:159, 1975.

Doran, T. A., and Thompson, D. W.: Malignant cells in the peripheral blood of patients with endometrial adenocarcinoma. Am. J. Obstet. Gynecol., 94:985, 1966.

Eisenfeld, A. J.: Estrogen receptors. Clin. Obstet. Gynecol., 19:767, 1976.

Factor, S. M.: Papillary adenocarcinoma endometrium with psammoma bodies. Arch. Pathol., 98:201, 1974.

Gardner, W. U., Allen, E., Smith, G. M., and Strong, L. C.: Carcinoma of cervix in mice receiving estrogen. J.A.M.A., 10:1182, 1938.

Geisler, H. E., Huber, C. P., and Rogers, S.: Carcinoma of endometrium in premenopausal women. Am. J. Obstet. Gynecol., 104:657, 1969.

Gore, H., and Hertig, A. T.: Premalignant lesions of the endometrium. Clin. Obstet. Gynecol., 5:1148, 1962.

Gore, H., and Hertig, A. T.: Carcinoma in situ of the endometrium. Am. J. Obstet. Gynecol., 94:134, 1966.

Graham, J.: The value of preoperative or postoperative treatment by radium for carcinoma of the uterine body. Surg. Gynecol. Obstet. 132:855, 1971.

Gravlee, L. C., Jr.: Jet-irrigation method for diagnosis of endometrial adenocarcinoma: its principle and accuracy. Obstet. Gynecol., 34:168, 1969.

Gray, P. H., Anderson, C. T., Jr., and Monnell, E. W.: Endometrial adenocarcinoma and ovarian agenesis. Obstet. Gynecol., 35:513, 1970.

Greene, J. W.: Feminizing mesenchymomas and endometrial carcinoma. Am. J. Obstet. Gynecol., 74:31, 1957.

Gurpide, E., et al.: Estrogen metabolism in normal and neoplastic endometrium. Am. J. Obstet. Gynecol., 129:809, 1977.

Gusberg, S. B.: The individual with high risk endometrial carcinoma. Am. J. Obstet. Gynecol., 126:535, 1976.

Gusberg, S. B., and Hall, R. E.: Precursors of corpus cancer. III. The appearance of cancer of the endometrium in estrogenically conditioned patients. Obstet. Gynecol., 17:397, 1961.

Gusberg, S. B., and Hall, R. E.: Precursors of corpus cancer. IV. Adenomatous hyperplasia as stage 0 carcinoma of the endometrium. Am. J. Obstet. Gynecol., 87:662, 1963.

Gusberg, S. B., and Yannopoulos, D.: Therapeutic decisions in corpus cancer. Am. J. Obstet. Gynecol., 88:157, 1964.

Gusberg, S. B., et al.: Endometrial cancer: factors influencing the choice of treatment. Gynecol. Oncol., 2:308, 1974.

Henriksen, E.: The lymphatic dissemination in endometrial carcinoma. Am. J. Obstet. Gynecol., 123:570, 1975.

Hertig, A. T., and Sommers, S. C.: Genesis of endometrial carcinoma. I. Study of prior biopsies. Cancer, 2:946, 1949.

Hofmeister, F. J., and Vondrak, B. F.: Endometrial carcinoma in patients with bilateral oophorectomy or irradiation castration. Am. J. Obstet. Gynecol., 107:1099, 1970.

Homesley, H. D., Boronow, R. C., and Lewis, J. L., Jr.: Treatment of adenocarcinoma of the endometrium at Memorial—James Ewing Hospitals, 1949–1965. Obstet. Gynecol., 47:100, 1976.

Jackson, R. L., and Dockerty, M. B.: Stein-Leventhal syndrome and endometrial cancer. Am. J. Obstet. Gynecol., 73:161, 1957.

Jafari, K., et al.: Endometrial carcinoma and the Stein-Leventhal syndrome. Obstet. Gynecol., 51:97, 1978.

Johnson, F. L.: Adenocarcinoma of the endometrium. Obstet. Gynecol., 27:622, 1967.

Jones, H. O., and Brewer, J. I.: Studies of ovaries and endometriums of patients with fundal adenocarcinoma. Am. J. Obstet. Gynecol., 42:207, 1941.

Jones, H. W., III: Treatment of endometrial adenocarcinoma. Obstet. Gynecol. Surv., 30:147, 1975.

Julian, C. G., et al.: Adenoepidermoid (squamous) carcinoma of the uterus. Am. J. Obstet. Gynecol., 128:106, 1977.

Karlen, J. R., et al.: Carcinoma of the endometrium coexisting with pregnancy. Obstet. Gynecol., 40:334, 1972.

Katayama, K. P., and Jones, H. W.: Chromosomes of atypical (adenomatous) hyperplasia and carcinoma of the endometrium. Am. J. Obstet. Gynecol., 97:978, 1967.

Kaufman, R. H., Abbott, J. P., and Wall, J. A.: The endometrium before and after wedge resection of the ovaries in the Stein-Leventhal syndrome. Reversibility of atypical endometrial hyperplasia. Am. J. Obstet. Gynecol., 77:1271, 1959.

Keller, W. B., et al.: Early endometrial carcinoma. Cancer, 33:1108, 1974.

Kelley, R. M., and Baker, W. H.: Progesterone for endometrial cancer. N. Engl. J. Med., 264:216, 1961.

Kelley, H. W., et al.: Endometrial carcinoma following sequential oral contraceptives. Obstet. Gynecol., 47:200, 1976.

Kennedy, B. J.: Progesterone for treatment of advanced endometrial cancer. J.A.M.A., 184:102, 1963.

Kistner, R. W.: The effects of progestational agents on hyperplasia and carcinoma in situ of the endometrium. Int. J. Obstet. Gynecol., 8:561, 1970.

Kistner, R. W.: Estrogens and endometrial carcinoma. Obstet. Gynecol., 48:479, 1976.

Kistner, R. W.: Estrogen therapy. Obstet. Gynecol., 48:479, 1976.

Knab, D. R.: Estrogen and endometrial carcinoma. Obstet. Gynecol. Surv., 32:267, 1977.

Kurman, R. J., and Scully, R. E.: Clear cell carcinoma of the endometrium, an analysis of 21 cases. Cancer, 37:872, 1976.

Lewis, J. L., Jr.: Symposium on endometrial carcinoma. Cont. Obstet. Gynecol., 6:106, 1975.

Liggins, G. C., and Way, S. A.: A comparison of the prognosis of adenoacanthoma and adenocarcinoma of the corpus uteri. J. Obstet. Gynaecol. Brit. Emp., 62:294, 1960.

Lipsett, M. B.: Estrogen use and cancer risk. J.A.M.A., 237:1112, 1977.

Lucas, W. E.: Endocrine-metabolic variables with endometrial carcinoma. Obstet. Gynecol. Surv., 29:507, 1971.

Lyon, F. A.: Endometrial abnormalities occurring in young women on long-term sequential oral contraception. Am. J. Obstet. Gynecol., 123:299, 1975.

Lyon, F. A., and Frisch, M. J.: The development of adenocarcinoma of the endometrium in young women receiving long-term sequential oral contraception. Obstet. Gynecol. 47:639, 1976.

Mack, T. M., et al.: Estrogens and endometrial carcinoma in a retirement community. N. Engl. J. Med., 294:1262, 1976.

Malkasian, G. D., Jr., et al.: Progesterone treatment of recurrent endometrial carcinoma. Am. J. Obstet. Gynecol., 110:15, 1971.

Marnett, L. D., et al.: Recent trends in the incidence and mortality of cancer of the uterine corpus in Connecticut. Gynecol. Oncol., 6:183, 1978.

McDonald, T. W., et al.: Endometrial cancer with feminizing ovarian tumor and polycystic ovaries. Obstet. Gynecol., 49:654, 1977.

McDonald, T. W., et al.: Exogenous estrogen and endometrial carcinoma. Am. J. Obstet. Gynecol., 127:572, 1977.

McGarrity, K. A., and Scott, G. C.: A review of cancer of the corpus uteri in New South Wales. J. Obstet. Gynaecol. Brit. Commonw., 75:14, 1968.

McLennan, M. T., and McLennan, C. E.: Estrogenic action of postmenopausal women by vaginal smear. Obstet. Gynecol., 37:325, 1971.

Meissner, A., Sommers, S. C., and Sherman, G.: Endometrial hyperplasia, endometrial hyperplasia, and endometriosis produced experimentally by estrogens. Cancer, 10:505, 1957.

Merriam, J. C., Easterday, C. L., McKay, D. G., and Hertig, A. J.: Experimental production of endometrial carcinoma in the rabbit. Obstet. Gynecol., 16:253, 1960.

Morrison, D. L.: Adenoacanthoma of the uterine body. J. Obstet. Gynaecol. Brit. Commonw., 73:605, 1966.

Muggia, F. M., et al.: Doxorubicin (Adriamycin)-cyclophosphamide for advanced endometrial carcinoma. Am. J. Obstet. Gynecol., 128:314, 1977.

Ng, A. B. P., et al.: Mixed adenosquamous carcinoma at the endometrium. Am. J. Clin. Pathol., 59:765, 1973.

Nolan, J. F., Donough, M. E., and Anson, J. H.: The value of preoperative radiation therapy in stage I cancer of the corpus. Am. J. Obstet. Gynecol., 98:663, 1967.

Novak, E., and Rutledge, F.: Atypical endometrial hyperplasia simulating adenocarcinoma. Am. J. Obstet. Gynecol., 55:46, 1948.

Novak, E., and Yui, E.: Relation of endometrial hyperplasia to adenocarcinoma of uterus. Am. J. Obstet. Gynecol., 32:674, 1936.

Novak, E. R.: Uterine adenocarcinoma in a patient receiving estrogens. Am. J. Obstet. Gynecol., 62:688, 1951.

Novak, E. R.: Postmenopausal hyperplasia. Am. J. Obstet. Gynecol., 71:1312, 1956.

Novak, E. R., Goldberg, B., Jones, G. S., and O'Toole, R. V.: Enzyme histochemistry of the menopausal ovary associated with normal and abnormal endometrium. Am. J. Obstet. Gynecol., 93:669, 1965.

Novak, E. R., and Mohler, D. I.: Ovarian stromal changes in endometrial cancer. Am. J. Obstet. Gynecol., 65:1099, 1953.

Novak, E. R., and Nalley, W. B.: Uterine adenoacanthoma. Obstet. Gynecol., 9:396, 1957.

Novak, E. R., and Villa Santa, U.: Factors influencing the ratio of uterine cancer in a community. J.A.M.A., 174:1395, 1960.

O'Neill, R. T.: Pregnancy following hormonal therapy for adenocarcinoma of the endometrium. Am. J. Obstet. Gynecol., 108:318, 1970.

Quint, B. C.: Changing patterns in endometrial carcinoma. Am. J. Obstet. Gynecol., 122:498, 1975.

Peterson, W. F., and Novak, E. R.: Endometrial polyps. Obstet. Gynecol., 8:40, 1956.

Procopé, B. J.: Studies on the urinary excretion, biological effects and origin of estrogens in postmenopausal women. Acta Endocrinol. 60(Suppl. 135):9–101, 1968.

Randall, C. L., Birtch, P. K., and Harkins, L. L.: Ovarian function after the menopause. Am. J. Obstet. Gynecol., 74:719, 1957.

Richardson, G. S.: Endometrial cancer as an estrogen-progesterone target. N. Engl. J. Med., 286:645, 1972.

Rome, M., et al.: Oestrogen excretion and pathology in the postmenopausal woman. Br. J. Obstet. Gynaecol., 84:88, 1977.

Rubin, B. L., et al.: Estrogen dependence of endometrial carcinoma. Am. J. Obstet. Gynecol., 114:660, 1972.

Rutledge, F.: Radical hysterectomy in endometrial carcinoma. Gynecol. Oncol., 2:331, 1974.

Ryan, K. J.: Carcinoma risk and estrogens. N. Engl. J. Med., 293:1199, 1975.

Sartwell, P. E.: Estrogen replacement therapy and endometrial carcinoma. Clin. Obstet. Gynecol., *19*:817, 1976.

Schwartz, P. E., et al.: Hysterography in endometrial carcinoma. Obstet. Gynecol., *45*:376, 1975.

Scully, R. E., and Barlow, J. F.: "Mesonephroma" of ovary. Cancer, *20*:1405, 1967.

Seltzer, V. L., et al.: Squamous carcinoma of the endometrium. Obstet. Gynecol., *49*:345, 1977.

Shah, C. A., and Green, T. H.: Evaluation of current management of endometrial carcinoma. Obstet. Gynecol., *39*:489, 1972.

Siiteri, P. K., et al.: Estrogen receptors and the estrone hypothesis in endometrial carcinoma. Gynec. Oncol., *2*:130, 1974.

Silverberg, S. G., and Makowski, E. L.: Endometrial carcinoma in young women taking oral contraceptive agents. Obstet. Gynecol., *46*:503, 1975.

Smith, D. C., et al.: Exogenous estrogen and endometrial carcinoma. N. Engl. J. Med., *293*:1164, 1975.

Smith, J. P., Rutledge, F., and Soffar, S. W.: Progestins in the treatment of patients with endometrial adenocarcinoma. Am. J. Obstet. Gynecol., *94*:977, 1966.

Stanley, M. A., and Kirkland, J. A.: Cytogenetic studies of endometrial carcinoma. Am. J. Obstet. Gynecol., *102*:1070, 1968.

Steiner, G. J., Kistner, R. W., and Craig, J. M.: Histologic effects of progestins on hyperplasia and carcinoma in situ of the endometrium—further observations. Metabolism, *14*:356, 1965.

Sugimoto, O.: Hysteroscopic diagnosis of endometrial carcinoma. Am. J. Obstet. Gynecol., *121*:105, 1975.

Taylor, H. C., Jr.: Endometrial hyperplasia and carcinoma of body of uterus. Am. J. Obstet. Gynecol., *23*:309, 1932.

Thompson, N. J., and Graham, J. B.: Carcinoma of corpus and endocervix. Obstet. Gynecol., *24*:144, 1964.

Tweedale, D. N., Early, L. S., and Goodsitt, E. S.: Endo-metrial adenoacanthoma. Obstet. Gynecol., *23*:611, 1964.

Twiggs, L. B., et al.: Gravlee jet irrigator. J.A.M.A., *235*:2745, 1976.

Underwood, P. B., et al.: Carcinoma endometrium; surgery post-irradiation. Am. J. Obstet. Gynecol., *128*:106, 1977.

Varga, A., and Henriksen, E.: Urinary excretion assays of pituitary luteinizing hormone (LH) related to endometrial cancer. Obstet. Gynecol., *22*:129, 1963.

Wade, M. E., Kohorn, E. I., and Morris, J. M.: Adenocarcinoma of the endometrium. Am. J. Obstet. Gynecol., *99*:869, 1967.

Wall, J. A., Franklin, R. R., and Kaufman, R. H.: Reversal of benign and malignant endometrial changes with clomiphene. Am. J. Obstet. Gynecol., *88*:1072, 1964.

Wall, J. A., Franklin, R. R., Kaufman, R. H., Kaplan, R. H.: The effects of clomiphene citrate on the endometrium. Am. J. Obstet. Gynecol., *93*:842, 1965.

Weiss, N. S., et al.: Increasing incidence of endometrial carcinoma. N. Engl. J. Med., *294*:1259, 1976.

Welander, C., et al.: Staging and treatment of endometrial carcinoma. J. Reprod. Med., *8*:41, 1972.

Woll, E., Hertig, A. T., Smith, G. Van S., and Johnson, L. C.: Ovary in endometrial carcinoma. Am. J. Obstet. Gynecol., *56*:617, 1948.

Woodruff, J. D., and Julian, C. G.: Multiple malignancies of upper genital tract. Am. J. Obstet. Gynecol., *103*:810, 1969.

Young, P. C. M., et al.: Progesterone binding in endometrial carcinoma. Am. J. Obstet. Gynecol., *125*:353, 1976.

Ziel, H. K., and Finkle, W. D.: Increased risk of endometrial carcinoma among users of conjugated estrogens. N. Engl. J. Med., *293*:1167, 1975.

Ziel, H. K., and Finkle, W. D.: Estrone and endometrial carcinoma. Am. J. Obstet. Gynecol., *124*:735, 1976.

Chapter 10

ENDOMETRITIS AND OTHER BENIGN CONDITIONS OF THE ENDOMETRIUM

ENDOMETRITIS

Etiology

The cause of endometritis is usually bacterial, and the organisms most frequently responsible are various strains of the gonococcus, streptococci (often anaerobic), staphylococci, and bacteroides, as noted in articles by Ledger and by Sweet. Tuberculosis is uncommon in most well-developed areas although it may be seen in certain ethnic groups in the United States (Klein et al.). Such unusual organisms as coccidioiomycosis or actinomycosis in conjunction with use of an IUD may be encountered infrequently. The specific role of mycoplasma is uncertain.

The causative organisms are characteristically associated with one of two chief clinical types of the disease. The *pyogenic* organisms are concerned with the cases of puerperal endometritis, following full term delivery or abortion.

On the other hand, *gonorrheal* endometritis is encountered in association with gonorrheal infection of the lower genital tract, especially of the cervix. This is rarely a clinical problem until salpingitis ensues. The majority of cases, therefore, are of either the gonorrheal or the puerperal type, though endometritis may be due to other causes, such as tuberculosis, submucous myoma, and, in recent years, use of various intrauterine contraceptive devices (IUD).

It is becoming increasingly apparent that inflammatory disease may be caused by organisms other than the gonococcus (or that there is secondary invasion). There is growing evidence that *Chlamydia trachomatis* may play an important role in acute pelvic infection.

Acute Endometritis

This is far less frequently encountered pathologically than is the chronic form, partly because of the relative infrequency with which either curettage or hysterectomy is performed in the acute stage of any pelvic inflammatory disease, although some clinics advocate high dosage of antibiotics followed by immediate evacuation of the uterine contents. In such instances microscopic evidence of acute endometritis may be present (Fig. 10–1).

Puerperal. The most severe form is that in which the acute inflammation of the endometrium, usually with other pelvic structures as well, is seen in association with acute puerperal sepsis, following abortion or full term delivery. The severity of the local reaction depends upon the virulence of the infecting organisms. In the milder forms, the endometrium is swollen, hyperemic, and edematous, with marked infiltration of leukocytes, chiefly of the polymorphonuclear variety.

In the more virulent types, the destructive effects of the bacterial toxin bring about necrosis of the endometrium and sometimes frank ulceration (Fig. 10–2). The inflammatory infiltration usually invades the myometrium and often the parametrium as well. In

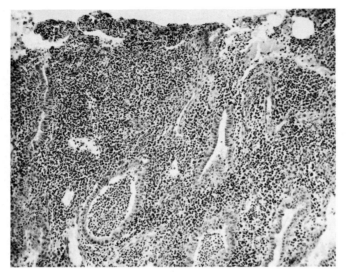

Figure 10–1. Acute endometritis, with marked leukocytic infiltration. Note exudate in glands.

Figure 10–2. Acute postabortive infection. Uterus is large and edematous. There is necrosis of uterine wall at placental site. Remnant of retained placental tissue is present, and there is bilateral thrombosis of uterine veins.

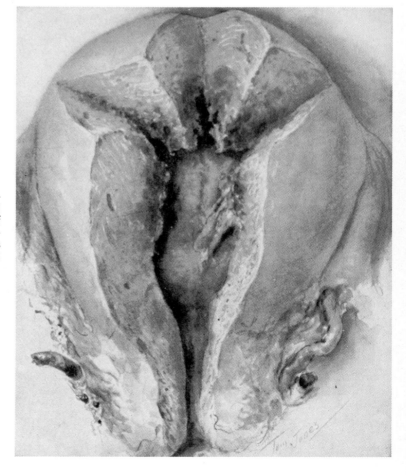

the milder forms, the gland lumina contain an exudate made up of polymorphonuclear leukocytes and dead epithelial cells, and the blood vessels are prominent and injected. In the severe forms, *thrombophlebitis* of the uterine and pelvic vessels may be a prominent feature; in the pre-antibiotic days, septic emboli would incur multiple abscesses—subdiaphragmatic, hepatic, and the like—with a considerable mortality (Fig. 10–3). Today these are unusual sequelae of postpartum or abortal endometritis, which generally responds promptly to appropriate antibiotic therapy, although clostridium infections may lead to septicemia and even death. The significant role of *Bacteroides fragilis* (anaerobic) as a cause of septic emboli following thrombophlebitis has been recognized only recently and may lead to delayed postoperative or postabortal infections.

Gonorrheal. In gonorrheal invasion of the lower genital canal, the organism makes its way to the tubes by way of the endometrium, so that acute gonorrheal endometritis must be a part of the frequently encountered acute gonorrheal pelvic inflammatory disease. Yet, for reasons already mentioned, one only occasionally encounters such acute inflammatory phases in laboratory material. The tendency, moreover, is to rather rapid subsidence, though a residue of chronic endometritis may persist for a considerable time. Use of the Thayer-Martin or Transgrow culture has led to the detection of many unsuspected cases of female gonorrhea, even in the upper class low-risk patient; fortunately, concentrated high dosage treatment with penicillin, tetracycline, and other

antibiotics is generally curative. Many other secondary organisms may be involved, such as *Mycoplasma, Chlamydia,* and so forth, so that other suitable agents must be utilized as supplemental therapy (Monif and Welkos).

Intrauterine Device

There seems little doubt that the IUD may be associated with pelvic infection, and Faulkner and Gray find that a febrile PID is five times as common in the IUD user. A very recent Federal Drug Administration (FDA) Drug Bulletin notes that IUD users are 3 to 5 times more likely than nonusers to develop pelvic inflammatory disease. Undoubtedly this begins with an endometritis with subsequent adnexal involvement.

The frequency of unilateral (tubo-)ovarian abscess as recorded by Taylor and associates suggests a very real infectious stimulus. There seems little doubt from many studies that use of an IUD is associated with inflammatory disease at a significantly increased rate (Eschenbach). The high incidence of actinomycosis (even fatal) has been noted by Hager and Majmudar. Indeed, in the well-motivated patient with no medical problems who does not object to the pill (or use of a diaphragm) there is little need for the IUD. In this area most of the medicolegal problems arise from complications from the IUD or laparoscope.

Chronic Endometritis

Incidence. The chronic phases of inflammation are far more frequently observed in the endometrium than the acute phases. However, the incidence of chronic endome-

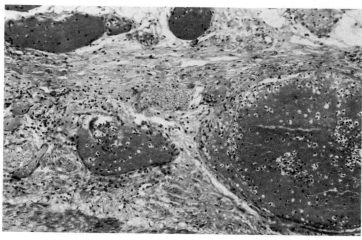

Figure 10–3. All vessels are occluded by septic thrombi in patient with induced abortion.

tritis is probably greater than that found many years ago, partly because of the more widespread use of the IUD, which is frequently associated with an inflammatory response. This may merely represent an immune reaction, for culture is often negative. However, bacteriologic studies of uteri at varying days after placement of an IUD frequently show a positive culture initially, followed by a subsequent drop-off, suggesting an improved immune response.

In the normal endometrium, especially in certain phases of the cycle, one may find a sprinkling of infiltrating mononuclear leukocytes, so that it is often the degree of this infiltration that may influence one in the diagnosis of chronic inflammation.

Just before menstrual desquamation and bleeding begin, there is a rather massive pseudoinflammatory infiltration of the endometrium as an entirely normal feature, and one familiar with this will not be apt to make the mistake of diagnosing endometritis. However, even a trained pathologist may have difficulty in establishing a diagnosis of endometritis if the material was obtained in the premenstrual era.

Microscopic Appearance. The microscopic diagnosis must be based upon the criteria of chronic inflammation in general. Most important is round cell and plasma cell infiltration (Fig. 10–4), although in advanced cases one may find fibroblast formation, new blood vessels, and even at times the appearance of granulation tissue areas.

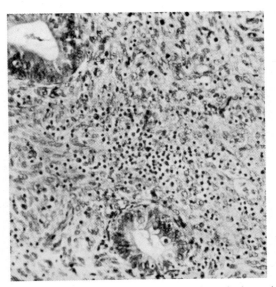

Figure 10–4. Chronic endometritis, with marked round cell and plasma cell infiltration.

The presence of plasma cells has been emphasized as essential to a diagnosis of chronic endometritis, although there is some question about this. Our own opinion is that their presence is not necessary to establish the diagnosis, although they are often present.

Although the interstitial changes of chronic endometritis are the primary ones, there is often considerable distortion of the glands, so that the lumina may be distended in some places and compressed in others. Not infrequently there is a rather angular outline to many of the lumina, but they only occasionally show any exudate.

Course and Effect upon Menstrual Cycle

The tendency of endometritis is toward resolution, in all except the virulent forms of puerperal origin. Two factors seem to be responsible for this capacity of the endometrium to throw off infection. One is the usually good downhill drainage of the uterine canal, like that of a bottle turned upside down. Even more important seems to be the monthly desquamation of menstruation which gradually decreases the infectious process. In a study of chronic endometritis, Vasudeva and co-workers have reaffirmed the fact that is is frequently nonspecific, often self-limited, and responsive to such minor forms of treatment as curettage. They also stress the importance of plasma cells in the diagnosis.

In the early stages the brunt of the infection falls upon the upper functional layers of the endometrium. With the occurrence of the first menstrual desquamation, however, much of the infected layer is cast off, the infection being thus attenuated and entrenching itself in a diluted form in the deeper layers of the endometrium, so that after a few cycles the endometrium may purge itself of the infection.

This explains why even in chronic pelvic inflammatory disease of very long standing one most frequently finds the uterine mucosa normal, though it originally served to convey the infection to the tubes. This, however, is by no means always the case, for the course of chronic pelvic inflammatory disease is ordinarily punctuated with exacerbations or reinfections, and with recurrence of inflammatory lesions in the endometrium, which may be a sequel to refractory disease persisting in the (endo)cervix. The milder forms of endometritis appear to exert little or no effect upon menstruation, but in the more severe forms, acute or chronic, the endometrial responsiveness to the ovarian hormones is impaired, and abnormalities of menstrual rhythm or amount may occur. Bleeding or a bloody discharge may be a symptom, though certainly not characteristic.

From a practical laboratory standpoint, *one should never diagnose chronic endometritis without thorough study of the sections for a possible explanation of the cause.* One should think especially of the possibility of *retained gestational tissue* or *tuberculosis,* both of which are causes of chronic endometritis. Not infrequently a cluster of degenerated chorionic villi, or islands of hyalinized or well formed decidual cells, point to recent incomplete abortion as the cause of the chronic inflammation. In other cases the finding of tubercles, with or without giant cells, points to a probable tuberculous etiology of the infection. Giant cells are merely suggestive of an acid-fast infection, for other granulomatous lesions, foreign bodies, etc., may produce these. In the Middle and Far East such diseases as schistosomiasis must always be considered as a possibility.

Another frequent association of endometritis, of either the acute or the chronic type, is with *submucous myoma.* The mucous membrane over the submucous growths is characteristically thin, and prone to infection from the genital canal. The inflammatory process may extend deeply into the substance of the tumor. When round cell infiltration of the superficial portions of the tumor is intense, it may lead to the erroneous diagnosis of sarcoma.

Very similar changes may be noted as a sequel to the use of various *intrauterine contraceptive devices,* as noted earlier. The study by Ober and co-workers shows a frequent associated epidermidalization (Fig. 10–5). Moyer and Mishell prefer to believe that the tissue reaction to the IUD represents a sterile foreign body reaction, and is instrumental in producing the contraceptive effect.

Finally, in the *senile endometritis* which so often is superimposed on postmenopausal atrophy, the endometrium is thin and heavily infiltrated with round and plasma cells. Patches of squamous metaplasia may be seen replacing the normal columnar epithelium (Fig. 10–6), and in rare cases the entire corporeal surface may be covered with a be-

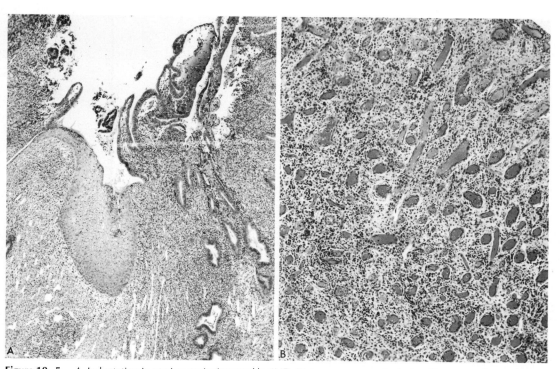

Figure 10–5. *A,* Indentation in uterine cavity incurred by IUD. Note squamous metaplasia with surrounding endometritis. *B,* Long-standing use of IUD (3 years) has led to replacement of endometrium by granulation tissue at insertion site.

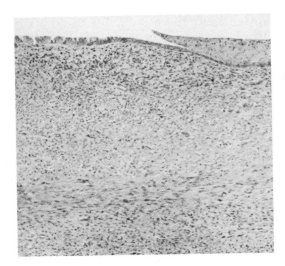

Figure 10–6. Senile endometritis, with so-called squamous metaplasia. Note the atrophy and the chronic inflammatory infiltration of the endometrium.

Figure 10–7. So-called ichthyosis uteri, the entire endometrium being replaced by stratified squamous epithelium. This section is from the fundus.

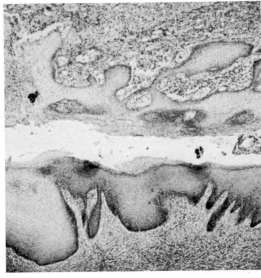

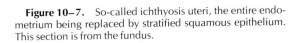

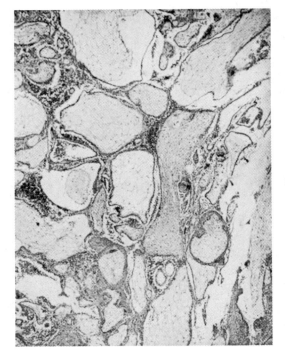

Figure 10–8. Well preserved chorionic villi. The surrounding endometrium shows chronic endometritis.

nign stratified squamous epithelium (*ichthyosis uteri*) (Fig. 10–7). Ulceration of the surface is common with senile endometritis, and is a frequent cause of postmenopausal bleeding, which must be distinguished from that due to adenocarcinoma.

Postabortal Endometritis

This is not nearly so frequent today since liberal abortion laws have minimized illegal abortion, but it may occur after either spontaneous or induced abortion despite an aseptic hospital environment. It is easy to understand the occurrence of endometrial infection, which may on occasion be caused by *Clostridium perfringens,* with overwhelmingly septic gas gangrene. It is important to remember, however, that even in spontaneous abortion the uterine cavity within a very short time is invaded by organisms from the vaginal canal, so that some degree of endometritis invariably follows. With this is associated, in a certain proportion of cases, a retention of some of the gestational products, with bleeding as the common clinical symptom.

As a matter of fact, bleeding due to incomplete abortion is one of the most common indications for uterine curettage, and one of the frequent problems presented to the pathologist is to determine whether uterine bleeding is due to the retention of chorionic tissue. When large masses of placental tissue are present, the diagnosis is obvious (Fig. 10–8). However, in many cases the abortion has occurred many weeks before the curetting, or there is doubt as to whether there has been a pregnancy, so that the amount or appearance of the curetted material may throw no light on the cause of the bleeding.

If curettage is necessary, it should not be so vigorous as to remove all of the endometrium down to and including the basalis. Jones suggests that this may lead to "traumatic intrauterine adhesions" as a result of a denuded anterior and posterior uterine wall. This, in conjunction with infection and associated cervical stenosis, may lead to the so-called Asherman's syndrome, characterized by persistent amenorrhea.

Prostaglandin is a relatively new abortifacient drug, the precise mechanism of which is still uncertain. In the few cases studied there was rather intense endometritis with necrosis and sloughing immediately postabortion; curettage at a later date revealed varying degrees of hyalinization and fibrosis of any residual decidua and villi in nonspecific fashion.

The point to emphasize is that in every case of chronic endometritis the pathologist should make careful microscopic search for the cause of the endometritis. Sometimes, as has been mentioned, he finds an unsuspected tuberculosis. Far more frequently, however, the search reveals such gestational products as chorionic villi or decidual cells, although it must be understood that the latter are of maternal origin and merely suggestive of pregnancy (Fig. 10–9).

When clearly demonstrable, chorionic villi are of course absolutely pathognomonic of a previous intrauterine pregnancy. They may be well preserved and abundant, so that their recognition is simple. Under such circumstances they show the characteristic two-layered trophoblast of the young villus, with the typical light-textured stroma.

More often, however, they show degenerative changes, usually in the nature of fibrosis or hyalinization (ghost villi). In the latter case, especially, they may be difficult to distinguish from the organized thrombi which are not rare with certain endometrial conditions (Fig. 10–10). The distinction between the two can generally be made by the fact that even in old villi one often finds at

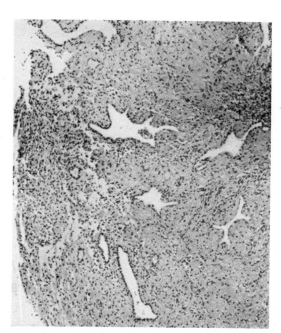

Figure 10–9. Large field of decidual cells found in association with chronic endometritis.

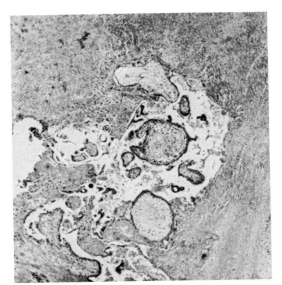

Figure 10–10. Degenerated chorionic villi such as these may be found in association with chronic endometritis.

shows at least a vestige of the cell structure of the villous stroma. Bone is a rare finding and usually suggests an old missed abortion (Fig. 10–11 A). An earlier implantation site is shown in Figure 10–11 B.

Since decidual cells are of maternal origin, and since they can occasionally be simulated by other cells, they cannot be considered as pathognomonic of pregnancy as are trophoblastic cells (Fig. 10–12) or villi, which are definitely fetal. The appearance of cytotrophoblast approximates decidua; the presence of syncytium is decisive. When large fields of typical decidual cells are seen, there can be little doubt of pregnancy, although one could not be sure, on the basis of decidual cells alone, whether the pregnancy had been intrauterine or extrauterine, unless villi are also found. Yet when an old decidual reaction is present and associated with an inflammatory overlay, it is probably representative of an old abortus, although demonstrable villi are absent. Obviously exogenous progesterone can produce a decidual reaction.

Furthermore, it should be remembered that in the premenstrual endometrium of the nonpregnant woman, the stromal cells ap-

least a degenerated or atrophic epithelial covering (the trophoblast), while this is lacking in thrombi. The latter usually take a homogeneous eosin stain, and show little or no cell structure, whereas the hyalinized villus takes little or no eosin stain, and usually

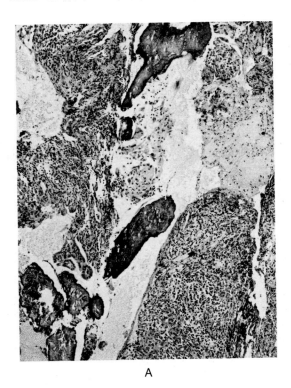

A

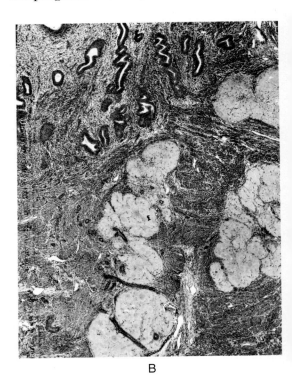

B

Figure 10–11. A, Fragments of bone with subacute and chronic endometritis probably represent an old missed abortion rather than metaplasia, although the latter can occur. B, Old implantation site noted at hysterectomy.

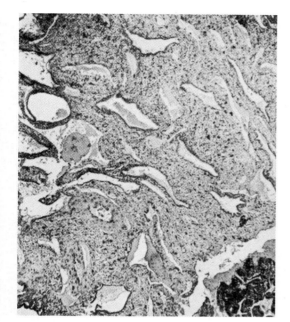

Figure 10–12. Decidual cells, interspersed with trophoblastic cells.

proximate decidual cells to a greater or lesser degree, and on this criterion alone it is often impossible to be sure, in the absence of villi or trophoblast, whether one is dealing with a marked predecidual reaction in the nonpregnant woman, or with the genuine decidua of very early pregnancy. If there is a clinical suspicion of the latter, numerous sections should be studied in order to demonstrate villi if they are present. The progestational change in the nonpregnant woman is most marked in the stroma, the cells of which may at times become so large and hypertrophic that they cannot be distinguished from genuine decidual cells. At somewhat later stages, however, the decidual characteristics are so outspoken that there can be little doubt of pregnancy. When only scattered patches of decidua are found, they are most apt to be seen surrounding blood vessels whose walls show considerable hyalinization, with frequently adjacent patches of diffusely eosin-staining fibrinoid material. In most cases a reasonably certain diagnosis is justified on the basis of such areas alone, particularly if there is an associated inflammatory reaction.

What has been said as to the qualified significance of decidual cells applies even more to the gland pattern. The premenstrual reaction of the nonpregnant woman may produce a high degree of tortuosity and secretory activity of the glands, so that they cannot be distinguished from those of very early pregnancy. Later they lose their tortuosity and are lined by a very flat epithelium. Moreover, it should not be forgotten that in the long-standing cases of incomplete abortion, in which bleeding has been present for many weeks, the glands may have retrogressed, or that their cyclical activity has been resumed even though rests of chorionic tissue are still present somewhere in the uterus. The Arias-Stella reaction has been commented on elsewhere.

Placental Polyp

Although true placental polyps may occur (Fig. 10–13), they are generally more apparent than real, consisting of a chunk of retained placenta. Should hysterectomy be done, the lesion may grossly resemble choriocarcinoma; far more often, operation reveals old villi and decidua and thus is indistinguishable from a mere incomplete abortion. Dyer and Bradburn suggest that such polyps may arise from a focal placenta accreta; HCG was generally negative in the few cases studied (Fig. 10–14).

Tuberculous Endometritis

Almost without exception, tuberculosis of the endometrium is secondary to tubercu-

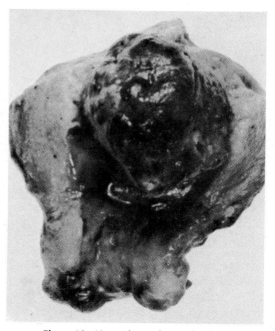

Figure 10–13. A large placental polyp.

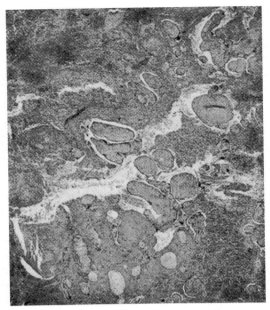

Figure 10–14. Structure of placental polyp. Degenerated and "shadow" villi in a groundwork of blood clot.

losis of the tube, and indeed pelvic tuberculosis is uniformly a sequel to tubal disease. *Granulomatous endometritis*, even with a negative acid-fast stain and culture, is generally presumed to be of tuberculous origin although theoretically there are other possible agents, such as sarcoid or foreign body reactions. Adnexal involvement usually follows extragenital tuberculosis, which is commonly pulmonary but occasionally os-

seous or of another type. Since it is not always easy to demonstrate tubal tuberculosis even when it is present, one is justified, when tuberculous endometritis is revealed by curettage, in suspecting that tuberculous tubal disease likewise exists, even though no clinical evidence of the latter can be elicited (Fig. 10–15). (It is occasionally helpful to take cultures prior to curettage, although these and acid-fast studies are usually negative.) Certain newer viewpoints on this general question are discussed in Chapter 15.

A number of authors (Sharman, Sutherland, and others) have reported the finding of unsuspected tuberculosis in 5 per cent of endometria obtained by biopsies done in routine sterility studies in Scotland, Israel, and other countries, usually with no clinical suspicion of tubal tuberculosis. Although certain cases of unsuspected endometrial tuberculosis occur in ostensibly normal women, the incidence of this finding is far less than the 5 per cent cited, perhaps because of the better nutritional and physical standards of the American woman. It seems probable that tuberculous endometritis is almost 100 per cent proof of tubal tuberculosis even without clinical or palpable evidence of adnexal disease. There has been more than one patient whose curettage has revealed evidence of an unsuspected acid-fast involvement of the endometrium; even though no adnexal disease was apparent, tubo-ovarian masses became apparent months later despite antibiotic therapy.

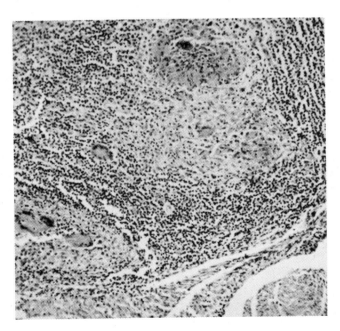

Figure 10–15. Typical tubercles and chronic inflammation replacing endometrium and extending toward myometrium (below).

Nevertheless, it is in this group of women with unsuspected endometrial tuberculosis often detected by curettage in the course of a sterility study that medical treatment has enjoyed its greatest vogue (Fig. 10–16). There is no objection if the patients have patent tubes, are afebrile, and have no palpable tender masses. At the same time, it should be remembered that *very* few normal full term pregnancies have followed antibiotic therapy of genital tuberculosis, as noted by Sutherland. Patients so treated should be kept under close observation lest their silent tuberculosis gradually extend with the advent of peritonitis or a miliary process.

The report by Snaith and Barns records six full term pregnancies among 158 treated patients, and Stallworthy records an 18 per cent conception rate with 10 per cent term pregnancy, which seems overly high. Schaefer has critically analyzed cases of full term pregnancy following genital tuberculosis when such an analysis was possible. His careful critique makes it seem apparent that in many reported cases the diagnosis of tuberculosis was far from absolute, and without histologic or culture proof of acid-fast disease. Schaefer states that "less than 100 of 7357 patients with genital tuberculosis had full term intrauterine pregnancies. The exact number is difficult to ascertain," for in many cases the diagnosis of tuberculosis was uncertain. The author adds that in the infrequent cases of pregnancy following genital tuberculosis, the end result is usually an abortion or an ectopic pregnancy, as indicated by Halbrecht. He further emphasizes the failure of tubal plastic surgery after antituberculous therapy, and points out that extensive degrees of genital infection lead to permanent infertility. This scholarly review should emphasize the extreme infrequency of normal term pregnancy in the woman with treated pelvic tuberculosis, and it is best to appraise the patient of this fact before institution of therapy.

Sutherland points out that about 20 per cent of women with pelvic tuberculosis ultimately come to surgery because of persistent pain due to adnexitis, adnexal masses, recurrent endometritis, or bleeding. At least 18 months of continuous drug therapy is carried out with surgical intervention *only* if there is failure of response. Schaefer believes that surgery, preceded by chemotherapy, should be standard treatment for the older parous woman, and we are in complete accord. The same author notes six patients with *postmenopausal* tuberculous endometritis (although this is uncommon) who were treated by chemotherapy with and without surgery.

In early cases of tuberculous endometritis one may find only an occasional tubercle or cluster of tubercles, with the characteristic epithelioid and giant cells. With this one may find marked chronic inflammatory infiltration with perhaps even a granulomatous appearance in some areas. When the disease is extensive, such infiltration is pronounced, tubercles are numerous, and caseation is apt to be present to a greater or lesser degree. In the milder cases the glandular structure may

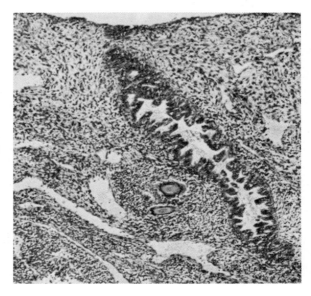

Figure 10–16. Another section of granulomatous endometritis, showing typical tubercles. A secretory pattern is obvious.

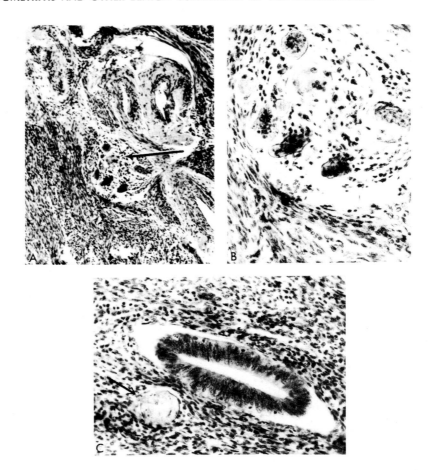

Figure 10–17. *A* and *B*, Bilharzial ova in myometrium. *C*, Bilharzial ovum in endometrium. (Courtesy of M. Fathalla, Assuit University, Cairo, Egypt.)

be almost intact, but in the more advanced stage it is almost completely destroyed, with often extensive surface ulceration.

When a granulomatous endometritis is present, it is probably tuberculous; however, in areas of the Middle and Far East where *bilharziasis* is endemic, the characteristic ova should be searched for. These may involve both the myometrium and endometrium (Fig. 10–17).

MYOMETRITIS

Both acute and chronic forms may occur in conjunction with endometrial infections. Myometrial involvement is more intense with the puerperal streptococcus than with gonococcal disease, and marked edema, muscle hypertrophy, leukocytic infiltration, and other signs of infection are more extensive (Fig. 10–18).

Chronic myometritis is characterized by

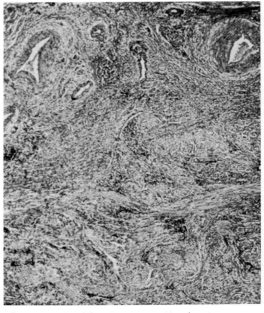

Figure 10–18. Chronic myometritis, showing scattered and clumped round and plasma cells.

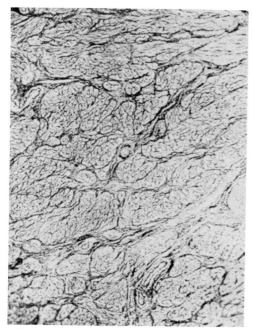

Figure 10–19. Chronic myometritis, with marked increase in connective tissue (orcein–van Gieson stain). Black areas are connective tissue.

an infiltration of plasma cells and frequent inlays of fibrous tissue between muscle bundles. Such differential stains as the orcein-van Gieson are necessary to distinguish between fibrous and muscle cell components. Grossly, the fundus may be enlarged and boggy, with resultant irregular and often profuse bleeding (Fig. 10–19).

MYOMETRIAL HYPERTROPHY

The condition in which there is an enlarged symmetric uterus (in the absence of adenomyosis) has been in a sense a "dumping ground," dignified by such nomenclature as fibrosis uteri or chronic passive congestion. Although in many instances the terminology may represent an attempt by an overenthusiastic surgeon to slip a normal parous uterus past an alert tissue committee, on occasion the grossly but diffusely enlarged uterus seems to represent a valid symptom-producing entity which Lewis and associates have chosen to call *myometrial hypertrophy*. Normal uterine weight varies from 30 to 50 grams.

They arbitrarily utilize a weight of more than 120 grams as a diagnostic index, and point out that the increased size is due to

smooth muscle hypertrophy. It is suggested that over 5 per cent of uteri removed warrant this designation, which is associated with excessive menstrual bleeding. Although the authors seem loath to assign a cause and effect basis, it would seem that the mere increase in size of the uterus might be expected to incur more profuse periods, aided in part by an overstretched if hypertrophic myometrium that might be incompetent and unable to exhibit adequate contraction, so that the periods are prolonged and heavy.

Although uncommon, such hypertrophic uteri do occur with bleeding so profuse as to lead to frank anemia and even shock. The pathologist must be cognizant of the occasional clinical problems associated with these "normal" but oversized uteri, but such degrees of myometrial hypertrophy are rarely seen and poorly understood. In any case, even a histologically normal uterus weighing more than 150 to 200 grams seems to be at least a potentially pathologic uterus. The recent study by Hanzlik and Leissring of "parametrial phlebectasia" would seem to provide rather persuasive evidence that this is an entity and closely approximates myometrial hypertrophy.

SUBINVOLUTION OF UTERUS

The Normal Involution of the Uterus

This process is often referred to as the most striking instance of very rapid atrophy occurring in the human body. Within a period of about 8 weeks the uterus shrinks from a weight of about 2 pounds to 1 or 2 ounces. The expulsion of the placenta and membranes is followed by the formation of a line of demarcation on the denuded surface of the uterus. This line serves to mark off the tissue which is to be shed from that which will serve to regenerate the new mucous membrane. The division becomes evident as early as the second day (Fig. 10–20).

By the end of the second week the necrotic material has practically all been cast off and the regeneration of the new endometrium is well on the way. As in postmenstrual regeneration, it is from the stumps of the endometrial glands in the basalis that the new surface is restored. On the other hand, the regeneration of the placental site takes place much more slowly, often requiring 6 weeks or more. Williams believes that the process

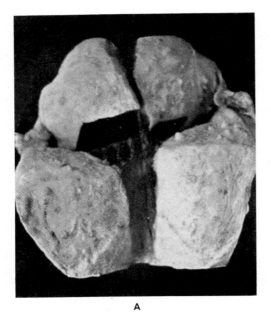

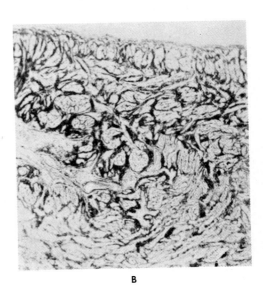

A   B

Figure 10–20. *A*, Gross structure of chronic subinvolution, showing the thickness of the uterine wall and the bumpy appearance due to enlarged blood vessel walls. *B*, Chronic subinvolution of uterus (outer third of wall), showing old dead, swollen, unabsorbed elastic tissue between muscle bundles.

here is one of exfoliation "brought about by the undermining of the placental site by the growth of endometrial tissue" (Fig. 10–21).

As for the enormous shrinkage of the muscular mass of the uterus, there is still a difference of opinion as to whether this is brought about only by a great reduction in the cyto-plasm of the individual cells, or whether there is an actual diminution in the number of cells. Autolysis is believed to play an important part, as well as fatty degeneration.

The blood vessel changes have been the subject of much study, and much of this has been concerned with the distribution and

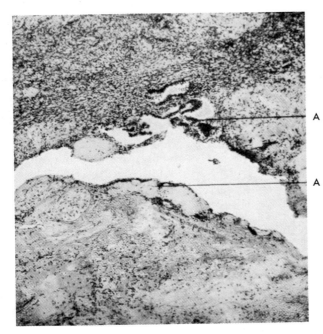

A

A

Figure 10–21. Section of wall of uterus 5 weeks postpartum. *A*, Regenerating endometrium.

amount of elastic tissue. Normally the latter is represented in the multiparous uterus only by a thin layer corresponding to the internal elastic lamina of the blood vessels. There is essential agreement among those who have studied the subject that with increasing parity, there is an increased amount of elastic tissue around the blood vessels, this being due not to an increased deposit but to imperfect absorption or involution during the puerperium. This would substantiate the view that new blood vessels are formed within the lumina of the old blood channels (Fig. 10–22).

Subinvolution of the Uterus

When the process of involution is for any reason incomplete, the amount of elastic tissue is increased, with exaggerated fibrous tissue elements, and often edema and congestion. Important factors in inhibiting normal involution are displacements—especially the marked retroflexion so frequent after childbirth—and infection.

Grossly, the subinvoluted uterus is larger than normal, sometimes considerably so. Its consistency is soft and boggy, and the serous coat may be of bluish hue and sometimes mottled. The cut surface shows the greatly thickened uterine walls, with the thickened blood vessels often projecting somewhat above the surface, giving it a bumpy appearance.

While subinvolution is a definite entity, it seems to be receiving less attention today. Perhaps more complete pathologic examination is revealing adenomyosis or other forms of pathology formerly thought to represent subinvolution.

PYOMETRA

On occasion an inflammatory process may involve the endometrium with a concomitant stenosis of the cervix. If the infection is sufficiently virulent, the endometrial cavity may become filled with pus, and so softened and enlarged that a pregnant uterus or an ovarian cyst may be mimicked (Fig. 10–23). Frequently there may be no systemic indication of any infection.

The finding of a pyometra is strongly suggestive of a cervical or fundal cancer, but is also found as a sequel of such benign processes as adhesive vaginitis, cervical amputation, or radium therapy. The finding of pus in

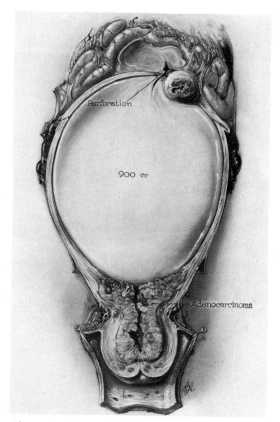

Figure 10–23. Pyometra with adenocarcinoma of cervix. Spontaneous perforation of uterus with walled-off abscess has occurred. (Courtesy of Dr. Erle Henriksen, Los Angeles.)

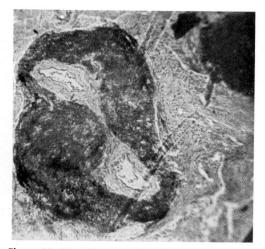

Figure 10–22. Chronic subinvolution, showing formation of new arteries within the old (orcein–van Gieson stain). Old blood vessel collars take dark stain. Section from inner third of uterine wall.

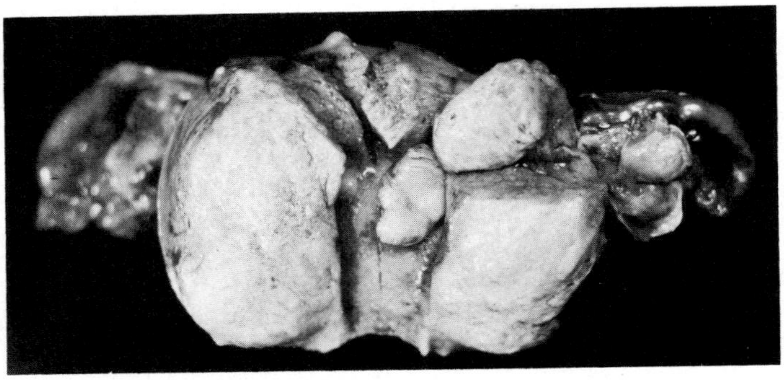

Figure 10–24. Gross appearance of rather large endometrial polyp (previous amputation of cervix).

the uterine cavity following dilatation of the cervix is a firm contraindication to curettage or intracavitary radium for fear of a subsequent pelvic cellulitis. Such an edematous and softened uterus is easily perforated, with dire results. Pyometra rarely occurs in the menstrual era as a sequel to the usual forms of endometritis. It is usually a combination of malignancy plus secondary infection.

ENDOMETRIAL POLYP

Introduction

The term *polyp* is a clinical rather than a pathologic one, referring simply to a growth which is attached by a pedicle or stem, and not indicating in any way its histologic characters (Fig. 10–24). For example, a myoma may be polypoid, and so may a carcinoma or sarcoma. The most common variety, however, is that in which the polyp has a structure like that of the endometrium itself, consisting simply of a localized heaping up of

the latter. Polyps of this structure may be single or multiple (Fig. 10–25), small or large enough to fill the uterine cavity. The pedicle may be short, or so long that the body of the polyp protrudes through the cervix into the vagina or even to the outside of the body. We have recently seen a case in which a large pedunculated endometrial polyp protruded out the introitus, and the patient was referred for correction of a uterine prolapse. Unquestionably, many polyps are so badly macerated by curettage that specific diagnosis is impossible; for this reason it is impossible to assess their frequency.

Clinical Symptoms

The smaller polyps, being well protected from trauma by the thick walls of the uterus, usually produce no bleeding or other symptoms (Fig. 10–26). Most of them are revealed only accidentally, either on curettage or in the routine laboratory examination of uteri removed at operation for other reasons. When the polyp is large, however, and espe-

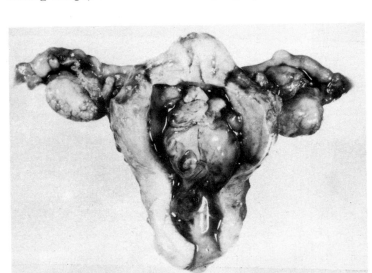

Figure 10–25. Multiple endometrial polyps in association with myomatous uterus.

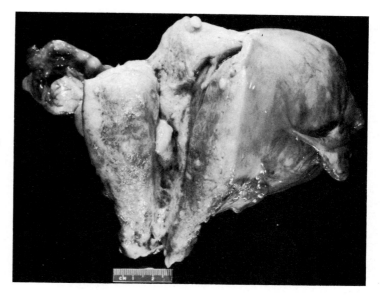

Figure 10–26. Endometrial polyp in myomatous uterus.

cially when a long pedicle permits it to obtrude itself into the cervix or vagina, ulceration and degeneration occur, with clinical bleeding. The latter may be only slight and occasional, but with the large polyps it may be much freer and more persistent (Fig. 10–27).

Histologic Types of Endometrial Polyps

Since the endometrial polyp is made up of endometrial tissue, it might be expected that

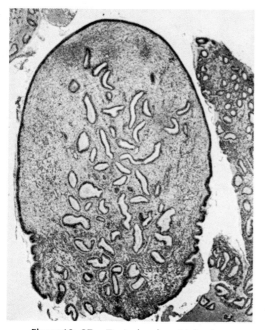

Figure 10–27. Typical endometrial polyp.

it would exhibit the cyclic histologic changes that characterize the uterine mucosa from which it springs. This, however, is by no means always the case. As a matter of fact, from the standpoint of responsiveness to the ovarian hormones, we may distinguish two types of endometrial polyps.

1. *Polyps made up of functional endometrium* (Fig. 10–28), in which the endometrium of the polyp responds just as does the general corporeal endometrium to the ovarian hormones. In such growths a progestational picture parallels the secretory response of the surrounding endometrium, and so with the other phases of the normal cycle. The endometrial tissue of the polyp is of a mature functioning type and is responsive to the effects of both estrogen and progesterone. The dependent portion of the polyp often shows a prominent "vascular core" with marked injection of the vessels, hemorrhage into the stroma, inflammatory changes, and not infrequently ulcerative loss of the surface layers.

2. *Polyps made up of immature endometrium* (Fig. 10–29), in which the constituent endometrial tissue is apparently responsive only to the growth effect of estrogen, but exhibits no progesterone response even when the surrounding endometrium is in a phase of marked secretory activity. The endometrium of such polyps usually shows a stationary hyperplastic pattern, often of the Swiss-cheese type. Frequently, too, the crowding of the glands in the polyp produces an adenomatous pattern, and this, together with the

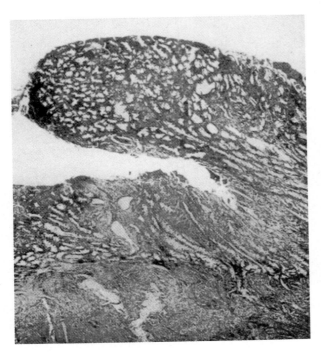

Figure 10–28. Endometrial polyp made up of functioning endometrium, with secretory picture corresponding to that of surrounding endometrium.

dark-staining and perhaps stratified epithelium, produces a picture which may be easily mistaken for adenocarcinoma. This variety of polyp is far more common than that made of ripe, fully functioning endometrium (Fig. 10–28).

Such nonresponsive polyps commonly

show the same types of hyperplastic patterns as the endometrium in general (Fig. 10–29). A cystic glandular, a retrogressive, or an atypical adenomatous architecture may be found in either the menstrual or the postmenopausal era (Fig. 10–30). Varying combinations of these are common; on occasion

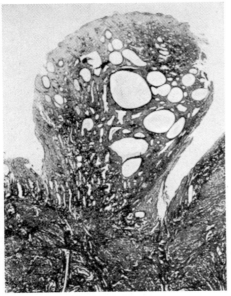

Figure 10–29. Endometrial polyp showing hyperplastic, nonfunctioning structure. This is much more common than the functioning type.

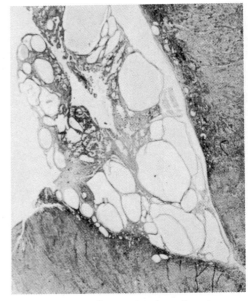

Figure 10–30. Endometrial polyp of postmenopausal woman, showing retrogressed hyperplastic pattern.

there is very real difficulty in distinguishing the proliferative microscopic patterns from genuine adenocarcinoma.

It seems quite certain that a not inconsiderable proportion of cases of supposed malignant degeneration of endometrial polyps have really been instances of this pseudomalignant hyperplastic activity in polyps made up of endometrium capable only of proliferation and not of functional differentiation. In some polyps of this type it is possible to trace the immature endometrium of the polyp downward as a broad zone to the basalis, which itself is made up similarly of an immature type of endometrium. The impression one gets in such cases is that patches of unripe endometrium have herniated through the functionalis and become polypoid.

A third type of endometrial polyp, much less common than those already described, is composed not only of endometrial elements but shows in addition a variable, but at times considerable amount of involuntary muscle tissue. This variety is properly called *adenomyomatous polyp*, and, as might be expected, is often associated with adenomyosis of the uterus.

Genesis of Endometrial Polyps

In discussing endometrial hyperplasia, Schroeder also speculates as to the occurrence of small endometrial adenomas arising from the basalis portion of the endometrium. They tend to protrude into the functional zone of the endometrium, but are not shed at menstruation. In time they press upward and present into the cavity as polyps. As they become extruded and push inward, they are enveloped by a layer of the functional endometrium. This enveloping blanket may rarely be thick and complete; more commonly it is extremely thin and sloughed with menstruation. Most polyps generally exhibit a basalis-like refractory hormonal pattern to even a biphasic cycle.

Malignant Changes

Actual malignant degeneration may occur in endometrial polyps, especially in those which reach large size. It is sometimes difficult to distinguish between adenocarcinomatous degeneration of a primarily benign endometrial polyp and a polypoid adenocarcinoma, for the latter may begin as a sharply localized polypoid growth. The differentiation can usually be made by careful study of

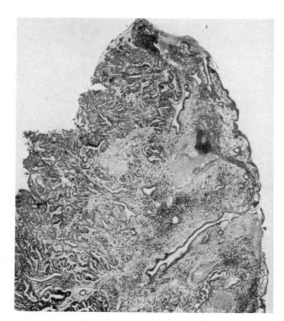

Figure 10–31. Endometrial polyp, showing malignant changes (adenocarcinoma of intermediate grade) on left edge of field.

the polyp base. When the entire polyp, including its base and perhaps the immediately adjacent uterine surface, shows adenocarcinoma, there is little doubt that one is dealing with an adenocarcinoma of polypoid type. When, on the other hand, adenocarcinoma is found only in one segment of an otherwise benign polyp, with no adenocarcinoma at the base, it can be assumed that one has to deal with malignant changes in a primarily benign growth (Fig. 10–31).

Finally, attention may be called to the fact that in cases of hyperplasia of the endometrium the latter may be the seat of a *multiple polyposis*, constituting the so-called polypoid hyperplasia. The endometrium in polypoid hyperplasia is like that in the far more common nonpolypoid form. Sarcoma may also occur (Fig. 10–32).

Associated Malignancy

Although malignant degeneration of a benign polyp is a rather rare occurrence, co-association of a benign polyp with other malignancy is by no means uncommon. A study by Peterson and Novak finds that, in the postmenopausal era, there is a 15.5 per cent malignancy associated with benign polyps. The vast majority of these are carcinomas involving the adjacent endometrium, although the polyp itself may be benign. This of course

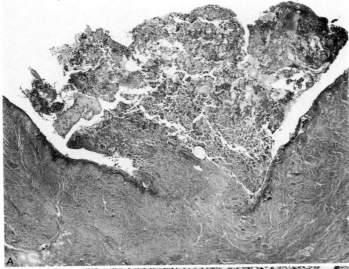

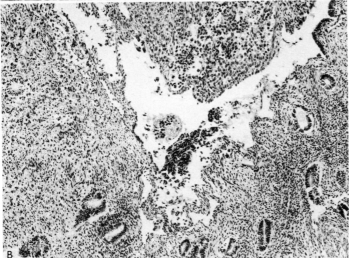

Figure 10–32. *A*, Endometrial polyp with sarcomatous change. *B*, Higher power of base of polyp showing normal endometrium with sarcoma in polyp (top).

suggests the importance of endometrial polyps in the genesis of fundal cancer, as noted in the preceding chapter, and has been emphasized by Armenia, who finds a ninefold increase of endometrial cancer in patients who have had a previous polyp. It also warns that the finding of only a benign endometrial polyp in the woman with postmenopausal bleeding is no guarantee that the polyp represents the sum total of pathology. Wolfe and Mackles have more recently confirmed our observations.

REFERENCES

Armenia, C. S.: Sequential relationships between endometrial polyps and carcinoma of the endometrium. Obstet. Gynecol., *30*:524, 1967.

Bahary, C. M., Ovadia, Y., and Neri, A.: Schistosoma mansoni of the ovary. Am. J. Obstet. Gynecol., 98:290, 1967.

Burkman, R. T., et al.: Untreated gonorrhea and endometritis following abortion. Am. J. Obstet. Gynecol., *126*:648, 1976.

Cadena, D., et al.: Chronic endometritis. A clinicopathologic study. Obstet. Gynecol., *41*:733, 1973.

Chalvardgian, A.: Sarcoidosis of the genital tract. Am. J. Obstet. Gynecol., *132*:78, 1978.

Chow, A. W., et al.: The bacteriology of acute pelvic inflammatory disease. Am. J. Obstet. Gynecol., *122*:876, 1975.

Dawood, M. Y., and Birnbaum, S. J.: Unilateral tubo-ovarian abscess and intrauterine contraceptive devices. Obstet. Gynecol., *46*:429, 1975.

Dyer, I., and Bradburn, D. M.: An inquiry into the etiology of placental polyps. Am. J. Obstet. Gynecol., *109*:858, 1971.

Eschenbach, D. A.: Pathogenesis of acute pelvic inflammatory disease. Am. J. Obstet. Gynecol., *128*:838, 1977.

Fathalla, M. F., Assuit University, Cairo, Egypt. Personal communication.

Faulkner, W. L., and Ory, H. W.: Intrauterine devices and acute pelvic inflammatory disease. J.A.M.A., 235:1851, 1976.

Federal Drug Administration Drug Bulletin, Pelvic inflammatory disease in IUD users. Vol. 19, May–July, 1978.

Gibbs, R. S., and Weinstein, A. J.: Puerperal infection in the antibiotic era. Am. J. Obstet. Gynecol., 124:769, 1976.

Gibbs, R. S., et al.: Puerperal endometritis: a prospective microbiologic study. Am. J. Obstet. Gynecol., 121:919, 1975.

Golde, S. H., et al.: Unilateral tubo-ovarian abscess. Am. J. Obstet. Gynecol., 127:807, 1977.

Hager, W. D., and Majmudar, B.: Pelvic actinomycosis in women using IUD. Am. J. Obstet. Gynecol. 133:60, 1979.

Haines, M.: Genital tuberculosis in the female. J. Obstet. Gynaecol. Brit. Emp., 59:721, 1959.

Halbrecht, I.: Endometrial and tubal sequelae of latent nonspecific infections. Int. J. Fertil., 121:121–126, 1965.

Hall, W. L., Sobel, A. L., Jones, C. P., and Parker, R. T.: Anaerobic postoperative pelvic infections. Obstet. Gynecol., 30:1, 1967.

Hanzlik, H., and Leissring, J. C.: Parametrial phlebectasia. Am. J. Obstet. Gynecol., 125:431, 1976.

Heaton, F. C., and Ledger, W. J.: Postmenopausal tubo-ovarian abscess. Obstet. Gynecol., 47:90, 1976.

Henderson, D. N., Harkins, J. L., and Stitt, J. F.: Pelvic tuberculosis. Am. J. Obstet. Gynecol., 94:630, 1966.

Israel, S. L., Roitman, H. B., and Clancy, C.: Infrequency of unsuspected endometrial tuberculosis. J.A.M.A., 183:63, 1963.

Jones, W. E.: Traumatic intrauterine adhesions. Am. J. Obstet. Gynecol., 89:304, 1964.

Josey, W. E., and Cook, C. C.: Septic pelvic thrombophlebitis. Obstet. Gynecol., 35:891, 1970.

Kadner, M. L., and Anderson, G. V.: Septic abortion (with special reference to Clostridium welchii infection). Obstet. Gynecol., 21:86, 1962.

Klein, T. A., et al.: Pelvic tuberculosis. Obstet. Gynecol., 48:99, 1976.

Ledger, W. J.: Anaerobic infections. Am. J. Obstet. Gynecol., 123:111, 1975.

Lewis, P. L., Lee, A. B. H., and Easler, R. E.: Myometrial hypertrophy. Am. J. Obstet. Gynecol., 84:1032, 1962.

Lomax, C. W., et al.: Actinomycosis of the female genital tract. Obstet. Gynecol., 48:341, 1976.

March, P., et al.: Chlamydia trachomatis infection in acute salpingitis. N. Engl. J. Med., 296:1377, 1977.

McNamara, M. T., and Mead, P. B.: Diagnosis and management of the pelvic abscess. J. Reprod. Med., 17:299, 1976.

Mead, P. B., et al.: Incidence of infections associated with the intrauterine contraceptive device in an isolated community. Am. J. Obstet. Gynecol., 125:79, 1976.

Monif, G. R. G.: Clinical response to doxycycline. Am. J. Obstet. Gynecol., 129:614, 1977.

Monif, G. R., and Welkos, S. L.: Infectious morbidity due to Bacteroides fragilis in obstetric patients. Clin. Obstet. Gynecol., 19:131, 1976.

Monif, G. R., et al.: Cul-de-sac isolates from patients with endometritis-salpingitis-peritonitis and gonococcal endocervicitis. Am. J. Obstet. Gynecol., 126:158, 1976.

Moyer, D. L., and Mishell, D. R., Jr.: Reactions of human endometrium to the intrauterine foreign body. II. Long-term effects on the endometrial histology and cytology. Am. J. Obstet. Gynecol., 111:66, 1971.

Ober, W. B., Sobrero, A. J., Korman, R., and Sold, S.: Endometrial morphology and polyethylene intrauterine devices; a study of 200 endometrial biopsies. Obstet. Gynecol., 32:782, 1968.

Peterson, W. F., and Novak, E. R.: Endometrial polyps. Obstet. Gynecol., 8:40, 1956.

Pocheco, J. C., and Kempers, R. D.: Etiology of postmenopausal bleeding. Obstet. Gynecol., 32:40, 1968.

Rivlin, M. E., and Hunt, J. A.: Ruptured tubo-ovarian abscess. Obstet. Gynecol., 50:518, 1977.

Rubenstein, P. R., et al.: Colpotomy drainage of pelvic abscess. Obstet. Gynecol., 48:142, 1976.

Saw, E. C., et al.: Female genital coccidioidomycosis. Obstet. Gynecol., 45:199, 1975.

Schaefer, G.: Tuberculosis of the female genital tract. Clin. Obstet. Gynecol., 112:681, 1972.

Schaefer, G.: Female genital tuberculosis. Clin. Obstet. Gynecol., 19:223, 1976.

Schiffer, M. A., et al.: Actinomycosis infections associated with intrauterine contraceptive devices. Obstet. Gynecol., 45:67, 1975.

Schroeder, R.: Endometrial hyperplasia in relation to genital function. Am. J. Obstet. Gynecol., 68:294, 1954.

Schwarz, R. H.: Management of postoperative infections in obstetrics and gynecology. Clin. Obstet. Gynecol., 19:97, 1976.

Sharman, A.: Endometrial tuberculosis in sterility. Fertil. Steril., 3:144, 1952.

Snaith, L., and Barns, T.: Fertility in pelvic tuberculosis. Lancet, 1:712, 1962.

Stallworthy, J.: Fertility and genital tuberculosis. Fertil. Steril., 14:284, 1963.

Stearns, H. C., and Sneeden, V. D.: Observations on the clinical and pathologic aspects of the pelvic congestion syndrome. Am. J. Obstet. Gynecol., 94:718, 1966.

Sutherland, A. M.: The place of surgery in the treatment of genital tuberculosis in women. Acta Obstet. Gynecol. Scand., 44:163, 1965.

Sweet, R. L.: Anaerobic infections of the female genital tract. Am. J. Obstet. Gynecol., 122:891, 1975.

Taylor, E. S., et al.: The intrauterine device and tubo-ovarian abscess. Am. J. Obstet. Gynecol., 123:338, 1975.

Taylor, H. C., Jr.: Pelvic pain based on vascular and autonomic nervous system disorder. Am. J. Obstet. Gynecol., 67:1177, 1954.

Vasudeva, K., Thrasher, T. V., and Richart, R. M.: Chronic endometritis: a clinical and electron microscopic study. Am. J. Obstet. Gynecol., 112:749, 1972.

Whitelaw, P. F., and Hanletti, J. D.: Pyometra: a reappraisal. Am. J. Obstet. Gynecol., 109:108, 1971.

Williams, J. T., and Kinney, G. D.: Myometrial hypertrophy. (So-called fibrosis uteri.) Am. J. Obstet. Gynecol., 47:380, 1944.

Willson, J. R., Ledger, W. J., and Andros, G. J.: The effect of an intrauterine contraceptive device on the histological pattern of the endometrium. Am. J. Obstet. Gynecol., 93:802, 1965.

Wolfe, S. A., and Mackles, A.: Malignant lesions arising from benign endometrial polyps. Obstet. Gynecol., 20:542, 1963.

Chapter 11

MYOMA AND OTHER BENIGN TUMORS OF THE UTERUS

Introduction

One of the most common human tumors, and much the most frequent uterine neoplasm, is the myoma. Autopsy studies have shown that approximately 20 per cent of women over 30 harbor uterine myomas of various sizes, though often there have been no symptoms produced. Myomas have been reported in females as young as 11 years of age.

These tumors are quite generally spoken of as "fibroids" of the uterus. Since they are definitely of muscle tissue origin, this term is incorrect. However, it is so thoroughly entrenched through long usage that it would be difficult to dislodge, and it need not be considered objectionable as a clinical designation for these tumors. Indeed, we use the terms interchangeably.

General Characteristics

The *size* of uterine myomas is exceedingly variable. They may appear as tiny, microscopic growths (seedling myomas) or they may reach huge proportions. As a group they are not apt to attain the enormous size and weight of the occasional giant ovarian cysts, but weights of 100 pounds and more have been reported. The tumors may be single or, more frequently, multiple.

The position of the tumors in the uterus may be *corporeal* or *cervical*, the latter constituting only a small fraction of the total number. When the tumor is in the cervix, the posterior wall of the cervix is the most com-

mon location (Fig. 11–1), though the lateral or anterior wall may also be involved. When the cervical tumor grows anteriorly, it often displaces the bladder and impinges on the urethra, with resultant retention of urine. Large cervical tumors constitute difficult surgical problems, the cervical mass being impacted in the pelvis, so that its removal is technically difficult and associated with danger of damaging such important structures as

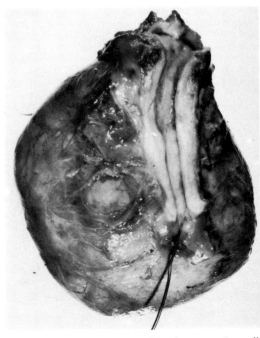

Figure 11–1. Large myoma arising from posterior wall of cervix. (Probe in os.)

260

the ureters and bladder. In such large cervical tumors the small uninvolved uterine body may be perched like a small cap on top of the tumor mass.

The usual subdivision of the corporeal tumors is into the *subserous*, the *interstitial* or *intramural*, and the *submucous* varieties, according to whether the growth is located just beneath the serous wall, within the substance of the uterine muscular wall, or just beneath the mucosa, respectively.

The subserous growths may present as knobby excrescences, or as masses which have developed distinct pedicles, the so-called *pedunculated myomas*. Not infrequently, lateral growths may extend outward between the folds of the broad ligament. Such *intraligamentary* tumors, when of large size, may burrow far outward and form retroperitoneal masses (Fig. 11–2).

The omentum frequently becomes adherent to subperitoneal growths, especially when there is an associated pelvic inflammatory disease. The tumors thus acquire an additional blood supply from the adherent omentum. Gradually more and more nutrition comes from the omentum and less and less from the pedicle, which becomes thinner. The tumor may thus be completely weaned away from the uterus by the omentum, becoming a floating solid tumor which

receives all its nutrient blood supply from the latter. This is the relatively rare *parasitic* type of myoma, which may give rise to interesting clinical problems. Ascites, due to increased transudation from partial torsion and obstruction of the omental vessels, may occur but, paradoxically, without the frequency with which ovarian fibroma may coexist with ascites and hydrothorax (Meigs's syndrome).

The intramural growths, when of small size, may cause no change in the contour of the uterus. When larger, they produce an enlargement of the organ, and give it a hilly or nodular contour. In the majority of such cases, moreover, some of the interstitial growths become subserous or submucous, this being the tendency with intramural growths as they increase in size (Fig. 11–3).

Although the *submucous* tumors constitute the least frequent group numerically (about 5 per cent), they are perhaps the most important clinically, and may be considered a rather specific group. Whereas other myomas attain large size with frequently no symptomatology, even a small tumor in a submucous location may impinge on the blood vessels of the endometrium and produce free bleeding. As they grow in size they bring about a domelike protrusion into the uterine cavity, with impingement on the op-

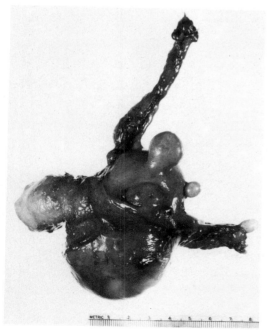

Figure 11–2. Multinodular myomatous uterus with large intraligamentary tumor (below).

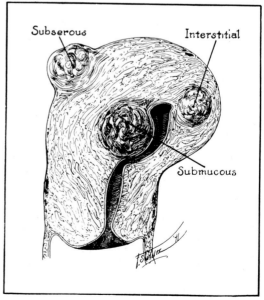

Figure 11–3. Cut surface of myomas showing characteristic whorl-like appearance.

posite uterine wall and marked distortion and enlargement of the cavity of the uterus (Fig. 11–4). Most submucous myomas, even of small size, ultimately necessitate hysterectomy because of continued bleeding, but it should never be assumed that just because a woman has myomas any bleeding must be due to these. Preoperative smear with possible curettage and biopsy should be routine, although examination of the opened uterus at the time of hysterectomy is probably just as informative to any pathologically oriented gynecologist. Much larger intramural and subserous tumors may never require surgery. Submucous tumors can usually be noted at curettage by feeling the curette "bump over" the protruding fibroid, although it is usually too firmly embedded for removal; we do not routinely utilize hysterograms, as is advocated by some.

As with the subserous variety, many of the submucous group develop pedicles, which may become so long that the tumors may protrude into the cervix or vagina, or even beyond the vaginal orifice (*pedunculated submucous myoma*). Infection and ulceration are common concomitants of such growths, and the circulatory disturbances caused by constriction of the pedicle may bring about sloughing and necrosis (Fig. 11–5 A). Uterine inversion may occur rarely (Fig. 11–5 B).

Etiology

Little or nothing is known as to the underlying cause for the development of uterine myoma. *Heredity* does not appear to be an important factor. It is generally accepted that the black race is more prone to the development of uterine myoma than the white.

The relation of *sterility* to these growths has been the subject of much discussion. Some believe that sterility may be a causative factor in the development of the tumors; others hold that the tumors are responsible for the sterility. Certainly a large proportion (from 25 to 35 per cent) of patients with myomas suffer from sterility, and myoma is admittedly common in unmarried women.

The mechanical factors entailed by the size of the tumors and the uterine distortion

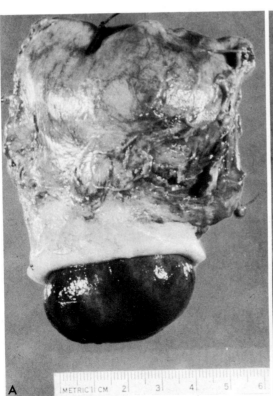
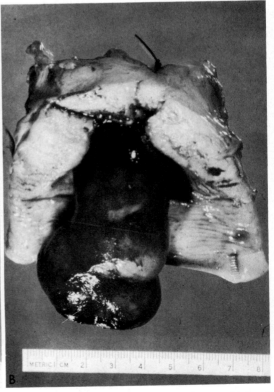

Figure 11–4. *A,* Cervix distended (as in abortion) by large submucous myoma. *B,* Opened uterus showing thick stalk of grossly necrotic tumor. Vaginal myomectomy might have been extremely complicated.

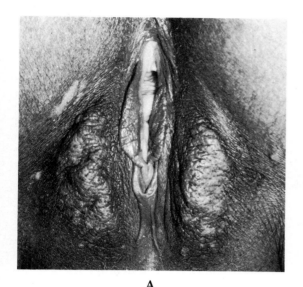 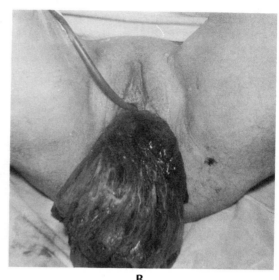

A

B

Figure 11–5. *A*, Degenerative submucous myoma, resembling sarcoma. *B*, Uterine inversion (nonpuerperal) with submucous myoma. (*B*, Courtesy of L. S. Pinheiro, São Paulo, Brazil.)

which they produce would not seem sufficient to explain the high incidence of sterility, though such factors might logically be considered important in explaining the increased tendency to abortion which most authors believe to exist in the presence of uterine myoma. On the other hand, in a considerable proportion of cases, fertility seems to be unimpeded, and pregnancy often goes on to full term. Abitbol believes that submucous fibroids are rarely compatible with term pregnancy, for they usually lead to failure of implantation or early abortion. He also discusses the complications incurred by concomitant pregnancy and submucous myoma (Fig. 11–6).

This question is bound up with that of the possible role of the *ovarian hormones* in the etiology of uterine myoma. The fact that these tumors occur during the reproductive era and retrogress after the menopause has been offered to substantiate this claim. It is possible, however, that such retrogression can be as logically attributed to the diminished blood supply accompanying cessation of ovarian function as to withdrawal of the hormones themselves.

Although the role of estrogen as actually inciting the development of myoma must be regarded as uncertain, it seems fair to state that the continued growth of these tumors is dependent upon a continued hormonal stimulus, either directly or via increased vascularity. There is also reason to believe that

adenomyosis of the uterus, which is not a true tumor but is apparently due to an exaggerated proliferative activity of the uterine mucosa, might be due to abnormal functional activity of the ovaries, though even this is not scientifically established.

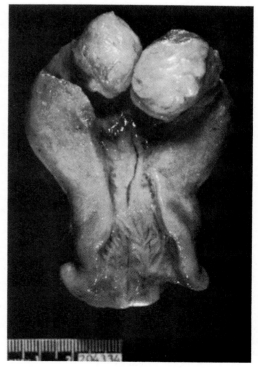

Figure 11–6. Solitary submucous myoma.

In the case of uterine myoma, the circumstantial evidence for ovarian responsibility must be considered very inadequate. More weight can be attached to efforts to produce uterine myomas experimentally by the injection of huge dosage of estrogenic hormones. Multiple tiny subperitoneal nodules have been thus produced, but in such cases neither the structure nor the distribution of such nodules was similar to those of uterine myoma. In only one or two instances (Nelson) has such experimental estrogenic treatment apparently produced an interstitial nodule resembling myoma. Moreover, it must be remembered that the ovaries present no characteristic histologic pattern, and that in a large proportion of cases cyclic activity is normal and there is no evidence of estrogenic excess. Although this hypothesis of an ovarian hormonal causation of myoma is of interest and certainly merits further study, there is as yet no complete justification for its acceptance.

The interesting studies of Lipschütz, demonstrating a marked fibromatogenic effect of estrogen in certain animals, especially the guinea pig, would at first appear to have a bearing upon this question. However, the tumor-like masses produced in these animals not only involve the uterus but are extensively distributed throughout the peritoneal cavity and, moreover, they apparently are not genuine tumors, since they disappear after the withdrawal of the estrogen or on administration of progesterone. The antagonistic effects of estrogen and progesterone seem apparent. Finally, the estrogen-induced masses are made up of fibrous and not muscle tissue.

Histogenesis

It is now quite generally accepted that the source of uterine fibroids is muscle tissue rather than the fibrous elements of the uterus. There have been differences of opinion as to whether the mature muscle fibers of the uterus, or certain immature or indifferent elements in the musculature, are the starting point of tumor formation, and also as to whether or not the tumors arise from muscle elements in the blood vessel walls (Fig. 11-7).

These questions cannot be answered arbitrarily, but the viewpoint of Meyer, based on the study of tiny microscopic growths, has been rather generally accepted. According to this, myoma arises from immature muscle cells in the uterine wall, but the blood vessels of these proliferative centers enter from

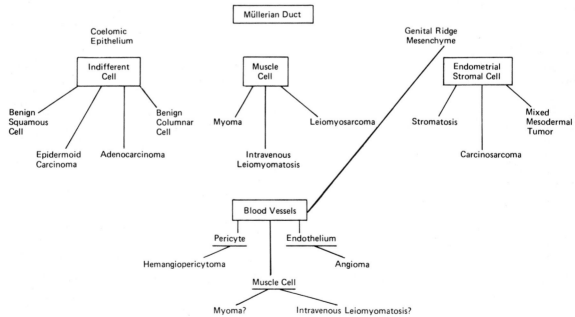

Figure 11–7. Schematic outline of the embryonic origin of mesenchymal tumors of the uterus. The müllerian duct is formed by invagination of the coelomic epithelium into the mesenchyme of the genital ridge. The left side of the diagram represents epithelial development of the müllerian derivatives. The right side illustrates the *mesenchymal* origins of the primitive muscle cells, blood vessel components, and endometrial stroma. (Courtesy of M. S. Baggish: Clin. Obstet. Gynecol., *17*:51, 1974.)

the outside, being derived from the muscle layers of blood vessels in the adjoining area.

Studies by Miller and Ludovici have utilized tissue culture in differentiating and observing the growth of myoblast and fibroblast. These authors have also published results of studies on the role of frequent anovulation with myomas and believe that it is the anovulation rather than the myoma itself which may lead to the common problem of sterility. The possible role of estrogen is apparent, but most gynecologists accept the concept with some reluctance, since ovulation and pregnancy are common in women who develop myomas.

Gross Pathology

The nodular gross appearance of myoma has already been described in the discussion of subperitoneal, interstitial, and submucous growths. The consistency of the nodules is very firm, so that they can be readily palpated in the softer wall of the uterus even though they are not visible. They may be exceedingly hard and stony when calcification is marked; on the other hand they may be soft or elastic with other forms of degeneration. Especially characteristic is the appearance of the cut surface, which is whitish in color, as might be expected from the poor blood supply of such tumors. The surface presents a characteristic whorl-like, trabeculated appearance. In the larger growths, especially, this pattern may be blotted out in areas corresponding to the very common hyaline degeneration, which imposes an amorphous, homogeneous appearance on the involved areas.

Although there is no definite capsule to the myomatous nodules, they are usually separated from the surrounding uterine muscle by a thin pseudocapsular layer of light areolar tissue, so that the tumors can be readily enucleated from the uterine wall. The retraction of the myomatous uterine wall causes the tumor nodules to project somewhat above the surrounding surface. The nutrient vessels penetrate the pseudocapsule, there usually being only one rather large artery, while the remaining vessels are very small and often not readily demonstrable.

Microscopic Appearance

The essential histologic element, from the standpoint of the classification of the tumor as a myoma, is the unstriated muscle cell. Bundles of cells of this type are seen running in all directions, but tending always toward the characteristic whorl-like pattern (Fig. 11–8). The nuclei of these cells are rodlike in shape, with rather rounded extremities. They are strikingly uniform in size and shape, if one makes proper allowance for the fact that they are cut at all possible angles. When a muscle bundle is cut transversely, for example, the cells appear rounded or polyhedral, with abundant cytoplasm and with central round nuclei. In longitudinal section the spindle shape of the cells and the elongation of the nuclei are more clearly evident. Mast cells are not rare but seemingly have no significance.

In spite of the intrinsic muscular character of myoma, there is always, except in the tiniest growths, some admixture of connective tissue elements. As a matter of fact, these fibrous tissue cells may preponderate over the muscle. Since the muscle origin of the entire group is apparently established, the fibrous elements are to be looked upon as an adventitious diluent of the muscle cells, and the term *myoma* is applicable to the entire group. The cellular variety of myoma is characterized by a preponderating richness of muscle cells, with very little connective tissue (Fig. 11–9). Such tumors, because of their compactness of structure, have a superficial resemblance to spindle cell sarcoma, and this diagnosis is often incorrectly made, as will be discussed in Chapter 13.

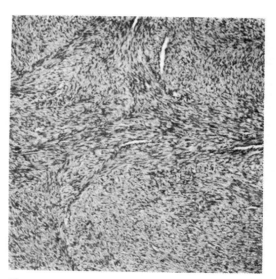

Figure 11–8. Microscopic appearance of myoma of uterus.

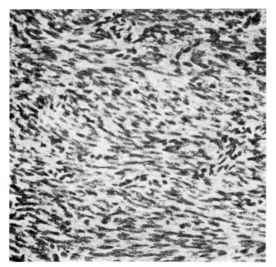

Figure 11–9. Cellular but entirely benign myoma, which has sometimes been mistaken for spindle cell sarcoma.

Intravenous Leiomyomatosis

Intravenous extension of benign myomatous tumor into the pelvic veins is a rare finding (see Figs. 13–11 to 13–13). In observing this occurence Harper and Scully note the difficulty in distinguishing it from certain malignant processes as (endometrial) sarcoma or stromatosis, but indicate a favorable prognosis. Idelson and Davids, Ariel and Trinidad, and Clark and Weed describe benign but metastasizing myoma and review the literature on this infrequent problem; it would seem difficult to exclude the possibility of sarcoma in some area of the tumors despite the extensive studies by the authors to establish this fact. However, the only fatal case (Steiner) died of cor pulmonale, not tumor. Wolfe and Mackles have described certain uncommon tumors of the generative tract, and have noted various blastomatous lesions, as well as neoplasms containing striated muscle, perhaps a variant of the mixed mesodermal tumor.

Extrauterine Myomas

In discussing *leiomyomatosis peritonealis disseminata* (LPD), Taubert and co-workers have noted histologically benign myomatous implants in the omentum and peritoneum. That this represents a low-grade infiltrating sarcoma or parasitic myoma seems possible. Two of the three patients concerned were pregnant, and some type of en-

docrine stimulus must be considered (as in Lipschütz's animal studies). In any event, all of the patients concerned have remained well. More recent studies by Parmley and Woodruff suggest that the presumed leiomyomatosis is really ectopic decidua, but electron microscopic studies by Goldberg and associates would dispute this; it seems agreed that there is some type of hormonal influence with LPD (Fig. 11–10).

Secondary Changes in Uterine Myoma

Both the macroscopic and microscopic features which characterize the typical myoma, as previously described, may be greatly altered by certain secondary degenerative processes, as indicated in the article by Novak. Among these secondary changes may be enumerated the following: hyaline or cystic degeneration; calcification; infection and suppuration; necrosis, including the so-called red degeneration; fatty changes; and sarcomatous degeneration.

Hyaline Degeneration. Hyaline degeneration of some degree or other is an almost invariable feature of all except the tiniest myomas. Even in the very cellular growths, made up almost entirely of muscle cells, small scattered areas of hyaline degeneration are usually seen. Since the connective tissue elements of myoma seem to be first and most extensively attacked, this form of degeneration is more apt to be present in marked degree in the less cellular varieties. The degenerated areas may occur as scattered patches, or as large and often interlacing fields throughout the tumor (Fig. 11–11).

Grossly the occurrence of hyaline degeneration is indicated by a loss of the normal whorl-like appearance characterizing the cut surface, the degenerated areas having a homogeneous character and a softer consistency. They do not, however, have the pultaceous character and the necrotic tendency which characterize sarcomatous degeneration.

Under the microscope, with the ordinary hematoxylin-eosin stain, the hyalinized areas take a diffuse bright pink stain, standing out quite sharply from the well-preserved muscle tissue of the myoma. All sorts of bizarre pictures may be produced when hyaline change is pronounced. Frequently only scattered islands of muscle cells are left intact in broad expanses of hyaline degeneration, whereas in other cases large areas of

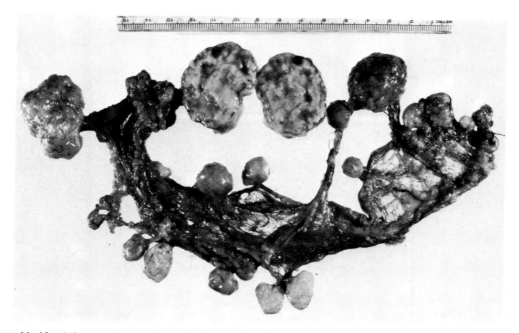

Figure 11–10. Leiomyomatosis peritonealis disseminata (LPD). Multiple resected benign omental myomas. (Courtesy of M. F. Goldberg et al.: Obstet. Gynecol., 49:465, 1977.)

the original myoma may undergo a diffuse hyaline transformation.

A peculiar type of what is apparently a hyaline degeneration produces the so-called "rhythmic" pattern, the nuclei being arranged in rather regular and more or less palisaded rows, as shown in Figure 11–12. It would seem possible that such a pattern may be linked up with the distribution of blood vessels, but Meyer believes at least some of

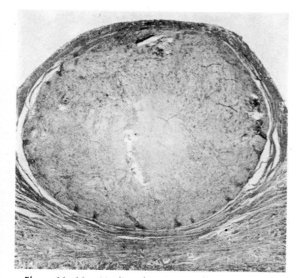

Figure 11–11. Hyaline change in small myoma.

the rare tumors presenting this peculiar rhythmic structure are probably to be classified as neurinomas (nerve sheath blastomas).

Cystic Degeneration. A discussion of this type of degeneration should naturally follow that of hyaline degeneration, because the tendency of the latter is toward liquefaction, with the production of cystic cavities of varying size. Wherever hyaline degeneration is extensive, this melting-down tendency is quite sure to be seen. Sometimes only small irregular cavities filled with gelatinous material may be seen, but with continuing liquefaction large cysts are formed. This mechanism then produces a variety of uterine cyst (Fig. 11–13). When the cystic myoma is symmetric, its shape and the elastic consistency may simulate pregnancy perfectly.

More frequently the cystic liquefaction is incomplete, the tumor presenting a variegated appearance because of the presence of ragged cystic cavities, between whose walls are to be seen remnants of intact or only partly degenerated tumor tissue. Cystic degeneration may occasionally be a sequel of forms of degeneration other than hyaline, such as necrosis. Hyaline and cystic degeneration may be seen in patients who are taking contraceptive pills; however, since such changes also occur in the absence of these hormones, it seems unrealistic to incrimi-

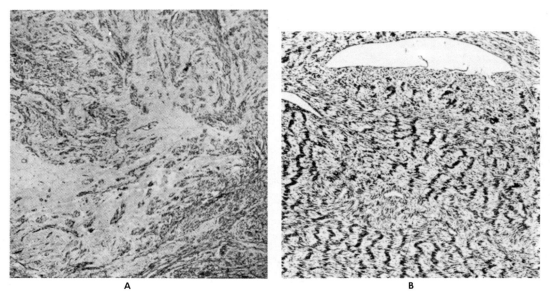

Figure 11–12. *A,* Hyaline degeneration of myoma. Note diffuse hyalin material (staining a bright pink with hematoxylin-eosin stain) between the muscle bundles. *B,* Peculiar rhythmic pattern with palisading of nuclei, seen in rare cases of apparent myoma, but possibly of neurinomatous origin.

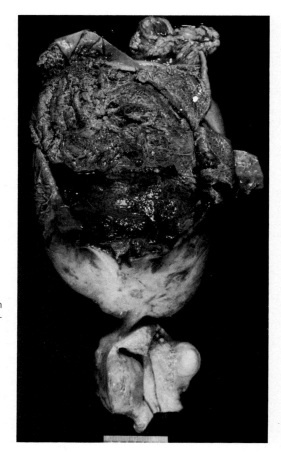

Figure 11–13. Subserous pedunculated myoma with marked cystic degeneration and necrosis, although no torsion of the pedicle. (Fundus below.)

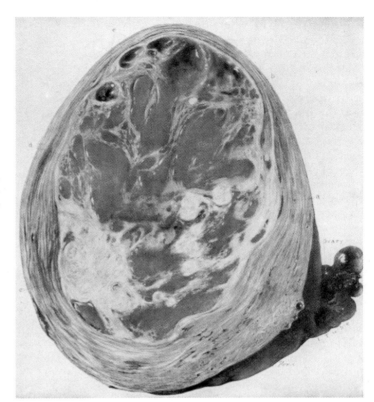

Figure 11–14. Hyaline and cystic degeneration of myoma. (From Kelly and Cullen: Myomata of the Uterus. Philadelphia, W. B. Saunders Company.)

nate the pills as a causative factor (Fig. 11–14).

Calcification (Calcareous Degeneration). Since calcification is usually an evidence of degeneration, it is to be expected that it is most apt to occur when there has been circulatory impairment, such as in the myomas of postmenopausal women, or in subserous myomas with small pedicles. It is practically never seen in the submucous variety of growth. The calcium is deposited in the tissue in the form of carbonate and phosphate. When the calcareous areas are small and scattered, they may pass unnoticed, except that a gritty resistance is encountered on cutting into the tumor. When the calcification is extreme, the tumor is converted into a stony mass, constituting the "womb-stone" as it is called by older authors (Fig. 11–15).

Histologically, the calcified areas appear in the form of lamellated deposits, large or small, rounded or irregular, and take a dark blue hematoxylin stain. Occasionally frank

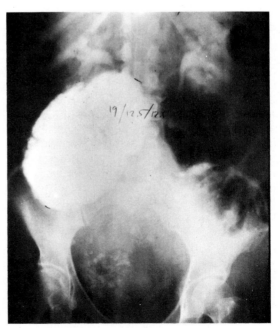

Figure 11–15. Intravenous pyelogram showing large calcified myoma.

osteoid material may be found, generally as a sequel to an old missed abortion, but occasionally as a metaplastic phenomenon.

Infection and Suppuration. The type of myoma most prone to infection is the submucous, because it offers such obvious portals of entry to infectious organisms from the genital tract. The overlying mucosa is characteristically thinned out, and almost invariably its infection is evident in the inflammatory changes seen microscopically. The mucosa may be lost over considerable areas through ulceration, and the infectious process may penetrate deeply into the substance of the myoma. Suppuration may occur, and in rare instances abscesses have been noted in the substance of the tumor. Such infectious processes may have their inception in such operations as uterine curettage, and they are prone also to develop after miscarriage or parturition in uteri containing myomas of the submucous variety.

When infection is of a virulent type, extensive sloughing of the tumor may occur, with evidences of general sepsis. Subserous and interstitial tumors are less frequently infected than the submucous variety. The former, however, may be involved in inflammatory diseases of the adnexa, the tumors showing marked inflammatory changes which begin on the peritoneal surface and penetrate the tumor to varying degree.

Necrosis. This may occur in any variety of myoma, and is commonly due to impairment of the blood supply or to severe degrees of infection. Pedunculated tumors may undergo torsion of the pedicle, with resulting necrosis and sometimes *gangrene*. Tumors that are the seat of extensive hyaline degeneration may likewise show areas of necrosis, although small areas of necrosis are seen in many tumors, with no assignable cause other than poor circulatory and nutritional conditions. Such areas are more apt to be in the central portions of the tumor, in which the circulation is most likely to be inadequate (Fig. 11–16).

Necrotic areas are often recognizable grossly through the absence of the whitish color and the firm trabeculated myoma pattern in such areas, which instead have a yellowish white hue and a soft pultaceous consistency, with at times the presence of small ragged degeneration cavities.

A special variety of necrosis which has received more attention in the British than the American literature is the so-called *carneous*

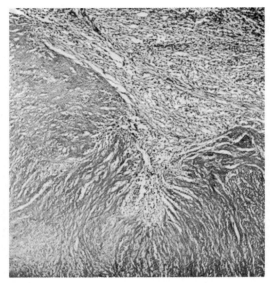

Figure 11–16. Section of myoma undergoing necrosis.

degeneration. It occurs most characteristically in conjunction with pregnancy, but may be observed in the nonpregnant uterus. The designation is expressive of the gross appearance of the degenerated tumors, which on section have the dull reddish hue and appearance of partly cooked beef. Although the mechanism is not entirely clear, it is believed that the lesion is an aseptic degeneration associated with local hemolysis. The latter is believed to take place within the lumina of blood vessels which, like the surrounding tissue, have undergone degeneration, bringing about thrombotic and hemolytic changes. Others believe that extravasation of blood is responsible for the reddish color, though this seems unlikely in view of the diffuseness of the hemorrhagic appearance.

Fatty Changes. These are rare in myoma, but may occur under one of two conditions. In the first place, *fatty degeneration* may occur as a sequel to or concomitant with the late stages of hyaline degeneration or necrosis. In such cases fat may be demonstrable only on differential staining, although at times droplets may coalesce to form yellowish areas visible macroscopically. In the other variety of fatty change, much less common, large areas of yellowish fatty appearance may be seen with the naked eye. These not only give the chemical reactions of fat, but microscopic examination reveals genuine adipose tissue cells. It is possible that in

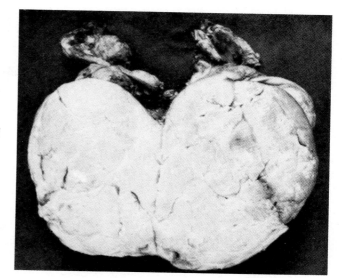

Figure 11–17. Lipoma of uterus. (Courtesy of Dr. Ellis Kellert.)

such cases there has been a metaplasia of tumor cells into fat cells, but it seems more probable, as has been suggested by various authors, that such cases represent mixed tumors, arising from immature cells of multiple differentiating potency. Still other hypotheses have been suggested to explain the rare cases of *lipoma* of the uterus, of which fewer than 50 cases have been reported (Figs. 11–17 to 11–19).

Sarcomatous Proliferation. For a full discussion of the incidence, as well as the gross and microscopic characteristics, of this important variety of secondary change in uterine myoma (Fig. 11–20), the reader is referred to Chapter 13. In this chapter there is also a discussion of the relatively rare recurring fibroid, in which histologically benign tumors assume many of the clinical characteristics of malignancy.

On exceptional occasions myomata may be the site of metastatic spread of cancer. The recent report by Banooni and co-workers summarizes the literature and adds a case of breast carcinoma with metastasis to a myoma. There have been only rare such cases in our own material, although we have observed a few cases of myomatous involvement by adjacent pelvic tumors.

Relation of Myoma to Uterine Cancer

Previous editions of this text have always suggested that the proportion of corporeal to cervical cancer is very much higher in myomatous than in nonmyomatous uteri. Others, however, could not substantiate this. In an analysis of cervical and endometrial cancer, we have noted no difference in the occurrence of fibroids with these two types of neoplasm. It seems that myomas are dependent on estrogen for continued growth; it is possible that estrogen is also a factor in endometrial cancer. Thus, one might anticipate the association of these two. On the other hand, myomas are more frequent in the black race, in which epidermoid cancer is common.

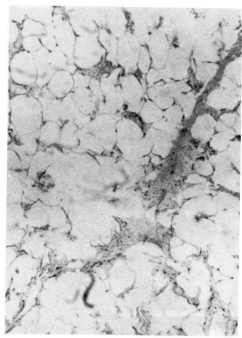

Figure 11–18. Microscopic appearance of lipoma shown in Figure 11–17.

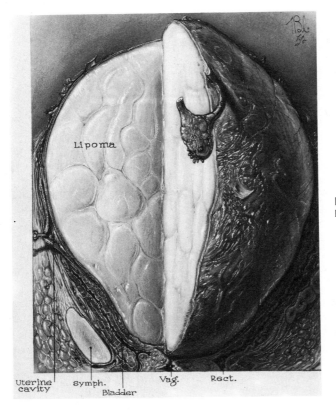

Figure 11–19. Semidiagrammatic view of uterine lipoma with anatomic relationships. (Courtesy of Dr. Erle Henriksen, Los Angeles.)

Thus, the two sets of coincidences tend to equalize one another.

Effects of Myoma on Uterus

Small tumors, and even larger tumors of the subperitoneal variety, produce little or no effect upon the musculature of the uterus or the size of the organ. Interstitial growths, when large, bring about an increased development of the uterine muscle, as a result of the richer blood supply. The chief factor in the often enormous size of the myomatous uterus, however, is the size of the tumors

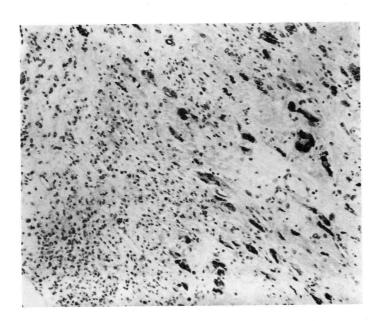

Figure 11–20. Sharp line of demarcation between myoma (left) and sarcoma with many giant cells (right).

themselves. Small submucous tumors may cause no change in the size or shape of the uterus, but the larger ones may bring about a definite increase in the size and vascularity of the organ.

The shape and size of the uterine cavity may undergo marked alteration from the presence of myomas. For obvious reasons this applies least of all to the subserous type. With interstitial tumors, the increasing size brings about a deepening and enlarging of the uterine cavity, while the presence of submucous tumors produces with increasing growth a marked distortion of the cavity.

Endometrial Changes

Especially interesting is the condition of the endometrium in association with myoma. It may show little or no departure from the normal, and the histologic sequence of cyclic changes may occur just as it does in the ovulatory cycle of nonmyomatous patients.

On the other hand, in a considerable proportion of cases one finds an association of the nonovulatory type of cycle with myoma, with frequently a hyperplasia of the endometrium of more or less marked degree (see Chapter 8). This is another way of saying that in at least some cases of myoma the abnormal bleeding may be of dysfunctional origin and is not due to the presence of the myoma. Those who believe in the endocrine etiology of myoma are inclined to invoke an endocrine causation for the bleeding in most cases of myoma, but there is no scientific support for this view. A recent study of Farrer-Brown and associates suggests that it is dilatation and congestion of myometrial and endometrial venous plexuses, caused by the expanding tumors, that lead to bleeding (rather than intrinsic vascular patterns within the tumors).

When intramural tumors are present, there may be marked thickening, hypertrophy, and edema of the endometrium, especially in the depressions between tumor nodules. The mucosa over submucous tumors, on the other hand, characteristically exhibits atrophy and thinning, so that the glands may disappear entirely and only a very thin stromal layer is left, with a flattened epithelial layer covering it. The great frequency of infection with this form of myoma has already been stressed. Chronic or subacute endometritis is a common finding, and acute exacerba-

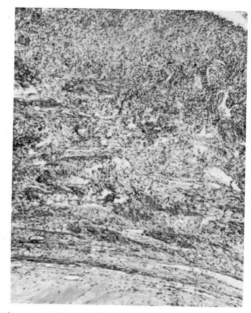

Figure 11–21. Hyalinized submucous myoma (below); endometrium is barely recognizable because of the intense inflammatory reaction.

tions are not rare. The mucosa may be lost entirely, and the infection may extend deeply into the underlying tumor tissue (Fig. 11–21).

Myomas and Pregnancy

As a rule, myomas increase in size during pregnancy, but diminish again after the pregnancy is terminated. Some believe that they may even disappear, but this is not the usual experience. During pregnancy they frequently undergo degeneration, especially of the carneous type, and this may be associated with acute symptoms, such as pain, tenderness, and fever. On the other hand, pregnancy is often undisturbed by even large tumors. There is only slight hypertrophy of the muscle fibers of a myoma during pregnancy, but usually marked edema of the connective tissue elements (Fig. 11–22).

We believe that myomectomy should occasionally be considered as treatment for the sterile woman in whom all other causes of infertility have been excluded. Although no one can explain the mechanism, it seems that myomectomy may benefit the barren patient. Ingersoll has fully discussed the status of myomectomy.

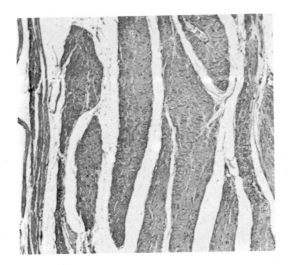

Figure 11–22. Myoma in pregnant uterus, showing moderate hypertrophy of cells and the edema separating the muscle bundles.

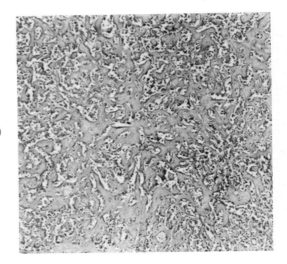

Figure 11–23. Lymphangioma (possibly mesothelioma) of uterus.

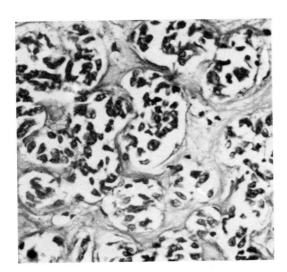

Figure 11–24. High power view of section shown in Figure 11–23.

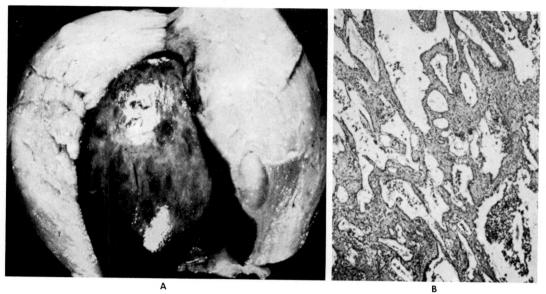

Figure 11–25. *A*, Large polypoid hemangioma of uterus, a rare lesion. *B*, High power of hemangioma shown in *A*. (Courtesy of Dr. Casper G. Burn, Brooklyn, N.Y.)

Other Benign Tumors

Figure 11–7 indicates the potential origin of various uterine tumors, as previously noted.

Lymphangioma is a rare uterine lesion, and the term should not be applied to the marked lymphangiectasis seen at times in association with myomas. The pattern of lymphangioma is not always the same, being of rather compact variety in some tumors, and of cavernous type in others (Figs. 11–23 and 11–24). These *adenomatoid* tumors seem more common in the tube than in the uterus. Most tumors of this group have run a clinically benign course. Irwin has noted the prevalence of lymphoid tissue in the endometrium (and even reported an apparently primary lymphoma arising as a polyp from the endometrium).

Hemangioma is even more of a rarity than lymphangioma, and it likewise is benign. Articles by Pedowitz and coworkers (Fig. 11–25) are recommended for a complete review of benign and malignant vascular tumors of the uterus. The authors believe that such vascular tumors as hemangiomas are more common that those of lymphoid origin, and are usually benign. They emphasize the importance of differential stains in establishing the diagnosis, as well as stressing the benign course of hemangiopericytoma as opposed to the more malignant hemangiosarcomas. Even more uncommon than these

adenomatoid tumors is *melanoma*, but Lamoureux has reported a single case apparently confined to the endometrium.

Hemangiopericytoma is a rather new tumor in gynecologic parlance, being first noted by Stout in 1949 (Fig. 11–26). It is a

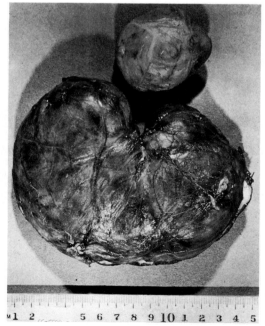

Figure 11–26. Large intraligamentary hemangiopericytoma (below) with myomatous uterus (above). (Courtesy of Dr. Albert Brown, Wilmington, N.C.)

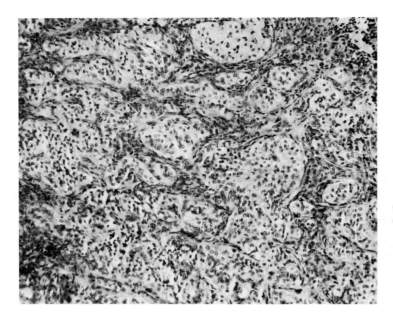

Figure 11–27. Hemangiopericytoma with concentric pericapillary arrangement of pericytes.

vascular lesion not unlike the glomus tumor and may be distinguished by a tendency toward concentric arrangement of pericytes around capillaries (Fig. 11–27). Special stains (such as Masson's, silver, and reticulum) are frequently helpful in distinguishing this rather benign tumor from other malignant growths of endothelial or mesothelial origin. Pedowitz and co-workers note a rather low malignancy of 20 to 25 per cent in the 16 cases reported in the literature, but Zeigerman has noted at least 10 fatal cases in a more recent review of the literature. On occasion there is considerable difficulty in distinguishing between this and endome-

trial stromatosis or sarcoma (Fig. 11–28). The recent report by Wilbanks and associates considers a large series of cases.

Plexiform Tumorlets

A rare myometrial lesion is the so-called plexiform tumor of the uterus, a term coined by Larbig, although certain authors disagree with the proposed endometrial stromal origin. Budinger and Green had earlier referred to it as a distinctive myometrial tumor of undetermined origin. Patchefsky notes 19 such cases in the literature, and indicates that these lesions are generally small incidental

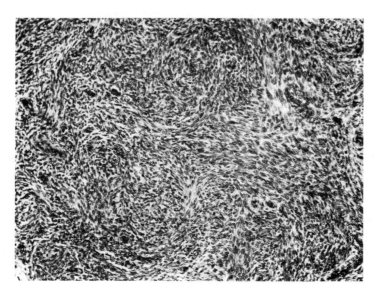

Figure 11–28. Probable hemangiopericytoma rather than cellular myoma or stromatosis; differentiation is often difficult.

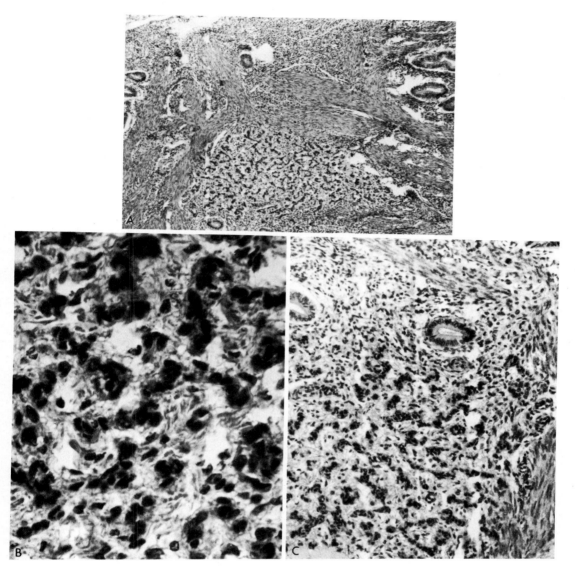

Figure 11–29. Isolated plexiform tumorlet. *A*, Low power; *B*, high power; *C*, intermediate power. (Courtesy of Dr. A. S. Patchefsky, Philadelphia.)

findings, frequently associated with myomas, although seemingly not a mere degenerative change.

The lesion is well encapsulated and generally less than 1 cm. There is a distinct cordlike pattern with no discernible lumen, surrounded by an eosinophilic matrix. The cells are characterized by scant cytoplasm and a large hyperchromatic nucleus simulating the endometrial stromal cell (Fig. 11–29). Clinically there is no evidence of malignancy.

Patchefsky points out that the differential diagnosis must include adenomatoid tumors, hemangiopericytoma, stromatosis,

endometrial or mixed mesodermal sarcoma, and various other rare lesions.

Retroperitoneal Fibrosis

Unrelated to the myomatous uterus either anatomically or histologically, but sometimes confused clinically, is the poorly understood *idiopathic retroperitoneal fibrosis* in which there may be dense retroperitoneal accumulation of hyalinized connective tissue. Pelvic tumors may be present and there is often obstructive uropathy. The cause is uncertain, but recent reviews by Ormond and by Symmonds and colleagues discuss the possibilities, which include collagen disease and hypersensitivity. A considerable number of cases have followed methysergide maleate treatment for migraine, which may have led to a vasculitis secondary to drug sensitivity.

REFERENCES

Abitbol, M. A.: Submucous fibroids complicating pregnancy, labor and delivery. Obstet. Gynecol., *10*:529, 1957.

Ariel, I. M., and Trinidad, S.: Pulmonary metastases from a uterine "leiomyoma," Am. J. Obstet. Gynecol., *94*:110, 1966.

Baggish, M. S.: Mesenchymal tumors of the uterus. Clin. Obstet. Gynecol., *17*:51, 1974.

Banooni, F., Labes, J., and Goodman, P. A.: Uterine leiomyoma containing metastatic breast carcinoma. Am. J. Obstet. Gynecol., *111*:427, 1971.

Barber, H. R. K., and Graber, E. A.: Gynecological tumors in childhood and adolescence. Obstet. Gynecol. Surv., *28*:357, 1973.

Barter, R. H., and Parks, J.: Myoma uteri associated with pregnancy. Clin. Obstet. Gynecol., *1*:519, 1958.

Brown, J. M., Malkasian, G. D., Jr., and Symmonds, R. E.: Abdominal myomectomy. Am. J. Obstet. Gynecol., *99*:126, 1967.

Budinger, J. M., and Greene, R. R.: A distinctive myometrial tumor of undetermined origin. Cancer, *17*:1155, 1964.

Clark, D. H., and Weed, J. C.: Metastasizing leiomyoma. Am. J. Obstet. Gynecol., *127*:672, 1977.

Courpas, A. S., Morris, J. D., and Woodruff, J. D.: Osteoid tissue in utero. Obstet. Gynecol., *23*:636, 1964.

Edwards, D. L., and Peacock, J. F.: Intravenous leiomyomatosis of the uterus. Obstet. Gynecol., *27*:176, 1966.

Farrer-Brown, G., Beilby, J. O. W., and Tarbit, M. H.: The vascular patterns in myomatous uteri. J. Obstet. Gynaecol. Brit. Commonw., *77*:917, 1970.

Farrer-Brown, G., Beilby, J. O. W., and Tarbit, M. H.: Venous changes in the endometrium of myomatous uteri. Obstet. Gynecol., *38*:743, 1971.

Fox, J. E., and Abell, M. R.: Mast cells in uterine myometrium and leiomyomatous neoplasms. Am. J. Obstet. Gynecol., *91*:413, 1965.

Goldberg, M. F., et al.: Leiomyomatosis peritonealis disseminata. Obstet. Gynecol., *49*:46S, 1977.

Green, R. R., Gerbie, A. B., Gerbie, M. V., and Eckman, T. R.: Hemangiopericytomas of the uterus. Am. J. Obstet. Gynecol., *106*:1020, 1970.

Harper, R. S., and Scully, R. E.: Intravenous leiomyomatosis of the uterus. Obstet. Gynecol., *18*:519, 1961.

Henriksen, E.: Lipoma of uterus. West J. Surg., *60*:609, 1952.

Honore, L. H.: Leiomyoma with hemangiopericytoma. Am. J. Obstet. Gynecol., *127*:891, 1977.

Idelson, M. G., and Davids, A. M.: Metastasis of uterine fibroleiomyomata. Obstet. Gynecol., *21*:78, 1963.

Ingersoll, F. M.: Myomectomy and fertility. Fertil. Steril., *14*:596, 1963.

Irwin, J. B.: Lymphoid apparatus of endometrium with

primary lymphoma. Am. J. Obstet. Gynecol., *72*:915, 1956.

Jonas, H. S., and Masterson, B. J.: Giant uterine tumors. Obstet. Gynecol., *50*:25, 1977.

Kelly, H. A., and Cullen, T. S.: Myomata of uterus. Philadelphia, W. B. Saunders Company, 1909.

Kimbrough, R. A.: Symposium on fibromyomas of the uterus. Clin. Obstet. Gynecol., *1*:407, 1958.

Lamoureux, C.: Melanome de l'uterus. Un. Med. Canada, *99*:282, 1970.

Larbig, G. G., Clemmer, J. J., Koss, L. G., et al.: Plexiform tumorlets of endometrial stromal origin. Am. J. Clin. Pathol., *44*:32, 1965.

Lipschütz, A.: Steroid Hormones and Tumors. Baltimore, Williams & Wilkins Co., 1950.

Lock, F. R.: Multiple myomectomy. Am. J. Obstet. Gynecol., *104*:642, 1969.

Marshall, J. F., and Morris, D. S.: Intravenous leiomyomatosis of the uterus and pelvis. Ann. Surg., *149*:126, 1959.

Meyer, R.: Die pathologische Anatomie der Gebärmutter. Henke-Lubarsch Handbuch der spezielle pathologische Anatomie und Histologie. Bd. vii, Erster Theil. Berlin, Julius Springer, 1930.

Miller, J. N.: Pregnancy and intravenous leiomyomatosis. Am. J. Obstet. Gynecol., *122*:485, 1975.

Miller, N. F., and Ludovici, P. P.: Origin and development of uterine fibroids. Am. J. Obstet. Gynecol., *70*:720, 1955.

Nelson, W. O.: Atypical uterine growths produced by prolonged administration of estrogenic hormones. Endocrinology, *24*:50, 1939.

Nelson, W. O.: Endometrial and myometrial changes, including fibromyomatous nodules induced in the uterus of the guinea-pig by prolonged administration of estrogenic hormones. Anat. Rec., *68*:99, 1937.

Newman, H. F.: Clinical observation in patients with myoma of the uterus with particular regards to changes in size and indication for surgery. Am. J. Obstet. Gynecol., *68*:1489, 1954.

Novak, E. R.: Benign and malignant changes in uterine myoma. Clin. Obstet. Gynecol., *1*:407, 1958. (See Kimbrough.)

Novak, E. R., and Villa Santa, U.: Factors influencing the ratio of uterine cancer in a community. J.A.M.A., *174*:1395, 1960.

Ormond, J. K.: Idiopathic retroperitoneal fibrosis. An established clinical entity. J.A.M.A., *174*:1561, 1960.

Parmley, T. H., et al.: Leiomyomatosis peritonealis disseminata (LPD). Obstet. Gynecol., *46*:511, 1975.

Patchefsky, A. S.: Plexiform tumorlet of the uterus: report of a case. Obstet. Gynecol., *35*:592, 1970.

Pedowitz, P., Felmus, L. B., and Grayzel, D. M.: Vascular tumors of uterus: benign vascular tumors. Am. J. Obstet. Gynecol., *69*:1291, 1955.

Pedowitz, P., Felmus, L. B., and Grayzel, D. M.: Vascular tumors of uterus: malignant vascular tumors. Am. J. Obstet. Gynecol., *69*:1309, 1955.

Plaut, A.: Lymphangiocystic fibroma of uterus. Am. J. Obstet. Gynecol., *51*:842, 1946.

Sabbagh, M. L.: Lipoma of the uterus. Obstet. Gynecol., *4*:399, 1954.

Saidi, F., Constable, J. D., and Ulfelder, H.: Massive intraperitoneal hemorrhage due to uterine fibroids. Am. J. Obstet. Gynecol., *82*:367, 1961.

Steiner, P. E.: Metastasizing fibroleiomyoma; report of case and review of literature. Am. J. Pathol., *15*:89, 1939.

Stout, A. P.: Hemangiopericytoma. Cancer, *2*:1027, 1949.

Symmonds, R. E., Dahlin, D. C., and Engel, S.: Idiopathic retroperitoneal fibrosis. Obstet. Gynecol., *18*:591, 1961.

Taubert, H. D., Wissner, S. E., and Haskins, A. L.: Leiomyomatosis peritonealis disseminata. Obstet. Gynecol., *25*:561, 1965.

Wilbanks, G. D., et al.: Pelvic hemangiopericytoma. Am. J. Obstet. Gynecol., *123*:555, 1975.

Wolfe, S. A., and Mackles, A.: Uncommon myogenic tumors of the female generative tract. Obstet. Gynecol., *22*:199, 1963.

Wynn, K. J., et al.: Electron microscopic studies of leiomatosis peritonealis disseminata. Obstet. Gynecol., *48*:225, 1976.

Zeigerman, J. H.: Vascular tumors of the uterus: Benign or malignant. J.A.M.A., *176*:108, 1961.

Chapter 12

ADENOMYOSIS
(ADENOMYOMA) UTERI

Definition and General Characteristics

Adenomyosis of the uterus is a condition characterized by a *benign invasion of the endometrium* into the uterine musculature, associated with a diffuse overgrowth of the latter. The term is a better one than adenomyoma, since the suffix "-oma" refers to a tumor, and adenomyosis is not a tumor in the proper sense of the word, any more than is endometriosis.

From the standpoint of its endometrial constituent, adenomyosis, in common with pelvic endometriosis, is characterized by a diffuse ectopic growth of endometrium; it previously was often referred to as *endometriosis interna*, to distinguish it from endometriosis externa, or pelvic endometriosis. It differs. from the latter in the type of patient involved, women with adenomyosis characteristically being parous fourth or fifth decade patients as contrasted to the involuntarily sterile younger woman afflicted by endometriosis. Almost certainly there is a different etiology of the diseases, and indeed the only similarity is the common property of aberrant endometrial tissue which is dependent on sustained ovarian function.

Without meaning to overemphasize niceties of definition, the term *adenomyoma* should be limited to actual circumscribed tumors made up of endometrium and muscle tissue. Such growths are observed more frequently in the uterine ligaments than in the uterus although adenomyosis may be observed in certain endometrial polyps. Finally, a genuine endometriosis of the uterus, with little or no muscle admixture, is seen in cases in which a pelvic endometriosis attacks the uterus from without, involving most commonly its posterior serous surface and the immediately underlying muscularis, though such a lesion is only a part of a more general pelvic endometriosis.

Adenomyosis is found in 25 to 40 per cent of all hysterectomy specimens, although the recent publication by Bird and associates indicates that if sufficient sections are obtained, ectopic endometrium may be noted in nearly 62 per cent of uteri removed for all causes. It would appear that these authors are including very minor degrees of subbasal disease, in which we might not be inclined to make this diagnosis. Molitor's figure of 8.8 per cent seems more realistic, if on the low side.

Gross Characteristics

In adenomyosis the uterus may be slightly or markedly enlarged, though the increase in size never reaches the large proportions seen so often with myoma. As a matter of fact, the organ is rarely much larger than a large orange. However, it must be remembered that adenomyosis and myoma often coexist, the latter being responsible for the frequently large size of the uterus in such cases. The increase in size produced by adenomyosis is of diffuse type, and as a rule one wall, usually the posterior, is much thicker than the other, although sometimes there is a more or less symmetric thickening of both. In certain instances the thickness of the uterine wall may be several times that of the normal organ (Fig. 12–1).

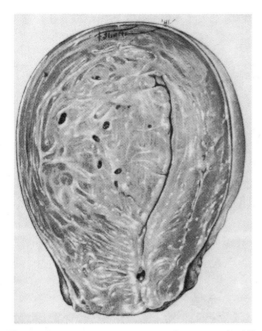

Figure 12–1. Gross appearance of uterus with diffuse adenomyosis, in sagittal section.

In some cases the uterus is adherent to surrounding organs, since the adenomyosis is often associated with pelvic endometriosis, the irritation of the menstrual hemorrhage exciting marked peritoneal reaction and the formation of adhesions. It is often difficult to know just when adenomyosis ends and endometriosis begins, but it is our own opinion that the two coexist in 40 per cent or more cases, excluding those in which minor degrees of microscopic adenomyosis are found, although Benson and Sneeden believe that an association occurs in less than 15 per cent. At times the fixation of the pelvic organs may be extreme, producing the "frozen pelvis" which so often makes the surgical problem a difficult one. On the other hand, the uterus may be quite free of surrounding adhesions, even when the uterine enlargement is marked. Most frequently the diagnosis is made purely from pathologic examination of uteri removed for other causes, as functional bleeding, prolapse, etc.

On section through the uterus, the striking feature is the diffuse symmetric increase in the thickness of the muscular wall, as already described. The cut surface presents a characteristic whorl-like, trabeculated appearance, but there is no tendency to form circumscribed nodules, as with myoma. A frequent but by no means constant feature is the presence of dark hemorrhagic or chocolate-colored areas, sometimes very tiny but sometimes many millimeters in diameter, scattered discretely throughout the musculature. These represent islands of endometrium in which menstrual hemorrhage has occurred, with retention of the menstrual blood. The endometrial layer of the uterus may be quite normal or it may be much thickened and perhaps polypoid in the not infrequent cases in which endometrial hyperplasia is associated with the adenomyosis (Fig. 12–2).

Microscopic Characteristics

The microscopic diagnosis of adenomyosis is based chiefly upon the finding of endometrial islands deep beneath the mucous surface, within the muscular layer. It is our belief that the diagnosis should not be made unless the endometrial tissue is *at least the distance of one high power field* below the basal endometrium. Normally the uterine mucosa is spread in an uneven layer of variable thickness over the muscularis, with no submucosal layer between, so that the tips of the glands, with the surrounding stroma, often dip into the muscle interstices for a short distance (Fig. 12–3). In adenomyosis, however, there is an invasion of otherwise normal endometrium far beyond its normal bounds, sometimes at least appearing to follow the lymphatics. In some cases the islands of mucosa may be found throughout the thickness of the uterine wall, extending to the serosa itself. On occasion the endometrium penetrates the uterus and infiltrates the rectum, giving rise to pelvic endometriosis and producing a firm welding of the uterus to the rectum. With this endometrial process is associated the hyperplasia of muscle tissue which produces the thickening of the uterine wall.

The islands formed by the invading endometrium show the typical glands and stroma of that structure, though there are interesting variations regarding functional activity. Occasionally the aberrant endometrium exhibits the cyclic functional responsiveness of normal endometrium (Fig. 12–4), but more often it is apparently of an immature or unripe variety. In the latter case, it is responsive only to the estrogenic stimulus, but not to progesterone. In such cases, even though the surface endometrium is in a phase of pre-

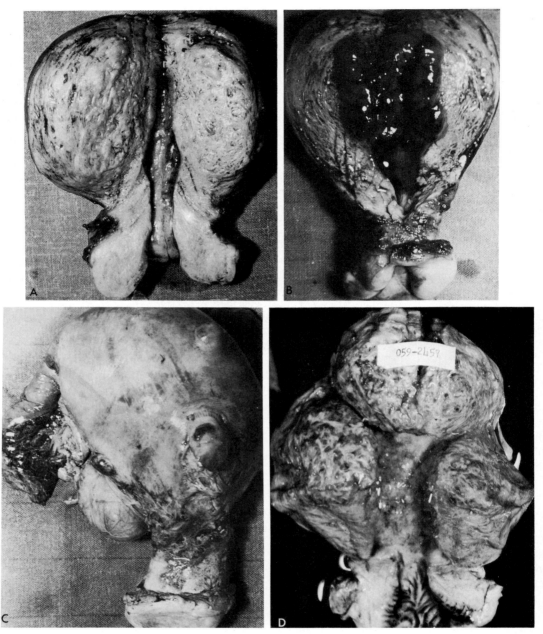

Figure 12–2. *A*, Extensive adenomyosis of posterior uterine wall. *B*, Marked endometrial hyperplasia with large uterus although with no significant adenomyosis. *C*, Adenomyosis and myomas. *D*, Extensive diffuse adenomyosis extending into cervix. (Courtesy of Emge, L.: Elusive adenomyosis of the uterus. Am. J. Obstet. Gynecol., *83*:1541, 1962. C. V. Mosby Co., Publishers.)

menstrual secretory activity, the aberrant endometrium may show not the slightest evidence of secretory activity, but instead a purely proliferative picture. Often it may show a striking Swiss-cheese hyperplastic pattern. In the frequent cases in which the surface endometrium shows hyperplasia,

the same picture is found in the islands of invading tissue (Figs. 12–5 and 12–6).

In other words, there are the same variations in functional response that are noted with endometrial polyps (see Chapter 10). As a matter of fact, the penetrating extensions of endometrial tissue seen in adeno-

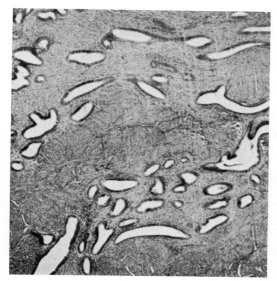

Figure 12–3. Microscopic appearance of adenomyosis, showing uterine glands and stroma invading musculature.

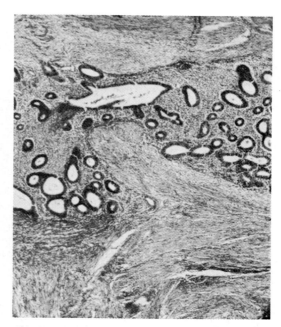

Figure 12–5. Adenomyosis, showing a nonfunctioning hyperplasia-like endometrial island.

myosis are much like inverted polyps and, like the latter, may be composed of either ripe and functioning tissue, or tissue which from the standpoint of full menstrual response is unripe and nonfunctioning. These variations explain why in some cases menstrual blood is found in the abnormal islands while in others it is absent (Fig. 12–7). In the former case the endometrial islands constitute miniature uterine cavities in which the same cyclic changes and the same bleeding take place as in the uterine cavity proper.

Not only the cyclic changes of menstruation (Fig. 12–8) but also the decidual

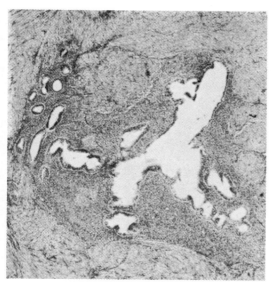

Figure 12–4. Adenomyosis, showing an island of functioning (secretory) endometrium.

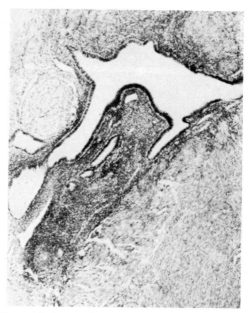

Figure 12–6. Nonfunctioning hyperplastic island of endometrium in a case of adenomyosis (compare with Figure 12–8).

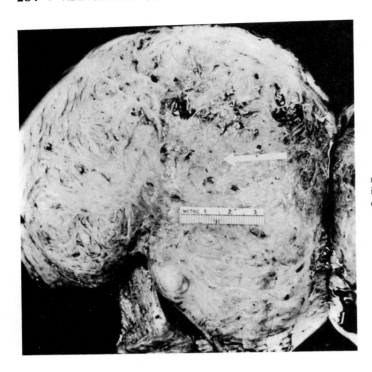

Figure 12–7. Extreme degrees of adenomyosis with obvious old blood in endometrial islands. (Courtesy of Dr. Ludwig Emge, San Francisco.

changes of pregnancy may be seen in the invading endometrium of adenomyosis. In such cases the glands first become highly convoluted and secretory, and later flattened and perhaps almost slitlike. The stromal cells assume the large size and the mosaic arrangement so characteristic of decidual cells (Fig. 12–9).

Adenomyosis not infrequently occurs in the region of the uterine cornua. In some of these cases the microscopic characteristics are like those already described. Stroma is often present, in which case distinction from salpingitis isthmica nodosa is generally possible (see Chapter 15). When this is absent, however, the difficulty may be extreme. As a

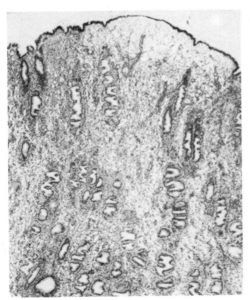

Figure 12–8. Surface endometrium of same uterus as in Figure 12–6, showing a typical progestational reaction.

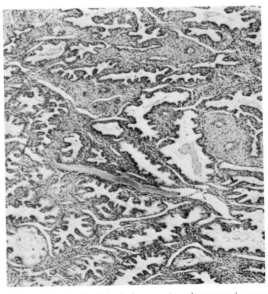

Figure 12–9. Decidual changes in adenomyosis associated with pregnancy.

rule, however, with adenomyosis the glands occur in clusters and are lined by a tall epithelium; with salpingitis isthmica nodosa the glandular acini are generally arranged sparsely and contain a lower epithelium.

Indeed, Benson indicates that salpingitis isthmica nodosa may represent a mere extension of uterine cornual adenomyosis in many cases. Although admitting that this sequence may occur, we still see a bona fide tubal pattern without evidence of uterine adenomyosis, and believe that the tubal disease is a specific entity, though often misdiagnosed.

Histogenesis

It has been definitely established, through the early work of Cullen and others, that adenomyosis has its source in the endometrium lining the uterine cavity. Formerly it had been hypothesized, chiefly by von Recklinghausen, that the endometrial islands arise from wolffian duct rests, and there are some who believe this explanation applies to the comparatively small group of cornual cases. The theory of origin from müllerian rests in the musculature has likewise been abandoned, and it is now universally accepted that the endometrium of the uterine cavity, because of some unknown growth stimulus, flows down like streams of lava between the muscle bundles (Fig. 12–10). Serial section often reveals the direct continuity of the aberrant islands with the surface, though often this connection has been nipped off by the muscle, thus isolating the deeper-lying endometrial areas. Often the basal layers of the endometrium can be seen pushing deeply into the myometrium to constitute adenomyosis (Fig. 12–11).

As to the underlying cause of this invasiveness of the endometrium, as well as of the increased proliferative activity of the muscle, there is little direct evidence. The facts that adenomyosis represents merely an increased growth activity of otherwise normal tissues, that it does not assume the circumscribed form so characteristic of genuine neoplasms, and that the immediate normal cause of endometrial and muscle growth is the estrogenic hormone of the ovary lend support to the belief that adenomyosis will be found to be due to an endocrine dysfunction of the ovary. It must be admitted, however, that experimental evidence is incomplete, although Marcus discusses the possibilities.

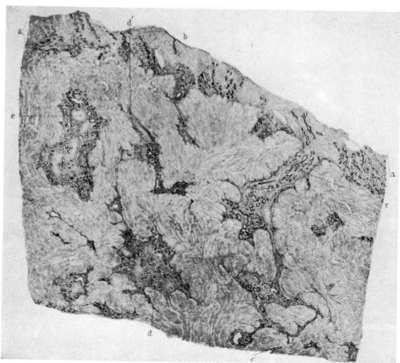

Figure 12–10. Low power section of wall of uterus shown in Figure 12–1, showing invasion of uterine musculature.

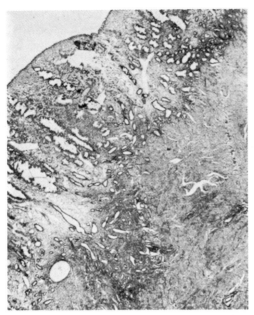

Figure 12–11. Endometrial basalis shown pushing deep into the muscularis in a case of adenomyosis.

Clinical Connotations

The special signs and symptoms of adenomyosis are explained quite adequately by the pathology of the lesion. Menorrhagia is very common, as might be expected, not only from the increased endometrial surface, but even more from the endocrine dysfunction manifested often histologically by the fact that the endometrium is the seat of well marked hyperplasia. Most authors believe, as do Emge, Benson and Sneeden, and Novak and deLima, that hyperplasia accompanies adenomyosis in about 25 per cent of cases, although Greenwood finds no correlation of adenomyosis with hyperplasia/adenocarcinoma.

Perhaps more characteristic is the colicky dysmenorrhea complained of by most patients suffering with adenomyosis, and explained by the menstrual swelling of islands of endometrium, under the tension entailed by their enclosure in the surrounding musculature, with therefore the production of painful contractions of the latter.

In a considerable proportion of cases, patients with adenomyosis complain of menstrual pain referred to the rectum or to the lower sacral or coccygeal region. This is explained by the frequent involvement of the uterosacral ligaments and perhaps the rectum itself. The premenstrual and menstrual swelling of endometrial islands in these regions explains the reference of the pain to the rectum or sacrococcygeal regions. The involvement of the uterosacral ligaments is also of much diagnostic importance, though it is not always present. When, however, pelvic examination does reveal a moderately enlarged, fixed uterus, with one or more definite nodules palpable in the uterosacral regions, especially when menorrhagia, colicky dysmenorrhea, and menstrual pain in the sacral or coccygeal regions are among the symptoms, a diagnosis of adenomyosis with pelvic endometriosis can be made with a reasonable certainty of its correctness.

The most outstanding critique of adenomyosis is that by Emge, who discusses comprehensively the history, etiology, and symptomatology of the disease. He further comments on the concurrence of adenomyosis and endometrial malignancy. Perhaps the most intriguing aspect of his study is the frequency of adenomyosis at the time of hysterectomy for fibroids (52 per cent), endometriosis (69 per cent), unselected hysterectomies (29 per cent), and corpus cancer (33 per cent), and in uteri removed at autopsy (53.7 per cent). Obviously the range of co-associations with other lesions is wide.

Malignant Degeneration

Although atypical hyperplasia is common in the deep islands of aberrant endometrium, it is astounding how infrequently primary adenocarcinoma is found in this area. We have seen a few such cases which showed a normal surface endometrium with an adenocarcinoma evolving in an island of hyperplastic adenomyosis. Colman and Rosenthal have published a report with review of the literature, and similar British publications are those of Cope and of Kumar and Anderson.

Perhaps this sequence is more common than can be recognized. Extension of malignant adenomyosis would naturally tend to creep up the gland lumina, the line of least resistance, with resultant endometrial involvement. The bleeding thus produced could easily be the first symptom leading to ultimate hysterectomy, but by this time the lesion would understandably be diagnosed as an endometrial adenocarcinoma with myometrial extension (Fig. 12–12).

On the other hand, a uterus removed because of a very definite endometrial adeno-

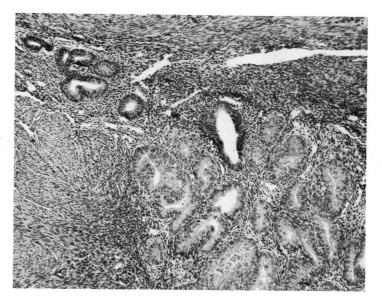

Figure 12–12. Endometrial surface toward top (not shown): early adenocarcinoma (lower right) with typical adenomyosis.

carcinoma may show islands of glands deep in the muscularis. It is often difficult to ascertain if this represents myometrial invasion by the surface malignancy, or whether there is a concomitant adenomyosis. This problem is intensified and sometimes impossible to solve if the surface lesion and myometrial "glands" are well differentiated. If, however, the endometrium shows a highly anaplastic tumor, and the myometrial islands are well differentiated, it is probable that there is merely an associated adenomyosis. This is not simply an academic exercise, for it is recognized that increasing degrees of myometrial invasion by endometrial adenocarcinoma progressively impair the prognosis (Fig. 12–13).

Stromal Endometriosis or Adenomyosis (Stromatosis)

A rather uncommon lesion, comparable to adenomyosis without glands, has been variously referred to as endolymphatic stro-

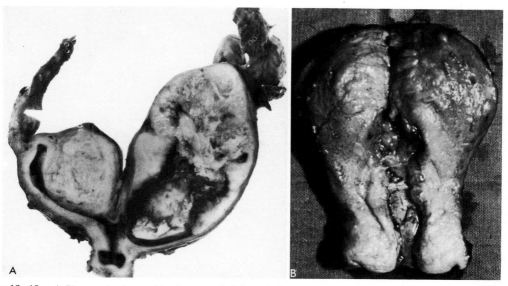

Figure 12–13. *A*, Bicornuate uterus with adenomyosis (left) and adenocarcinoma (right). (Courtesy of Drs. A. S. Duncan and A. H. John, Cardiff, Wales.) *B*, Endometrial adenocarcinoma with diffuse adenomyosis. (From Emge, L.: Elusive adenomyosis of the uterus. Am. J. Obstet. Gynecol., *83*:1541, 1962. C. V. Mosby Co., Publishers.)

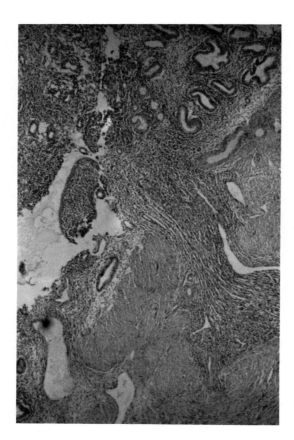

Figure 12–14. Beginning stromatosis.

Figure 12–15. Stromatosis or stromal adenomyosis of uterus, a variant of adenomyosis. In this case the invading stroma showed malignant characteristics (endometrial sarcoma).

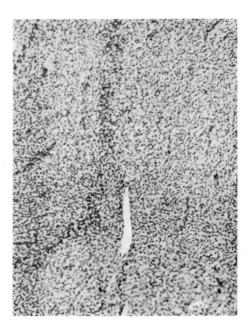

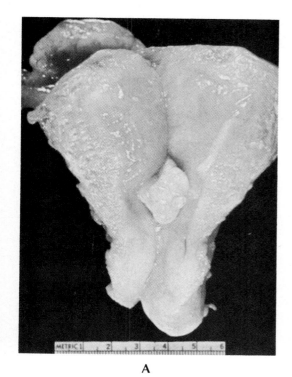

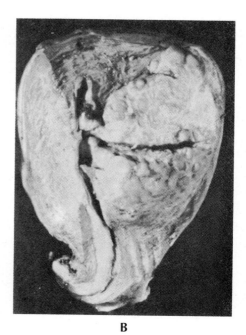

A   B

Figure 12–16. *A*, Benign stromatosis. (Courtesy of Dr. David Nichols.) Contrast lack of invasion with uterus shown in *B*. *B*, Gross appearance of uterus with malignant stromatosis. (Courtesy of Harper Hospital, Detroit, Mich.)

mal myosis, fibromyosis, stromal adeno-myosis or endometriosis, or stromatosis. In discussing the gross and microscopic pathology, Hunter and co-workers, in 1956, noted 94 cases reported.

It seems likely that in stromatosis the stromal cells extend into the myometrium, not with destruction and necrosis, but in an orderly manner along the course of the lymphatics and muscle bundles (Figs. 12–14 and 12–15). Hunter and associates question the impression of Pedowitz and his colleagues that the tumor is of vascular origin and akin to the hemangiopericytoma of Stout. Stearns points out that the disease is not dependent on ovarian activity and, in this respect, stromatosis is not comparable to adenomyosis.

When confined to the uterus, it is generally rather innocuous, but wormlike extension through the serosa into the leaves of the broad ligament may make it difficult to eradicate. The course of the disease is slow, and Hart and Yoonessi note that recurrence may be late; only occasional metastases have been noted, although the outcome may be fatal. Indeed, the study by Koss and associates may make one wonder if stromatosis is

an entity or a low grade type of endometrial sarcoma. Norris and Taylor distinguish between a malignant *infiltrating* and a benign *"pushing"* (Fig. 12–16) variety of this stromal disease. For further details, in particular about the fine distinction between this disease and endometrial sarcoma, see Chapter 13. A case with associated endometrial cancer has been recorded by Cope.

REFERENCES

Benson, R. C., and Sneeden, V. D.: Adenomyosis: A reappraisal of symptomatology. Am. J. Obstet. Gynecol., 76:1044, 1958.

Bird, C. C., McElin, T. W., and Manalo-Estrella, P.: The elusive adenomyosis of the uterus—revisited. Am. J. Obstet. Gynecol., 112:583, 1972.

Colman, H. I., and Rosenthal, A. H.: Carcinoma developing in areas of adenomyosis. Obstet. Gynecol., 14:342, 1959.

Cope, E.: Adenocarcinoma of the endometrium with malignant stromatosis. J. Obstet. Gynaecol. Brit. Emp., 65:58, 1958.

Cullen, T. S.: Adenomyoma of Uterus. Philadelphia, W. B. Saunders Company, 1908.

Cullen, T. S.: Distribution of adenomyomata containing uterine mucosa. Arch. Surg., 1:215, 1920.

Emge, L. A.: Problems in the diagnosis of adenomyosis uteri. West. J. Surg., 64:291, 1956.

Emge, L. A.: The elusive adenomyosis of the uterus. Am. J. Obstet. Gynecol., 83:1541, 1962.

Giammalvo, J. T., and Kaplan, K.: Endometriosis interna and endometrial adenocarcinoma. Am. J. Obstet. Gynecol., 75:161, 1958.

Greene, J. W., and Enterline, J. T.: Carcinoma arising in endometriosis. Obstet. Gynecol., 9:417, 1957.

Greenwood, S. M.: Adenomyosis. Am. J. Obstet. Gynecol., 48:68, 1976.

Hart, W. R., and Yoonessi, M.: Endometrial stromatosis. Obstet. Gynecol., 49:393, 1977.

Henderson, D. N.: Endolymphatic stromal myosis. Am. J. Obstet. Gynecol., 52:1000, 1946.

Hunter, W. C., Nohlgren, J. E., and Lancefield, G. M.: Stromal endometriosis or endometrial sarcoma. A reevaluation of old and new cases, with especial reference to duration, recurrences and metastases. Am. J. Obstet. Gynecol., 72:1072, 1956.

Koss, L. G., Spiro, R. H., and Brunschwig, A.: Endometrial stromal sarcoma. Surg. Gynecol. Obstet., 121:531, 1965.

Kumar, D., and Anderson, W.: Malignancy in endometriosis interna. J. Obstet. Gynaecol. Brit. Emp., 65:435, 1958.

Marcus, C. C.: Relationship of adenomyosis uteri to endometrial hyperplasia and endometrial adenocarcinoma. Am. J. Obstet. Gynecol., 82:408, 1961.

Meyer, R.: Über entzündliche heterotope Epithelwucherungen im weiblichen Genitalgebiete, etc. Virchows Arch. f. Path. Anat., 195:487, 1900.

Molitor, J. J.: Adenomyosis: a clinical and pathological appraisal. Am. J. Obstet. Gynecol., 110:275, 1971.

Norris, H. J., and Taylor, H. B., Jr.: Mesenchymal tumors of the uterus. I. A clinical and pathological study of 53 endometrial stromal tumors. Cancer, 19:755, 1966.

Novak, E., and deLima, O. A.: Correlative study of adenomyosis and pelvic endometriosis, with special reference to hormonal reaction of ectopic endometrium. Am. J. Obstet. Gynecol., 56:634, 1948.

Novak, E. R., and Woodruff, J. D.: Post-irradiation malignancy of the pelvic organs. Am. J. Obstet. Gynecol., 77:667, 1959.

Park, W. W.: Stromatosis. J. Obstet. Gynaecol. Brit. Emp., 56:755, 1952.

Park, W. W.: Nature of stromatous endometriosis. J. Obstet. Gynaecol. Brit. Emp., 56:759, 1959.

Pedowitz, P., Felmus, L. B., and Grayzel, D. M.: Vascular tumors of the uterus. II. Malignant vascular tumors. Am. J. Obstet. Gynecol., 69:1309, 1955.

Robertson, T. B., Hunter, W. C., Larson, C. P., and Snyder, G. A. C.: Benign and malignant stromatosis. Am. J. Clin. Pathol., 12:1, 1942.

Sandberg, E. C., and Cohn, F.: Adenomyosis in the gravid uterus at term. Am. J. Obstet. Gynecol., 84:1457, 1962.

Schiffen, M. A., and Mackles, A.: Stromal endometriosis. Obstet. Gynecol., 7:531, 1956.

Scott, R. B.: Adenomyosis and adenomyoma. Clin. Obstet. Gynecol., 1:413, 1958.

Stearns, H. C.: A study of stromal endometriosis. Am. J. Obstet. Gynecol., 75:663, 1958.

Stout, A. P.: Hemangiopericytoma. Cancer, 2:1027, 1949.

von Recklinghausen, F.: Die Adenomyome und Cystadenoma den Uterus und Tuberwandung: ihne Abkunft von Resten des Wolffschen Korpers. Berlin, August Hirschwald, 1896.

Winkleman, J., and Robinson, R.: Adenocarcinoma of endometrium involving adenomyosis. Cancer, 19:901, 1966.

Chapter 13

SARCOMA AND ALLIED LESIONS OF THE UTERUS

Classification

Ober has classified uterine sarcomas under six main headings, as follows:

1. Leiomyosarcoma, from myoma or normal myometrium
2. Mesenchymal (endometrial stromal or mixed mesodermal tumors)
3. Blood vessel sarcoma
4. Lymphoma
5. Unclassified sarcoma
6. Metastatic

The last four are uncommon, and thus, for practical purposes, sarcoma may be thought of as arising from (1) leiomyoma or basic myometrium, or (2) endometrial elements (e.g., stroma). The second group should be included under the general heading of the mixed mesodermal tumor, variants of which are carcinosarcoma, stromal sarcoma, and the mixed type lesion.

This approach, quite similar to Ober's, is used in our laboratory and is as follows:

Sarcoma and Allied Lesions

1. Smooth muscle
   a. Secondary in preexisting myoma
   b. Primary in myometrium
   c. Intravenous leiomyo-matosis (metastasizing myoma) } non-malignant
2. Endometrial
   a. Stromal sarcoma } usually mixed
   b. Carcinosarcoma } lesions
   c. Mixed mesodermal tumors
   d. Stromatosis (discussed in Chapter 12)
3. Others
   a. Vascular
      Hemangiopericytoma (see Chapter 11)
      Angioma and Lymphangiosarcoma
   b. Lymphoma
   c. Unclassified

LEIOMYOSARCOMA

Incidence

The incidence of uterine sarcoma is extremely difficult to compute, for there is considerable divergence of opinion among pathologists in establishing acceptable criteria for differentiating a low-grade sarcoma from a cellular myoma. The majority of uterine sarcomas apparently originate as a malignant alteration in a previously benign myoma. Despite the frequency of fibroids, the incidence of sarcomatous change is extremely low. Thornton and Carter found sarcoma in fewer than 1 per cent of nearly 2500 cases of fibromyoma. Corscaden and Singh noted an incidence of only 0.13 per cent, and in a series from our laboratory, Montague and coworkers reported 38 sarcomas in a 20 year period during which 13,000 fibromyomas were processed—an incidence of 0.29 per cent. The problems in diagnosis were emphasized in this group, since of 77 previously diagnosed leiomyosarcomas only 38 were finally acceptable. Included in the "nonacceptable" cases were cellular myomas, mixed tumors, hemangiopericytomas, and stromatosis.

Thus, although dogmatic statements regarding the frequency of uterine leiomyosarcoma seem unwarranted, it seems fair to state that the incidence of malignancy in myoma is less than 0.5 per cent. Primary uterine sarcoma is less common than that which arises in the leiomyoma.

Pathogenesis

Corpus or cervix may be the site of sarcoma, the former more frequently because of the predilection of myomas for this site. There has been speculation as to whether sarcoma arises from mature muscle cells of the uterine wall or of a myoma, or whether it evolves from nests of undifferentiated cells in the myometrium. Meyer and others believe that an origin from a fully differentiated muscle cell is unproved and unlikely. Ober, on the other hand, states categorically that leiomyosarcoma, the most frequently encountered form, is derived from adult smooth muscle.

This debate is purely academic, for all of the constituent elements of the uterus—muscle, connective tissue, epithelium, and blood vessels—are of mesodermal origin, and undoubtedly all neoplasms develop from undifferentiated cells. Thus, it might be expected that a pure sarcoma or a mixed tumor could arise from the basic element, the type depending on the lability of the originating cell. As will be noted, a multitude of diverse patterns are found in these unusual mixed uterine malignancies.

Although sarcoma may arise from muscle, connective tissue, vascular elements, and endometrial stroma, it is not always possible to be certain of the exact site of origin. The morphologic criteria are often insufficient for a precise classification. Such terms as spindle cell, round cell, mixed cell, or giant cell have been used as purely descriptive terms. It is more important, however, to label the tumor as to its cell of origin; thus, the so-called round cell sarcomas are probably examples of stromal malignancy rather than being of myometrial origin (Fig. 13–1), while the converse is true of the spindle cell variety. Various prefixes, such as lipo-, myxo-, rhabdo-, osteo-, and chondro-, while suggesting metaplasia, merely indicate the presence of the specified element, and this

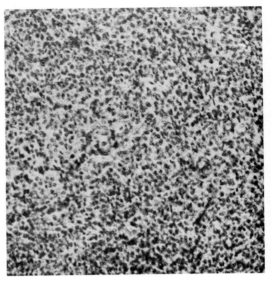

Figure 13–1. Round cell sarcoma of uterus, a lesion undoubtedly of endometrial stromal origin, therefore a variety of stromal sarcoma (see Fig. 13–20).

will be discussed more fully under mixed mesodermal tumors.

Gross Pathology

Leiomyosarcoma is rarely diagnosed preoperatively or at the operating table. It is occasionally recognized at gross pathologic examination, but most frequently is an unexpected finding at microscopic examination. Ideally every myomatous uterus should be opened in the operating room, but, practically speaking, section of every portion of a large multinodular uterus is not feasible.

Marked softening and grayish-blue discoloration of a myoma, especially if associated with a history of rapid or postmenopausal growth, should suggest malignant change. However, certain degenerative conditions in myomas simulate these malignant changes (Figs. 13–2 and 13–3). If, however, the operating surgeon should cut across a suspicious myoma and find a mushy, necrotic, "raw pork" appearance with hemorrhage, sarcoma should be suspected, and the surgeon may wish to extend the scope of surgery. Frequently the changes in the myoma are hyaline, cystic, or hemorrhagic, but occasionally malignant alteration is responsible.

Mural sarcoma or primary leiomyosarcoma generally arises in a diffuse pattern from the uterine wall, although at times it may be impossible to exclude the possibility

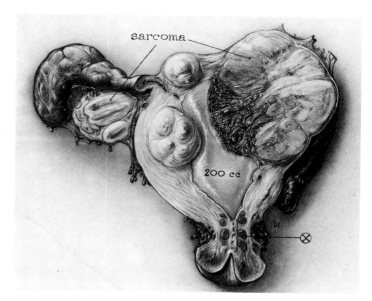

Figure 13–2. Leiomyosarcoma (in an infected submucous myoma) with pyometra and associated cervical stenosis. (Courtesy of Dr. Erle Henriksen, Los Angeles.)

of a preexisting myoma. The generalized enlargement of the uterine fundus is difficult to distinguish from adenomyosis or an intrauterine gestation. Fortunately, sarcoma arising in this fashion is unusual.

Microscopic Characteristics

A prime problem for the gynecologic pathologist is differentiation between a cellu-
lar but benign myoma and a low grade leiomyosarcoma. This may become almost insurmountable if there is associated necrosis and hemorrhage, as is so often true of the larger tumors (Fig. 13–4) and in fibroids of the patient who is taking oral contraceptives. In the latter, the initial alterations are edema and aseptic necrosis. Later the edema subsides, as does the relative size of the tumor, and reparation results in certain bi-

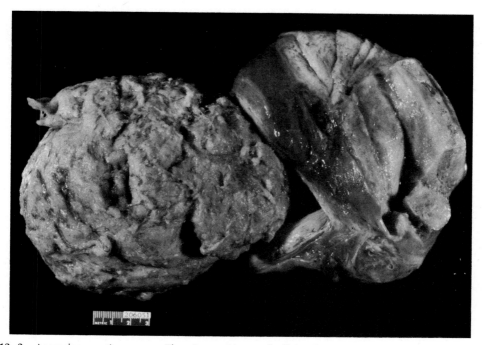

Figure 13–3. Large degenerating myoma. There is no evidence of cellular aberrations indicative of sarcoma.

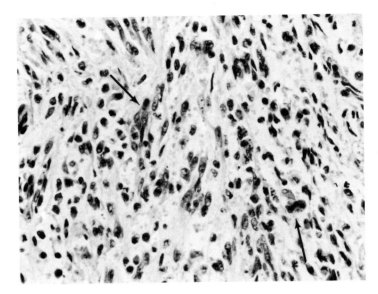

Figure 13–4. Bizarre cellular patterns (at arrows) associated with infection in myoma —lymphocytes scattered throughout the edematous tumor.

zarre but benign changes, predominantly the appearance of "symplasmic" giant cells and irregular chromatin aberrations.

It is important to study the individual cells carefully. Either the degenerative elements show no evidence of nuclear aberration, although more than one nucleus is present, or the dark masses are smudged and have no nuclear and often no cellular borders (Figs. 13–5 and 13–6). It is imperative to remember that although mitosis, regular or irregular, is the basic criterion for malignancy, nevertheless pleomorphism is the rule in the more anaplastic lesions (Fig. 13–7 A and B).

Invasion and breakthrough of the capsule are not theoretically necessary for proper diagnosis of sarcomatous degeneration, although Corscaden and Singh advocate this thesis. As noted previously, the usual criteria for assaying malignancy seem acceptable, namely, cellular atypia, mitotic activity, hyperchromatism, and giant cell formation (Figs. 13–8 to 13–10). Malignant change in a myoma most frequently occurs in the central portion of the fibroid. If no discernible myomatous nodule is present, and an alveolar pattern is present that suggests an attempt at the production of vascular channels, angio-

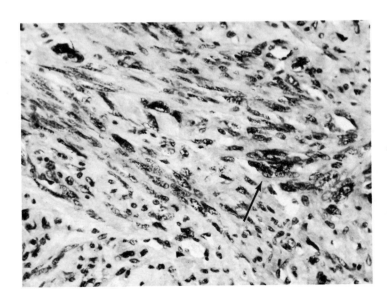

Figure 13–5. Degenerative changes in myoma with multinucleate figures.

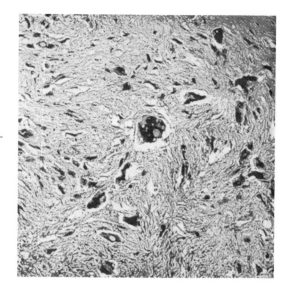

Figure 13–6. Giant cells of symplasmic type, due to degenerative process.

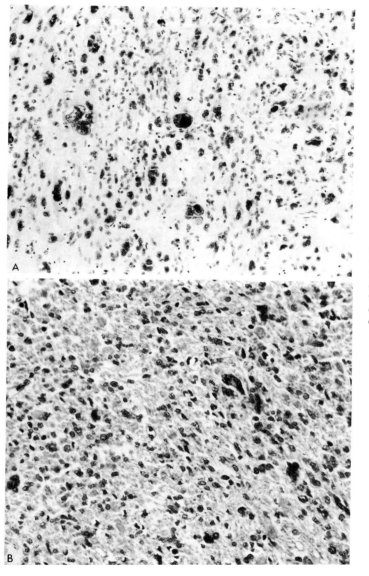

Figure 13–7. *A*, Bizarre nuclear figures, some apparently degenerative but others showing hyperchromatism and abnormal mitotic activity. *B*, Section from leiomyosarcoma showing tissue edema and degeneration with cellular pleomorphism. Undoubtedly some of the atypical nuclei are degenerative, but many are neoplastic.

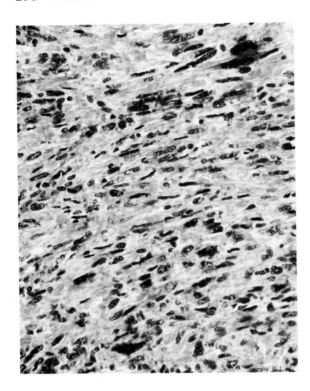

Figure 13–8. Atypical nuclei are evident in upper right and middle.

matous sarcoma may be suspected, although viability of cells adjacent to the vessels with intervening degeneration is the usual cause of such a pattern. When anaplasia, marked undifferentiation, and invasive properties are demonstrable, the diagnosis is obvious. Conversely, when there is only excessive cellularity and mild departure from cellular maturity, a diagnosis of sarcoma is rarely, if ever, justified.

Mitosis

Almost every author who has studied uterine sarcomas has been impressed with evaluation of mitoses in formulating a prognosis, as emphasized by Baggish. If fewer than 5 mitoses were found in any high power field, prognosis was generally good, but worsened progressively as more mitoses were apparent.

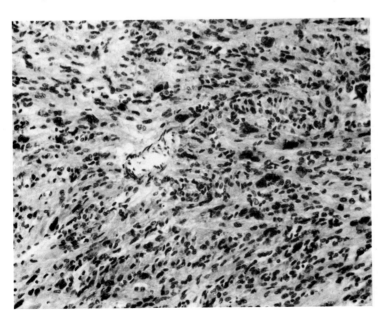

Figure 13–9. Variation in cellular patterns with leiomyosarcoma.

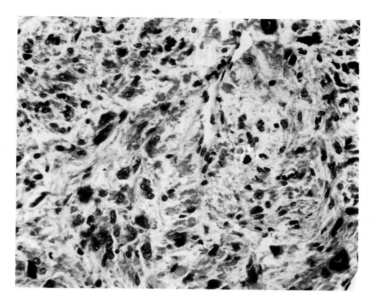

Figure 13–10. High power view showing abnormal cells with sarcoma.

Mitoses/HPF	No. of Cases	Per Cent Survival	
		1 Year	5+ Years
2 to 5	18	100	77
6 to 10	8	63	38
10+	3	0	0

Recurrent Fibroid

The so-called recurrent fibroid, a sequel of subtotal hysterectomy in which recurrent fibroids arose in the cervical stump, probably represents low grade sarcomatous change; nevertheless, such lesions may be simply leiomyomas developing in the cervix.

Occasionally sarcoma is found during the course of myomectomy, often in a young woman. The subsequent course of action depends on factors such as the activity of the tumor, age of the patient, and procreative desires.

Treatment and Salvage

Surgery, usually consisting of total hysterectomy and bilateral salpingo-oophorectomy, remains the primary therapy for uterine sarcoma. Nevertheless, the diagnosis is rarely suspected preoperatively or even at the operating table. Thus in certain instances, particularly in the young patient, the adnexa have been retained, which is probably of little prognostic importance. Unlike most sarcomas, the neoplasm that arises in the myoma kills by local extension rather than by widespread vascular dissemination. In our reported 38 cases, 14 of the 18 who succumbed to the neoplastic disease had gross extension beyond the uterus at the time of initial surgery. Consequently, when the tumor was confined to the fundus, regardless of the degree of cellular aberration, only 4 of 24 patients without extrauterine extension died of the tumor.

Of major concern is the young patient treated by myomectomy. In view of the frequency with which neoplastic changes seemingly involve not only the pseudoencapsulated myoma but also the adjacent myometrium, obviously the lesion may have been incompletely removed. Thus, it seems that if a diagnosis of uterine sarcoma has been confirmed, the safest procedure would be hysterectomy. Metastases as late as 18 years after surgery have been reported by Drake and Dobben. Unfortunately, adjunctive treatment with irradiation or chemotherapy has not proved efficacious, and Gilbert and co-workers have reached similar conclusions. In our series radiation seemed to produce adverse reaction; however, it must be noted that, for the most part, it was the hopeless case with extensive extrauterine disease that received such therapy.

Relating salvage to the position of sarcoma in the fundus, the best results were obtained with the intramural and submucous lesions; the neoplasm originating in the subserous area was more prone to early extrauterine extension. Finally, vascular invasion was a

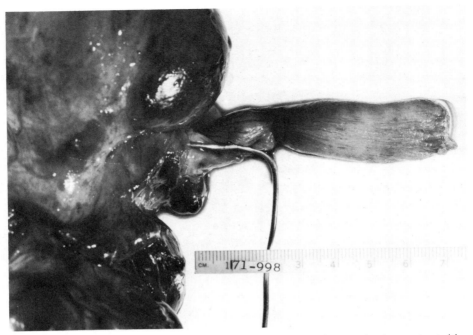

Figure 13–11. Intravenous leiomyoma. Probe is inserted into dilated channel. Tumor has been extracted from the broad ligament.

poor prognostic sign; however, 8 of 23 patients with microscopic evidence of such invasion survived 5 years.

INTRAVENOUS LEIOMYOMATOSIS

Although already discussed in Chapter 11, these bizarre "semimalignant" uterine lesions warrant repeat mention in this chapter. Usually designated as *intravenous leiomyomatosis*, the lesions present a rather typical gross appearance with cords of tumor extending through the myometrium and into the broad ligaments (Figs. 13–11 and 13–12). As noted by Miller and others, many cases are associated with pregnancy and a

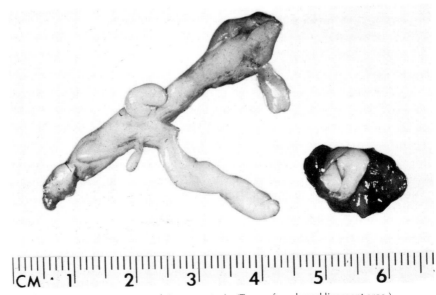

Figure 13–12. Gross patterns in intravenous leiomyomatosis. (Tumor from broad ligament area.)

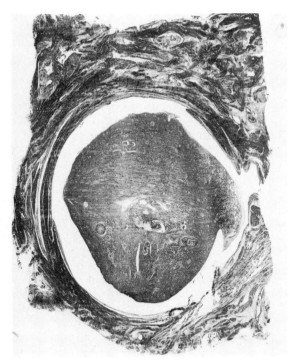

Figure 13–13. Myomatous lesion in broad ligament vessel.

possible impaired immune reaction to a usually very innocuous tumor.

Microscopically, the intravascular tumor is typical of the leiomyoma of the fundus (Fig. 13–13). In certain instances, the collagenous changes suggest an organized thrombus with revascularization. In the characteristic case, however, the smooth muscle pattern leaves no doubt as to the leiomyomatous nature of the tumor. It seems quite possible that this neoplasm actually arises from the muscularis of the vessel wall.

METASTASIZING MYOMA

Metastasizing myoma with pulmonary leiomyoma was reported by McEachern and co-workers. Following lobectomy this patient survived for more than $3\frac{1}{2}$ years without evidence of disease. Ariel and Trinidad have recently recorded a similar case in which the pulmonary lesions were microscopically benign, and the patient was alive 3 years postoperatively, although two small nodules had been demonstrated in the same lung.

Clark and Weed have recently reported an 8 year survivor; castration with no estrogen is their suggested therapy. The question as to terminology for such tumors is controversial; however, justification for use of the term leiomyosarcoma seems doubtful. It would appear more logical to assume that such lesions represented multiple primary tumors, all of which were benign. Leiomyomatosis peritonealis disseminata (Fig. 11–9) represents a similar localized process and has been discussed in Chapter 11.

ENDOMETRIAL SARCOMA AND MIXED TUMORS (MESENCHYMAL)

Incidence

These lesions are uncommon; however, when all varieties are grouped together the incidence approaches that of leiomyosarcoma. For example, Symmonds and Dockerty report 177 cases, including 105 leiomyosarcomas, 69 endometrial sarcomas, and 3 lymphosarcomas. The average age for the appearance of these tumors is identical to that of adenocarcinoma of the fundus, i.e., the middle of the sixth decade. Nevertheless, it must be recognized that the sarcoma botryoides of the cervix and upper vagina is a variant of the mixed tumor and occurs routinely during the first decade of life.

Histogenesis

The histogenesis of the mixed mesodermal tumors or mesenchymomas has always excited much speculation. Previous editions of this text have suggested a fusion of paramesonephric and mesonephric duct elements as an explanation for the various structures seen in these lesions. Symmonds and Dockerty emphasized that totipotent mesodermal elements can form a variety of structures. Studies by Taylor and by Williams and Woodruff offer persuasive evidence that metaplasia of the parent endometrial stromal cell is responsible for the bizarre inconsistent architecture. Indeed, the paper by Williams and Woodruff poses a close kinship, and frequent transition phases between polypoid endometrial cancer and mixed mesodermal tumors. A case report by Cope of an adenocarcinoma with a low grade endometrial sarcoma exemplifies this thesis. It is supported further by the appearance, in the same uterus, of multiple polyps demonstrating varying stromal and epithelial patterns (Fig. 13–14).

Mesenchymal sarcomas are uncommon,

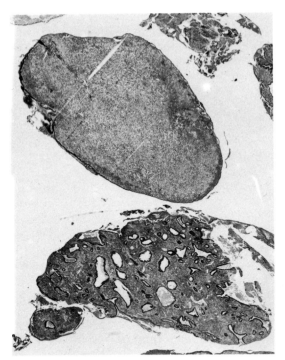

Figure 13–14. Multiple polyps—stromal hyperplasia above with stromal and epithelial elements below.

interest is the history of previous radiation therapy in one third of the collected series as well as in their own cases.

MÜLLERIAN ADENOSARCOMA

Clement and Scully have recently reported 10 cases of endometrial sarcoma that have contained a number of essentially hyperactive endometrial glands, and have regarded them as a specific entity. These *adenosarcomas* occur in older women and have a rather low degree of malignancy, with late local recurrence and only rare metastasis.

With all due respect to the authors, it is our own belief that they are drawing too fine a line in distinguishing these from the ordinary endometrial sarcoma, which may show occasional benign endometrial glands (see Fig. 13–17). Although fundal carcinoma is characterized by "back to back glandular crowding," with loss of stroma, some stroma is often apparent. Thus, why make an issue of endometrial sarcoma in which some normal glandular pattern is retained?

Gross Pathology

Endometrial sarcoma and mixed tumors present as a grayish-pink polypoid excrescence often extruding from the cervical os or the vaginal introitus (Figs. 13–15 and 13–16). Inversion of the uterus may develop as a complication, although frequently this is not recognized until surgery. Indeed, the

and Taylor accepts fewer than 150 of the previously reported cases as authentic. Of 40 patients available to him for study, he notes only six 4-year salvages, with rapid death due to both local recurrence and distant metastasis. Williams and Woodruff have collected 400 cases from the literature, and of

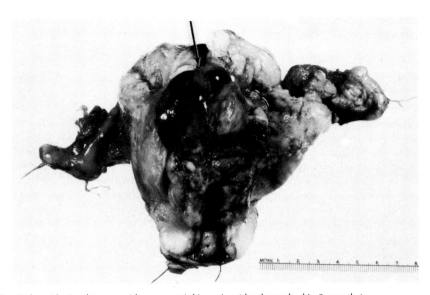

Figure 13–15. Polypoid mixed tumor with myometrial invasion (death resulted in 3 months).

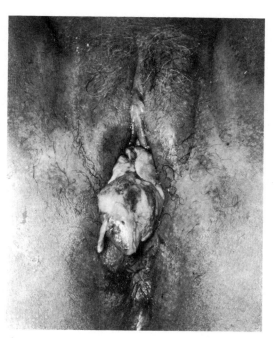

Figure 13–16. Polypoid mixed mesodermal tumor arising in the uterine cavity and projecting beyond the introitus.

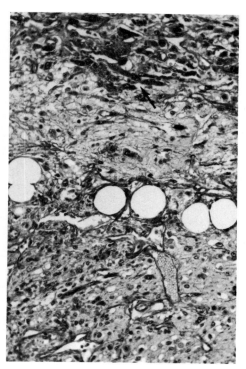

Figure 13–18. Mixed elements in mesodermal tumor—striated cell at arrow.

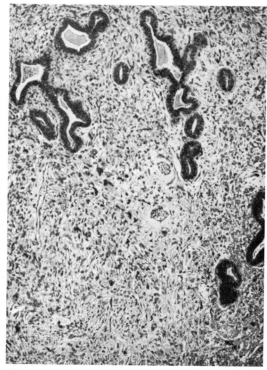

Figure 13–17. Endometrial sarcoma, showing marked nuclear hyperchromatosis.

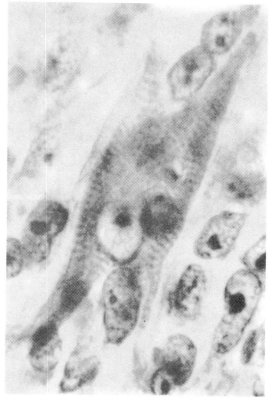

Figure 13–19. Striated muscle elements in a mixed mesodermal tumor. (Courtesy of Dr. P. Hartz.)

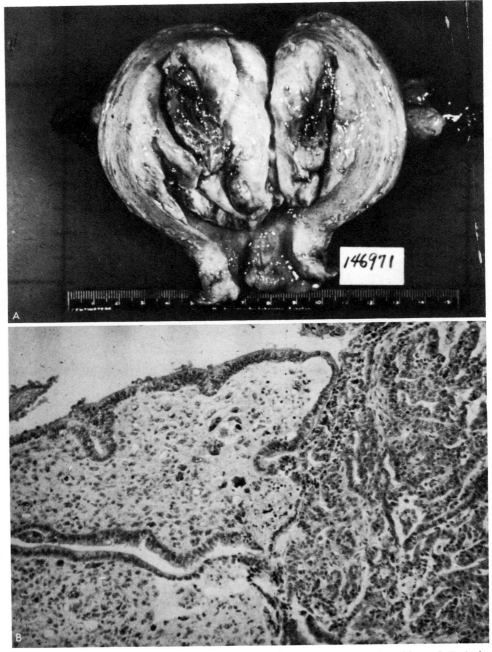

Figure 13–20. *A*, Frequently polypoid in appearance, endometrial sarcoma may project out of the os. *B*, Typical sarcoma at left with adenocarcinoma (carcinosarcoma) at right. Heterologous elements (bone, cartilage, striated muscle, etc.) may be found in mixed mesodermal tumor.

malignant nature of these polypoid lesions is generally not recognized unless excision or biopsy of the polyp is carried out.

Microscopic Pathology

Symmonds and Dockerty have carried out an extensive study of endometrial sarcoma, including carcinosarcoma, mixed mesodermal tumors, and benign but proliferative conditions of the endometrial stroma. These latter instances of so-called stromal hyperplasia and stromal endometriosis (benign stromatosis) pose interesting diagnostic problems, do not metastasize, but can kill the patient because of persistent locally invasive tendencies. Unfortunately, there is no sharp line of demarcation between the histologically benign and the malignant.

In another excellent résumé of mesenchymal lesions, Ober and Tovell emphasize that the common denominator of all these tumors is the endometrial stroma (Fig. 13–17). *Homologous* (indigenous to the uterus) or *heterologous* (foreign to the uterus, e.g., cartilage and striated muscle) elements may be found (Figs. 13–18 and 13–19). In the former instance, carcinosarcoma evolves (Fig. 13–20); in the latter, a mixed mesodermal tumor results (Fig. 13–21). It must be restated that these two lesions are clinically and histogenetically similar, and are variants of the same process.

Ober and Tovell also note the varying degrees of malignancy in neoplasms of endometrial stroma with all intermediate gradations between stromatous endometriosis and frank endometrial sarcoma. They point out that the low grade pure tumors are much more common in younger women, and are relatively innocuous. The heterologous and mixed sarcomas afflict an older age group, and the prognosis is much worse.

Many lesions demonstrate the association of various patterns in the same tumor (Fig. 13–14). Multiple polyps are often present and these may demonstrate benign epithelial and stromal elements, as noted in endometrial hyperplasia, with associated stromal and epithelial anaplasias, including metaplastic mesodermal elements.

Mixed mesodermal sarcoma is a variant of endometrial sarcoma, for in addition to sarcoma it exhibits the other heterologous elements noted previously. Bone, cartilage, striated muscle, and other mesodermal elements may be found, but it is no longer believed that the demonstration of rhabdomyoblasts (striated muscle cells) is necessary for diagnosis (Fig. 13–19). Nevertheless, rare malignancies of these elements, the rhabdomyosarcoma, osteosarcoma, chondrosarcoma, and liposarcoma, are variants of the mixed tumor.

Tumors of this mixed type have been divided into the composition, combination, and collision types. Actually, the distinction between composition and combination is impossible since both are varieties of lesions demonstrating different patterns but arising from the same base tissue. Collision tumors —two malignancies with an equivocal intermediate transition zone (as leiomyosarcoma merging with endometrial carcinoma)— should not, we believe, be accepted as true carcinosarcoma. The collision tumor is an uncommon type, and represents two distinct and dissimilar malignancies. In any case, these terms are becoming passé.

Course of Disease

Breakdown of this varied group of tumors into specific pathologic types is difficult since many authors believe that they are variants of the same disease. Although histologically this is undoubtedly true, nevertheless there are grades of malignancy similar to those noted with other tumors, and although the clinical course is dependent largely on the extent of the disease at time of therapy, the degree of anaplasia must play a role. The low grade endometrial sarcoma confined largely to the cavity, for example, offers a much better prognosis than the bizarre mixed mesodermal tumor that has extended into the adjacent tissues. Nevertheless, the overall salvage is poor, and early recurrences are the rule. In a collected series. Williams and Woodruff noted that, in the fatal cases, death occurred within 2 years in 92 per cent of the patients.

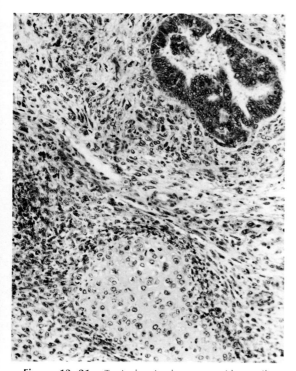

Figure 13–21. Typical mixed tumor with cartilage below.

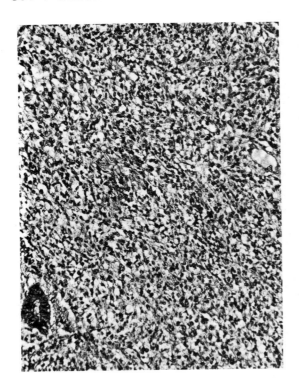

Figure 13–22. Intrauterine tumor—stromal sarcoma with rare epithelial element at lower left.

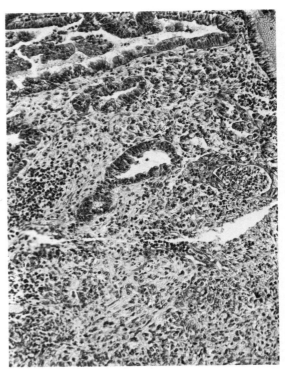

Figure 13–23. Recurrent lesion in vaginal vault showing carcinosarcoma 2½ years after removal of tumor in Figure 13–22.

It is of interest to note that regardless of the initial patterns, the metastatic lesions resemble adenocarcinomas in 75 to 80 per cent of cases, although the stromal component has often gone unnoted. Furthermore, the lesions clinically behave more as carcinomas than sarcomas, since they tend to invade and metastasize locally via lymphatics. An example of the former feature is provided by the following case:

Hysterectomy was performed on a 56 year old patient and an endometrial sarcoma was discovered (Fig. 13–22). Two and one half years later a recurrence developed in the vagina and the pattern was that of carcinosarcoma (Fig. 13–23). At death three months later (of a cardiovascular accident) the only residual tumor was adenocarcinoma.

Generally, therapy has consisted of surgery plus irradiation, although progesterone may be helpful. Iradiation has been given both preoperatively and postoperatively with little difference in the results. The best 5 year salvage has been approximately 26 to 28 per cent. A few cases have been treated initially by radical Wertheim hysterectomy, with seemingly excellent results. The num-

bers, however, are too small to be statistically significant.

Angioma, Lymphangioma, and Angiosarcoma

These lesions have been reported as arising in both the endometrium and myometrium. Generally they are incidental findings, although if present in the surface layers they may be associated with metrorrhagia.

REFERENCES

Aaro, L. A., Symmonds, R. E., and Dockerty, M. B.: Sarcoma of the uterus. Am. J. Obstet. Gynecol., 94:101, 1966.

Ariel, I. M., and Trinidad, S.: Pulmonary metastases from a uterine "leiomyoma." Am. J. Obstet. Gynecol., 94:110, 1966.

Carleton, C. C., and Williamson, J. W.: Osteogenic sarcoma of the uterus. Arch. Pathol., 20:378, 121, 1961.

Clank, D. H., and Weed, J. C.: Metastasizing leiomyoma. Am. J. Obstet. Gynecol., 127:672, 1977.

Clement, P. B., and Scully, R. E.: Müllerian adenosarcoma of the uterus. Cancer, 34:1138, 1974.

Cope, E.: Adenocarcinoma of the endometrium with

malignant stromatosis. J. Obstet. Gynaecol. Br. Emp., 65:58, 1958.

Corscaden, J. A., and Singh, B. P.: Leiomyosarcoma of the uterus. Am. J. Obstet. Gynecol., 75:149, 1958.

Drake, E. T., and Dobben, G. D.: Leiomyosarcoma of the uterus with unusual metastasis. J.A.M.A., 170:114, 1959.

Finn, W. F.: Sarcoma of uterus. Am. J. Obstet. Gynecol., 60:1254, 1950.

Gilbert, H. A., et al.: The value of radiation therapy in uterine sarcoma. Obstet. Gynecol., 45:85, 1975.

Goodfriend, M. J., and Lapan, B.: Carcinoma of uterus. N.Y. State J. Med., 50:1139, 1950.

Greene, R. R., Gerbie, A. B., Gerbie, M. V., and Eckman, T. R.: Hemangiopericytomas of the uterus. Am. J. Obstet. Gynecol., 106:1020, 1970.

Harper, R. S., and Scully, R. E.: Intravenous leiomyomatosis of the uterus. Obstet. Gynecol., 18:519, 1961.

Hunter, W. C., Nohlgren, J. E., and Lancefield, G. M.: Stromal endometriosis or endometrial sarcoma. Am. J. Obstet. Gynecol., 73:1072, 1957.

Johnson, C. E., and Soule, E. H.: Malignant lymphoma as a gynecological problem. Obstet. Gynecol., 9:149, 1957.

Kimbrough, R. A., Jr.: Sarcoma of uterus. Am. J. Obstet. Gynecol., 28:723, 1934.

Korn, G. W.: Mixed mesenchymal tumors of uterus with superimposed adenocarcinoma. J. Obstet. Gynaecol. Br. Emp., 63:887, 1956.

Krieger, P. D., and Gusberg, S. B.: Stromal myosis (Gr. I endometrial sarcoma). Gynec. Oncol., 1:299, 1973.

McEachern, C. G., Gitlin, M. M., and Sullivan, R. E.: Lobectomy for metastatic leiomyosarcoma of the uterus. J.A.M.A., 174:1734, 1960.

Meyer, R.: Uterussarkome. In Henke-Lubarsch Handb. d. spez. Path. Anat., Vol. 7. Berlin, Julius Springer, 1930.

Montague, A. C.-W., Swartz, D. P., and Woodruff, J. D.: Sarcoma arising in a leiomyoma of the uterus. Am. J. Obstet. Gynecol., 92:421, 1965.

Novak, E. R.: Benign and malignant changes in myoma. Clin. Obstet. Gynecol., 1:421, 1958.

Ober, W. B.: Uterine sarcomas: histogenesis and taxonomy. Ann. N.Y. Acad. Sci., 75:658, 1959.

Ober, W. B., and Tovell, H. M.: Malignant lymphoma of uterus. Bull. Sloane Hosp., 5:59, 1959.

Ober, W. B., and Tovell, H. M.: Mesenchymal sarcomas of the uterus. Am. J. Obstet. Gynecol., 77:246, 1959.

Schiffer, M. A., Mackles, A., and Wolfe, S. A.: Reappraisal of diagnosis in sarcoma. Am. J. Obstet. Gynecol., 70:521, 1955.

Steiner, P. R.: Metastasizing fibroleiomyoma of the uterus. Am. J. Pathol., 15:89, 1939.

Symmonds, R. E., and Dockerty, M. B.: Sarcoma and sarcoma-like proliferation of endometrial stroma. Surg. Gynecol. Obstet., 100:232, 1955.

Symmonds, R. E., Dockerty, M. B., and Pratt, J. H.: Sarcoma and sarcoma-like proliferation of the endometrial stroma. Am. J. Obstet. Gynecol., 73:1054, 1957.

Taubert, H. D., Wissner, S. E., and Haskins, A. L.: Leiomyomatosis peritonealis disseminata. Obstet. Gynecol., 25:561, 1965.

Taylor, C. W.: Mesodermal mixed tumors of the female genital tract. J. Obstet. Gynaecol. Br. Emp., 60:177, 1958.

Thompson, J. W., III, Symmonds, R. E., and Dockerty, M. B.: Benign uterine leiomyoma with vascular involvement. Am. J. Obstet. Gynecol., 84:182, 1962.

Thornton, W. N., Jr., and Carter, J. P.: Sarcoma of uterus, a clinical study. Am. J. Obstet. Gynecol., 62:294, 1951.

Webb, G. A.: Uterine sarcoma. Obstet. Gynecol., 6:38, 1955.

Williams, T. J., and Woodruff, J. D.: Similarities in malignant mixed mesenchymal tumors of the endometrium. Obstet. Gynecol. Surv., 17:1, 1962.

Wilson, L. A., Jr., Graham, J., Jr., Thornton, W. N., Jr., and Nokes, J. M.: Mixed mesodermal tumors. Am. J. Obstet. Gynecol. 66:718, 1953.

Wolfe, S. A., and Pedowitz, P.: Carcinosarcoma of the uterus. Obstet. Gynecol., 12:54, 1958.

Chapter 14

HISTOLOGY OF FALLOPIAN TUBES

Anatomically, the fallopian tube is commonly divided into four portions: (1) an *interstitial* portion, traversing the muscular wall of the uterine cornu from which the tube arises; (2) a narrow *isthmic* portion adjacent to the uterus (Fig. 14–1); (3) the *ampulla*, which is the widened middle and outer third of the tube (Fig. 14–2); and (4) the *fimbriated extremity* or *infundibulum*, representing the distal portion of the tube.

On histologic examination the tube has three coats: an outer *serous*, a middle *muscular*, and an inner mucosa. The *serous* coat is formed by the peritoneum which envelops the tube, and which is reflected as a double layer over the mesosalpinx from the lower border of the tube. The *muscular* layers consist of an outer longitudinal coat, basically an extension of the myometrium; a middle, circular layer, the true autochthonous muscle of the oviduct; and an inner, poorly defined, but important layer of fibers into the lamina propria. These fibers extend into the mucosal folds and may play a role in the transport of materials. The circular muscle is of major import since its segmental contractions assist in transport of the egg from infundibulum to the uterus. The interstitial or intramural portion is surrounded by the interlacing meshwork of cornual muscle tissue.

The mucosa or endosalpinx is disposed in longitudinal folds or rugae. Only three or occasionally four of these rugae are seen at the inner end of the tube, so that a cross section shows a narrow lumen shaped somewhat like a Roman cross. As the rugae pass outward, however, they divide and subdivide so that a cross section of the ampulla is much more intricate, and that of the fimbriated end is highly arborescent. Between the epithelium and the muscularis is seen a layer of connective tissue described as the lamina propria. This submucous layer is similar in many respects to the stroma of the endometrium, and it is in this area that decidua is recognized during pregnancy. Furthermore, being müllerian or paramesonephric in origin, it may demonstrate the metabolic and microscopic aspects of endometrial stroma.

The epithelium is composed of three distinct types of cells: (1) the ciliated cells (Fig. 14–3); (2) the nonciliated or secretory cells (Fig. 14–4); and (3) the intercalary or peg cells ("Stiftchenzellen"). In addition to these well-defined varieties, an indifferent cell, lying at the base of the epithelial layer,

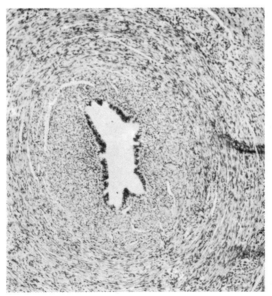

Figure 14–1. Section of isthmic end of the fallopian tube, close to uterus.

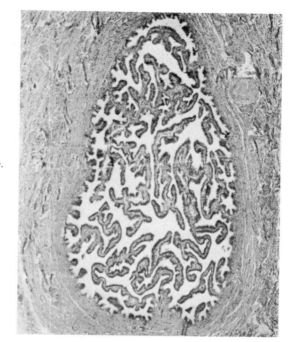

Figure 14–2. Section of outer third of the fallopian tube.

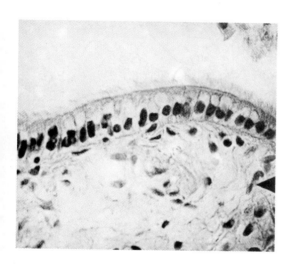

Figure 14–3. Ciliated epithelium on the fimbria ovarica, where this type is found almost exclusively.

Figure 14–4. Tubal epithelium at end of menstruation (postmenstrual). The cells are low, both the ciliated and the secretory. Note the dark rodlike peg cells at x.

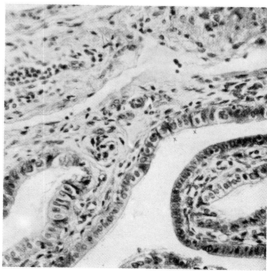

has been noted. The chief characteristics of these three main types and of the indifferent cells may be summarized as follows.

Ciliated Cells

These are most easily studied in the interval phase when they reach their greatest development (Figs. 14–5 and 14–6). At this stage they are both tall and broad, measuring often as much as 30 to 35 micrometers (μm.) in height, and as much as 12 μm. in breadth. The cytoplasm is very pale and almost refractile in appearance, especially that surrounding the nucleus where a clear "halo" may be seen. By oil-immersion study, however, it is found to show numerous fine granules, especially near the nucleus. The nucleus is quite large, and either round or slightly ovoid. Its long axis is not infrequently placed at right angles to the long axis of the cell. It is situated far above the basement membrane, often near the ciliated edge of the cell. This is in striking contrast to the nuclei of the nonciliated cells, which are much more

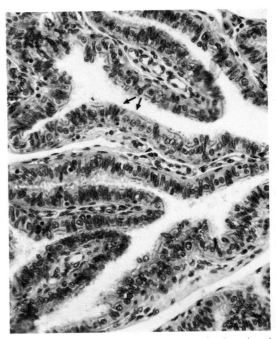

Figure 14–6. Interval phase showing the broad, pale ciliated cells (at right arrow) and the narrow, darker-staining secretory cells with the "cupola" effect (at left arrow).

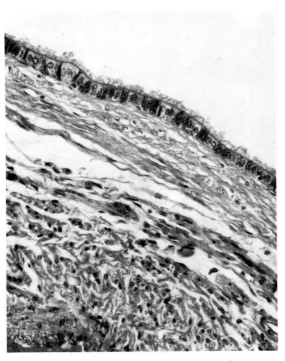

Figure 14–5. Classic tubal epithelium in isthmus near the ampullary-isthmic junction. Note the thin layer of circular muscle and the more prominent longitudinal fibers from the adjacent myometrium.

deeply placed near the basement membrane. This fact gives one, at first glance, the impression of a double layer of nuclei, the superficial belonging to the ciliated cells, the deeper to the nonciliated cells.

The differentiation of the two types is further facilitated by the difference in staining reaction, the nuclei of the ciliated cells taking a rather pale hematoxylin stain, as against the solid and darker stain of the nuclei of the nonciliated cells. The nine cilia are attached to a layer of basal granules, which, under proper magnification, stand out quite sharply. The cilia themselves, even in the microscopic section, are quite long and slender, often measuring 7 or 8 μm. in length. In fixed sections they show clumping and agglutination, and are recognized only as a layer of acidophilic material attached to the luminal surface of the cell.

In the immediately postmenstrual phase the ciliated cells are much shorter than in the interval (Fig. 14–4), but they rapidly increase in height. Perhaps even more striking is the increase in breadth in the interval as compared with the postmenstrual phase. Beyond the interval, the ciliated cells appear to become lower in contrast to the secretory cell, and the minimum height of both varieties is seen in association with pregnancy.

The simplest and most satisfactory manner of studying the cilia is in freshly removed unfixed tissue, and it was by this method that the presence of cilia in the uterine epithelium of the sow was first demonstrated. The simple technique consists of snipping off a tiny, thin bit of mucosa, placing it on a slide, flattening it out into a thin layer by pressure, and studying it under the ordinary high dry lens. The cilia are best seen with minimal illumination. They retain their vitality for a surprisingly long time after removal of the tissue from the body. For the first hour or two their motility is vigorous, but definite ciliary activity for as long as four hours after the operation at which the tissue was removed has been noted. The addition of the stain to the fluid almost immediately eliminates this activity.

Cilia are also found in the tubal epithelium before puberty and after the menopause. This suggests that they may have some function other than, or in addition to, that of assisting in the propulsion of the ova. Hartman suggests the very plausible explanation that their chief function may be merely that of keeping the tubal lumen cleansed of any foreign material.

Nonciliated or Secretory Cells

These cells have been the object of even more extensive investigation than the ciliated type. The secretions and their effects on sperm survival have been studied extensively by Mastroianni and others. From a morphologic standpoint, there can be no doubt as to the essential differences between the secretory and the ciliated elements. Like that of the ciliated cells, their height varies at different phases of the cycle. They are low immediately after menstruation (Fig. 14–4), become tall in the interval (Fig. 14–6), remain tall in the premenstrual period (Fig. 14–7), and again become lower during menstruation and pregnancy (Figs. 14–8 and 14–10). In the postmenstrual period they are, like the ciliated cells, of narrow cylindrical shape, so that at this time sharper scrutiny is required to differentiate them from the latter (Fig. 14–4). The chief points of distinction, aside from the presence or absence of cilia (with proper allowance for

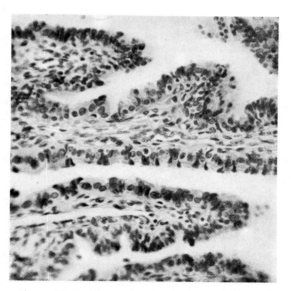

Figure 14–7. The premenstrual phase of the cycle, showing the difference in height between the ciliated and the secretory cells, the nuclei of the latter projecting far above the cell margins, producing an irregular epithelial edge. Note the extrusion of some of the nuclei.

absence due to imperfect preservation or preparation), are the shape, size, and staining qualities of the nuclei, as already described, the elongated shape of the cell, and the staining of the cytoplasm. The cytoplasm in the secretory cells is considerably darker

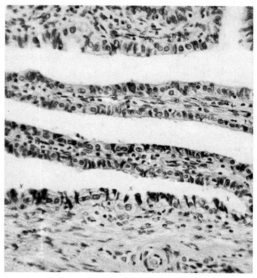

Figure 14–8. Tubal epithelium during menstruation (24 hours after onset), showing transition between premenstrual and postmenstrual pictures.

and more uniform than that in the ciliated cells.

In the interval phase the distinction between the two types is clearly marked (Fig. 14–6), partly by the increased width of the ciliated cells, their more easily recognized cilia, and the clear appearance of their cytoplasm, and partly by certain changes which now manifest themselves in the secretory cells. Whereas in an earlier phase these are narrow, almost rodlike in appearance, their free borders now become wider and slightly convex. There is thus produced an appearance suggesting a small cupola at the top of many of these cells, the cytoplasm appearing to herniate through the cell membrane. The cell as a whole changes shape, so that it becomes pear-shaped, or perhaps from compression of its center by surrounding cells, dumbbell-shaped (Fig. 14–6).

This variation in the shape and appearance of the nonciliated cells becomes more marked in the secretory phase of the cycle. The domelike cell extremities appear to break into the tube lumen, leaving the nucleus with little or no discernible cytoplasmic envelope. Frequently, too, the nucleus with the cytoplasmic secretion may be extruded into the lumen in a manner similar to that described by Hartman for the opossum (Fig. 14–7). Mitoses are almost never seen in the tubal epithelium, unlike the endometrium, where, during the postmenstrual phase, they are found in large numbers in both epithelium and stroma. Recent studies by Pauerstein suggest that the metabolic activity of the indifferent cell may offer an explanation for the continuing viability of the tubal epithelium in the absence of the usual evidences of cell replication.

In the premenstrual period, these secretory changes become more pronounced, and another striking feature is added. The free borders of the secretory cell often project for a considerable distance above their ciliated neighbors, presenting a striking and characteristic picture (Fig. 14–7). The bulging ends overhang the cilia, while extruded clumps of cytoplasm, often containing the cell nuclei, are to be seen, either matted to the cilia or lying free in the lumen.

Nuclei are often seen lying quite naked on the free border, the cytoplasm having been emptied into the lumen. Such nuclei are wedge-shaped or triangular, being dovetailed into the subjacent cells. They may have a small amount of cytoplasm suggesting that they retain a capacity for further cyclic change.

The changes in the secretory cells characterizing the premenstrual epoch are continued into the phase of actual menstruation, except that the cells become lower, and the cytoplasmic and nuclear extrusion is completed. At the end of menstruation these cells appear to consist almost entirely of nucleus, although some of them show a moderate cytoplasmic envelope (Fig. 14–4).

Intercalary or Peg Cells (Stiftchenzellen)

These cells are in many respects the least understood of the types to be found in the tubal epithelium. Their characteristics can perhaps best be studied in the premenstrual and menstrual periods, when they are present in largest number. At these periods they present a rather striking appearance, being interjected at frequent intervals between groups of cells of the other two types. At first sight they seem to consist of nothing but long, slender rodlike nuclei which are squeezed in between the adjoining cells (Fig. 14–4). It is for this reason that they may be spoken of as "peg cells" for they look not unlike slender pegs driven between the other cells. Throughout the literature they are rather commonly designated by the German term "Stiftchenzellen."

Although, with the ordinary hematoxylin-eosin stain, these cells most characteristically appear as intensely dark "lashes" between the neighboring cells, the nuclei not infrequently appear as wedgelike masses of nuclear material close to the basement membrane. By careful examination one often discerns a small amount of cytoplasm about the nucleus, at luminal and basel areas, giving the cell an almost dumbbell shape. Under these conditions, it cannot be distinguished from the secretory cell at a certain phase, as one will appreciate from the description already given of the latter cells. For example, in the menstruating phase, many of the secretory cells, emptied of their secretion, or, at any rate, deprived of the cytoplasm which has been thrown off into the tubal lumen, appear as peg cells.

For this reason, i.e., because we have been able to distinguish definite transition stages between these peg cells and the fully formed secretory cells, we believe that there is little doubt that the two represent different phases of the same life cycle.

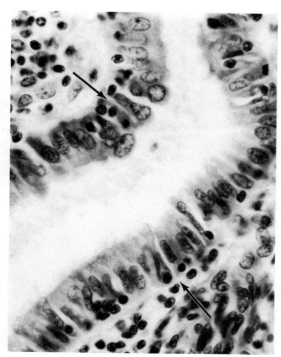

Figure 14–9. Indifferent cells can be seen at base of normal epithelial cell (at arrows) and also at other positions.

Indifferent Cells

The method of replication of the epithelial cell in the tube is not defined histologically (Fig. 14–9). The indifferent cell, lying at the base of the normal epithelium, has been described in textbooks; however, the relationship of this cell to the regeneration and stability of the layer is unknown. Nevertheless, as noted previously, this cell is metabolically more active than any of the other well documented cells, and may, in fact, be the progenitor of the epithelial and stromal elements.

PATHOPHYSIOLOGIC CHANGES IN THE TUBAL EPITHELIUM

The cyclic changes evidencing the paramesonephric origin of the oviduct have been described earlier, in the discussion of the individual varieties of cell types, each of which reacts to the hormonal milieu of the patient.

During pregnancy, the menstrual changes, characterized by a decrease in height of both varieties of cell types and an increase in the number of peg cells, are exaggerated. The epithelium is low and, al-

though the various cell types can be appreciated, secretory activity is essentially nonexistent. In a rare instance, a hypersecretory pattern suggestive of the Arias-Stella phenomenon has been recognized in the pregnant tube, but usually only in the earlier stages of gestation. A decidual reaction in the lamina propria is frequently seen, demonstrating the ability of the tubal stroma to react to the pregnancy hormones (Fig. 4–10).

In the immediate postpartum period there is a rather marked infiltration of the lamina with polymorphonuclear cells in 8 to 10 per cent of the tubes studied by Hellman. One might suspect that this nonbacterial infiltration could account for the instances of so-called "one-child sterility." Of interest are the findings in a group of patients who had been treated with estrogen to suppress lactation and were sterilized postpartum. No inflammatory reaction was found in the removed cornual section of the tube, suggesting that the proliferation produced by the estrogen may have prevented the process; conversely, the low, inactive epithelium, classic of pregnancy, was prey to local irritative phenomena.

Changes similar to those noted above are seen in the patient receiving oral contraceptives; however, they are never as dramatic, and in many instances are not demonstrable histologically.

The tubal epithelium associated with prolonged estrogenic stimulation, i.e., in the patient who has been receiving exogenous estrogens or who harbors an estrogen-producing ovarian neoplasm, is characteristically tall, pseudostratified, and proliferative; mitoses, however, are absent. There is no evidence of secretory activity; this, in addition to the epithelial stimulation noted above, suggests a reaction similar to that seen with endometrial hyperplasia—proliferation without the modifying effect of progesterone (Figs. 14–11 and 14–12).

The epithelium in *prepubertal* and *senile* tubes is low, but shows both chief types of cells. Cilia are sparse. In the fetus of 20 weeks or more, only two cilia per cell are noted as compared with the usual nine appreciated in the mature, ciliated cell (Fig. 14–13).

The epithelium of the *postmenopausal* tube may remain quite high for many years. Cilia, likewise, may persist for many years.

Text continued on page 315

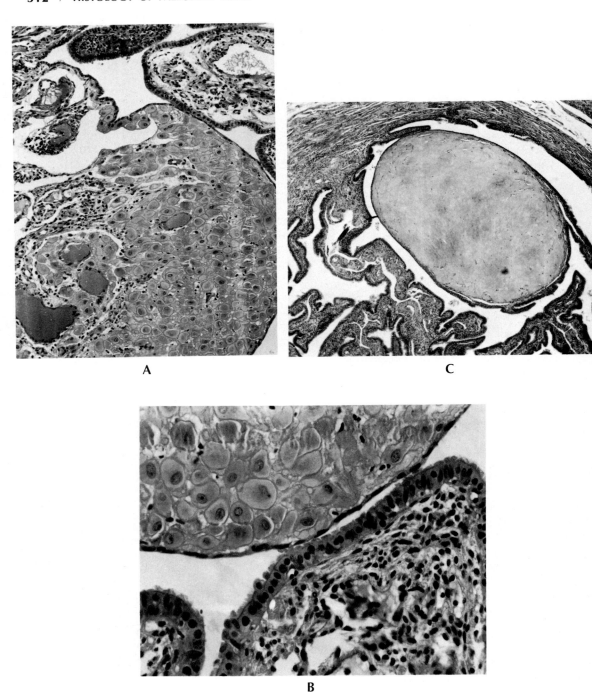

Figure 14–10. *A*, Marked decidual reaction in the fallopian tube associated with intrauterine pregnancy. The classic flattened epithelium of pregnancy is seen. *B*, High power view of decidual reaction in fallopian tube. Note inactive epithelium associated with pregnancy. Fibrosis of such foci may produce the appearance of a fibroma or fibromyoma (see C). *C*, Fibrosis with hyalinization in the lamina propria of a normal tube (?residue of decidua).

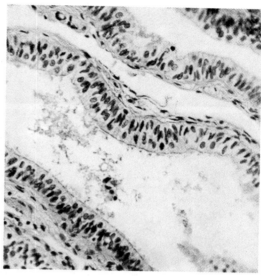

Figure 14–11. Tubal epithelium in a case of hyperplasia of the endometrium associated with functional bleeding. As might be expected, the epithelium shows an exaggeration of the interval picture.

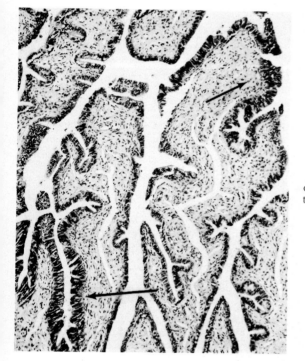

Figure 14–12. Epithelial proliferations (at arrows) associated with endometrial hyperplasia in postmenopausal patient.

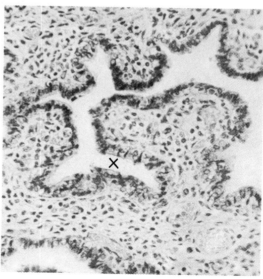

Figure 14–13. Tubal epithelium in infant born prematurely at six and one half months. The two types of cells can be distinguished, especially at x.

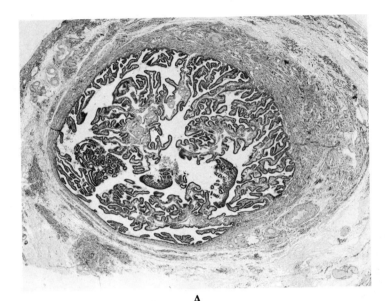

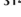

Figure 14–14. *A,* The tubal lumen containing fragments of endometrium. *B,* Desquamated fragments of menstruating endothelium in tubal lumen. Metaplasia of repair at arrow. Tubal mucosal folds are visible at upper right.

A

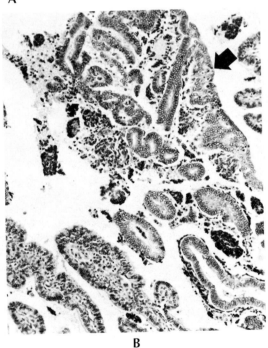

B

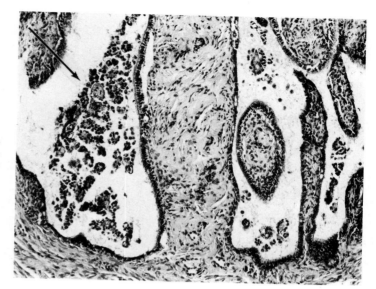

Figure 14–15. Cells from papillary serous tumor lying free in the lumen of the tube (at arrow). Ciliated cells lining the tube are obvious.

Eventually, the tubal folds become rounded and of fibrous appearance, the epithelium becomes low or even quite flat, and cilia, of course, disappear.

FUNCTIONS OF FALLOPIAN TUBE

The *oviduct* is no longer regarded as a simple conduit for the transport of ovum from ovary to uterus. Basically, its functions may be condensed into the following:

1. Sperm transport and capacitation.
2. Ovum transport and capacitation.
3. Zygote transport and maintenance.
4. Transport of particulate matter.

All of these functions are explained in depth for the interested student in the survey article by Pauerstein and Woodruff. The assistance of uterine and tubal activity in the transport of semen is recognized by the fact that sperm can be recovered in the tube 5 to 8 minutes after deposition in the vagina. Definite knowledge of capacitation is still incomplete; however, it is known that sperm must be in an atmosphere similar to that of the tube prior to its ability to fertilize the ovum. Pick-up and transport of the egg have been studied at length by numerous investigators —Westman, Doyle, Blandau and others. There seems to be little doubt that the fimbriae, with their predominance of ciliated cells and muscular activity, play the major role in engulfing the ovary and allowing for ovum pick-up. Of interest is the importance of the ampullar-isthmic junction. The con-

centration of adrenergic fibers here justifies the use of the term "sphincter" for this area, and it is well known that the egg, after moving from the fimbriated end to the isthmus in 20 to 30 minutes, must remain here for $1\frac{1}{2}$ days if satisfactory implantation is to occur.

From a pathologic point of view, the transport of particulate matter is of major import. The passage of endometrium from the cavity into the peritoneal cavity has been promoted as a basic cause of endometriosis (Fig. 14–14). Similarly, the transport of tumor cells from the abdominal cavity to the vagina allows for the diagnosis of intra-abdominal lesions by study of the vaginal cytology (Fig. 14–15).

HETEROTOPIC ALTERATIONS IN THE TUBE

As noted above, the tube is part of the paramesonephric system and as such reacts to the same local and systemic stimuli. Furthermore, the epithelium may demonstrate heterotopic alterations as may the epithelia of the cervix and endometrium, although less commonly. Patches of mucinous secreting cells, classic of those seen in the endocervix, may be recognized in the otherwise normal tube; squamous metaplasia is rarely noted (Fig. 14–16).

Most frequently endometrial type elements—both glands and stroma—are appreciated. A remarkable example of this is shown in Figure 14–17. The chief signifi-

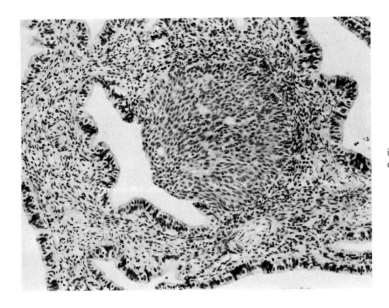

Figure 14–16. Squamous metaplasia in the center with typical tubal epithelium on both sides.

cance of this differentiation anomaly is in its possible bearing on the etiology of tubal pregnancy, as will be discussed in Chapter 28.

The presence of endometrium in the tubal lumen is not uncommon, and Rubin and co-workers found this in nearly 10 per cent of 200 cases in which tubes were also removed during hysterectomy (Fig. 14–18). This was more common in the isthmic portion of the tube and the incidence decreased toward the fimbriated end. Only one third of these cases showed evidence of pelvic endometriosis.

The normal tube may be subjected to a variety of traumas, of which inflammatory reactions are the most common (see Chapter 15).

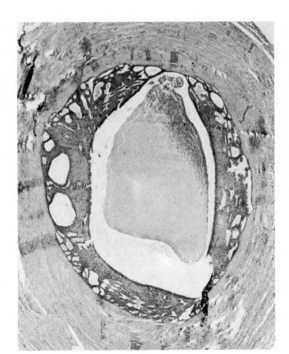

Figure 14–17. Unusual occurrence of typical endometrium surrounding the tubal lumen at about the middle third of the tube. (Courtesy of Dr. Herbert F. Traut, Cornell Medical School.)

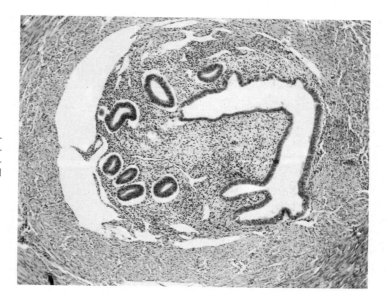

Figure 14–18. Tubal lumen with classic endometrial glands and stroma replacing the endosalpingeal epithelium. A relatively common finding in the cornual region.

Neoplasms are rare but interesting (see Chapter 16). These pathologic conditions alter the normal anatomy. Conversely, torsion may occur in an otherwise normal oviduct (Fig. 14–19). Furthermore, such traumas often result in auto-amputation. The surgeon may be confused when at the time of initial pelvic exploration only one adnexa is present and a calcified nodule may be found in the cul-de-sac. Trauma should be suspected if the tubal stump is present, a finding that differentiates the acquired from the congenital abnormality (the unicornuate uterus).

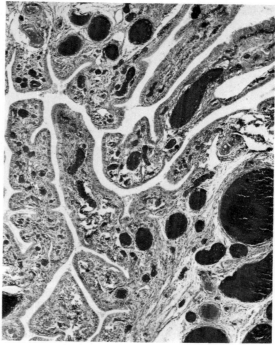

Figure 14–19. Torsion of fallopian tube. Congestion and edema are evident but architecture is otherwise normal.

REFERENCES

Andrews, M. C.: Epithelial changes in the puerperal fallopian tube. Am. J. Obstet. Gynecol., 62:28, 1951.

Blandau, R.: Follicular growth, mechanism of ovulation and egg transport. Symposium on the Physiology and Pathology of Reproduction.

Doyle, J. B.: Tubo-ovarian mechanism: observation at laparotomy. Obstet. Gynecol., 8:686, 1956.

Hartman, C. H.: Personal communication.

Hellman, L. M.: The morphology of human fallopian tube in the early puerperium. Am. J. Obstet. Gynecol., 57:154, 1949.

Mastroianni, L.: The structure and function of the fallopian tube. Clin. Obstet. Gynecol. 5:781, 1962.

Moore, J. W. et al.: Significance of proliferative epithelial lesions of the uterine tube. Obstet. Gynecol., 45:385, 1976.

Nassberg, S., McKay, D. G., and Hertig, A. T.: Physiologic salpingitis. Am. J. Obstet. Gynecol., 67:130, 1954.

Novak, E., and Everett, H. S.: Cyclical and other variations in the tubal epithelium. Am. J. Obstet. Gynecol., 16:499, 1928.

Pauerstein, C. J.: The Fallopian Tube: A Reappraisal. Philadelphia, Lea & Febiger, 1974.

Pauerstein, C. J., and Woodruff, J. D.: Cellular patterns in proliferative and anaplastic disease of the fallopian tube. Obstet. Gynecol., 95:486, 1966.

Pauerstein, C. J., and Woodruff, J. D.: The role of the "indifferent" cell of the tubal epithelium. Am. J. Obstet. Gynecol., 98:121, 1967.

Rubin, S. C., Lisa, J. R., and Trinidad, S.: Further observations of ectopic endometrium of fallopian tube. Surg. Gynecol. Obstet., 103:409, 1956.

Seitchik, J., Goldberg, E., Goldsmith, J. P., and Pauerstein, C. J.: Pharmacodynamic studies of the human fallopian tube in vitro. Am. J. Obstet. Gynecol., 102:727, 1968.

Smith, H. A., and Greene, R. R.: Physiologic endosalpingitis. Am. J. Obstet. Gynecol., 72:174, 1956.

Snyder, F. F.: Changes in the human oviduct during the menstrual cycle and pregnancy. Bull. Johns Hopkins Hosp., 35:141, 1924.

Suzuki, S., and Mastroianni, L.: In vitro fertilization of rabbit ova in tubal fluid. Am. J. Obstet. Gynecol., 93:465, 1965.

Sweeney, W. J.: The interstitial portion of the uterine tube—its gross anatomy, course, and length. Obstet. Gynecol., 19:3, 1962.

Westman, A.: Studies of function of fallopian tubes. Int. J. Fertil., 4:201, 1959.

WHO Symposium: Ovum transport and fertility regulation. Copenhagen, Scriptor, 1976.

Woodruff, J. D., and Pauerstein, C. J.: The Fallopian Tube. Baltimore, Williams & Wilkins Co., 1969.

Chapter 15

SALPINGITIS

PELVIC INFLAMMATORY DISEASE (PID)

Pelvic inflammatory disease has been defined as "a clinical syndrome consisting of a complex combination of symptoms and signs resulting from the ascending contiguous flow of an organism or organisms through the endometrium into the salpinx." Variations on this theme have been introduced by infections associated with pregnancy, use of the intrauterine contraceptive device, or local intra-abominal processes. Due to the importance of the fallopian tube in this sequence of events and the devastating results of tubal infection on subsequent fertility, the following discussion will deal primarily with *salpingitis*.

Etiology

The bacterial causes of salpingitis are primarily the gonococcus plus a host of other aerobic and anaerobic organisms. The tubercle bacillus, a common problem in the past, is today an infrequent cause of such infections in the United States, although still prevalent in some areas of the world.

In the last two decades it has been demonstrated by Ledger and others that, in addition to the commonly accepted organisms noted in previous reports (i.e., the gonococcus and the gram-negative bacilli and gram-positive cocci), anaerobic organisms are important, and often unrecognized, invaders of the tube and adjacent area.

The gonococcus is still the most important cause of pelvic inflammatory disease in the United States, the incidence among all cases varying from 25 to 80 per cent, depending on the geographic area. It is estimated that there are approximately 1 million new cases of gonococcal infection in the female per year (1978) and about 250,000 women are hospitalized with cases of pelvic inflammatory disease.

The gonococcus reaches the fallopian tube from the lower genital canal by way of the endometrium and produces initially an endometritis and a subsequent endosalpingitis. Since the tubal infection is primarily an endosalpingitis, the destructive effect of the infection upon the tubal mucosa often leads to tubal occlusion, a common cause of infertility in the United States. Studies of the intra-abdominal flora in cases of the lower genital canal infection, determined primarily by positive endocervical cultures, demonstrate that only approximately one third of the cases in which the endocervical culture is positive for the gonococcus will the intra-abdominal culture confirm the presence of the intracellular diplococci.

Although pelvic inflammatory disease is associated with other bacteria that may gain access to the pelvis by different pathways (Fig. 15–1), nevertheless the key to appropriate therapy is identification of the offending organism and institution of the appropriate therapy. With refined aerobic and anaerobic cultural techniques, such organisms as *Bacteroides*, the *Peptococcus*, and the *Peptostreptococcus* are found to be frequent invaders.

In recent years, adnexal disease associated with use of the intrauterine device has added a new entity to the long list of pelvic infections. The histopathologic findings are unique in our experience. Although the tube (both the endo- and perisalpinx) is involved, nevertheless the extensive oophoritis with actual abscess formation has been unusual in

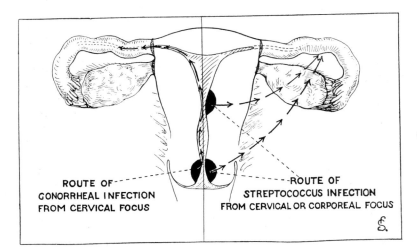

Figure 15–1. Schematic drawing of two chief routes of pelvic infection.

ROUTE OF
GONORRHEAL INFECTION
FROM CERVICAL FOCUS

ROUTE OF
STREPTOCOCCUS INFECTION
FROM CERVICAL OR CORPOREAL FOCUS

the past, excepting only the postoperative ovarian infections and rarely those related to granulomatous disease. Interestingly, both *Chlamydia* and *Actinomyces* have been identified as offending agents, particularly in the patient with an intrauterine device.

In some clinics, laparoscopy has become a routine diagnostic tool. Nevertheless, endocervical cultures and regular therapeutic regimens based on coverage of both aerobic and anaerobic organisms have proved to be effective in a great majority of the cases. Obviously, if the clinical findings suggest that a specific regimen has not been successful after trial for at least 72 hours, modifications in therapy should be seriously considered.

Post-PID Infertility

It has been appreciated in the past that the patient with pelvic inflammatory disease will have a high index of infertility in succeeding years. Recent studies have suggested that with the appropriate therapy for the initial attack, this instance of infertility should be greatly reduced. Most authors have reported that, following a single episode of pelvic inflammatory disease treated appropriately, the incidence of infertility should approximate 15 to 20 per cent. Conversely, with the second episode, this incidence increases to 30 to 35 per cent, and following third or subsequent attacks, infertility approaches 85 to 90 per cent. Again, the importance of early and appropriate therapy is demonstrated by the above figures.

As noted above, the recognition of specific organisms such as the *Bacteroides* (particularly *fragilis* species), anaerobes, and the peptostreptococcus in the adnexal lesion offers the possibility of instituting the most appropriate therapeutic regimen.

Granulomatous Disease

Tuberculous salpingitis is uncommon today. From 1920 to 1950, the tubercle bacillus accounted for 3.9 per cent of all salpingitis; however, less than 0.5 per cent of tubal infections in our laboratory is due to this bacterium. Nevertheless, in other countries, particularly the Far East, such lesions are more frequent. The adolescent is a not uncommon victim of the initial onslaught by the tubercle bacillus. Other infectious agents, such as Schistosoma, are common invaders of the adnexa in Egypt and South Africa. The possibilities exist that lymphogranloma venereum (LGV) and granuloma inguinale may involve the tube; however, definite proof is difficult to document.

ACUTE AND SUBACUTE SALPINGITIS

Acute Endosalpingitis (Gonococcal Type)

Grossly, the tube is red, swollen and turgid, the fimbriated orifice being still patent. From it can be expressed a purulent exudate. The increase in size is due largely to edema. Adhesions, if present, are fibrinous and easily separated.

Microscopically, the rugae of the mucous membrane are edematous because of the in-

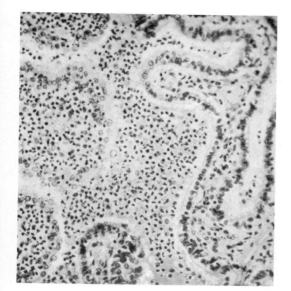

Figure 15–2. Acute salpingitis.

tense inflammatory reaction involving both the epithelium and the subepithelial lamina propria. The epithelium may not be altered; however, it may be denuded in certain foci. Beneath it the tissue is intensely infiltrated with leukocytes, chiefly of the polymorphonuclear variety, and the blood vessels show marked engorgement. The moderately distended lumen is filled with purulent exudate, consisting chiefly of leukocytes and epithelial cells. The leukocytic infiltration in this early stage may be limited almost entirely to the mucosa (Fig. 15–2). In the subacute phase there is more extensive mucosal involvement (Fig. 15-3A), which may eventuate in a panmural infection (Fig. 15–3 B). The escape of the purulent exudate into the peritoneal cavity produces a pelvic peritonitis and may give rise to a *pelvic abscess*. In other cases the extention of the purulent process to the adherent ovary may produce large abscesses involving both organs (*tubo-ovarian abscess*). In the later stages, rupture of such an abscess results in an extremely toxic and shocked patient with a high incidence of such serious complications as subdiaphragmatic or other intraperitoneal abscess, and septicemia. Even though the pus found in such surgical problems is probably gonococcal in origin, the culture is frequently sterile or secondary invaders are found.

As the inflammation tends to subside into a *subacute stage*, there is a greater admixture of mononuclear leukocytes and plasma cells in the inflammatory infiltrate. There is no doubt, however, that in some cases, particularly those of milder type, complete or al-

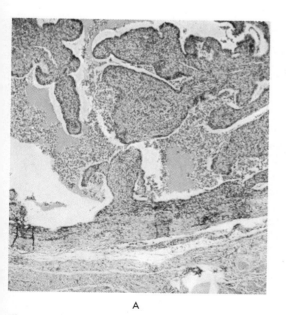

A

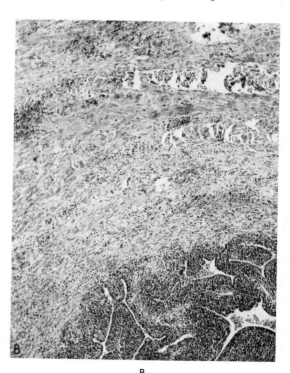

B

Figure 15–3. *A*, Subacute salpingitis. *B*, Severe salpingitis with extensive myosalpingian infiltration—panmural salpingitis.

most complete resolution takes place. This is indicated by the fact that in women in whom gonorrheal infection has been complicated by clinical salpingitis, subsequent operation for other indications has shown essentially normal tubes.

There is rather general agreement that the apparent chronicity of so many cases is due largely to reinfections, as has been suggested by Curtis and others. The elimination of foci in the lower genital canal and the avoidance of coitus with potentially infected partners are therefore of great importance in avoiding the exacerbations which so often mark the course of gonorrheal salpingitis. Even in the first attack, the destructive effect of the infection upon the mucous membrane may bring about occlusion of the tube, either at the fimbriated end or at various points along the course of the oviduct. As a result of such obstruction, the purulent exudate may distend the lumen with the eventual production of a pyosalpinx. More frequently, however, this sequel is noted in tubes in which repeated exacerbations have occurred.

Pyogenic Type

The enlargement of the tube in this type of infection is commonly much greater than with acute gonorrheal salpingitis. The fact that this enlargement is due to interstitial involvement rather than to distention of the lumen is apparent on cross section. The lumen is thus seen to be of normal or almost normal size, while the tube wall is enormously thickened and edematous.

Microscopically, the mucosa may show little more than a slight edema with an essentially normal epithelium. The muscularis, however, shows marked edema and an acute inflammatory infiltrate, often directly continuous with similar involvement of the mesosalpinx. There may be fine fibrinous peritoneal adhesions and these may at times cause matting down of the fimbriated end, with occlusion later. There are, however, numerous exceptions to this, as already mentioned.

CHRONIC SALPINGITIS

The chronic form of salpingitis may manifest itself in four chief forms, viz.: (1) pyosalpinx, (2) hydrosalpinx, (3) chronic interstitial salpingitis, and (4) follicular salpingitis. Previously (5) salpingitis isthmica nodosa was included in this category, but there is doubt

at present as to whether such alterations are the result of an inflammatory process. In rare instances the exudate in the lumen may be somewhat bloody (hematosalpinx), but hematosalpinx is far more frequently caused by tubal pregnancy or, much less often, by gynatresia.

Pyosalpinx

This condition is a sequel of gonorrheal salpingitis in the great majority of cases, though it may occur with other inflammatory processes. It is the result of blockage of the tubal lumen at the fimbriated orifice, combined with complete or partial blockage at the isthmus or at various other points in the tube. The accumulated purulent exudate is thus retained, producing tubal distention (Fig. 15–4). In order to induce such dilatation, the preceding inflammatory process must produce acute distention with obstruction, to the end that agglutination of the mucosal folds is reduced to a minimum. Such tubes are generally adherent to surrounding structures, because of the associated perisalpingitis.

Microscopically, the lumen is found to be distended with pus, while the folds are distorted and usually flattened from the pressure of the exudate in the lumen. The stroma is infiltrated with lymphocytes, leukocytes, and plasma cells, the involvement extending throughout the muscularis, sometimes diffusely, sometimes in scattered interstitial foci. The peritoneal involvement is demonstrated by the presence of organized adhesions, sometimes densely cicatricial. The peritoneal mesothelium beneath the adhesions often exhibits proliferations with adenomatous and papillary formations. These may at times be wrongly interpreted as representing endometriosis. Bizarre patterns, suggestive of malignancy, may develop when the mesothelial reaction produces not only adenomatous changes, but also agglutination of the cells with giant cell formation (Fig. 15–5). Psammoma bodies are frequent findings, as they are with any chronic irritative process, and do not indicate any atypical or neoplastic proliferation.

While pyosalpinx is usually indicative of a chronic tubal infection, acute exacerbations are common, so that the picture of an acute inflammatory flare-up may be superimposed on that of the chronic process characterizing most cases of pyosalpinx.

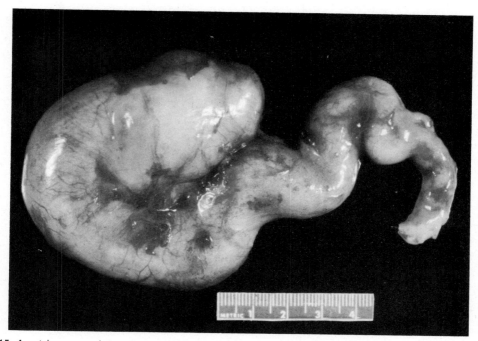

Figure 15–4. A large pyosalpinx. Patient had had recurrent bouts of pelvic pain and febrile reaction. On one occasion a pelvic abscess had been drained by colpotomy.

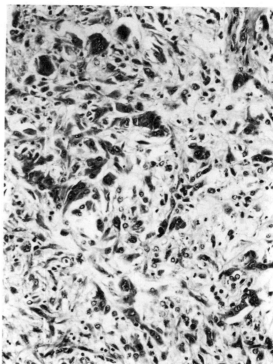

Figure 15–5. Bizarre mesothelial reaction with giant cell formation and adenoid areas in chronic adhesive salpingitis.

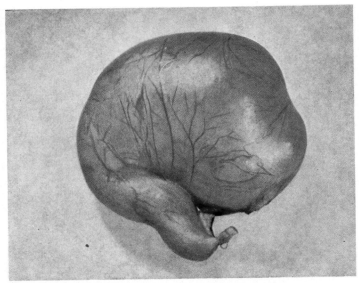

Figure 15–6. Large thin-walled hydrosalpinx.

Hydrosalpinx

Hydrosalpinx is practically always an end result of pyosalpinx. With resorption of the purulent exudate, a clear watery fluid remains. Hydrosalpinx, therefore, is especially apt to be encountered when there is a history of long-standing infection, with no exacerbations for many years. The tubal enlargement may be enormous, or relatively slight, with or without extensive adhesions. At times the lumen of the hydrosalpinx merges with the cavity of a cyst in the adjoining adherent ovary, giving rise to the so-called *tubo-ovarian cyst*. When the hydrosalpinx is very large, it tends to assume a characteristic retort-like shape (Fig. 15–6). Occasionally a hydrosalpinx may undergo torsion, like an ovarian cyst (Fig. 15–7).

The walls of a hydrosalpinx are thin and often translucent, so that the condition may be diagnosed grossly even before sectioning. The fimbriae are inverted and obliterated, with complete closure of the abdominal orifice, the end of the tube being rounded and bulbous. On cutting across the tube, one of two pictures will be encountered, leading to a subdivision into two varieties of hydrosalpinx.

Hydrosalpinx Simplex. In this variety the distended tube forms a single lumen, the tubal rugae being flattened out against the wall. Often they are so atrophied that only a few small folds project from the otherwise smooth surface. The epithelium is flattened, except for that of the small remaining folds, where the normal characteristics exist. Neither the mucosa nor the muscularis shows any appreciable evidence of the original inflammatory process, indicating the long du-

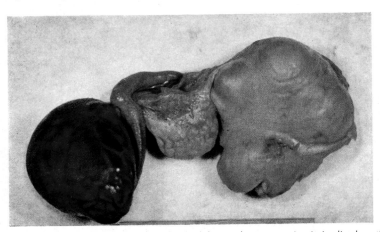

Figure 15–7. Moderate-sized hydrosalpinx which has undergone torsion in its distal portion.

ration and the relative quiescence of the condition.

Hydrosalpinx Follicularis. Here again the tubal lumen is distended with clear fluid, but instead of being unilocular, it is divided into many compartments by trabeculae which often present a complicated pattern, as seen on cross section. This type is explained by the fact that adjoining rugae have adhered and merged one with another, forming gutter-like compartments between them. This form of hydrosalpinx differs from follicular salpingitis only in the cystic overdistention characterizing the former (Figs. 15–8 and 15–9).

Chronic Interstitial Salpingitis

The tube is enlarged, sometimes enormously. The enlargement is due not so much to distention of the tube with exudate, but rather to the great thickness of the wall itself. The fimbriated extremity is completely or only partially closed, usually with inversion of the fimbriae, though some of the latter may still be visible externally. Very frequently the end of the tube, when completely sealed, is rounded and bulbous, and practically always the tube is adherent to surrounding structures (perisalpingitis), especially the

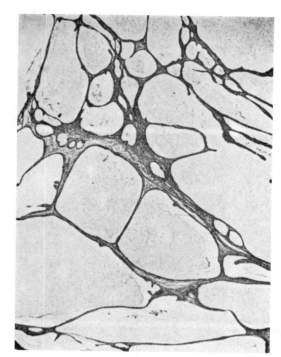

Figure 15–9.   Section of hydrosalpinx follicularis.

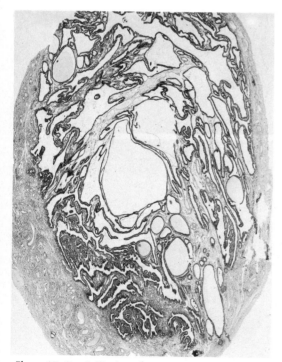

Figure 15–8.   Follicular salpingitis, with multilocular appearance produced by agglutination of folds.

ovaries and the posterior surface of the broad ligament (Fig. 15–10).

Microscopically, one finds extensive infiltration of all the tubal layers, but especially of the mucosa, usually with plasma cells and histiocytes. The epithelium is usually intact, with inflammatory adhesions between adjacent folds. At times the epithelium is proliferative and pseudostratified (Fig. 15–11). Increase in the number of indifferent cells is striking, but mitoses are not seen, thus differentiating these lesions from anaplastic change. Merging of rugae is often very marked; a cross section of the tube may present an intricate multilocular or adenoma-like pattern, giving rise to the designation of chronic *follicular salpingitis.* In addition to this adenomatous pattern, a pseudopapillary picture may result from this chronic recurrent inflammatory process (Fig. 15–12).

Tubal pregnancy may be due to a fertilized ovum wandering into the cul-de-sac of one of the gutter-like compartments between the adherent folds, presupposing that the tubal lumen is at least partially open to permit the meeting of the sperm and ovum.

Salpingitis Isthmica Nodosa

Salpingitis isthmica nodosa is a lesion presumably resulting from the residue of a

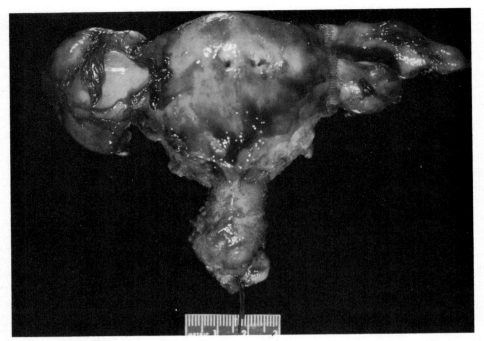

Figure 15–10. Chronic salpingitis with thickened tubes and associated periovarian and periuterine adhesions. Mesothelial reactions as noted in Figure 15–5 are common and sometimes confusing, particularly to the cytologist.

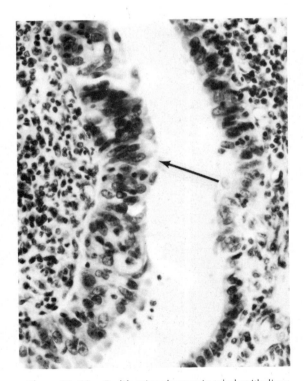

Figure 15–11. Proliferative changes in tubal epithelium associated with inflammatory disease. Pseudostratification is evident (at arrow). Mitoses are absent.

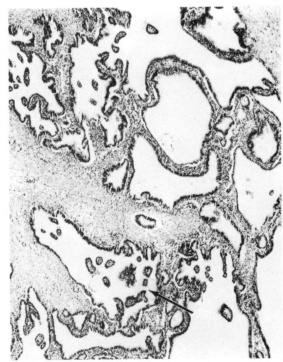

Figure 15–12. Adenomatous pattern with pseudopapillae associated with follicular salpingitis (at arrow).

chronic interstitial salpingitis. *Grossly*, this condition is characterized by the presence of one or more firm nodules in the isthmic portion of the tube and often involving the superior surface of the adjoining uterine cornu. These nodules may be no larger than a buckshot in some cases, but in others they may be large, perhaps as much as 2 cm. in diameter, so that they then have a definitely neoplastic appearance.

The *microscopic* appearance has given rise to much discussion. Aside from the great thickening of the muscularis, the striking microscopic feature suggests that the tubal lumen has apparently been split up into numerous small canals, so that in marked cases an adenomatous picture may be noted. As a rule the small tubal lumen can be identified, as well as many other epithelium-lined spaces scattered throughout the muscularis, at various distances between the lumen proper and the serosa. A mild inflammatory infiltrate may be noted in the lamina propria; however, this is frequently absent.

Although the name implies an inflammatory process, there are some who suggest that salpingitis isthmica nodosa results from a direct invasion of the muscularis by the epithelium, resembling the process similar to that associated with adenomyosis of the uterus. Mechanically, it is difficult to envision the agglutination of the few tiny mucosal folds of the isthmus with the resultant extensive muscular "invasion" by the adenomatous process. In the ampullary area such a sequence of events is easily demonstrable in the follicular salpingitis.

Investigators have suggested that these lesions represent endometriosis of the tube. Nevertheless, although it is not uncommon to find endometrium in the tube, being present either in the lumen, as noted in Chapter 14, in the wall near the cornua, or in the serosa as with generalized pelvic endometriosis, the presence of endometrial stroma is the key diagnostic feature, and this is generally absent in salpingitis isthmica nodosa. The presence of tubal epithelium in these adenomatous foci is not a deterrent to the diagnosis of endometriosis since endosalpingeal elements are common findings in the endometrium within the fundus. It is not uncommon to find a mixture of typical tubal and endometrial foci adjacent to one another in such cases (Figs. 15–13 and 15–14). On occasion, proliferative processes suggestive of those seen in the ovarian tumor of low ma-

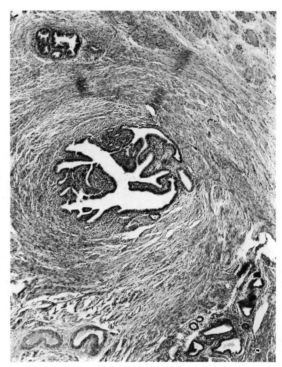

Figure 15–13. Salpingitis isthmica nodosa showing lumen with endometrium-like stroma and adenomatous nests in the muscle. Stroma can be recognized surrounding the glands in the myosalpinx.

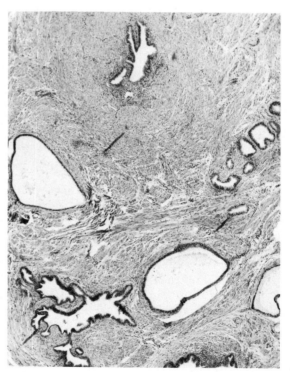

Figure 15–14. Section taken at another level in same lesion as in Figure 15–13. Adenomatous structures are lined by tubal epithelium and stroma is missing.

lignant potential may be recognized in one or more of the intramuscular inclusions. This may be associated with other demonstrations in tube, ovary, and adjacent peritoneum of such mesothelial hyperactivity similar to those seen in many irritative reactions in the pelvic peritoneum.

GRANULOMATOUS SALPINGITIS

TUBERCULOUS SALPINGITIS

Incidence

The major type of granulomatous salpingitis is that produced by the tubercle bacillus. This important but at present infrequent form of tubal disease at one time constituted almost 5 per cent of all cases of salpingitis, but in recent years, the incidence of such infections in the pelvic organs has diminished due to control of the infectious processes.

Modes of Infection

As noted by many authors, such as Tovell and Ganem, pelvic tuberculosis is commonly a reflection of systemic disease, and behaves as such. Tubal tuberculosis is always secondary to a focus elsewhere in the body; however, it is almost always the primary seat of tuberculosis in the female genital organs. In fact, if there is involvement of endometrium, cervix, or lower genital tract, one can say with almost 100 per cent assurance that there is primary tubal disease, and various studies bear out this thesis.

The tubercle bacilli reach the tube by one of several routes, most frequently by the bloodstream from a distant focus, generally the lung, but occasionally the urinary tract or abdominal cavity. The primary pulmonary disease may be in an active stage, but frequently it is quiescent. Sometimes the pulmonary focus heals with no residua, and the secondary process may remain dormant in the tube for years to flourish at a later date. In a postmortem study of patients dying of pulmonary tuberculosis, 4 to 5 per cent were found to have an unsuspected tubal infection.

Gross Characteristics

The macroscopic appearance of the tuberculous tube is not distinctive, so that in the majority of cases the diagnosis is not made until microscopic examination. There are, however, instances in which the tubal peritoneum, like the peritoneum generally, may be studded with tubercles, thus identifying the process as being of granulomatous origin, especially if there is an associated ascites. Nevertheless, much more frequently the gross picture of tuberculous salpingitis may be similar to that of chronic salpingitis of nontuberculous nature, presenting as a chronic interstitial salpingitis, a pyosalpinx, a follicular hydrosalpinx, or a salpingitis isthmica nodosa. When tuberculous pyosalpinx exists, a cross section of the tube may reveal a cheesy necrotic exudate and caseation of the tubal wall. In the occasional case of tuberculous salpingitis isthmica nodosa, the distal portion of the tube may seem essentially normal.

There is one gross characteristic which points to the probability of tuberculosis, though it is noted in only about half of the cases. In the common chronic gonorrheal salpingitis, the fimbriated end of the tube is characteristically closed and bulbous, with inversion and obliteration of the fimbriae. In the tuberculous tube, on the other hand, there is a tendency for the fimbriae to remain everted, with patency of the orifice even when the tube proper is much enlarged and distended (Fig. 15–15 and 15–16). There is thus produced the characteristic tobacco-pouch appearance, and when this is noted, there is justification for suspecting the probability of tuberculosis.

The fact that the tubal orifice tends to remain open explains the frequent exacerbations which mark the clinical course of tubal tuberculosis, and which are often due to periodic expulsion of exudate into the pelvic cavity, with flare-up of fever and pain.

On the other hand, pelvic and (thereby) tubal tuberculosis is frequently asymptoniatic and represents a chance finding in sterility work-ups. Rubin's test is frequently successful and the endometrium often shows a secretory pattern though riddled with tuberculosis. These cases of so-called "silent pelvic tuberculosis" represent the greatest indication for medical treatment. Halbrecht found 21 of 31 pregnancies following medical treatment to be extrauterine, with five others terminating in abortion. In addition, the chance of advanced acid-fast disease must always be considered. Although the initial reports on pregnancy following

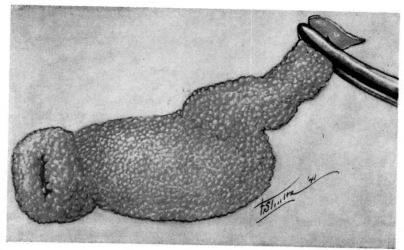

Figure 15–15. Gross appearance of tuberculous salpingitis, in this case associated with tuberculous peritonitis.

medical treatment were discouraging, recent studies are more promising. Consequently, most authorities propose long-term antibiotic-chemotherapy regimes. It must be recognized that persistent adnexal masses should be removed, and further, that there may be an occasional case that flares up during therapy.

Microscopic Diagnosis

The microscopic diagnosis of tubal tuberculosis may be easy or difficult. In advanced cases, the extensive granulomatous reaction in the tubal folds, with caseation, and the presence of typical tubercles establishes the diagnosis. The tubercles and the chronic inflammation involve the muscularis and serosa as well as the mucosa (Figs. 15–17 and 15–18). Special stains and cultures are needed to confirm the diagnosis; however, since in many cases the process is quiescent, these studies may be negative.

In most cases, however, the disease is occult, only an occasional tubercle being found in the mucous membrane, which otherwise

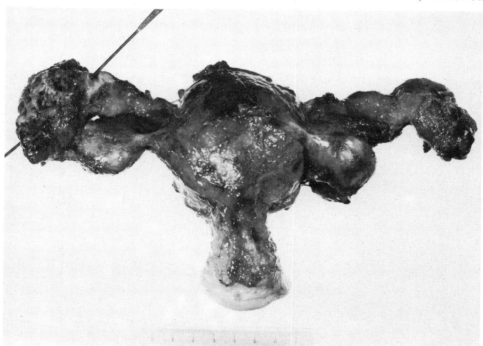

Figure 15–16. Tuberculous salpingitis. Probe shows edematous but patent fimbriated end.

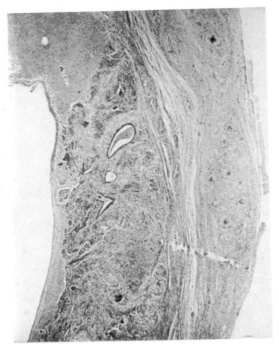

Figure 15–17. Advanced tuberculosis of tube, with tuberculous infiltration and caseation of mucosa, and tubercles, with giant cells, on the serosa (at right).

blocks of the tube, with the study of many sections, may be necessary before one finds telltale evidence in the form of characteristic tubercles.

Attention must be directed to the microscopic picture, which should always make one highly suspicious of tuberculosis, even if tubercles or extensive epithelioid reaction is not seen. The striking adenomatous pattern frequently produced by the proliferative changes in the rugae, and the tendency of the folds to merge, so that an intricate glandlike picture is produced suggestive of adenocarcinoma (Figs. 15–19 and 15–20). As a matter of fact, some cases reported as adenocarcinoma of the tube have really been instances of this exaggerated form of follicular salpingitis seen in many cases of tubal tuberculosis. Therefore, whenever such a picture is encountered, tuberculosis should be suspected, and very thorough study of sections from all parts of the tube should be made.

OTHER GRANULOMATOUS DISEASES

Obviously, tuberculous infection must be suspected with the patterns just described; however, proof lies only in the demonstration of the tubercle bacillus in tissue or by cultural techniques. Other diseases, such as the lymphogranuloma, syphilis, fungus, schistosomiasis (Fig. 15–21 A, B), and sar-

presents an appearance not different from chronic gonorrheal salpingitis. Moreover, it should be remembered that there is a strong regenerative tendency, so that in longstanding cases the tube presents the ordinary microscopic appearance of chronic salpingitis, most often of the follicular type. Numerous

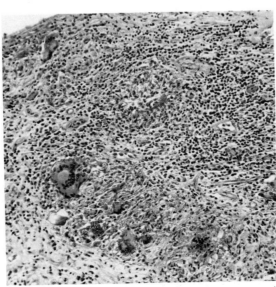

Figure 15–18. Granulomatous reaction on peritoneal surface of tube.

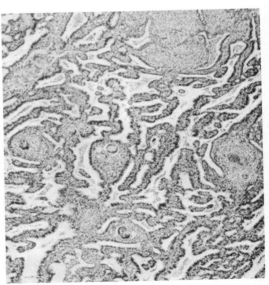

Figure 15–19. Tubal tuberculosis, with typical tubercles and giant cells, and marked proliferation of the tubal folds.

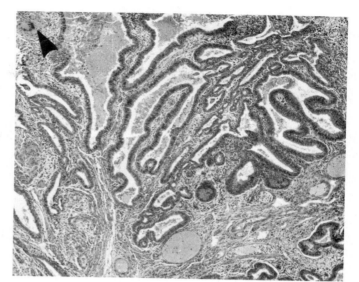

Figure 15–20. Adenomatous reaction associated with tuberculosis tubercle at arrow.

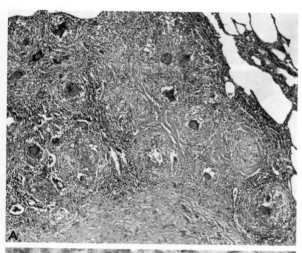

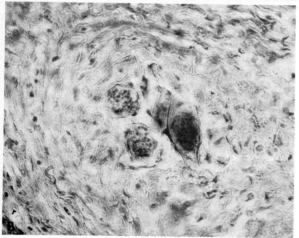

Figure 15–21. *A*, Bilharzial infection in fallopian tube. Note the granulomatous reaction. *B*, High power view of bilharziasis with classic granuloma.

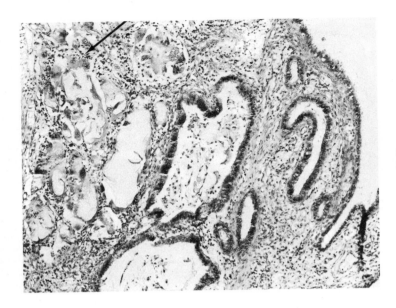

Figure 15–22. Salpingitis due to foreign body (oil) in tube with giant cell formation (at arrow).

coid, may produce similar microscopic pictures.

Although the granulomatous diseases, such as lymphogranuloma, syphilis, and granuloma inguinale, are well documented infections in the lower genital canal, there has been little interest in studying their upper canal manifestations. In Egypt and South Africa, schistosomiasis is common and adnexal involvement is well known. The careful pathologist should be aware of such possibilities since treatment is more effective if a positive diagnosis can be rendered. Two cases of actinomycosis in tubo-ovarian inflammatory disease have been recognized in our laboratory in the past 24 months.

Giant cells may result from foreign bodies, such as suture material from previous operative procedures or nonabsorbable material, such as iodized oil, introduced into the tube for diagnostic study (Fig. 15–22).

PERISALPINGITIS

Perisalpingitis may be found in association with a variety of pelvic and intra-abdominal infections. Not uncommonly, the acutely infected appendix or diverticulum may lie in the pelvis and the tube be involved by direct extension. The postabortal pelvic abscess similarly may produce a marked perisalpingitis. Interestingly, the high incidence of infertility associated with endosalpingitis is not true in those patients with a purely perisalpingian infection.

REFERENCES

Blinick, G.: Gonorrheal disease in the female. Clin. Obstet. Gynecol., 2:492, 1959.

Bobrow, M. L., Winkelstein, L. B., and Friedman, S.: Streptomycin in advanced pelvic tuberculosis. Obstet. Gynecol., 8:299, 1956.

Bromberg, Y. M., and Rozin, S.: Pregnancies in cases of endometrial tuberculosis treated by streptomycin. J. Obstet. Gynaecol. Br. Emp., 61:121, 1954.

Brown, A. B., Gilbert, C. R. A., and TeLinde, R. W.: Pelvic tuberculosis. Obstet. Gynecol., 2:476, 1953.

Chalvardgian, A.: Sarcoidosis of the genital tract. Am. J. Obstet. Gynecol., 132:78, 1978.

Collins, C. G., and Jansen, F. W.: Treatment of pelvic abscess. Clin. Obstet. Gynecol., 2:512, 1959.

Collins, C. G., Nix, F. G., and Cerha, H. T.: Ruptured tubo-ovarian abscess. Am. J. Obstet. Gynecol., 72:820, 1956.

Curtis, A. H.: Chronic pelvic infections. Surg. Gynecol. Obstet., 42:6, 1926.

Curtis, A. H.: Bacteriology and pathology of fallopian tubes removed at operation. Surg. Gynecol. Obstet., 33:621, 1921.

Earn, A. A.: Living births following drug therapy for infertility associated with proven genital tuberculosis. J. Obstet. Gynaecol. Br. Emp., 65:739, 1958.

Frost, O.: Bilharzia of the fallopian tube. S. Afr. Med. J., 49:1201, 1975.

Gardner, G. H.: The more common pelvic infections, their etiology, pathology, differential diagnosis, treatment and prevention. Northwest Med., 34:417, 1935.

Golde, S. H., Israel, R., and Ledger, W. J.: Tubo-ovarian abscess, unilateral: a distinct entity. Am. J. Obstet. Gynecol., 1127:807, 1902.

Greenberg, J. P.: Tuberculous salpingitis, a clinical study of 200 cases. Johns Hopkins Hosp. Rev., 21:1921.

Haines, M.: Genital tuberculosis in the female. (Discussion by Stallworthy, J., Ten Berge, B. S., Sharman, A., Sutherland, A. M. et al.) J. Obstet. Gynaecol. Br. Emp., 59:721, 1952.

Halbrecht, I.: Latent genital tuberculosis in women, its

early diagnosis and treatment. Tuberk.-Arzt, *12*:712, 1958.

Hedberg, E., and Spetz, S. O.: Acute salpingitis; views on prognosis and treatment. Acta Obstet. Gynecol. Scand., *37*:131, 1958.

Kistner, R. W., Hertig, A. T., and Rock, J.: Tubal pregnancy complicating tuberculous salpingitis. Am. J. Obstet. Gynecol., *62*:1157, 1951.

Ledger, W. J.: Infection in the Female. Philadelphia, Lea & Febiger, 1977.

Pauerstein, C. J.: Reappraisal of Fallopian Tube. Philadelphia, Lea & Febiger, 1974.

Pauerstein, C. J., and Woodruff, J. D.: The Fallopian Tube. Baltimore, Williams & Wilkins Co., 1969.

Schaefer, G.: Tuberculosis as a cause of female sterility. Am. Rev. Tuberc., *70*:1096, 1954.

Schaefer, G.: Treatment of female genital tuberculosis. Proc. Roy. Soc. Med., *52*:947, 1959.

Schenken, J. R., and Burns, E. L.: Diverticula of tubes, study and classification of nodular lesions: "salpingitis isthmica nodosa." Am. J. Obstet. Gynecol., *45*:624, 1943.

Sharman, A.: Endometrial tuberculosis in sterility. Fertil. Steril., *3*:144, 1952.

Siegler, A. M.: Tuberculosis of the uterine tubes. Obstet. Gynecol., *6*:188, 1955.

Studdiford, W. S.: Pregnancy and pelvic tuberculosis. Am. J. Obstet. Gynecol., *69*:379, 1955.

Sutherland, A. M.: Female genital tuberculosis: a critical review of literature from 1940 to 1949. Glasg. Med. J., *31*:279, 1950.

Sutherland, A. M.: Genital tuberculosis in women. Am. J. Obstet. Gynecol., *79*:486, 1960.

Tovell, H. M. M., and Ganem, K. J.: Pelvic tuberculosis: Review of 87 cases. N.Y. State J. Med., *57*:2367, 1957.

Vermeeren, J., and TeLinde, R. W.: Intra-abdominal rupture of pelvic abscesses. Am. J. Obstet. Gynecol., *68*:402, 1954.

Westrom, L.: Effect of acute pelvic inflammatory disease on fertility. Am. J. Obstet. Gynecol., *121*:707, 1975.

Westrom, L., Skude, G., and Mradh, P. A.: Peritoneal fluid isoamylases in acute salpingitis. Am. J. Obstet. Gynecol., *126*:657, 1976.

Chapter 16

TUMORS OF THE TUBE, PAROVARIUM, AND UTERINE LIGAMENTS

Primary tubal neoplasms, except for "tumors" of inflammatory origin, are rare. Secondary involvement of the tube, however, from lesions arising in the adjacent organs is common. Consequently, a preoperative diagnosis of true tubal tumor is uncommon.

BENIGN TUMORS

The rarity of benign lesions is recognized in such reports as that of Roberts and Marshall, who in 1961 could accumulate only 54 cases of fibromyoma, one of which weighed 2 kg. Zelinger and co-workers in 1960 collected 33 instances of dermoid cyst of the tube. The experience in our laboratory has shown that most such neoplasms have arisen in either the adjacent ovary or the fundus and involved the tube secondarily. Microscopically, these tumors resemble in every respect the similar lesions described elsewhere in the pelvis.

The adenomatoid tumors are the most notable of the benign tubal neoplasms (Fig. 16–1). These are found in the broad ligament and fundus as well as in the tube, and have been reported by Teel in the homologous areas of the male genital tract, i.e., the epididymus and cord. Electron microscopic studies have documented that these tumors are of mesothelial origin. Undoubtedly the term adenomatoid was applied to such lesions because of the lack of unanimity of opinion as to

pathogenesis. Grossly, the tumors are rarely more than 1 to 2 cm. in greatest dimension; however, multiple foci may be seen, particularly near the cornua of the fundus. They are not diagnosed preoperatively or even at surgery in most instances due to their unimpressive gross characteristics. Microscopically, the tumor is made up of a mass of small tubules lined by a flattened or low cuboidal epithelium (Fig. 16–2). The cytoplasm of the epithelial cell contains minor amounts of mucopolysaccharide and is therefore periodic acid–Schiff (PAS) positive. Mitoses are absent, and thus, although the lesions suggest malignancy because of the marked adenomatous appearance and disturbance of

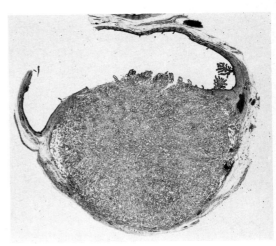

Figure 16–1. Adenomatoid tumor.

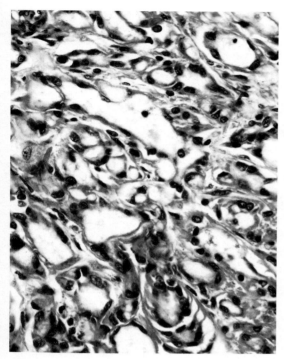

Figure 16–2. High power view of adenomatoid tumor.

the tubal architecture, they do not cause necrosis of the involved tissue, nor do they metastasize.

TUBAL POLYPS AND PAPILLOMAS

Tubal polyps and papillomas have been described intermittently, but accurate histology of such lesions has not been documented. The apparent finding of polypoid lesions in the cornua by hysterosalpingography is unsatisfactory evidence of their existence. There has not been a documented instance of such a lesion in the files of the Gynecologic Pathology department at the Johns Hopkins Hospital. Nevertheless, the malignant counterpart, papillary carcinoma, is well known, if rare; however, histologic study of such lesions does not suggest the development in a polyp.

ENDOMETRIOSIS

Endometriosis may be seen in the interstitial portion of the tube, usually as an exten-

sion of endometrium from the cavity of the uterus. In the occasional case, however, it appears to originate in this region, and Sampson has described endometriosis arising in the stumps of amputated tubes. Recent experience suggests that recanalization of the tube following tubal sterilization may result from such a process, with penetration of the muscularis by the endometrial invasion.

Unless characteristic uterine glands and stroma are found in the tubal walls, one should hesitate in applying the designation of endometriosis; nevertheless, extensive involvement may be appreciated in both lumen and musculature (Fig. 16–3 A). Nodular alterations in the cornual and isthmical portions of the tube have been most frequently alluded to as salpingitis isthmica nodosa (Fig. 16–3 B); the arguments as to histogenesis are discussed more fully in Chapter 15.

CARCINOMA OF THE TUBE

Primary Carcinoma

This is a comparatively rare lesion; approximately 1000 cases are to be found in the literature. Approximately 0.2 to 0.5 per cent of all primary malignancies of the genital canal arise in the tube, the variations in frequency ranging from 0.15 to 1.8 per cent. In the 230 cases accumulated by Sedlis, the mean age was 52 years, the tumor was bilateral in 26 per cent of the cases, and the 5 year salvage was a surprisingly high 34 per cent.

Chronic inflammation of the tube has been suggested as an important predisposing factor; however, the great frequency of the latter as contrasted to the rarity of tubal carcinoma would incline one to doubt such a relationship. The same doubt exists as to the possible influence of tubal tuberculosis, which, in a number of instances, has been found to coexist with carcinoma. It is probable that in at least some of the latter the combination was wrongly interpreted because of the adenocarcinoma-like picture seen in some cases of tuberculous salpingitis, as described in the preceding chapter.

Carcinoma of the tube is almost never diagnosed preoperatively. Adnexal enlargements generally are interpreted as ovarian neoplasia, inflammatory disease, or pedunculated leiomyomatosis. Goetz reports that

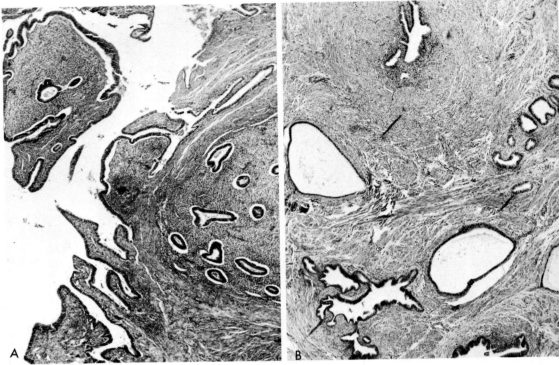

Figure 16–3. *A,* Diffuse endometriosis in both lamina propria and muscularis. *B,* Salpingitis isthmica nodosa simulating endometriosis.

in only 2 of 577 cases was a correct diagnosis rendered before surgery.

Diagnosis and Differential Diagnosis

Because of the infrequency of these lesions and the nonspecific nature of the physical findings, the correct preoperative diagnosis of tubal malignancy rarely is made. The palpable mass is usually diagnosed as an ovarian tumor or tubo-ovarian inflammatory mass.

Salpingography has been suggested as an aid in differentiating adnexal lesions. Because of the possibility of mechanically spreading the disease, this procedure has not been widely accepted. Cytopathologic study of vaginal smears has led to the early diagnosis of an occasional tubal malignancy. Fidler and Lock, and Brewer and Guderian, recorded isolated instances of the positive diagnosis of tubal cancer by this method. These reports serve to emphasize the value of routine cytologic investigation. Laparoscopy may play a role in evaluating the "negative pelvis" of a patient with recurrent postmenopausal bleeding, and ultrasonog-

raphy may define a nonpalpable mass. Nevertheless, in the patient with any suspicion of intrapelvic disease, laparotomy with definitive therapy is the most appropriate approach to the problem.

Gross Pathology

In the advanced case the macroscopic appearance of primary tubal carcinoma is quite characteristic. The tube is enlarged and sausage-shaped, and gives the impression of a huge pyosalpinx, except that, unlike the latter, adhesions to surrounding structures (Fig. 16–4) are rare except in the advanced case. The external surface is usually quite smooth. Most frequently the disease arises in the middle or outer third of the tube. When the neoplasm is encountered in an earlier stage, only a localized nodular enlargement at the involved area may be noted, though there may be dilation of the proximal tube as a result of the retention of a serosanguineous or actually bloody exudate (Fig. 16–4). The tubal wall itself may be normal in thickness or thinner than normal even with large growths.

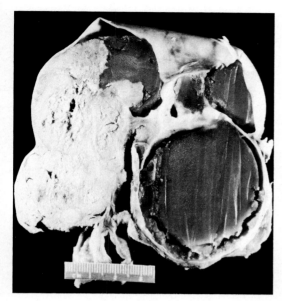

Figure 16–4. Primary carcinoma of the tube showing the dilated lumen on the right filled with coagulated fluid and the solid tumor mass on the left. (Smooth, thinned tubal musculature is grossly free.)

The fimbriated ends are either patent or occluded in approximately equal numbers of cases. Similarly, bilateral involvement is present in about half the lesions. For the most part, the latter finding represents tumor arising in "paired organs," and thus is not an example of lymphatic or direct extension, as previously reported (Fig. 16–5).

Microscopic Appearance

Tubal carcinoma presents generally as a papillary or an alveolar type of histologic appearance, although an admixture is frequent. Classifications have been suggested by various authors:

Sanger and Barth
  a. Papillary carcinoma
  b. Papillary alveolar carcinoma (corresponding to adenocarcinoma of the uterus)

Hu, Taymor, and Hertig
  a. Papillary (Fig. 16–6)
  b. Papillary alveolar (Fig. 16–7)
  c. Alveolar medullary (Fig. 16–8)

The papillary type is more common and characteristic, and the papillary alveolar pattern probably results from the fusion of adjoining papillae, simulating a glandular pattern (Fig. 16–7A).

In the differential histopathologic diagnosis of tubal carcinoma, especially of the papillary alveolar variety, it is worth reemphasizing that tubal tuberculosis may produce a highly adenomatous picture which can be mistaken for carcinoma (Chapter 15).

The microscopic appearance of the common papillary variety is very characteristic. Springing from the wall of the tube are tree-like papillae, which tend to fill the lumen (Fig. 16–6A, B). Instead of the normal tubal epithelium, the papillae are covered with a multilayered atypical epithelium (Fig. 16–7B). Mitoses are frequent but not bizarre. The increased number of indifferent cells is dramatic. Nevertheless, the muscular wall of the tube is involved only late in the disease (Fig. 16–7A). Consequently, even in the latter stages of the disease with extensive local

Figure 16–5. Large tubal carcinoma on the right with smaller, pyosalpinx-like lesion on left. Tumor had begun at various points in the left tube.

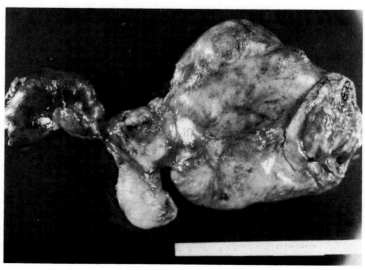
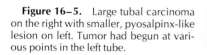

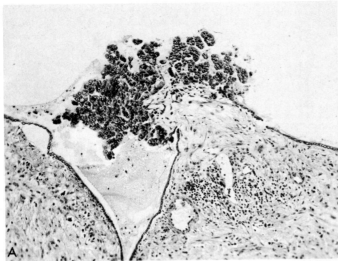

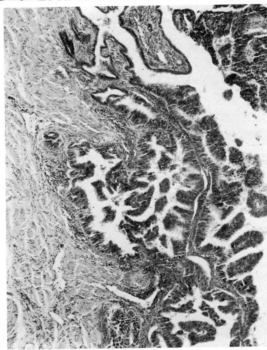

Figure 16–6. *A*, Small papillary lesion adjacent to a more proliferative papillary alveolar carcinoma. *B*, Early lesion showing origin from normal tubal epithelium and demonstrating classic papillary pattern.

proliferation, the common demonstration of early stromal invasion in other malignancies is often absent. In view of the above, staging is difficult and cannot be evaluated as for other pelvic neoplasias.

In many cases, both tube and ovary are involved by cancer, and since ovarian carcinoma commonly presents a histologic appearance identical to tubal malignancy, the tendency is to consider that the tubal lesion is secondary. When, however, there is only superficial involvement of the gonad, and when the characteristic alveolar papillary architecture coexists with extensive intratubal disease, the diagnosis of a primary tubal tumor must be seriously entertained (Fig. 16–8).

Carcinoma In Situ

Several cases of carcinoma in situ have been reported and generally have been microscopic findings. Such malignant alterations consist of multilayered epithelium with individual cell neoplasia. In the well-

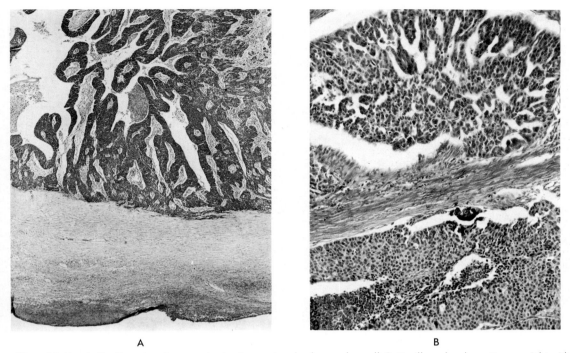

A   B

Figure 16–7. *A*, Papillomatous tumor springing from uninvolved muscular wall. *B*, Papillary alveolar pattern on right with alveolar medullary tumor on left.

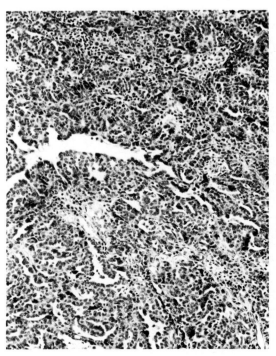

Figure 16–8. Tubopapillary mesothelioma of tube(?)—tumor diffuse throughout pelvis.

differentiated lesion, cilia may be appreciated, as is consistent with the changes seen in the low grade papillary tumor of the ovary. Of interest is the occasional in situ malignancy of the tube associated with primary ovarian or endometrial cancer. These concomitant findings suggest the presence of a common stimulating agent affecting epithelia of similar embryologic origin at multiple sites (Fig. 16–9).

It is important to remember that proliferations of the tubal epithelium are noted with inflammatory disease and with excess estrogen stimulation. These are not anaplastic alterations. The only valid evidence of malignancy, as suggested by Pauerstein and Woodruff, is the presence of mitoses, rarely noted in the normal tube.

Malignancy and Mode of Extension

Primary carcinoma of the tube is known as a very malignant tumor because of the low 5 year salvage. Thorough evaluation of these lesions, however, suggests that the problem is late diagnosis rather than high degree of malignancy. In one reported case, a tumor had been palpated 18 years prior to surgery for the lesion. Furthermore, the extent of the intratubal lesion compared to the evidence of invasion of the wall is not indicative of early and rapid spread.

The disease may extend through the open tubal orifice into the peritoneum; however, in more invasive lesions the lymphatics play an important role in the dissemination of the disease. Perhaps a previous salpingitis resulting in closed fimbriae may be a blessing in militating against spread into the peritoneal cavity. Metastases to the peritoneum and omentum are common, while the uterus and ovary are also frequently involved because of their intimate lymphatic relations to the tube. In addition to this, lymphatic extension to the iliac and lumbar glands often occurs, as in carcinoma of the uterine fundus or ovary.

As appreciated in the evaluation of ovarian neoplasms, a careful clinicopathologic study of the abdominal cavity is imperative if an adequate prognosis is to be given and a realistic therapeutic regimen is to be recommended. Although the CCABC (Cancer Control Agency of British Columbia) has proposed an alternative clinical classification, most students have accepted the FIGO groupings, as noted below:

FIGO Classification

STAGE O   Carcinoma in situ limited to the tubal mucosa.

STAGE I   Tumor extending into the submucosa or muscularis but not penetrating to the serosal surface of the fallopian tube.

STAGE II   Tumor extending to the serosa of the fallopian tube.

STAGE III   Direct extension of the tumor to the ovary or endometrium.

STAGE IV   Extension of tumor beyond the reproductive organs.

Secondary or Metastatic Carcinoma

Secondary neoplasia is much more common than primary cancer due to the frequency of ovarian and fundal malignancy. With either of the latter, emboli of cancer cells may be seen in the subepithelial lymphatics or vascular channels or the adjacent mesosalpinx (Figs. 16–10 and 16–11). Direct implantation of cancer cells upon the tubal mucosa may occur but the presence of superficial neoplastic epithelial changes may represent new growths. Multicentric foci of epi-

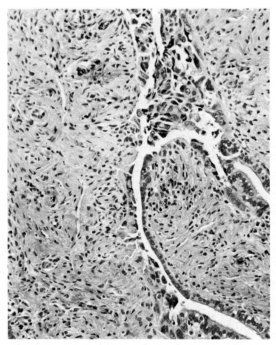

Figure 16–9. Surface neoplastic changes in tube associated with ovarian malignancy.

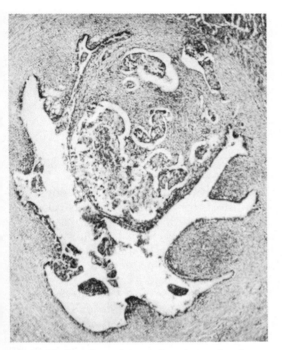

Figure 16–10. Secondary tubal carcinoma showing carcinomatous area beneath intact tubal epithelium, though later loss of the epithelium would give impression of implantation of cancer on surface instead of spread via lymphatics.

thelial neoplasia in the upper genital canal are well documented and the tube may take part in such regional disease (Fig. 16–10). Instances of in situ carcinoma have been seen in the tubal epithelium in association with both fundal and ovarian malignancies.

OTHER TUMORS OF THE TUBE

Choriocarcinoma

Choriocarcinoma may occur as a primary tubal neoplasm in view of the great frequency of tubal pregnancy. A collected series of 15 such cases has been reported by Cope and Kettle. It is interesting to note that there are more recorded cases of choriocarcinoma than of hydatiform mole. This may be an incorrect statistic, since the villus distortion associated with an eccyesis may not be recognized as molar transformation. It must be appreciated that the term *tubal mole* referred to a mass of blood clot and trophoblastic tissue, not to a hydatiform mole.

The secondary variety of choriocarcinoma is the result of extension from a primary tumor of the ovary or uterus. In the latter circumstances the lesion is often found in the cornual portion of the tube or uterus, and the clinical picture is that of ruptured extrauterine pregnancy. The pathologic characteristics are like those described for the latter (Chapter 34). A rare case of choriocarcinoma of the tube in conjunction with a viable intrauterine pregnancy has been reported by Crisp. Therapy is similar to that used in the treatment of the gestational lesion.

Sarcoma

Sarcoma is likewise an extremely rare and highly malignant primary neoplasm of the

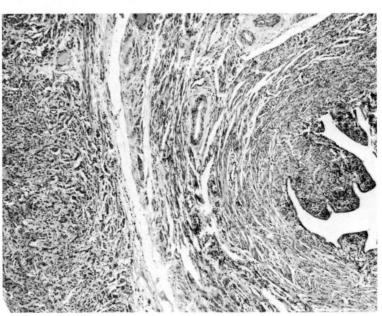

Figure 16–11. Normal fallopian tube with metastatic breast cancer on the left.

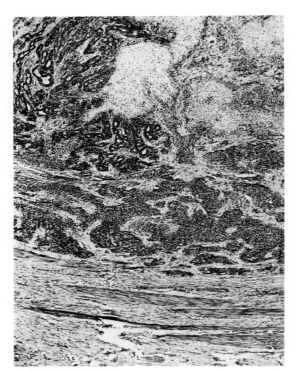

Figure 16–12. Microscopic pattern of mixed tumor showing muscle wall below and luminal tumor with adenomatous, stromal, and metaplastic (cartilaginous) components.

with the mixed type of lesion elsewhere in the paramesonephric system, is poor. Surgery is the primary therapy of choice. Exenteration procedures have been proposed for the fundal type of mixed tumor, and although the numbers treated in such a manner are small, the results seem to warrant further application in selected cases.

PAROVARIAN CYSTS

The parovarium (epoophoron, organ of Rosenmuller), representing the vestigial remnant of the wolffian body, is situated in the mesosalpinx, between the tube and the hilum of the ovary. Its main duct is the wolffian or mesonephric duct. In its persisting form, it is often described as Gartner's duct. Tiny cystic structures or hydatids may arise from dilatation of mesonephric duct or its tubules; however, the largest, often pedunculated from the tip of the tube, is of müllerian or paramesonephric origin (Fig. 16–13). This structure, as well as most parovarian cysts, represents a blind accessory lumen of the oviduct. Such cysts are of no especial clinical significance except in the very rare

tube. In a survey of the literature, Abrams and co-workers note only 31 cases. The lesions are generally diagnosed as leiomyosarcomas and as might be expected for such lesions elsewhere, the prognosis is poor.

Mixed Mesodermal Tumors

Since the tube is of paramesonephric origin, these rare mixed tumors may occur here. The gross appearance simulates that of the solid carcinoma, the mass filling the lumen, and often the wall seems relatively free of disease. They present the same microscopic patterns as seen in the similar tumors of the fundus (Fig. 16–12).

Microscopically, in addition to the papillary alveolar pattern of the epithelial elements, there is a stromal malignancy and other mesodermal tissues, most frequently cartilage and striated muscle cells, can often be recognized. The differences in malignant potential of the various elements have been debated; however, in the only case recorded in our laboratory, both compounds were present in the metastases. The prognosis, as

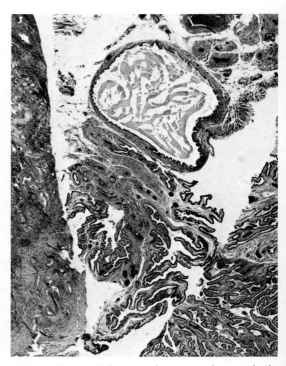

Figure 16–13. Dilatation of accessory lumen of tube with formation of hydatid.

case in which the long, thin, and cordlike pedicle may produce intestinal angulation and obstruction, or more frequently torsion and acute abdominal pain.

From the main mesonephric duct a group of 12 to 16 tubules extends toward and sometimes into the hilum of the ovary and the mesosalpingeal border of the tube. These tubules are often seen in sections of the tube, appearing singly or in small clusters. They are recognized by the central lumen lined by a single layer of cuboidal epithelium, around which there is always to be seen a well-marked layer of muscle tissue.

Gross Pathology

As noted above, cysts of various sizes may develop from the mesonephric duct or its tubules; however, when one recognizes the striking muscular coat of the tubules and the relative lack of secretory activity of the lining cells, it seems unlikely that perceptible dilatation could take place. Conversely, the hydatid and most gross cystic lesions are of paramesonephric origin and undoubtedly represent dilatation of diverticular or accessory lumina of the tube. These are more common than previously suspected and are found near the infundibulum where the developing tube is compressed by the large mesonephric body and the regressing pronephros. Such structures may dilate readily since they are lined by typical tubal epithelium. Thus, a majority of parovarian cysts are, in truth, hydrosalpinges, and the so-called papillae are residual mucosal folds, a

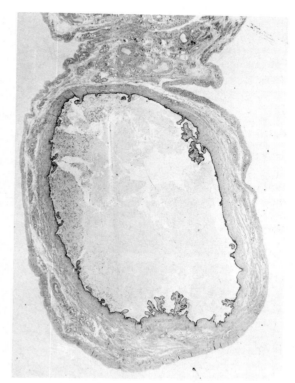

Figure 16–14. Hydrosalpinx: a parovarian cyst showing the changing significance of the tubal diverticula or accessory lumen, or both.

situation that is replicated in the hydrosalpinx simplex (Figure 16–14) (see Chapter 15). In Figure 16–15 an essentially normal tubal lumen can be seen on one side, with a smaller, slightly dilated lumen on the opposite aspect.

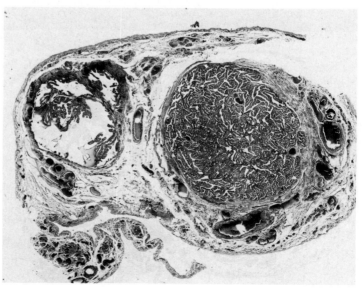

Figure 16–15. Note the normal lumen on one side (right) with the smaller, slightly dilated one on the opposite aspect. Mucosal folds in the latter appear as papillae.

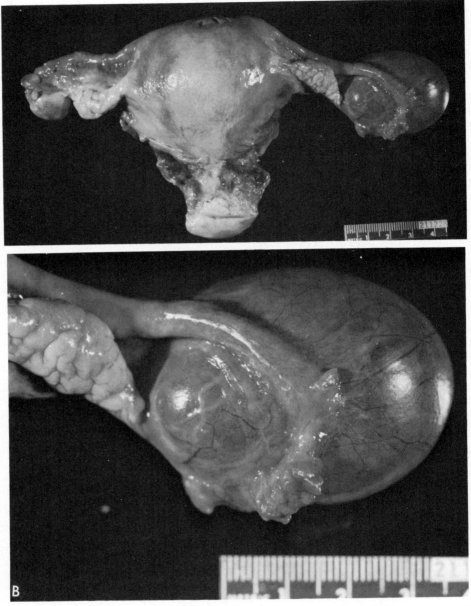

Figure 16–16. *A*, Bilateral parovarian cysts. Note the accessory tiny dilatation on the superior surface of tube at left. Multiple fimbriae can be noted on either side. *B*, Parovarian cyst—higher power view of *A*.

The parovarian cyst can be recognized by its position between the tube and the ovary. The latter is intact, while the tube may be elongated and stretched over the upper border of the tumor. The cyst is ovoid in shape, with extremely thin walls, and is enclosed between the widely spread layers of the mesosalpinx (Figs. 16–16 *A*, *B*). Simple slitting of this covering peritoneum will often permit the surgeon to enucleate the cyst from its bed.

The cavity of the cyst is usually unilocular, and it is filled with a clear fluid of very low specific gravity. In some of the smaller cysts, however, there is a definite papillomatous tendency, as noted in the common tubal dilatations.

Microscopic Appearance

The lining epithelium is of cuboidal or columnar variety, arranged in a single layer. A variety of cells are present, including ciliated and secretory types, the latter often containing clear, neutral cytoplasm. As noted by Gardner and co-workers a basement membrane may be demonstrated beneath the mesonephric epithelium (Fig. 16–17), although such a layer is usually absent in the paramesonephric structures. When the cyst is large, the epithelium may be flat. Beneath the epithelium is a thin layer of connective tissue and smooth muscle. The presence of the latter has suggested that the origin of the larger cysts is, in truth, paramesonephric rather than mesonephric.

A review of 116 cases of parovarian cysts from the Gynecologic Pathology Laboratory at the Johns Hopkins revealed that only three of the lesions appeared to arise from mesonephric elements. The remainder represented either mesothelial inclusions or diverticulae or accessory lumina of the tube. Since the epithelia of both latter types may be similar (mesothelial metaplasia) (Fig. 16–18), only the wall of either smooth muscle or connective tissue could be used to identify the correct designation. Often the latter was attenuated by the pressure and thus no definite assessment of the histogenesis could be determined.

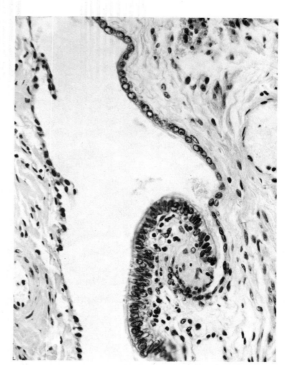

Figure 16–18. Transition from mesothelium to typical tubal type in the parovarian area.

Malignant alteration in parovarian cysts is rare and was found in only 4 of the 116 cases. Most commonly the neoplasm was of the papillary serous type similar to that seen in both tube and ovary; consequently, it is imperative to carefully rule out such associations (Fig. 16–19). Nevertheless, since the cyst is of paramesonephric origin, such lesions may arise de novo as was true of four tumors reported above, and all have had no recurrences to date. In one instance the tumor was endometrioid, of low malignant potential, and again there has been no recurrence.

Mesonephric Duct Tumors

Novak and colleagues found the so-called Schiller type of mesonephroma and the clear cell adenocarcinoma described by Saphir and Lackner arising in the parovarian area, suggesting a mesonephric origin for certain of these lesions. Similarity between such tumors and those arising in the kidney promotes this opinion. Actually the cases showed various admixtures of these two tumors, frequently in the same section.

Schiller's mesonephroma is characterized by a glomerulus-like architecture with a tu-

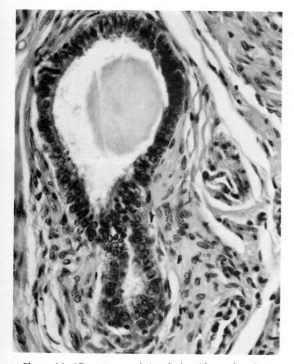

Figure 16–17. Mesonephric tubule with nondescript cuboidal epithelium.

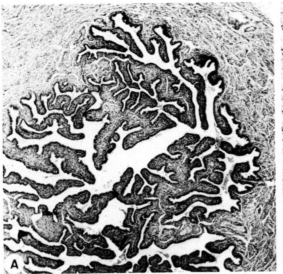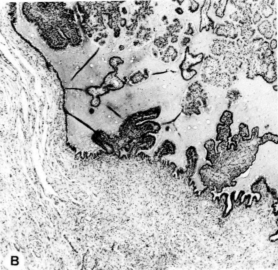

Figure 16–19. Normal tube on left with papillary cystadenocarcinoma of low malignant potential in parovarian cyst.

bular pattern featuring a low cuboidal lining epithelium with frequent peglike budding into the lumen, and simulates the embryonic mesonephric glomerulus. This is frequently associated with the clear cell, hypernephroid tumor, as reported by Saphir and Lackner. This lesion, regardless of its location in the genital tract, demonstrates varying degrees of malignancy. Further discussion will be found in Chapter 21, for such tumors generally involve the ovary and most frequently arise from the paramesonephric epithelium.

TUMORS OF THE PARA-ADNEXAL STRUCTURES

(INCLUDING PERITONEUM, LIGAMENTS, AND EMBRYONIC REMNANTS

Lesions arising in the para-adnexal structures may be classified as follows:

Primary

A. Connective Tissue Origin
1. Benign
a. Myoma and fibromyoma
b. Lipoma
c. Adenomyoma
2. Malignant
a. Leiomyosarcoma, fibrosarcoma, etc.

B. Vascular
1. Angioma, lymphangioma
2. Varices, varicocele
C. Mesothelial
1. Benign (parovarian cysts)
a. Paramesonephric (including hydatid)
b. Mesonephric
c. Mesothelial (peritoneal inclusion)
2. Malignant
a. Papillary serous
b. Endometrioid
c. Mesonephroid
D. Embryonic Remnant Origin
1. Hilar cell tumor
2. Adrenal tumor
3. Dermoid cyst
E. Non-neoplastic
1. Inflammatory
2. Hernia
3. Extrauterine pregnancy
4. Hematoma

Secondary

A. Endometriosis and leiomyomatosis peritonealis disseminata
B. Inflammatory—salpingitis, endometritis, etc.
C. Neoplastic—benign and malignant (of genital or extragenital origin—ovary, uterus, tube, and intestine).

The round, uterosacral, cardinal, utero-ovarian, and broad ligaments are the common ligaments of the internal genitalia. The round and uterosacral varieties are those most involved in both primary and secondary pelvic neoplasia. The uterosacral and cardinal ligaments are part of the same anatomic structure; however, defining the tumors arising in the cardinal ligament is essentially impossible, since it actually lies in the base of the broad ligament.

As a result of the above comments, the first section of the discussion will be directed primarily to lesions arising in or involving the round and uterosacral ligaments.

ROUND LIGAMENT

Since Wells' initial description of a myoma of the round ligament in 1865, few such lesions have been reported, as noted by Breen and Neubecker's collection of only 257 cases in 1962. Only five leiomyomas and endometriosis involving the ligament were diagnosed in the Gynecologic Pathology Laboratory between the years 1971 and 1975. Furthermore, certain lesions, specifically endometriosis and dermoid cysts, are not justifiably designated as tumors of the ligaments but are only lesions involving the ligament and arising from adjacent structures.

BENIGN TUMORS

Fibromyoma

These lesions have generally been divided into intra-abdominal and extra-abdominal (inguinal canal or labial) types. The former are generally indistinguishable from pedunculated uterine or ovarian tumors and are therefore rarely diagnosed preoperatively (Fig. 16–20). The extra-abdominal tumors are commonly detected by the patient, and therefore are reported frequently. They may be mistaken for endometriosis, lipoma, cyst of the canal of Nuck (hydrocele), hernia, varicocele, or enlarged lymph node.

The tumors are most frequently unilateral and single, with no increased predilection for one ligament. They are generally small, averaging from 1 to 7 cm.; however, the largest intra-abdominal tumor weighed 13.6 kg. (30 lb.), and the largest extra-abdominal (labial) lesion 14 kg. (31 lb.). The latter hung to the patient's knees.

Microscopically, the neoplasms are similar to those of the uterus, being composed of interlacing bundles of fibrous and muscle tissue with varying types of degenerative change (Fig. 16–21). Among the 257 cases reported by Breen and Neubecker were 17 cases of sarcoma.

Adenomyoma and Endometrioma

These lesions, similar to the fibromyomas, occur in the intra-abdominal or inguinal portion of the round ligament. Endometriosis should not be considered a primary lesion of the round ligament but one that represents an alteration in the overlying mesothelium induced by the regurgitated endometrium. As noted by Sampson in 1926, endometriosis also may develop by transplantation of the endometrium through lymphatic or vascular channels.

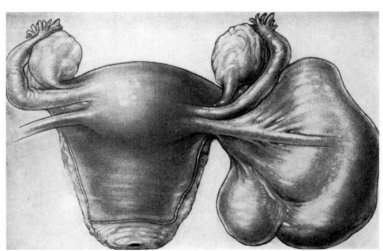

Figure 16–20. Myoma of round ligament.

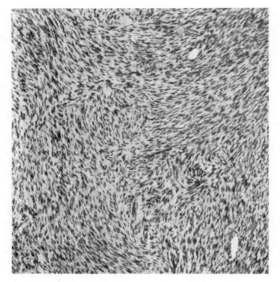

Figure 16–21. Myoma of round ligament.

The use of the term adenomyoma in this extrauterine position may be questioned. Since adenomyosis, as demonstrated by Cullen in 1896, represents a direct invasion of the myometrium from the basalis of the endometrium, it is difficult to justify such a de-velopmental process in the round ligament. Nevertheless, the reaction set up by the invading endometrium often produces a nodularity and growth into the fibromuscular elements of the ligament could be termed adenomyoma (Fig. 16–22). Pathologically, these lesions are similar to those found elsewhere in the pelvis and identified by the presence of endometrial glands and stroma (Fig. 16–23). In the end stage, the fibrotic reaction may have destroyed the classic histologic pattern and only small, epithelium-lined cavities with pigment-laden macrophages in the underlying tissue (siderophagic cysts) are visible. Grossly, these cavities contain old blood or yellow cheesy material. Physiologic and pathologic alterations may be appreciated in certain foci. Conversely, fibrosis of the decidualized subperitoneal nodule may be diagnosed as leiomyomatosis peritonealis disseminata.

Cysts

A majority of the cysts occurring along the round ligament are found in the inguinal canal. They are actually circumscribed dila-

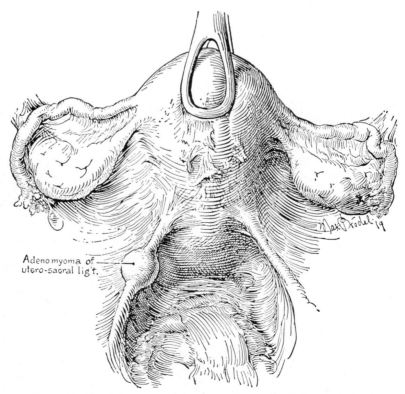

Adenomyoma of utero-sacral lig't.

Figure 16–22. Adenomyoma of uterosacral ligament. (Cullen: Arch. Surg.)

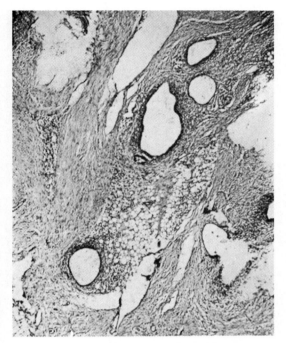

Figure 16–23. Adenomyoma of round ligament.

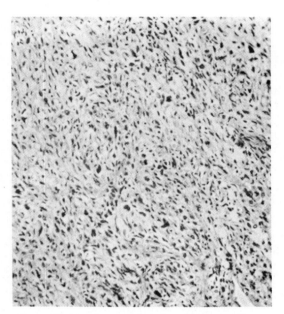

Figure 16–24. Sarcoma (spindle cell) of round ligament (leiomyo- or fibrosarcoma).

tions of the peritoneal investment of the ligament or cysts of the canal of Nuck (hydrocele). The flattened lining epithelium is mesothelium. These lesions may present at any point along the ligament even into the labia majora, and may be quite difficult to distinguish from inguinal hernias. At the time of surgical excision it is wise to repair the canal in view of the frequently associated inguinal hernia. Occasionally a papillary serous tumor may arise de novo from the peritoneum of the inguinal canal in the absence of a primary ovarian neoplasm; however, the presence of the latter must be ruled out by careful evaluation of the internal genitalia, pelvis, and general peritoneal cavity.

MALIGNANT TUMORS

Sarcoma

The majority of sarcomas of the round ligament undoubtedly represent instances of malignant change in a preexisting benign tumor (Fig. 16–24). The problems of microscopic differentiation between the degenerative changes commonly noted in myomas at any site (symplasmic giant cells) and the malignant pleomorphic and multinucleate cells are well known. Furthermore, nodular fasciitis, instances of which have been reported in the round ligament, is an example of confusing benign pathology characterized by bizarre cellular aberrations. Other malignancies arising at extrapelvic sites may involve the ligament and adjacent pelvic structures, but these rarely focus specifically on the round ligament.

Carcinoma

Such lesions arise from adjacent embryonic structures (mesonephric), from initially benign endometriosis, or from the mesothelium. The latter are usually of the papillary serous variety; all of them are rare. Whereas primary carcinoma is uncommon, secondary involvement of the ligament from the adjacent organs is common. Both by direct extension and by lymphatic spread, the ligament may be involved from lesions primary in the ovary and fundus.

Surgery is the definitive therapeutic approach to lesions of the uterine ligaments.

TUMORS OF THE BROAD LIGAMENT

Tumors *of* the broad ligament are, for the most part, tumors *in* the broad ligament. The anterior and posterior leaves of this ligament encase the round ligaments, the fallopian tubes, and the remnants of the mesonephric system. In the loose connective and adipose tissue lie the major vessels, lymphatics, and nerves that supply and drain much of the genital canal. The ureter courses through the base of the ligament and at least two lymph nodes are found in this general area. Anteriorly the peritoneum is reflected over the bladder and posteriorly over the cul-de-sac, the adjacent uterosacral ligaments, and the rectum. Consequently, all retroperitoneal tumors arising from these structures represent tumors in the broad ligament.

Diagnosis of Broad Ligament Tumors

The findings on abdominal, vaginal, and rectovaginal examination must be correlated. Of the various diagnostic approaches, the rectal study is probably the most informative. The absence of cul-de-sac bulge and the ability to separate the fundus and adnexa from the lesion suggest the broad ligament as the site of origin. Such a lesion limits the motility of the uterus more than similar sized tumors of the fundus and ovary. A tumor presenting in the buttock, with a mass in the pelvis on the corresponding side, should be considered as possibly arising from the broad ligament.

Cystoscopy is important in evaluating possible bladder involvement. Intravenous pyelograms aid in determining ureteral obstruction and displacement as well as ruling out pelvic kidney. Barium enema assists in eliminating diverticulitis and rectosigmoid tumors.

Leiomyoma is the most common solid tumor in the broad ligament. In the majority of the cases reported these lesions have arisen in the fundus as subserous tumors, and have become divorced from the organ of origin to lie unattached between the leaves of peritoneum, since the lesion is extraperitoneal. Stroheker collected 204 cases from the literature; of these he felt that probably not more than 50 were primary in the broad ligament (Fig. 16–25).

The symptoms are due largely to the pressure of the tumor on the surrounding structures. Lesions developing anteriorly often displace the bladder, while those growing posteriorly may cause pressure on the colon or rectum. They may grow downward into the vagina or through the obturator foramen. There may be pressure on the nerves, producing pain; on the bladder, pro-

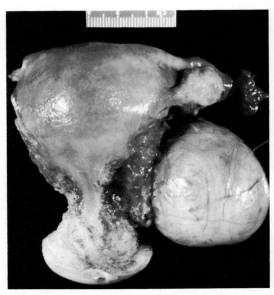

Figure 16–25. Intraligamentary myoma probably of uterine origin.

ducing frequency; or on the rectum, producing constipation. Edema of one extremity without ascites and pain in the renal region due to ureteral compression are suggestive evidences of retroperitoneal tumor.

In 1949 only 19 *lipomas* could be collected from the literature. Their presentations are similar to those described for the leiomyoma.

A variety of *other neoplasms* in the broad ligament have been recorded in the literature, including lymphangioma, angioma, and sarcoma. Most of these lesions have been described as incidental findings.

Hystopathology

The microscopic appearance of these various lesions in the broad ligament does not vary from that of similar tumors elsewhere in the pelvis. Degeneration is common because the blood supply may be compromised by compression of the vascular tree. Malignant alterations are uncommon but, again, histopathologically simulate those sarcomas occurring secondarily in leiomyomas of the uterus. Retroperitoneal sarcomas, on the other hand, may arise de novo and dissect into the pelvis with the first presentation being a posterior mass. Such lesions may represent a variety of histologic entities, including lymphoma and tumors of the paraganglion system.

Tumors by Extension from Other Organs

As noted above, most broad ligament tumors arise from the uterus, the ovaries, or the oviduct, and become secondarily incarcerated into the broad ligament. Thus, it is necessary to demonstrate that the tumor does not arise from one of these structures before it can be considered as primary in the broad ligament. Whereas primary tumors arising de novo in this area are rare, secondary malignant disease is common. Most such neoplasia originates in the cervix, although the fundus, ovary, bladder, and intestinal tract may be primary sites. Staging of cervical disease depends to a degree on evaluation of broad ligament involvement. Furthermore, after radiation therapy, differentiation of malignant invasion from radiation scarring and cellulitis may present major problems. Needle biopsy may be of value in establishing a correct diagnosis.

The Pelvic Congestion Syndrome

Varicosities, even of great size, often are encountered in the broad ligament during operations for pelvic pathology. In the absence of the latter, varicosities undoubtedly occur; however, there is reasonable doubt that they cause significant symptoms. Dwight directed attention to this condition in 1887, and subsequently there have been numerous reports on the subject. Retroposition of the uterus, lowered vitality, and other vague explanations have been cited as possible etiologies. The usual indication for surgery has been pain or pressure in the pelvis. The subjective improvement following the operation may well be due to the improved health of the patient, as well as to the correction of minor pelvic pathology. Thus the pelvic congestion syndrome as a cause of specific pelvic distress is not a widely accepted concept.

Whereas the uncomplicated pelvic varices questionably produce symptoms, pelvic thrombophlebitis may be life-endangering. Usually resulting from parametritis and most commonly seen in association with or following pregnancy, particularly induced abortion, such problems may be due to postoperative pelvic infections. The thromboses may extend upward from the ovarian vein into the renal vein on the left or the vena cava on the right. Rarely they form a recognizable pelvic mass and, on occasion may be palpated abdominally. A rectovaginal examination is essential, even if difficult, in fixing the location in the broad ligament. The mass may be more easily palpated if the patient is examined in the standing position.

In contrast to thrombophlebitis, a broad ligament hematoma rarely presents as a clinically definable entity. Probably, postoperative hematomas are common following hysterectomy but seldom cause significant symptoms and are gradually absorbed. Rarely, if bleeding cannot be controlled, internal iliac artery ligation may be a life-saving procedure.

Tumors Arising in Embryonic Rests

The embryonic remnants in the broad ligament region are primarily of mesonephric origin. It is well known that the mesonephric (wolffian) duct, mesonephric tubules, and glomeruli are first recognized at about 3 to $3\frac{1}{2}$ weeks of embryonic life. The mesonephric glomeruli are functionless in the human animal, but remnants can be recognized easily in section through the hilar area (parovarium) of the normal ovary. Cystic dilatations at the terminus of the broad ligament, the hydatid of Morgagni, are of paramesonephric origin. Although rarely of clinical importance, torsion of the pedicle may produce acute pain and necessitate surgical intervention.

Also present in this area, associated with the remnants of the mesonephric system, are the interesting hilar cells described by Berger as sympathicotropic, since they are routinely found in the vicinity of the hilar nerves. Recent studies suggest, however, that these are actually interstitial or Leydig type cells, and the finding of Reinke crystalloids confirms this opinion.

Hilar Cell and Adrenal Rest Tumors

These lesions develop in the broad ligament, and the classic cell rests from which they arise can frequently be recognized in routine sections through the parovarian region. The tumors commonly are hormonally active and are described in detail later (Chapter 27).

Echinococcus Cyst

Such cysts may develop in the broad ligament in the course of hydatid disease. These may rupture and the contents collect in the cul-de-sac and broad ligament, giving rise to secondary cysts. Primary cysts of this type have been observed, although only five cases had been reported up to 1950. It is important to recognize that lesions developing from parasitic disease are rare in this country but not infrequent in other areas of the world; for example, Schistosoma infections in the ovary are not uncommon in Egypt. Two views have been advanced to explain their presence in the ovary: (1) by direct invasion from the intestinal tract or (2) via the circulation. The former route seems more probable as the embryos can, without a doubt, perforate the intestinal peritoneum. The second theory has been practically abandoned.

In the broad ligament the cyst may develop slowly over a period of years without any characteristic symptoms. Dystocia has been recorded as the first indication of the presence of such a tumor. When the cyst involves the bladder, it may cause urinary symptoms.

In rare instances the cysts have attained a size of 30 cm. They are usually round, firm, and elastic but rarely fluctuant. The diagnosis is usually not made preoperatively; however, if the condition is suspected, serologic tests can be of great assistance. A positive diagnosis can be confirmed by demonstration of the hooklets and membranes in the fluid obtained by drainage or after spontaneous rupture of the cyst in a hollow viscus. Suppuration occasionally occurs.

Tumors of Trophoblastic Origin—Choriocarcinoma, Hydatidiform Mole; Invasive Mole (Chorioadenoma Destruens)

Most cases represent direct invasion by a primary uterine neoplasm, although the rare oviductal lesion may extend into the ligament. The histopathology is described in Chapter 33.

Ectopic Pregnancy

Uncommonly a tubal pregnancy ruptures into the broad ligament. The amount of blood lost is limited by the available space, but immediate surgery is indicated if there is evidence of intraperitoneal hemorrhage, as demonstrated by precipitous fall in hematocrit and the clinical signs of impending shock. Conversely, many patients with a

tubal rupture into the broad ligament do not present with acute symptoms leading to the correct diagnosis and treatment. Some have survived this accident and the pregnancy has continued. King, in his review of 262 cases of advanced extrauterine pregnancies, added 12 cases of his own, four of which were intraligamentous. He stated that the incidence of the latter is only exceeded by that of secondary abdominal pregnancies.

Nevertheless, not all tubal pregnancies that survive rupture into the broad ligament progress to term. The residual tumor mass may remain for months. Mummification and/or calcification may occur, and rupture of the residua into the bowel, bladder, or vagina has been reported.

Inflammatory Processes

Broad ligament cellulitis is most frequently diagnosed in the patient with postpregnancy endometritis, specifically after induced abortion. It has been stated that such infections develop after intrauterine manipulation or curettage, especially when fundal or endocervical malignancy is present. Rarely such cellulitis is associated with severe subacute cervicitis.

The acute stages are characterized by pelvic pain and the usual signs, symptoms, and laboratory changes seen with infections. Again, a rectovaginal examination is essential in the diagnosis.

The usual treatment is palliative, with the use of broad spectrum antibiotics. If an inguinal abscess develops, extraperitoneal drainage through an inguinal incision above Poupart's ligament is the procedure of choice. Conversely, the abscess may occur in the cul-de-sac of Douglas, and vaginal drainage is the proper approach.

REFERENCES

Abrams, J., Kazal, H. L., and Hobbs, R. E.: Primary sarcoma of the fallopian tube; review of the literature and report of one case. Am. J. Obstet. Gynecol., 75:180, 1958.

Andrews, H. R.: A case in which torsion of a hydatid of Morgagni during pregnancy without torsion of tube or ovary caused urgent symptoms. J. Obstet. Gynaecol. Br. Emp., 22:220, 1912.

Benedet, J. L., White, G. W., Fairey, R. N., and Boyes, D. A.: Adenocarcinoma of the fallopian tube. Obstet. Gynecol., 50:654, 1977.

Berger, L.: La glande sympathicotrope du hile de l'ovaire. Arch. Anat. Histol. Embryol., 2:255, 1923.

Bernstine, J. B., and Breckenridge, R. L.: Sarcoma of

round ligament. Am. J. Obstet. Gynecol., 63:1367, 1952.

Breen, J. L., Lukeman, J. M., and Neubecker, R. D.: Modular fascitis of the round ligament: report of a case. Obstet. Gynecol., 19:397, 1962.

Breen, J. L., and Neubecker, R. D.: Tumors of the round ligament; a review of the literature and a report of 25 cases. Obstet. Gynecol., 19:771, 1962.

Bret, A. J., and Grepinet, J.: Endometrial polyps in the intramural part of the tube (relation to sterility and endometriosis). Sem. Hôp. Paris, 43:183, 1967.

Brewer, J. I., and Guderian, A. M.: Diagnosis of uterine-tube carcinoma by vaginal cytology. Obstet. Gynecol., 8:664, 1956.

Cope, V. Z., and Kettle, E. H.: A case of chorionepithelioma of the fallopian tube, following extrauterine gestation. Proc. Roy. Soc. Med., 6:247, 1912–13.

Crisp, W. E.: Choriocarcinoma of the fallopian tube coincident with viable pregnancy. Am. J. Obstet. Gynecol., 71:442, 1956.

Crissman, J. D., and Handwerker, D.: Leiomyoma of the tube. Am. J. Obstet. Gynecol., 126:1046, 1976.

Cullen, T.: Distribution of adenomyomas containing uterine mycosa. Am. J. Obstet. Gynecol., 80:130, 1919.

Cullen, T. S.: Adenomyoma of the round ligament. Bull. Johns Hopkins Hosp., 7:112, 1896.

Dede, J. A., and Janovski, N. A.: Lipoma of the uterine tube. Obstet. Gynecol., 22:461, 1963.

Devi, A. L.: Primary choriocarcinoma of the tube. J. Int. Coll. Surg. 44:62, 1965.

Dodson, M. G., Ford, J. H., and Averette, H. E.: Carcinoma of the tube. Obstet. Gynecol., 36:935, 1970.

Downing, W., and O'Toole, L.: Parovarian cysts complicating pregnancy; report of case causing dystocia; review of the literature. J.A.M.A., 112:1798, 1939.

Fidler, H. K., and Lock, D. R.: Carcinoma of the fallopian tube detected by cervical smear. Am. J. Obstet. Gynecol., 67:1103, 1954.

Flickinger, F. M., and Masson, J. C.: Lipomas of broad ligament extending beyond confines of pelvis. Am. J. Obstet. Gynecol., 52:681, 1946.

Gardner, G. H., Greene, R. R., and Peckham, B.: Normal and cystic structures of broad ligament. Am. J. Obstet. Gynecol., 55:917, 1949.

Gardner, G. H., Greene, R. R., and Peckham, B.: Tumors of the broad ligament. Am. J. Obstet. Gynecol., 73:536, 1957.

Genadry, R., Parmley, T. H., and Woodruff, J. D.: The origin and behavior of parovarian tumors. Am. J. Obstet. Gynecol., 129:873, 1977.

Goldman, J. A., Gans, B., and Eckerling, B.: Hydrops tubae profluens; symptom in tubal carcinoma. Obstet. Gynecol., 18:631, 1961.

Govender, N. K., and Goldstein, D. P.: Metastatic tubal mole and coexisting intrauterine pregnancy. Obstet. Gynecol., 49:675, 1977.

Green, T. H., and Scully, R.: Tumors of the fallopian tube. Clin. Obstet. Gynecol., 5:886, 1962.

Grubisic, S.: Primary chorionepithelioma of the tube consequent to tubal pregnancy. Clin. Obstet. Gynecol., 58:159, 1956.

Henderson, S. R., Harper, R. C., Salazar, O. M., and Rudolph, J. H.: Primary carcinoma of the fallopian tube. Gynecol. Oncol., 5:168, 1977.

Hu, C. Y., Taymor, M. L., and Hertig, A. T.: Primary carcinoma of the fallopian tube. Am. J. Obstet. Gynecol., 59:58, 1959.

Ireland, K., and Woodruff, J. D.: Masculinizing ovarian tumors. Obstet. Gynecol. Surv., 31:83, 1976.

Kaloyerides, N.: Torsion and gangrene of a hydatid of Morgagni. Obstet. Gynecol., 21:464, 1963.

Kershner, D., and Shapiro, A. L.: Multilocular serous cysts of round ligament simulating incarcerated hernia; report of three cases. Ann. Surg., 117:216, 1943.

Kinzel, G. E.: Primary carcinoma of the fallopian tube. Am. J. Obstet. Gynecol., 125:816, 1976.

Koff, A. K.: Development of the vagina. Carnegie Contrib. Embryol. 24:140, 1933.

Kulka, E. W.: True bone formation in the fallopian tube. Am. J. Obstet. Gynecol., 44:384, 1942.

Lang, W. R., and Bland, C. B.: Bilateral broad ligament lipomata; report of case and review of literature. Ann. Surg., 130:281, 1949.

Malinak, L. R., Miller, G. V., and Armstrong, J. T.: Primary squamous cell carcinoma of the fallopian tube. Am. J. Obstet. Gynecol., 95:1067, 1966.

Mayo, C. W., and Schunke, G. B.: Leiomyoma of the round ligament. Arch. Surg., 41:637, 1940.

Mazzarella, P., Okagaki, T., and Richart, R. M.: Teratoma of the uterine tube. A case report and review of the literature. Obstet. Gynecol., 39:391, 1972.

Meigs, J. V.: Endometriosis. Ann. Surg., 127:795, 1948.

Nagel, W.: Parovarial cyste von 33 Liter Inhalt. Ztschr. Geburtsh. Gynäk., 52:505, 1904.

Novak, E.: Pelvic endometriosis; spontaneous rupture of endometrial cysts, with report of three cases. Am. J. Obstet. Gynecol., 22:826, 1931.

Novak, E., Woodruff, J. D., and Novak, E. R.: Probable mesonephric origin of certain female genital tumors. Am. J. Obstet. Gynecol., 68:1222, 1954.

Okagaki, T., and Richart, R. M.: Neurilemoma of the fallopian tube. Am. J. Obstet. Gynecol., 106:929, 1970.

Orthmann, E. J.: Ueber Carcinoma Tubae. Ztschr. Geburtsh. Gynäk., 15:212, 1888.

Parmley, T. H., Woodruff, J. D., and Winn, K.: The histogenesis of leiomyomatosis peritonealis disseminata. Obstet. Gynecol., 46:511, 1975.

Pauerstein, C. J., and Woodruff, J. D.: Cellular patterns in proliferative and anaplastic disease of the fallopian tube. Am. J. Obstet. Gynecol., 96:486, 1966.

Pauerstein, C. J., Woodruff, J. D., and Quinton, S. W.: Developmental patterns in "adenomatoid lesions" of the fallopian tube. Am. J. Obstet. Gynecol., 100:1000, 1968.

Ragins, A. B., and Crane, R. D.: Cavernous hemangioma of the fallopian tube. Am. J. Obstet. Gynecol., 54:883, 1947.

Ray, H. N.: Echinococcal cyst of broad ligament. Indian Med. Gaz., 85:88, 1950.

Riggs, J. A., Wainer, A. S., Hahn, G. A., and Farell, D. M.: Extrauterine tubal choriocarcinoma: a case report and review of recent literature. Am. J. Obstet. Gynecol., 88:637, 1964.

Roberts, C. L., and Marshall, H. K.: Fibromyoma of the fallopian tube; report of a case and review of the literature. Am. J. Obstet. Gynecol., 82:364, 1961.

Roscher, W.: Primary tubal sarcoma. Zbl. Gynäk. 78:1063, 1956.

Ryan, G. M., Jr.: Carcinoma in situ of the fallopian tube. Am. J. Obstet. Gynecol., 84:198, 1962.

Rubenstein, M. W., and Kurzon, A. M.: Adenomyoma of the round ligament in pregnancy. Am. J. Obstet. Gynecol., 63:458, 1952.

Sampson, J. A.: Endometriosis of the sac of a right inguinal hernia, associated with pelvic peritoneal endometriosis and an endometrial cyst of the ovary. Am. J. Obstet. Gynecol., 12:459, 1926.

Sapan, I. P., and Solberg, N. S.: Prolapse of the uterine

tube after abdominal hysterectomy. Obstet. Gynecol., 42:26, 1973.

Saphir, O., and Lackner, J. E.: Adenocarcinoma with clear cells (hypernephroid) of ovary. Surg. Gynecol. Obstet., 79:539, 1944.

Schnedorf, J. G., and Orr, T. G.: Five tumors of round ligament of the uterus—one a capillary hemangioma. Surgery, 10:642, 1941.

Segal, S., et al.: Choriocarcinoma of the fallopian tube. Gynecol. Oncol., 3:40, 1975.

Seidner, H. M., and Thompson, J. R.: Fibroma of the fallopian tube. Am J. Obstet. Gynecol., 79:32, 1960.

Strong, L. W.: Lymphangioma of the fallopian tube. Am. J. Obstet. Gynecol., 10:853, 1925.

Sweet, R. L., et al.: Malignant teratoma of the uterine tube. Obstet. Gynecol., 45:553, 1975.

Taussig, F. G.: Sarcoma of the round ligament of the uterus. Surg. Gynecol. Obstet., 19:218, 1914.

Teel, P.: Adenomatoid tumors of the genital tract. Am. J. Obstet. Gynecol., 75:1347, 1958.

Turunen, A.: Diagnosis and treatment of primary tubal carcinoma. Int. J. Gynacol. Obstet., 7:294, 1969.

Wallenburg, H. C. S., and Go, D. M. D. S.: Vaginal cytology as aid in diagnosis of carcinoma of the fallopian tube. Nederl. T. Verlosk, 70:1, 1970.

Wells, S.: Fibromyoma of the round ligament of the uterus. Path. Soc. London, 17:188, 1860–1866.

Williams T. J., and Woodruff, J. D.: Malignant mesenchymal tumors of the uterine tube: report of a case. Obstet. Gynecol., 21:618, 1963.

Woodruff, J. D., and Julian, C. G.: Multiple malignancy in the upper genital canal. Am. J. Obstet. Gynecol., 103:810, 1969.

Woodruff, J. D., and Pauerstein, C. J.: The Fallopian Tube. Baltimore, Williams & Wilkins, 1969.

Zelinger, B. B., Grinvalsky, H. T., and Fields, C.: Simultaneous dermoid cyst of the tube and ectopic pregnancy. Obstet. Gynecol., 15:340, 1960.

Chapter 17

EMBRYOLOGY AND HISTOLOGY OF OVARIES

EMBRYOLOGY

In order to understand the pathophysiology of the ovary, one should have at least an elementary idea of its embryology. The reproductive and urinary systems of both sexes are formed almost in entirety from the mesonephric and paramesonephric ducts adjacent to the wolffian body, a large and important structure occupying the posterior or dorsal portion of the primitive peritoneal cavity.

Important embryologic factors that aid in the understanding of ovarian neoplasia include the following:

1. Significance of differential development of ovary and testes
2. Significance of mesothelium
   a. Of mesodermal origin—i.e., stroma and epithelium of same origin
   b. Urogenital canal epithelium of similar origin
3. Significance of germ cell
   a. Site of origin and migratory vagaries
   b. Relationship to germ cell tumors

Undifferentiated Phase

The anlage of the sex gland, either testis or ovary, appears very early in fetal development as an aggregation of cells on the anterior aspect of the wolffian body, covered by the primitive peritoneal or coelomic epithelium. It should be emphasized that in its earlier stage it is impossible to determine from histologic examination whether this cellular mass is to become a testis or an ovary. Development of the sex glands in a male or female direction is determined systemically

by the genetic makeup of the fetus and locally by an enzyme of the polypeptide group, both of which play major roles in the final decision. Certainly the development of the gonad is dependent on the migration of the germ cell from the original site in the wall of the yolk sac, later the mesentery of the hindgut, into the gonadal area (Fig. 17–1). Studies by Witschi and associates and by Pinkerton and co-workers have demonstrated the presence of typical germ cells

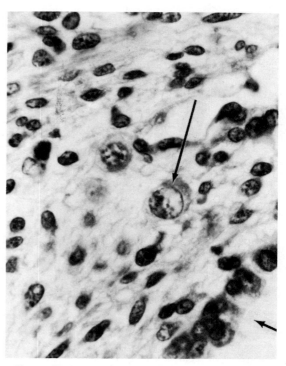

Figure 17–1. Germ cells in mesentery at top arrow, showing coelomic epithelium at arrow in lower right. (Embryo of 5½ weeks.)

in the epithelium of the gut, the coelomic epithelium, and the mesentery. Glycogen granules and positive reaction for alkaline phosphatase have been prominent findings in differentiating the germ cell from surrounding tissues, as noted by McKay and co-workers. The absence of germ cells is the significant feature in gonadal agenesis. The "streak gonad" contains an embryonic stroma, which does not develop in the absence of the proliferating germ cell.

STAGE OF DIFFERENTIATION

The early undifferentiated phase of male gonadal development is soon followed by one in which the primitive Sertoli cells are arranged into sex cords, the embryonic seminiferous tubule of the testes. These converge toward the hilus (Fig. 17–2) and link up with the mesonephric structures to complete the framework of the male testicular apparatus. The epididymis is formed by the mesonephric tubules and the mesonephric duct, the latter becoming the vas deferens.

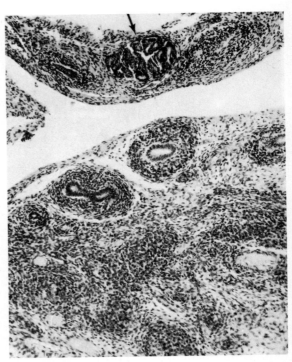

Figure 17–3. Rete (at arrow) and mesonephric tubules (in center).

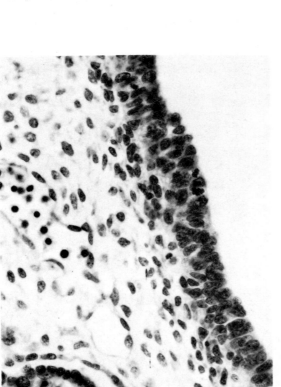

Figure 17–2. Gonadal ridge at 5 weeks of embryonic life. Stromal and surface epithelium show same histology. Germ cells are present in the mesothelium.

In the male gland a fibrous capsular layer forming beneath the germinal epithelium between the tenth and twelfth week of embryonic life becomes the tunica albuginea.

In the female, definable sex cords are not present; however, remains of the mesonephric ductile system are seen in the hilus, amid the rete ovarii (Fig. 17–3). Further differentiating phenomena soon make themselves evident in the cells of the sex gland. These cells lose their original mesothelial character and become mesenchymal in appearance; thus, both the epithelial (granulosal) and stromal (thecal) elements arise from the same basic anlage (Fig. 17–4).

Origin of Granulosa and Theca

The studies of Gillman indicate that the cell columns previously described in both the first and second waves of differentiation originate from the germinal epithelium, and this opinion has been accepted by most observers. Fischel, Meyer, Politzer, and others suggest that the granulosa is formed by differentiation from the ovarian mesenchyme in situ. According to this viewpoint, the mesenchymal cells may develop into either

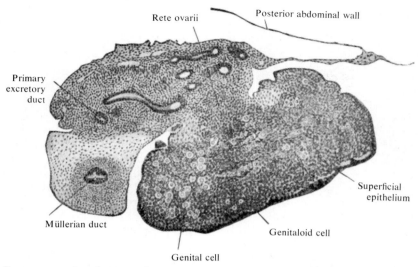

Figure 17–4. Transverse section of a 50 mm. human embryo showing relation of ovary and rete ovarii to mesonephros and müllerian duct. (From collection of Prof. R. Meyer.)

granulosa (epithelial) or theca (connective tissue) cells, and this concept explains certain characteristics of the granulosa cell and theca cell tumors, as well as the common stromal component of the epithelial ovarian tumors.

HISTOLOGY

Coelomic Epithelium

Covering the ovary is the coelomic mesothelium. The term "germinal epithelium" is no longer acceptable since there is no evidence that germ cells are formed in or by this epithelium. It is very perishable and is usually entirely or almost entirely lacking in sections of the adult ovary, though it is often well preserved in the ovaries of young children (Fig. 17–5). It consists of a single layer of cuboidal and sometimes peglike epithelial cells. This epithelium, or more specifically, mesothelium, is of mesodermal origin. It is also from this mesothelium, by invagination at $5\frac{1}{4}$ to 6 weeks of embryonic life, that the paramesonephric duct is formed. Consequently, there is similarity in lesions arising in the upper genital canal, the ovary, and adjacent peritoneum.

Germ Cell

As noted above, most investigators accept the theory that the germ cells migrate by

their own amoeboid activity, as noted by Witschi and others, along a "Keimbahn" from the base of the mesentery to their final positions in the gonad. Failure of this process may lead to gonadal agenesis or to the development of extragonadal germ cell tumors.

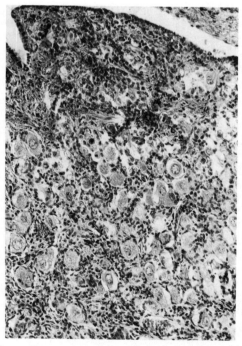

Figure 17–5. Many primordial follicles in the ovary at birth. Note the well-preserved germinal epithelium at the top of section. The underlying stromal cells are prominent at this point.

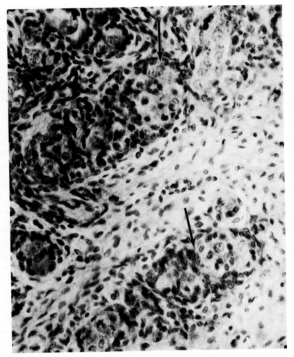

Figure 17–6. Aggregates of germ and stroma cells (at arrows) with primordial follicles at top. (Embryo of 20 weeks.)

The germ cell arrives in the gonadal ridge as early as 4 weeks postovulation according to the studies of Witschi. Since it originally lies directly beneath the mesothelium, it may become encapsulated and then progress toward the luteum. It is recognized, however, that during the stages of development,

many germ cells do not become encapsulated by primitive granulosa but present aggregates of both germ cells and stromal cells that simulate dysgerminoma (Fig. 17–6). Mitoses may be seen until encapsulation is complete, usually at 7 months of embryonic life; however, in many instances this process has not been completed at the time of birth. Furthermore, polyovular follicles are commonly found at this stage of development (Fig. 17–7).

At completion of the differentiative processes, 800,000 to 2 million primordial follicles are present (Fig. 17–5). The prevailing viewpoint is that no new ova are formed in the postembryonic era. Evans and Swezy have suggested, on the basis of animal studies, that the process of ovum formation may go on throughout reproductive life. In the human, however, there has been no evidence to support this view. Studies by Baker suggest that a majority of the 6 million germ cells present in the embryo at the age of 6 to 7 months degenerate, resulting in 400,000 to 600,000 available oocytes at the menarche.

Cortex and Medulla

The ovary is divisible into the cortex and the medulla. During reproductive life the cortex is broad, constituting from one half to two thirds of the depth of the ovary, and thus the ovary, in contrast to the testis, is primarily a cortical structure. It consists of a very characteristic stroma in which are found the follicular elements of the ovary. The

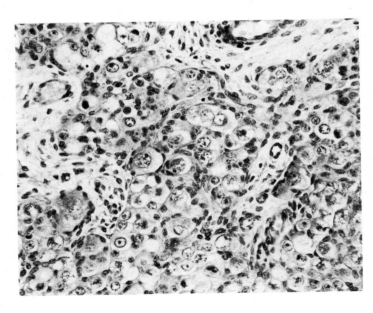

Figure 17–7. Ovary at birth showing many polyovular follicles (upper center) with some unencapsulated germ cells.

stroma is made up of spindle-celled connective tissue cells. There is only slight superficial condensation of this connective tissue into a layer called the *tunica albuginea,* however, this layer is never a well-defined structure in the ovary. Only a few involuntary muscle fibers are found, chiefly around the larger blood vessels.

The ovarian medulla consists primarily of a connective tissue matrix surrounding the major ovarian blood vessels and lymphatics. It may also contain such structures as the rete ovarii and hilus cells; for this reason many consider the medulla as potentially androgenic, stressing the medullary nature of the testes, in contrast to the estrogenic role of the cortex, wherein may be found the follicles and the granulosa and theca cells.

The Follicles and Their Derivatives

Scattered throughout the cortical zone are the graafian follicles and their derivative structures. In the ovaries of children and younger women large numbers of primordial follicles are to be seen (Fig. 17–5), though at later phases of reproductive life their number is progressively less, and they are entirely absent after the menopause. In the "senile" ovary, the cortex is represented by a rather narrow zone of dense fibrous tissue which stands out in sharp contrast to the relatively large inner or medullary zone of loose connective tissue, containing numerous thick-walled blood vessels.

In addition to the primordial follicles, the cortex during reproductive life contains numbers of follicles that have progressed to varying stages of maturation: blighted atretic follicles or corpora fibrosa, corpora lutea or their residue, corpora albicantia or corpora lutea hematomas. The characteristics of these various structures can best be described by tracing the life history of a follicle from its earliest stages to full maturation, and of the corpus luteum from the time of ovulation to its terminal stages.

The *primordial* follicles, found in such large numbers in the cortex, consist of a central *germ cell* or *ovum* encircled by a flattened or low cuboidal layer of epithelium, which constitutes the follicle epithelium or *membrana granulosa* (Fig. 17–8). Polyovular follicles may be recognized, particularly in early life. As the follicle grows, the granulosa becomes definitely cuboidal and later stratified, showing at first two and later several layers of cells. The follicle now begins to show a central cavity or antrum, the ovum being placed at one pole and surrounded by a peninsula-like accumulation of granulosa cells, the *cumulus oophorus* or *discus proligerus* (Figs. 17–9 and 17–10). No blood vessels are to be seen in the granulosa, which is dependent for its nutrition upon the highly vascular *theca interna,* which surrounds it externally. The cells of the theca interna, although stromal in appearance, as noted above are derived from the mesothelium and are very sensitive to hormonal influences, which at various phases give them an epithelial appearance (theca lutein cells). Strassmann has shown that a cone or wedge of theca cells, the *theca cone,* is formed at one portion of the follicle, apparently directing the growth of the latter toward the surface. Finally, external to the theca interna is a layer of rather condensed ovarian stroma, the *theca externa,* which under certain circumstances, such as trophoblastic disease and metastatic tumors, may demonstrate its ability to react (become luteinized), with the resultant hormone production.

The Mature Follicle. The mature graafian follicle is a structure of considerable size, though rarely exceeding 8 mm. in diameter.

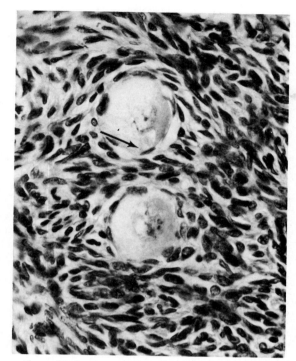

Figure 17–8. Primordial follicles—germ cells with flattened, primitive granulosa (at arrow).

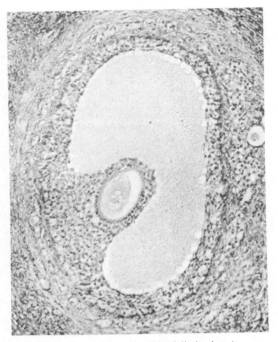

Figure 17–9. Maturing graafian follicle showing ovum embedded in cumulus oophorus.

It does not usually protrude to any extent above the surface of the ovary, as is the case in many of the lower animals. Nor does it present any external characteristics which enable one to distinguish it from other cystic structures frequently seen on the surface of the ovary, particularly the degenerated or atretic follicles. From without inward it shows the following elements:

1. *Theca externa,* which, as already mentioned, represents a layer of condensed ovarian mesenchyme.

2. *Theca interna,* made up of a zone of cells of specialized mesenchymal tissue and highly susceptible to both normal and abnormal hormonal influences. In the mature follicle the cells show marked hypertrophy and are rich in lipid before and after ovulation. The theca interna is very vascular, the blood vessels forming a wreath about the granulosa (perigranulosal vascular wreath).

3. The *membrana granulosa* of the mature follicle consists of a number of layers of characteristically round or polyhedral cells, compactly placed, and showing darkly staining central nuclei with frequent mitoses (Fig. 17–11). As the granulosa grows, it not infrequently shows tiny vacuolar areas of cystic degeneration, with clear central cavities surrounded by a layer of granulosa cells (Figs. 17–12 and 17–13), the so-called Call-Exner bodies. These arrangements are characteristic of granulosa growth, a point of importance in the diagnosis of the granulosa cell tumor. At this stage, the large ovoid central cavity or *antrum* is filled with a clear fluid, the *liquor folliculi.*

4. *The germ cell area.* At one pole is the large and well developed *cumulus oophorus* or *discus proligerus,* an aggregation of granulosa cells in which the ovum is embedded (Fig. 17–9). The innermost layer of granulosa cells, those immediately surrounding the ovum, are disposed in radial fashion, constituting the *corona radiata.* Within the latter is an amorphous refractile membrane, the *zona pellucida.* Between this and the

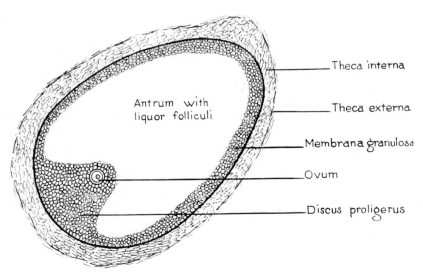

Antrum with liquor folliculi

Theca interna

Theca externa

Membrana granulosa

Ovum

Discus proligerus

Figure 17–10. Diagrammatic drawing of chief constituent elements of mature follicle.

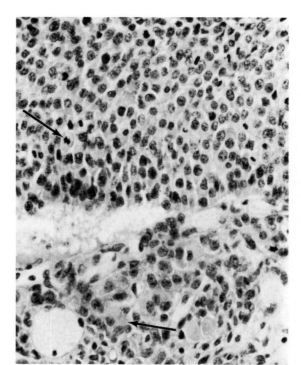

Figure 17–11. Mature follicle, showing mitoses in unluteinized granulosa above and vascularization of luteinized theca below.

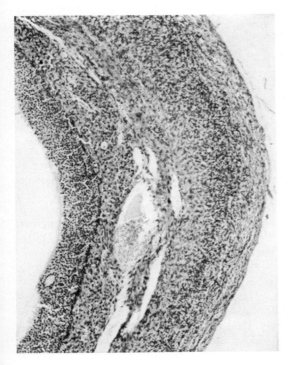

Figure 17–12. Wall of mature follicle. Note the well developed theca interna beneath the granulosa.

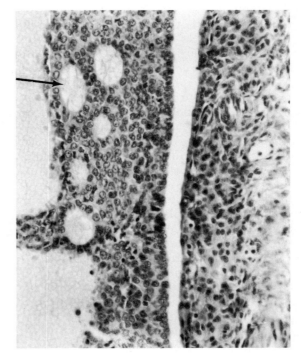

Figure 17–13. High power view showing Call-Exner bodies in the granulosa layer (at arrow).

ovum is a very small *perivitelline space*. The cell wall of the ovum is the *vitelline membrane*, its nucleus the *germinal vesicle*, and its nucleolus the *germinal spot*.

A histochemical study of the adult human ovary, which is profusely illustrated and heartily recommended, is that of McKay and co-workers, who describe the histology and function of the ovary throughout the cycle.

The Corpus Luteum of Menstruation

The life history of the corpus luteum begins immediately after ovulation, although it is impossible to distinguish a recently ruptured follicle from an early corpus luteum until luteinization becomes apparent in the transformed granulosa cells. The exact hormonal mechanism of the ovulation suggests a delicate balance between the pituitary gonadotropic hormones, with a "luteinizing hormone surge" that is of key importance. The local mechanism in the ovary is not well defined. The increasing tension of the follicular fluid, the contraction of questionably present involuntary muscle fibers surrounding the follicle, and a local enzyme-like erosion effect upon the ovarian tissue overlying the follicle have all been suggested, though the last of these is now commonly accepted as the most important. Possibly prostaglandin is the key enzyme in this process. Strassmann has stressed the fact that ovulation is facilitated by wedgelike thickening of the theca interna at the distal pole of the follicle.

Very Early Corpus Luteum (Stage of Proliferation or Hyperemia). With the extrusion of the egg, at approximately the midinterval period, the follicle collapses and its wall undergoes more or less crumpling (Fig. 17–14). The small opening from which the egg escapes (the stigma) soon becomes plugged with fibrin and then a light cicatricial tissue. In its earliest stages the corpus luteum is not a conspicuous structure and is in most instances demonstrated only on section of the ovary. Bleeding does not characteristically occur with ovulation, contrary to the belief of ovulatory bleeding as a cause of "Mittelschmerz." In this early stage the corpus luteum presents as a collapsed vesicle whose wall is thin, not convoluted, and has a grayish-yellow hue instead of the brilliant yellow of later phases.

As might be expected, the microscopic appearance of the wall just after ovulation does

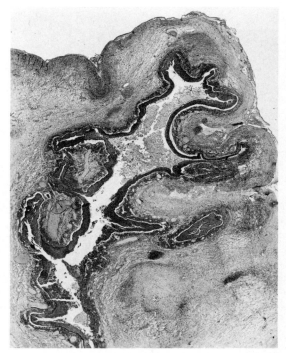

Figure 17–14. Crumpling of mature follicle which has just ruptured.

not differ very materially from that of the follicle just before rupture, so that the distinction is not easily made. The granulosa is not thrown off at ovulation, though the ovum carries with it the zona pellucida and a portion of the cells of the cumulus, probably utilizing these for nutritional purposes in its passage through the tube, and in certain animals as a necessary complement for ovum "pick-up." The major portion of the granulosa remains, and the characteristic lutein cells of the corpus luteum are formed from a modification of these remaining granulosa cells. Within a matter of hours the beginning of this transformation is seen, though in the early stages the theca interna cells resemble lutein cells far more than do the granulosa cells (Figs. 17–15 and 17–16).

In this early stage (stage of proliferation or hyperemia), the histologic picture represents only a slight advance over that characterizing the mature follicle. The characteristic features are the as yet untransformed granulosa, the large ovoid or polyhedral theca cells laden with lipid, the absence of blood vessels in the granulosa as contrasted with the vascularity of the theca, and the fact that the lumen of the corpus as yet contains little or no blood.

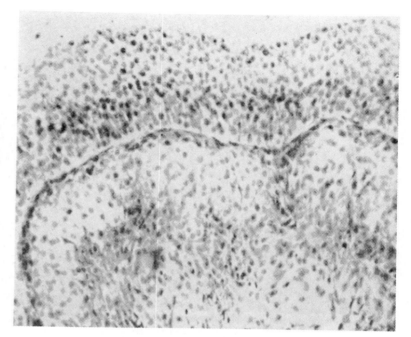

Figure 17–15. High power view of corpus luteum. Granulosa layer above; theca below, though marked luteinization is as yet not apparent.

Stage of Vascularization. By rapid transition, however, the corpus passes into its second phase, that of vascularization. The chief feature is a penetration of the granulosa by thin-walled blood channels arising from the vessels of the theca. These pass vertically through the granulosa toward the lumen,

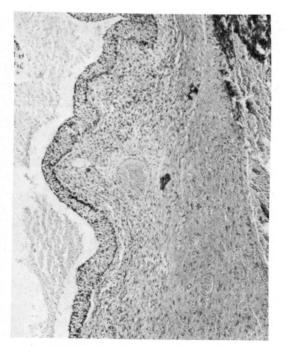

Figure 17–16. Another very early corpus luteum.

often opening into the latter and filling it at least partially with blood. The granulosa cells have in the meantime become large and polyhedral. The cytoplasm is abundant and acidophilic. The small dark nuclei show mitoses until the eighteenth day of the normal 28-day cycle. The hemorrhage into the lumen is usually of a zonal type, a layer of blood being seen adjacent to the lutein zone. In some cases, however, bleeding is much freer, so that the entire lumen is distended with blood (Fig. 17–17). When the bleeding is extremely free, a corpus luteum hematoma may be produced (see Chapter 20). Immediately after the bleeding phase, a layer of fibroblasts forms over the inner surface of the lutein cells. The age of this layer aids in determining the age of the corpus luteum. Degeneration begins on about the twenty-second or twenty-third day of the cycle and is recognized by the appearance of vacuoles in the lutein cells, the "mulberry cells." These changes have been well described by Corner.

The theca interna, so prominent in the earlier stage, undergoes regression, the cells becoming much smaller and losing their lipoid content. The theca begins to push down with the blood vessels into the lutein layer, forming wedgelike trabeculae, which later divide the lutein zone into compartments. The stage of vascularization is sometimes divided into two stages, early and late vascu-

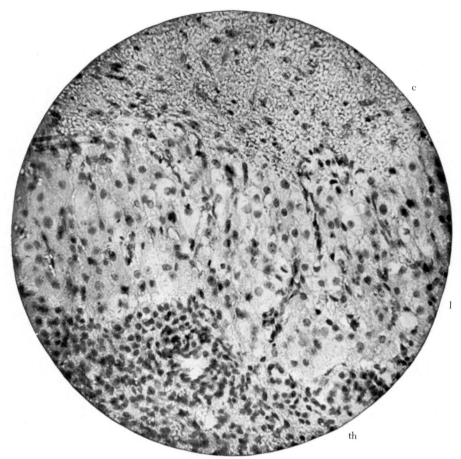

Figure 17–17. Wall of corpus luteum in stage of early vascularization (sixteenth day). Blood vessels from the theca are pushing into the granulosa layer (*l*) which now shows definite lutein characteristics. The theca cells (*th*) have undergone retrogression. The blood now in the cavity (*c*) is beginning to be invaded by endothelial cells.

larization, differing from one another only in degree. On occasion intraperitoneal hemorrhage may occur (this may present a clinical picture identical with ectopic pregnancy, especially when bleeding occurs from the corpus luteum in the gravid patient).

During this phase the corpus is usually easily recognizable on the surface of the ovary. It may form a dark reddish mound rising above the surface, but in other cases it is entirely beneath the surface. Surrounding the hemorrhagic corpus one frequently sees intensely injected blood vessels converging toward it. On cutting into the corpus, the now definitely festooned and bright yellowish lutein zone stands out in sharp contrast to the blood within the lumen.

Stage of Maturity. With the approach of the menstrual period the corpus reaches the stage of maturity. This phase may be arbi-

trarily considered to begin about 10 days or so preceding the menstrual flow, though there is no sharp histologic line of demarcation between this and the preceding phase. The lutein zone is now a very broad one, traversed by trabeculae of theca interna containing numerous blood vessels. The theca cells become definitely epithelioid in appearance, and frequently somewhat alveolar in arrangement (Figs. 17–18 and 17–19). The endocrine significance of these *theca lutein* or *paralutein cells* is related apparently to estrogen production. They are highly developed in the early corpora lutea of early pregnancy. The so-called luteoma of pregnancy will be discussed in a later chapter.

As the corpus matures, there is gradual resorption of the blood within the cavity, though its disappearance is rarely complete. A delicate layer of fibroblastic tissue is de-

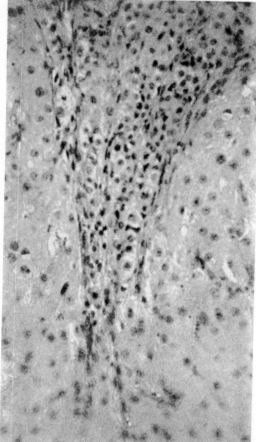

Figure 17–18. Contrast between the granulosa lutein and the theca lutein or paralutein cells near top of septum (labeled *p* in Figure 17–19).

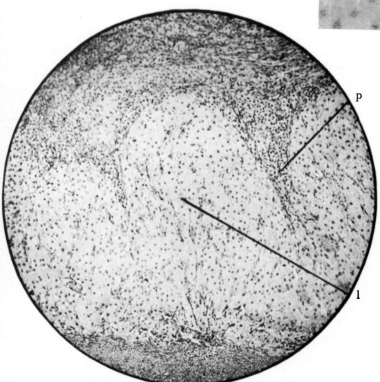

Figure 17–19. Wall of mature corpus luteum (twenty-seventh day), showing lutein (*l*) and theca lutein or paralutein (*p*) cells.

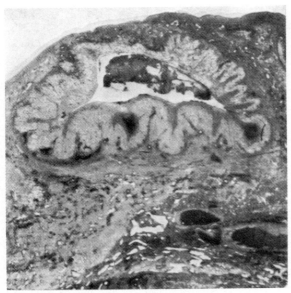

Figure 17–20. Mature corpus luteum near surface of ovary.

posited along the lumen edge of the lutein zone at about the eighteenth day, shutting off the blood vessels.

The mature corpus luteum is a large structure, measuring at least 1 to 1.5 cm. in diameter. It may be easily visible on the ovarian surface, but sometimes it is below the surface, so that it is exposed only on cutting into the ovary (Figs. 17–20 and 17–21). Its cavity is sometimes large and filled with light yellowish fluid, though more often the cavity is small, partly organized with light connective tissue, with a small amount of clear or bloody fluid. The lutein zone is broad and heavily festooned, of bright carrot-like hue. Various

shades of yellow may be observed in different corpora, probably due to different oxidation products of the pigment carotin, upon which the yellowish color depends.

Stage of Retrogression. The retrogressive phase of the corpus luteum begins, not at the onset of menstruation, but probably on about the twenty-second or twenty-third day of the cycle, according to the studies of Brewer. Corner, on the basis of extensive studies in the rhesus monkey, is inclined to place the beginning of retrogression at about four or five days before the onset of menstruation, i.e., the twenty-third to twenty-fourth day of the "normal" menstrual cycle.

Retrogression is characterized by increase of lipids and increasing fibrosis of the lutein zone, followed after some weeks by hyalinization (Fig. 17–22). With these changes is associated an increasing cicatrization and shrinkage of the core, so that after a few months the structure, now known as a *corpus albicans*, is characterized by an amorphous, convoluted, completely hyalinized center surrounding a plug of cicatricial tissue (Fig. 17–23). It is of interest that even in its fossilized, hyalinized state the original lutein zone is sharply marked off from the cicatricial mass filling the original lumen. The yellowish color of the retrogressive corpus may persist for as long as 4 to 6 months. Ultimately, as indicated by the work of Joel and Foraker, the corpus albicans is completely resorbed by the ovarian stroma.

Corner has also called attention to the observation that while corpora lutea of the standard type undergo the retrogressive changes described, an alternative mode of

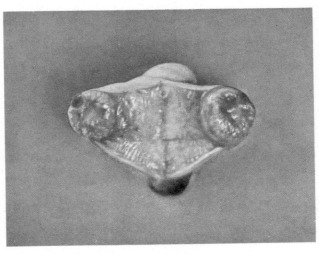

Figure 17–21. Mature corpus luteum.

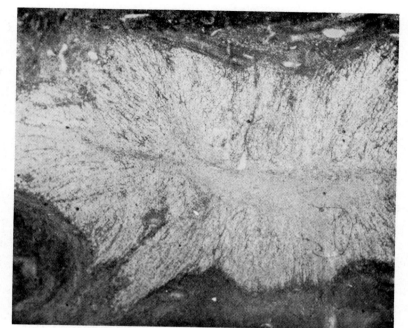

Figure 17–22. Corpus luteum showing beginning retrogression.

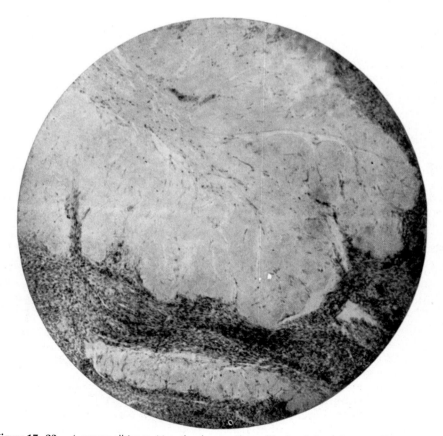

Figure 17–23. A corpus albicans. Note the sharp outline of the hyalinized, festooned lutein layer.

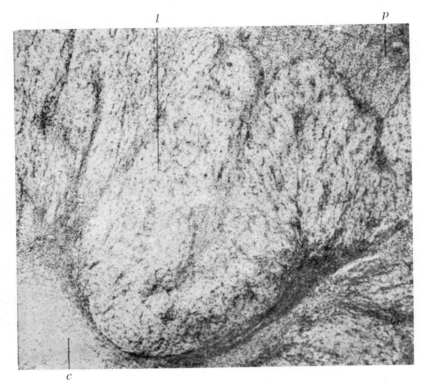

Figure 17–24. Corpus luteum of early pregnancy, showing lutein cells (*l*), paralutein cells (*p*), and organization along inner wall of lutein layer (c).

retrogression sometimes occurs in the rhesus monkey. Retrogression in the monkey involves *corpora aberrantia*, which after the menstrual period enter into a phase of prolonged existence somewhat like that of the corpus luteum of pregnancy, although there is no knowledge as to the mechanism and time of their ultimate disappearance. Corner also speaks of the occasional occurrence in monkeys of *herniation* or *eversion of the corpus luteum*, the lutein layer being widely everted on the surface of the ovary, forming a conspicuous cauliflower crater.

The Corpus Luteum of Pregnancy

In the event of pregnancy the corpus luteum does not retrogress, but becomes even larger, to form the corpus luteum of pregnancy (Fig. 17–24). This structure may make up a third or more of the ovarian substance. Not infrequently it has a rather large cystic content (Fig. 17–25). In such cases the festooning of the lutein zone is less marked, although in others, with more cicatricial tissue within the lumen, the convolution of the lutein zone may be marked. Paralutein cells may be prominent, largely dependent on the stage of the pregnancy. During the early weeks the high levels of chorionic gonado-

tropin produce alterations which mimic the extreme proliferation that may occur with hydatidiform mole or choriocarcinoma. Thus theca lutein cysts similar to those found with trophoblastic disease may occur in conjunction with normal pregnancy.

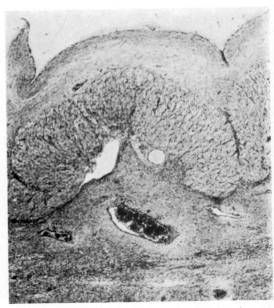

Figure 17–25. Another corpus luteum of early pregnancy.

Atresia Folliculi

Of the many primordial follicles in the ovary at birth, only a very small proportion run the entire gamut of changes described. The vast majority die long before full maturation, and with every cycle many follicles are thus blighted, only one as a rule going on to complete maturation and corpus luteum formation. And yet many start to mature at the beginning of each cycle, degenerating at various stages of development through the process known as atresia folliculi. The death of the ovum undoubtedly is the immediate cause of the death of the follicle, being followed by degeneration of the satellite follicle epithelium.

In the *cystic stage* of atresia (Fig. 17–26), therefore, one finds a follicle of varying size lined by degenerating granulosa or a fibrotic core, in which case the theca interna forms the wall. Numerous tiny follicular cysts, or microcysts, are found in most ovaries. In some cases they may become large enough to be classified as a non-neoplastic cyst (see Chapter 20). Under certain pathologic conditions, and also during pregnancy, the ovary may be studded with these cystic atretic follicles.

The cystic stage is followed by one of *cicatricial obliteration* (Fig. 17–27). A layer of cicatricial tissue develops just within the theca, with often a dense, refractile layer marking the basement membrane of the granulosa. With increasing cicatrization the cavity becomes completely obliterated, the cicatrix being surrounded by a wavy hyalinized layer of connective tissue. The end product thus left is known as the *corpus fibrosum*. It is easily distinguishable from the corpus albicans, chiefly by its small size and the much narrower hyalinized connective tissue zone. Follicles of varying degrees of maturation and atresia are frequent in the youthful premenarchal female.

Ovarian Changes in Pregnancy

The most conspicuous feature of the ovary in early gestation is the presence of the *corpus luteum of pregnancy*, already described. It begins to retrogress after about $2\frac{1}{2}$ months.

Decidual changes are quite common, patches of decidual cells being found just beneath the surface of the ovary (Fig. 17–28). They are not to be interpreted as representing decidual changes in a proceeding endometriosis, though this may also occasionally be seen. Characteristically such ectopic ovarian decidua is not associated with glandular elements and, like the ectopic decidua regularly seen in the pelvis, it is apparently due to the sensitivity of the submesothelial stroma to the pregnancy hormones. These foci of decidua classically fibrose and disappear; however, in large groups, the fibrosis may produce a tumorlike projection, known erroneously as leiomyomatosis peritonealis disseminata.

Although *ovulation* usually *ceases* during pregnancy, *numerous atretic follicles* are seen throughout the ovaries, the follicles being thus blighted at an early stage of development. The paper by Nelson and Greene adequately summarizes pregnancy changes in the ovary.

Medulla of Ovary

The medulla of the ovary is made up of a rather loosely arranged connective tissue quite different from the closely packed spindle cells of the cortex. At the hilus, where the ovarian vessels, lymphatics, and nerves enter and leave, the arrangement is especially loose (Fig. 17–29). In this region one often finds remnants of certain early embryonic structures, especially the *rete ovarii*

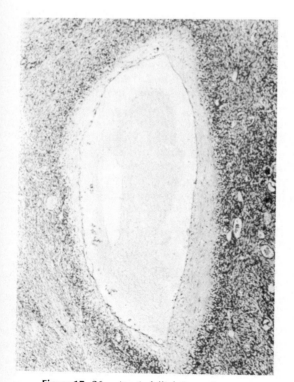

Figure 17–26. Atretic follicle in cystic stage.

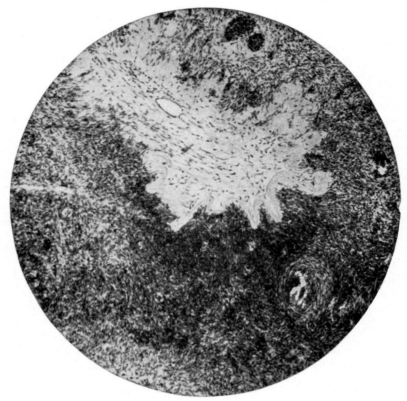

Figure 17–27. The obliterative stage of atresia folliculi, the cavity being practically obliterated by fibrous tissue (corpus fibrosum).

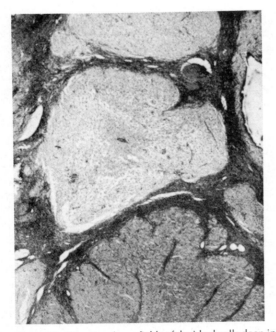

Figure 17–28. Two large fields of decidual cells deep in ovary, with corpus luteum of pregnancy below. Ectopic ovarian decidua is more frequently found on or just beneath surface.

and the *parovarian tubules* (Fig. 17–30). The latter are of wolffian (mesonephric) origin. They appear usually as clusters of small lumina lined by cuboidal epithelium and always surrounded by a thick muscular zone. The rete, on the other hand, appears as narrow, slitlike tubules, often zigzag in arrangement and frequently anastomosing. They are lined by a flat epithelium and show no surrounding muscle tissue. Occasionally a papillary-like invagination into one of these cystic spaces is representative of the mesonephric glomerulus.

Sympathicotropic or Hilus Cells

In 1923, Berger described islands of so-called sympathicotropic cells, which are not infrequently found in the hilus of the ovary, sometimes only as small perineural rests, but occasionally forming large fields. These cells vary somewhat in size and shape, but are usually polyhedral or ovoid, and arranged in somewhat mosaic fashion (Fig. 17–31). They are undoubtedly present in

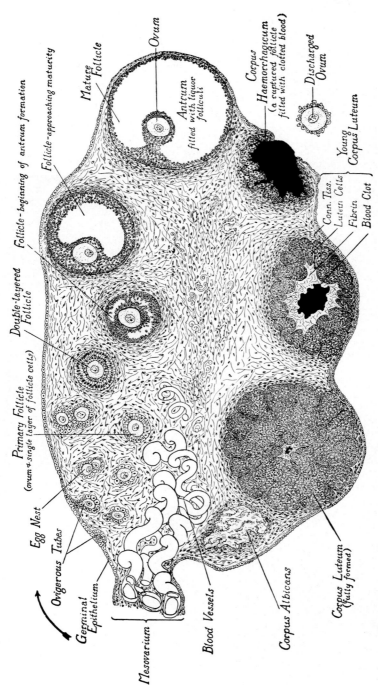

Figure 17–29. Schematic drawing of mammalian ovary showing sequence of events in origin, growth, and rupture of ovarian follicle, and retrogression of corpus luteum. (From Patten: Embryology of the Pig. P. Blakiston's Son & Co., Inc., Publishers.)

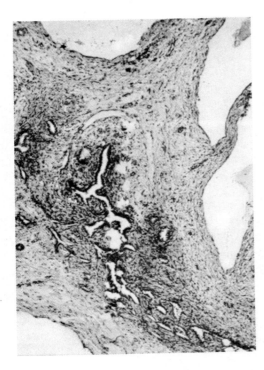

Figure 17–30. Tubules of rete ovarii in hilus of ovary.

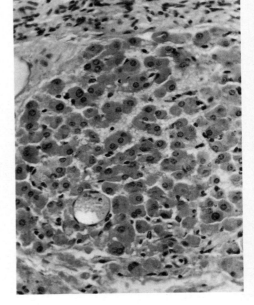

Figure 17–31. A large nest of hilus cells, formerly called sympathicotropic, in hilus of ovary, considered to be homologues of testicular interstitial cells of Leydig.

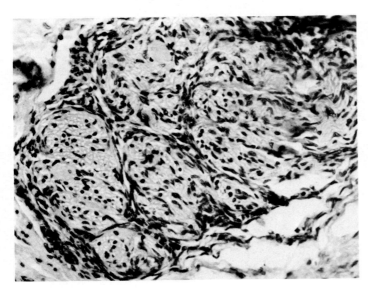

Figure 17–32. Nerve in hilus of ovary with stromal cells divided into compartments (unluteinized hilus cells?).

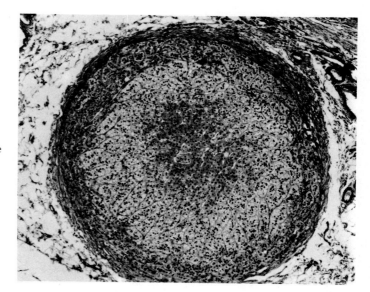

Figure 17–33. Adrenal rest found in the parovarian region.

the hilus of all ovaries as "stroma-like" elements (Fig. 17–32); however, as with most gonadal mesenchyme, only when luteinization occurs is the cell unique. The cells seem to be histologically and functionally related to the interstitial or Leydig cells of the testicle, particularly since the so-called Reinke crystals are also found in the ovarian hilus cells. As a matter of fact, a small number of tumors arising from these cells have been reported as producing virilizing effects similar to those found with arrhenoblastoma (see Chapter 28).

In the same area, often more closely associated with the tube, are found adrenal rests (Fig. 17–33). These, too, may give rise to tumors that can produce any of the alterations in the host that are ascribed to adrenal lesions in the normal, suprarenal locale. Masculinization has been the most frequent manifestation of such neoplasms to which the literature has alluded.

REFERENCES

Baker, T. G.: Development of the ovary and oogenesis. Clin. Obstet. Gynecol., *3*:26, 1976.

Baker, T. G.: A quantitative and cytological study of germ cells in human ovaries. Proc. Roy. Soc. Med., 56:417, 1963.

Beck, F., Moffatt, D. B., and Lloyd, J. B.: Human embryology and genetics. Oxford, England, Blackwells, 1973.

Berger, L.: La glande sympathicotrope du hile de l'ovaire; ses homologies avec la gland interstitielle du testicule. Les rapports nerveuses des deux glandes. Arch. Anat., *2*:255, 1923.

Brewer, J. I.: Studies of the human corpus luteum. Am. J. Obstet. Gynecol., *44*:1063, 1942.

Corner, G. W.: Development, organization and breakdown of the corpus luteum in the rhesus monkey. Contrib. Embryol., *31*:117, 1945.

Corner, G. W., Jr.: Histologic dating of corpus luteum of menstruation. Am. J. Anat., *98*:377, 1956.

Curtis, E. M.: Normal ovarian histology in infancy and childhood. Obstet. Gynecol., *19*:444, 1962.

Evans, H. M., and Swezy, O.: Ovogenesis and the normal follicular cycle in adult mammalia. Mem. Univ. Calif., *9*:119, 1931.

Felix, W.: Development of the urogenital organs. *In* F. Keibel and F. P. Mall (Eds.): Manual of Human Embryology. Vol. 2. Philadelphia, J. B. Lippincott Co., 1912, p. 752.

Fischel, A.: Uber die Entwicklung der Keimdrusen des Menschen. Z. ges. Anat., Abt. 1, *92*:43, 1930.

Fraenkel, L.: Die Funktion des Corpus Luteum. Arch. Gynäk., *68*:438, 1903.

Gillman, J.: The development of the gonads in man with a consideration of the role of fetal endocrines and the histogenesis of ovarian tumors. Contrib. Embryol., *32*:81, 1948.

Gillman, J., and Stein, H. B.: Human corpus luteum of pregnancy. Surg. Gynecol. Obstet., *72*:129, 1941.

Gondos, B.: Surface epithelium of the developing ovary. Am. J. Pathol., *81*:303, 1975.

Gruenwald, P.: Development of sex cords in gonads of man and mammals. Am. J. Anat., *70*:359, 1942.

Joel, R. V., and Foraker, A. G.: Fate of the corpus albicans. A morphologic approach. Am. J. Obstet. Gynecol., *80*:314, 1960.

Jones, W. J., and Huston, J. W.: Bilateral theca lutein cysts associated with an apparently normal pregnancy. Am. J. Obstet. Gynecol., *81*:1033, 1961.

Lynch, M. J. G., Kyle, P. R., Raphael, S. S., and Bruce-Lockhart, P.: Unusual ovarian changes (hyperthecosis) in pregnancy. Am. J. Obstet. Gynecol., 77:335, 1959.

Marcotty, A.: Uber das Corpus luteum menstruationis und das Corpus luteum graviditatis. Arch. Gynäk., *103*:63, 1914.

McKay, D. G., Pinkerton, J. H. M., Hertig, A. T., and

Danzigen, S.: The adult human ovary—a histochemical study. Obstet. Gynecol., *18*:13, 1961.

Meyer, R.: Uber Corpus Luteumbidlung beim Menschen. Zbl. Gynäk., *35*:1206, 1911.

Meyer, R.: Uber das Stadium proliferationis s. Hyperaemicum sowie uber den Bergriff und die Abgrenzung des Blutstadiums des Corpus Luteum beim Menschen. Arch. Gynäk., *149*:315, 1932.

Nelson, W. W., and Green, R. R.: Histology of human ovary during pregnancy. Am. J. Obstet. Gynecol., *76*:66, 1958.

Novak, E.: The corpus luteum; its life cycle and its role in menstrual disorders. J.A.M.A., *67*:1285, 1916.

Pinkerton, J. H. M., McKay, D. G., Adams, E. C., and Hertig, A. T.: Development of the human ovary using differential stains. Obstet. Gynecol., *18*:152, 1961.

Politzer, G.: Die Keimbahn des Menschen. Z. Anat. Entwicklungagesch., *100*:331, 1933.

Pratt, J. P.: Human corpus luteum. Arch. Pathol., *19*:380, 1935.

Rosenthal, A. H.: Rupture of the corpus luteum. Am. J. Obstet. Gynecol., *79*:1008, 1959.

Strassmann, E. O.: The theca cone and its tropism toward the ovarian surface, a typical feature of growing human and mammalian follicles. Trans. Am. Assn. Obstet. Gynecol., *53*:11, 1940.

Wallart, J.: Uber Fruhstadien und Abortivformen der Corpus Luteumbildung. Arch. Gynäk., *103*:544, 1914.

Witschi, E.: Migration of the germ cells of human embryos from the yolk sac to the primitive gonadal folds. Contrib. Embryol., *32*:67, 1948.

Chapter 18

INFLAMMATORY DISEASES
OF THE OVARY

Etiology

In the overwhelming majority of cases, inflammatory lesions of the ovary or more accurately on the peritoneal surfaces of the ovary, are secondary to inflammation of the tube, with which the ovary is in such intimate contact. The organisms concerned, therefore, are those responsible for salpingitis, including the gonococcus, the streptococcus, *Bacteroides*, and a variety of both aerobic and anaerobic organisms. The colon bacillus may be either a primary or a secondary invader, as is the case when adnexal disease is secondary to such conditions as acute appendicitis or sigmoid diverticulitis. Hematogenous infection is rare but may be associated with mumps or, less frequently, the acute exanthemas of children.

Basically the body of the ovary appears to be relatively resistant to involvement with the common pelvic inflammatory disease. To a major degree the peritoneal surface demonstrates a perioophoritis with adhesion formation. The associated peritoneal inclusions, often with mesothelial proliferation and formation of psammoma-like concretions, suggest the development of the common papillary serous cystadenoma. Nevertheless, malignancy resulting from such chronic inflammatory reactions must be rare, since the tube rarely demonstrates the classic results of chronic infection in cases of ovarian neoplasia.

ACUTE OOPHORITIS

This is far less frequently encountered than the chronic form because operations are rarely performed for the common acute pelvic inflammatory disease. In this acute phase the inflammation is limited to its most superficial portion, appearing as a serofibrinous or fibrinous acute perioophoritis. Grossly, this is characterized by a light fibrinous deposit upon the surface of the ovary, with evidences of an acute inflammatory process in the immediately subepithelial fibrous tissue, but with little tendency to penetrate more deeply. On the other hand, in the occasional severe acute pelvic infection, the ovarian involvement may be much more pronounced, the whole organ being edematous and hyperemic.

The ovarian surface at certain cyclic phases may offer inviting portals of entry to infectious organisms from the tubal orifice, and extensive inflammatory involvement or tubo-ovarian abscess formation may result. Similarly, the ovary is involved through its proximity or fixation to an acutely inflamed appendix or sigmoid. More frequently, however, the acute process is mild and superficial, disappearing with the subsidence of the acute tubal inflammation with which it is most frequently associated, leaving only a chronic perioophoritis and its associated adhesive disease.

ABSCESS OF THE OVARY

True abscess formation in the ovary appears to be a rare entity. Even with severe salpingitis and its associated peritonitis, the body of the ovary is relatively free of deep-seated disease and continues to function with remarkable regularity, the associated menstrual irregularities probably resulting

375

from acute exacerbations of endometritis. Nevertheless, such deep-seated infections may be seen with pelvic tuberculosis in which hematogenous spread of the infection has occurred.

Ovarian abscess, without tubal involvement, may develop under a variety of circumstances, as noted by Willson and Black, in patients who have undergone hysterectomy, usually vaginal. In such cases direct infection of the ovary, often lying against the vaginal cuff, seems to be the mode of spread of organisms into the stroma. It was originally suggested that patients operated on at the time of ovulation were more prone to develop such abscesses, but subsequent studies have not confirmed this impression. Obviously lymphatic and hematogenous spread of infectious agent may play a role in the development of such abscesses, though the associated systemic reaction is minimal.

More commonly, ovarian infection is a sequel to tubal disease, a pyosalpinx, in which the tube fuses with the ovary forming a tubo-ovarian abscess. Such abscesses are frequently bilateral. A corpus luteum abscess is rarely a discrete entity, although a tubo-ovarian abscess may involve the recent site of ovulation. More frequently, the yellowish-gray color of the inflammatory mass creates an erroneous gross impression. Added to this is the microscopic appearance of pseudoxanthoma cells, which mimic the color of lutein tissue.

Recent studies of pelvic infections associated with use of intrauterine devices suggest that the ovarian stroma is the site of foci of acute infection in the absence of extensive tubal disease. The possibility exists that repeated "bursts" of infected material from the tubal ostium into the operculi created by ovulation may be the modus operandi in the genesis of such lesions.

Microscopic Appearance

Under the microscope, the wall of an ovarian abscess presents the picture of an acute or chronic inflammatory process, depending upon the age of the lesion. In the acute abscess, especially the interstitial variety, the purulent exudate, consisting of polymorphonuclear leukocytes and cellular detritus, is surrounded by ovarian stroma showing an acute inflammatory reaction in the immediate vicinity of the infected tube but little evidence of widespread involvement of the ovarian stroma. More frequently one sees the abscess in a chronic or quiescent stage. Under these conditions, the abscess wall is found to consist of granulation tissue or, in still later stages, a layer of fibroblastic or even dense, fully formed connective tissue, with considerable hyalinization (Fig. 18–1). Deposits of cholesterol crystals are common findings in the adjacent tissue. Even with such extensive reaction, the gonadal stromal elements remain remarkably normal and cyclic function persists. Actually the evidence is lacking that such common inflammatory processes cause destruction of functioning elements and early menopause.

The large phagocytic leukocytes or pseudoxanthoma cells found in the walls of abscesses of any type, as previously noted, may be mistaken for lutein cells (Fig. 18–2). These likewise may be arranged in a tilelike manner. They are often larger than the lutein cells, and the classic lobular arrangement of the old corpus luteum is usually lacking; occasionally, however, an absolute differentiation between the two processes is impossible.

Finally, in the uncommon tuberculous ab-

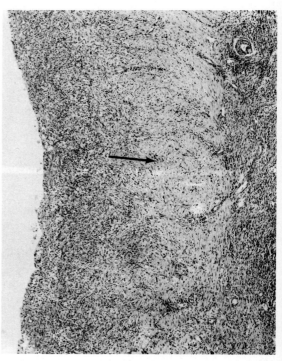

Figure 18–1. Wall of tubo-ovarian abscess. Upper layer of chronic inflammatory cells has few polymorphonuclear leukocytes; beneath this is a layer of scar tissue with hyalinization (at arrow). Developing follicle is seen in upper right.

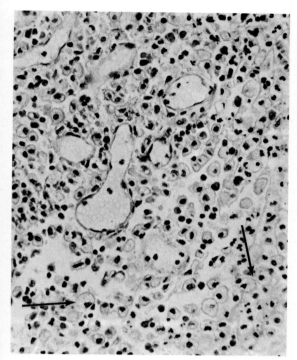

Figure 18–2. Pseudoxanthoma cells (at arrows) simulating lutein cells.

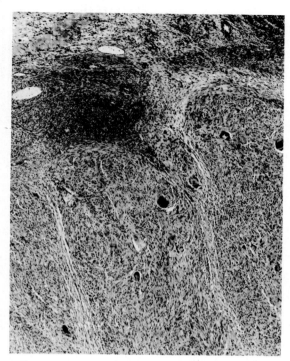

Figure 18–3. Granulomatous perioophoritis with fibrosis and tubercle formation. Ovarian stroma above.

scess, the microscopic diagnosis must depend upon the finding in the wall of the abscess or in the immediately adjoining ovarian tissue of such characteristic features as tubercles with giant cells and the infecting organisms (Fig. 18–3). The diagnosis rarely presents any difficulty, since ovarian tuberculosis is practically always the result of tubal tuberculosis, usually in an advanced stage (Chapter 16). Bilharzial infections are uncommon in our culture, but in Egypt, ovarian stromal reactions suggestive of thecosis have been reported.

CHRONIC PERIOOPHORITIS

The most frequent finding in old pelvic inflammatory disease is chronic perioophoritis. To translate this statement into clinical terms, an adherent but otherwise essentially normal ovary is the most common finding in cases of chronic pelvic inflammatory disease. There is difference of opinion as to whether the presence of dense surrounding adhesions, with thickening of the tunica albuginea, plays an important part in preventing the extrusion of ova at ovulation. Theoretically, this would seem to be

possible when the adhesions are dense and extensive, but practically, this is probably not the cause of the accompanying sterility.

Again, the role of this factor in the production of the cystic ovary must be considered, though it is probably much less important than is believed by many. Certainly it is not rare to find even densely adherent ovaries that are not at all cystic, just as it is common to find polycystic ovaries in the entire absence of adhesions.

Microscopically, chronic perioophoritis appears as a layer of newly formed connective tissue, in various stages of organization, involving the ovarian surface, sometimes quite diffusely and sometimes in small scattered areas. An interesting picture that is frequently encountered, and which may confuse the pathologist, involves the metaplastic changes in the surface epithelium of the peritoneum in the presence of chronic inflammation. The flat mesothelial cells often become cuboidal or columnar, with secretory and ciliated elements.

Invaginations of this modified peritoneum are often seen beneath and between ovarian adhesions, presenting as irregular epithelium-lined clefts that resemble glands (Fig. 18–4). Indeed, a common error is to mistake

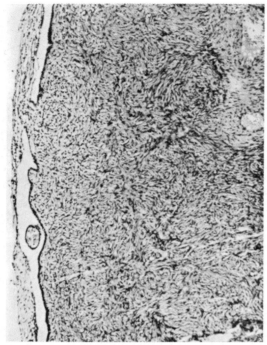

Figure 18–4. Chronic perioophoritis showing metaplasia of surface of ovarian epithelium and peritoneum beneath adhesions on surface.

such glandlike spaces for endometriosis, though no stroma is present except in genuine endometriosis, which is usually seen on the ovarian surface. Such proliferations with psammoma bodies simulate the patterns and cell types seen in the papillary serous tumors of the ovary, and may be construed as neoplastic alterations (Fig. 18–5).

In some cases the coelomic epithelium or the peritoneum included beneath the surface may show a squamous type of metaplasia, with the production of plaques of squamous epithelium characteristic of the so-called Walthard islands. Frequently, the central cavity remains, with the resultant tiny cysts lined by epithelium that is flat or cuboidal in some places and stratified in others.

CHRONIC OOPHORITIS

This term applies to a chronic inflammatory involvement of the entire ovarian structure. It is a rather poorly defined pathologic entity. In spite of the frequency of chronic perioophoritis, the ovary itself seems resistant to the low grade type of infection seen in most cases of pelvic inflammatory disease. However, one does find in some cases a diffuse chronic inflammatory infiltration of the ovarian stroma. Advanced forms of chronic inflammation are described as resulting in ovarian sclerosis, though it would seem difficult to distinguish between this and the sclerotic changes that may result from purely atrophic processes.

One must distinguish between the Stein-Leventhal polycystic ovary and that associated with infection, but it should be noted that with the latter there is frequent evi-

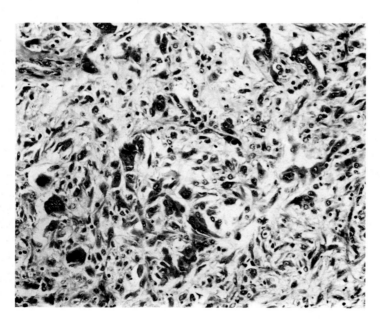

Figure 18–5. Mesothelial proliferations simulating neoplasia.

dence of tubal disease. In addition, the ovary is often adherent, there may be bilateral enlargement, and there is often evidence of one or more corpora lutea. Finally, the classic clinical finding of anovulation is absent in the patient with chronic pelvic infection.

REFERENCES

Amstey, M. S., and Monif, G. R. G.: Genital herpes infection in pregnancy. Obstet. Gynecol., 44:394, 1974.

Black, W. T.: Abscess of ovary. Am J. Obstet. Gynecol., 31:487, 1936.

Curtis, A. H.: Chronic pelvic infections. Surg. Gynecol. Obstet., 42:6, 1926.

Davis, C. H.: Contribution to etiological study of ovaritis. Surg. Gynecol. Obstet., 23:560, 1916.

Hartman, C. G.: Origin of ovarian adhesions from organized liquor folliculi in rhesus monkey. Surg. Gynecol. Obstet., 98:391, 1944.

Ledger, W. J.: Infection in the Female. Philadelphia, Lea & Febiger, 1977.

Niebyl, J., Parmley, T. H., Spence, M., and Woodruff, J. D.: Unilateral ovarian abscess associated with intrauterine device. J. Obstet. Gynecol. (in press).

Novak, E., and TeLinde, R. W.: Pathological anatomy of corpus luteum (abscess, cyst, hematoma and neoplasm). Johns Hopkins Hosp. Bull., 34:289, 1923.

Willson, J. R., and Black, J. R.: Ovarian abscess. Am. J. Obstet. Gynecol., 90:34, 1964.

Chapter 19

CLASSIFICATION OF OVARIAN TUMORS

Classification has been defined as a method, possibly the simplest one, for producing order in any scientific system. Thus, classifications should be practical and understandable to clinician, pathologist, and therapist alike.

A variety of clinical classifications of ovarian tumors have been suggested. Helsel's simple but workable grouping is as follows: Group I, completely removable without extension; Group II, completely removable despite extension; Group III, incompletely removable because of local extension; Group IV, extreme extension or distant metastasis.

The Mayo and the Munnell classifications are similar to that of Helsel except that they include all bilateral tumors in Group II. The Iowa classification, although widely used, has the disadvantage that Group III comprises "recurrent tumors," a rather nebulous term because primary evaluation is a basic feature in staging all malignancies, and reclassification is considered unacceptable.

The accurate staging of carcinoma of the ovary demands careful evaluation of the entire abdominal cavity at the time of initial exploration. Not only must all resectable tumor be removed, but in addition the omentum, lateral gutters of the cavity, dome of the liver, undersurfaces of the diaphragm, and retroperitoneal nodes must be explored.

The pathologic classifications are many and varied; however, as noted above, any classification of ovarian tumors must have a simple skeletal pattern based on the fundamental gross features (cystic or solid) and the microscopic evaluation (benign or malignant).

Of historic interest and comparison with present classifications, the following, devised by Emil Novak, was used in our laboratory for many years:

TUMORS OF THE OVARY

Benign Tumors

    I. Cystic
        A. Non-neoplastic
            1. Follicle
            2. Lutein
                a. Granulosa
                b. Theca
            3. Stein-Leventhal (polycystic with theca luteinization)
            4. Germinal inclusion
        B. Epithelial
            1. Epithelial
                a. Mucinous (see FIGO, page 381)
                b. Serous (see FIGO)
                c. Endometrial
                    (1) Endometriosis (see FIGO)
                    (2) Siderophagic cyst (see FIGO)
            2. Dermoid (benign cystic teratoma)
    II. Solid
        A. Fibroma
        B. Brenner
        C. Others (lymphangioma, mesothelioma, osteochondroma, and assorted rare lesions)

Malignant Tumors

    I. Cystic
        A. Cystadenocarcinoma (see FIGO)

   1. Mucinous
   2. Serous
   B. Carcinoma (epidermoid) arising
      in dermoid
II. Solid
   A. Carcinoma
      1. Papillary
      2. Nonpapillary
   B. Endometrioid (including carcino-
      sarcoma)
   C. Mesonephroma   (metamesone-
      phroma)
III. Other malignant lesions (rare)
   A. Teratoma (including choriocar-
      cinoma, melanoma, etc.)
   B. Lymphoma
   C. Others
IV. Tumors with endocrine potential
    (low malignant potential)
   A. Dysgerminoma—generally inert
   B. Granulosa theca (with or without
      luteinization), generally feminiz-
      ing
   C. Arrhenoblastoma ⎫
   D. Adrenal   ⎬ generally
   E. Hilus   ⎭ virilizing
 V. Metastatic or by extension—pattern
    similar to primary lesion or Kruken-
    berg tumor

A classification based on the fundamental
embryonic features of the ovary and its adjacent structures with the additional of the
common inflammatory and physiologic alterations is as follows:

CLASSIFICATION OF OVARIAN TUMORS BASED ON PATHOPHYSIOLOGY AND EMBRYOLOGY

I. Non-neoplastic lesions
   A. Inflammatory—including adhe-
      sive disease due to subacute or
      chronic infections; peritoneal in-
      clusions and cystic dilatation of
      anomalous paramesonephric struc-
      tures
   B. Physiologic—including granulosa
      and theca lutein cysts; diffuse or
      focal proliferations (thecosis, cor-
      tical granulomas, ?stromal hyper-
      plasia, etc.)
      Stein-Leventhal ovary, luteoma
II. Mesothelial lesions (stromal and epi-
    thelial)
   A. Primarily mesothelial (epithelial),

serous, mucinous, and endometrioid, mesonephroid and clear
cell tumors, mesothelioma: *benign*, borderline (of low malignant
potential), or *malignant* (varying
degrees)
   B. Primarily stromal
      1. Low functional potential—
         fibroadenoma,   cystadenofi-
         broma, Brenner tumor: *benign*,
         borderline (of low malignant
         potential); *malignant* (varying
         degrees)
      2. High functional potential—
         granulosa-theca cell and Ser-
         toli-Leydig tumors; gonadal
         stromal tumors with varying
         degrees of differentiation (see
         Chapter 27)
   C. Stromal (mesenchymal) tumors
      (variable functional potential)—
      fibroma, fibrothecoma, thecoma,
      ?luteoma, gonadal stromal tumors,
      and sarcoma
   D. Metastatic tumors
III. Germ cell tumors
   A. Dysgerminoma
   B. Teratoma
      1. Extraembryonal—endodermal
         sinus; choriocarcinoma, poly-
         vesicular vitelline (yolk sac);
         mixed (?embryonal carcinoma)
      2. Embryonal
         a. Polymorphic (benign tera-
            toma or dermoid cyst)
         b. Monomorphic
            (1) Struma ovarii
            (2) Carcinoid
            (3) Mucinous (benign)
         c. Immature—primarily neuro-
            blastic (?polyembryoma)
         d. Secondary—squamous car-
            cinoma, mucinous cysta-
            denocarcinoma, malignant
            struma,   leiomyosarcoma,
            etc.
      3. Mixed types (specify)
   C. Dysgenetic   gonads—common
      sites for the development of germ
      cell tumors (gonadoblastoma and
      other aberrant gonads in which
      the XY mosaicism is present)
IV. Parovarian lesions
   A. Cysts and hydatids, etc.
   B. Mesonephroma (also known as
      metamesonephroma)
   C. Hilar cell

D. Adrenal rest
E. Arrhenoblastoma
V. Other tumors (rarely primarily ovarian)
   A. Lymphoma, hemangiopericytoma, myoma, angioma

In 1964 at Mar del Plata, the Cancer Committee of the International Federation of Gynecology and Obstetrics adopted the following classification of primary carcinoma of the ovary. Although this classification covers only the epithelial tumors, it is a step in the direction of uniformity, and clarifies the position of the hitherto nebulous group of endometrioid lesions. Further standardization of the many complicated neoplasms must be forthcoming.

Histologic Classification of the Common Primary Epithelial Tumors of the Ovary

I. Serous cystomas
   A. Serous benign cystadenoma
   B. Serous cystadenomas with proliferating activity of the epithelial cells and nuclear abnormalities, but with no infiltrative destructive growth (low potential malignancy)
   C. Serous cystadenocarcinomas
II. Mucinous cystomas
   A. Mucinous benign cystadenomas
   B. Mucinous cystadenomas with proliferating activity of the epithelial cells and nuclear abnormalities, but with no infiltrative destructive growth (low potential malignancy)
   C. Mucinous cystadenocarcinomas
III. Endometrioid tumors (similar to adenocarcinomas in the endometrium)
   A. Endometrioid benign cysts
   B. Endometrioid tumors with proliferating activity of the epithelial cells and nuclear abnormalities but with no infiltrative destructive growth (low potential malignancy)
   C. Endometrioid adenocarcinomas
IV. Mesonephric tumors
   A. Benign mesonephric tumors
   B. Mesonephric tumors with proliferating activity of the epithelial cells and nuclear abnormalities but with no infiltrative destructive growth (low potential malignancy)
   C. Mesonephric cystadenocarcinomas
V. Concomitant carcinomas, unclassified carcinomas (tumors which cannot be allotted to one of the Groups I, II, or III)

These broad classifications are generally acceptable, although Group V needs further classification and germ cell tumors must be added for completeness.

Clinical staging of the ovarian tumor is as significant as the pathologic grading. The accepted FIGO staging is as follows:

FIGO CLASSIFICATION

Based on findings at clinical examination and surgical exploration.

Stage I	Growth limited to the ovaries.
Stage IA	Growth limited to one ovary; no ascites.
Stage IB	Growth limited to both ovaries; no ascites.
Stage IC	Growth limited to one or both ovaries; ascites present with malignant cells in the fluid (or rupture at operation).
Stage II	Growth involving one or both ovaries with pelvic extension.
Stage IIA	Extension and/or metastasis to the uterus and/or tubes only.
Stage IIB	Extension to other pelvic tissues.
Stage III	Growth involving one or both ovaries with widespread intraperitoneal metastasis to the abdomen (the omentum, small intestine and its mesentery).
Stage IV	Growth involving one or both ovaries with distant

metastasis outside the peritoneal cavity.

Special Category   Unexplored cases which are thought to be ovarian carcinoma (surgery, explorative or therapeutic, not having been performed).

Note: The presence of ascites will not influence the staging for Stages II, III, and IV.

Recently a WHO classification has been devised, as follows:

WHO CLASSIFICATION

A. Serous Tumors
1. Benign
   a. Cystadenoma and papillary cystadenoma
   b. Surface papilloma
   c. Adenofibroma and cystadenofibroma
2. Of borderline malignancy (carcinomas of low malignant potential)
   a. Cystadenoma and papillary cystadenoma
   b. Surface papilloma
   c. Adenofibroma and cystadenofibroma
3. Malignant
   a. Adenocarcinoma, papillary adenocarcinoma, and papillary cystadenocarcinoma
   b. Surface papillary carcinoma
   c. Malignant adenofibroma and cystadenofibroma
B. Mucinous Tumors
1. Benign
   a. Cystadenoma
   b. Adenofibroma and cystadenofibroma
2. Of borderline malignancy (carcinomas of low malignant potential)
   a. Cystadenoma
   b. Adenofibroma and cystadenofibroma
3. Malignant
   a. Adenocarcinoma and cystadenocarcinoma

b. Malignant adenofibroma and cystadenofibroma
C. Endometrioid Tumors
1. Benign
   a. Adenoma and cystadenoma
   b. Adenofibroma and cystadenofibroma
2. Of borderline malignancy (carcinomas of low malignant potential)
   a. Adenoma and cystadenoma
   b. Adenofibroma and cystadenofibroma
3. Malignant
   a. Carcinoma
      (1) Adenocarcinoma
      (2) Adenoacanthoma
      (3) Malignant adenofibroma and cystadenofibroma
   b. Endometrioid stroma sarcomas
   c. Mesodermal (müllerian) mixed tumors, homologous and heterologous
D. Clear Cell (Mesonephroid) Tumors
1. Benign: adenofibroma
2. Of borderline malignancy (carcinoma of low malignant potential)
3. Malignant: carcinoma and adenocarcinoma
E. Brenner Tumors
1. Benign
2. Of borderline malignancy (proliferating)
3. Malignant
F. Mixed Epithelial Tumors
1. Benign
2. Of borderline malignancy
3. Malignant
G. Undifferentiated Carcinoma
H. Unclassified Epithelial Tumors

This classification is of no value to the clinician since the various subgroups of the benign tumors, those of low malignant potential, and those that are malignant follow the same clinical course. The prognosis and therapy depend on the neoplastic potential of the individual cell type and the extent of the disease at the time of initial exploration.

Thus, the FIGO clinical and pathologic classifications are recommended to correlate the clinical and pathologic aspects of the specific tumor. Only by acceptance of a standard classification can the results of therapy be evaluated accurately and a prognosis be afforded to the patient and her family.

REFERENCES

Bassis, M. L.: An embryologically derived classification of ovarian tumors. J.A.M.A., *174*:170, 1960.

Emge, L. A.: Classifying ovarian tumors. Am. J. Obstet. Gynecol., *68*:348, 1954.

Helsel, E. V.: Ovarian cancer. Am. J. Obstet. Gynecol., *52*:435, 1946.

Heyman, J.: Experience with radiological treatment of cancer of uterus and ovaries. Acta Radiol., *13*:329, 1932.

International Federation of Gynecology and Obstetrics: Classification and staging of malignant tumours in the female pelvis. J. Int. Fed. Gynecol. Obstet., *3*:204, 1965.

MacKinlay, C. J.: Male cells in granulosa cell ovarian tumors. J. Obstet. Gynaecol. Br. Emp., *64*:512, 1957.

Nokes, J. M., Claiborne, H. A., and Reingold, W. N.: Thecoma with associated virilization. Am. J. Obstet. Gynecol., *78*:722, 1958.

Scully, R. E.: World Health Organization Classification and Nomenclature. Natl. Cancer Inst. Monogr., *421*:5, 1975.

Shippel, S.: Ovarian theca cell. J. Obstet. Gynaecol. Br. Commonw., *57*:362, 1950.

Teilum, G.: Classification of ovarian tumors. Acta Obstet. Gynecol. Scand., *31*:292, 1952.

Teter, J.: A new concept of classification of gonadal tumors arising from germ cells (gonocytoma) and their histogenesis. Gynecologia, *150*:84, 1960.

Turner, J. C., Jr., ReMine, W. H., and Dockerty, M. B.: Clinicopathological study of 172 patients with primary carcinoma of ovary. Surg. Gynecol. Obstet., *109*:198, 1959.

Warner, N. E., Friedman, N. B., Bomze, E. J., and Masin, F.: Comparative pathology of experimental and spontaneous androblastomas and gynoblastomas of the gonads. Am. J. Obstet. Gynecol., *79*:971, 1960.

Chapter 20

NON-NEOPLASTIC LESIONS OF THE OVARY

Introduction

The ovarian tumor represents the major diagnostic and therapeutic challenge to the gynecologist today. Fundamentally, it is enigmatic that the degree of neoplasia is inversely proportional to the symptomatology. Thus, the inflammatory and dysfunctional enlargements commonly produce pain or menstrual irregularities, whereas the neoplastic lesions are associated with rare clinical manifestations which might lead to their early diagnosis.

INFLAMMATORY "TUMORS"

The most common of the non-neoplastic lesions involving the ovary are those of inflammatory origin and have been described previously. The tubo-ovarian and peritoneal inclusion cysts are the direct result of adhesive disease in which the ovary has become cystic because of its proximity to the infected tube and its adherence to the adjacent peritoneum.

The tubo-ovarian inflammatory mass is usually composed of an adherent tube with a thickened fibrous ovarian capsule. The wall of the inflammatory cyst is composed of a dense mass of organized granulation tissue with glandular elements (Fig. 20–1B). The latter represent the remains of the adherent tubal fimbriae.

The peritoneal or mesothelial inclusion cyst commonly develops as the result of adhesive disease following pelvic surgery and represents the most frequent cyst for which a second pelvic procedure is performed. Nevertheless, it is impossible in most instances to differentiate the neoplastic from the non-neoplastic tumor; thus, surgery is necessary.

FOLLICLE CYSTS

The most frequent but, from a neoplastic standpoint, the least important variety of ovarian cyst is that which arises from the ovarian follicles through the process called atresia folliculi. Every month a number of follicles undergo atresia, with death of the ovum. They appear as tiny, often microscopic, cysts lined by one or more layers of granulosa cells. If the granulosa disintegrates, which may occur as a result of its inherent lack of blood supply, the cyst becomes lined by theca. As might be expected, the clear fluid content of such cysts shows little or no estrogenic activity.

Although the cystic atretic follicles are usually very tiny, and are found in considerable numbers even in normal ovaries, they may attain sizes of up to 8 to 10 cm. Rarely they then become of clinical importance, producing discomfort in the pelvis, and are subject to the same possibility of torsion as are neoplastic cysts. They cannot be distinguished from the latter by pelvic examination. Generally they resorb and disappear within a few days. Such would not be the case for a true neoplastic lesion. Repeat examination is always desirable in the young female, especially if the commonly related menstrual irregularities, such as a prolonged interval or prolonged episode

385

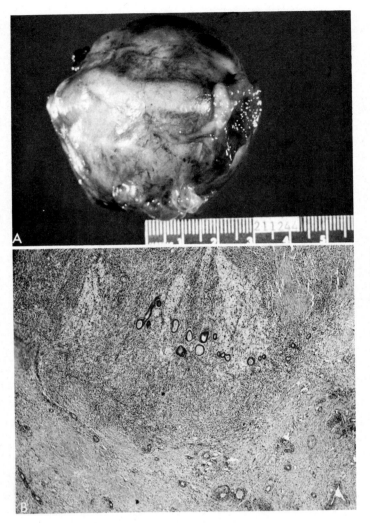

Figure 20–1. *A,* Tubo-ovarian inflammatory mass. Note tube adherent to underlying mass with fimbriae to far left. *B,* Wall of a tubo-ovarian abscess. Note small cystic inclusions of tubal epithelium in wall of inflammatory mass.

of bleeding, are associated with ovarian enlargement. Cyclic medications have been used effectively by some observers in an effort to produce withdrawal bleeding and the "hoped for" degeneration of the granulosa in the persistent follicle. Nevertheless, most such follicle cysts regress spontaneously without medical intervention. In the older and especially the postmenopausal woman, procrastination is unsafe and is not warranted because of the increased incidence of cystic malignancy.

Although the *microscopic diagnosis* of the follicular cyst is usually very easy, there may be occasional difficulty with those of larger size, in which a single layer of cuboidal or low columnar epithelium lines the cyst wall. It is sometimes impossible to be sure whether the cyst is of follicular type or a small serous cyst. If one can demonstrate the remains of the cumulus oophorus or the surrounding theca lutein cells, there is little doubt of the follicular origin. If not, the distinction may be impossible. In such cases the designation of "simple cyst" of the ovary is often employed and when there is uncertainty of the exact source, this diagnosis seems justifiable. Such cysts are, however, of either follicular or coelomic epithelial origin (Chapter 21).

Although the follicle cyst usually represents a follicle which has degenerated, under certain conditions large cystic follicles are encountered in which the ovum and granulosa are well preserved, and in which the fluid content is rich in estrogenic hormone. This applies especially to the primarily pituitary dysfunction associated with excessive follicle ripening activity, which clinically is manifested by functional bleeding.

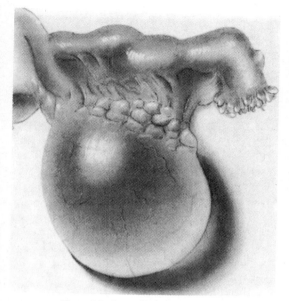

Figure 20–2. Follicle cyst of ovary.

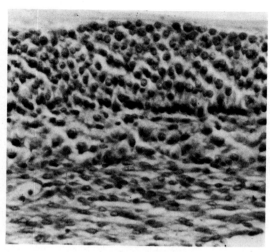

Figure 20–3. Wall of follicle cyst, showing contrast between granulosa (above) and theca (below).

In this syndrome, one of two conditions is found in the ovary. There may be, in one ovary or the other, a moderately large cyst, which represents a persistent follicle, or both ovaries may be of the polycystic variety, studded with many small but actively functioning cystic follicles. Grossly, such polycystic ovaries resemble the polycystic ovaries found so often in association with chronic inflammatory disease, but their histologic appearance and functional significance are quite different. In the latter condition the cysts show degenerated granulosa and loss of hormonal activity.

Finally, it must be noted that the follicle cyst is the most common finding in the child with precocious puberty (Fig. 20–2). In many instances the cyst is interpreted as a granulosa cell tumor and surgery is performed. Nevertheless, these cysts spontaneously regress in most instances, as do the evidences of precocity. It must be assumed that a surge of pituitary gonadotropic hormone has occurred that is transient and thus self-limiting.

Follicle Hematoma

Hemorrhage into the cavity of a cystic atretic follicle is common, producing the so-called follicle hematoma. The source of the bleeding is the perifollicular blood vessels in the theca (Fig. 20–3). These often are seen to be distended with blood, and they not infrequently break into the follicle cavity, filling it with blood (Figs. 20–4 and 20–5). Such hematomas are usually very small, but may occasionally reach a diameter of several centimeters. They should not be confused with endometrial cysts merely because like

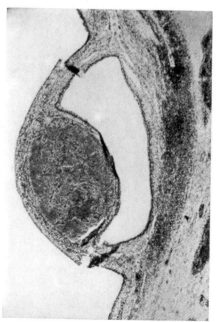

Figure 20–4. Perifollicular hemorrhage, which, by breaking into cavity, produces hematomas.

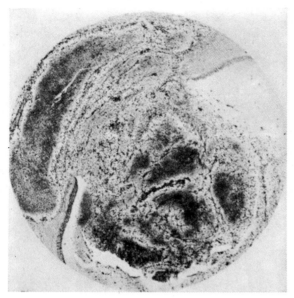

Figure 20–5. Blood breaking into follicle from perifollicular hemorrhage, giving rise to hematoma.

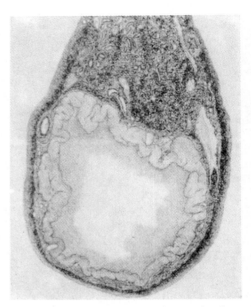

Figure 20–6. Unusually large and cystic, but functionally normal, mature corpus luteum making up at least half the transverse section of the ovary.

the latter they may show a dark chocolate-colored bloody content. Unlike the endometrial cyst, however, the lining of the follicle hematoma does not resemble endometrium but consists of fibrous and hyaline tissue.

LUTEIN CYSTS

(LUTEINIZED GRANULOSA-THECA CYSTS)

Both the granulosa and the theca cells are capable of undergoing luteinization under the influence of the luteinizing gonadotropic hormones of the anterior pituitary. The most perfect example of granulosa luteinization is seen in the normal corpus luteum, for here the luteinized granulosa cells form the great bulk of the yellow festooned lutein wall that characterizes the mature corpus. Even in the latter, however, evidences of theca luteinization are seen in the theca lutein or paralutein cells (see Chapter 17).

Lutein cysts of the ovary, therefore, may be divided into a granulosa and a theca variety, depending on the origin of the luteinized cells that line the cyst.

Granulosa Lutein Cysts

By far the most frequent cyst of this group is the corpus luteum cyst (Fig. 20–6). A dis-

tinction may be drawn between cystic corpora lutea and genuine corpus luteum cysts, although this is academic and they are frequently spoken of collectively as lutein cysts.

There are marked individual variations in different corpora lutea during the stage of maturity. Young corpora lutea have a central core that consists of light, newly formed connective tissue with little or no fluid, whereas others show a large central cavity filled with clear or bloody fluid. When the latter is the case, the lutein wall is thinner and less festooned than when the corpus is of the solid type, but in either case the functional activity appears to be the same.

The corpus luteum of pregnancy, apart from its relatively large size, is apt to be cystic, so that it may be mistaken at operation for a neoplastic cyst (Fig. 20–7). If it is removed, there is risk of producing abortion. *Microscopically,* the earliest corpus luteum of pregnancy is similar to that of the normal cycle. Later, during the second and third months, the theca luteinization is striking, probably because of the large quantity of chorionic gonadotropin; however, in late pregnancy this layer becomes attenuated. At term, although the mass may be large, if the theca is proliferative, abnormal activity must be suspected, as noted by Greene.

At times, there is continued function of the apparently normal corpus luteum, the so-

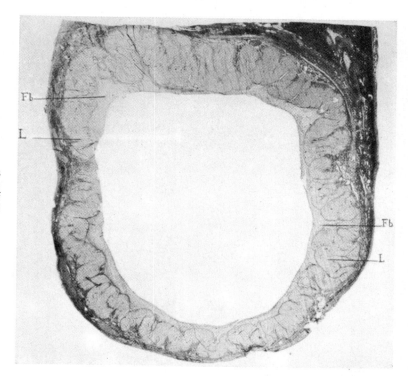

Figure 20–7. Large cystic corpus luteum of pregnancy. *L*, Lutein layer; *Fb*, fibrous tissue. Other corpora of pregnancy may be much smaller and much less cystic.

called *corpus luteum persistens*. Clinically, it may produce a delay of menstruation followed by persistent bleeding. Since the latter symptoms are associated with the presence of the unilateral tender mass, it is not surprising that the diagnosis of tubal pregnancy is often made. Massive hemoperitoneum may occur, as noted by Rosenthal. The endometrium in such cases may show a decidua-like transformation as a result of the abnormally prolonged progesterone influence. As a matter of fact, there are some who believe that in such cases one actually is dealing with a gestation in which the fertilized egg succumbs at a very early, perhaps even preimplantation, phase. Others look upon the syndrome as analogous to the phenomenon of pseudopregnancy in the lower animals.

In the great majority of cases lutein cysts may be considered to be sequelae of *corpus luteum hematomas*. In the hemorrhagic or vascularization phase of the corpus luteum, hemorrhage normally takes place into the lumen. Usually this is of limited amount, but in some cases the cavity of the corpus is inundated with blood, giving rise to hematomas that may be of considerable size. The lining of such hematomas is formed by the thinned-out, bright yellow lutein zone. The gradual resorption of the blood elements may take

many weeks, leaving a cavity filled with a clear fluid, i.e., a lutein cyst.

In its early stages the lutein cells may be well preserved, but fatty degeneration and fibrosis soon begin, so that later it is only with difficulty that one can recognize the probable lutein character of the cyst wall. In the later stages, too, a layer of light connective tissue is deposited along the inner margin of the lutein zone, and finally the latter may be buried deeply beneath a heavy cicatricial layer (Fig. 20–8).

The *corpus albicans cyst* is considered to be a variant or sequel of the corpus luteum cyst (Fig. 20–9). As with the normal corpus, the lutein layer of the cyst may ultimately undergo complete hyalinization, producing the appearance of a large corpus albicans whose cavity is distended with fluid, in contrast to the cicatricial core of the normal corpus albicans. It is possible, however, that a corpus albicans cyst may be the end result of a corpus luteum cycle which is quite normal except in the persistence of an abnormally large amount of fluid in the late stages of retrogression. This is suggested by the histologic appearance of some corpus albicans cysts.

To summarize, therefore, granulosa lutein cysts, as they present themselves, may be of various types: (1) cystic but normally func-

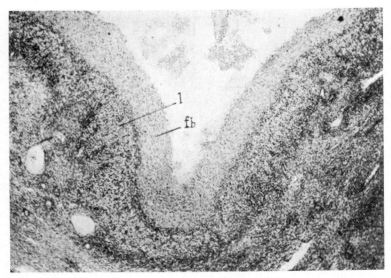

Figure 20–8. Wall of older corpus luteum cyst, showing lutein layer (*l*) and fibrous tissue (*fb*).

tioning corpora lutea of menstruation or of pregnancy; (2) cystic corpora lutea in which overdistention is associated with cessation or disorder of function; (3) corpus luteum cysts resulting from partial or complete resorption of the blood elements in corpus luteum hematomas, the contents being clear or hemorrhagic in various degrees, and the function being sometimes impaired, sometimes not.

Theca Lutein Cysts

Extremely large cystic ovaries are frequently found in conjunction with hydatidiform mole and choriocarcinoma (Fig. 20–10), and rarely in conjunction with a normal pregnancy (Jones and Huston) (Fig. 20–11). Theca luteinization under the latter circumstances may be dramatic, particularly in the early stages when the chorionic gonado-

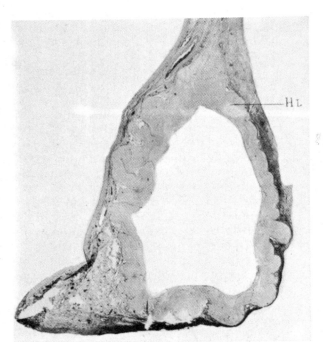

Figure 20–9. Corpus albicans cyst showing hyalinized lutein layer (*HL*).

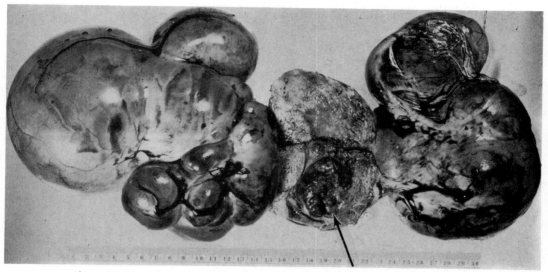

Figure 20–10. Bilateral theca lutein cysts with trophoblastic tumor in uterus (at arrow).

tropin levels are highest. Cysts may develop at this stage of pregnancy but regress spontaneously, and thus temporary conservatism is in order, recognizing always the potentiality of neoplastic alteration.

The lutein cysts associated with trophoblastic disease may attain the size of a man's

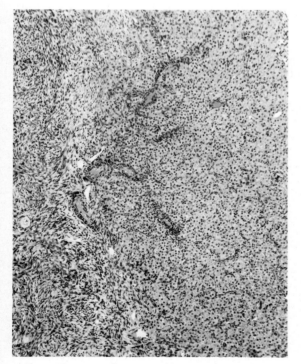

Figure 20–11. Diffuse stromal luteinization with normal pregnancy.

head, but following termination of the pregnancy they slowly regress over the course of months. Almost certainly these cysts represent a response to the large amounts of gonadotropin which are present in the trophoblastic disease, and indeed such changes can be induced in animal ovaries by the injection of interstitial–cell–stimulating hormone (ICSH) (LH) or chorionic gonadotropin.

These *theca lutein* cysts show marked luteinization of the theca zone. The granulosa layer is usually present but is not prominent (Fig. 20–12). Usually the ovary is polycystic. Fuller discussion of these ovarian changes can be found in Chapter 33. It should be mentioned that lutein-like changes in the surface of the ovary may occur in the complete absence of pregnancy. In discussing this so-called "pseudodeciduosis," Bassis believes that it represents a response to some type of endocrine dysfunction, and is a different process from theca lutein cysts. Indeed, deciduosis or pseudodeciduosis may occur in a normal-sized noncystic ovary.

Stein-Leventhal Ovary

In 1928 Dr. Irving Stein published his first paper on an infrequent but important entity characterized by such symptoms as oligoamenorrhea, anovulation, infertility, and occasionally mild virilism, hirsutism, and enlarged clitoris. In this and subsequent papers, he was careful to emphasize that this

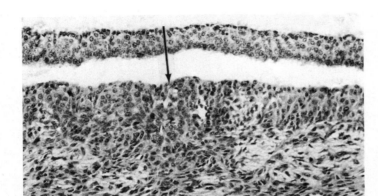

Figure 20–12. Theca lutein cyst with granulosa above and luteinized theca (at arrow).

syndrome is associated with a characteristic bilateral ovarian enlargement. If wedge resection of these ovaries is carried out, there is an 85 to 90 per cent chance that ovulation with normal menses and pregnancy may occur. The excellent results from wedge resection suggest that the primary problem lies in the ovary, and there is evidence of local enzymatic abnormality. Incubation of ovarian tissue with steroid precursors often demonstrates the presence of excess amounts of androgen. Nevertheless, recent studies indicate that the effect of these androgens on the hypothalamus allows for release of the acyclic variety of ICSH and results in anovulation.

Grossly, the true Stein-Leventhal ovary is at least twice the size of the normal ovary, oyster gray in color, with a firm, smooth cortex, showing no evidence of corpus luteum formation but studded with small bluish cysts (Figs. 20–13 and 20–14). The tunica may be so thickened and fibrosed that resection demonstrates a tough gritty capsule on scalpel incision. The thickened, fibrotic cortical tunica contains myriads of seemingly "trapped" primordial follicles (Fig. 20–15). Below it are many follicles in all stages of maturation and atresia, although no evidences of corpora lutea are found (Fig. 20–14). Marked hyperplasia of the theca interna cells in the walls of atretic follicles is frequent (Figs. 20–16 and 20–17). It has been suggested by some (Shippel) that these cells are actively androgenic and respon-sible for the virilism. Gonadotropins will cause a marked increase in the size of the Stein-Leventhal ovary and are useful as a diagnostic adjuvant, although rupture with intraperitoneal bleeding may occur.

Although Stein and others have suggested that wedge resection removes a fibrotic cortex, which serves as a mechanical barrier to ovulation, there have been other suggestions as to the rationale of the good results achieved by wedge resection of the ovary. Lipschütz's proposal of the "law of follicle constancy" has been mentioned, i.e., a given amount of gonadotropin has a lesser amount

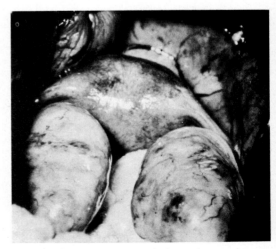

Figure 20–13. Stein-Leventhal ovaries as large as fundus.

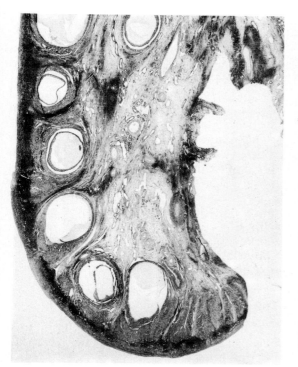

Figure 20–14. Multiple cysts in cortex of Stein-Leventhal ovary (no recent or old corpora lutea).

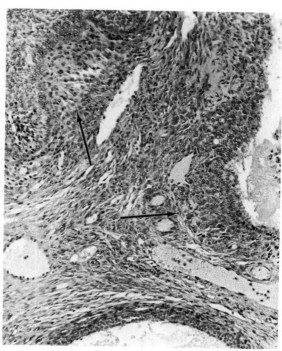

Figure 20–16. Marked theca luteinization in adjacent follicles (at arrows).

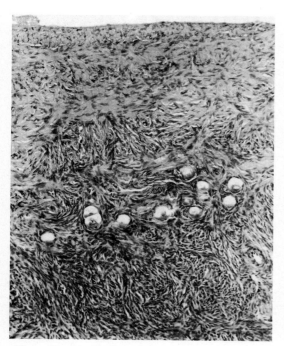

Figure 20–15. Thickened capsule with numerous primordial follicles—ovarian mesenchyme below.

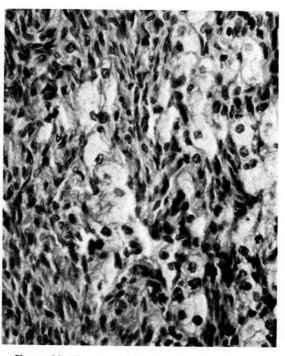

Figure 20–17. Stromal luteinization (lipoid cells) in Stein-Leventhal ovary.

of ovarian substance to stimulate following resection and can thereby "beat" the ovary into ovulating. As noted, recent studies suggest that increased androgen production by the gonadal stroma results in inhibition of the cyclic ICSH and anovulation. Whatever hypothesis is correct, the fact remains that critical clinicians such as Stein and others achieve excellent results in *properly selected women*.

The "large edematous ovary syndrome," often associated with masculinization, is a variant on the polycystic ovary or Stein-Leventhal syndrome and in the author's opinion results from chronic or repeated torsion of the enlarged gonad. The large luteinized cells are similar to those in Figures 20–17 and 21–19.

We have recently tried to compare ovarian tissue removed at wedge resection with ovaries removed in conjunction with hysterectomy performed for recurrent menorrhagia due to repeated anovulation. They have much in common, such as a thick cortex, many developing follicles with an absence of corpora lutea, and frequent proliferation of the theca. Frankly, we could not distinguish any histologic differences in many cases, and we wonder if the only distinction is quantitative—the enlarged Stein-Leventhal ovary. This, of course, would be highly compatible with the opinion (Evans and Riley) that the Stein-Leventhal syndrome is merely an advanced degree of ovarian anovulation.

Evans and Riley have reported two cases of thecoma (one with granulosa elements) in conjunction with polycystic disease of the ovaries. They believe that this represents an ovarian response to a (pituitary) gonadotropin similar to the experiments of the Biskinds (see Chapter 26).

In a number of articles, as summarized by Jackson and Dockerty, the authors have attempted to relate the Stein-Leventhal syndrome to endometrial adenocarcinoma. Kaufman and associates have noted the frequency of hyperplasia with the Stein-Leventhal syndrome. Most cases in their series responded to wedge resection with reversion of the endometrium to a secretory pattern; however, atypicality is irreversible in the occasional patient. Anovulation and consequently unopposed estrogen might be considered to be a common denominator, but at present the association must be regarded only as speculative. Confirmation seems necessary before the preliminary work of these Mayo Clinic authors is accepted unequivocally. It is interesting to note that both the Stein-Leventhal syndrome and many cases of endometrial cancer are apt to be associated with rather profound metabolic and endocrine effects, which of course suggests a potential pituitary role.

Other tumors have been reported in cases of Stein-Leventhal syndrome. In our laboratory, approximately 10 per cent of the cases have had a coexistent dermoid cyst. The range in age of the patients with this condition is, of course, similar to that of patients with the cystic teratoma. Betson and co-workers have reported an associated arrhenoblastoma, and one similar case has been noted in our laboratory.

Mesothelial Inclusion Cysts

These cysts are of no clinical importance because they are tiny—most frequently of microscopic size—and present in most ovaries. They are the result of invaginations of the mesothelium, seen in the ovaries of all women who have ovulated. These may be important in the genesis of ovarian neoplasia. It is proposed by several investigators

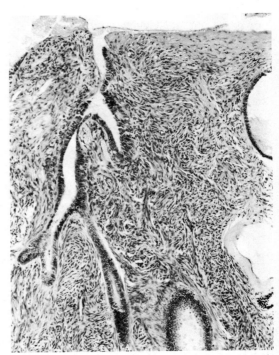

Figure 20–18. Invaginations of mesothelium with inclusion cysts at right.

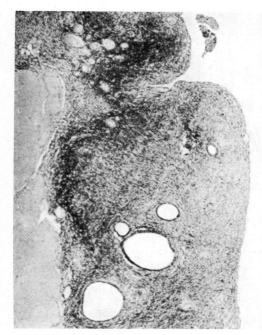

Figure 20–19. Mesothelial inclusion cysts.

that the ovulating woman of low fertility is at higher risk for developing epithelial tumors. Conversely, the anovulatory patient (the woman on long-term oral contraceptives or with polycystic ovarian disease) is at lower risk (Figs. 20–18 and 20–19). The indentations of the surface epithelium may be nipped off or blocked by the surrounding stroma, with the formation of tiny cysts. They are lined by the cuboidal germinal epithelium, which, however, exhibits frequent metaplastic transformation into a variety resembling that of either the endometrium or the endosalpinx.

Endometrial Cysts

These are discussed in full in Chapter 29.

REFERENCES

Allen, W. M., and Woolf, R. B.: Medullary resection of ovaries in Stein-Leventhal syndrome. Am. J. Obstet. Gynecol., 72:826, 1959.

Bassis, M. L.: Pseudodeciduosis. Am. J. Obstet. Gynecol., 72:1029, 1956.

Betson, J. R., Marshall, R. A., and Chiffelle, T. L.: Scleropolycystic (Stein-Leventhal) ovary with arrhenoblastoma of the opposite gonad. Am. J. Obstet. Gynecol., 83:93, 1962.

Buxton, C. L., and Van de Wille, R.: Wedge resection for polycystic ovaries. N. Engl. J. Med., 251:293, 1954.

Dutoit, D. A. H.: Polycystic Ovaries—Menstrual Disturbances and Hirsutism. Leyden, Kroese, 1951.

Evans, T. N., and Riley, G. M.: Polycystic ovarian disease: a clinical experimental study. Am. J. Obstet. Gynecol., 80:873, 1960.

Evans, T. N., and Riley, G. M.: Thecoma and polycystic disease of the ovaries. Obstet. Gynecol., 18:52, 1961.

Goodall, J. F.: Tumors of ovary. In Curtis' Obstetrics and Gynecology. Vol. II. Philadelphia, W. B. Saunders Company, 1933.

Greene, R. R., Holzwarth, D., and Roddick, J. W.: Luteomas of preganancy. Am. J. Obstet. Gynecol., 88:1001, 1964.

Haas, R. S., and Riley, F. M.: Polycystic ovaries and amenorrhea. Obstet. Gynecol., 5:657, 1955.

Hofner, H., and Young, J. J.: Hyperreactio luteonalis. Obstet. Gynecol., 6:285, 1955.

Ingersoll, F. M., and McDermott, W. V., Jr.: Bilateral polycystic ovaries, Stein-Leventhal syndrome. Am. J. Obstet. Gynecol., 60:17, 1950.

Jackson, R. L., and Dockerty, M. B.: Stein-Leventhal syndrome and endometrial cancer. Am. J. Obstet. Gynecol., 73:161, 1957.

Jones, W. J., and Huston, J. W.: Bilateral theca lutein cysts associated with an apparently normal pregnancy. Am. J. Obstet. Gynecol., 81:1033, 1961.

Kaufman, R. H., Abbott, J. P., and Wall, J. A.: Endometrium before and after wedge resection of the ovaries in the Stein-Leventhal syndrome. Am. J. Obstet. Gynecol., 77:1271, 1959.

Keetel, W. C., Bradbury, J. T., and Stoddard, F. J.: Unusual ovarian changes in pregnancy. Am. J. Obstet. Gynecol., 73:954, 1957.

Klinefelter, H. F., Jr., and Jones, G. E. S.: Amenorrhea due to polycystic ovaries (Stein-Leventhal syndrome). J. Clin. Endocr., 14:1247, 1954.

Leventhal, M. L.: The Stein-Leventhal syndrome. Am. J. Obstet. Gynecol., 76:825, 1958.

Novak, E., and TeLinde, R. W.: Pathological antomy of corpus luteum (abscess, cyst, hematoma and neoplasm). Bull. Johns Hopkins Hosp., 34:289, 1923.

Rosenthal, A. H.: Rupture of the corpus luteum, including four cases of massive intraperitoneal hemorrhage. Am. J. Obstet. Gynecol., 79:1008, 1959.

Shippel, S.: Ovarian theca cell. J. Obstet. Gynaec. Br. Commonw., 57:632, 1950.

Stein, I. F.: The Stein-Leventhal syndrome. West. J. Surg., 63:319, 1955.

Stein, I. F., and Leventhal, M. L.: Amenorrhea as associated with bilateral polycystic ovaries. Am. J. Obstet. Gynecol., 29:181, 1935.

Chapter 21

OVARIAN NEOPLASIA: MESOTHELIAL; STROMOEPITHELIAL LESIONS— PRIMARILY EPITHELIAL (BENIGN, OF LOW MALIGNANT POTENTIAL, AND MALIGNANT) (SEROUS, MUCINOUS, ENDOMETRIOID, MESONEPHROID, MESOTHELIAL)

The ovary is the third most common site of primary malignancy in the femal genital canal, in most series constituting approximately 12 to 20 per cent of all such neoplasms. In 1978 these lesions will cause approximately 11,000 deaths in the United States. Thus, although cervical cancer is three to four times more common than ovarian neoplasia, it is estimated that more deaths result from ovarian than from cervical and endometrial carcinoma combined. Ovarian cancers are the fifth leading cause of death from cancer in women at present. They are more common in the white than the black race although the differential between the two has been reduced in the past two decades. The incidence is higher in industrialized areas (the exception being Japan), a rate of 15 per 100,000 being reported in the Scandinavian countries, 7 to 8 per 100,000 in the United States, and as low as 0.1 per 100,000 in Paraguay. It is more common in women of low parity (two or fewer pregnancies) and is less frequent in patients who have used oral contraceptives for several(?) years. Furthermore, rare cases have been reported in women with unresolved polycystic ovary disease.

It is of interest that, in spite of the number of ovariotomies performed between McDowell's epoch-making procedure of 1809 and the beginning of the twentieth century, there were few, if any, reports of ovarian malignancy in these patients; e.g., Emmett in 1880 stated that, in the observation of more than 100 cases of ovarian cysts, he had not seen one case of cancer. Although there are many factors to be considered, it is possible that the malignant ovarian neoplasm is a disease of our century, and is related directly to contamination of the pelvic viscera by persistently irritative agents.

The ovary is a striking exception to the Virchow's dictum that organs that are frequently the site of primary cancer are rarely involved in secondary malignancy, and vice versa. Both primary and secondary carcinomas of the ovary are relatively frequent, and show an astounding variety of pathologic patterns. These tumors may present as solid or cystic lesions, but most consist of an admixture of the two gross features, the cystic portion being due either to secretory activity or to degeneration.

Unfortunately, the malignant potential of the primary ovarian tumor is inversely proportional to the symptomatology. Whereas the inflammatory and physiologic enlargements routinely produce either pain or menstrual disturbances, the true neoplasm is silent and found most commonly only on pelvic examination or because a mass has been felt or local discomfort has brought the patient to the physician. Menstrual disturbances are infrequent and acute pain is rare unless torsion or rupture takes place. Consequently, many of the malignant ovarian tumors have had variable periods of time to grow and often involve the adjacent organs before any symptoms develop or recognition takes place.

In many instances, the term ovarian cancer may be a misnomer in that the ovary is only involved in a diffuse *intra-abdominal neoplastic process*. For example, it is often stated that the common papillary serous cystadenoma of low malignant potential is a tumor that becomes implanted although the histology describes a lesion composed of mature cells. Such an implantation theory seems questionable although widely accepted. Possibly a more logical explanation for the widespread nature of such process would be a diffuse intra-abdominal response to a local agent or tumor arising in multicentric foci.

STROMOEPITHELIAL LESIONS

Approximately 75 per cent of all primary ovarian malignancies arise from the basic coelomic epithelium or *mesothelium*. Fundamentally, these epithelial tumors are unique in that they are of mesodermal origin and could be designated mesotheliomas, differentiated or undifferentiated, with varying amounts and activities of the gonadal mesenchyme. The latter, commonly known as ovarian stroma, contains two elements, both of mesodermal origin—namely, the potentially functioning theca and the supporting connective tissue. Thus, all ovarian tumors are potentially hormone producing, since an integral element of each lesion is the basic gonadal stroma. The vagaries of the individual groups will be discussed under separate headings, in an attempt to follow our proposed, and the FIGO, classifications (see Chapter 19).

Group I

(FIGO GROUPS I-IV)

MESOTHELIAL

   I. Differentiated mesotheliomas
      A. Serous (endosalpingeal)
      B. Mucinous (endocervical)
      C. Endometrioid
      D. Mesonephroid (clear cell, etc.)

It was stated by Goodall more than half a century ago that the ovaries of all women over the age of 35 years contain inclusion cysts lined by tubal, endometrial, or endocervical epithelia. These differentiated coelomic or mesothelial cysts are the sites of origin of many of the larger lesions, the size undoubtedly related to the secretory and proliferative activities of the lining cells. The stimulant for the increased fluid production is unknown, but some variable must be present, since some cysts increase rapidly in size while others seem to remain small and nonpalpable. Both local and systemic agents have been suggested, and both may be at work; however, the proliferation of the cell population is a function of the predominant cell type and obviously varies whether the cyst is serous, mucinous, endometrioid, or mesonephroid. Furthermore, it has been demonstrated by the electron microscope that multiple cell types may be present in the same tumor if differentiation is adequate enough to identify the specific variants.

SEROUS LESIONS (FIGO HISTOLOGIC GROUP I)

(FIGO HISTOLOGIC CLASSIFICATION GROUP I)

The largest group of ovarian cystomas of the epithelial or stromoepithelial variety have been classified as serous, primarily because the cystic fluid is rich in the serum proteins—albumin and globulin. However, as in the mucinous variety, the laboratory diagnosis is made on the character of the epithelium and on certain characteristics of the growth pattern. Generally the serous cysts do not attain the enormous size sometimes acquired by the mucinous variety, although individual tumors may fill the abdominal cavity. The incidence of the two varieties is approximately the same in our laboratory, al-

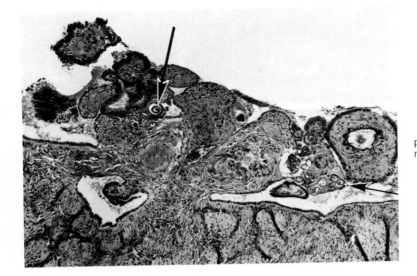

Figure 21–1. Surface papillary projections on a normal ovary. Foreign material may be seen at arrows.

though if the simple cysts are included, the balance would favor the serous variety.

Histogenesis

There can be no doubt but that the origin of the serous tumor is the surface epithelium (mesothelium) of the ovary. The chief evidence for the validity of this statement is demonstrated by the finding of all possible histologic gradations of tumor growth from simple invaginations of the coelomic epithelium to the fully formed serous papillary cystadenoma. In fact, small superficial papillomatous outgrowths of the coelomic epithelium are commonly seen on the normal ovary (Fig. 21–1). These surface papillomas may at times attain large proportions, with no cystic cavities, and on rare occasions fill the entire pelvis. These, although multiple, are often histologically and clinically benign (Fig. 21–2 A,B).

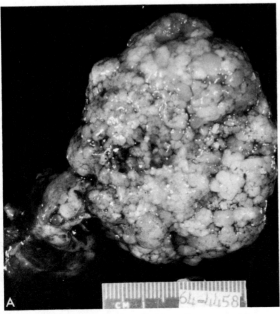

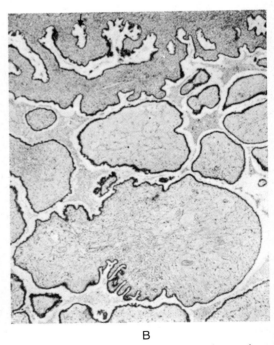

Figure 21–2. *A*, Large papillary ovarian tumor with no cystic component. *B*, Marked papillary proliferations from surface of ovary. Note small invaginations into ovarian stroma (arrow)—*not* a sign of stromal invasion! The epithelium is benign.

Another interesting variation of the invasiveness that may be assumed by germinal epithelium is seen in the so-called fibroadenoma of the ovary. In such conditions, the surface epithelium invades the cortex in long branching tubules, producing a picture quite similar to that seen in the fibroadenoma of the breast. These invasions or *invaginations* may be the result of ovulation and the associated rupture of the capsule (Fig. 21–3).

When many of the glandlike invaginations become cystic, the designation of the cystadenofibroma might be more appropriate. Psammoma bodies are frequently associated with these invaginations and may be found in response to irritative phenomena that produce adhesion formation and the entrapment of the surface epithelium. In many instances, the normal ovary will reveal multiple adenomatous foci with surrounding concentrations of stroma, suggesting the use of a term such as adenosis or fibroadenosis. In rare cases, squamous metaplasia may develop suggestive of the alterations noted in the *Walthard islands* (Fig. 21–4 *A,B*). This

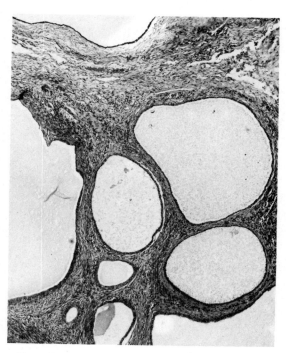

Figure 21–3. "Fibroadenoma" of the ovary. Cysts are lined by a low, flat, inactive mesothelium.

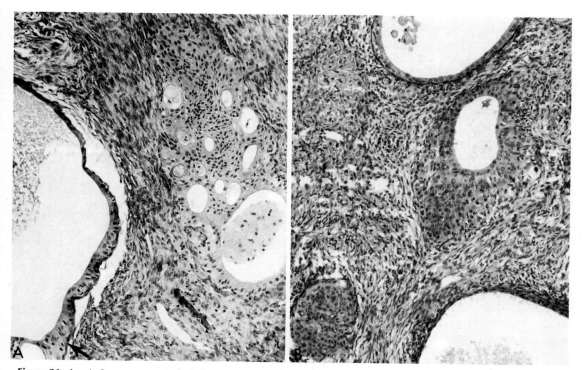

Figure 21–4. *A*, Squamous metaplasia in a serous cystadenoma. Note beginning change in larger cavity (arrow). *B*, More definite Brenner type changes in a serous adenoma.

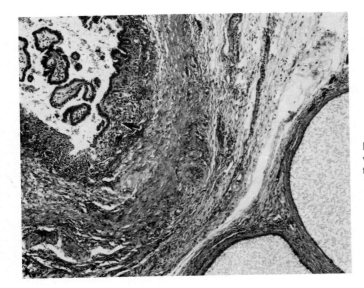

Figure 21–5. Inclusion cysts. Two in right lower area are lined by flat, inactive epithelium, while that in upper left shows papillary proliferations and an endometrium-like stoma (arrow).

topic will be described extensively in Chapter 23.

One may find in the wall of these mesothelial invaginations definite papillary ingrowths constituting the early stages in the development of a papillary serous cystadenoma. Of interest are the variations in proliferation of these mesothelial inclusions. Several foci may be lined by flattened inactive epithelium while adjacent cavities demonstrate papillary excrescences. One must wonder as to the agent present in one cavity and not in another (Fig. 21–5). It must be assumed that ovarian cysts, if related to ovulation, must have been present since time immemorial; conversely, proliferating agents that produce neoplastic alterations may be additions of the last century. Finally, even in the smaller cysts; one can see evidence of the differentiative capacity of germinal epithelium in the presence of cuboidal, ciliated, or mucus-secreting epithelium (Fig. 21–6).

Gross Characteristics

It is not always possible to distinguish grossly between the serous and mucinous lesions, for the appearance may be similar and the consistency of the fluid contents is an unsafe criterion. In a large proportion of cases, however, one can be reasonably sure of the classification because of the common tendency of the serous variety to form papillary excrescences into the cyst cavities and not infrequently on the external surfaces.

Consequently there is much more variation in the gross appearance of the serous than of the mucinous cyst (Figs. 21–7 A,B, and 21–8).

The simplest variety of ovarian cyst is a unilocular structure, usually lined by a layer of flattened or cuboidal epithelium. In small cysts it is often extremely difficult to distin-

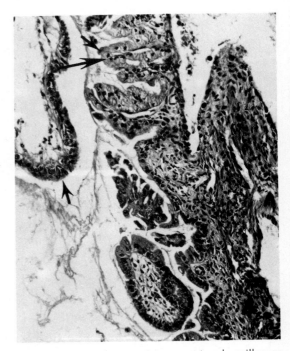

Figure 21–6. Mucinous (two arrows) and papillary serous epithelia (single arrow) adjacent to each other. Endometrial alterations are present elsewhere in the same lesion.

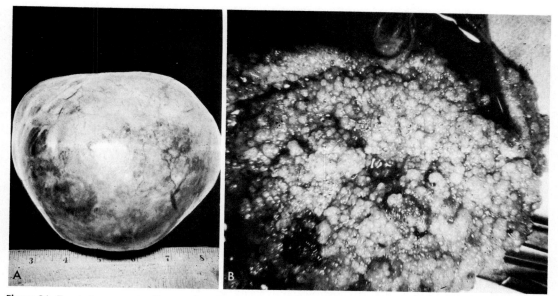

Figure 21–7. *A,* Serous cyst with smooth surface. *B,* Same tumor—on section inner surface is found to be studded with papillary excrescences.

guish between the follicular and the serous varieties, as either may be lined by such nondescript elements. This latter variety has been commonly designated a simple cyst.

The larger serous cysts are usually lobulated and multilocular, similar to the mucinous variety, though the contained fluid is more watery and less viscid than in the latter, and may be brownish or chocolate-colored from the admixture of blood. When the serous cyst is opened, papillary outgrowths from the lining are often found in one or more of the compartments. Some of the latter may practically fill the smaller cavities, whereas in other cases only a tiny warty ex-

crescence may be noted here and there. Moreover, the external surface of the tumor itself is often covered with masses of papillae which, although extensive, maybe histologically benign (Fig. 21–8). The ratio of cystic and papillary elements, extra- or intracystic, exhibits the widest variation.

At times, the exophytic papillary growth may be so dominant that the tumor, for all practical purposes, is properly designated a solid papilloma (Fig. 21–2). These may form enormous cauliflower growths filling the entire pelvis and infringing on the surrounding organs, even when the cellular evidence of malignancy is absent. Since there are so

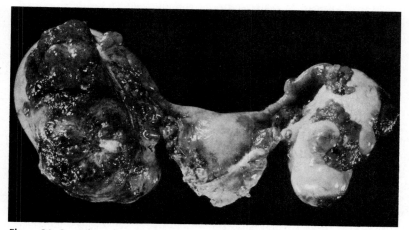

Figure 21–8. Bilateral papillary serous cystadenocarcinomas with external papillae.

many variations on the cystic, papillary, and stromal components with the same malignant potential, clinically there is little, if any, need for the complex classification proposed by WHO (Chapter 18). Unfortunately, it is difficult, and often impossible, to distinguish grossly between the degrees of proliferation; thus, frozen section is of importance, particularly in the young woman desirous of maintaining her fertility. Fortunately, the cellular alterations in the papillary serous tumors usually remain constant from one area to the next. Such is not true for malignancy arising in other cell types.

Microscopic Characteristics

The epithelia that characterize the serous lesion are more variable than that of the mucinous neoplasm. This is not surprising in view of its more generally accepted origin from the coelomic epithelium, which notoriously is possessed with a magnificent degree of metaplastic totipotency. Therefore, the epithelium both on the surface and in the invaginations may resemble the flattened platelike or the round cells with its abundant acidophilic cytoplasm, classic of the mesothelium (Fig. 21–9). In contrast, it may replicate the epithelia of the fallopian tube, showing both the ciliated and secretory elements (Figs. 21–10A,B); however, classically there is a combination of these three cell types. On rare occasions mucus-secreting or endometrioid elements may be present. It is interesting that such invaginations demonstrating their cellular variations are present not only in the ovary but may be found in any area of the abdomen and are particularly confusing if seen within a lymph node. It should be appreciated that even in such situations, if the epithelium is normal, it does not represent a neoplastic alteration (Fig. 21–11).

The fact that so many of the epithelial cells are ciliated has led to the designation of these tumors by German authors as cystadenoma cilioepitheliale. Rarely, however, is a ciliated cell predominant, and in most instances the tuftlike pseudociliary cytoplasmic projections of flat or rounded mesothelial cells is the common finding. In the frankly benign growths, the epithelium is one cell thick, although an appearance of stratification may be given by tangential section through the wavy or papillary layers. Vacuolization in or impinging on the nu-

cleus in some papillary lesions is reminiscent of the changes noted in the cervical or vulvar condyloma and thus is suggestive of a virus associated lesion (Fig. 21–12).

A unique histologic feature of the serous cystadenoma, as well as the tumor of low malignant potential, is the frequent finding of tiny calcified granules (calcospherites), the so-called psammoma bodies. These apparently represent gradual degeneration and calcification in small papillae or inclusions, and may be seen frequently on or near the surface of the otherwise normal ovary in the absence of any neoplasia (Fig. 21–13). Their finding is highly suggestive, but not pathognomonic, of the papillary serous tumor but may occur with other types of papillary lesions in other locales, such as the thyroid. Aure, Hoeg, and Kolstad felt that they may represent evidences of tissue resistance to the tumor growth, since they were more commonly seen in the low grade lesions. On occasions foreign material may be found in these psammoma bodies, suggesting that an irritant, such as talc, may be the agent producing the atypical proliferation seen in the neoplasm. The alterations noted in Figure 21–14 (A,B) were found in a patient who had had hysterectomy and bilateral salpingo-

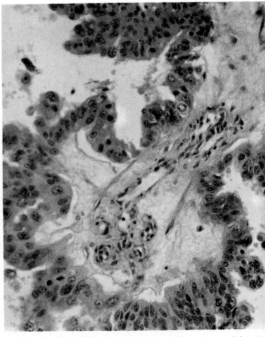

Figure 21–9. Serous tumor. Round, proliferating mesothelial cells on papillary frond. Small, dark nuclei of indifferent cells are frequently noted.

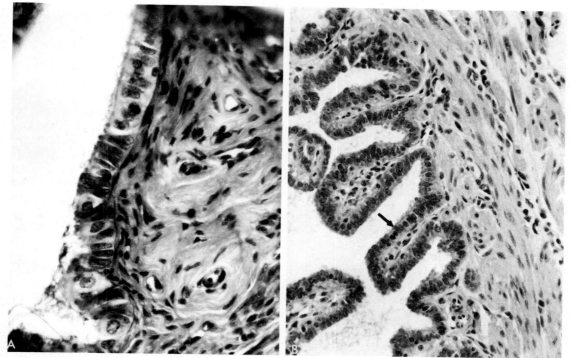

Figure 21–10. *A,* Classic tubal epithelium with secretory and ciliated cells. *B,* Papillary fronds with classic tubal-type epithelium. Ciliated and secretory cells are seen at arrow.

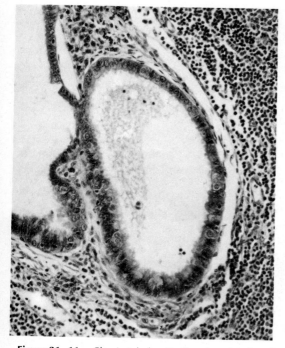

Figure 21–11. Classic tubal epithelium in pelvic lymph node. There was no ovarian tumor.

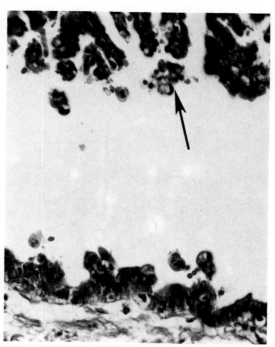

Figure 21–12. Papillary tumor of low malignant potential. Note intranuclear inclusions(?) at arrow.

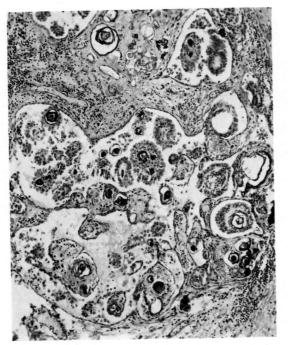

Figure 21–13. Ovary with many psammoma bodies · with papillary fronds. No true tumor was present.

oophorectomy 9 years previously for inflammatory disease.

Malignant Alterations

The papillary structure in many of these tumors is, from a histologic standpoint, benign with no suggestion of overactivity in the epithelium and with a sharp demarcation between it and the stroma, even though the latter is elevated into arborescent projections with intricate patterns (Fig. 21–15 A,B). In the tumor of low malignant potential an occasional mitosis may be seen but never more than one per high power field. In a study of 64 cases of these papillary tumors of low malignant potential (FIGO Histologic Grade IB), more than 50 per cent of the patients were under the age of 40 years. Furthermore, when the pattern was uniform—i.e., when the cells were of the three classic histologic types described above—and there was one or fewer mitoses per high power field, the 5 year salvage was 100 per cent if the tumor was confined to the ovaries and/or the adja-

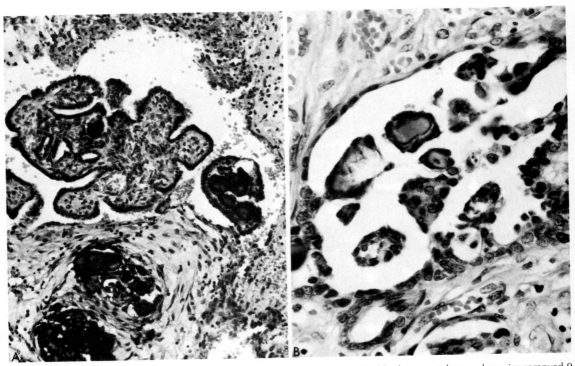

Figure 21–14. *A*, Papillary tumor with psammoma bodies in patient who had had uterus, tubes, and ovaries removed 9 years previously. *B*, Omental lesion removed from patient with pelvic lesion seen in *A*. Foreign material(?) is observed in papillae. Patient underwent exploration for intestinal obstruction 9 years after hysterectomy and removal of tubes and ovaries.

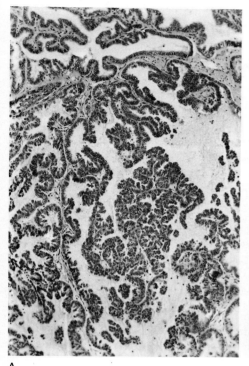
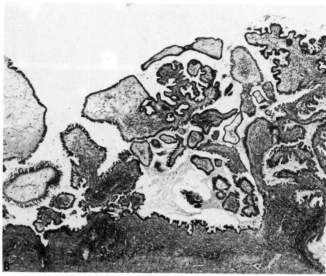

A

Figure 21–15. *A*, Tumor of low malignant potential, such as is often found in omentum and the right hemidiaphragm. Lining cells simulate the mesothelium, thus justifying use of the term mesothelioma in certain instances. *B*, In this section there are varying degrees of papillary proliferation but no mitotic activity. Note tumor arising from the mesothelial surface of the ovary.

cent genital organs (FIGO Clinical Stages IA, IB, and IIA). Even when the neoplasm had spread throughout the abdomen, surgical excision of as much tumor as possible was accompanied by excellent survival (Table 21–1). Thus, careful histologic evaluation of numerous sections is important to rule out other associated cell types if an accurate prognosis is to be provided. Finally, if the lesion proves to be uniform, as noted above, conservative therapy, without adjunctive radiation or chemotherapy, is the treatment of choice in the young patient, an important consideration since the neoplasm is often found in the third decade of life. It should be appreciated that the actual proliferating agent is not known, and thus these patients are always at risk for the development of

Table 21–1 SURVIVAL RATES IN OVARIAN SEROUS TUMORS OF LOW MALIGNANT POTENTIAL

FIGO Stage	Number of Cases	No Evident Disease	Dead from Tumor	Living With Tumor	Dead from Other Cause	Per Cent 5-Year Salvage (Relative)
IA	25	24	—	—	1	100
IB	9	9	—	—	—	100
IC	0	0	—	—	—	—
IIA	7	7	—	—	—	100
IIB	7	4	1	1	1	86
III	11	7	2	1	1	82
IV	5	2	1	1	1	80
Total	64	53	4	3	4	92

tumor in, or on, the opposite ovary, or in the abdominal cavity in general. Therefore, it would seem wise to suggest that the patient have her family and after that submit to more thorough excision of the tissues at highest risk.

In some of these histologically benign cases, multiple foci of neoplasia (so-called implants) are associated with ascites, intestinal obstruction, and a massive omental "cake." Patients with such widespread disease may succumb to cachexia, as is true of the classic mesothelioma; furthermore, extra-abdominal metastases are rare, although fluid from the pleural cavity may contain positive cells.

When overt malignancy develops in the papillary lesion, there is a proliferation of the cells lining the papillae. This proliferation, with disparity of cellular pattern and nuclear activity, may still be differentiated enough to define the basic cell as one of the serous variety (Fig. 21–16 A,B). In the latter situation, the pathologist is confronted with the same problem as that encountered in evaluating the papilloma of the bladder, namely of differentiating benign and proliferating lesions

from the true malignancy. In our experience, this group is identified by increased mitotic activity (2 to 5 mitoses in the poorest high power field). Conversely, the poorly differentiated carcinoma, containing six or more mitoses per high power field, is difficult to identify as a serous tumor (Fig. 21–17 A,B). Simply because there is a papillary formation, one should not attempt to identify a specific cell type (Fig. 21–18). It would seem wiser in such situations to classify such lesions as mesotheliomas with the modifying pathologic pattern of either papillary or solid. A comparison of the clinical and pathologic grades of the papillary ovarian tumors identifies the prognosis on the basis of mitotic count (Table 21–2). These lesions undoubtedly make up the great majority of the FIGO Group E. Of interest in this category of poorly differentiated serous papillary lesions is the tumor in which the papillary fronds have agglutinated to form a papillary-alveolar pattern. The latter is the type most classically seen in the fallopian tube (Fig. 21–18 A,B). The similarity again suggests the frequency with which tumors of the upper genital canal (i.e., endocervix, endo-

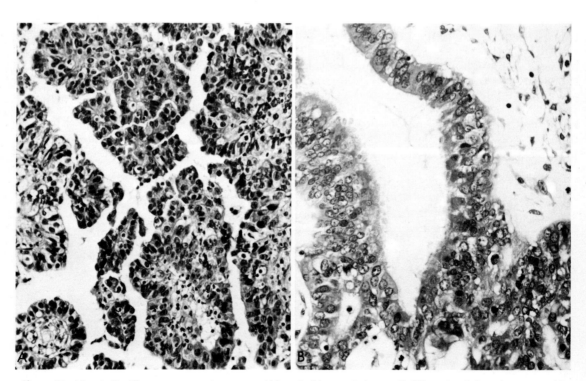

Figure 21–16. *A*, Papillary serous ovarian tumor. Although this type is less well differentiated than the tumor of low malignant potential, individual cell types can still be identified. *B*, Increased proliferation with two or more mitoses per high power field but still a serous tumor.

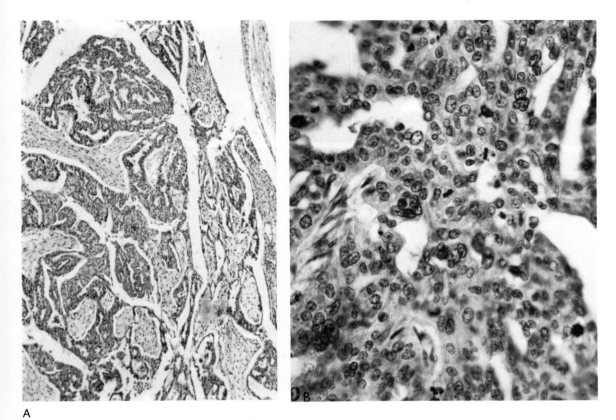

Figure 21–17. *A*, Marked cellular proliferation in a largely papillary serous tumor (tubopapillary pattern). Proliferative cell here is mesothelial. In other areas, only a single cell layer was present. *B*, Multiple mitoses in a poorly differentiated ovarian tumor.

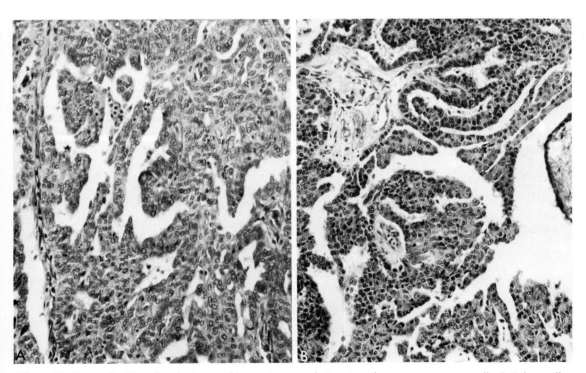

Figure 21–18. *A*, Papillary-alveolar tumor. This is not a serous lesion since there are no secretory cells. *B*, Tubopapillary ovarian tumor similar to that seen in the fallopian tube.

407

Table 21–2 SURVIVAL OF 162 PATIENTS WITH PAPILLARY OVARIAN NEOPLASIA

Mitoses Per High Power Field	Total	No Evident Disease	Living With Tumor	Dead from Tumor	Dead from Other Cause	Per Cent 5 Year Survival
0–1	64	53	3	4	4	92
2–5	10	5	—	5	—	50
6+	78	7	—	71	—	9

metrium and endosalpinx) simulate those seen in the ovary (Fig. 21–6).

The stroma of the serous ovarian tumor, as noted above, is composed of both the basic supporting connective tissue and the potentially functioning tissues. Classically it is edematous and loose-textured resembling Wharton's jelly. Functional activity of the stroma in these lesions is clinically uncommon. Nevertheless, it should be appreciated that the potentiality exists. The foci of luteinized cells described by Sternberg in the edematous ovary syndrome is appreciated in Figure 21–19. The stroma is edematous as a result of torsion and the nests of luteinized cells are easily identified. There was no evidence of clinical masculinization or feminization in this specific case. Consequently the

reaction may be associated with the mechanical feature of torsion.

Clinical Course

As noted previously, the serous ovarian tumor, regardless of its microscopic degree of differentiation, is relatively asymptomatic until the lesion has reached palpable size or has involved other intra-abdominal structures.

The prognosis depends on the clinical stage and the histologic grade of the lesion. Consequently, careful staging should be performed at the time of initial exploration. Since the papillary serous tumor is frequently multifocal in origin and often involves not only the ovary but peritoneal surfaces elsewhere, palpation of the entire abdominal cavity, particularly the right hemidiaphragm, the lateral gutters, and the omentum, with sampling of the latter, is of major importance. The lymph nodes of the pelvis, mesentery, and periaortic areas should be investigated, since penetration of the tumor through the peritoneal surface will permit spread to the nearest lymphatic reservoir. In our autopsy material, for example, the mesenteric nodes were more commonly involved with tumor than were the pelvic or periaortic lymphatics. It has been noted repeatedly that a thorough study of the peritoneal cavity in referred material has resulted in an upstaging of the original clinical classification in as many as 40 to 50 per cent of the cases. Obviously, it is patently impossible to compare survival statistics if the original lesion has not been correctly evaluated.

In spite of the importance of clinical staging, the degree of cell proliferation and mitotic activity is equally, if not more, significant. As noted above, the lesion exhibiting one or fewer mitoses per high power field has an excellent prognosis regardless of the clinical stage. Conversely, the tumor demon-

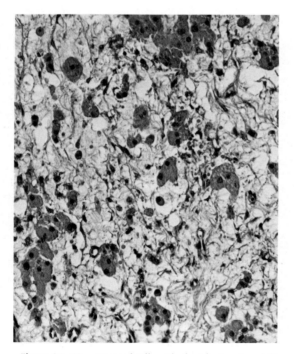

Figure 21–19. Nests of cells with abundant eosinophilic cytoplasm simulating luteinization in edematous stroma of a papillary serous tumor.

strating no tendency to differentiate into a specific cell type, basically a mesothelioma, and demonstrating more than 5 mitoses per high power field, is associated with a low survival rate (Table 21–2).

Therapy

The basic treatment for all ovarian tumors regardless of histologic type, is surgery, which is necessary not only to establish the correct diagnosis and staging, but also for the fundamental purpose of excising as much neoplastic tissue as possible without jeopardizing the life of the patient. Adjuvant therapy depends on the histologic grade, the clinical stage, and the amount of residual tumor. For the Stage IA lesion of low malignant potential, adjuvant therapy is not indicated. The use of intraperitoneal radioisotopes is the therapy of choice if small foci of residual disease remain and the peritoneal cavity is relatively clear so that the radioactive material will not be loculated.

Chromic phosphate (^{32}P) is the isotope of choice in our opinion and 15 mc. may be injected approximately 7 to 10 days postoperatively.

With more extensive or anaplastic disease, chemotherapy is the most accepted adjuvant therapy. A variety of treatment schedules have been proposed with a change of agent if the original protocol seems ineffective or if after a period of time, there is regrowth of the lesion. A 30 to 50 per cent response rate (i.e., a reduction in tumor mass) may be anticipated in most cases, but the 5 year survival rate has not been significantly improved with any treatment protocol in the past 25 years. Nevertheless, there has been prolonged survival time and an improved quality of life in a small group of cases.

It is important to appreciate the potential hazards of long-term chemotherapy. Beyond the routine associated toxicities, well outlined in most investigative programs, there are recent reports of nonlymphocytic leukemias occurring in patients on long-term therapy, more specifically those using alkylating agents. Consequently, in the patient with good initial response, a second-look operation is indicated after 18 months of treatment or 10 to 12 courses of the agent so that the chemotherapeutic agents may be discontinued in favorable cases or other agents may be employed as indicated.

MUCINOUS TUMORS

(FIGO GROUP II)

These lesions, basically cystic with loculi lined by mucus-secreting epithelium, contain fluid previously described as "pseudomucin," thus explaining the earlier designation of pseudomucinous cysts. This specific secretory product was thought to differ from mucin in a number of respects, specifically in its reaction to acetic acid. It seems apparent, however, from the studies of Fisher and others that the so-called pseudomucin is similar to mucin despite individual differences in the percentages of glycoproteins, carbohydrates, and serum proteins, as noted by Odin.

Tumors of this group may reach an enormous size, filling the entire abdominal cavity (Fig. 21–20). Most of the reported giant cysts, i.e., those weighing more than 68.1 kg (150 lb.), fall into this category, the largest being that reported by Spohn as weighing 149 kg (328 lb.).

Although there is a variation in reported

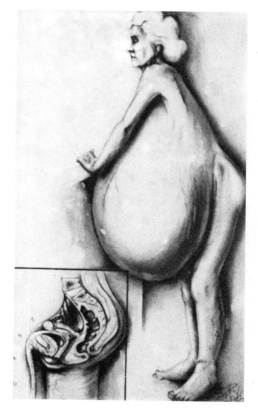

Figure 21–20. Enormous enlargement and compression of abdominal viscera produced by large mucinous cyst. (Courtesy of Dr. Erle Henriksen, Los Angeles, Calif.)

statistics as to the comparative frequency of mucinous and serous cysts, the majority of observers consider the mucinous variety to be less frequent than the serous.

Histogenesis

The mucinous epithelium in the tumor developing in the patient over the age of 40 years generally derives from the mesothelium by heterotopic alteration (Fig. 21–21 A, B). Demonstration of multiple histologic cell types in many such ovarian tumors confirms the validity of this thesis. Conversely, in the younger patient, the mucinous cyst is frequently of teratoid origin. It has been suggested that approximately 15 to 20 per cent of benign adult teratomas are found to contain mucinous epithelium if many sections are made. Furthermore, other elements of germ cell derivation may be discerned in the mucinous lesion; nevertheless, the excessive secretion from these secretory elements may eliminate other teratoid tissues. Finally, it should be appreciated in such lesions that there may be malignancy in the associated teratoid elements, and this association may explain the reported poor survival rates in the younger patients with the malignant mucinous tumors (Fig. 21–22). Certainly the patient in the late second or early third decade of life is prone to develop teratomas, and often these contain embryonal or extraembryonal elements. Such tumors are well known for their aggressiveness and associated poor survival rates (see Chapter 25).

Furthermore, the kinship of the epithelium of the mucinous cyst with other endodermic epithelium is demonstrated by the mucocele of the appendix, which may be associated with a similar lesion in the ovary. In such instances, the derivation of the epithelium in the ovarian cyst may be identified by the use of argentaffin stains. Nevertheless, the absence of argentophilic granules is not proof that the elements in the ovarian lesion are not of endodermal origin.

PATHOLOGY

Gross Characteristics

Mucinous tumors, unlike the serous variety, are, in 95 to 98 per cent of cases, intraovarian and rarely papillary. They are charac-

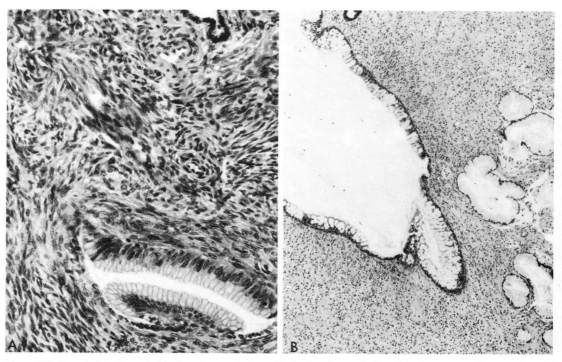

Figure 21–21. *A,* Mucinous epithelium in association with flattened mesothelium found in a normal ovary. *B,* Benign mucinous epithelium in a ovarian cystadenoma.

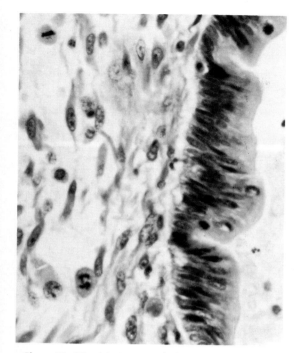

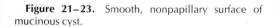
Figure 21–22. Mucinous epithelium in a tumor removed from 19 year old female. The underlying stroma shows rhabdomyosarcoma, accounting for the early demise.

teristically lobulated, with a smooth outer surface (Fig. 21–23). Adhesions are uncommon unless the cyst has leaked, degenerated, or become malignant. The wall of the cyst is usually thin, often translucent, and whitish or blue-white in appearance. As the tumor grows, it completely replaces the ovary, so that rarely is there a trace of normal ovarian tissue retained. Because of the size, the ovarian vessels become hypertrophied and a well-defined pedicle develops. The latter is not infrequently the site of torsion, especially in the case of the freely movable tumor of moderate size.

When the cyst is opened, the contents are usually found to be thick and viscid. Fluid of thinner consistency suggests the association of other epithelia in certain locules. The fluid is frequently light blue or straw-colored; however, when intracystic bleeding occurs, it may be hemorrhagic or brownish.

Characteristically, the cyst is composed of locules or compartments separated by thin septa of fibrous tissue. Because of the latter feature, the tumors are often called multilocular, although one large compartment

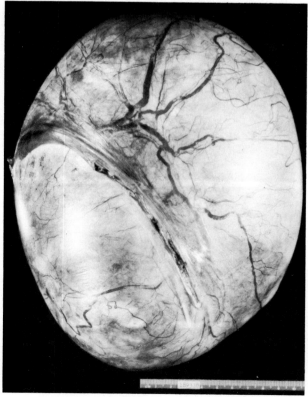

Figure 21–23. Smooth, nonpapillary surface of mucinous cyst.

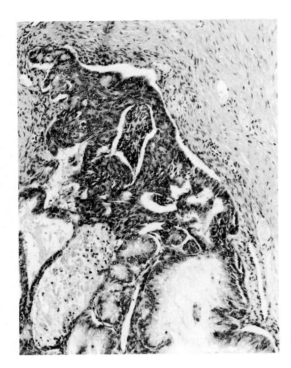

Figure 21–24. Mucinous cystadenoma with squamous metaplasia at top. Similar alterations are seen in the Brenner tumor.

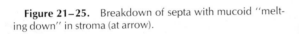

Figure 21–25. Breakdown of septa with mucoid "melting down" in stroma (at arrow).

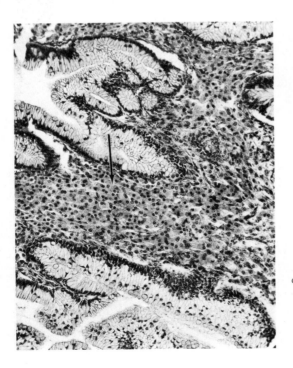

Figure 21–26. Leydig-like change in stroma of mucinous cyst (at arrow) with clinical masculinization.

may result from a merger of smaller locules produced by pressure atrophy of the intervening fibrous septa. Remains of the latter usually persist as raised or sickle-shaped ridges running along the inner walls of the cyst and at times are misinterpreted as papillae.

Although the cyst wall is generally thin, it is not unusual to find thickened or knobby areas. Such localized foci should always attract the special attention of the pathologist, since in these areas evidence of malignancy may be found and metaplasia occurs, often simulating the alterations associated with the Brenner tumor and its stromal proliferation (Fig. 21–24). The latter theca-like hyperplasia is probably responsible for the hormonal effect occasionally noted with these tumors. Finally, as noted previously, in the younger patient these tumors are often of teratoid origin, and diagnostic elements of the teratoma may be recognized in these firm nodules.

Microscopic Characteristics

The most distinctive feature of the mucinous lesions, and the one upon which the diagnosis is based, is the characteristic tall columnar epithelium (Fig. 21–21) with a clear, refractile cytoplasm and dark-staining, basally placed nucleus. Breakdown of the septa that separate the locules may result in extravasation of mucoid material into the stroma. This so-called "melting down" process produces a loss of the normal pattern (Fig. 21–25). Goblet cells may be seen in the well-differentiated tumor, although these elements are not as dramatic as those present in the gastric neoplasm. The epithelial lining is basically a single layer of the uniform tall columnar cell, although a pseudostratified appearance may be seen in loci because of the characteristic undulation of the epithelium and because tangential sectioning is common. Squamous metaplasia may be seen in the mucinous epithelium. The resultant pattern is similar to that noted in the Brenner tumor, and the pathogenesis of the latter lesion can be recognized in such metaplastic changes (Chapter 22).

The capsule and the interlocular trabeculae are of ovarian stromal origin which in some areas is quite compact but more frequently is loose textured and often edematous or myxomatous. This stromal component has evidenced its ability to react as the totipotent ovarian mesenchyme with resultant hormone production and associated alterations in the host—i.e., feminization, as noted by Brown and co-workers, or masculinization, as has been reported during pregnancy (Fig. 21–26). It is of interest to recognize that masculinization is associated with luteinization of the stroma in the mucinous cyst and the Krukenberg tumor in the pregnant patient, whereas estrogen production is noted in similar situations during the postmenopausal period. In view of this unique ability of the ovarian stroma to respond to the proliferating epithelium or its secretion in either the primary or secondary mucinous tumors, care must be taken not to mistake a metastatic tumor with the arrhenoblastoma because of the similar clinical picture.

In the benign as well as most malignant mucinous tumors, the demarcation between the lining epithelial cells and the adjacent stroma is sharp. Unlike the serous variety of cystadenoma, there is very little tendency to papillary proliferation of the epithelium. True papillae are treelike and demonstrate epithelial proliferation and potentially malignant alterations similar to the significance of the villous polyp of the bowel. Similarly, adenomatous patterns often suggest anaplastic change in the loss of the classic tall mucus-secreting element (Fig. 21–27 A,B); nevertheless, the adenomatous alterations are generally less ominous than the true papillary proliferations.

Malignancy developing in primarily benign mucinous cysts occurs in 5 to 10 per cent, according to most reported series. The ovarian neoplasm may be cystic from the outset and therefore one must not necessarily assume that the malignancy represents secondary neoplastic alteration (Fig. 21–28). Conversely, when carcinoma is found in only a small area of a largely benign cystadenoma whose existence has been known for many years, the evidence for the secondary nature of the neoplastic alteration is unimpeachable.

In a study of 78 mucinous cystadenocarcinomas, it was determined that mitotic count in the most anaplastic areas (usually papillary) was of major prognostic significance. Although the numbers in each group were small, the 5 year survival was only 60 per cent in the Clinical Stage IA tumors with more than 4 mitoses per high power field in the most malignant foci (Table 21–3).

The incidence of mucinous carcinoma of

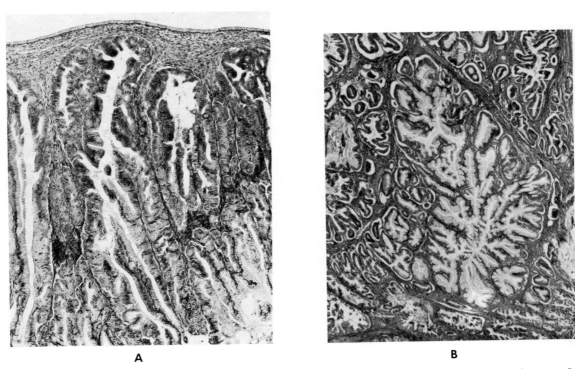

A
B

Figure 21–27. *A*, Early cellular anaplasia in papillary adenomatous lesion—piling up of cells with occasional mitoses. *B*, Very adenomatous area in a mucinous cystadenoma without cellular anaplasia.

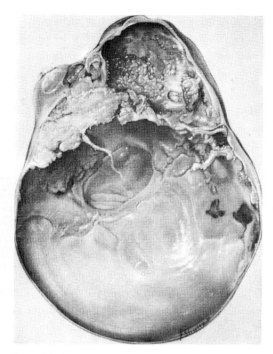

Figure 21–28. Mucinous cystadenocarcinoma of ovary, arising in mucinous cystadenoma.

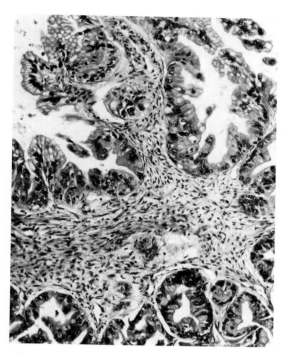

Figure 21–29. Early malignant alterations in mucinous cystadenocarcinoma simulating the similar lesion of the endocervix.

the ovary is less, in our experience, than that of the serous or endometrioid types. Among 192 consecutive ovarian cancers only 18 (9 per cent) were mucinous. Obviously, when the neoplastic cell loses its ability to differentiate, it becomes difficult to define the initial cell of origin. In certain instances the early malignant changes simulate the carcinoma in situ of the endocervix, again demonstrating the similarity between lesions of the upper genital canal and those of the ovary (Fig. 21–29). Finally, it must be reemphasized that although papillary proliferations are much less common in the mu-

cinous than in the serous tumors, nevertheless such alterations are basic evidences of atypical proliferation and it is in these foci that the true mitotic activity of the mucinous carcinoma can be most accurately identified.

Whereas in the papillary serous lesions of low grade malignancy, it is common to find a rather uniform pattern from section to section, such is not true in the mucinous tumors. Frequently well-differentiated and benign mucinous epithelium is found immediately adjacent to a poorly differentiated focus (Fig. 21–30 A,B). Consequently it is much more important to make multiple sections from many areas in the mucinous tumor in order to identify the most significant anaplastic alteration. Special stains, even in the very anaplastic appearing tumor, will identify the presence of mucin, and such techniques should be used routinely if there is a suspicion that the lesion basically arose from mucin-secreting epithelium. Furthermore, it should be appreciated that metastatic lesions from the gastrointestinal tract may simulate the primary ovarian mucinous tumor. Consequently, careful search should be made if there is any question as to the primary nature of the lesion. Primary ovarian

Table 21–3 SURVIVAL RATES OF 65 PATIENTS WITH MUCINOUS OVARIAN NEOPLASIA

Mitoses per High Power Field	Total	Clinical Stage				Per Cent Survival
		I	II	III	IV	
0–1	6	6	0	0	0	100
2–3	24	16	1	7	0	63
4–5	22	14	4	3	1	58
5+	13	5	3	4	1	23

A Simple serous cyst. Both external and internal surfaces are smooth.

B Papillary serous cystadenocarcinoma. The external surface appears smooth but numerous papillary projections are found on section.

C Multilocular mucinous cystadenoma. Firm areas at upper pole need serious microscopic study.

D Mucinous fluid evacuated from abdominal cavity of patient with pseudomyxoma peritoneii.

E Bilateral "endometrioid" carcinoma of the ovary. Old blood was present in cystic areas and transition from endometriosis to cancer could be seen.

F Bilateral fibrocystadenoma showing both cystic and solid components.

G Poorly differentiated tumor of both ovaries with multiple histologic patterns (mesothelioma) and omental cake.

H Mixed mesodermal tumor of ovary. Friable aggressive lesion with stromal and epithelial components.

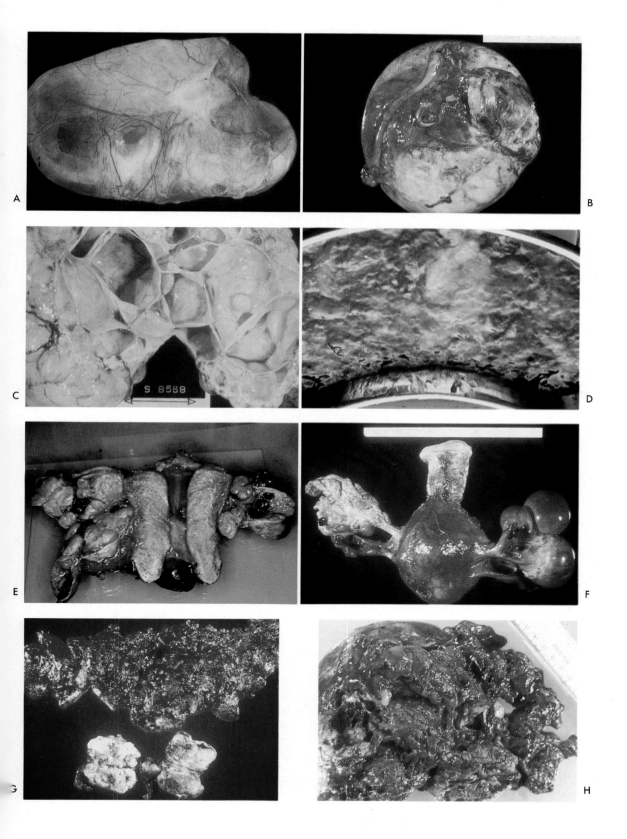

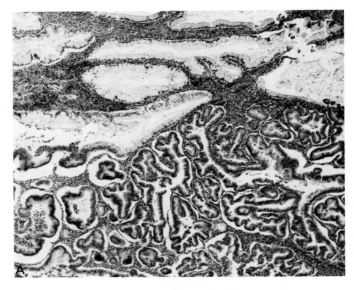

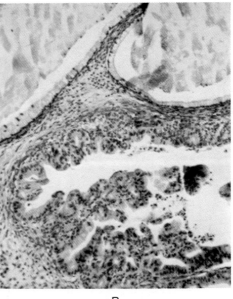

Figure 21–30. *A*, Well-differentiated mucinous epithelium in the upper section, with low grade adenocarcinoma in the lower segment. *B*, High power of transition between benign (top) and papillary proliferations of early malignant change (bottom).

neoplasms rarely metastasize to the mucosa of the bowel, although they commonly involve the serosa, whereas gastrointestinal lesions frequently are metastatic to the ovary (Fig. 21–31 *A,B*).

PSEUDOMYXOMA PERITONEI

Of major concern are those mucinous cysts that perforate spontaneously. In such situa-

tions there is intra-abdominal transformation of the peritoneal mesothelium into a mucin-secreting type, a reaction similar to that which initiates primary alteration in the ovarian coelomic epithelium of the cyst. This altered peritoneal mesothelium continues its mucus secretion with the gradual intraperitoneal accumulation of huge amounts of gelatinous material, constituting the so-called pseudomyxoma peritonei (Figs. 21–32 and 21–33). Evacuation of

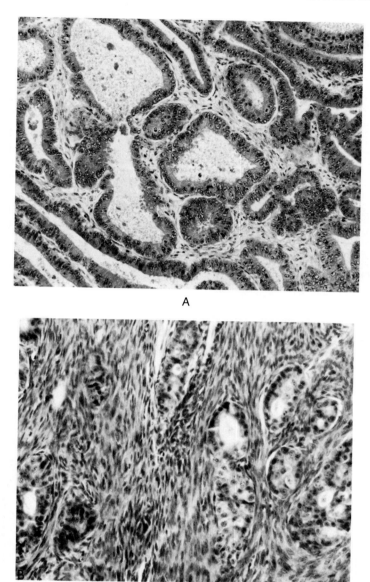

Figure 21–31. *A*, Mucinous carcinoma of the ovary associated with intestinal cancer. The primary focus would be difficult to establish through cell pattern alone. *B*, Metastatic mucinous tumor to the ovary. Patient was masculinized and diagnosis was arrhenoblastoma on basis of tubular tumor with stromal reaction.

this material at surgery is almost invariably followed by reaccumulation because of the impossibility of altering the secretion of the mucinous epithelium lining the cavity.

The previously suggested implantation of cells through rupture of the mucinous cyst at surgery has not proved to be a valid consideration. Nevertheless, when feasible, these tumors should be removed intact, even if an extended incision is necessary. Certainly careful toilet of the cavity at the termination

of the procedure is imperative, especially if the cyst has ruptured at surgery.

Among 13 cases of pseudomyxoma, Shanks noted that 10 cases originated in benign and two in malignant ovarian tumors, whereas one was associated with an appendiceal mucocele (Fig. 21–34). Of seven survivors, two had recurrences after 14 and 16 years, respectively. In a recent series Sandenbergh and Woodruff noted that, although only one of nine patients with pseudomyx-

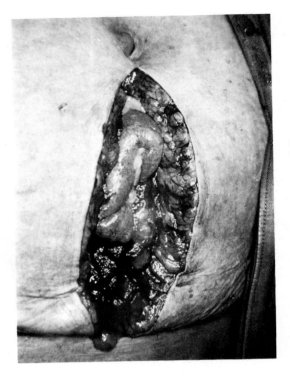

Figure 21–32. Pseudomyxoma peritonei. Note mucinous liquid dripping from the lower end of incision (fourth operation for this patient over a period of 12 years).

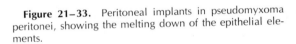

Figure 21–33. Peritoneal implants in pseudomyxoma peritonei, showing the melting down of the epithelial elements.

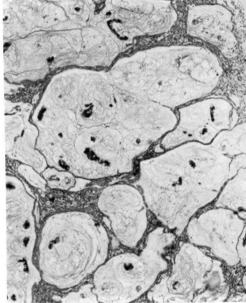

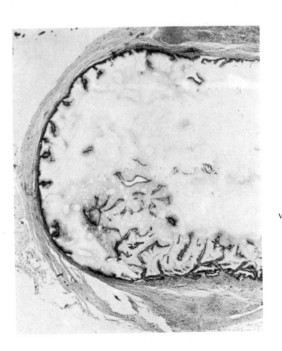

Figure 21–34. Mucocele of the appendix in association with pseudomyxoma peritonei.

oma peritonei survived, the tumor was still intraperitoneal at the time of demise. A review of the literature revealed only one case of extra-abdominal disease among the reported incidences of pseudomyxoma.

Treatment of this condition remains a persistent problem. Irradiation to the abdominal cavity has proved to be totally ineffective. A variety of chemotherapeutic agents have been used but again none has been associated with reduction in incidence of reaccumulation of mucin, with the possible exception of hexamethylmelamine. The use of intra-abdominal dextrose has been reported to reduce liquefaction of the mucin so that paracentesis is more effective. Barber has suggested the use of intraperitoneal ether at the time of evacuation of the mucinous material. He does note that this produces a rather severe reaction initially.

Clinical Course and Treatment

The mucinous tumors behave quite differently than the serous lesions. Bilateral development occurs in 8 to 10 per cent of the cases in our experience, whether the lesion is benign or malignant. This figure obviously does not include those cases in which there is widespread pelvic disease from extension of the tumor through the capsule into the adjacent cavity. Furthermore, the mucinous lesions are intraovarian in 95 yo 98 per cent of our cases, in contrast to the common multifocal intraperitoneal neoplasia associated with the papillary serous tumors. Finally, whereas the latter lesions cause death by widespread intra-abdominal growth and repeated bouts of intestinal obstruction, the malignant mucinous tumor often metastasizes 5 to 10 years after the initial procedure, and the metastases often are found in the pulmonary system. Despite this, massive intraperitoneal disease may be associated with poorly differentiated tumor, although it should be appreciated that in many instances the identification of the mucinous cell may be impossible, and thus such tumors should not be included among the mucinous, but rather with the poorly differentiated, or mesothelial, tumors.

As with all ovarian neoplasia, the initial procedure is surgery for diagnosis and staging. Adjunctive treatment for extensive intra-abdominal disease is usually chemotherapeutic. Use of intraperitoneal radioisotopes, sometimes quite effective for the serous

tumor with multiple implants, has not been effective for the mucinous lesion. As noted above, reoperation is important in cases of pseudomyxoma, although reaccumulation of the mucinous ascites is common.

ENDOMETRIOID NEOPLASIA

(FIGO GROUP III)

Endometriosis is extremely common, as noted in many publications. FIGO IIIA lesions include all the benign demonstrations of endometriosis and will be discussed in detail in Chapter 29.

In 1925, Sampson suggested that certain cases of adenocarcinoma of the ovary probably arose in areas of endometriosis. His criteria were so strict that few cases were reported in the literature since he demanded that both typical endometriosis and typical adenocarcinoma with a transition between the two must be identified. Obviously such a transitional zone may be eliminated totally by the aggressive malignancy. Nevertheless, in a small group of cases, such an origin has been demonstrated beyond any question (Fig. 21–35). In these cases the tumors were almost identical to those seen in the uterine

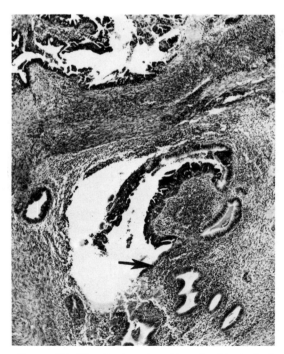

Figure 21–35. Carcinoma arising in histologically demonstrable endometriosis (arrow).

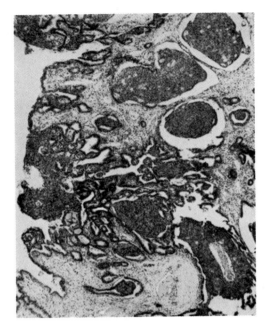

Figure 21–36. Adenoacanthoma developing in wall of endometrial cyst.

Figure 21–37. Transition from a low cuboidal to a taller endometrioid type.

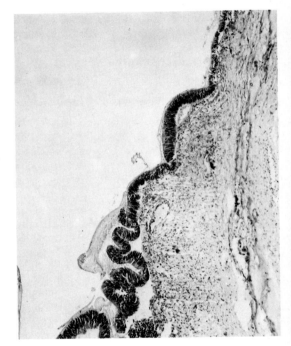

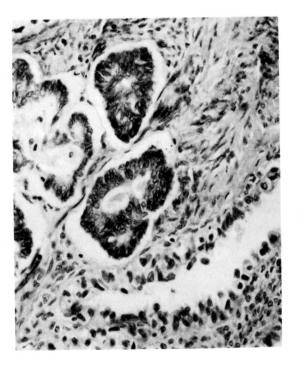

Figure 21–38. Mixed epithelial elements with organized glandular components—endometrioid and "hobnail" patterns.

cavity and approximately 50 per cent were classified as adenoacanthomas (Fig. 21–36). Basically these lesions were low grade malignancies, rarely metastasized, and were associated with excellent prognosis. Andrews and Larsen noted the infrequency with which ovarian endometriosis undergoes malignant alteration (less than 1 per cent of cases in their series).

The genesis of endometriosis is still debated (Chapter 29). Conversely, the transition from the ovarian mesothelium (coelomic epithelium) to an endometrioid variety (Fig. 21–37) and the finding of such an epithelium in association with other metaplastic elements is readily demonstrable (Figs. 21–38 and 21–39). In view of these recognizable transitions, the term endometrioid was accepted by FIGO in 1961. The incidence of these lesions among all ovarian malignancies is reported as approximately 5 to 10 per cent. Nevertheless, there are so many varied patterns with an adenoid component that it is difficult to be accurate in assessing this figure.

Clinical Features

Whereas endometriosis is commonly found in the third and fourth decades of life, endometrioid carcinoma develops most frequently, as do the majority of ovarian malignancies, in the fifth and sixth decades. Interesting cases of postmenopausal activation of endometriosis with associated malignancy have been reported in the past decade. Such

sequences would only suggest that, as with most neoplasms, it takes time for the benign alterations to become malignant—that is, if they ever do. In most cases, one would suspect that the endometriosis "burns out" or fibroses without ever developing into a carcinoma.

There are no specific symptoms of the endometrioid tumor unless it develops in endometriosis, certainly a rare occurrence. In the latter circumstance, the symptom would be that of the parent endometriosis, namely pelvic discomfort, pressure, and dyspareunia.

PATHOLOGY

Gross Characteristics

Malignancies arising in endometriosis may demonstrate the hemorrhagic foci characteristic of benign lesions. Conversely, the neoplasms developing de novo from the mesothelium are not distinctive.

Microscopic Characteristics

As noted above, benign endometriosis may be demonstrated in association with the neoplastic alterations. The endometrioid tumors, however, are characterized only by an adenocarcinomatous pattern with potentially all the variations seen in the uterus (Fig. 21–40A,B). Adenoacanthoma, often reported with definable endometriosis, is asso-

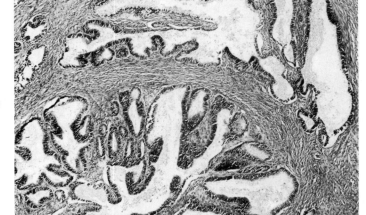

Figure 21–39. Transition of mucinous to endometrioid epithelium in benign cyst.

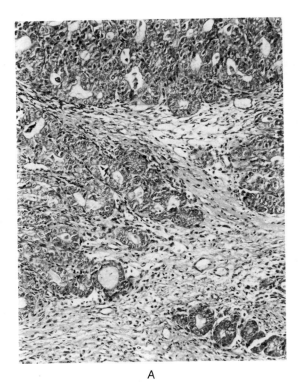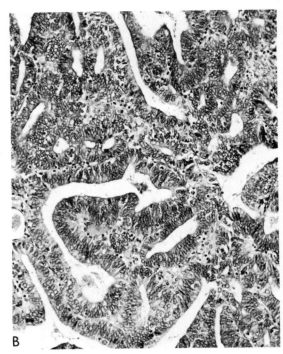

A

Figure 21–40. *A*, Endometrioid carcinoma with no evidence of endometriosis. *B*, Classic endometrioid carcinoma in the ovary simulating accurately the well-differentiated lesion seen in the fundus.

ciated, as in the fundus, with an excellent prognosis (Fig. 21–36). Conversely, patients with adenosquamous and mixed tumors have a very low survival rate (Figs. 21–41 and 21–42).

It must be recognized that histogenetic differentiation of ovarian malignancy is of more than academic interest today. With the widespread use of chemotherapeutic agents as adjunctive treatment to surgery, it becomes imperative to use the correct agent for the specific neoplasm. Whether any other than the well-differentiated endometrioid lesion will respond to progestational agents still remains a question; nevertheless, it is obvious that such treatment should be entertained if the tumor is classified as endometrioid. In contrast, the tumor of multiple patterns or the poorly differentiated lesion should be treated with other agents. Whether the use of radiation therapy is more effective for the endometrioid tumor than for other histologic types is equivocal, although there is certainly more basis for its use in view of its effectiveness in the treatment of uterine carcinoma.

MESONEPHROID CANCER (CLEAR CELL CARCINOMA)

(FIGO GROUP IV)

In 1939 Schiller applied the term mesonephroma to a group of tumors which, because of certain histologic attributes, he believed originated in mesonephric structures. Other authors have published reports of cases conforming to those described by Schiller (Figs. 21–43 and 21–44). There seems to be general agreement that they constitute a definite pathologic group, though practically all who have studied the question express skepticism concerning Schiller's concept of the histogenesis of these growths. Teilum reported a series of teratoid lesions in which the classic pattern of the endodermal sinus simulated that noted in two of the original cases described by Schiller. Undoubtedly there may be difficulty in separating these lesions, and certain of Schiller's original cases were in truth teratomas (see Chapter 25).

In 1944 Saphir and Lackner described a

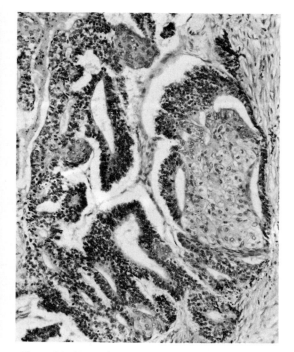

Figure 21-41. Adenosquamous carcinoma in ovary.

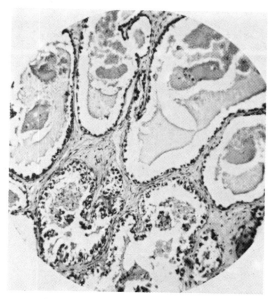

Figure 21-43. Mesonephroid tumor demonstrating hobnail epithelium and papillary infolding (lower left center).

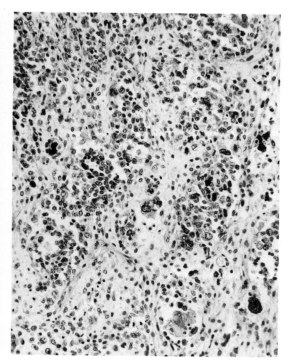

Figure 21-42. Mixed mesodermal tumor primary in the ovary.

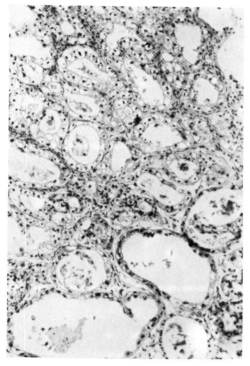

Figure 21-44. At bottom is the typical Schiller pattern with a clear cell adenocarcinoma at top. This admixture is common and suggestive of a similar basic origin.

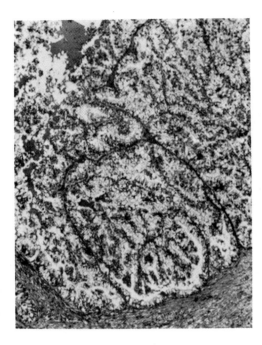

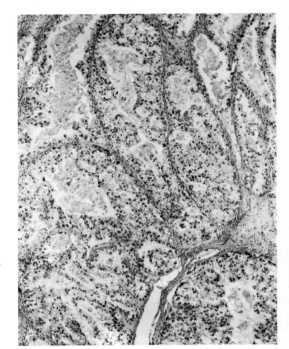

Figure 21–45. So-called clear cell adenocarcinoma, probably of mesonephric origin.

Figure 21–46. Mesonephroid tumor with clear cell component mixed with the hobnail areas.

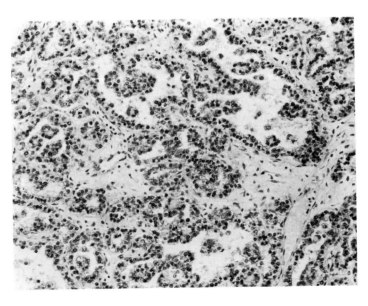

Figure 21–47. Mesonephroid tumor simulating the Teilum tumor. However, there is a uniformity of pattern, no true endodermal sinus and no mesoblastic stromal component. There is a poor clear cell component.

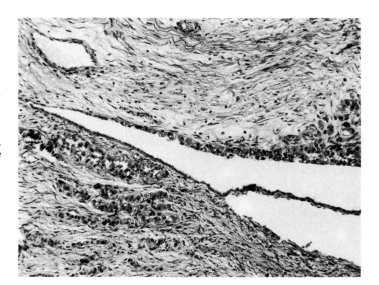

Figure 21–48. Mesothelioma of the ovary. Origin of the tumor directly from the surface mesothelium.

clear cell carcinoma which they designated a mesonephroma since it histologically corresponded to the nephric clear cell carcinoma (Fig. 21–45). In succeeding years the combination of the two patterns of hobnail and clear cell in an ovarian tumor earned it the title "metamesonephroma," an effort to associate the classic glomerulus-like tufting and hobnail epithelium of the mesonephric glomerulus with the clear cell or hypernephroid lesion of the kidney (Figs. 21–46 and 21–47). Furthermore, these tumors may arise at any point in the pelvis where the primitive mesonephric duct once existed, from the lower vagina to the parovarian region. Thus, certain mesonephromas of the ovary are not really ovarian tumors; however, the originating cells lie in such close proximity to the gonad that the latter may be completely replaced by tumor.

Scully in his studies of the clear cell ovarian tumor has noted the similarity between the histologic characteristics of this lesion and certain endometrial cancers. The occurrence of endometriosis with the mesonephroid tumor has added weight to the thesis that these neoplasms are paramesonephric rather than mesonephric in origin. Finally, others have recognized that mesonephroid tumors may arise de novo from the coelomic epithelium. Since the latter and the endometrium are of the same embryologic origin, the question as to the individual cell of origin is academic (Fig. 21–48).

The incidence of the mesonephroid carci-

noma among all ovarian malignancies is difficult to assess, although most authors quote figures of 5 to 8 per cent. A major problem in identifying an accurate figure is the frequency with which the mesonephroid pattern is associated with other patterns (Fig. 21–49).

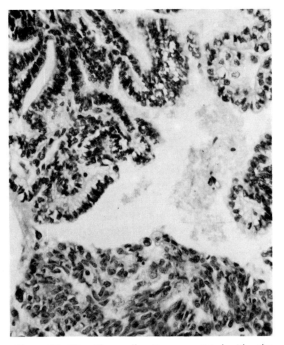

Figure 21–49. Clear cell pattern associated with other elements.

Clinical Features

Of 95 cases of mesonephroid neoplasm collected from the files of the Ovarian Tumor Registry, more than 75 per cent of the patients were over the age of 40 years. In spite of the size of many lesions (e.g., rising to the level of the umbilicus), approximately two thirds were Stage IA tumors and the prognosis was excellent. As might be expected in patients with Stages III and IV tumors, the survival, regardless of therapy, was essentially nil.

Clinically these tumors are the most common ovarian neoplasm associated with hypercalcemia. Furthermore, unexplained hyperpyrexia may herald the presence of this mesonephroid tumor. Other than these occasional unique features, this neoplasm, like most ovarian tumors, is asymptomatic until the mass becomes palpable or produces pelvic discomfort.

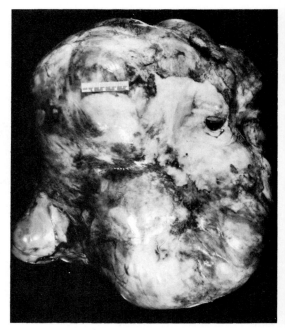

Figure 21–50. Gross appearance of mesonephroid lesion—not distinctive of any specific variety.

PATHOLOGY

Gross Characteristics

These tumors, as noted above, are commonly large and unilateral, with a smooth surface unless the malignancy has extended beyond the confines of the ovary (Fig. 21–50). Cystic and solid components are commonly present, the proportions obviously dependent on the amount of stroma, the secretory activity, and degrees of degeneration.

Microscopic Characteristics

Two basic histologic patterns are present in the mesonephroid tumor, the clear cell and the hobnail. The tall clear cells with basophilic nuclei at various positions within the cytoplasm are interspersed with elements containing essentially no cytoplasm and a cell membrane collapsed about the nucleus (hobnail). Whether these actually represent variations on a theme is not definitely known; however, there is every reason to expect that such a thesis is valid (Fig. 21–51). Mitoses are infrequent and a differentiation in malignant potential between the two histologic types was not identified in our series.

Finally, it is not uncommon to find clear cell foci in an ovarian tumor demonstrating a variety of histologic features—e.g., papillary, adenomatous, and undifferentiated. In such situations, it is important to diagnose the tumor as one with multiple patterns, and the malignant potential of the most aggressive element should be identified, for it is the latter upon which the prognosis will be based. Treatment of the mesonephroid tumors follows the same pattern as that for the malignant ovarian neoplasm. No special therapy has been more effective for the mesonephroid tumor than for other ovarian malignancies.

MESOTHELIAL REACTIONS AND THE MESOTHELIOMA

Mesothelial proliferations in and around the ovary are common reactions to a variety of local irritants, infectious and neoplastic (Fig. 21–52), and the benign is frequently difficult, if not impossible, to differentiate from the malignant (Figs. 21–53 and 21–54). This differentiation becomes more complicated when it is appreciated that all epithelial

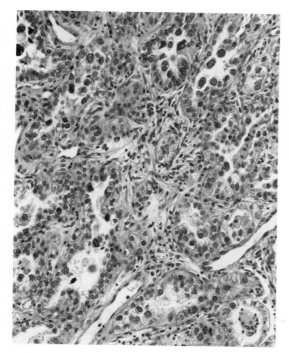

Figure 21–51. Mesonephroid carcinoma showing hobnail pattern with interspersed clear cells similar to the vaginal lesion developing in the young woman exposed to DES.

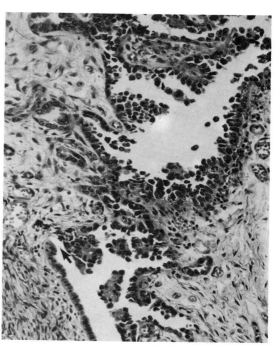

Figure 21–53. Mesothelial lesion arising from surface of gonad (arrow). Cells found in vaginal cytologic preparation. Cells are similar to those seen in Figure 21–52.

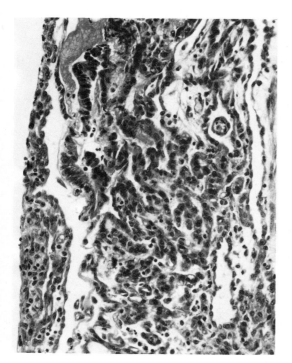

Figure 21–52. Mesothelial reaction in patient with endometriosis.

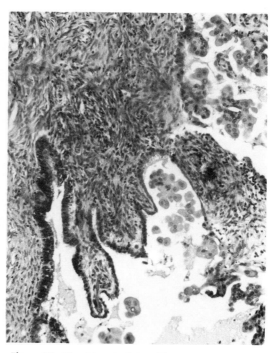

Figure 21–54. Mesothelial proliferation associated with a papillary lesion of low malignant potential. Cells appear histologically benign, and the tumor was found at many sites. Patient living without tumor 5½ years later.

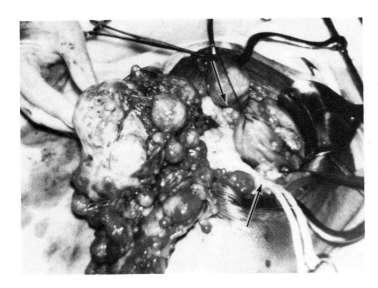

Figure 21–55. Intra-abdominal mesothelial tumor. Ovaries are involved (arrows) but majority of tumor is in omentum.

ovarian tumors are variations on the mesothelial "theme." Nevertheless it is imperative that the histologically identifiable lesion be so designated (i.e., serous, mucinous, or endometrioid), since prognosis and therapy are so dependent on such histopathologic identities.

In spite of these well-known varieties, there are ovarian or, better, intra-abdominal, neoplasms (Fig. 21–55) in which the

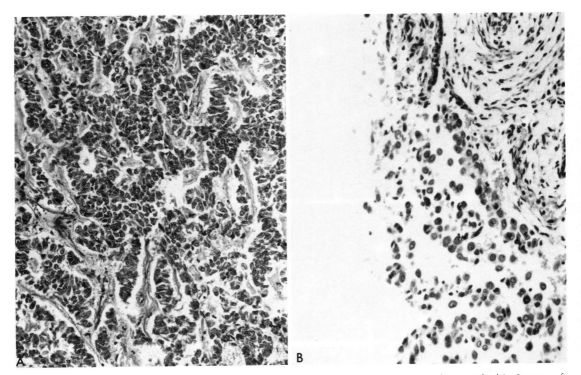

Figure 21–56. *A*, Alveolar mesothelioma. Patient had diffuse intra-abdominal disease and succumbed in 8 years, after multiple procedures had been performed. *B*, Mesothelial proliferation found in omentum. Cells are shed into vaginal pool and found in lumen of tube and on endometrial surface, but not in or on the ovary. Patient living and well 5 years postsurgery with no adjunctive therapy.

mesothelial cell predominates (Fig. 21–56 A,B). In these lesions, the round or ovoid cell with abundant finely granular cytoplasm and a round, lightly basophilic nucleus may be arranged in a variety of patterns. Since the stroma and epithelium are of mesothelial origin, both elements may be involved in the tumefactions (Fig. 21–57) and simulate those described in the pleural cavity (Fig. 21–58 A,B) as:

1. Stromal (fibrosarcomatous)
2. Tubopapillary (papillary-alveolar)
3. Mesothelial
4. Mixed histologic patterns

Careful evaluation of a number of poorly differentiated ovarian tumors reveals that many fell into one or another of these categories, particularly those classified as FIGO Histologic Group E. In certain instances, only the mesothelial cell is present. Often, in such cases, the tumor appears to have begun at many foci in the abdomen and the ovary is involved only with surface tumor (Fig. 21–59). The prognosis for such tumors is poor, although prolonged remissions may be achieved by chemotherapy and multiple operative procedures.

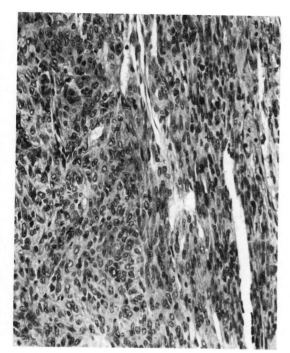

Figure 21–57. Mesothelioma found at multiple foci in abdominal cavity. Stromal and epithelial(?) components are difficult to distinguish. Patient succumbed to disease.

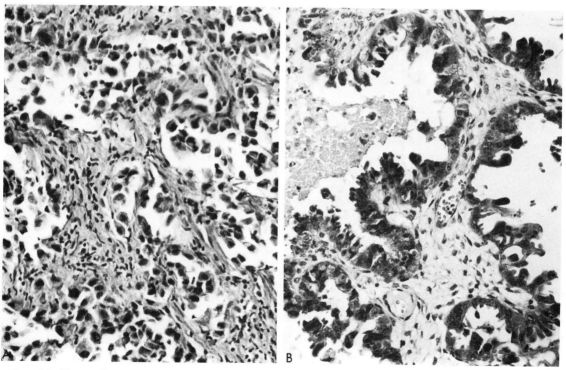

Figure 21–58. *A*, Pleural mesothelioma in male. *B*, Papillary mesothelioma—pattern is similar to the pleural mesothelioma in *A*.

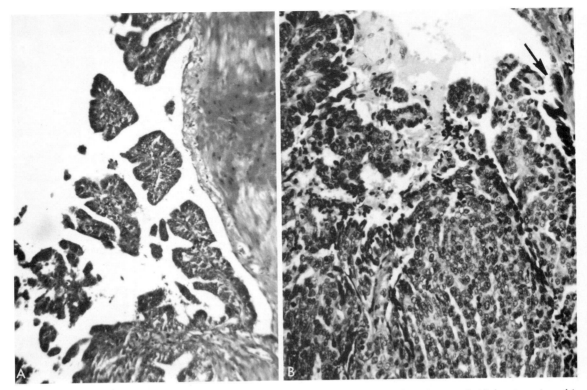

Figure 21–59. *A*, Papillary mesothelioma arising from surface of ovary. Diagnosis by Pap smear. *B*, High power view of *A*. Papillary mesothelioma arising from the surface of the ovary (at arrow). Note absence of mitoses. Patient asymptomatic, had a "normal pelvis." There were multiple intra-abdominal lesions and patient died within 18 months.

UNSPECIFIED DESIGNATIONS— UNDIFFERENTIATED CARCINOMA (PRIMARY SOLID CARCINOMA OF OVARY)

The use of the terms *solid* or *undifferentiated* in the discussion of ovarian neoplasia is unsatisfactory and unrealistic. Classifications of tumors in other areas often are based upon general pathologic considerations— e.g., the pattern of the growth and the proportion of epithelium versus connective tissue; however, the ovary represents a unique situation, since the majority of epithelial tumors arise from a basic mesothelial cell. The latter may differentiate into a variety of cell-specific tumors, may be totally mesothelial, and may or may not have a stromal component. Thus, the histologic descriptions adenocarcinoma and papillary, medullary, scirrhous, alveolar, and plexiform tumors are of no significance, since different patterns may coexist in different areas of the same tumor. For this reason these terms should not be included as an integral part of any

tumor classification, but instead the tumors should be identified as having multiple patterns and then the most malignant element and predominant cell type determined.

EXTENSION AND METASTASIS OF OVARIAN CARCINOMA

Uterus

As noted previously, the coexistence of ovarian and uterine adenocarcinoma is not uncommon and the primary site in such situations is often a matter of conjecture—if indeed these lesions are really metastatic and not representative of multicentric foci of origin (Fig. 21–60 *A,B*). In contrast, the serosa of the uterus may be involved by direct extension from the ovarian growth, and in such instances the primary ovarian origin is easily established.

The endometrial involvement may show itself in the form of superficial deposits on an otherwise normal endometrium, in which

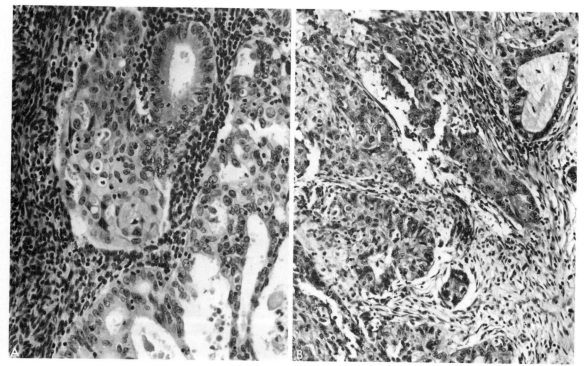

Figure 21–60. *A*, Adenosquamous carcinoma of endometrium. *B*, Adenosquamous carcinoma in ovary. There is no evidence of myometrial invasion of uterine cancer and no evidence of ovarian capsular or lymphatic invasion.

circumstance implantation has been invoked as the method of deportation of tumor tissue. Nevertheless, there is difference of opinion as to the frequency or even the possibility of such implantation. In such instances, it seems quite possible, as will be discussed in Chapter 24, that the same carcinogenic agent may affect both the endometrial and ovarian epithelia.

Tube

The tube is frequently involved in ovarian cancer, most commonly by direct involvement of the serosa. Implants or multicentric foci of the papillary lesion may be seen in many widely separate areas. Such involvement of the tube by a tumor of low malignant potential has not altered the prognosis in our experience (Fig. 21–61*A,B*).

In certain cases a direct surface transition from the normal tubal epithelium to the atypically proliferate pattern of the ovarian cancer can be recognized (Fig. 21–62). There is no evidence of lymphatic invasion in many such cases, and it seems possible that the tubal epithelium may be responding to the

same stimulus as that which produced the ovarian neoplasia and represent true carcinoma in situ.

Contralateral Ovary

In ovarian neoplasia, the contralateral ovary is a frequent site of tumor formation. The incidence depends largely on the histologic variety of neoplasm. The mucinous tumors demonstrate bilateral development in 8 to 10 per cent of the cases while the papillary serous tumor, commonly a surface lesion, often demonstrates bilateral involvement. Obviously, the very anaplastic tumor often involves the pelvic viscera by direct extension. Lymphatic extension is an unlikely explanation for involvement of the contralateral gonad, since there is no evidence that the lymphatics extend directly from one adnexa to the opposite.

Peritoneum

Perhaps the most common secondary site of tumor involvement is the visceral or parietal peritoneum, and this occurs in most can-

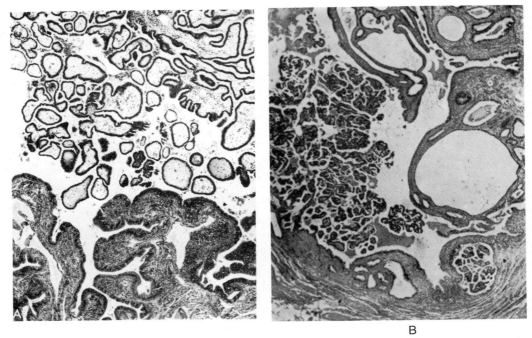

B

Figure 21–61. *A*, Papillary serous tumor of low malignant potential in tubal lumen. At separate areas, psammoma bodies were seen in tubal fronds. *B*, Large carcinoma particles from ovarian cancer migrating through tube. Note the apparent change in tubal morphology to conform to that of transported tumor (arrow). Also, there is a nest of tumor in agglutinated mucosal folds in right lower.

cers in which there is breakthrough of the capsule, or papillary seeding. The peritoneal extension may be manifested by the formation of nodules on the anterior parietal wall, the omentum (Fig. 21–63), the surface of any portion of the intestine, the right hemidiaphragm, and almost any of the abdominal viscera. In advanced cases the umbilicus may show metastatic nodules (Fig. 21–64). Ascites is a frequent accompaniment of peri-

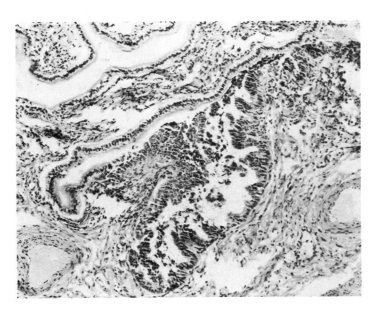

Figure 21–62. Fimbria of the tube showing transition from the normal ciliated cells to neoplastic alterations in the center and lower middle. Patient had ovarian cancer. Note that there are areas of normal tubal epithelium in the midst of the atypical proliferations.

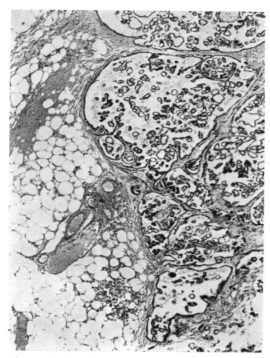

Figure 21–63. Omental tumor associated with similar low grade lesion of the ovary.

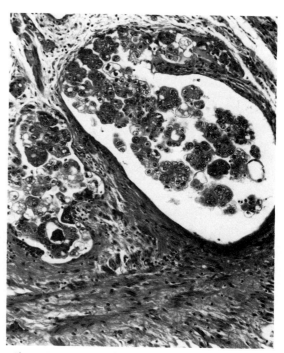

Figure 21–65. Lymphatic invasion from ovarian tumor.

toneal carcinomatosis, and malignant cells can usually be demonstrated in the ascitic fluid.

Lymph Nodes

In many cases, especially in the later stages, the lymphatic glands are the site of metastases (Fig. 21–65). Again, the histopa-

thology of the lesion is significant in determining the extent of such involvement. The anaplastic lesions invade the peritoneum at any site and thus the regional nodes, often the mesenteric chain, will be focus for such extension. From the ovary, the paraortic lymphatics are commonly involved. Later, distant nodal groups, such as the inguinal, mediastinal, and supraclavicular, may be involved. Finally, invaginations of mesothelium directly into the node may simulate lymphatic invasion (Fig. 21–6); however, in such cases the prognosis is much better than those instances of true invasive cancer.

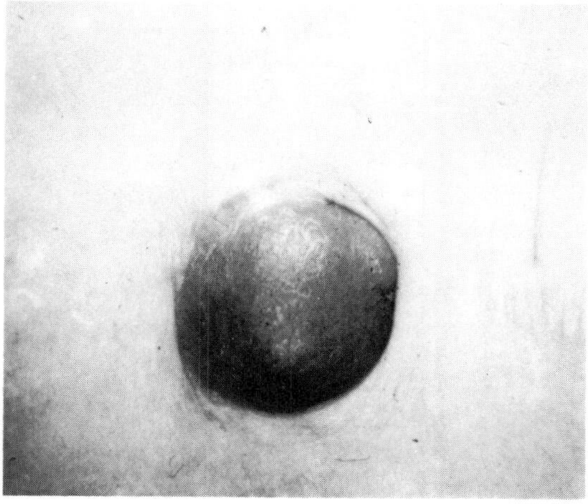

Distant Organs

Among the distant organs which may be involved with ovarian carcinoma are the liver, gallbladder, pancreas, the gastrointestinal tract, lungs, pleura, ribs, and occasionally the long bones.

TREATMENT AND SALVAGE OF OVARIAN CANCER

Adequate surgery for ovarian cancer is a hysterectomy with removal of both adnexa

Figure 21–64. Metastatic ovarian tumor in umbilicus.

except for those special cases noted previously. The extent of the procedure beyond the genital organs demands careful evaluation. Resection of the omentum is commonly necessary, particularly in the papillary lesions. Resection of an involved loop of intestine is often justified; however, multiple resections with obvious widespread disease must be looked upon askance.

The use of intraperitoneal radioactive isotopes has been effective as adjunctive therapy for small foci of residual tumor (2 to 3 mm.) or with positive findings from the peritoneal cytologic preparation. Chromic phosphate (^{33}P) has minimal penetrability, but presumably delivers 6000 to 7000 rads of beta irradiation to the total peritoneal surface, and avoids the untoward side effects of radioactive gold, which has a gamma component and a very short half life (3.5 days) compared with phosphorus (14.5 days).

Chemotherapeutic agents have largely supplanted the use of external beam irradiation, which cannot deliver effective dosage, especially to the upper abdomen, without damage to vital intra-abdominal organs. A majority of clinics are employing alkylating agents, e.g., Alkeran, as first line therapy, with changes to such medications as hexamethylmelamine and cis-platinum when recurrences or nonresponse becomes evident by the size of tumor mass. Triple and even quadruple therapeutic regimens have been and are being tried; however, the toxicity is prohibitive in many cases and the results to date have not justified the risks.

Finally, more serious, life-threatening side effects are now being reported, particularly with the use of long-term therapy with the alkylating agents. Regrettably, in some instances, patients dying of nonlymphocytic leukemia, apparently resulting from the chemotherapy, have been found at autopsy to be free of the original disease. As a consequence, many investigators are suggesting that after 10 to 12 courses of the agent (approximately 18 months) the patient should be subjected to a "second look" procedure by laparotomy or laparoscopy. Further therapy would be dependent on the findings at the exploratory procedure.

Above all, it seems important to remove the parent (pelvic) tumor. Even when there has been extensive tumor, removal of the pelvic lesion has occasionally been followed by a remarkable regression of the generalized process. Omentectomy minimizes recurrent ascites, and peritoneal lavage at the time of surgery, with cytopathologic study, is of prognostic importance and may also indicate specific therapy (Moore et al.).

Despite prompt and adequate therapy, salvage with ovarian cancer is extremely poor. Approximately 60 per cent of the cases are inoperable when initially seen. The distressing nature of the disease is that it is asymptomatic until adjacent organs are involved. Five year salvage in most series of all epithelial neoplasia approximates 30 per cent.

In our laboratory, breakdown of the cases of papillary tumors according to mitotic count has increased our ability to prognosticate on survival. Clinical stage must be included, particularly in the more anaplastic lesions, if the statistics are to be accurate.

Little advance has been made in early diagnosis of ovarian malignancy. Nevertheless, shed cells may be transported through the tube and may be recovered from the vaginal pool. According to Frost (see Chapter 35), vaginal smears from about one third of the cases of ovarian cancer demonstrate malignant cells cytologically. In the postmenopausal patient, it has been recognized that, regardless of the variety of the tumor, a hormone may be produced by the ovarian mesenchyme as a result of the mechanical stimulation of the proliferating lesion. As a consequence, a shift to the right in the vaginal Maturation Index, in the absence of use of exogenous estrogen, should increase the clinician's index of suspicion and demand further study of the pelvic viscera. Finally, Graham has suggested that abnormal cells may be picked up by culdocentesis in the suggestive case. Regrettably, these studies are commonly positive when a tumor is already clinically present. As a screening procedure, for example, to diagnose the early lesion, these techniques, particularly culdocentesis, have been inadequate and the latter is often an uncomfortable one.

Finally, in the author's opinion, more studies are necessary to identify possible carcinogenic agents. An appreciation of the facts that this lethal tumor occurs more frequently in urban areas, has been correlated with persistent ovulation, and apparently was seen rarely prior to the last century should focus our attention on potential carcinogenic processes. Certainly in a neoplasm that is so lethal, that cannot as yet be diagnosed early, and that has responded poorly to current therapeutic modalities, an ounce of prevention is worth a good deal more than a pound of cure.

Immunology

At present, the study of the immunology of the ovary tumor is in its infancy; however, the investigations Barber, DiSaia, and others suggest that this approach may offer great promise in the future.

REFERENCES

Abel, S.: Ovarian carcinoma; diagnosis and treatment. Miss. Med., 54:523, 1957.

Andrews, W. C., and Larsen, G. D.: Endometriosis. Am. J. Obstet. Gynecol. 118:643, 1974.

Aure, J. C., Hoeg, K., and Kolstad, P.: Clinical and histologic studies of ovarian carcinoma. Obstet. Gynecol., 37:1, 1971.

Bassis, M. L.: Classification of ovarian tumors. J.A.M.A., 174:170, 1960.

Beck, R. P., and Latour, J.P.A.: Review of 1019 benign ovarian neoplasms. Obstet. Gynecol., 16:1019, 1960.

Betson, J. R., and Golden, M. L.: Primary carcinoma of the ovary co-existing with pregnancy. Obstet. Gynecol., 12:589, 1958.

Bigelow, B., and Demophoulos, R. I.: Endometrioid carcinoma arising in an unusual ovarian cyst. Gynecol. Oncol., 4:391, 1976.

Bowles, H. E., and Tilden, I. L.: Mesonephric carcinoma of the ovary. Obstet. Gynecol., 9:64, 1957.

Brooks, J. J., and Wheeler, J. E.: Malignancy arising in extragonadol endometriosis. Cancer, 40:3065, 1977.

Brown, J. B., Kellar, R., and Matthew, G. D.: Preliminary observations on urinary oestrogen excretion in certain gynecologic disorders. J. Obstet. Gynaecol. Br. Emp., 66:177, 1959.

Bullock, W. K., Houts, R. E., and Gilrone, J. J.: Ovarian tumor. Arch. Surg., 71:153, 1955.

Caricker, M., and Dockerty, M. B.: Mucinous cystadenomas and cystadenocarcinomas. Cancer, 7:302, 1954.

Carler, G. J., and Frodey, R. J.: Primary ovarian cancer. Obstet. Gynecol., 9:71, 1957.

Chan, L. K. C., and Prothrop. K.: Mucinous cystadenoma with virilization during pregnancy. Am. J. Obstet. Gynecol., 107:946, 1970.

Corscaden, J. A.: Gynecologic Cancer. 2nd Ed. Baltimore, Williams & Wilkins Co., 1956.

Czernobilsky, B., Silverman, B. B., and Enterline, H. T.: Clear cell carcinoma of the ovary. Cancer, 25:762, 1970.

Davis, B. A., Latour, J. P. A., and Philpott, N. W.: Primary carcinoma of the ovary. Surg. Gynecol. Obstet., 102:565, 1956.

Decker, D. G.: Prognostic importance of histologic grading in ovarian carcinoma. Natl. Cancer Inst. Monogr., 42:9, 1975.

Dockerty, M. B.: Ovarian neoplasms (collective review). Int. Abstr. Surg., 81:179, 1945.

Doshi, N., et al.: Primary clear cell carcinoma of the ovary. Cancer, 39:2658, 1977.

Dougal, D.: Pseudomyxoma of ovary and appendix. J. Obstet. Gynaecol. Br. Emp., 38:729, 1931.

Dyson, J. L.: Factors influencing survival in ovarian carcinoma. Br. J. Cancer, 25:237, 1971.

Ewing, J.: Neoplastic Diseases. 3rd Ed. Philadelphia, W. B. Saunders Company, 1928.

Fenoglio, C. M., Puri, S., and Richart, R. M.: The ultrastructure of endometrioid carcinomas of the ovary. Gynecol. Oncol., 6:152, 1978.

Ferencz, A., Okagaki, T., and Richart, R. M.: Para-endocrine hypercalcemia in ovarian neoplasm. Cancer, 27:427, 1971.

Fisher, E. R.: Pseudomucinous cystadenoma: A misnomer? Obstet. Gynecol., 4:616, 1954.

Frankl, O.: Zur Pathologie und Klinik des Fibroma ovarii adenocysticum. Arch. Gynäk., 131:325, 1927.

Garnett, J. D.: Primary adenoacanthoma of ovary. Am. J. Obstet. Gynecol., 60:1374, 1950.

Henderson, D. N., and Bean, J. L.: Results of treatment of primary ovarian malignancy. Am. J. Obstet. Gynecol., 73:657, 1957.

Julian, C. G., and Woodruff, J. D.: The role of chemotherapy in the treatment of primary ovarian malignancy. Obstet. Gynecol. Surv., 24:1307, 1969.

Julian, C. G., and Woodruff, J. D.: The biologic behavior of low-grade papillary serous carcinoma of the ovary. Obstet. Gynecol., 40:860, 1972.

Kazancigil, T. R., Laqueur, W., and Ladewig, P.: Mesonephroma of ovary. Am. J. Cancer. 40:199, 1940.

Kent, S. W., and McKay, D. G.: Primary cancer of ovary. Am. J. Obstet. Gynecol., 80:430, 1960.

Kurman, R. J., and Craig, J. M.: Endometrioid and clear cell carcinomas of the ovary. Cancer, 29:1653, 1972.

Legros, R., and Fain-Giono, J.: Post-menopausal activation of endometriosis. Rev. Fr. Gynecol. Obstet., 68:25–33, 1973.

MacFarlane, K. T.: Management of ovarian tumors. Can. Med. Assoc. J., 71:440, 1954.

Malpas, P.: Pseudomyxoma peritonei. J. Obstet. Gynaecol. Br. Emp., 66:247, 1959.

Masson, J. C., and Hannick, R. O.: Pseudomyxoma peritonei of ovarian origin, analysis of 30 cases. Surg. Clin. N. Amer., 101:61, 1930.

Masson, J. C., and Hannick, R. O.: Pseudomucinous cystadenoma. Surg. Gynecol. Obstet., 50:752, 1932.

Masterson, B. J.: Multiple threat: second primary malignancies in patients with ovarian carcinoma treated with radiation and chemotherapy. J. Kans. Med. Soc., 78:283, 1977.

Meyer, R.: Handbuch der spezielle pathologische Anatomie und Histologie. F. Henke and O. Lubarsch, Eds. Berlin, J. Springer, 1930.

Meyer, R.: Zur Histogenese und Einteilung der Ovarialkystome. Mschr. Geburtsh. Gynäk., 44:302, 1916.

Montgomery, T. L., Bowens, P. A., and Kittleberger, W. C.: The diagnosis and management of breast cancer. Obstet. Gynecol., 17:19, 1960.

Moore, G. E., Sako, K., Kondo, T., Badillo, J., and Burke, E.: Assessment of the exfoliation of tumor cells into the body cavities. Surg. Gynecol. Obstet., 112:469, 1961.

Munnell, E. W., Jacox, H. W., and Taylor, H. C., Jr.: Treatment and prognosis in cancer of the ovary. Am. J. Obstet. Gynecol., 74:1187, 1957.

Morton, D. G., Moore, J. G., and Chang, N.: The clinical value of peritoneal lavage for cytologic examination. Am. J. Obstet. Gynecol., 81:1115, 1961.

Novak, E.: Pseudomyxoma peritonei. Bull. Johns Hopkins Hosp., 33:182, 1922.

Novak, E.: Ovarian metastasis with cancer of the uterine body. Am. J. Obstet. Gynecol., 14:470, 1927.

Novak, E.: Adenoacanthoma of ovary arising from endometrial cyst, with report of case. J. Mt. Sinai Hosp., 14:529, 1947.

Novak, E. R., and Woodruff, J. D.: Mesonephroma of the ovary. Amer. J. Obstet. Gynec., 77:632, 1959.

Novak, E., Woodruff, J. D., and Novak, E. R.: Probable mesonephric origin of certain femal genital tumors. Am. J. Obstet. Gynecol., 68:1222, 1954.

Odin, L.: Studies on the chemistry of ovarian cyst contents. Acta Soc. Med. Ups., 64:25, 1959.

Pankamaa, P.: Pseudomyoma peritonei. Ann. Chir. Gynaecol. Fenn., 47:1, 1958.

Parker, T. M., Dockerty, M. B., and Randall, L. M.: Mesonephric clear cell carcinoma, a clinical and pathological study. Am. J. Obstet. Gynecol., 80:430, 1960.

Parmley, T. H., and Woodruff, J. D.: The ovarian mesothelioma. Am. J. Obstet. Gynecol., 120:234, 1974.

Pearse, W. H., and Behrman, S. J.: Carcinoma of ovary. Obstet. Gynecol., 3:32, 1954.

Piver, M. S., Lele, S., and Barlow, J. J.: Pre-operative and intra-operative evaluation of ovarian malignancy. Obstet. Gynecol., 48:312, 1976.

Radisavljevic, S. V.: The pathogenesis of ovarian inclusion cysts and cystomas. Obstet. Gynecol., 49:424, 1977.

Randall, C. L., and Hall, D. W.: Treatment of ovarian malignancies. Am. J. Obstet. Gynecol., 63:497, 1952.

Randall, J. H.: Treatment of ovarian cancer. Obstet. Gynecol., 5:445, 1955.

Rogers, L. W., Julian, C. G., and Woodruff, J. D.: Mesonephroid carcinoma of the ovary. J. Gynecol. Oncol., 1:76, 1972.

Roth, L. M., and Ehrlich, C. E.: Mucinous cystadenocarcinoma of the retroperitoneum. Obstet. Gynecol., 49:345, 1977.

Sampson, J. A.: Endometrial carcinoma of ovary. Arch. Surg., 10:1, 1925.

Sampson, J. A.: Carcinoma of tubes and ovaries secondary to carcinoma of body of uterus. Am. J. Pathol., 10:1, 1934.

Sandenberg, H. A., Woodruff, J. D.: Histogenesis of pseudomyxoma peritonei. Obstet. Gynecol., 49:339, 1977.

Saphir, O., and Lackner, J. E.: Adenocarcinoma with clear cells (hypernephroid) of ovary. Surg. Gynecol. Obstet., 79:539, 1944.

Schiller, W.: Mesonephroma ovarii. Am. J. Cancer, 35:1, 1939.

Schiller, W., Rilke, F., and Degna, A. T.: Parvilocular cystomas of the ovary. Obstet. Gynecol., 10:28, 1957.

Scott, R. B.: Serous adenofibromas and cystadenofibromas of ovary. Am. J. Obstet. Gynecol., 43:733, 1942.

Scully, R. E., and Barlow, J. F.: "Mesonephroma" of the ovary. Tumor of müllerian nature related to endometrioid carcinoma. Cancer, 20:1405, 1967.

Seski, A. G., and Amirikia, H.: Starch granuloma syndrome. Obstet. Gynecol., 48:605, 1976.

Shanks, H. G. I.: Pseudomyxoma peritonei. J. Obstet. Gynaecol. Br. Commonw., 68:212, 1961.

Shaw, W.: Pathology of ovarian tumors. J. Obstet. Gynaecol. Br. Emp., 39:13, 234, 1932.

Slye, M., Holmes, H. F., and Wells, H. G.: Primary spontaneous tumors of the ovary. Cancer Res., 5:205, 1920.

Smith, G. V.: Ovarian tumors: with special reference to some unexpectedly good outcomes in treatment of cancer of ovary. Am. J. Surg., 95:336, 1958.

Spohn, W.: Cited by Lynch, F. W., and Maxwell, A. F.: Pelvic Neoplasms. New York, D. Appleton and Company, 1922.

Steinberg, L., Rothman, D., and Drey, N. W.: Mullerian cyst of the retroperitoneum. Am. J. Obstet. Gynecol., 107:963, 1970.

Stromme, W. B., and Traut, H. F.: Mesonephroma or teratoid adenocystoma of ovary. Surg. Gynecol. Obstet., 76:296, 1943.

Taylor, C. W.: Pathology of malignant ovarian tumors. J. Obstet. Gynaecol. Br. Emp., 57:328, 1951.

Taylor, H. C., and Long, M. E.: Problems in papillary adenocarcinoma of the ovary. Am. J. Obstet. Gynecol., 70:753, 1935.

Taylor, H. C.: The diagnosis and treatment of ovarian carcinoma. Clin. Obstet. Gynecol., 1:1078, 1958.

Teilum, G.: Carcinoma arising in ovarian endometriosis. Acta Obstet. Gynec. Scand., 25:377, 1945.

Teilum, G.: Classification of ovarian tumors. Acta Obstet. Gynecol. Scand., 31:292, 1952.

Teilum, G.: Mesonephric tumors of female and male genital system. Acta Pathol. Microbiol. Scand., 34:431, 1954.

Teilum, G.: Endodermal sinus tumors of the ovary and testis. Cancer, 12:1092, 1959.

Thompson, J. D.: Ovarian adenoacanthoma. Obstet. Gynecol., 9:403, 1957.

Towers, R. F.: Note on the origin of the pseudomucinous cystadenoma of the ovary. J. Obstet. Gynaecol. Br. Emp., 63:253, 1956.

Turner, J. C., Remine, W. H., and Dockerty, M. B.: Primary ovarian carcinoma. Surg. Gynecol. Obstet., 109:198, 1959.

Weiss, N. S., and Silverman, D. T.: Laterality and prognosis in ovarian cancer. Obstet. Gynecol., 49:421, 1977.

Weiss, N. S., et al.: Incidence of histologic types of ovarian cancer. Gynecol. Oncol., 5:161, 1977.

West, R. H.: Survival in ovarian cancer. Quart. Bull. Northw. Univ. Med. Sch., 29:256, 1955.

Williams, T. J.: Status of the contralateral ovary in encapsulated low grade malignant tumors of the ovary. Surg. Gynecol. Obstet., 143:763, 1976.

Woodruff, J. D.: The histology and histogenesis of ovarian neoplasia. Cancer, 38 (Suppl. 1):411, 1976.

Woodruff, J. D., and Novak, E. R.: Papillary serous tumors of the ovary. Am. J. Obstet. Gynecol., 67:1112, 1954.

Woodruff, J. D., Bie, L. S., and Sherman, R. J.: Mucinous tumors of the ovary. Obstet. Gynecol., 16:699, 1960.

Woodruff, J. D., and Julian, C. G.: Explorations into the genesis of ovarian cancer. Int. J. Gynecol. Obstet., 8:587, 1970.

Woodruff, J. D., Genadry, R., and Parmley, T. H.: Mucinous cystadenocarcinoma. Obstet. Gynecol., 51:483, 1978.

Chapter 22

OVARIAN NEOPLASIA: STROMOEPITHELIAL LESIONS— PRIMARILY STROMAL (BRENNER TUMORS, FIBROTHECOMAS, SARCOMAS, ETC.)

All epithelial ovarian tumors have a basic stromal component. Nevertheless, the latter is not a prominent feature of most such neoplasms, although some are composed mainly of gonadal mesenchyme. The epithelial component in these lesions varies from the simple mesothelium of the surface fibromatous papillomas (Fig. 22–1) to the stratified metaplastic epithelium of the Brenner tumor. The common inclusions of the peritoneal epithelium often produce an apparent stromal reaction, with a resultant fibroadenosis (Fig. 22–2) in an otherwise grossly normal ovary. Conversely, these stromoepithelial tumors may become quite large. With the exception of the Brenner tumor, they are rarely associated with clinical evidences of hormone production. The reason for the differences in activity remains obscure; however, there seems to be a definite association between mucus-secreting epithelium and stromal reactivity, as noted in the Krukenberg tumor and mucinous cysts.

In addition to the minor changes noted above, i.e., the surface papillomas and the fibroadenosis, there are those lesions which attain palpable size and have variously been

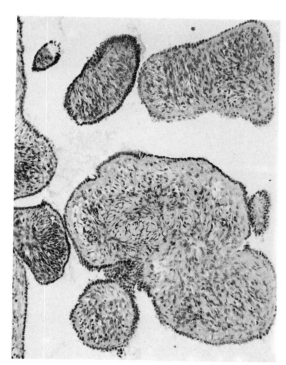

Figure 22–1. Surface fibromatous nodules on a normal ovary. Note the absence of epithelial proliferations and thus essentially no malignant potential.

437

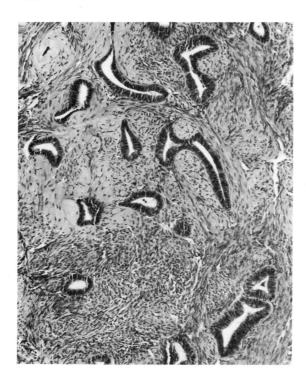

Figure 22–2. Ovary in which both epithelial and stromal components are proliferate, producing a picture of fibro-adenosis.

termed cystadenofibromas or fibrocystaden-omas (Figs. 22–3 and 22–4 *A,B*). For the most part, these lesions are composed of go-nadal stroma and supporting connective tis-sue through which are dispersed cystic structures of varying sizes. Most commonly these cysts are lined by tubal type epithe-lium or mesothelium, or both; and, as in other ovarian lesions with similar lining cells, papillae may develop. Other cell types, particularly the mesonephroid type, may be recognized if careful search is made (Fig. 22–5). On occasion, squamous meta-plasia may occur in one or more of the cystic components, thus simulating the alterations that take place in the Brenner tumor (Fig. 22–6). Malignancy developing in these fi-brocystadenomas is extremely uncommon;

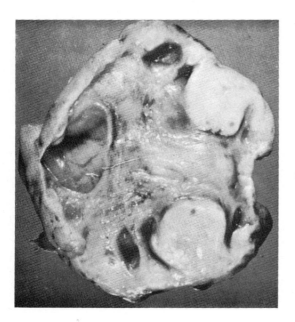

Figure 22–3. Gross appearance of cystadenofibroma.

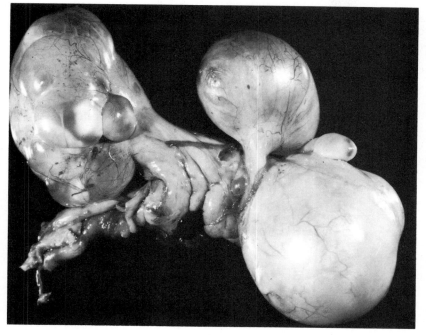

A

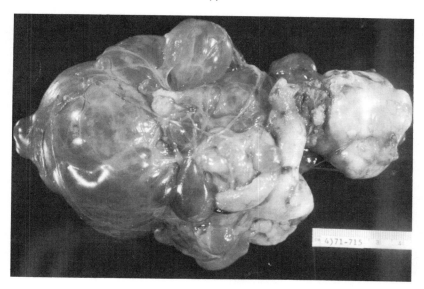

B

Figure 22–4. *A,* Multifaceted ovarian tumor. Sections showed patterns that varied from cystadenofibroma to the simple cyst—a variant of the stromoepithelial neoplasm. *B,* Cystadenofibroma of the ovary showing separate cystic and solid components at either end of the specimen and admixture in the center.

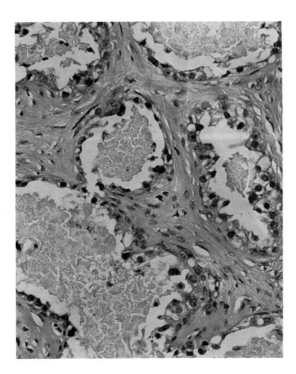

Figure 22–5. Mesonephroid epithelium in primarily stromal lesion.

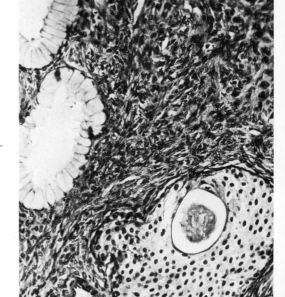

Figure 22– 6. Metaplasia in mucinous cystadenoma simulating changes that take place with Brenner tumors.

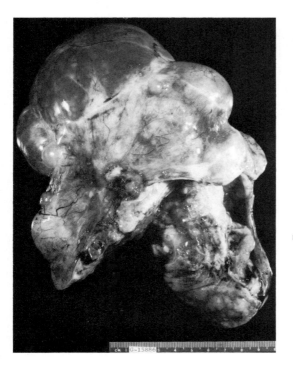

Figure 22–7. Mucinous cystadenofibroma with malignant alterations found only on permanent sections.

however, obviously numerous sections should be made to rule out such alterations (Fig. 22–7).

BRENNER TUMORS OF THE OVARY

The most interesting of these stromoepithelial lesions is the Brenner tumor. Described in 1907 by Brenner under the designation of oophoroma folliculare, it was considered by the author to be related to granulosa cell lesions. Meyer in 1932 redescribed the pathologic and histogenetic characteristics of the Brenner tumor; however, in light of the studies of Greene and of Reagan, it appears likely that there is more than a single histogenesis.

As noted above, Brenner believed the lesion to be a variety of granulosa-theca cell tumor because of the ovum-like structures seen so often within the cell rests, and because of the superficial resemblance of the latter to follicles. The condensed ovarian tissue around the cell islands was interpreted as representing the theca folliculi. Meyer believed that the tumor arose from the islands of indifferent cells first described by Walthard in 1903.

The Walthard inclusions may be found in the subserosal portion of the ovaries, the tubes, and the uterine ligaments (Fig. 22–8). They consist of nests of cells resembling squamous epithelium, often showing a central cystic cavity (Fig. 22–9) lined by mesothelium or any variety of epithelium found in the upper canal, most frequently of tubal type. In other words, the transmutations of the epithelium are much like those exhibited by the epithelial nests in Brenner tumors, constituting at least circumstantial evidence of similarity of origin of these elements.

The co-association of Brenner and mucinous tumors is accepted, although there is uncertainty as to the sequential origin. Can one assume that there is mucinous transition in a Brenner tumor, or should the epithelioid changes be construed as representing metaplasia in a preexisting mucinous tumor, just as squamous metaplasia may involve the tall columnar endocervical epithelium? Woodruff and Acosta make a rather strong case for the latter possibility, and stress that any epithelial alteration might be expected to progress from an undifferentiated reserve to an epithelioid type of cell.

Greene's classic discussion of Brenner

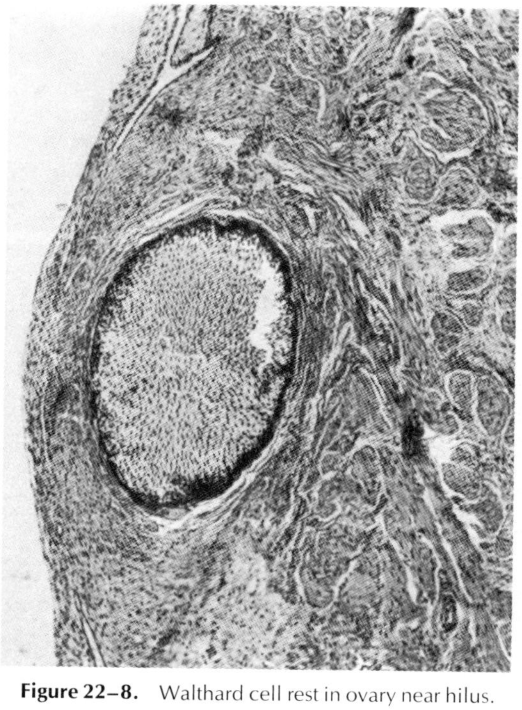

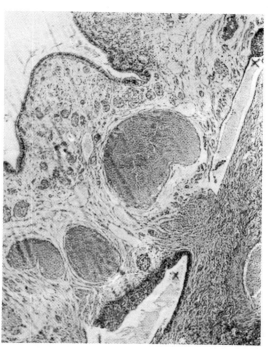

Figure 22–8. Walthard cell rest in ovary near hilus.

Figure 22–9. Metaplastic epithelial areas (x) which resemble Walthard islands, especially as latter often show the central cavity of the preexisting peritoneal inclusion.

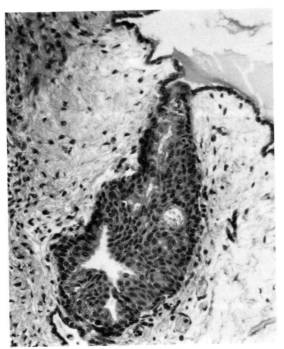

Figure 22–10. Metaplasia in an invagination of peritoneal epithelium. This appears like transitional epithelium; however, it is in reality squamous cell metaplasia, an early stage in the development of the "Walthard cell rest."

tumors points out clearly the many sources of metaplastic epithelium of the rete and the ovarian stroma. Genesis from the rete would undoubtedly account for many of the small lesions found in the hilus of the ovary. Actually, very early changes may be recognized in such epithelia without the formation of a true tumor (Figs. 22–8 and 22–9). Also as a result of this proposal, Sneeden has likened the alterations seen in these tumors to the

epithelium of the urogenital system—i.e., a transitional variety (Fig. 22–10).

In carefully performed reconstructions Arey rather conclusively has demonstrated that Brenner rests and tumors are not isolated islands but branching treelike sprouts of invaginated mesothelium. The similarity between metaplasia in such inclusions of the coelomic epithelium and urothelium is easily appreciated (Fig. 22–10). Although such patterns simulate transitional epithelium, it must be understood that the Brenner tumor is not derived from rests or modifications of endodermal epithelium.

Although previous reports suggested that the Brenner tumor was extremely rare (1 in 1200 to 1500 cases of ovarian neoplasia) a more careful study of ovarian lesions has revealed that small focal fibrothecomas often contain epithelial rests with squamous metaplasia. These may not be true tumors; however, the incidence of such foci is not unusual in the otherwise normal ovary.

PATHOLOGY

Gross Characteristics

The size of the tumor varies widely, in one third of our cases being 2 cm. or less in diameter; thus they are primarily microscopic findings, often in the hilus of the ovary (Fig. 22–11). Conversely, they may reach major proportions; that reported by Averbach and co-workers weighed over 8.6 kg. (19 lb). The gross appearance of the solid tumors is quite similar to that of fibroma (Fig. 22–12). There is very little tendency to ne-

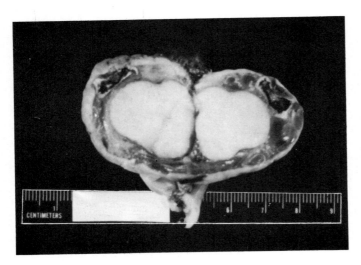

Figure 22–11. Brenner tumor arising from medullary or hilar area. Note intact cortex.

STROMOEPITHELIAL—PRIMARILY STROMAL—TUMORS / **443**

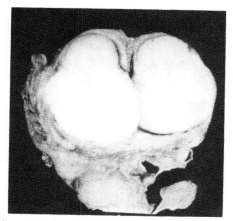

Figure 22–12. Gross appearance of Brenner tumor.

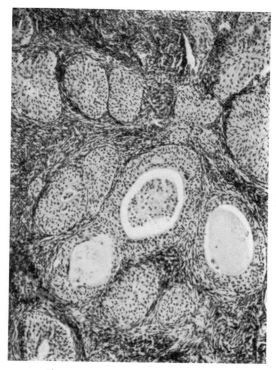

Figure 22–13. Typical Brenner tumor.

crosis or cystic degeneration in the solid variety, and hemorrhage is uncommon. The capsule is poorly defined, although the surrounding ovarian stroma is more or less compressed. In rare instances Brenner tumors may be bilateral. Furthermore, it is not uncommon to find a Brenner tumor in one ovary and a fibroma or fibroadenoma in the contralateral organ.

Microscopic Characteristics

From a microscopic standpoint there are two essential constituents—viz., the characteristic nests of epithelial cells and the concentration of mesenchymal tissue surrounding the epithelial islands (Fig. 22–13). Both features must be present to justify the diagnosis of Brenner tumor, a fact overlooked by some authors, who apply the term to the epithelial Walthard rests.

The epithelial elements of the Brenner tumors may be round or cylindrical, very small or extremely bulky. A striking characteristic is the uniformity of the cells. In the classic benign tumor, the cells are large, often flattened, with abundant pale, almost agranular cytoplasm and small, regular nuclei with coarse chromatin. Danforth and Arey have called attention to a peculiar longitudinal grooving of nuclei (Fig. 22–14), the "coffee-bean nucleus," a characteristic finding in the cells of the Walthard islands, sequelae of squamous metaplasia in peritoneal inclusions. Similar nuclear patterns are seen in squamous metaplasia elsewhere in the pelvis and in the granulosa cells. It must be appreciated that, in the large tumor, numerous sections should be made to eliminate the possibility of the missing ma-

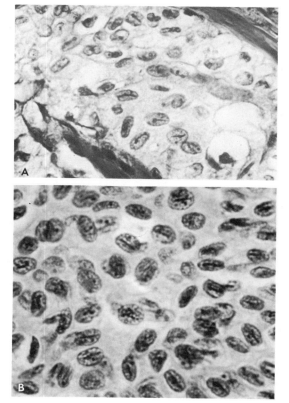

Figure 22–14. Characteristic longitudinal grooving to produce "coffee bean" pattern. (Courtesy of Dr. John MacKinlay, Glasgow, Scotland.)

lignant change, as in all epithelial ovarian tumors.

In most tumors some evidence of the tubular or cystic structure from which metaplastic epithelium has arisen still remains as a central cavity. These small cavities superficially resemble ova, and were interpreted by Brenner as oophoroma folliculare (Fig. 22–15 A). The slightly condensed surrounding ovarian tissue layer was thought to represent theca (Fig. 22–15A,B).

The central cavity may contain desquamated, degenerated material as the result of maturity of the metaplastic epithelium, a process that in some instances simulates a "keratin plug or inclusion cyst." Conversely, the epithelium of the original cystic cavity in which metaplasia took place may continue to secrete and maintain a central core. In a small proportion of cases the superficial epithelium may be of a columnar, mucus-secreting variety, quite like that which

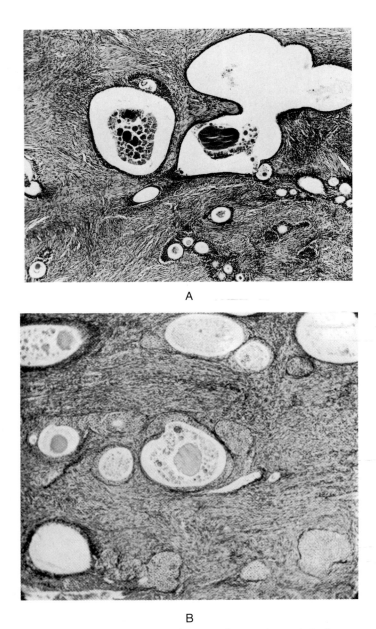

A

B

Figure 22–15. Different patterns in the Brenner tumor with varying degrees of metaplasia. Some nests are solid, while others show only a single layer of mesothelium. The superficial similarity to ova is seen in the lower portion of A. Stromal reaction is also quite variable.

characterizes the ordinary mucinous cystadenoma (Fig. 22–6).

In the same section are found solid epithelial nests, those with a superficial layer of mucinous epithelium lining the small central cavities, and areas in which the mucinous epithelium alone lines glandlike spaces and perhaps large cystic cavities. The latter presents the characteristic picture of mucinous cystadenoma, and such tumors may show small areas of metaplasia simulating the common squamous metaplasia of the endocervical epithelium (Fig. 22–16).

Fibromas have been reported with epithelial aggregations that have been variously interpreted, but these are properly construed as Brenner tumors in which the characteristic connective tissue response has assumed major proportions. The gross picture of Brenner tumors is quite similar to that of the fibromas, and there is little doubt that a careful study of many supposedly simple ovarian fibromas would show them to be of the Brenner variety (Fig. 22–17).

Of both histopathologic and clinical importance is the stroma of the Brenner tumor. Commonly this portion of the lesion is fibro-

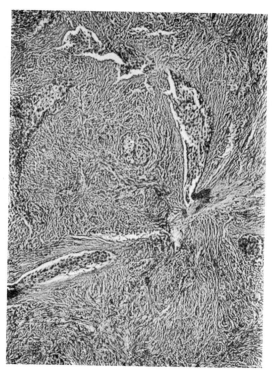

Figure 22–17. Large ovarian fibroma of Brenner origin. Note characteristic epithelial rests.

matous and often almost acellular. Myxomatous and hyaline changes with an occasional focus of calcification are similar to those seen in the fibroma. In contrast, this stromal component may demonstrate evidence of theca-like alterations with abundant, slightly eosinophilic cytoplasm and a large, pale nucleus with a well-defined nucleolus. These changes are classically noted adjacent to the epithelium and may demonstrate the presence of lipid. Histochemical stains reveal that these cells are similar to the theca and thus may be steroid producing. It has been noted previously that the stroma of the mucinous lesions demonstrates similar features.

Degree of Malignancy

A majority of Brenner tumors are benign, but in recent years an increasing number of both proliferating (intraepithelial) and invasive malignancies have been reported. The probable reason for this change is the more careful classification of many neoplasms formerly diagnosed as poorly differentiated carcinomas or squamous cell cancer originating in teratomas or adenocarcinoma. However,

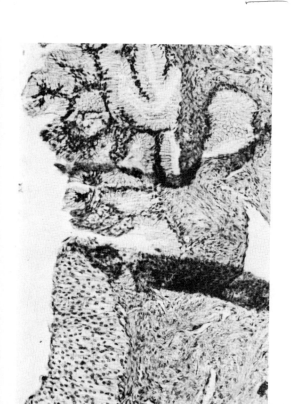

Figure 22–16. Sharp transition between proliferating metaplastic and mucinous epithelia (at ink mark).

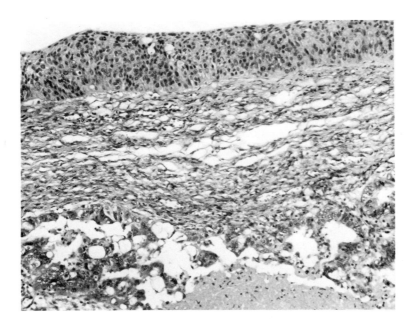

Figure 22–18. Multilayered neoplastic epithelium (above) simulating carcinoma in situ with neoplasia in mucin-secreting epithelium below.

as noted in previous editions, many so-called malignant Brenner tumors represented neoplasia arising in a preexisting cystic lesion (Fig. 22–18).

A recent review revealed six instances of proliferating or intraepithelial carcinoma and 12 cases of malignancy. All of the six proliferating tumors (Figs. 22–19, 22–20) demonstrated classic loss of stratification in the metaplastic epithelium with the finding

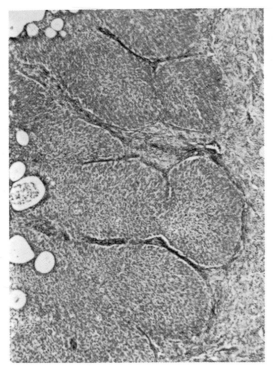

Figure 22–19. Beginning malignancy in Brenner tumor. High power microscopic study confirms the malignant properties of the Brenner cells. Proliferating Brenner tumor.

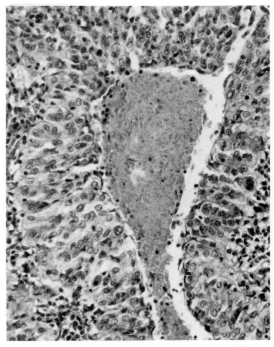

Figure 22–20. Proliferating Brenner tumor, showing changes simulating in situ neoplasia of the cervix.

of a pseudo-squamocolumnar junction (Fig. 22–16). One patient had bilateral ovarian tumors, both showing similar epithelial alterations, associated with carcinoma in situ in the cervix!

The carcinomas demonstrated a variety of histopathologic patterns. True squamous cancer with maturation of the epithelial elements was rare, in contrast to the more poorly differentiated epidermoid neoplasia. It could be argued that in the latter circum-

stance, the diagnosis of malignant Brenner tumor is in doubt; however, careful review of the sections revealed an origin of the multi-layered, neoplastic epithelium from the basic mesothelium, and such tumors may develop in multiple sites in the upper genital canal (Fig. 22–21 A,B,C).

Neoplasia arising in the stromal component of the Brenner tumor (a stromal sarcoma) is rare, since either the neoplastic stroma or the epithelium obscures the alter-

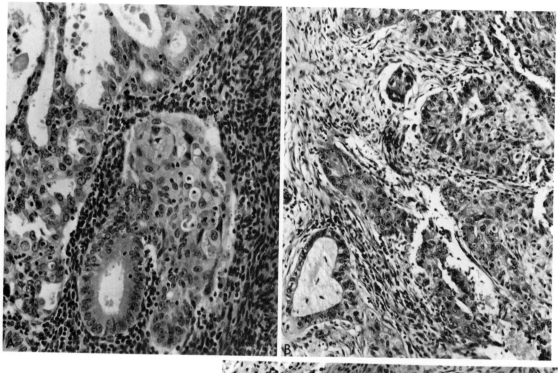

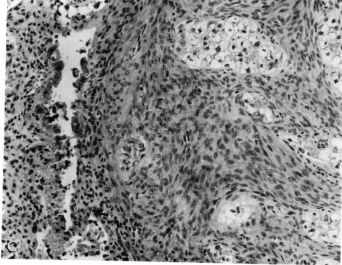

Figure 22–21. *A,* Adenosquamous carcinoma of endometrium with similar alterations in ovary. *B,* Adenosquamous carcinoma in ovary with adenosquamous cancer in uterus and malignant Brenner tumor in opposite ovary. *C,* Malignant Brenner tumor showing atypical mature cells with reactive stroma on right and adenomatous element with beginning atypical metaplasia on left (at arrow).

nate component. Nevertheless a low grade malignancy may recur and thus demonstrate the multiple stromoepithelial potentialities (Fig. 22–22 A, B). The two elements are difficult to identify in this case, but careful survey of the two parts of the figure demonstrates the proliferation of primarily the stroma in the case of recurrent disease over a period of 7 years. Both elements can be recognized, but the difficulty in differentiating stroma from epithelium is evident.

General Clinical Characteristics

Brenner tumors of the ovary occur most frequently in women beyond the menopause; more than 50 per cent are reported in the sixth decade of life. Nevertheless in a series of 90 cases from the Emil Novak Ovarian Tumor Registry, 30 per cent of the patients were between the ages of 20 and 40 years and 50 per cent were under the age of 50 years. The growth of Brenner tumors, like that of their fibrothecomatous counterpart, is likely to be slow. Furthermore, it produces no characteristic symptoms, so that the high

incidence in elderly women loses some of its significance because the excised tumors might well have been present for many years. Ascites is rare, but on occasion it may be associated with hydrothorax (Meigs' syndrome). The menstrual history is not characteristic; nevertheless, as already noted, the stromal component may histologically and functionally resemble theca with all of the endocrine capacities of this specific cell.

Surgery is recommended for both diagnosis and therapy. Since most such tumors are benign, conservative unilateral adnexectomy is advised for the young woman. Nevertheless, in the patient who has had her family or is over the age of 40 years, total hysterectomy and bilateral salpingo-oophorectomy is the treatment of choice. Furthermore, it must be appreciated that bilateral solid tumors are commonly found to be metastatic, and the complete preoperative work-up should include a survey for a primary site if both ovaries are enlarged. If malignancy is found in the sections, adjunctive therapy is indicated, either irradiation or chemotherapy.

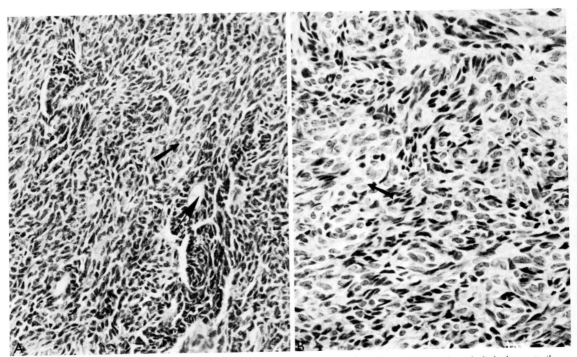

Figure 22–22. *A*, Malignant Brenner tumor removed in 1971. Note relatively well-defined epithelial elements (larger arrow) and indefinite stromoepithelial(?) component (smaller arrow). *B*, Recurrence 7 years after initial surgery of tumor seen in A. Note the epithelial(?) component at arrow with "coffee bean" nuclei. Again there is difficulty in differentiating stroma from epithelium.

Endocrine Influence

The capacity of the granulosa cell tumors to produce hyperplasia of the endometrium and menstruation-like bleeding in postmenopausal women is well known, and is readily explainable by their capacity to produce estrogenic hormone. Similarly, Schifferman and others have reported on the association of hyperplasia and adenocarcinoma of the endometrium with Brenner tumors.

It is, however, well known that hyperplasia of the endometrium may at times be found in postmenopausal women in the absence of any tumor, and thus such associations are but presumptive evidence of cause and effect. Nevertheless, in view of the increasing number of reported cases of apparent endometrial stimulation and the theca-like reaction of the periepithelial stroma, the potentiality of hormone production by some Brenner tumors must be appreciated. Furthermore, our histochemical studies, as noted previously, lend support to this thesis.

Ullery and co-workers have studied extensively a Brenner tumor that was associated with testosterone synthesis. Indeed, there has been increasing recognition of the ability of various ovarian tumors to produce steroids, which may be predominantly estrogenic or androgenic; however, sometimes an admixture is produced so that no overt hormone pattern predominates.

TUMORS WITH FUNCTIONING MATRIX

Morris and Scully have noted that certain ovarian tumors, notably but not exclusively cystadenofibromas and Brenner tumors, might exert an estrogenic action, although morphologically they were not of the classic feminizing lesions.

As noted, the Brenner tumor, in addition to the epithelioid nests, features a dense mesenchymal matrix that simulates that of the perifollicular theca. A number of authors have reported single cases, and Farrar and co-workers have compiled the results of the many studies. Of 376 Brenner tumors, adequate information about the endometrium was available in only 65 cases (17 per cent), including those cases previously reported by Teoh, MacKinlay, Eton, and Parker. Of the 402 cases, an estrogenic effect was thought to exist in 7.5 per cent. Nevertheless, the endometrium was available for study in only about one fifth of the cases, and when this could be studied, estrogen effect was present in close to 50 per cent. Furthermore, the absence of abnormal bleeding is no proof of the inactivity of the tumor.

The authors, with many others, agree that the hormone production arises from the theca-like cells in the stroma of Brenner tumors. Tighe found one adenocarcinoma and six cases of hyperplasia among 19 endometria associated with ovarian Brenner tumors, and his conclusions approximate those of Ming and Goldman and of Woodruff and Acosta.

An androgen effect has been observed with a number of different ovarian tumors, not classically of the endocrine variety. In addition to Brenner tumors, mucinous, Krukenberg, and other neoplasms have been noted to produce virilism, and references to these will be noted in Chapter 25.

REFERENCES

Arey, L. B.: Nature and significance of grooved nuclei of Brenner tumors and Walthard cell islands. Am. J. Obstet. Gynecol., 45:614, 1943.

Arey, L. B.: The origin and form of Brenner tumors. Am. J. Obstet. Gynecol., 81:743, 1961.

Averbach, L. H., Promin, D., and Hanna, G. C., Jr.: Brenner tumor of the ovary: a case of unusually large size. Am. J. Obstet. Gynecol., 74:207, 1957.

Balasa, R. W., Adcock, L. L., Prem, K. A., and Dehner, L. P.: The Brenner tumor. Obstet. Gynecol., 50:120, 1977.

Bamforth, J., Dempster, K. R., and Garland, G. W.: Brenner tumors of the ovary. J. Obstet. Gynaecol. Br. Emp., 63:344, 1956.

Bovard, R. E., Schaefer, F. C., and Behringer, F. R.: Malignant Brenner tumor. Am. J. Obstet. Gynecol., 74:977, 1957.

Brenner, F.: Das Oophoroma folliculare. Frankfurt. Z. Path., 1:150, 1907.

Chalvardjian, A., and Scully, R. E.: Sclerosing ovarian stromal tumor. Cancer, 31:664, 1973.

Chang, S. H., Roberts, J. M., and Homesley, H. D.: Proliferating Brenner tumor. Obstet. Gynecol., 49:489, 1977.

Danforth, D. N.: Cytologic relationship of Walthard cell rest to the Brenner tumor of the ovary and to the pseudomucinous cystadenoma. Am. J. Obstet. Gynecol., 43:984, 1942.

Dubrauszky, V.: Ein weiterer Fall aines verkrebsten Brenner-Tumors. Geburtshilfe Frauenheilkd., 9:473, 1949.

Eton, B., and Parker, R. A.: Endometrial abnormalities including carcinoma associated with ovarian Brenner tumors. J. Obstet. Gynaecol. Br. Emp., 65:95, 1958.

Farrar, H. K., Elesh, R., and Libretti, J.: Brenner tumors and estrogen production. Obstet. Gynecol. Surv., 15:1, 1960.

Farrar, H. K., and Greene, R. R.: Bilateral Brenner tumors of the ovary. Am. J. Obstet. Gynecol., 80:1089, 1960.

Fauvet, E.: Zur Klinik und Genese der Brenner-Tumoren. Arch. Gynäk., 159:585, 1935.

Fischel, A.: Uben die Entwicklung der Kelmdrusen des Menschen. Zeitschr. ges. Anat. 92:34, 1930.

Foda, M. S., and Shateek, M. A.: Malignant Brenner tumor. Obstet. Gynecol., 13:226, 1959.

Freda, V., and Montimurro, J. A.: Coexistence of mucinous cystadenoma and Brenner tumors of the ovary. Am. J. Obstet. Gynecol., 77:651, 1959.

Greene, R. R.: The diverse origin of Brenner tumors. Am. J. Obstet. Gynecol., 64:878, 1952.

Hameed, K.: Brenner tumor of ovary with Leydig cell hyperplasia. Cancer, 30:945, 1972.

Idelson, M. G.: Malignancy in Brenner tumors of the ovary, with comments on histogenesis and possible estrogen production. Obstet. Gynecol. Surv., 18:246, 1963.

Jennings, R. C., and Irwin, W. R.: Interstitial cell hyperplasia of ovary with Brenner tumor. J. Obstet. Gynaecol. Br. Emp., 63:914, 1956.

Jonas, E. G.: Functioning Brenner tumor. J. Obstet. Gynaecol. Br. Emp., 66:141, 1959.

Jondahl, W. H., Dockerty, M. B., and Randall, L. M.: Brenner tumors of ovary. Am. J. Obstet. Gynecol., 60:160, 1950.

Kendall, B., and Bowers, P. A.: Bilateral Brenner tumors of the ovary. Am. J. Obstet. Gynecol., 80:439, 1960.

MacKinlay, C. J.: Brenner tumors of the ovary. J. Obstet. Gynaecol. Br. Emp., 63:58, 1956.

Meyer, R.: Der Tumor Ovarii Brenner. Zentralbl. Gynaekol., 56:770, 1932.

Ming, S., and Goldman, H.: Hormonal activity of Brenner tumors in postmenopausal women. Am. J. Obstet. Gynecol., 83:666, 1962.

Morris, J. M., and Scully, R. E.: Endocrine Pathology of the Ovary. St. Louis, C. V. Mosby Company, 1958.

Novak, E., and Jones, H. C.: Brenner tumors of ovary, with report of 14 new cases. Am. J. Obstet. Gynecol., 38:872, 1939.

Postoloff, A. V., and Sotto, L. S.: Secondary changes in Brenner tumor. Obstet. Gynecol., 8:704, 1956.

Pratt-Thomas, P. B., Kreutner, A., Jr., Underwood, P. B., and Dowdeswell, P. H.: Proliferative and malignant Brenner tumors of the ovary. Gynecol. Oncol., 4:176, 1976.

Rawson, A. J., and Helman, M. R.: Malignant Brenner tumors. Am. J. Obstet. Gynecol., 69:429, 1956.

Reagan, J. W.: Ovarian Brenner tumor; its gross and microscopic pathology. Am. J. Obstet. Gynecol., 60:1315, 1950.

Robinson, T. G.: Extra-ovarian Brenner tumor. J. Obstet. Gynaecol. Br. Emp., 57:890, 1950.

Roth, L. M.: The Brenner tumor and the Walthard cell nest. Lab. Invest., 31:15, 1971.

Roth, L. M., and Sternberg, W. H.: Proliferating Brenner tumors. Cancer, 27:687, 1971.

Schifferman, J.: Postklimakterische Blutung und Brennerscher Ovarialtumor. Arch. Gynäk., 150:159, 1932.

Shaabar, A. H., Tabline, F. A., and Youset, A. F.: Functioning Brenner tumor of the ovary, J. Obstet. Gynaecol. Br. Emp., 67:138, 1960.

Shay, M. D., and Janovski, N. A.: Malignant Brenner tumor associated with endometrial adenocarcinoma. Obstet. Gynecol., 22:246, 1963.

Sirsat, M. V.: Malignant Brenner tumor of the ovary. J. Obstet. Gynaecol. India, Vol. 6, June 1956.

Stohr, G.: Relationship of Brenner tumors to the rete ovarii. Am. J. Obstet. Gynecol., 72:389, 1956.

Teoh, T. B.: Histogenesis of Brenner tumors of ovary. J. Pathol. Bacteriol., 66:441, 1953.

Tighe, J. R.: Brenner tumors of the ovary. J. Obstet. Gynaecol. Br. Commonw., 68:292, 1961.

Ullery, J. C., et al.: Testosterone synthesis by a Brenner tumor. Am. J. Obstet. Gynecol., 86:1015, 1963; Part III, 87:463, 1963.

Velasco, A. R., and Munoz, N.: Brenner tumors. Bol. Soc. Chil. Obstet. Gynecol., 21:30, 1956.

Von Szathmary, Z.: Über Brennersche Tumoren in der Wand grosserer Ovarialcystome. Arch. Gynäk., 154:390, 1933.

Woodruff, J. D., and Acosta, A. A.: Variations in the Brenner tumor. Am. J. Obstet. Gynecol., 83:657, 1962.

Woodruff, J. D., Williams, T. J., and Goldberg, B.: Hormone activity of some common ovarian neoplasms. Am. J. Obstet. Gynecol., 87:679, 1963.

Chapter 23

OVARIAN NEOPLASIA: PRIMARILY STROMAL LESIONS (FIBROMA, FIBROTHECOMA INCLUDING THE MIXED MESODERMAL TUMORS)

STROMAL TUMORS

These are far less common than the benign and malignant primarily *epithelial* neoplasms. It has been suggested in fact that if bilateral solid tumors of the ovary are encountered they routinely will be found to represent metastatic disease. Also, it is stated that bilateral solid tumors must be looked on askance, and the patient should be studied carefully to rule out a possible extragenital primary lesion. This statement is patently an exaggeration since fibromas, Brenner tumors, and similar solid lesions may occupy both gonads.

FIBROMA (FIBROTHECOMA)

Clinically, the fibroma—or more accurately, the fibrothecoma—occurs most commonly in the fifth and sixth decades of life, although smaller tumors have been reported in much younger patients (Figs. 23–1 and 23–2). Obviously, unless symptoms occur or the tumors become palpable, they may be present for many years without being recognized. Consequently, most lesions are found on routine examination, although pressure

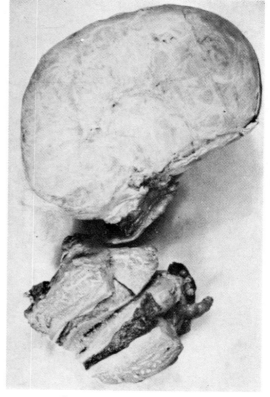

Figure 23–1. Fibroma of ovary.

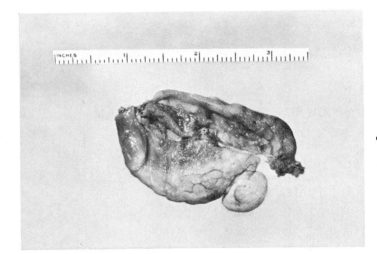

Figure 23–2. Small fibroma on surface of ovary.

Figure 23–3. Fibrothecoma of the ovary. This section is characterized by cells with abundant cytoplasm and dark or light nuclei; thus, there are undoubtedly both connective tissue and ovarian stromal components.

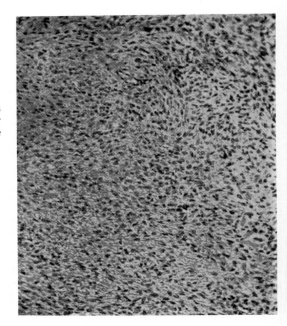

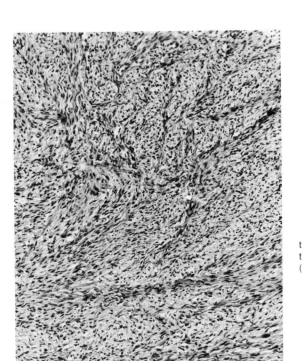

Figure 23–4. Fibrothecoma of the ovary. The majority of the tumor is made up of connective tissue, in contrast to the tumor in Figure 23–3, but interwoven are stromal elements (larger cells).

and discomfort may appear if the tumor becomes large or if torsion occurs. On rare occasions there may be associated evidences of hormone production, with a clinical picture simulating that seen with the Stein-Leventhal syndrome, and masculinization has been described in patients with large and calcified lesions (Figs. 23–3 and 23–4).

PATHOLOGY

Gross Characteristics

The fibroma may reach an enormous size, weighing as much as 22.7 kg (50 lb.). In such lesions, identifiable elements of the original ovary often cannot be recognized. On the other hand, small fibromas are more common, occurring either on the surface of the ovary as polypoid growths or in the ovarian substance as firm, whitish, well-circumscribed nodules of various sizes. Although generally dense and solid, the larger tumors may show areas of degeneration with cystic cavities of considerable size. The cut surface is whitish, at times with a yellowish tinge, and hemorrhagic foci may be recognized. The surface is usually very homogeneous but is more apt to be trabeculated, and thus differing from the whorl-like pattern so characteristic of uterine myoma.

The larger tumors often develop distinct pedicles. Because of the weight and solidity of the tumors, twisting of the pedicle may occur, with resultant infarction. More frequently, the venous return in the pedicle is only partially occluded, owing to partial twisting or the weight of the tumor. This causes increased transudation from the veins, so that ascites is an occasional accompaniment of such tumors.

Meigs' syndrome, initially associated with the ovarian fibroma, is characterized by hydrothorax and ascites. There has been speculation as to the mechanism by which the fluid is produced, especially the hydrothorax. It seems probable that, as Meigs has stated, the fluid finds its way into the thorax by permeation through the diaphragmatic lymphatics; Meigs demonstrated this passageway by intraperitoneal injections of India ink.

Although the syndrome was thought at first to be characteristically associated with fibroma, its occurrence has been noted also in combination with other solid ovarian lesions (Brenner tumor, granulosa cell tumor, thecoma, etc., as well as carcinoma). It is difficult to understand why large subserous myomas do not produce ascites and hydrothorax, but such associations are not recorded.

The transmission of abdominal fluid into the pleural cavity through the diaphragm is probably best demonstrated by those cases in which the right hemidiaphragm is involved with intra-abdominal neoplasia of ovarian origin(?), as commonly noted with the tumor of low malignant potential.

Histopathology

Microscopically, the fibroma or fibrothecoma is composed of both elements that make up the matrix of the ovarian cortical tissues, i.e., the supporting connective tissue and the true gonadal mesenchyme (Fig. 23–3). These elements, whether in the normal ovary or in the tumor, may be difficult to differentiate from one another; however, the functional cell is often more fusiform, with abundant cytoplasm and a pale nucleus, suggesting metabolic activity. In other areas the tissue may be more compact and the cells are spindle-shaped with small, round, dark nuclei resembling fibrocytes. Thus, although undoubtedly pure fibromas do develop from the supporting matrix of the so-called capsule or the perivascular or perineural connective tissues, more frequently there is an admixture of ovarian stroma (the theca-like element) and the fibrous tissue (Figs. 23–3 and 23–4). Stains for lipid may demonstrate the potential hormone production in such lesions. Obviously the opposite of the pure fibroma would be the pure thecoma, a lesion well known for its ability to produce steroids. In rare instances muscle bundles may be demonstrable. Much less common than the fibrothecoma are such mixed connective tissue growths as fibrochondroma, osteoma, and myxoma. As noted in Chapter 22, the Brenner tumor appears grossly as a solid fibromatous lesion, and the epithelial elements may be difficult to identify unless many sections are cut (Fig. 23–5).

Degenerative changes are common, particularly in the larger tumors, and are similar to those described for the leiomyoma of the uterus. Hyalinization is frequent even in the smaller lesions. Calcification and even bone formation occur, particularly in the larger

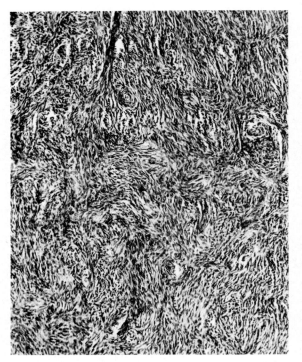

Figure 23–5. Brenner tumor. The arrangement of the stroma in concentric bundles is suggestive but the epithelial component is difficult to identify in this section.

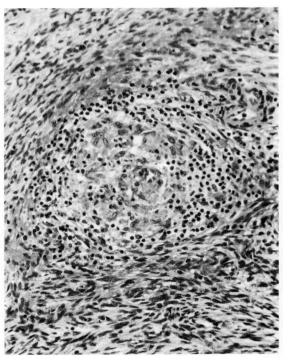

Figure 23–7. Cortical granuloma. The central focus with its lymphocytes is surrounded by a concentric thecal reaction.

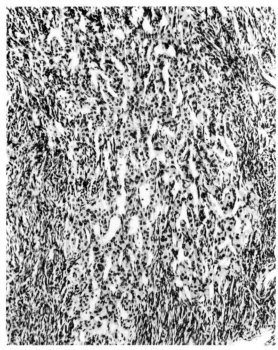

Figure 23–6. Diffuse but organized thecosis in a normal postmenopausal ovary. Note the lymphatic distention of the vessels adjacent to the luteinized cells.

neoplasm, and small areas of cystic change develop when liquefaction takes place in foci of degeneration.

Careful inspection of the noninvolved portion of the gonad may reveal evidence of focal thecosis. Furthermore, study of the opposite, often normal appearing, ovary will be rewarded by the finding of cords or strands of luteinized stromal cells (Fig. 23–6) or cortical granulomas (Fig. 23–7). The presence of such stromal alterations is probably more related to hormonal aberrations than is the presence of the tumor itself.

The cause of such stromal reactions is difficult to identify; however, in the postmenopausal patient, the elevated pituitary gonadotropins could play the stimulating role (Fig. 23–6) as they do for the hilar cell. The most dramatic response of the gonadal stroma to hormonal stimuli is demonstrated in the luteoma of pregnancy (Fig. 23–8). Although Greene felt that these lesions were examples of luteinization in a preexisting fibrothecoma, and such a tumor undoubtedly is possible (Fig. 23–9), nevertheless, a majority of observers feel that such tumors rep-

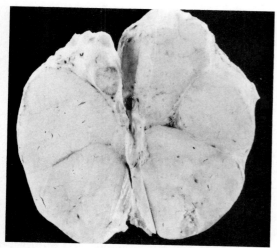

Figure 23–8. Luteoma of pregnancy. Note the apparent focal tumor isolated from the cortex.

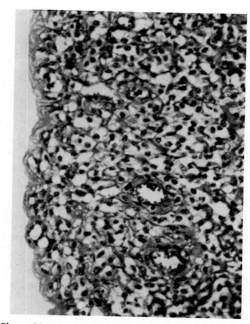

Figure 23–10. Wall of cystic lymphangioma of ovary.

resent abnormal responses of gonadal stroma to chorionic gonadotropin (see Chapter 25).

OTHER SOLID TUMORS

Other benign solid tumors, such as angioma, lymphangioma, and neuroma, may

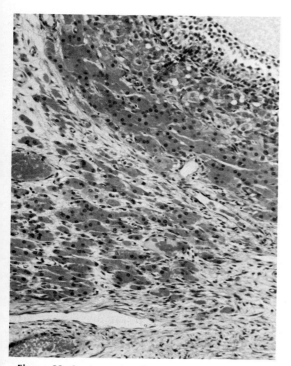

Figure 23–9. Luteoma of pregnancy showing diffuse stromal luteinization as well as the characteristic perifollicular alterations.

occur in the ovary, but they are exceedingly rare (Fig. 23–10). As for lymphangioma, although it is probable that it may occasionally occur, some believe that most of the tumors so designated are really adenomatoid tumors. These have been discussed more fully in the chapter dealing with tubal neoplasms (Chapter 16).

OVARIAN SARCOMAS

Sarcoma of the ovary is rare; its incidence compared to carcinoma is generally reported as 1 to 40. It may occur at any age; however, many of the cases reported in past years as ovarian sarcoma in children were really instances of teratoma, granulosa cell tumor, or dysgerminoma. Sarcoma is more common in the adult than in the young child. It is usually primary, but may be the result of secondary malignant change in a fibroma or teratoma. In a study of 47 such lesions from the Ovarian Tumor Registry, Azoury and Woodruff divided ovarian sarcomas into three groups: teratoid, mesenchymal, and mixed tumors.

Teratoid Sarcomas

Generally, these lesions are found in patients under the age of 25 years. Definable teratoid elements may be recognized in a

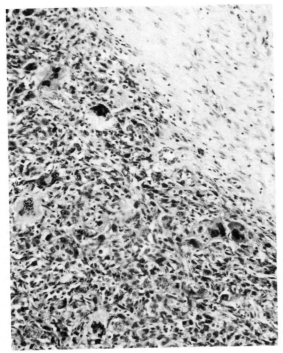

Figure 23–11. The bizarre nuclei of a stromal sarcoma are quite apparent. Such aberrations may be noted in the unusual teratoid lesions or in the myosarcoma.

majority of the cases, but in many instances the lesions are so undifferentiated that it is difficult to identify specific elements (Fig. 23–11). The youth of the patient strengthens the diagnosis of teratoma, since it is uncommon to find an admixture of such bizarre tissues representing histologic variations from all germ layers in the older patient. Myxomatous elements, rhabdomyoblasts, and teratoid bodies assist in establishing the genesis of these lesions. The teratoid bodies are identified as large cells with an eosinophilic homogeneous cytoplasmic mass displacing the nucleus to the periphery of the cell. In some instances the nucleus may be eliminated completely. These eosinophilic bodies may contain enzymes that are found in more specific varieties of teratoma, such as the endodermal sinus tumor and the choriocarcinoma (see Chapter 25).

On rare occasions sarcoma develops in a preexisting benign adult or mature teratoma. Generally, these are leiomyo- or fibrosarcomas. The teratoid origin may be established in some instances by the identification of mature elements, such as mucus-secreting epithelium in the adjacent area. In such lesions the malignancy probably arose in the smooth muscle of the gut (Fig. 23–12). The prognosis in these lesions is extremely poor, and in the cases reviewed from the Ovarian Tumor Registry there were no survivors.

Stromal Cell Sarcoma or Fibroleiomyosarcoma

Malignancies arising in these fibromas, fibrothecomas or thecomas have been classified as (1) stromal cell sarcoma and (2) fibroleiomyosarcoma. The stromal cell variety is generally found in the younger patient. Five of the seven cases in this category occurred in patients 20 years of age or younger. Histology suggested that these arose from the ovarian mesenchyme or the supporting connective tissue. Five of the seven tumors were of the low grade variety and mitoses were sparse (Fig. 23–13). Four of the five patients were living and well, and one could not be traced. Conversely, the two cases in which there was increased pleomorphism succumbed rapidly to the malignancy.

In the second group of fibroleiomyosarcomas, the tumors were found in the older patient, only one being under the age of 40 years. In all of these cases the cellular evi-

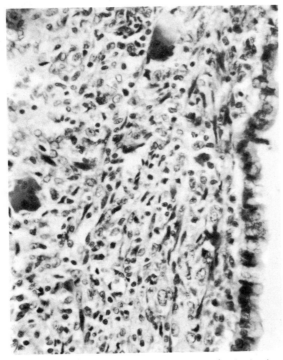

Figure 23–12. Probable leiomyosarcoma beginning in a previously benign teratoma. Patient was 56 years of age.

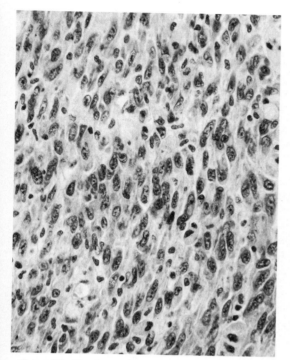

Figure 23–13. Stromal sarcoma. An unusual neoplastic proliferation of the gonadal stroma. The nuclei are larger and more irregular; nevertheless, individual cell atypism is rare.

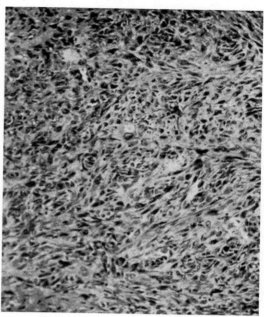

Figure 23–14. Spindle cell sarcoma of ovary—probably fibroleiomyosarcoma.

dence of malignancy was striking, and the outcome was fatal in all, although one patient survived 8 years (Fig. 23–14). The tendency for local recurrence rather than widespread extra-abdominal metastases makes repeat surgical excision the secondary treatment of choice. Adjunctive chemotherapy may be used for widespread disease, local or elsewhere.

Müllerian or Paramesonephric Sarcomas

There were 23 cases in this group and, as with similar lesions in the endometrium, an attempt was made to divide them into carcinosarcomas or mixed mesodermal tumors. As has been our experience in studies of the intrauterine lesion, no difference was found in the clinical features, and the outcome was fatal in all but a single case. Final diagnosis in the latter instance was stromatosis and the clinical course was similar to that described for uterine stromatosis, with long-term survival but also a tendency for local recurrence (Fig. 23–15). Treatment for such lesions should be progestational agents.

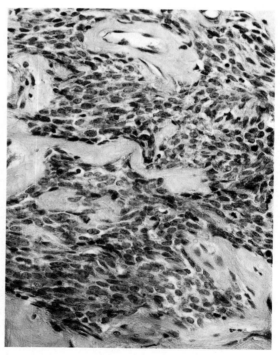

Figure 23–15. Stromatosis of ovary recurrent in pelvis 8 years after initial surgery. Stromatosis was not found in any other structure at original investigation.

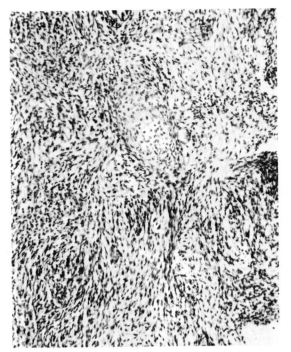

Figure 23–16. Stromal neoplasia primary in the ovary. Attempt at cartilage formation can be seen in the center.

23–16 and 23–17). Rare cases of abnormally proliferating stroma with benign glands (adenosarcoma) have been reported. In our experience these lesions tend to follow the clinical course of stromatosis and thus the initial postoperative therapy should be progestational agents.

In five instances a direct origin from well-defined endometrial tissue could be appreciated. In four of the five, there was the association of the ovarian neoplasm with other malignancies of the upper genital canal. In two cases the endometrium contained a lesion similar to that found in the ovary, and thus the ovarian tumor may possibly have represented a metastasis. In the three additional cases there was associated adenocarcinoma in the uterus, tube, or endocervix. In these cases, multicentric foci of origin must be considered as a theory for the genesis of the alternate lesion.

LYMPHOMA

With a few rare exceptions, the lymphoma of the ovary is secondary, usually to a primary lesion in the gastrointestinal area. Occasionally, as noted by Johnson and Soule, it is a gynecologic complaint that first sends the patient for medical advice.

In a study of 35 cases of lymphoma from the files of the Ovarian Tumor Registry, there was only one patient found who lived

The histologic findings in the mixed tumor were essentially those characteristic of the intrauterine lesions, i.e., there was a stromal and epithelial component or there were mixed mesodermal elements, including cartilage, bone, and striated muscle (Figs.

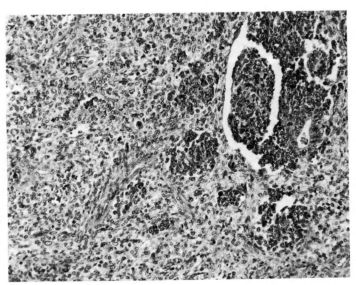

Figure 23–17. Bizarre epithelial neoplasia on the right is associated with the undifferentiated stromal reaction on the left. This combination in the endometrium justifies the terminology of mixed mesodermal tumor.

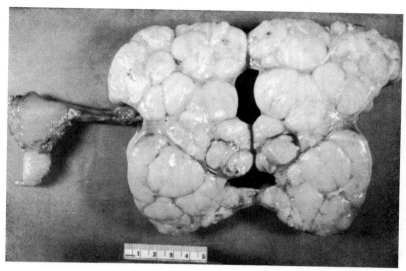

Figure 23–18. Lymphoma of ovary, secondary to primary disease in cecum in girl of 16 years. (Case of Dr. D. M. Grayzel.)

more than 5 years. Furthermore, in all instances save that of the sole survivor, there was evidence of systemic disease. All varieties of lymphoma in the ovary, including Hodgkin's disease and Burkitt's tumor, have been described (Figs. 23–18 and 23–19). All may represent a real diagnostic problem, especially if systemic disease is not recognized (Fig. 23–20). In a review of the unclassified tumors of the Ovarian Tumor Registry, the lymphomas represented a major proportion of lesions that could not be categorized because of inherent morphologic difficulties.

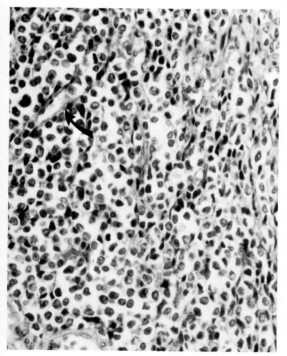

Figure 23–19. Histiocytic lymphoma of the ovary in 34 year old patient. Note the clinging of the cells to the stromal elements (arrow).

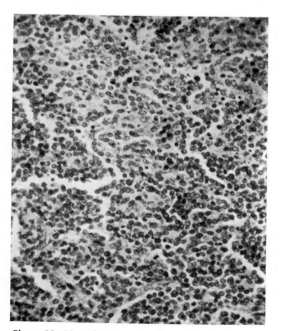

Figure 23–20. This type of lesion, previously designated as a round cell sarcoma, may represent a stromal sarcoma. Actually it is difficult to be sure the proliferating cells are not epithelial, thus producing an undifferentiated carcinoma.

REFERENCES

Aiman, J., Edman, C. D., Worley, R. J., Vellios, F., and MacDonald, P. C.: Androgen and estrogen formation in women with ovarian hyperthecosis. Obstet. Gynecol., 51:1, 1978.

Azoury, R. S., and Woodruff, J. D.: Primary ovarian sarcomas. Obstet. Gynecol., 37:920, 1971.

Burket, R. L., and Rauh, J. L.: Gorlin's syndrome: ovarian fibromas at adolescence. Obstet. Gynecol., 47:435, 1976.

Czernobilsky, B., et al.: Cystadenofibroma of the ovary. Cancer, 34:1971, 1974.

Dehner, L. P., Norris, H. J., and Taylor, H. B.: Carcinosarcomas and mixed mesodermal tumors of the ovary. Cancer, 27:207, 1971.

Dockerty, M. B., and Masson, J. C.: Ovarian fibroma: a clinical and pathological study of 283 cases. Am. J. Obstet. Gynecol., 47:741, 1944.

Giere, J. W., and Binder, R. H.: Burkitt's lymphoma involving the ovary and jaw. Obstet. Gynecol., 48:635, 1976.

Hernandez, W., DiSaia, P. J., Morrow, C. P., and Townsend, D. E.: Mixed mesodermal sarcoma of the ovary. Obstet. Gynecol., 49:595, 1971.

Hughesdon, P. E.: The endometrial identity of benign stromatosis of the ovary and its relation to other forms of endometriosis. J. Pathol., 119:201, 1976.

Johnson, C. E., and Soule, E. H.: Malignant lymphoma as a gynecological problem. Obstet. Gynecol., 9:149, 1957.

Meigs, J. V.: Fibroma of ovary with ascites and hydrothorax. Am. J. Obstet. Gynecol., 67:962, 1954.

Meigs, J. V., Armstrong, S. H., and Hamilton, H. H.: Further contributions to the syndrome of fibroma of the ovary with fluid in abdomen and chest. Meigs' syndrome. Am. J. Obstet. Gynecol., 46:19, 1943.

Morrison, C. S., and Woodruff, J. D.: Fibrothecoma and associated ovarian stromal neoplasia. Obstet. Gynecol., 23:344, 1964.

Nelson, G. A., Dockerty, M. B., Pratt, J. H., and Remine, W. H.: Malignant lymphoma involving the ovaries. Am. J. Obstet. Gynecol., 76:861, 1958.

Neubecker, R. D., and Breen, J. L.: Embryonal carcinoma of the ovary. Cancer, 15:546, 1962.

Nissen, E. D.: Consideration of the malignant carcinoid syndrome. Obstet. Gynecol. Surv., 14:459, 1959.

Noguchi, T. T., and Lonser, E. R.: Unusual teratoma of the ovary with implantation in the abdominal cavity. Am. J. Obstet. Gynecol., 82:381, 1961.

Novak, E. R.: Solid teratoma of the ovary, with report of 5 cases. Am. J. Obstet. Gynecol., 56:300, 1948.

Novak, E. R., Woodruff, J. D., and Linthicum, J. M.: Evaluation of the unclassified tumors of the Ovarian Tumor Registry. Am. J. Obstet. Gynecol., 87:999, 1963.

Richardson, G. S., and Ulfelder, H.: Problems presented by benign solid ovarian tumors. Clin. Obstet. Gynecol., 4:834, 1961.

Roth, L. M.: Massive ovarian edema with stromal luteinization. Am. J. Clin. Pathol., 55:757, 1971.

Williamson, H. O., and Moore, M. P.: Ovarian and paraovarian adenomatoid tumors. Am. J. Obstet. Gynecol., 90:388, 1964.

Woodruff, J. D., Noli Castillo, R. D., and Novak, E. R.: Lymphoma of the ovary. Am. J. Obstet. Gynecol., 85:912, 1963.

Zeigerman, J. H., Imbriglia, J., Makler, P., and Smith, J. J.: Ovarian lymphosarcoma. Am. J. Obstet. Gynecol., 72:1351, 1956.

Chapter 24

OVARIAN NEOPLASIA: METASTATIC LESIONS

Metastatic ovarian cancer is not uncommon, and presents some of the most challenging and controversial clinical and pathologic pictures. Basically, the problems consist of (1) differentiating the primary from the metastatic lesion, and (2) interpreting the sometimes bizarre (though sometimes absent) symptoms.

Of the two chief varieties of carcinoma that have a tendency to metastasize to the ovary, there are (a) those arising primarily in the genital canal, and (b) those arising at an extragenital site.

TUMORS ARISING IN THE GENITAL CANAL

Adenocarcinoma of the endometrium is the most common form of pelvic neoplasia to be associated with an ovarian malignancy. Of 147 cases from the Gynecologic Pathology Laboratory at the Johns Hopkins Hospital, seven (4.8 per cent) demonstrated ovarian disease. In a larger group of 518 cases, Gusberg and Yannopoulos found ovarian involvement in 60 (nearly 12 per cent).

Of interest is the occurrence of ovarian and uterine carcinomas as a demonstration of multicentric foci of origin in the upper genital canal. In a series of 120 secondary ovarian malignancies from the Emil Novak Ovarian Tumor Registry, there were 38 in which associated neoplasia was present in the fundus. The 5 year survival in this group was an amazing 50 per cent, certainly not the clinical course for most metastatic lesions. Furthermore, there was frequently a difference of opinion among observers as to which lesion was the primary. In view of these features, it seemed quite conceivable that the two lesions had arisen in separate foci and did not represent metastatic disease but, in truth, were two separate tumors. Often these multiple primary tumors revealed similar histopathologic patterns (Fig. 24–1 A,B).

In spite of this interesting facet of tumors arising at separate foci from tissues of the same embryologic origin (i.e., the upper genital canal) there are unquestioned instances of vascular spread of the malignancy from a primary to a secondary site (Fig. 24–2). In a majority of such cases in which the endometrium harbors the initial lesion, there is evidence of extensive myometrial invasion. Furthermore, the ovarian metastases are commonly noted in the vascular channels of the gonad rather than apparently representing a more characteristic primary lesion (Fig. 24–2).

Carcinoma of the lower genital canal rarely metastasizes to the ovary. As noted in Table 24–1, only 4 of the 120 secondary ovarian malignancies were associated with a cervical primary (Fig. 24–3) and there was no example of a vulvovaginal malignancy with ovarian involvement. If such relationships develop, the mode of spread is generally by direct extension. Other tumors arising in the adjacent pelvic structures (e.g., retroperitoneal sarcoma and teratoma) may invade the ovary by continuity. Carcinoma of the tube may involve the ovary. It should be appreciated that similarly to the endometrial and ovarian associations, when the tube and ovary are involved in a neoplastic process it

461

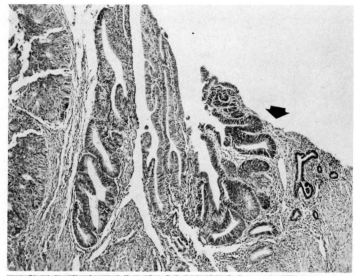

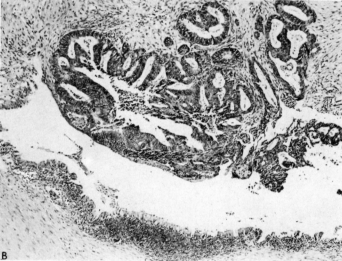

Figure 24–1. *A,* Adenocarcinoma of the endometrium associated with endometrioid carcinoma of the ovary. *B,* Carcinoma of the ovary beginning in endometriosis(?). (From J. D. Woodruff et al.: Metastatic ovarian tumors. Am. J. Obstet. Gynecol., *107*:202, 1970. Courtesy of C. V. Mosby Co.)

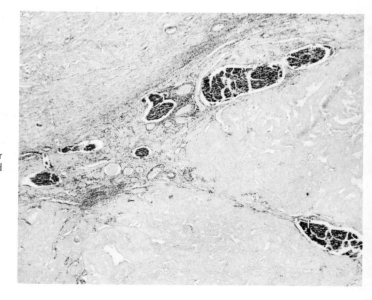

Figure 24–2. Classic metastatic cancer showing vascular channels in the ovary filled with tumor.

Table 24–1 SECONDARY OVARIAN MALIGNANCY

Primary Site	Total Cases		Dead	Present Status			
	No.	Per Cent		Living 5 yr. with Recurrence	Living < 5 yr., No Recurrence	Living > 5 yr., No Recurrence	No Follow-up
Adenocarcinoma of endometrium	32	27	5	2	3	15	7
Sarcoma of endometrium Stromatosis	6	5	3			2	1
Cancer of breast	16	14	10	1	1		4
Gastrointestinal tract (including 2 carcinoid)	24	20	18			2	4
Others	23	19	20				3
? Site	19	16	18			1	
Total	120	100	74	3	4	20	19

is frequently difficult to identify the specific organ of origin. Among 18 primary tubal cancers, the ovary was involved in 50 per cent and there was disagreement in 4 of the 9 cases as to the site of the initial malignancy (see Chapter 16).

Gross and Microscopic Characteristics

The metastatic ovarian lesion is often small, and may be found only on microscopic examination. Conversely, the ovarian tumor may be dominant, so that it overshadows the primary lesion, and there may be difficulty in determining the original site of the malignancy. The microscopic characteristics of the ovarian metastasis may resemble those of the original carcinoma; however, primary tumors in the breast and gastrointestinal tract—e.g., the Krukenberg tumor—produce strikingly atypical patterns in the ovary.

In contrast to the true metastatic lesion, the tumors representing multicentric foci of origin are generally of the same histologic type, with minor variations, such as adenocarcinoma versus adenoacanthoma (Fig. 24–4A,B).

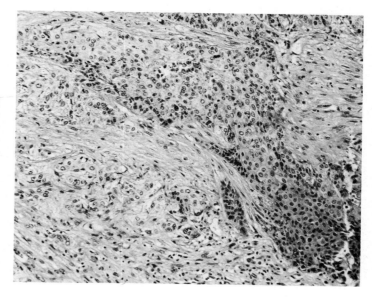

Figure 24–3. Epidermoid carcinoma of the cervix metastatic to the ovary, an uncommon site. (From J. D. Woodruff et al.: Metastatic ovarian tumors. Am. J. Obstet. Gynecol., *107*:202, 1970. Courtesy of C. V. Mosby Co.)

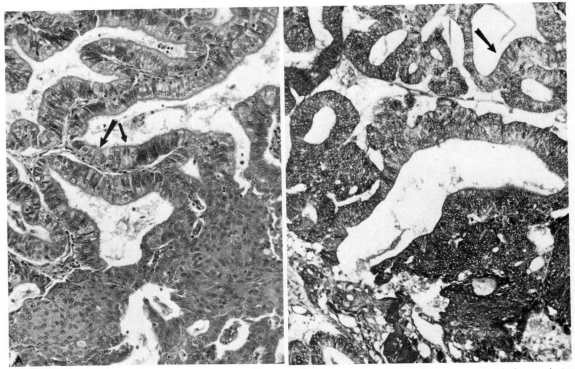

Figure 24–4. *A,* Adenoacanthoma in endometrium. Note tubal metaplasia at arrows (squamous and tubal metaplasias related to estrogen stimulation?). *B,* Adenocarcinoma of ovary with pattern similar to that in *A.* There is tubal metaplasia at arrow.

METASTATIC LESIONS WITH AN EXTRAGENITAL PRIMARY TUMOR

As noted in Table 24–1, a variety of extragenital malignancies may metastasize to the ovary. Of major interest are the breast and gastrointestinal tumors.

Breast Primary Tumor

Kasilag and Rutledge and others have noted that in women with *recurrent* breast tumor, therapeutic castration has revealed ovarian metastasis in 25 per cent of cases in which ovariectomy was performed. As with most metastatic lesions, both ovaries are invaded in 70 to 80 per cent of the cases. Classically, the tumors are solid, freely mobile, and bosselated. Cystic areas are degenerative.

Microscopically, a variety of patterns can be expected. The appearance may suggest the primary breast lesion to the extent that, without prior knowledge of the tissue source, the ovary would not be suspected (Fig. 24–5). Conversely, the more common cellular arrangement is that characterized by small columns of the metastatic cancer filtering into the ovarian stroma, "Indian file" (Fig. 24–6). Since in 25 to 30 per cent of the cases there is no gross enlargement of the gonad, the malignant elements may be missed, particularly if they are encased in the dense ovarian stroma. Furthermore, the cortical portion is most frequently involved and the neoplastic cells appear to melt into the mesenchyme (Fig. 24–7). In rare instances, the arrangement may suggest that seen in the Krukenberg tumor, with the classic signet cell occupying the myxomatous stroma, as will be discussed later. Finally, a pattern suggestive of lymphoma may develop, and the epithelial elements are difficult to identify (Fig. 24–8).

It is of interest to note the differences in the potential hormone production of the various metastatic ovarian tumors. Whereas there are frequent reports of such reactions in the patient with the so-called Krukenberg tumor, this has not been the case when the primary lesion was in the breast. The explanation for this discrepancy is not clear; however, it seems possible that the difference

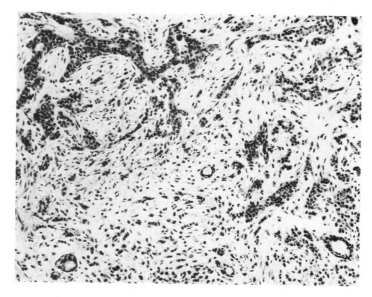

Figure 24–5. Carcinoma of the breast metastatic to ovary; pattern very suggestive of lobular cancer with diffuse stromal infiltration. (From J. D. Woodruff et al.: Metastatic ovarian tumors. Am. J. Obstet. Gynecol., *107*:202, 1970. Courtesy of C. V. Mosby Co.)

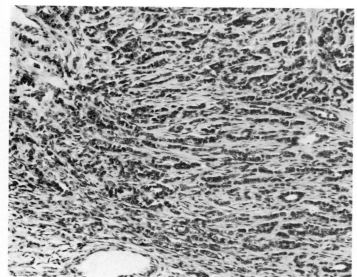

Figure 24–6. "Indian file" pattern characteristic of metastatic ovarian cancer, usually primary in the breast. Occasionally mistaken for tubular variety of arrhenoblastoma. (From J. D. Woodruff et al.: Metastatic ovarian tumors. Am. J. Obstet. Gynecol., *107*:202, 1970. Courtesy of C. V. Mosby Co.)

Figure 24–7. Diffuse infiltration into dense stroma of the cortex by metastatic breast tumor. Difficulty may be encountered in defining the tumor cells from the proliferating mesenchyme. (From J. D. Woodruff et al.: Metastatic ovarian tumors. Am. J. Obstet. Gynecol., *107*:202, 1970. Courtesy of C. V. Mosby Co.)

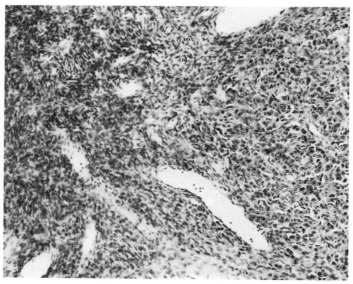

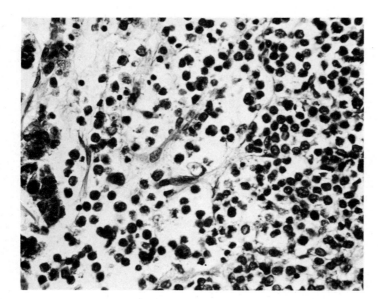

Figure 24–8. Lymphoma-like pattern in metastatic breast cancer. Few epithelial cells can be seen on the left.

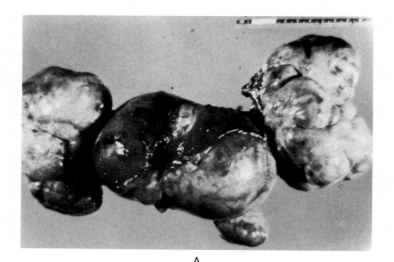

A

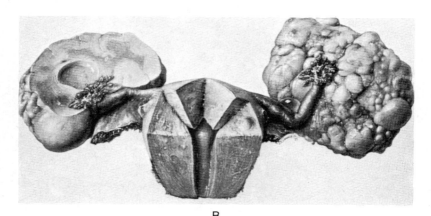

B

Figure 24–9. *A*, Bilateral ovarian tumors secondary to gastrointestinal malignancy. Myomatous uterus present in the center. *B*, Bilateral Krukenberg tumors secondary to gastric cancer.

lies in the secretory activity of the invading elements.

Gastrointestinal Primary Tumor

These metastatic tumors, like those primary in the breast, are largely solid, bilateral, lobulated, and free. They may attain tremendous size, weighing 2000 grams or more, and completely overshadowing the primary gastrointestinal tumor (Fig. 24–9 A,B). The practical lesson from the surgeon's standpoint, therefore, is never to overlook careful examination of the abdominal organs—especially the pylorus—in every case of ovarian cancer, particularly when the latter is bilateral.

In contrast to the metastatic breast lesion, the secondary disease from a gastrointestinal primary tumor may be cystic, particularly if the original tumor arose from the large bowel. The cystic component is generally related to the secretory nature of the invading epithelium. The unique Krukenberg tumor will be described in detail later in this chapter.

As with the lesions arising primarily in the breast, there is a wide variety of microscopic patterns. Of major difficulty is the lesion that replicates accurately an ovarian primary tumor (Fig. 24–10). Whereas there is little difficulty in suggesting that the ovarian tumor is secondary when associated with a breast malignancy, the same does not hold true for the primary intestinal tumor. Since

ovarian carcinoma may be mucinous, the pattern can be quite similar to that of the intestinal neoplasm (Fig. 24–11 A,B), and, as with uterine and ovarian lesions, the original site of origin may be ambiguous (Fig. 24–12 A,B). Furthermore, even the primary ovarian malignancy may produce an infiltration suggestive of that seen in the Krukenberg tumor. Finally, both primary and secondary mucinous lesions may produce a stromal reaction with subsequent hormone production (Fig. 24–13 A,B).

On rare occasions, the intestinal carcinoid may metastasize to the gonad. Conversely, such lesions may be primary in the ovary, as will be noted in the chapter on teratomas (Chapter 25). Whereas the latter is usually unilateral, the metastatic lesions are bilateral in the great majority of cases. The microscopic picture of such lesions may be confused at first glance with that seen in the granulosa cell tumor and the arrhenoblastoma. Closer inspection usually reveals areas in which true acini are formed. Silver stains, if positive, assist in differential diagnosis; however, the absence of argentophilic cells does not rule out carcinoid (Fig. 24–14).

Lymphoma in the ovary is most commonly metastatic. As with other such lesions, both ovaries are involved. A variety of histologic types of lymphoma have been described, including the so-called Burkitt's tumor. Frequently the latter as well as other types are found in patients during the early decades of life. The lymphomas have been classically

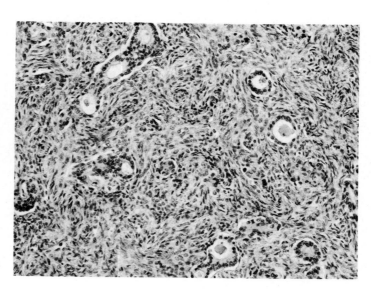

Figure 24–10. Metastatic carcinoma from the intestinal tract. The pattern is quite similar to a fibroadenoma of the ovary with a mucus-secreting component. (From J. D. Woodruff et al.: Metastatic ovarian tumors. Am. J. Obstet. Gynecol., 107:202, 1970. Courtesy of C. V. Mosby Co.)

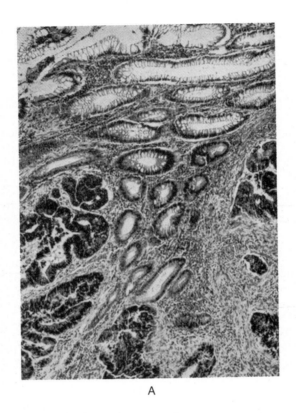

A

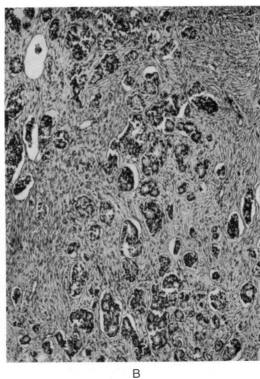

B

Figure 24–11. *A*, Carcinoma of sigmoid associated with Krukenberg tumor shown in *B*. *B*, Section of Krukenberg tumor. Primary lesion was in sigmoid colon.

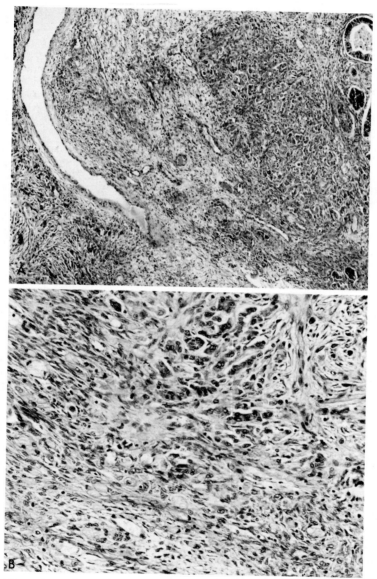

Figure 24–12. *A*, Metastatic carcinoma from stomach—multiple patterns with adenomatous foci on right and infiltrative foci in center and left. *B*, Higher power of metastatic carcinoma from stomach.

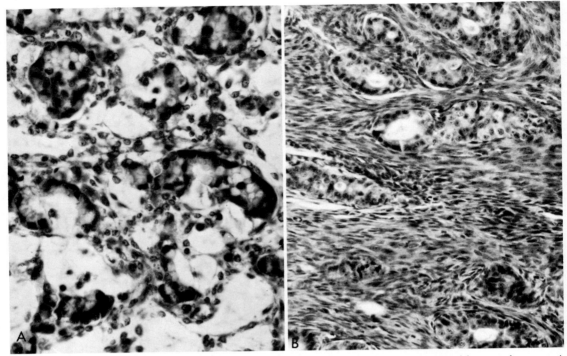

Figure 24–13. *A*, Metastatic mucin-producing tumor with virilization. *B*, Metastatic carcinoma of the ovary from gastrointestinal tract (marked stromal reaction). Diagnosed as arrhenoblastoma because of virilization of host.

confused with dysgerminomas and arrhenoblastomas.

Other Extragenital Sites

Metastatic disease from a variety of primary sites has been reported in the ovary. The primary kidney tumor often presents a difficult diagnostic problem, since the pattern often simulates the clear cell, or mesonephroid, tumor of the gonad (Fig. 24–15). On rare occasions, pulmonary, thyroid and bone tumors have been associated with metastatic ovarian disease.

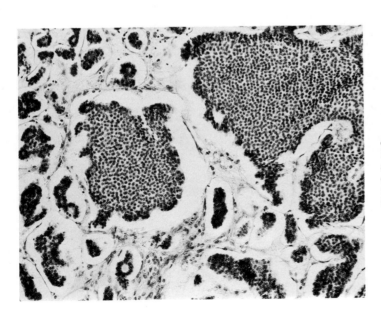

Figure 24–14. Carcinoid metastatic to ovary. Some areas simulate granulosa cell lesion but adenoid pattern is also apparent in areas. (From J. D. Woodruff et al.: Metastatic ovarian tumors. Am. J. Obstet. Gynecol., *107*:202, 1970. Courtesy of C. V. Mosby Co.)

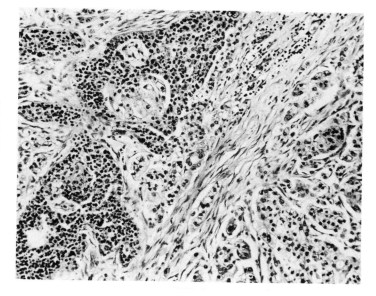

Figure 24–15. Metastatic tumor from the kidney. Clear cell area may be seen in lower right. (From J. D. Woodruff et al.: Metastatic ovarian tumors. Am. J. Obstet. Gynecol., *107*:202, 1970. Courtesy of C. V. Mosby Co.)

THE KRUKENBERG TUMOR OF THE OVARY

Definition

A most interesting secondary ovarian malignancy, particularly from the microscopic and clinical points of view, is the Krukenberg tumor. The definition of this neoplasm may seem vague; however, the term should be limited to the pathologic entity described by Krukenberg in 1896, making allowance only for his misinterpretation of its real nature. The tumor was originally described as a *sarcoma ovarii mucocellulare carcinoma-todes,* but Krukenberg's description of its gross and microscopic pathologic characteristics was quite accurate. The marked stromal reaction, together with the sparseness of the epithelial elements in many cases, led Krukenberg into the error of designating these tumors as sarcomas (Fig. 24–16).

This mistake was corrected by Schlagenhaufer, who deserves the credit for establishing the epithelial nature of the tumor, and for demonstrating that in most instances it is secondary to carcinoma elsewhere, most often in the gastrointestinal tract. This latter statement is responsible for the loose con-

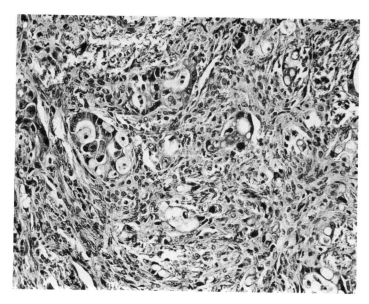

Figure 24–16. Beginning Krukenberg pattern showing some intact glandular acini with beginning breakdown into end picture (Figure 24–17). Note sarcomatoid pattern of adjacent stroma.

cept that all ovarian cancers secondary to gastrointestinal cancer are Krukenberg tumors, a concept which becomes apparent if one analyzes the cases in the literature; however, other primary sites, such as the breast, have been associated with the classic Krukenberg pattern. The definition must be much more circumscribed than this, and, if we are to continue this eponymic designation, it should be limited only to those tumors, whether secondary or primary, which assume the histologic characteristics first described by Krukenberg.

Gross Characteristics

Grossly, as is true for most metastatic lesions, the tumors are solid, usually of moderate size, almost always bilateral (approximately 80 per cent in our own series), and retain the general shape of the ovary (Fig. 24–9 A,B). The external surface is smooth, with a well-developed capsule, similar to most metastatic ovarian malignancies. On section, the cut surface is commonly of rather variegated appearance, some parts being quite firm, others finely spongy, still others degenerated, hemorrhagic, or cystic, although areas of gelatinous appearance are also common.

Microscopic Characteristics

These variations in the gross appearance of the cut surface parallel and are due to corresponding differences in the miscroscopic structure of the tumor. The *stroma* in some areas is firm and richly cellular, whereas in other areas it is edematous or genuinely myxomatous.

The *epithelial elements* may occur as clusters of well-marked acini, though always, in the true Krukenberg tumor, show various degrees of mucoid change. Often this is so extreme that the epithelial cells are completely liquefied, leaving only the shadows of the original gland framework (Fig. 24–17 A). The mucoid material may break through the gland wall and permeate the surrounding stroma, so that differential staining reveals mucin not only in the glands but also in the stroma.

The mucoid changes explain the occurrence of usually large numbers of *signet cells*, in which the nucleus is flattened out against the cell wall by the accumulated secretion within the cell (Fig. 24–17 B). These

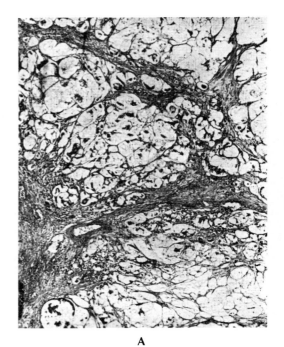

A

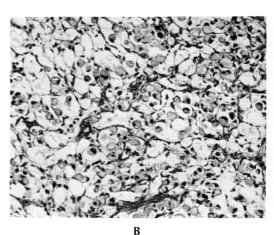

B

Figure 24–17. *A*, Mucoid liquefaction of epithelium in a Krukenberg tumor (carcinoma mucocellulare). *B*, Mucoid liquefaction with many typical signet ring cells. (Higher magnification.)

cells have suggested the very apt designation of *carcinoma mucocellulare* (Fig. 24–18). They are not specific and may be found in any mucus-secreting tumor.

Transition Forms

All gradations may be seen between a pure adenocarcinoma and the tumor in which all traces of an acinous structure are lost. In

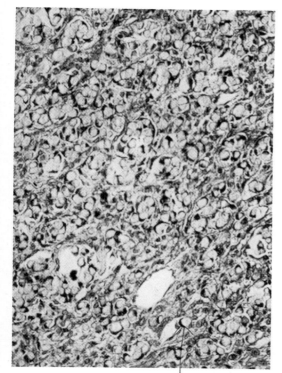

Figure 24–18. Characteristic signet cells in a Krukenberg tumor.

Lymphatic extension has been the most widely accepted theory of cancer dissemination, but there has been no convincing demonstration of the transportation of cancer cells from the stomach via the retroperitoneal glands to the ovarian lymphatics.

The transportation of tumor via vascular channels has not been emphasized sufficiently in previous discussions of the Krukenberg tumor or any other epithelial neoplasm. Nevertheless, there are those who believe that bloodstream transportation more often explains Krukenberg tumors than does lymphatic dissemination. Certainly this concept deserves more serious consideration, particularly in light of the frequency of breast tumor metastases to the gonad and the initial finding of tumor cells in the cortex where circulating cells could be filtered out and lodged in the fine transitional vessels.

Direct Extension. Little need be said about the few cases in which the ovarian involvement has been explainable by direct extension from a gastrointestinal carcinoma, usually in the rectum or sigmoid, which has become adherent to the pelvic organs.

other words, one finds transitional pictures, which suggest that the Krukenberg tumor may be only the end product of a mucoid adenocarcinoma which, in the environment of the ovary, assumes the features that we look upon as characteristic of the Krukenberg tumor.

Dissemination to Ovary

Four possible routes of dissemination to the ovary have been considered: (1) direct implantation of cancer cells on the ovarian surface, transported by the peritoneal fluid from the primary lesion into the pelvis; (2) lymphatic metastasis; (3) transportation of cancer cells by the vascular channels; and (4) extension by direct continuity from an adherent intestinal cancer. To accept the theory of direct implantation, we would have to conceive of the penetration of the intestinal wall by the invading neoplasm and the ability of the cells to implant on the ovary alone, since the adjacent peritoneum is rarely involved. This unique, historic theory is not valid in reality, since an intact ovarian capsule does not support surface implantation.

PRIMARY KRUKENBERG TUMORS

In 1960 Woodruff and Novak reported a study of 48 cases of Krukenberg tumors from the files of the Emil Novak Ovarian Tumor Registry, of which 10 appeared to be primary lesions. Of these 10 patients, four were alive and well 5 years and one was alive 2 years postoperatively. Of the additional five patients, there was no evidence of a primary lesion at the time of death; however, the postmortem examinations are not documented in four of these five cases. In spite of this experience, it must be assumed that most Krukenberg tumors are secondary to bowel lesions.

As with most true metastatic diseases, the prognosis is poor, only one patient surviving over 5 years with both a gastric and ovarian malignancy. In the series mentioned above, death usually occurred less than 2 years postoperatively. Conversely, with the primary tumor, a better prognosis is anticipated. Primary development of a Krukenberg tumor in the ovary should occasion no surprise; indeed, we have seen a number of mucinous tumors which exhibited a Krukenberg tendency in certain restricted areas (Fig. 24–19).

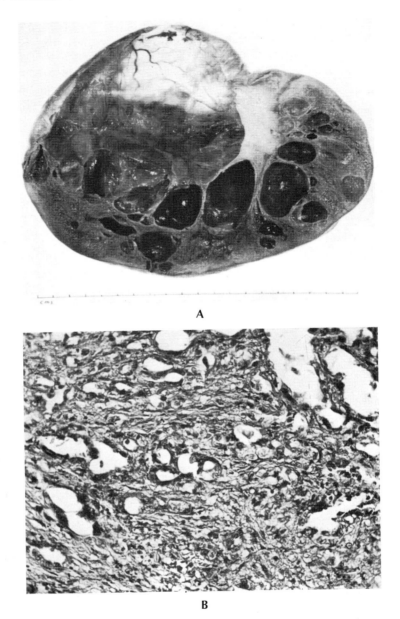

Figure 24–19. *A*, Gross appearance of primary unilateral Krukenberg tumor. (Courtesy of Dr. Agnes Scott, Dumfries, Scotland.) *B*, Microscopic appearance of primary Krukenberg tumor.

Endocrine Activity

In the study referred to above, there were no cases evidencing endocrine activity; however, it has been adequately documented elsewhere that the Krukenberg tumor may be associated with hormone function.

Turenen discussed the feminizing capa-

bilities of Krukenberg tumors in a study of postmenopausal patients harboring such lesions. Pre- and postoperative estrogen excretion, the vaginal Maturation Index, and associated endometrial hyperplasia attested to the validity of the thesis. Incubation and enzyme histochemical studies suggest that the hormone-producing cell is of ovarian mesenchymal and not neoplastic origin (Fig.

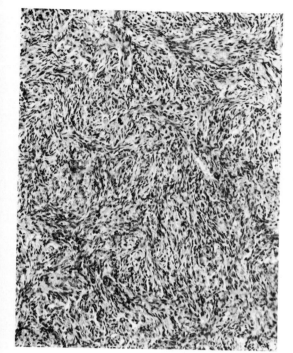

Figure 24–20. Metastatic ovarian tumor from primary lesion in stomach. Signet cells are present but difficult to distinguish because of marked stromal hyperplasia. Patient underwent masculinization during pregnancy.

24–20). Interestingly, this tumor, when associated with pregnancy, has proved to have a masculinizing effect on both the host and the fetus, as noted by Spadoni and others.

REFERENCES

Bachman, E.: Paradoxical metastasis and transpulmonary cancer spread. Am. J. Roentgenol., 72:499, 1954.

Bruegge, C. F. V.: Ovarian metastasis from renal adenocarcinoma. Obstet. Gynecol., 9:198, 1957.

Doucette, J. W., and Estes, W. B.: Primary ovarian carcinoid tumors. Obstet. Gynecol., 25:94, 1965.

Evans, G. M.: Vaginal metastasis from carcinoma of the ovary. J. Obstet. Gynaecol. Br. Emp., 59:82, 1952.

Ewing, J.: Neoplastic Diseases. 3rd Ed. Philadelphia, W. B. Saunders Company, 1928.

Fox, L. P., and Stamm, W. J.: Krukenberg tumor complicating pregnancy. Am. J. Obstet. Gynecol., 92:702, 1965.

Gusberg, S. B., and Yannopoulos, D.: Therapeutic deci-

sions in corpus cancer. Am. J. Obstet. Gynecol., 88:157, 1964.

Israel, S. L., Helsel, E. V., and Hausman, D. H.: The challenge of metastatic ovarian carcinoma. Am. J. Obstet. Gynecol., 93:1094, 1965.

Johnson, C. E., and Soule, E. H.: Malignant lymphomas as a gynecological problem. Obstet. Gynecol., 10:1049, 1957.

Karsh, J.: Secondary malignant diseases of ovary. Am. J. Obstet. Gynecol., 61:154, 1951.

Kasilag, F. B., Jr., and Rutledge, F. N.: Metastatic breast carcinoma in the ovary. Am. J. Obstet. Gynecol., 74:989, 1957.

Krukenberg, F.: Fibrosarcoma ovarii mucocellulare. Arch. Gynäk., 1:287, 1893.

Krukenberg, F.: Uber das Fibrosarcoma ovarii mucocellulare (carcinomatodes). Arch. Gynäk., 50:287, 1896.

Lawrence, W. D., Larson, P. N., and Hauge, E. T.: Primary Krukenberg tumor of the ovary in pregnancy. Obstet. Gynecol., 10:54, 1957.

McDuff, H. C.: Metastatic Krukenberg tumor of ovary, primary in breast. Rhode Island Med. J., 33:589, 1950.

Meyer, R.: Handbuch der spezielle pathologische Anatomie und Histologie. F. Henke and O. Lubarsch, Eds. Berlin, Julius Springer, 1930, p. 396.

Novak, E., and Gray, L. A.: Krukenberg tumors of the ovary. Clinical and pathological study of 21 cases. Surg. Gynecol. Obstet., 66:157, 1938.

Ober, W. B., Pollak, A., Gerstmann, K. E., and Kupperman, H. S.: Krukenberg tumor with androgenic and progestational activity. Am. J. Obstet. Gynecol., 84:739, 1962.

Rabe, M. A.: Krukenberg tumors. Ann. Surg., 22:86, 1956.

Robboy, S.: Carcinoid metastatic to ovary. Cancer, 33:798, 1974.

Schiller, W., and Kozoll, D. D.: Primary signet-ring cell carcinoma of ovary. Am. J. Obstet. Gynecol., 41:70, 1941.

Schlagenhaufer, F.: Uber das metastatische Ovarialkarzinom nach Krebs des Magens, Darmes und anderer Bauchorgane. Mschr. Geburtsh. Gynäk., 15:485, 1902.

Soloway, I., Latour, J. P. A., and Yound, M. H. V.: Krukenberg tumors of the ovary. Obstet. Gynecol., 8:636, 1956.

Spadoni, L. R., Kindberg, M. C., Mottet, N. K., and Herrmann, W. L.: Virilization coexisting with Krukenberg tumor during pregnancy. Am. J. Obstet. Gynecol., 92:981, 1965.

Turenen, K.: Hormonal secretion of Krukenberg tumors. Acta Endocrinol., 20:50, 1955.

Webb, M. J.: Cancer metastatic to ovary. Obstet. Gynecol., 45:391, 1975.

Wolfe, S. A.: Metastatic carcinoid tumors of the ovary. Am. J. Obstet. Gynecol., 70:563, 1955.

Woodruff, J. D., and Novak, E. R.: Krukenberg tumors of the ovary. Obstet. Gynecol., 15:351, 1960.

Woodruff, J. D., Murthy, Y. S., Bhaskar, T. N., Bordbar, F., and Tseng, S. S.: Metastatic ovarian tumors. Am. J. Obstet. Gynecol., 107:202, 1970.

Chapter 25

GERM CELL TUMORS

Part I

DYSGERMINOMA OF THE OVARY

Germ cell tumors include those lesions composed of germ cells—i.e., the dysgerminoma and the teratoid neoplasms. The WHO classification is as follows:

GERM CELL TUMORS

A. Dysgerminoma
B. Endodermal Sinus Tumor
C. Embryonal Carcinoma
D. Polyembryoma
E. Choriocarcinoma
F. Teratomas
   1. Immature
   2. Mature
      a. Solid
      b. Cystic
         (1) Dermoid cyst (mature cystic teratoma)
         (2) Dermoid cyst with malignant transformation
   3. Monodermal and highly specialized
      a. Struma ovarii
      b. Carcinoid
      c. Struma ovarii and carcinoid
      d. Others
G. Mixed Forms

From this classification one might suspect that lesions such as the endodermal sinus tumor, choriocarcinoma, and polyvesicular vitelline tumor are not teratoid. To the authors, a more realistic approach would be to use the terms embryonal and extraembryonal to describe the teratomas and to indicate the degree of maturation of the tissues in the embryonal tumors. Consequently, the following classification is proposed.

GERM CELL TUMORS AND PRECURSORY CONDITIONS

I. Dysgerminoma
II. Teratoma
   A. Embryonal
      1. Immature
         a. Embryoid body (mesoblastic?)
         b. Undifferentiated (single or multiple cell types)
      2. Mature (benign teratoma)
         a. Polyplastic
         b. Monoplastic—struma ovarii, etc.
      3. Mixed (immature and mature)
   B. Extraembryonal
      1. Endodermal sinus
      2. Polyvesicular vitelline (yolk sac)
      3. Choriocarcinoma
      4. Embryonal carcinoma(?)
      5. Mixed
III. Dysgenetic Gonads—non-neoplastic conditions with high neoplastic potential

476

GERM CELL*
|
Preimplantation stage of development

Extraembryonal pathway / *Embryonal pathway*

Placenta, cord, membranes, and yolk sac:
trophoblasts, mesoblasts, yolk sac, and
amnion epithelium

Embryo ⟶ Adult:
ectoderm, mesoderm, and endoderm in
various stages of maturation

GERM CELL* -----> Germinoma (Dys Germinoma)

Extraembryonal pathway / *Embryonal pathway*

Extraembryonal teratomas:
endodermal sinus tumor
choriocarcinoma
polyvesicular vitelline tumor

Teratomas:
immature
mature
struma ovarii

Simply, the genesis of teratomas may be explained by comparing normal development of the fertilized egg with the abnormal, as described by Jimerson and Woodruff.

DYSGERMINOMA (GERMINOMA)

These tumors are found in both sexes and morphologically the lesions generally are indistinguishable whether in the gonad or at an extragonadal site, literally from the pineal gland to low midline (Fig. 25–1).

Histologically these tumors represent abnormal growth patterns of the basic germ cell. Actually all female gonads during the early embryonic stages of development microscopically simulate the dysgerminoma. The germ cells are noted in large or small aggregates separated by stroma (Fig. 25–2). In the apparently normal gonad, many primordial follicles are noted in the adjacent area. In either sex, the germ cells continue undergoing mitosis until organized in either the seminiferous tubules of the male or the encapsulating primitive granulosa of the female. Since there are no sex cords in the female gonad, a dysgerminoma, such as the seminiferous seminoma, is not seen in the ovary. In the latter, the germ cells are encapsulated (the primordial follicle) at birth and the unencapsulated or free cells die. Nevertheless, if either of the latter processes fails, it is conceivable that the germ cell could free itself of its normal control and multiply indiscriminately.

Another circumstance suggesting the validity of the above theory is the frequent occurrence of such tumors in individuals with subnormal gonadal development or hermaphrodites. It cannot be too strongly emphasized, however, that in such cases the tumor has nothing to do with the development of the sex anomaly, which persists even after removal of the tumor. A female hermaphrodite in whose ovary a dysgerminoma develops shows no reversion of the ambiguous sexual status after removal of the tumor. This is to be expected in view of the asexual nature of the constituent cells. Taylor and co-workers indicate the importance of karyotype study, and many variations, including mosaicism, have been recorded in patients with these lesions.

Schellhas and associates noted the frequency of germ cell tumors with XY gonadal

* From Jimerson and Woodruff: Am. J. Obstet. Gynecol., 127:73, 1977.

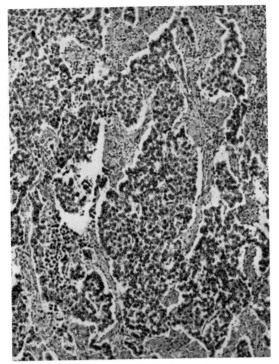

Figure 25–1. Seminoma of the testis, identical in histologic appearance to dysgerminoma of the ovary.

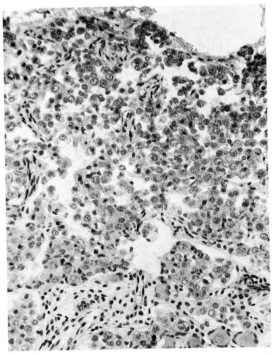

Figure 25–2. Aggregates of unencapsulated germ cells separated by fibrous strands—in normal female embryonic gonad. Note encapsulated germ cells (primordial follicles) in left lower quadrant.

Table 25–1 CLINICAL CHARACTERISTICS OF DYSGERMINOMA

Age
 Before age 20, 40–45 per cent
 Before age 30, 80–85 per cent

Symptoms
 "Abdominal pain"
 Menstrual history, normal (90 per cent)
 "Somatic sexual" changes, 10–15 per cent
 Fertility, normal

Operative Findings
 Ascites, rare
 Bilaterality, 10–15 per cent
 Intact capsule, 80–90 per cent
 Rupture capsule, 10 per cent (poor prognosis)
 Tumor free, 60 per cent
 Tumor adherent, 40 per cent

Tumor Spread
 None: limited to one ovary, 80 per cent
 Spread (in order of frequency), 20 per cent
  (1) Peritoneum, adjacent tube, omentum
  (2) Lymph nodes (retroperitoneal), uterus, other
      ovary (?)
  (3) Bowel, liver, lung, etc.
 Note: tumors <15 cm. localized; >15 cm. extended

Recurrence Most Likely
  (1) Young age group, <20 years
  (2) Spillage or bilateral tumors
  (3) Large tumors, >15 cm.
  (4) Vascular
  (5) Associated with teratoma

Salvage, 70–75 per cent overall
 "Pure," unilateral, 90 per cent
 Mixed (with teratoma, choriocarcinoma, etc.)
  25–30 per cent
 Unilateral SO with biopsy of contralateral
  gonad
 Radiosensitive even with "metastases"

dysgenesis, characterized by (1) female phenotype, (2) hypoplastic müllerian duct structures, (3) rudimentary or absent gonads, (4) absent menarche, and (5) 46, XY karyotype. Thus, when "streak ovaries" are present, the karyotype is of obvious importance in evaluating malignant potentialities and the disposition of the ovaries. Malignant changes occur in approximately 15 per cent of streak ovaries when a Y chromosome is present. Ninety-five to 98 per cent of tumors develop after the menarche, and thus many feel that the child should be allowed to ma-

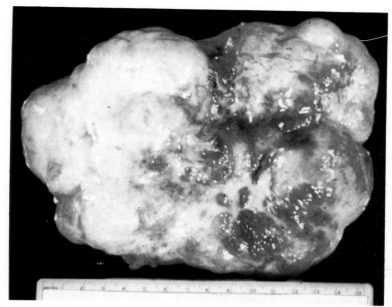

Figure 25–3. Gross appearance of dysgerminoma with smooth, slightly nodular capsule.

ture prior to excision of the gonad at risk. Nevertheless, there are dysgerminomas recorded prior to this critical age.

Gross Characteristics

The size of dysgerminomas varies widely, some measuring only a few centimeters in diameter, others filling the abdominal cavity. Characteristically, they are capsule-smooth, although the contour may be nodular (Fig. 25–3). The consistency of the tumor, which is essentially solid, has frequently been described as "doughy" or rubbery. The cut surface is grayish-pink, with foci of brownish-yellow areas.

Areas of necrosis, degeneration, and hemorrhage are not uncommon, although there is little tendency toward formation of cysts unless the tumor is associated with teratoid elements, and in the latter, the associated teratoma is generally solid. The tumors are generally unilateral, bilaterality being found grossly in about 8 to 10 per cent. Nevertheless involvement of the contralateral ovary may be microscopic and biopsy of the other gonad is mandatory. Ascites is observed on rare occasions, and a few cases have presented with torsion of the pedicle. The combination of dysgerminoma and pregnancy may be encountered, since 80 per cent of

the patients harboring these lesions are classically under the age of 30 years.

Microscopic Characteristics

Few tumors of the ovary present such distinctive histologic characteristics as does the dysgerminoma (Fig. 25–4). This applies to both the cell type and the general architecture of the tumor. For this reason, the microscopic recognition is usually easy. There is far more variation in the histology of the granulosa cell tumor or arrhenoblastoma. The large round, ovoid, or polygonal cells of dysgerminoma are responsible for the former designation of this tumor as the "large-cell carcinoma." The cytoplasm is abundant, clear, very pale-staining, and often translucent. The nucleus is also large and irregular in both contour and dispersion of the chromatin. Mitotic figures are seen in varying numbers, although they are not usually numerous.

Just as characteristic as the cell is the arrangement of the elements in alveoli or nests separated by fibrous trabeculae, which may show some degree of hyalinization, but which often are extensively infiltrated with lymphocytes (Fig. 25–5). Commonly the cells are arranged in long columns or strands, especially toward the periphery of the tumor.

only 10% Bilateral

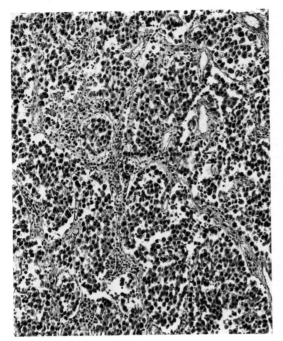

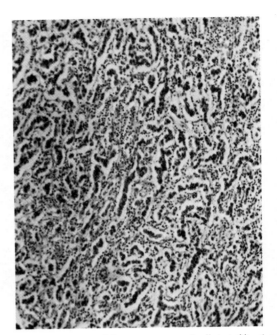

Figure 25–6. Cordlike arrangement of cells in infiltrative portion of dysgerminoma.

Figure 25–4. Ovarian dysgerminoma showing nests of large, round cells with connective tissue septa and lymphocytic infiltration.

In some tumors the septa are abundant and thick, and the cell nests are relatively sparse (Fig. 25–6). Others are characterized by foci with marked cellularity and atypical nuclei. Careful evaluation of many sections is neces-

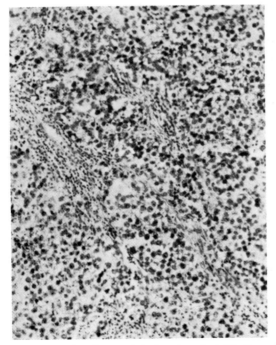

Figure 25–5. Characteristic lymphocytic infiltration of fibrous septa in dysgerminoma.

sary in order to make the correct assessment of the tumor and avoid designating an undifferentiated mesothelioma as dysgerminoma (Fig. 25–7). Although the latter would seem to indicate greater degree of malignancy, such has not proved to be true. Actually breakthrough of the capsule, bilaterality, and the presence of lymph node extension are the only poor prognostic signs. Consequently study of the para-aortic nodes and contralateral ovary is imperative. So-called teratoid bodies, cells containing eosinophilic bodies, which appear to either displace the nucleus or compress the remaining chromatin, are constant histologic findings but do not seem to be of prognostic significance. Within the stromal septum and its lymphocytic infiltrate, giant cells are recognized occasionally (Fig. 25–8). It has been suggested that both of these findings are evidences of cellular immunity and are thus good prognostic signs, but this has not proved to be true in our own series. On the basis of the finding of giant cells, the coexistence of tuberculosis has been suspected; however, true granulomas are not present and the clinical association is absent. Furthermore, there has been no proof that such cells are of trophoblastic origin.

It is of interest to note that sex chromatin may be found in malignant tumors although to a lesser degree than in normal females or

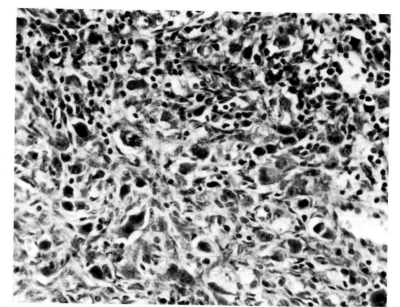

Figure 25–7. Atypical dysgerminoma. Large bizarre germ cells with lymphocytic infiltrate are seen above.

those with benign tumors. With dysgerminoma, however, Heinz found that the majority of his 10 cases showed a negative (male) pattern, although this discrepancy between the sex karyotype of tumor and that of host was not present in the cases of testicular seminoma. In many instances, these tumors are found in patients with an ambiguous phenotype and an equivocal karyotype. Furthermore, with the peculiarities of the chromatin distribution, there may be difficulties in identification of a true Barr body.

The reported survival rates for dysgerminoma are more varied than for most other specific groups of ovarian tumors. Mueller and co-workers, Pedowitz and associates, and others have quoted gloomy statistics, with a 25 to 30 per cent 5 year survival. Conversely, Malkasian and Symmonds, deLima, Assadourian and Taylor, and others have recorded an 85 to 90 per cent 5 year salvage for unilateral encapsulated lesions. Several facts may explain these discrepancies. In deLima's series and in our own study of teratomas, it was noted that if a teratoid lesion coexisted with the dysgerminoma, a 25 to 30 per cent survival could be expected. Furthermore, the incidence of bilaterality was not thoroughly evaluated in many earlier series, and if such exists, the mortality is high, particularly if adequate therapy is not instituted. Finally, para-aortic nodal involvement is of major importance. The latter does not necessarily predict death, for if the nodes are treated, long-term survivals can be expected. Late recurrence (or contralateral disease) may occur as many as 15 years after initial surgery (Chauser et al.).

From a clinical standpoint, three general groups of cases may be described: (1) those

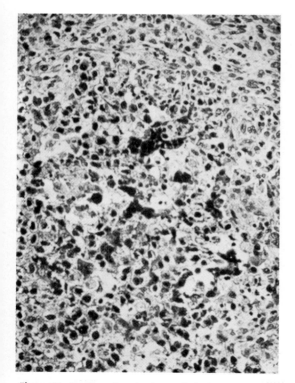

Figure 25–8. Symplasmic giant cells in dysgerminoma.

in which the tumor capsule is intact, with no extension beyond the ovary; (2) those in which there is infiltration, at times massive, of other pelvic viscera; (3) those in which extensive metastasis is seen.

The first of these groups, especially those in which the tumor is small, naturally offers the most favorable prognosis. Unilateral operations have been successful in curing 90 per cent of the cases. Consequently, conservative therapy (i.e., unilateral adnexectomy) should be the treatment of choice in the young patient after thorough exploration and biopsy of the contralateral gonad. Even in the second and third groups, long-term survivals have been recorded with adequate radiation therapy since the germ cell is known to be extremely radiosensitive. For example, in a child of 7 years with a huge infiltrating dysgerminoma that was incompletely removed, irradiation produced marked temporary shrinkage. Intra-abdominal recurrence was treated with additional irradiation, and the patient was alive more than 20 years later without evidence of disease. Nevertheless, it is in these patients that both late, local recurrences and distant metastasis must be anticipated.

In separate articles, Brody and Thoeny and co-workers indicate the radiosensitive nature of dysgerminoma. Nevertheless, we do not recommend radiation if only conservative surgery is performed, if thorough study revealed no extraovarian disease, and if the patient desires to maintain her reproductive potential.

Other clinics advise more stringent treatment, such as routine postoperative irradiation (with or without shielding of the residual ovary), but we believe that this can be withheld unless there is evidence of recurrence. Triple drug therapy may be a further therapeutic modality for recurrent disease, although the reports are inadequate for accurate evaluation at present.

Associated Teratoid Elements

Since the dysgerminoma is a germ cell tumor and parthenogenesis (stimulation of the germ cell) is probably the most commonly accepted genesis for the more immature teratomas, it would seem only logical that these two varieties of tumor would coexist (Fig. 25–9 A,B). Choriocarcinoma (Fig.

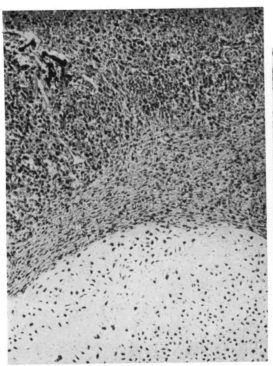
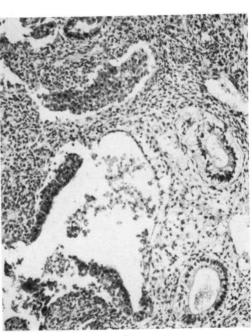

A **B**

Figure 25–9. *A,* Dysgerminoma combined with teratoma. Note large area of cartilage. *B,* Higher magnification of dysgerminoma and teratomatous elements.

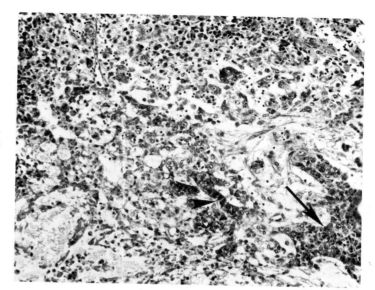

Figure 25–10. Dysgerminoma with extraembryonal teratoma, the latter simulating trophoblast, at arrows.

25–10) appears to be the most common associate of the dysgerminoma, although the endodermal sinus tumor and other extraembryonal lesions have been recorded. In a series of 97 malignant teratomas, dysgerminoma was found in 27, or nearly 30 per cent. DeLima also noted that the 5 year survival was approximately 75 per cent for all dysgerminomas but only 27 per cent in the combined teratoma-dysgerminoma patients. This association should be appreciated, since survivals of 25 to 30 per cent are recorded when these lesions coexist. Furthermore, therapy must be modified in these circumstances. Irradiation is of no value in the treatment of the teratoma and, as yet, triple chemotherapy has not been the treatment of choice for the dysgerminoma. Consequently, the correct histopathologic diagnosis leads to the correct therapy and improved results.

Age

Dysgerminoma is preeminently a tumor of early life, thus justifying the appellation of *carcinoma puellarum*. It is common in children before puberty, and likewise in young adolescents. It should be remembered, however, that it is occasionally found in adult women. More than 85 per cent of deLima's cases from the Ovarian Tumor Registry were found in women under 30 years of age. Abell and co-workers also have noted the frequency of this tumor in young women (under

20 years old), although it is less common than the teratoma.

Associated Developmental and Sex Changes

In the past, great stress has been placed on the frequent occurrence of dysgerminoma in pseudohermaphrodites and patients with sexual underdevelopment. However, this association is not the result of the tumor, but rather the neoplasm develops in patients with gonadal dysgenesis. For example, it is prevalent in the cryptorchid testes and in the female with gonadoblastoma. Thus, the presence of the Y chromosome in the phenotypic female constitutes a threat for the formation of germ cell tumors, primarily dysgerminoma. Nevertheless, it has become apparent that most dysgerminomas develop in "normal" women, usually in the third or early fourth decade of life.

In a review of 100 ovarian tumors associated with pregnancy, dysgerminoma was present in 19 cases and 13 were alive and well 5 or more years without disease, three were alive with recurrence, and three were dead. This would reemphasize the relatively favorable nature of such lesions.

Endocrine Aspects of Dysgerminomas

It has been stressed that dysgerminoma is usually biologically inert; thus, should it be found in a pseudohermaphrodite, reversion to normal sex status does not occur in the

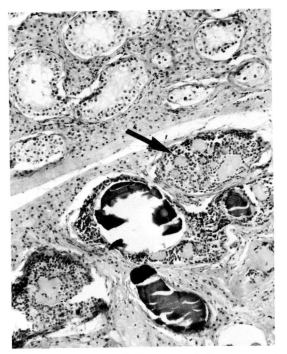

Figure 25–11. Gonadoblastoma—tubules are present on left. Folliculoid structures are seen at arrow. Calcifications are obvious.

postoperative era. This is true in the vast majority of cases, but there are exceptions.

Positive Pregnancy Test. A few cases of dysgerminoma have been associated with positive pregnancy tests, presumably because of a concomitant choriocarcinoma, although it has not always been possible to demonstrate trophoblast or evidence of pregnancy. It must be appreciated that there are literally thousands of patients with a variety of tumors in whom an elevated chorionic gonadotropin titer has been documented. Nevertheless, the presence of trophoblast with germ cell tumors impairs the prognosis, since nongestational trophoblastic disease has not responded to chemotherapy as readily as the gestational variety. However, Goldstein and Piro report improved results with combination drugs, such as methotrexate, actinomycin D, and chlorambucil. Of 11 patients, a substantial remission was noted in five, although only two of the 11 patients were female. It must be appreciated that elevated levels of HCG have been reported with many tumors containing no semblance of trophoblast.

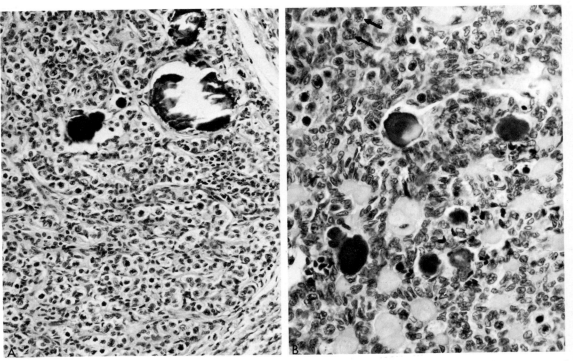

Figure 25–12. *A*, Calcifications seen in a dysgenetic gonad associated with dysgerminoma. *B*, Variety of dysgenetic gonad with pseudotubule formation, calcifications and germ cells (at arrows). There is karyotypic abnormality (both XX and XY).

GONADOBLASTOMA

In 1953 Scully reported two cases which he designated as gonadoblastoma, presumably of both germ cell and sex cord or mesenchymal origin (Fig. 25–11) with frequently discrete areas of calcification. The source of the steroid hormone is difficult to determine, but Scully believes that it lies in the gonadal stroma cells. Teter prefers to utilize the term gonocytoma for dysgerminoma in the fashion of Teilum, and recognizes various combinations of these germ cell tumors and admixtures of sex cord and mesenchymal elements with all kinds of hormonal end effects, and many of these neoplasms are bilateral.

Scully reviewed 74 cases of gonadoblastoma, most of which arose in gonads of "unknown" nature. The hormonal effect was generally androgenic, and chromatin-negative nuclei were present in 90 per cent. The largest lesion was 8 cm., and the lesions seemed generally benign, although a dysgerminoma may be superimposed. Talerman has noted combined dysgerminoma and gonadoblastoma in siblings with dysgenetic gonads and records two other similar cases. All combinations of germ cell and stromal tumors may occur (Fig. 25–12).

Part II

OVARIAN TERATOMAS

On referring to the classification of germ cell tumors it will be appreciated that Group II comprises the teratomas, both extraembryonal and embryonal. Rather than suggest that the choriocarcinoma, endodermal sinus tumor, and so forth, are not teratomas it would seem wiser to correlate all lesions with the tissues seen in the differentiation of elements arising from the normally fertilized egg and the comparable but malignant tissue developing from the germ cell, either by atypical maturation or parthenogenesis. The finding of both embryonal elements, mature and/or immature with extraembryonal (trophoblast, yolk sac, etc.) in the same tumor supports this classification.

The teratoma (Gk., teratos, "monster," and onkoma, "swelling") is one of the truly fascinating neoplasms of the body. Robbins has suggested that these lesions are "compound tumors, composed of cells from more than one germ layer." This definition emphasizes the origin of teratomas from cells retaining totipotency—i.e., the ability to differentiate into any of the three embryonic germ layers or into extraembryonic tissues, or both. Thus, it may be stated that the teratoma is a true neoplasm which contains tissues arising from more than one germ cell layer and foreign to the organ in which it resides.

Incidence

Approximately 15 per cent of all primary ovarian tumors fall into the category of the teratoma. The most common site of origin is the gonad, and lesions arising at this site are usually benign and cystic, with a peak incidence in the reproductive years. If such tumors are found during the postmenopausal years, it must be assumed that they have been present for many years and only recently appreciated because of symptomatology or in the course of a routine examination. The extragonadal lesions usually arise in the midline of the body, most commonly appear in the first two decades of life, and 60 to 70 per cent are benign. Extragenital tumors containing primarily trophoblastic tissue have been reported in the lung but probably do not represent true teratoid lesions. Furthermore, the so-called fetus in fetu should not be classified as a true teratoma.

Approximately 95 to 98 per cent of all teratomas are of the benign or adult variety; thus, approximately 2 to 5 per cent are malignant. The majority of the latter had been classified as secondary malignancies developing in a primarily benign teratoma. In the last decade, lesions composed primarily of immature embryonal or extraembryonal elements have become more prevalent, in our experience, and the basic demonstration of malignancy is the inability of the tissue to mature rather than the presence of individual cell anaplasia, the usual criterion for malignancy in the adult. This unique aspect of malignancy is demonstrated by an absence of aneuploidy in the few cases that have been studied.

Histogenesis

Two basic theories have been promoted to explain the histogenesis of the teratoma. The blastomere theory, supported by Marchand and Willis, suggests that the basic blastomere, when segregated at an early phase of embryonic life, may in later years develop into a bizarre form of the human being—i.e., a teratoma. A second theory proposes the germ cell as the basic element involved in the genesis of such neoplasms. This latter theory is championed by a majority of observers today. Initially, the germ cell theory is supported by the common midline or gonadal positions of the teratoma, the two sites at which this unique cell is found in the embryo and adult (Fig. 25–13). Circumstantial evidence is noted in the close association of teratomas with the primary germ cell tumor, the dysgerminoma.

Ashley has proposed four possible geneses, namely, (1) segregation of undifferentiated elements during embryonic life, (2) parthenogenetic development of the germ cell, (3) included twins or fetus in fetu, (4) union of haploid cells.

The frequency of the adult teratoma in the ovary in contrast to its rarity in the male gonad suggests a difference in genesis, although the basic germ cell is undoubtedly the key element. The possible union of haploid cells within the commonly seen polynuclear follicle (Fig. 25–14), after the second stage of meiotic division, is a potential explanation for this discrepancy. Since the polar bodies contain the haploid number of chromosomes but little cytoplasm, the union of these nuclei with reduced nutrient material may result in the development of a structure with normal chromosomal complement but reduced differentiating capacity. Studies by Linder have noted that tissues from teratomas are routinely homozygous while those

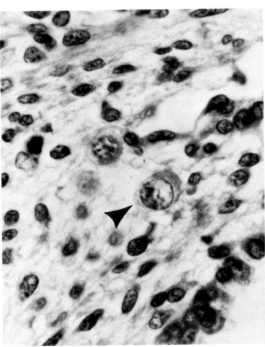

Figure 25–13. The germ cell (at arrow) in transit in the mesentery of the hindgut at approximately 5 weeks of embryonic life.

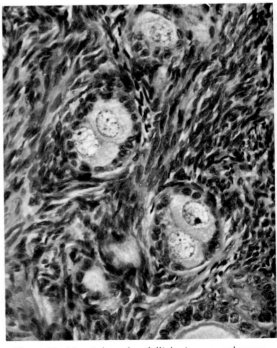

Figure 25–14. Polynuclear follicles in a normal ovary.

from the host are heterozygous in 30 per cent of the elements investigated. He suggests therefore that the teratoma must arise from a single germ cell. Nevertheless, the results do not eliminate the above proposal since the germ cells within the same capsule (polynuclear) may well result in the development of a homozygous structure. Jones has suggested that the union of such haploid cells may explain the origin of the chimera.

Actually, the maturity or immaturity of the tissues in the teratoma is easily explained if the tumors are correlated with the stages of normal fetal and adult development. Cytogenetic studies confirm this normalcy in that practically 100 per cent of ovarian teratomas and about 40 per cent of testicular teratomas have an XX sex chromosomal complement and a normal autosomal number of 44.

Terminology

The terms dermoid cyst and teratoma have been used to differentiate the two fundamental varieties of teratoma, i.e., the benign and the malignant. Previous points of distinction have been: (1) the dermoid cyst is largely cystic while the teratoma is fundamentally solid; (2) the dermoid is characterized by mature, ectodermal elements, although tissues from the other two germ layers are invariably present, while the teratoma is composed of immature elements derived from all germ layers; and (3) the dermoid cyst is classically benign while the teratoma has generally been malignant.

It would seem much wiser to differentiate these neoplasms into mature adult or immature tumors, the latter composed of embryonic or extraembryonic elements. This differentiation is used in the proposed classification noted above.

MATURE TERATOMAS

The majority of ovarian teratomas are benign and cystic, and the predominant element is usually of ectodermal origin—i.e., the tumor commonly known as the dermoid cyst. Grossly, these lesions are characterized by a smooth tense capsule beneath which is the major cystic component (Fig. 25–15). The size varies from those found only by the microscope to those filling the lower abdomen and weighing as much as 7.7 kg. (15½ lb.), as reported by Chalmers and Kurrein. The predominant content of this cyst is sebaceous material usually mixed with hair. The sebaceous contents, although liquid at body temperature, tend to solidify on removal. It is of major importance to recognize that the contents of the cyst may be clear. The clear fluid originates from one of many sources; however, it is occasionally cerebrospinal since neural tissue and its excretory element, the choroid plexus, are common components of the mature teratoma. Most such neoplasms are unifocal, although as many as nine individual tumors have been found in one gonad. The lesion often contains a solid prominence, Rokitansky's protuberance, located usually at the point of contact with the residual ovarian tissue. It is here that such structures as teeth and bone are commonly found, and this is also the area from which sections should be made, since here the greatest variation in the cellular elements will be recognized. As noted pre-

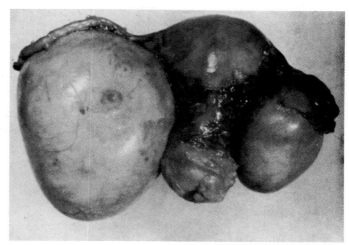

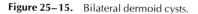

Figure 25–15. Bilateral dermoid cysts.

viously, microscopic examination reveals that, although the ectodermal derivatives are most common, tissues of mesodermal and endodermal origin are found in almost all cases. The most prominent elements are stratified squamous epithelium and its appendages (Fig. 25–16 A). Respiratory epithelium with its associated peribronchial glands and cartilage can be demonstrated in 50 to 75 per cent of the tumors (Fig. 25–16 B). Neural elements and endodermal epithelium are recognized in many cases. Unusual findings that may be present in the absence of any definable tissues are the sievelike areas resulting from the infiltration of sebaceous material into the solid portions of the lesion, and characterized by microscopic

cystic spaces containing foreign body giant cells (Fig. 25–17).

As noted earlier, the tumors may vary greatly in size. Peterson reported that 75 per cent of the mature teratomas were 10 cm. or less, while fewer than 4 per cent were more than 20 cm. in diameter. Various statistics indicate that approximately 15 to 20 per cent are bilateral (Fig. 25–13). It is extremely difficult to arrive at a realistic figure for bilaterality, since so commonly the patients are young and a unilateral procedure is performed. It would be necessary to have a careful follow-up of all these patients in order to accurately determine the incidence of bilaterality. Nevertheless, the possibility must be recognized, and the other ovary inspected

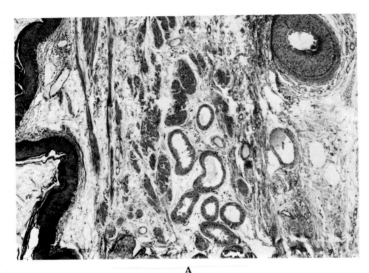

A

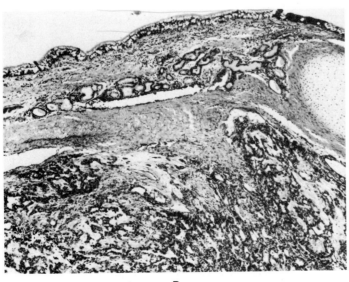

B

Figure 25–16. A, Classic findings in "dermoid cyst"—stratified epithelium and appendages (dilated apocrine glands in center). There are few muscle fibers beneath epithelium. A more acceptable term is "benign adult teratoma." B, Respiratory epithelium at the top of section with underlying cartilage and peribronchial glands. Remainder of tumor is of extraembryonal origin.

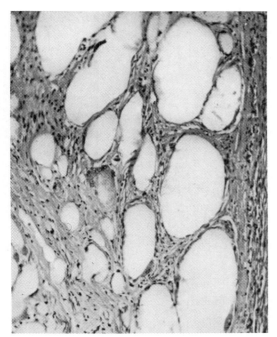

Figure 25–17. Sievelike area near dermoid cyst, showing foreign body giant cells. Such areas are produced by the penetration of fatty material through the wall of the cyst.

carefully when conservative procedures are performed.

In spite of the high incidence of bilaterality (15 to 18 per cent), the routine bisection of the contralateral ovary is a question-

able procedure, since an incision into the capsule may result in the development of adhesive disease and inclusion cysts. Furthermore, if the original tumor is benign, the development of a malignant teratoma in later life has not been reported, although it undoubtedly could occur.

Symptomatology

Most frequently the mature teratoma is asymptomatic, although if of sufficient size it may cause pressure and vague abdominal discomfort, and on rare occasions the patient appreciates the presence of a lower abdominal mass. Menstrual irregularities are unusual, and since many of these lesions are recognized during pregnancy, it seems obvious that infertility is rarely a presenting complaint. Frequently the tumors are found on routine examination or on x-ray of the abdomen for nonpelvic indications (Fig. 25–18). It has been estimated that calcifications or teeth or both are found in approximately one third of the adult teratomas, whereas masses of increased density and definite contour may be noted in the absence of calcification. Ultrasound is frequently capable of differentiating the echoes within the teratoid lesion from those associated with other adnexal lesions.

The complications occurring in the adult teratoma consist of torsion, rupture, infec-

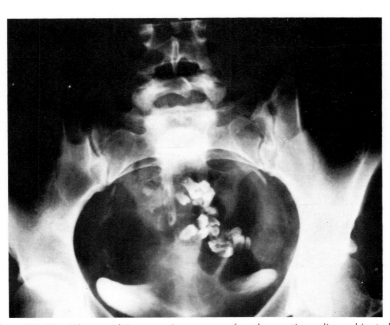

Figure 25–18. Fifteen teeth in an ovarian teratoma, found on routine radiographic study.

tion, or malignancy. Torsion is by far the most common and probably relates to the weight of the tumor and the frequency with which it occurs anterior to the broad ligament. Torsion and resultant infarction may lead to rupture, with distribution of the sebaceous contents into the general abdominal cavity, particularly during delivery. Regardless of the time, such an occurrence presents major problems due to the resultant peritonitis and occasional fistula formation. Spontaneous drainage of the contents of the teratoma through bladder, bowel, or vagina has been reported. Surgery is extremely complicated at the time of acute rupture; however, it is usually worse in the chronic phase since the peritoneal cavity may be virtually obliterated by the resultant granulomatous peritonitis. The infection is undoubtedly related to leakage of the sebaceous material with subsequent reactive "chemical peritonitis"; nevertheless, a variety of bacterial agents have been cultured from the abdominal cavity in such cases.

Malignant change in the benign cystic teratomas has been recorded as occurring in 1 to 3 per cent of cases. In our own experience this figure is high, and more realistically approximates 0.25 to 0.5 per cent. Such secondary malignancies should be differentiated from the immature variety of teratoma since the pathologic pictures, the ages of the patients, and the clinical courses are strikingly different. The most common malignancy developing in the initially benign teratoma is squamous cell carcinoma, although other neoplasias, including melanoma, a variety of sarcomas, and undifferentiated carcinoma, have been reported.

Most of these lesions occur in the fifth and sixth decades of life, in contrast to the immature variety, which has its peak incidence in the middle of the second decade. Since a majority of these secondary malignancies are found only after extension has taken place, the salvage rate is poor. Nevertheless, 5 year survivals of 50 per cent or more have been recorded when the capsule is intact. Treatment consists of primary surgery followed by appropriate adjunctive therapy.

Special Forms of Mature Teratoma (Monodermal)

As noted previously in the discussion of mucinous tumors, a certain percentage of such lesions undoubtedly represent tera-

tomas in which the proliferation of the single component has overgrown other tissues. Our own experience and that of others proposes that approximately 4 to 5 per cent of mucinous lesions are associated with other cellular elements consistent with the diagnosis of teratoma. The association of such epithelium with an underlying muscular layer suggests the reproduction of a segment of bowel, and malignancies arising in either the mucinous or the muscle elements have been recorded. The latter myosarcoma may be the reason for the reported poorer survival of patients with mucinous tumors in the early decades of life. (Fig. 25–19.) Nevertheless, most mucinous tumors represent heterotopic alteration of the totipotent coelomic epithelium or mesothelium.

Struma Ovarii

It has been noted by several observers that adult teratomas contain thyroid tissue in approximately 12 to 15 per cent of cases (Fig. 25–20). Such an occurrence does not justify a diagnosis of struma ovarii. It has been suggested that the latter diagnosis should be made only if the thyroid tissue is dominant or if there are evidences of either neoplasia or hormonal function in the evaluation of the individual case. The neoplastic alterations in struma may be confusing, and in certain instances a carcinoid pattern has been associated with the struma (Fig. 25–21 A,B,C).

Classically, the struma in gross appearance is grayish-brown in color and of spongy consistency. Most such lesions are recognized in the fifth and sixth decades of life. Large cystic areas may be present, either as a part of the struma or as an associated teratoid structure such as a mucinous cyst (Fig. 25–22). The microscopic appearance is usually that of essentially normal thyroid tissue. A variety of abnormal features have been described, including the so-called thyroiditis, fetal adenoma, and classic varieties of malignancy. Metastases have been reported in adjacent areas as well as in the lung. On rare occasions the metastases may demonstrate more maturity than the original lesion.

As noted earlier, hormone function has been appreciated in a small percentage of the strumas. Unfortunately, the pelvic tumor is not suspected as a cause of the patient's symptomatology, and thus thorough studies of abnormal thyroid function have been car-

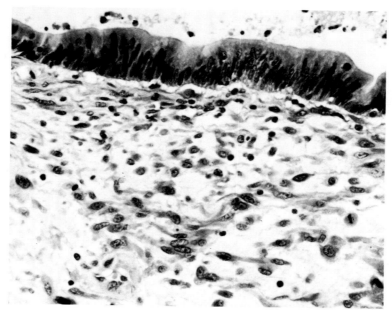

Figure 25–19. Mucinous carcinoma with rhabdomyosarcoma.

ried out in very few patients; nevertheless, the clinical picture has been classic in numerous instances. The regression of the symptoms postoperatively is circumstantial evidence of the activity of the pelvic struma. On rare occasions, abnormalities of the thyroid in the neck have been associated with the pelvic lesion, and surgical removal of the former followed by oophorectomy has been succeeded by the development of *hypo*thyroidism.

Carcinoid

Primary ovarian carcinoid has been accepted as a demonstration of unilateral development in a teratoma. As noted above, such neoplasms have been associated with struma as well as other teratoid elements, or may be metastases from an intestinal primary (see Chapter 24). The latter are commonly bilateral. This tumor has been mistaken histologically for either granulosa-cell tumor or arrhenoblastoma because of the cord-like or tubular arrangement of the cells (Fig. 25–23 A,B). The use of argentophilic stains may be helpful in differentiating these lesions since the carcinoid arises from neural crest elements and thus may show a positive reaction in the basal level of the epithelium with the silver stain. It is of interest to recognize that the carcinoid arising in the gastro-

intestinal tract has not been associated with the classic carcinoid syndrome unless the liver has been involved with metastatic disease. Conversely, there have been several cases of ovarian carcinoid in which the characteristic symptoms have been present with-

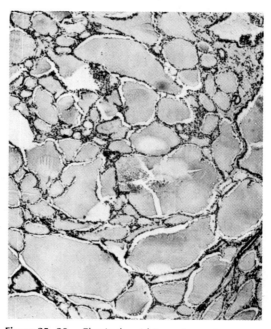

Figure 25–20. Classic thyroid tissue in ovarian struma.

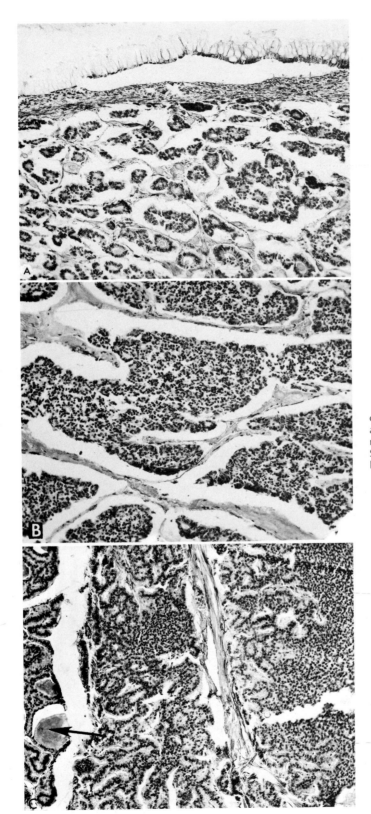

Figure 25–21. *A*, Dermoid cyst with mucinous epithelium above and malignant thyroid adenoma below. *B*, Higher magnification of thyroid carcinoma showing carcinoid pattern. *C*, Strumal carcinoid. Ribbon pattern with few colloid-filled follicles to the far left (arrow).

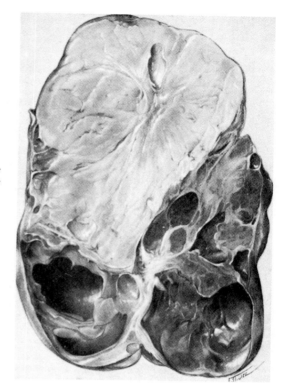

Figure 25–22. Gross specimen of a struma ovarii. The lower portion of the drawing represents thyroid tissue in the ovary, and a mucinous cyst.

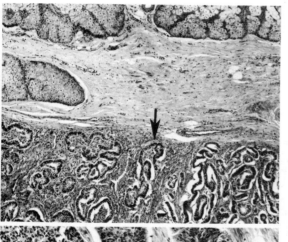

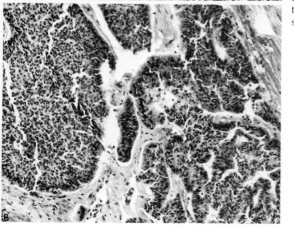

Figure 25–23. *A*, Carcinoid (at arrow) associated with classic sebaceous glands above. *B*, Carcinoid showing patterns simulating granulosa cell tumor (left) or a tubular lesion (right).

out metastatic disease. It is suspected that the difference in the venous drainage of the ovary may account for these variations in symptomatology.

IMMATURE TERATOMAS (EMBRYONAL)

To understand the various elements present in the ovarian teratoma, it is of basic importance to return to the fertilized egg and to recognize the tissues derived therefrom. Be-

ginning with the blastocyst, differentiation may be directed toward extraembryonal elements, classically the trophoblast, or the characteristic tissues derived from the three germ layers—ectoderm, mesoderm, and endoderm. Similarly, in any teratoma, one or all of these elements may be present in either mature or immature forms (Fig. 25–24 A,B). Thus, of fundamental importance in the study of the teratoma is a recognition of the ability of the tissues to mature. If maturation continues along normal processes, the mature or adult teratoma results, and the

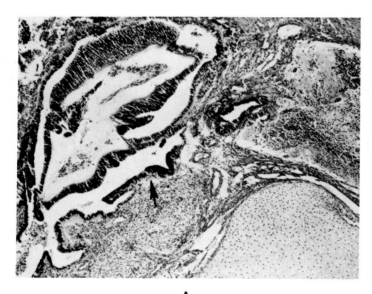

A

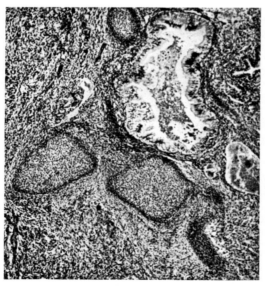

B

Figure 25–24. *A*, Teratoma with differentiated and undifferentiated neural elements. Neural tube is seen in upper left and an attempt at formation of choroid plexus in lower left. Retinal anlage with pigment is noted at arrow. Cartilage is present in lower right. *B*, Teratoma of ovary, showing cartilage and a cavity lined by endodermic epithelium like that seen in a mucinous cystadenoma.

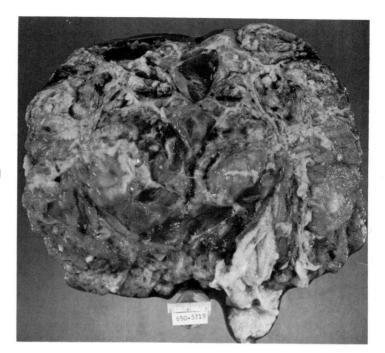

Figure 25–25. Poorly differentiated "embryonal" teratoma.

prognosis is excellent. Conversely, the inability of the elements to attain normal maturation culminates in an undisciplined growth that often eventuates in the death of the patient.

Teratomas containing immature elements fortunately are rare, constituting approximately 0.2 per cent of all ovarian tumors. They are usually solid; however, areas of degeneration are quite common because of the rapidity of the growth (Fig. 25–25). Microscopically the most immature is that tumor which replicates the embryoid body with its surrounding mesoblast (the polyembryoma). In the lineage of the normally developing fertilized egg, this tumor probably represents the stage immediately following the formation of the blastocyst (Fig. 25–26). An example of the biology of this lesion is represented by the tumor in a 5 year old child who died within 3 months after initial recognition of the lesion, which showed undifferentiated stroma and primitive embryoid bodies.

Among the tumors showing an embryonal element, those containing neural tissue most clearly demonstrate the importance of the ability to mature (Fig. 25–27). Fortt and Mathie have described 13 cases of gliomatosis peritonei—i.e., ovarian teratomas containing immature neural tissue with diffuse peritoneal spread, but with maturation oc-

curring in the metastases (Fig. 25–28). It is interesting to note that a majority of these patients have survived when this disseminated tissue has been able to mature. Conversely, in a study of 97 teratomas from the

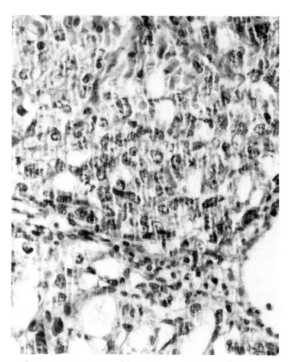

Figure 25–26. Mesoblastic tissue. Note similarity to cytotrophoblast.

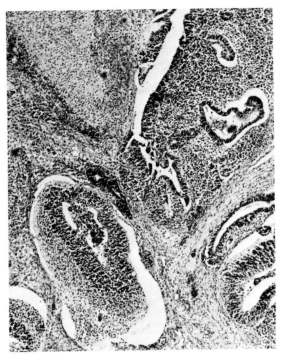

Figure 25–27. Mature and immature neural tissue in ovarian tumor—attempt at formation of a neural tube.

Ovarian Tumor Registry, it was noted that, with a predominance of immature neural tissue in the ovarian tumor, the prognosis must be guarded, since 50 per cent of the patients succumbed to the lesion.

A determination of the amount of undifferentiated glial tissue seems to be helpful in prognosis. Those lesions in which more than two thirds of the neural elements are immature, often demonstrating primitive neural tube formation, have a poorer survival rate. It is of further interest to appreciate that recurrences and extensions of these tumors are commonly local—i.e., within the peritoneal cavity—and repeat laparotomy with excision of the local disease is of more importance than adjunctive therapy. This is true whether the elements are glial or of other origin. Recently, improved survivals have been reported with the use of triple chemotherapy (DiSaia); nevertheless, the significant feature in improved salvage is the ability of the elements to mature, whether intra- or extraovarian, and of the surrounding tissues to confine the growth.

It is of major import to recognize that there are numerous undifferentiated stromal tissues present in many of these lesions, and that it may be impossible to categorize the specific elements. In many such cases the stromal component is probably mesoblast. One of the major difficulties encountered in such lesions is the absence of cellular aberrations that are generally associated with malignancy. It must be reemphasized that the malignant feature of the majority of these tumors is the inability to mature.

EXTRAEMBRYONAL TERATOMAS

Probably the most classic example of the extraembryonal teratoma is the endodermal sinus or yolk sac tumor described by Teilum. Superficially such lesions reveal patterns

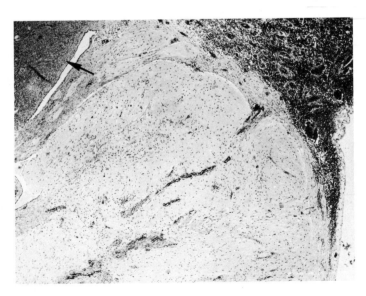

Figure 25–28. Mature neural tissue in lower part of section "implanted" on normal ovary (at arrow) found one year after removal of contralateral ovary for a teratoma containing immature neural tissue. (From Woodruff et al.: Ovarian Teratomas. Courtesy C. V. Mosby Co.)

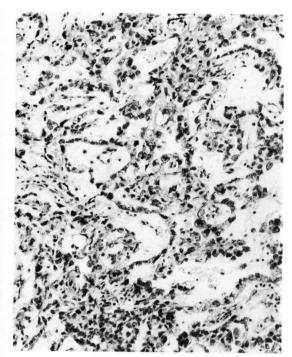

Figure 25–29. Typical endodermal sinus tumor with some resemblance to mesonephroma but showing characteristics noted by Teilum.

suggestive of the mesonephroid tumor (Fig. 25–29), and in Schiller's original publication on the ovarian mesonephroma, at least two of the tumors represent examples of the endodermal sinus teratoma. These lesions classi-

cally occur in the young female, the average age being approximately 16 to 17 years. Symptomatically most patients complain of abdominal pain, often acute, due to the rapidly growing tumor, with occasional torsion or rupture. In a few instances the mass has been noted on routine pelvic examination. The tumors grow extremely rapidly, and until the advent of triple chemotherapy, the only survivors were five patients in whom only unilateral adnexectomy had been performed. The use of VAC (vincristine, actinomycin D, and Cytoxan) in the pulse therapy regime has resulted in a few 5 year survivors and several patients living and well 2 or more years later. Rarely, if ever, are such extraembryonal teratomas bilateral, in contrast to the embryonal lesions; consequently, unless the tumor has spread, total pelvic "clean-out" is not indicated in such cases. This is in contrast to the relative frequency of bilaterality with embryonal teratomas.

The gross picture is that of a soft pultaceous tumor of grayish-brown color. Cystic areas due to degeneration are present in the rapidly growing lesions (Fig. 25–30). The capsule has been described as intact in a majority of cases (Stage IA); nevertheless, most patients have succumbed to the disease.

Microscopically, the characteristic feature is the endodermal sinus (Schiller-Duval body). The cystic space is lined by a layer of flattened or irregular endothelium into

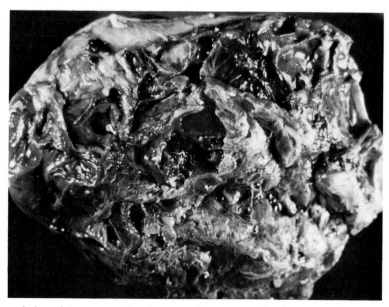

Figure 25–30. An endodermal sinus tumor. There is a general appearance of malignancy with focal areas of cystic necrosis.

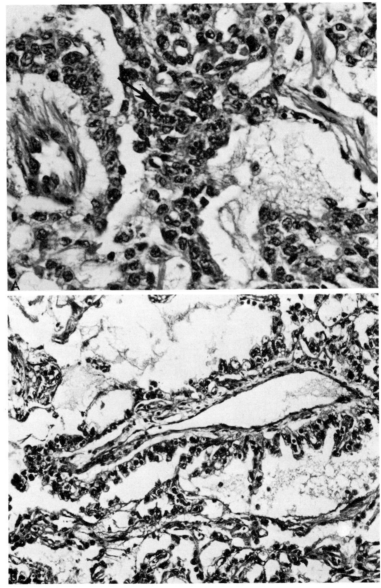

Figure 25–31. *A,* Endodermal sinus to left with "teratoid body" at arrow. Cells are poorly differentiated and mesoblastic(?) at center. *B,* Endodermal sinus cut longitudinally with central vessel and mantle of "endoderm" showing clear cells and hobnail cells.

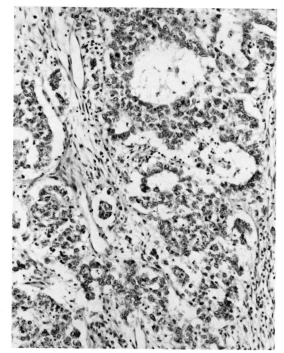

Figure 25–32. Extraembryonal teratoma with mesoblast and attempted formation of endodermal sinus.

which projects a glomerulus-like tuft with a central vascular core (Fig. 25–31 A,B). These structures vary throughout the tumor and the solid areas undoubtedly represent undifferentiated mesoblast (Fig. 25–32). The lining of the papillary infolding and the cavity is irregular with the occasional cell containing clear, glassy cytoplasm, simulating the hobnail appearance of the epithelium in the cystic structures of the mesonephroid tumors. In spite of this similarity, however, careful review of the section will reveal the classic features with the mesoblastic elements and the latter teratoid bodies (eosinophilic intracytoplasmic structures) frequently displacing the nuclei to the periphery of the cell (Fig. 25–33). Again the association of the teratoma with dysgerminoma must be emphasized if diagnosis and therapy are to be optimal (Fig. 25–34).

The marker for the endodermal sinus tumor is alpha fetoprotein (AFP). This can be demonstrated in the tumor by the use of immunoperoxidase staining, and in the patient by the determination of elevated serum AFP. Following surgical removal of the tumor, levels of AFP often disappear; however, reappearance of positive AFP is not sufficiently early to aid significantly in therapy, since the tumor is usually demonstrable clinically prior to laboratory documentation. It must be appreciated that levels of the marker (AFP) over the normal high of 20 ng/ml may be found in a variety of nonteratoid lesions. The patient with endodermal sinus tumor generally reveals higher titers than those with other ovarian tumors.

The yolk sac or polyvesicular vitelline tumor is rare and may be associated with the endodermal sinus lesion. This association is probably more common than appreciated, since the formation of the primary and secondary yolk sac may be quite bizarre and indefinite (Fig. 25–35). The associated mesoblast may be fibrous in appearance or quite immature and suggestive of poorly differen-

Figure 25–33. Endodermal sinus or yolk-sac tumor. Central tufting simulating the "glomerulus" structure, and often containing a small vessel—the endodermal sinus—is seen at the center and right border (arrowheads). Teratoid bodies in lower left at small arrows.

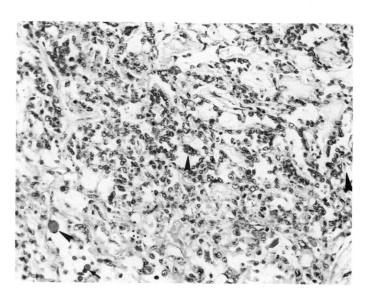

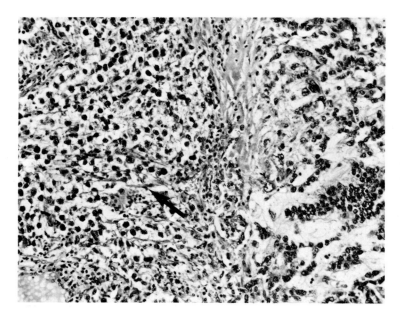

Figure 25–34. Endodermal sinus tumor on right with dysgerminoma at arrow.

tiated sarcoma. The prognosis is poor in such cases but with the advent of triple chemotherapy, improvement may be expected.

Included among the extraembryonal teratomas is the choriocarcinoma (Fig. 25–36). Although a few tumors composed solely of trophoblast have been reported, the majority show a variety of elements, some of which have matured. It is important to recognize that the classic cell by which trophoblast can be distinguished is the syncytial or mature element. The undifferentiated cytotrophoblast is quite difficult to evaluate, since although the cells in association with the syncytium seem quite diagnostic (Fig. 25–37), alone it is often indistinguishable from mesoblast. Thus, in some instances, a large ovarian tumor may be associated with a positive pregnancy test and yet histologically demonstrate none of the more mature and diagnostic trophoblastic elements.

Obviously the tumor marker in such cases

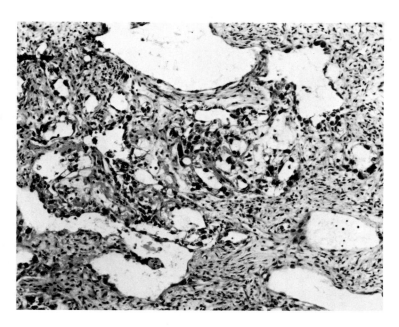

Figure 25–35. An extraembryonal teratoma—polyvesicular vitelline tumor. Bizarre attempt at the formation of a primary and secondary yolk sac. Trophoblast (?) in the center.

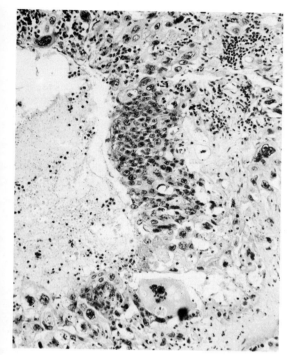

Figure 25–36. Teratoma with extraembryonic trophoblast. Both syncytium and cytotrophoblast are recognizable.

is chorionic gonadotropin (HCG) and, as with AFP, can be demonstrated by immunoperoxidase staining. Interestingly, AFP may also be positive in these tumors, suggesting the presence of other elements such as the endodermal sinus tumor. Again, it should be appreciated that both AFP and HCG may be found in association with tumors in which there are no apparent extraembryonal elements.

Recently the term *embryonal carcinoma* has been reintroduced into the classification of the ovarian teratomas. It is noteworthy that the definable element in such lesions by immunoperoxidase staining is HCG, thus suggesting that such elements are related to trophoblast, and histologically these tissue fragments resemble syncytial and cytotrophoblastic cells. These findings, plus the positive AFP marker in several cases, suggest that the tumor falls into the category of the extraembryonal teratomas. In a small series of cases, Kurman and Norris noted minor differences in the ages of the patients (16 years for endodermal sinus tumor and 18 years for embryonal carcinoma) and survival rates.

Finally, it must be noted that both mature and immature embryonal and extraembryonal elements may be present in the same tumor. It is of major importance, therefore, to investigate numerous sections in order to give an accurate prognosis in the individual case.

REFERENCES

Abell, M. R., and Holtz, F.: Ovarian tumors in childhood and adolescence II. Am. J. Obstet. Gynecol., 93:850, 1965.

Abell, M. R., Johnson, V. J., and Holtz, F.: Ovarian neoplasms in childhood and adolescence. Am. J. Obstet. Gynecol., 92:1059, 1965.

Abell, M. R., Johnson, V. J., and Holtz, F.: Dysgerminoma. Current opinions on clinical problems. Am. J. Obstet. Gynecol., 86:693, 1963.

Abitbol, M. M., Pomerance, W., and Mackles, A.: Spontaneous intraperitoneal rupture of benign cystic teratomas. Obstet. Gynecol., 13:198, 1959.

Alerover, R. L.: Squamous cell carcinoma arising in benign cystic teratoma of ovary. Am. J. Obstet. Gynecol., 65:1238, 1953.

Assadourian, L. A., and Taylor, H. B.: Dysgerminoma. Obstet. Gynecol., 33:370, 1969.

Blackwell, W. J., Dockerty, M. B., Masson, J. C., and Mussey, R. D.: Dermoid cysts of ovary; clinical and pathological significance. Am. J. Obstet. Gynecol., 51:151, 1946.

Blocksma, R.: Bilateral dysgerminoma with pseudohermaphroditism. Am. J. Obstet. Gynecol., 69:879, 1955.

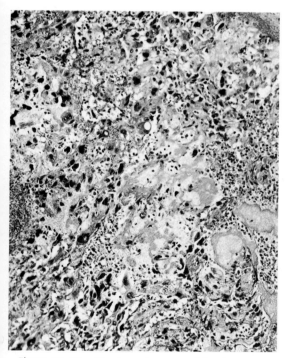

Figure 25–37. Choriocarcinoma evolving in teratoma. Many dark-staining syncytial cells with cytotrophoblast at right.

Booth, R. T.: Ovarian tumors in pregnancy. Obstet. Gynecol., 21:189, 1963.

Borushek, S., Berger, I., Echt, C., and Gold, J. J.: Functioning malignant germ cell tumor of the ovary in a 4½ year old girl. Cancer, 18:1485, 1965.

Breen, J. L., and Neubecker, R. D.: Malignant teratoma of the ovary. Obstet. Gynecol., 21:669, 1963.

Brody, S.: Clinical aspects of dysgerminoma of the ovary. Acta Radiol., 56:209, 1961.

Burgess, G. F., and Shutter, H. W.: Malignancy originating in ovarian dermoids. Obstet. Gynecol., 4:567, 1954.

Chalmers, J. A., and Kurrein, F.: A giant dermoid cyst. J. Obstet. Gynaecol. Br. Commonw., 68:315, 1961.

Chauser, B. M., Green, J. P., and Klein, H. Z.: Bilateral metachronous dysgerminoma with a 15-year interval. Cancer, 27:939, 1971.

DeLima, F. O. A.: Disgerminoma do ovario, contribucao para o seo estudo anatomo-clinico. São Paulo, Brazil, 1966.

Dominguez, C. J., and Greenblatt, R. B.: Dysgerminoma of the ovary in a patient with Turner's syndrome. Am. J. Obstet. Gynecol., 83:674, 1962.

Doss, N. E., Jr., Forney, J. P., Vellios, F., and Nalick, R. H.: Covert bilaterality of mature ovarian teratomas. Obstet. Gynecol., 50:651, 1977.

Danforth, D. N.: Endodermal sinus tumor. Obstet. Gynecol., 51:233, 1978.

DiSaia, P. J., et al.: Chemotherapeutic reconversion of immature teratoma. Obstet. Gynecol., 49:346, 1977.

Fortt, R. W., and Mathie, L. K.: Gliomatosis peritonei caused by ovarian teratomas. J. Clin. Pathol., 22:348, 1969.

Garcia-Bunuel, R., et al.: Luteomas of pregnancy. Obstet. Gynecol., 45:407, 1975.

Gerbie, M. V., et al.: Primary ovarian choriocarcinoma. Obstet. Gynecol., 46:720, 1975.

Goldstein, D. P., and Piro, A. J.: Combination chemotherapy in the treatment of germ cell tumors containing choriocarcinoma in males and females. Surg. Gynecol. Obstet., 134:61, 1972.

Groeber, W. R.: Ovarian tumors during infancy and childhood. Am. J. Obstet. Gynecol., 86:1027, 1963.

Heinz, H. A.: Investigations on the determination of the sex of dysgerminomas from the morphology of the cellular nuclei. Geburtshilfe Frauenheilkd., 21:144, 1961.

Hughesdon, P. E.: Structure, origin, and histological relationships of dysgerminoma. J. Obstet. Gynaecol. Br. Emp., 66:566, 1959.

Jakobovitz, A.: Hormone production by miscellaneous ovarian tumors. Am. J. Obstet. Gynecol., 85:90, 1963.

Jimerson, G. K.: Germ cell tumors of the ovary. Clin. Obstet. Gynecol., 17:229, 1974.

Jimerson, G. K., and Woodruff, J. D.: I. Endodermal sinus tumor. Am. J. Obstet. Gynecol., 127:73, 1977.

Jimerson, G. K., and Woodruff, J. D.: Ovarian extraembryonal tumor. Am. J. Obstet. Gynecol., 127:302, 1977.

Krepart, G., Smith, J. D., and Rutledge, F. N.: Treatment of dysgerminoma of the ovary. Cancer, 41:986, 1978.

Kurman, R. J., and Norris, H. J.: Endodermal sinus tumor of the ovary. Cancer, 38:2404, 1976.

Kurman, R. J., and Norris, H. J.: Embryonal carcinoma of the ovary. Cancer, 38:2420, 1976.

Kelley, R. R., and Scully, R. E.: Cancer developing in dermoid cysts of the ovary. Cancer, 16:989, 1960.

Liebert, K. I., and Stent, L.: Dysgerminoma of the ovary with chorion epithelioma. J. Obstet. Gynaecol. Br. Emp., 77:627, 1960.

Linder, D., and Power, J.: Further evidence for postmeiotic origin of teratomas in the human female. Ann. Hum. Genet., 34:21, 1970.

Malkasian, G. D., Jr., and Symmonds, R. E.: Treatment of unilateral encapsulated ovarian dysgerminoma. Am. J. Obstet. Gynecol., 90:379, 1964.

Meyer, R.: The pathology of some special ovarian tumors and their relation to sex characteristics. Am. J. Obstet. Gynecol., 22:697, 1931.

Mueller, C. W., Topkins, P., and Laff, W. A.: Dysgerminoma of ovary. An analysis of 427 cases. Am. J. Obstet. Gynecol., 60:153, 1950.

Norris, H. J., et al.: Immature teratoma of the ovary. Cancer, 37:2359, 1976.

Novak, E. R., et al.: Ovarian tumors in pregnancy. Obstet. Gynecol., 45:401, 1975.

Pedowitz, P., Felmus, L. B., and Grayzel, D. M.: Dysgerminoma of ovary. Am. J. Obstet. Gynecol., 70:1284, 1956.

Peterson, W. F.: Solid histologically benign teratomas of the ovary. Am. J. Obstet. Gynecol., 72:1094, 1956.

Peterson, W. F.: Malignant degeneration of benign cystic teratomas of ovary. Collective review of literature. Obstet. Gynecol. Surv., 12:793, 1957.

Robboy, S. J., et al.: Primary trabecular carcinoid of the ovary. Obstet. Gynecol., 49:202, 1977.

Roth, L. M., and Sternberg, W. H.: Proliferating Brenner ovarian tumors. Cancer, 27:687, 1971.

Sandenbergh, H. A., and Woodruff, J. D.: Pseudomyxoma peritonei. Obstet. Gynecol., 49:339, 1977.

Schellhas, H. F., Trujilo, J. M., Rutledge, F. N., and Cork, A.: Germ cell tumors associated with XY gonadal dysgenesis. Am. J. Obstet. Gynecol., 109:1197, 1971.

Schiller, W.: Mesonephroma ovarii. Am. J. Cancer 35:1, 1939.

Scully, R. E.: Gonadoblastoma. Cancer, 6:455, 1953.

Scully, R. E.: Gonadoblastoma. A review of 74 cases. Cancer, 25:1340, 1971.

Sherrer, C. W., Gerson, B., and Woodruff, J. D.: The incidence and significance of polynuclear follicles. Am. J. Obstet. Gynecol., 128:6, 1977.

Sirsat, M. V., Vakil, V. V., Motashaw, N. D., and Talwakan, G. V.: Gonadoblastoma of the ovary. Indian J. Pathol. Bacteriol., 8:77, 1965.

Smith, A. H., and Ward, S. V.: Dysgerminoma in pregnancy. Obstet. Gynecol., 28:502, 1966.

Sternberg, W. H., and Roth, L. M.: Stromal ovarian tumors with Leydig cells. I. Cancer, 32:940, 1973.

Talerman, A.: Gonadoblastoma and dysgerminoma in two siblings with dysgenetic gonads. Obstet. Gynecol., 38:416, 1971.

Taylor, H., Barter, R. H., and Jacobson, C. B.: Neoplasms of dysgenetic gonads. Am. J. Obstet. Gynecol., 96:816, 1966.

Teilum, G.: Homologous tumors in ovary and testis. Acta Obstet. Gynecol. Scand., 24:480, 1944.

Teilum, G.: Endodermal sinus tumors of the ovary and testis. Cancer, 12:1092, 1959.

Teilum, G.: Classification of endodermal sinus tumor and so-called embryonal carcinoma of the ovary. Acta Path. Microbiol. Scand., 64:407, 1965.

Teter, J.: A new concept of classification of gonadal tumors arising from germ cells (gonocytoma) and their histogenesis. Int. Monthly Rev. Obstet. Gynecol., 150:84, 1960.

Teter, J.: A mixed form of feminizing germ cell tumor (gonocytoma). Am. J. Obstet. Gynecol., 84:722, 1962.

Thoeny, R. H., Dockerty, M. B., Hunt, A. B., and Childs, D. S., Jr.: Study of ovarian dysgerminoma with emphasis on the role of radiation therapy. Surg. Gynecol. Obstet., 113:692, 1961.

Thurlbeck, W. M., and Scully, R. E.: Solid teratoma of the ovary. Cancer, 13:804, 1960.

Watson, S. L.: Dysgerminoma complicating labor. Am. J. Obstet. Gynecol., 72:1177, 1956.

Woodruff, J. D., and Markley, R. L.: Struma ovarii. Obstet. Gynecol., 9:707, 1957.

Woodruff, J. D., Rauh, J. T., and Markley, R. L.: Ovarian struma. Obstet. Gynecol., 27:194, 1966.

Woodruff, J. D., Protos, P., and Peterson, W. F.: Ovarian teratomas. Relationship of histologic and ontogenic factors to prognosis. Am. J. Obstet. Gynecol., 102:702, 1968.

Woodruff, J. D., et al.: Mucinous cystadenocarcinoma. Obstet. Gynecol., 51:483, 1978.

Chapter 26

GONADAL STROMAL TUMORS— FEMINIZING (GRANULOSA AND THECA CELL)

HISTOGENESIS

Some idea of the early embryology of the ovary is essential for an understanding of the histogenesis of this group of tumors. This has been discussed in Chapter 17, although it must be understood that many phases of early gonadal development are not clearly defined by embryologists.

We believe that both the theca and the granulosa cell evolve from the mesenchyme, and that the germinal (coelomic) epithelium plays no determining role, as was suggested earlier by Gillman. Whether the originating cell in granulosa-theca cell tumors is a reserve cell, as indicated by Warner and associates, or an adult cortical stromal cell, as suggested by Sternberg and Gaskill, seems of only academic importance. From this common mesenchymal stem cell arise various epithelial (granulosal) and connective tissue (thecal) elements, and various admixtures of both are present in most feminizing tumors, which seems further proof of a common ancestry. Hence, we suspect that the *ovarian stromal cell* may be stimulated to tumorogenesis and steroid function of diverse types, as has been noted frequently with certain nonendocrine tumors with a functioning matrix and an observed hormonal effect (see Chapter 27).

This concept has replaced the older concept of Meyer, who postulated that granulosa cell tumors arise from rests of redundant granulosa cells (granulosaballen) left over in the process of follicle formation. Such rests

(Fig. 26–1) may be found at times in the ovaries of young children, and even occasionally in those of adult women. However, this affords no explanation for the histogenesis of the other type of feminizing tumor, which may occur as a discrete thecoma but is more frequently associated with granulosa

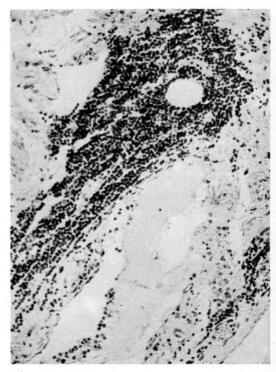

Figure 26–1. Granulosa cell rest in ovary of young adult woman.

504

cell elements. Failure to adequately explain these thecomatous changes seems to afford a serious challenge to Meyer's concept.

Experimental evidence is afforded by the studies of Geist and his co-workers, as well as others, who produced granulosa cell and thecal cell tumors at different phases following radiation of rodents. This method of approach to the problem seems to offer possibilities in determining the origin of similar tumors occurring spontaneously in the human female. In any case, the proposal by McKay and others (originally promulgated in 1930 by Robinson) that granulosa and theca cell tumors arise from blighted atretic follicles has met with little general enthusiasm.

It seems preferable to utilize a single term to adequately designate the various combinations of granulosa and theca cells that make up this type of tumor. In view of the mesenchymal origin of both cell types, the term *mesenchymoma* was coined by Ingram and Novak. The term *gonadal stromal* tumor is equally descriptive and perhaps less tongue-twisting. Because many functioning ovarian tumors of the endocrine-secreting variety probably originate from the mesenchyme or stroma, either term should be appropriate.

Previous editions of this text have always emphasized that the histologic appearance of any tumor should be the criterion for diagnosis. Today, however, there is increased recognition of the impossibility of adequate correlation of tumor morphology and endocrine effect. Typical examples are the characteristic folliculoid granulosa cell tumor with well studied androgenic function (Giuntoli et al.), or the typical hilus cell tumor with an estrogenic effect (Goodwin et al.). Therefore, because many of these lesions evolve from mesenchyme, there is a growing tendency to utilize such generic names as *mesenchymoma* or *gonadal stromal tumor*, qualified by such terms as *feminizing, virilizing,* and *inert,* as the case may be. This should be regarded as a realistic appraisal of the difficulties inherent in distinguishing between certain histologically similar tumors rather than as a defeatist complex. Indeed, the next generation may consider such designations as granulosa or theca cell tumor and arrhenoblastoma to be archaic; nor is it necessary to consider these tumors as dysontogenetic, since they *may* originate from mature gonadal stroma. This

is discussed more fully at the end of Chapter 27.

At present, we shall adhere to the time-honored designation of granulosa-theca cell tumor, which implies an almost inevitable admixture of epithelial and connective tissue elements, although relatively pure forms may be found. Falck has adequately demonstrated that only the theca cell produces estrogen, and that even predominantly granulosa cell tumors are estrogenic because of the invariable presence of theca cells. Fathalla suggests that the ovarian stromal cells are stimulated to produce estrogen by adjacent neoplastic granulosal or thecal cells; however, we have seen recurrent tumor following ablation of all ovarian tissue with evidence of profound estrogen excretion.

At the same time it seems expedient to subdivide these tumors in the subsequent paragraphs as if they were distinct and separate entities. Indeed, the architecture of predominantly granulosa cell or thecomatous neoplasms exhibits such an astounding variety of patterns that it might lead to confusion if they were all grouped under a single heading. Every conceivable combination of epithelioid and connective tissue pattern may be present in a single feminizing mesenchymoma (or gonadal stromal tumor).

PATHOLOGY OF GRANULOSA CELL TUMOR

Gross Characteristics

There are wide variations in size of the granulosa cell tumors that have been reported (Fig. 26–2). The smallest have been only a few millimeters in size, although others have filled the abdominal cavity, weighing approximately 69 kg. (150 lb.) (Robertson and Miller), considerably larger than the 15 kg. (34 lb.) tumor noted earlier by Dockerty, or the 20 kg. (44 lb.) thecoma reported by Krieger. As a rule, the tumors are almost always unilateral, are rarely larger than a grapefruit, and are more or less ovoid or kidney-shaped, with a smooth outer surface, though often lobulated (Fig. 26–3). On cut section, the tumors may be solid, especially if they are small, or they may show one or many cystic cavities (Fig. 26–4). The latter are usually of moderate size but may be very large. The solid portions of the tumor are granular, frequently trabeculated, and often

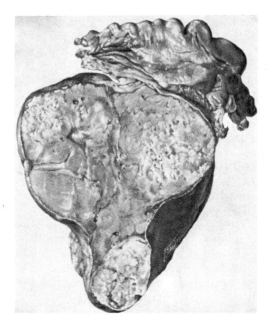

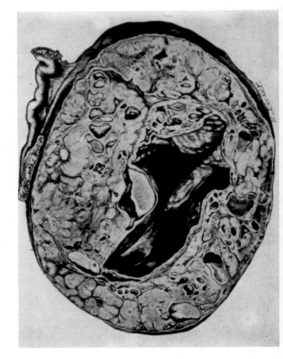

Figure 26–2. Gross appearance of granulosa cell carcinoma of the ovary.

Figure 26–3. Gross appearance of granulosa cell carcinoma with cystic and hemorrhagic degeneration.

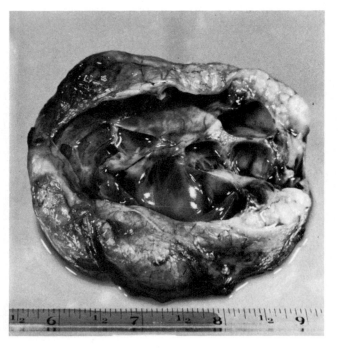

Figure 26–4. Feminizing granulosa–theca cell tumor in 2 year old girl. (Courtesy of Dr. John Updegrove, Easton, Pa.)

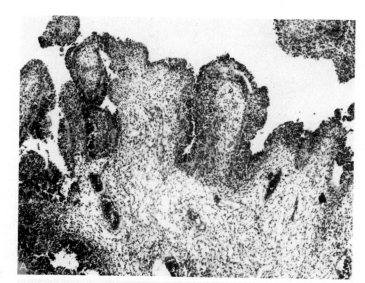

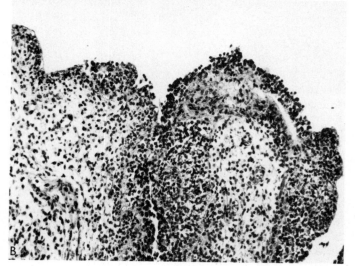

Figure 26–5. *A*, Rare papillary cystic lesion (note lining granulosa cells). *B*, Higher magnification of *A*.

show areas of yellowish hue. Recently we have seen a few primary cystic papillary lesions (Fig. 26–5). Norris and Chorlton have suggested that these may be associated with virilism, but we have not been impressed by this association.

Microscopic Characteristics

The extreme variability of the microscopic pattern is chiefly responsible for the confusion of nomenclature and classification of a number of ovarian tumors. Indeed, certain tumors of a seemingly sarcoma-like pattern, with little or no resemblance to granulosal tissue, must apparently be classed under this head. In the great majority of cases, the morphologic resemblance of the constituent cells to granulosa cells and the evidences of growth characteristics identical to those of granulosal tissue constitute the most important criteria for diagnosis.

The variability of microscopic patterns exhibited not only by different tumors but also by one tumor in different parts makes it very important to study numerous blocks, with multiple sections, to derive a comprehensive impression of the tumor. In perhaps the most common variety, the granulosa cells show a prevailing tendency to arrange themselves in small clusters or rosettes around a central lumen, so that there is a resemblance to primordial follicles (Fig. 26–6).

At times, large masses of granulosa cells may be seen surrounded by a theca-like capsule of stroma. Often there are found in these

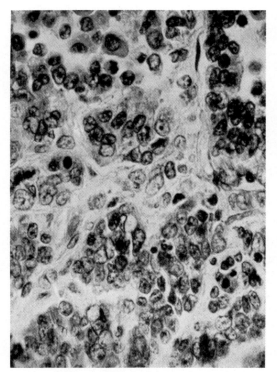

Figure 26–6. High power view of granulosa cell carcinoma showing tendency to formation of small clusters and rosettes.

epithelial masses numerous small areas of cystic liquefaction, resembling the Call-Exner bodies characteristic of granulosa cells in general (Fig. 26–7). The cells around the small cystic cavities are frequently arranged in a curious antipodal fashion, the nuclei of the inner layer being placed close to the central lumen, those of the outer layer away from it, toward the periphery. Between the two there may be only a thin zone of degenerated cytoplasm, or there may be a number of layers of well-preserved cells.

The content of the cystic cavities often superficially resembles the primordial egg, with which it was commonly confused by earlier writers. It is now generally agreed that it represents a degenerative liquefying process as with other types of ovarian cancer. Occasionally there may be a large central cystic cavity surrounded by perhaps many layers of granulosa, so that there is a decided resemblance to large graafian follicles (*folliculoma malignum*) (Fig. 26–8). In still other cases, the cystic cavities may again be large but with perhaps only a thin layer of granulosal epithelium. Rarely, the whole tumor may be cystic.

While a great many histologic patterns

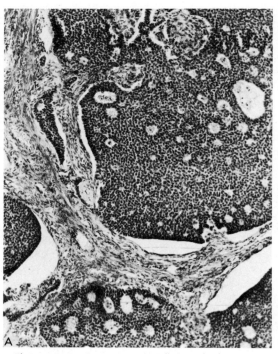

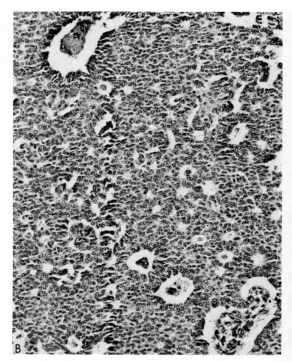

Figure 26–7. *A*, Numerous Call-Exner bodies are present in this folliculoid tumor. *B*, Higher magnification. Note the tendency to the formation of cystic spaces, with surrounding rosette-like arrangement of cells.

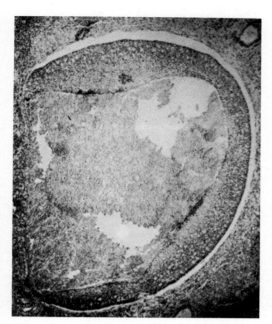

Figure 26–8. Folliculoma malignum type of granulosa cell carcinoma.

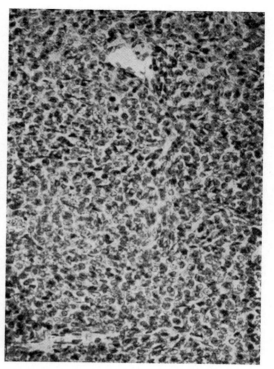

Figure 26–9. Diffuse variety of granulosa cell carcinoma.

have been described, most granulosa cell tumors present as predominantly (a) folliculoid, (b) diffuse, (c) cylindroid, or (d) pseudo-adenomatous, with a frequent admixture. *Folliculoid* tumors may exhibit either a finely follicular (*microfolliculoid*) appearance resembling primitive follicles or a *macrofolliculoid* picture like that of large mature follicles, with either solidly epithelial, cystic, or partly cystic content. Occasionally granulosa cell tumors present large diffuse fields of granulosa cells, with often no suggestion of a folliculoid pattern, so that this variety may well be spoken of as the *diffuse* or *parenchymatous* type (Fig. 26–9).

Where the folliculoid pattern is exaggerated the growth may even present a distinctly *pseudo-adenomatous* appearance, the thin epithelial strands showing an involved arrangement resembling adenoma (Fig. 26–10). In any of these types one often finds long cordlike or tubular columns, sometimes resembling the sex cords of early gonadal development, but often distinguished by a characteristic palisade-like arrangement of the epithelial cells.

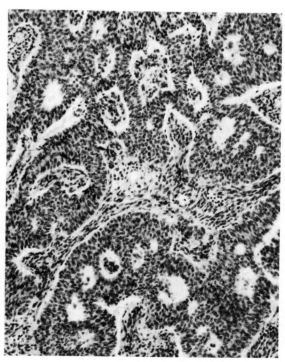

Figure 26–10. Pseudo-adenomatous pattern of granulosa cell carcinoma.

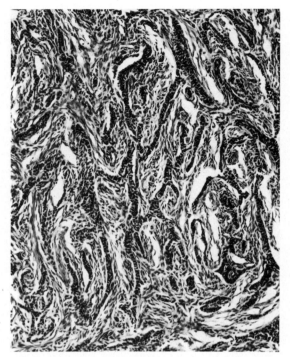

Figure 26–11. Cylindroid type of granulosa cell carcinoma.

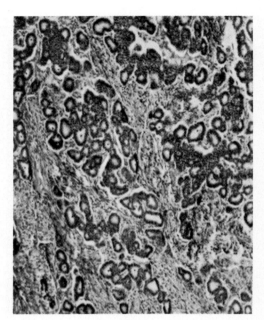

Figure 26–12. Rare tubular type of granulosa cell carcinoma, similar to Sertoli cell tumor. (This must be considered an uncertain entity.)

A very common pattern is produced by connective tissue invasion of the granulosal masses, producing the tumor type which has been designated as *cylindroid* (Fig. 26–11). This type is characterized by a splitting up of the epithelial masses into cylinders or columns of various sizes, often anastomosing with each other. It is usual to find some evidence of connective tissue overgrowth, with hyaline degeneration, in granulosa cell carcinoma, and the extent of this accounts for many of the variations presented by these tumors. The *cylindroid* pattern, therefore, is extremely common. All sorts of bizarre patterns may be encountered. In some cases the invasive connective tissue overgrowth splits up the epithelium into narrow zigzag cords, and in still other instances the epithelial growth presents the appearance of an elaborate scrollwork.

A rare variety of tumor generally included in the granulosa group is the *folliculoma lipidique* described by Lecène in 1910. Such tumors are of tubular or adenomatous (Fig. 26–12) pattern, the tubules being lined by clear-looking cells of low columnar type, which on differential staining are seen to be

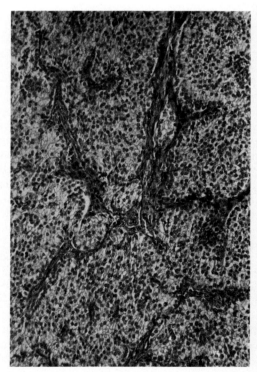

Figure 26–13. Folliculoma lipidique of solid consistency although generally of tubular pattern. (Ovarian Tumor Registry consensus.)

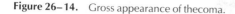

Figure 26–14. Gross appearance of thecoma.

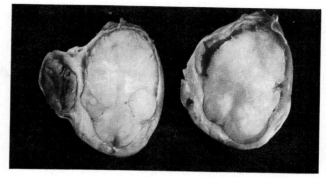

rich in lipid (Fig. 26–13). Teilum believes that this tumor type is homologous with the Sertoli cell tumor of the testis, which like the folliculoma lipidique produces estrogen, but there is still uncertainty as to the exact nature of the latter and its relation to other types of granulosal tumor. More will be said about Teilum's analogy between certain ovarian and testicular tumors, including their hormonal properties, in Chapter 27.

Scully has described certain tubular lipid sex cord tumors (which may bear a great resemblance to folliculoma lipidique) with associated *intestinal polyps* and *melanin spots* on the oral mucosa and skin: the so-called *Peutz-Jeghers* syndrome, which may have a familial basis. Another study, by Dozois, suggests that the ovarian tumor noted in this syndrome is not necessarily a sex cord tumor, but may be a simple cystic lesion instead. Christian, quoting various embryologic works, suggests that granulosa cells may evolve from certain endodermal sources. Some uncertain defect leads to both intestinal and gonadal tumors, although testicular lesions have not been a part of this syndrome.

PATHOLOGY OF THECOMA

Gross Characteristics

In a considerable proportion of cases, a fibroma-like character may be given to the histologic picture by the presence of many connective tissue elements. It is to this fibroma-like group that the term thecoma has been applied. Such tumors are commonly firm and fibrous, although they may, like the granulosal variety, show a tendency to cystic degeneration. They are often of yellowish hue (Fig. 26–14), and are usually unilateral.

Microscopic Characteristics

Microscopically, they are described as distinguished especially by the presence of broad spindle cells, which are epithelioid in appearance, distributed in an irregular interlacing manner throughout the tumor, and separated by varying sized bands of connective tissue and often hyaline plaques (Fig. 26–15). Actually, they are almost identical to fibroma, and frequently the only clue to their identity is the suggestion of clinical estrogen effect. This should, of course, suggest a fat stain which may show the presence of much

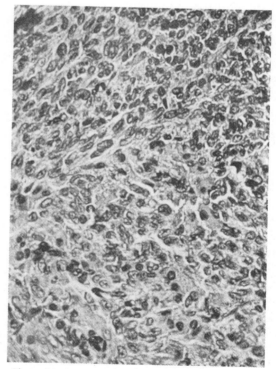

Figure 26–15. Microscopic appearance of thecomatous type of tumor shown in Figure 26–14.

doubly refractile fat within the cells and to a lesser extent in the surrounding connective tissue, although there is invariably an admixture of fibrous tissue cells.

In these thecal tumors, however, one often finds areas of what are apparently definite granulosal cells, so that one must question the advisability of too sharp a division between the granulosal and thecal tumors, especially in view of their identical endocrine effects. This belief is further supported by studies of the reticulum of thecal and granulosal tumors by using the Foot silver stain, as suggested by Traut and colleagues. These authors found that in the well-differentiated or folliculomatous type of granulosa cell tumors, both granulosal and thecal elements are present, and the same thing is true of thecomas.

Diverse patterns may be found in different parts of the same tumor, and mingling of epithelial and connective tissue elements is frequent, lending support to the concept of a common origin from the ovarian mesenchyme. In some cases there may be difficulty in distinguishing thecoma from fibroma. In the latter the connective tissue cells are often longer, with considerable intercellular tissue, although in the more cellular fibromas the cells are spindle shaped, like those of unstriped muscle. The cells of thecoma are ordinarily of a plumper, fusiform type, and it is common to find an admixture of apparent granulosal elements. Fat stains are usually necessary for distinction. The so-called *sclerosing stromal tumor*, as described by Chalvardjian and Scully, seems a rather uncertain entity but is apparently closely related to a luteinized stromal neoplasm.

DIFFUSE THECOSIS

A considerable number of authors believe that when a thecoma is present in one ovary, there is apt to be a diffuse thec(omat)osis (or stromal hyperplasia) in the contralateral ovary (Fig. 26–16). This ovarian stromal hyperplasia seems disproportionately common in ovaries in which the endometrium has been afflicted by adenocarcinoma.

Many authors, such as Woll and co-workers, Novak and Mohler, and Schneider and Bechtel, have been impressed with the possible importance of thecosis in the production of or in association with fundal, breast,

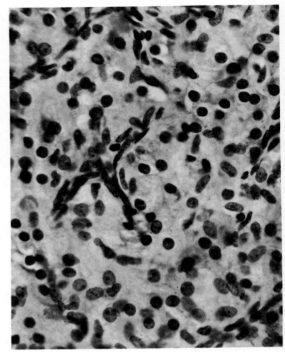

Figure 26–16. Postmenopausal stromal hyperplasia or thecomatosis (thecosis). The stromal cells, normally small, dark, and spindly, are plump, show a pale cytoplasm with an ovoid nucleus, and appear indistinguishable from theca cells.

and (to quote Sommers and co-workers) many types of female cancer. The possible relation of ovarian stromal hyperplasia and endometrial adenocarcinoma is discussed more fully in Chapter 9.

A generalized diffuse hyperplasia of the theca or ovarian stromal cell is observed with a variety of gynecologic pathologic problems. It may be quite apparent with the Stein-Leventhal syndrome, along with a thick fibrotic hyalinized cortex, an absence of corpora lutea, and many follicles in all stages of maturation and atresia with proliferation of the theca interna. It is felt by many that the theca cell may be androgenic and responsible for the hirsutism, oligo-amenorrhea, clitoral enlargement, and other virilizing features noted on occasion with polycystic ovarian disease. Givens and associates suggest that there may be a familial tendency to hyperthecosis.

On other occasions the theca cell may seem associated with an estrogenic stimulus, as with thecoma or diffuse thecosis, in association with a postmenopausal hyperplasia or endometrial adenocarcinoma. Shippel, however, in an exhaustive series of studies, suggests an androgenic form of stimulation.

It would seem that the stromal cell may be activated to various types of steroid production by a number of unknown stimuli, as may occur with certain ovarian tumors not classically associated with endocrine production. An estrogen, androgen, or even a progesterone influence may occur with various tumors with a functioning matrix, and we can only speculate as to why any certain steroid is produced. There is, however, so little difference in the biochemical structures involved as to make it seem reasonable to assume that many types of steroids may be produced, with one particular form dominating and leading to any observed clinical effect. Aiman and associates have recorded a marked increase in ovarian androgens with hyperthecosis.

That ovarian thecosis may occur in the adrenal gland has been reported by Wong and Warner and by Warner and associates. Embryologically these glands are in close juxtaposition, and adrenal rests are observed in the ovary on occasion. There is less frequent opportunity to review the adrenal gland from a pathologic standpoint, but it would seem that theca lutein cells may be present in the region of the adrenal. This would seem at least a possible site for extra-ovarian estrogen, even in the postmenopausal woman.

LUTEINIZATION OF GRANULOSA CELL TUMORS AND THECOMAS

Another interesting histologic characteristic of this tumor type is that the constituent granulosa or theca cells may at times undergo a transformation into what are evidently typical lutein cells. We have seen a considerable group in which such a transformation is in progress, so that parts of the tumor have a luteinized appearance, although others are still typically granulosa-theca. In the occasional case the entire tumor is thus transformed.

We believe the classification of *luteoma* (except with pregnancy) should be completely discarded, for most tumors so diagnosed belong properly under other classifications. Furthermore, the term luteoma suggests an origin from a lutein cell and it seems that such an evanescent and temporary structure would be an unlikely source

of tumor formation. Many such lesions should properly be indexed under meso-nephroma, hilus cell, or adrenal tumor; when a lutein cell appearance occurs with a suggestive granulosal pattern, the term *luteinized granulosa-theca tumor* seems preferable.

In at least a small group of this latter type, progesterone effects upon the endometrium have been noted in such transformed tumors, differing from the purely estrogenic effects that characterize granulosa cell tumors in general (Fig. 26–17, *A,B*). In other luteinized tumors, it seems that the cells may be morphologically but not functionally like lutein cells, and that they are perhaps better spoken of as pseudolutein rather than lutein cells.

When a progestational or decidual pattern is found in the endometrium of a young girl, the realistic gynecologist should wonder if she has gained access to her mother's birth control pills. Several such cases have been noted in our own community.

EFFECTS OF GRANULOSA CELL TUMORS AND THECOMAS ON ENDOMETRIUM

When granulosa cell tumors develop in the postmenopausal years, as they so often do, the endometrium may exhibit proliferative activity as a result of the stimulation by the estrogen produced by the tumor. Characteristically this appears as a typical Swiss-cheese hyperplasia, but in some cases the hyperplastic pattern is absent in spite of the obvious proliferative picture, which in such cases is apt to resemble the interval phase of the endometrium in younger women.

When this frequent association of hyperplasia with granulosa cell tumors was first noted, it was generally believed that the finding of hyperplasia on curetting the postmenopausal woman was at least a priori evidence that a granulosa cell tumor or thecoma was present in the ovary, even though it might not be palpable. Today it would seem that no such assumption is justified, because of the frequent occurrence of postmenopausal hyperplasia in the absence of any overt ovarian pathology or exogenous hormones. However, if the hyperplasia shows an adenomatous pattern, laparotomy deserves strong consideration because of a potential progression to endometrial adenocar-

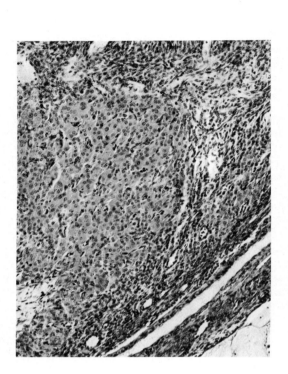 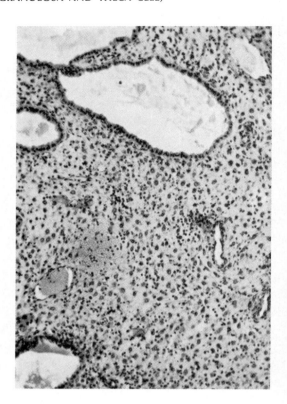

Figure 26–17. *A*, Thecoma with lutein-like transformation in central area. *B*, Decidual reaction produced by tumor in 5 year old girl with precocious puberty.

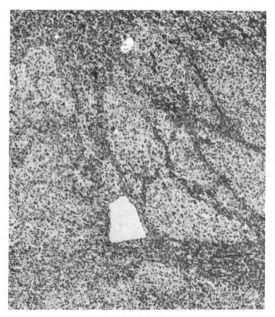 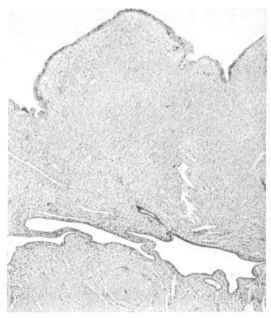

Figure 26–18. Granulosa cell carcinoma with partial luteinization of the tumor.

Figure 26–19. Decidual transformation of endometrium in association with tumor shown in Figure 26–18.

cinoma, especially if vaginal cytology and Maturation Index show a sustained shift to the right (in the absence of exogenous hormone therapy).

When the granulosal or thecal tumor has undergone partial or complete luteinization, one might expect to find evidences of a progesterone effect upon the endometrium, and, as a matter of fact, typical secretory endometria or even a decidual reaction has been observed in a few such cases, as already mentioned (Figs. 26–18 and 26–19). In most cases of luteinized tumors, however, the endometrium has failed to show progesterone effects, suggesting that the transformed tumor cells resemble lutein cells morphologically but not functionally.

LUTEOMA OF PREGNANCY

Sternberg and Barclay described a pregnancy luteoma as an ovarian enlargement (up to 12 cm.), which is generally solid, composed of eosinophilic, polyhedral cells, which are not a part of the corpus luteum of pregnancy, and may on occasion be bilateral (Fig 26–20). It originally was not certain whether this was a true neoplasm or merely a physiologic response to pregnancy.

Our impression is that they represent merely a profoundly exaggerated physiologic response of the ovary to the increased endocrine stimulus of gestation, and are similar to the theca lutein cysts or hyperreactio luteinalis seen with trophoblastic disease and (rarely) normal pregnancy. The *pregnancy luteoma,* however, is predominantly solid rather than cystic. It may be extremely difficult to exclude a hilus cell tumor on a purely morphologic basis, although the concomitant pregnancy and absence of Reinke crystalloids is helpful. Many of the cases of pregnancy luteoma have been associated with virilization of the mother or female fetus, or both. In a recent study of 20 cases, Garcia-Bunuel found evidence of masculinization in 40 per cent, although the cause is highly uncertain.

Most of these lesions regress spontaneously even after such inconclusive treatment as biopsy, which would further indicate a physiologic rather than a neoplastic origin. However, Barclay and co-workers report a case in which the lutein enlargement increased post partum and necessitated surgery (Fig. 26–21). We can only speculate whether true neoplasia followed a physiologic advent. It would seem, however, that most cases represent a mere response of the stromal cell to HCG, and we suspect that minor degrees of this "pseudo tumor" are often undiagnosed and occur frequently. More liberal abortion and sterilization statutes have allowed observation of many more pregnant uteri and ovaries, and it is apparent that focal stromal luteinization is common. This seems a logical stepping-stone to the

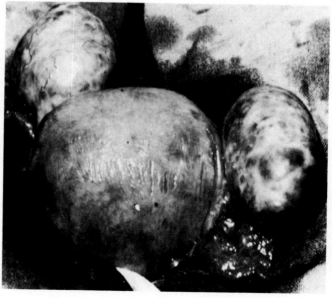

Figure 26–20. Bilateral ovarian enlargement with pregnant uterus—pregnancy luteoma. (Courtesy of Dr. D. L. Barclay, New Orleans, La.)

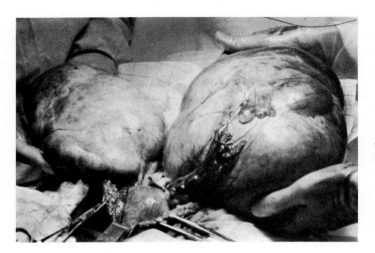

Figure 26–21. Massive postpartum lutein enlargement of ovaries that did not regress six weeks post partum. (Courtesy of Dr. D. L. Barclay, New Orleans, La.)

multinodular luteoma of pregnancy (Fig. 26–22).

ASSOCIATION OF ENDOMETRIAL ADENOCARCINOMA WITH FEMINIZING TUMORS

Of great interest is the fact that a considerable number of cases have been reported in which granulosa or theca cell tumors are associated with adenocarcinoma of the uterus, at once suggesting the possible predisposing role of the ovarian tumor in the production of the uterine carcinoma.

Various investigators have found that 15 to

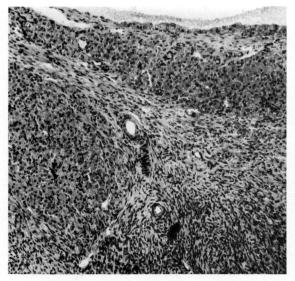

Figure 26–22. Note luteinization theca of follicle (at top) and lutein changes in stroma (lower left). Possible precursor to luteoma of pregnancy.

27 per cent of postmenopausal women with feminizing tumors of the ovary develop fundal carcinoma, although Stage and Grafton report a less than 10 per cent incidence. This association emphasizes the probable predisposing role of postmenopausal estrogen stimulation of the endometrium in the development of cancer, for the occurrence of these steroid-producing tumors and endometrial adenocarcinoma is much more frequent than the laws of chance would permit.

An interesting observation is that thecoma apparently exerts a much stronger carcinogenic effect on the endometrium than does granulosa cell carcinoma. In our own recent study of feminizing gonadal stromal tumors from the Ovarian Tumor Registry (414 cases, of which we studied the last 307 exclusively), it was possible to review the endometrium adequately in only 79 cases. Adenocarcinoma was present in 23 per cent of the cases, and hyperplasia in an additional 65 per cent, so that 88 per cent of the endometria studied showed evidence of an estrogen effect. Although thecomas were only slightly more common than granulosa cell tumors in our series, an abnormal endometrium occurred three times more commonly with a theca than with a granulosa cell lesion (Fig. 26–23). As noted in Chapter 9, the endometrial cancer patients with feminizing tumors seemingly have an improved prognosis.

The publication by Gusberg and Kardon concerning 115 patients with feminizing ovarian tumors where there was available endometrium reveals carcinoma in 21 per cent and cancer precursors in 43 per cent. The latter includes adenomatous hyperplasia and carcinoma in situ.

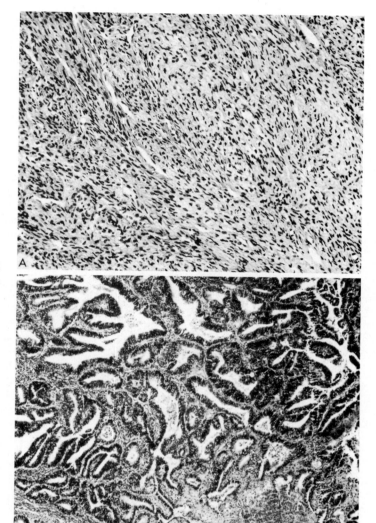

Figure 26–23. *A*, Well-differentiated benign fibrothecoma (positive fat stains). *B*, Associated endometrial adenocarcinoma.

EXPERIMENTAL PRODUCTION OF GRANULOSAL AND THECAL TUMORS

One of the most interesting developments of past years regarding this group of tumors is the demonstration of the possibility of their experimental production. Mention has been made that a number of investigators, especially Furth and Butterworth, have been able to produce granulosa cell tumors by light irradiation in mice (Fig. 26–24). At least two cases have been reported (Traut and Butterworth, McKay and co-workers) of the development of thecomas in previously irradiated patients, though such scattered observations have little statistical value, and clini-

cal evidence is against any assumption of such a hazard of irradiation.

Perhaps even more provocative are the results of ovarian transplantation experiments, which have been reported by Biskind and Biskind as well as Li and associates. After castration of mice, one of the ovaries is implanted in the spleen, so that the ovarian estrogen is carried through the portal circulation to the liver, where it is inactivated. Granulosa cell tumors, often luteinized (Figs. 26–24 to 26–26), are produced in the transplanted ovary, presumably because of the unopposed effect of pituitary gonadotropins upon the ovary. That tumors of this sort may be due to such endocrine imbalance introduces a new concept and suggests

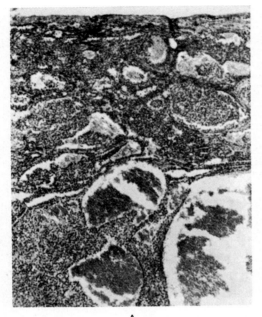

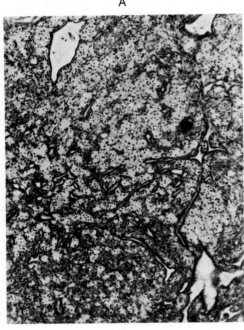

Figure 26–24. *A*, Granulosa cell tumor of mouse produced by irradiation. *B*, Luteinized granulosa cell tumor of mouse.

a continuance of such experimental studies, but it is too early to justify anything more than conjecture.

CLINICAL CHARACTERISTICS

Granulosa-theca tumors of the ovary may be considered a fairly common tumor, comprising probably about 10 per cent of all solid malignant ovarian neoplasms. On the other hand this represents the most common ovarian tumor in the canine and bovine species, as noted in the intriguing study of the animal ovary by Uyttenbroeck. These tumors may occur at any age—before puberty, during the reproductive epoch, or after the menopause. Although the larger tumors, like other ovarian neoplasms, may cause such symptoms as pain or discomfort, the more distinctive symptomatology is dependent upon the capability of the tumor cells to produce the estrogenic hormone. There have been, however, a considerable number of granulosa cell tumors in which rupture of the capsule has occurred, with massive intraperitoneal bleeding similar to tubal pregnancy, as noted by Gondos and Monroe. Such accidents have been reported in association with pregnant patients or very young children.

When the tumor occurs during reproductive life, as it does in a large proportion of cases, the clinical syndrome is not as striking as when it occurs against the background of the prepubertal or postmenopausal phases, during which there is normally little or no estrogen in the circulation. During the reproductive years, on the other hand, the tumor merely adds quantitatively to the cyclic hormonal content of the blood. No change would be expected in the secondary sex characters, for example, because these have long since been developed, although the effect upon menstruation would be merely a quantitative one, like that which characterizes the relative hyperestrinism that is associated with most cases of functional bleeding. Hyperestrinism may be associated with normal menstruation, with hypermenorrhea, or with long periods of amenorrhea, and these varying effects upon menstruation are noted with granulosa cell carcinoma. Tables 26–1, 26–2, and 26–3 illustrate our own findings in a recent study of 307 cases of granulosa-theca cell tumors. Twenty-seven cases of pregnancy associated with granulosa-theca cell tumors have been tabulated by Gillibrand, and in a recent review of 100 Ovarian Tumor Registry cases of pregnancy with associated ovarian cancer, 11 per cent were granulosa-thecal in type.

Creasman and associates concur that with Clinical Stage Ia germ cell or stromal tumors, *conservative (unilateral) operation* with preservation of the (pregnant) uterus is feasible. Although unilateral salpingo-oophorectomy is permissible in the young female,

Table 26–1 TYPE OF TUMOR—307 PATIENTS

Type	Incidence	Associated Lesions with All 307 Cases
Granulosa	71 (23%)	Thecosis (17)
Thecoma	87 (29%)	(9 cases bilateral)
Granulosa-theca	114 (37 %)	4 breast carcinoma 6 other carcinoma
Luteinized granulosa-theca	35 (11%)	
Total	307	

Table 26–3 PREDOMINANT SYMPTOMS— 307 PATIENTS*

	Granu-losa	Granu-losa-theca	The-coma	Lutein-ized Granu-losa-theca	Total
Bleeding	48	48	43	23	162
Oligo-amenor-rhea	10	12	11	5	38
Pregnancy	1	3	3	6	13
Ascites	14	19	11	0	44
Other					50
Virilism—14 cases					

* Certain cases had multiple symptoms.

complete operation should be performed in the older parous woman. Treatment is discussed more completely in Chapter 27.

When, on the other hand, such tumors occur in children, long before the inauguration of the normal estrogenic function of the ovary, the clinical manifestations of precocious puberty are evoked, viz., precocious menstruation, and the premature appearance of secondary sex characters, such as hypertrophy of the breasts and uterus, the appearance of axillary and pubic hair, and pubertal development of the external genitalia. With the removal of the tumor, these manifestations promptly regress, thus constituting a crucial biologic demonstration of the direct causal role of the tumor in the production of the symptoms. As a matter of fact, instances are recorded in which, after removal of a unilateral tumor and disappearance of the abnormal symptoms, a recurrent tumor has developed in the remaining ovary, with again the production of precocious pubertal symptoms with disappearance after the removal of the tumor. Recurrence need not involve a retained ovary, however.

It is of interest to note that the precocious menstruation of this syndrome is the anovulatory, purely follicular type. Thus, it differs from the so-called constitutional type of precocious puberty and menstruation, in which ovulation occurs. In the latter group insemination might theoretically bring about fertilization at abnormally early ages.

In the postmenopausal group of cases, again, occurring at a life phase at which little or no estrogen is found in the blood, the tumors produce a reestablishment of periodic menstruation-like bleeding and also a hypertrophy of the uterus. No effect is seen upon secondary sex characters, presumably because of their higher threshold or unreceptivity at this phase of life. With the removal of tumors at this age, the abnormal menstruation of course ceases, and, interestingly enough, the patient may experience a second menopause from the standpoint of the characteristic vasomotor phenomena.

Malignancy

Busby and Anderson have pointed out that if the tumor is confined to the ovary, 5 year mortality is 11.2 per cent; if there is extraovarian extension, the mortality is 42.8 per cent. They note little difference between the malignant properties of granulosa and theca cell tumors, although one frequently reads that thecomas are almost uniformly benign (Fig. 26–25). The same authors believe that they can prognosticate, according to the degree of differentiation, between early (Grades I and II) granulosa-theca cell tumors and advanced (Grades III and IV) lesions. In the early group, mortality is about 10 per cent; in the advanced, 65 per cent, giving an overall mortality of 22 per cent.

We believe that it is difficult, if not impossible, to evaluate the malignant trends of *any*

Table 26–2 AGE GROUP—307 PATIENTS

Decade	Granu-losa	Granu-losa-theca	The-coma	Lutein-ized Granu-losa-theca	Total (Percent-age)
1–20	4	11	4	9	28 (9%)
21–40	22	38	27	12	99 (32%)
41–60	26	42	33	12	111 (36%)
60	19	23	23	2	69 (22%)
TOTAL	71	114	87	35	307

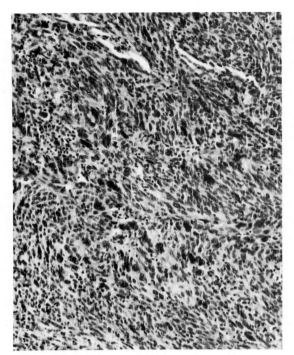

Figure 26–25. Malignant thecoma—note bizarre hyperchromatic anaplastic cells.

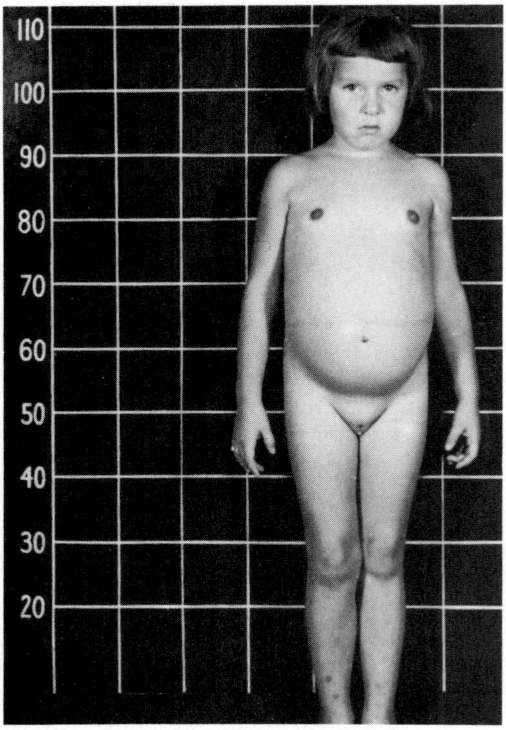

of the "special" tumors by mitosis count or any close scrutiny of the individual tumor cells. In any case, malignancy seems less likely in the younger female (Figs. 26–26 and 26–27).

Goldston and co-workers have performed a recent study consisting of 41 cases of granulosa cell tumors, and they are inclined to separate these from thecal lesions, one justification being the differences in biologic behavior of the two tumors. They note a 20 per cent mortality for the granulosal cell tumor as opposed to a 5 per cent mortality with thecal tumors. Their salvage is somewhat better than our own report with Ovarian Tumor Registry cases; although it is apparent that predominantly thecomatous tumors seem much more benign, there are certain exceptions. For reasons already expressed we feel it is expedient to consider these neoplasms jointly as feminizing gonadal stromal tumors.

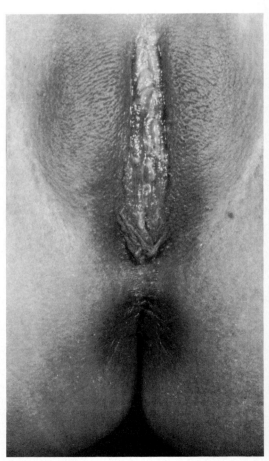

Figure 26–26. Five year old girl with large granulosa–theca cell tumor (luteinized). Note beginning breast development, prominent labia, and abdominal distention.

Figure 26–27. Adult labia in 5 year old child (Fig. 26–26).

It seems likely, therefore, that we must reckon with grades of malignancy in this as in other tumors. From the study of 414 cases from the Ovarian Tumor Registry, with as yet an insufficiently long follow-up of many cases, we believe that there is salvage in over 78 per cent of the patients followed, which approximates the results of Fox and associates (70 per cent). Norris and Taylor report a figure approximating 95 per cent, but they were able to exclude deaths not due to tumor. Results are better when any series contains a large proportion of the more favorable thecoma. Stage and Grafton comment on the problem of late recurrence, so that a 5 year salvage may be insufficient. Lusch and co-workers have recently recorded an 18 year recurrence and note others of up to 27 years. Indeed, late recurrence is so common that Fox and co-workers believe that a five year salvage is not valid; a 15 to 20 year follow-up would show an approximately 50 per cent figure.

REFERENCES

Abell, M. R., and Holtz, F.: Ovarian neoplasms in childhood and adolescence. II. Non-germ cell origin. Am. J. Obstet. Gynecol., 93:850, 1965.

Aiman, J., et al.: Androgen and estrogen formation in women with ovarian hyperthecosis. Obstet. Gynecol., 51:1, 1978.

Anikve, C., et al.: Granulosa and theca cell tumors. Obstet. Gynecol., 51:214, 1978.

Barclay, D. L., Leverich, E. B., and Kemmerly, J. R.: Hyperreactio luteinalis: postpartum persistence. Am. J. Obstet. Gynecol., 105:642, 1969.

Beacham, W. D., Webster, H. D., Lawson, E. H., et al.: Uterine and/or ovarian tumors weighing 25 pounds or more. Am. J. Obstet. Gynecol., 109:1153, 1971.

Betson, J. R., and Eicher, P. M.: Isosexual precocity produced by an ovarian thecoma (in a 2½ year old girl). Obstet. Gynecol., 22:219, 1963.

Biskind, G. R., and Biskind, M. S.: Experimental ovarian tumors in rats. Am. J. Clin. Pathol., 19:501, 1949.

Burstein, R. W., Langley, F. A., and Woodcock, A. S.: Clinicopathological study of estrogenic ovarian tumors. Cancer, 7:522, 1954.

Busby, T., and Anderson, G. W.: Feminizing mesenchymomas of the ovary. Am. J. Obstet. Gynecol., 68:1391, 1954.

Chalvardjian, A., and Scully, R. E.: Sclerosing stromal tumors of the ovary. Cancer, 31:664, 1973.

Christian, C. D.: Ovarian tumors: an extension of the Peutz-Jeghers syndrome. Am. J. Obstet. Gynecol., 111:529, 1971.

Creasman, W. T., Rutledge, F., and Smith, J. B.: Carcinoma of the ovary associated with pregnancy. Obstet. Gynecol., 38:111, 1971.

Dockerty, M. B., and McCartney, W. C.: Granulosa cell tumor, with the report of a 34-pound specimen and review. Am. J. Obstet. Gynecol., 38:698, 1939.

Dozois, R. R., Kempers, R. D., Dahlin, D. C., et al.: Ovarian tumors with the Peutz-Jeghers syndrome. Ann. Surg., 172:233, 1970.

Falck, B.: Site of production of estrogen in rat ovary as studied in microtransplants. Acta Physiol. Scand. (Suppl. 163), 47:5, 1959.

Fathalla, M. F.: The occurrence of granulosa and theca tumors in clinically normal ovaries. J. Obstet. Gynaecol. Br. Commonw., 71:279, 1967.

Fathalla, M. F.: The role of the ovarian stroma in hormone production by ovarian tumors. J. Obstet. Gynaecol. Br. Commonw., 75:32, 1968.

Fox, H., et al.: A clinicopathologic study of 92 cases of granulosa cell tumor of the ovary with special reference to the factors influencing prognosis. Cancer, 35:231, 1975.

Francis, H. H.: Granulosa cell tumor of the ovary at the age of 85 years. J. Obstet. Gynaecol. Br. Emp., 64:274, 1957.

Furth, J., and Butterworth, J. S.: Neoplastic diseases occurring among mice subjected to general irradiation with x-rays. II. Ovarian tumors and associated lesions. Am. J. Cancer, 28:66, 1936.

Ganem, K., Friedell, G. H., and Sommers, S.: A study of ovarian thecomatosis. Calif. Med., 96:254, 1962.

Garcia-Bunuel, R., et al.: Luteomas of pregnancy. Obstet. Gynecol., 45:407, 1975.

Geist, S. H., Gaines, J. A., and Pollock, A. D.: Experimental biologically active ovarian tumors in mice. Trans. Am. Gynecol. Soc., 64:21, 1939.

Gillibrand, P. N.: Granulosa-theca cell tumors of the ovary associated with pregnancy. Am. J. Obstet. Gynecol., 94:1108, 1966.

Gillman, J.: The development of the gonads in man with a consideration of the role of fetal endocrines and the histogenesis of ovarian tumors. Contrib. Embryol. Carnegie Inst. Wash. Pub., 32:81, 1948.

Giuntoli, R. L., et al.: Androgenic function of a granulosa cell tumor. Obstet. Gynecol., 47:77, 1976.

Givens, J. R., Wiser, W. L., Coleman, S. A., et al.: Familial ovarian hyperthecosis: a study of two families. Am. J. Obstet. Gynecol., 110:959, 1971.

Goldston, W. R., et al.: Clinicopathologic studies in feminizing tumors of the ovary. Am. J. Obstet. Gynecol., 112:422, 1972.

Gondos, B., and Monroe, S. A.: Cystic granulosa cell tumor with massive hemoperitoneum. Obstet. Gynecol., 38:683, 1971.

Goodwin, J. W., Ehrmann, R. L., and Leavitt, T., Jr.: An apparently estrogenic hilum cell tumor of the ovary. Obstet. Gynecol., 19:467, 1962.

Gusberg, S. B., and Kardon, P.: Proliferative endometrial response to theca-granulosa cell tumors. Am. J. Obstet. Gynecol., 111:633, 1971.

Hughesdon, P. E.: The structure and origin of theca-granulosa tumors. J. Obstet. Gynaecol. Br. Emp., 65:540, 1958.

Hughesdon, P. E.: Thecal and allied reaction in epithelial tumors. J. Obstet. Gynaecol. Br. Emp., 65:702, 1958.

Ingram, J. E., and Novak, E.: Endometrial carcinoma associated with feminizing ovarian tumors. Am. J. Obstet. Gynecol., 61:774, 1951.

Kempson, R. L.: Ultrastructure of ovarian stromal cell tumors. Arch. Pathol., 86:492, 1968.

Koudstall, J., Bossenbrock, B., and Hardonk, M. J.: Ovarian tumors investigated by histochemical and enzyme histochemical methods. Am. J. Obstet. Gynecol., 102:1004, 1969.

Krieger, J. S.: In Beacham, W. D., Webster, H. D., Lawson, E. H., et al.: Uterine and/or ovarian tumors weighing 25 pounds or more. A review of the literature in English since 1946. Am. J. Obstet. Gynecol., 109:1153, 1971.

Langley, F. A.: "Sertoli" and "Leydig" cells in relation to ovarian tumors. J. Clin. Pathol., 7:10, 1954.

Lecène, P.: Les diagnostics anatomo-cliniques. Pt. 2. Appareil génital de la femme. Paris, P. Moulonquet, Masson, 1932, p. 305.

Lewis, P. D., and Percival, R. C.: Combined thecoma and teratoma. J. Obstet. Gynaecol. Br. Commonw., 72:447, 1965.

Li, M. H., Gardner, W. W., and Kaylan, H. S.: Effects of x-ray irradiation on development of ovarian tumors in intrasplenic grafts in castrated mice. J. Natl., Cancer Inst., 8:91, 1947.

Lusch, C. J., et al.: Delayed recurrence of a granulosa cell tumor. Obstet. Gynecol., 51:505, 1978.

MacKinlay, C. J.: Male cells in granulosa cell ovarian tumors. J. Obstet. Gynaecol. Br. Emp., 64:512, 1957.

Madden, J. D., and McDonald, P. C.: Estrogen and granulosa-theca cell tumors. Obstet. Gynecol., 51:210, 1978.

Malinak, L. R., and Miller, G. V.: Bilateral multicentric ovarian luteomas of pregnancy associated with masculinization of a female infant. Am. J. Obstet. Gynecol., 91:251, 1965.

Malkasian, G. D., Jr., et al.: Observations on chemotherapy of granulosa cell carcinomas and malignant ovarian teratomas. Obstet. Gynecol., 44:885, 1974.

Mansell, H., and Hertig, A. T.: Granulosa-theca cell tumors. Obstet. Gynecol., 6:385, 1955.

Maxwell, D. M. W.: Granulosa cell tumor producing symptoms 4 years following radium menopause. J. Obstet. Gynaecol., Br. Emp., 63:232, 1956.

McCormack, T. P., and Riddick, D. H.: Hormonal function of a granulosa cell tumor. Obstet. Gynecol., 48:185, 1976.

McDonald, T. W., et al.: Endometrial carcinoma with functioning ovarian tumor and polycystic ovarian disease. Obstet. Gynecol., 49:654, 1977.

McKay, D. G., Hertig, A. T., and Hickey, W. F.: Histogenesis of granulosa and theca cell tumors. Obstet. Gynecol., 1:125, 1953.

Meyer, R.: The pathology of some special ovarian tumors and their relation to sex characters. Am. J. Obstet. Gynecol., 22:697, 1931.

Morris, J. M., and Scully, R. E.: Endocrine Pathology of the Ovary. St. Louis, C. V. Mosby Co., 1958.

Morrison, C. W., and Woodruff, J. D.: Fibrothecoma and associated ovarian stromal neoplasia. Obstet. Gynecol., 23:344, 1964.

Nokes, J. M., Claiborne, H. A., and Reingold, W. N.: Thecoma with associated virilization. Am. J. Obstet. Gynecol., 78:722, 1958.

Norris, H. J., and Chorlton, I.: Functioning tumors of the ovary. Clin. Obstet. Gynecol., 17:189, 1974.

Norris, H. J., and Taylor, H. B.: Luteoma of pregnancy. J. Clin. Path., 47:557, 1967.

Norris, H. J., and Taylor, H. B.: Prognosis of granulosa-theca cell tumors of the ovary. Cancer, 21:255, 1967.

Novak, E. R., and Mohler, D. I.: Ovarian stromal changes in endometrial cancer. Am. J. Obstet. Gynecol., 65:1099, 1953.

Novak, E. R., Kutchmeshgi, J., Mupas, R. S., and Woodruff, J. D.: Feminizing gonadal-stromal tumors (analysis of the granulosa-theca cell tumors of the Ovarian Tumor Registry). Obstet. Gynecol., 38:701, 1971.

Novak, E. R., et al.: Ovarian tumors in pregnancy. Obstet. Gynecol., 46:401, 1975.

Robertson, M. G., and Miller, R. E.: Massive cystic granulosa-theca cell tumor. Report of a case. Am. J. Obstet. Gynecol., 110:407, 1971.

Schneider, G. T., and Bechtel, M.: Ovarian cortical stromal hyperplasia. Obstet. Gynecol., 8:713, 1956.

Scully, R. E.: Sex cord tumor with annular tubules: a distinctive ovarian tumor of the Peutz-Jeghers syndrome. Cancer, 25:1107, 1970.

Shippel, S.: The ovarian theca cell. J. Obstet. Gynaecol. Br. Emp., 62:321, 1955.

Simmons, R. L., and Sciarra, J. J.: Treatment of late recurrent granulosa cell tumors of the ovary. Surg. Gynecol. Obstet., 124:65, 1967.

Sommers, S. C., Gates, O., and Goodof, I. I.: Late recurrence of granulosa cell tumors. Obstet. Gynecol., 6:395, 1955.

Stage, A. H., and Grafton, W. D.: Ovarian thecal tumors. Obstet. Gynecol., 50:21, 1977.

Sternberg, W. H.: Non-functioning ovarian neoplasms. In The Ovary. International Academy of Pathologists Monograph No. 3. H. G. Grady and D. E. Smith (Eds). Baltimore, Williams & Wilkins Co., 1963, p. 209.

Sternberg, W. H., and Barclay, D. L.: Luteoma of pregnancy. Am. J. Obstet. Gynecol., 95:165, 1966.

Teilum, G.: Estrogen-producing Sertoli cell tumors (androblastoma tubulare lipoides) of the human testis and ovary; homologous ovarian and testicular tumors. J. Clin. Endocrinol., 9:301, 1949.

Thompson, J. P., Dockerty, M. B., and Symmonds, R. E.: Granulosa cell carcinoma arising in a cystic teratoma of the ovary. Obstet. Gynecol., 28:549, 1966.

Traut, H. F., and Butterworth, J. S.: Theca, granulosa and lutein cell tumor of human ovary and similar tumors of mouse's ovary. Am. J. Obstet. Gynecol., 34:987, 1937.

Uyttenbroeck, F.: A study of the animal ovary. Acta Zool. Pathol. Antwerp, 42:3, 1967.

Verkauf, B. S., et al.: Virilization of mother and fetus associated with luteoma of pregnancy: A case report with endocrinologic studies. Am. J. Obstet. Gynecol., 129:274, 1977.

Warner, N. E., Friedman, N. B., Bomze, E. J., and Masin, F.: Comparative pathology of experimental and spontaneous androblastomas and arrhenoblastomas of the gonads. Am. J. Obstet. Gynecol., 79:971, 1960.

Woll, E., Hertig, A. T., Smith, G. V. S., and Johnson, L. C.: Ovary in endometrial carcinoma. Am. J. Obstet. Gynecol., 56:617, 1948.

Wong, T. W., and Warner, N. E.: Ovarian thecal metaplasia in the adrenal gland. Arch. Pathol., 92:319, 1971.

Woodruff, J. D., Williams, T. J., and Goldberg, B.: Hormone activity of the common ovarian neoplasm. Am. J. Obstet. Gynecol., 87:679, 1963.

Chapter 27

GONADAL STROMAL TUMORS—VIRILIZING (ARRHENOBLASTOMA, ADRENAL, AND HILUS CELL)

ARRHENOBLASTOMA

HISTOGENESIS AND TYPES

By contrast with the feminizing tumors, the masculinizing tumors, represented chiefly by arrhenoblastoma, are rare. However, by 1960, Pedowitz was able to report 240 cases, although there may be some duplication. Nevertheless it seems that this lesion is being recognized more frequently. In past years it has always been emphasized that virilization is not necessary for a diagnosis; the tumor may exist without endocrine effect, and today we might be inclined to designate this as an *inert gonadal stromal* tumor.

Various pathologists refer to arrhenoblastomas as *Sertoli-Leydig* tumors, but we prefer to avoid such terms, as these cell types are not part of the normal ovary and would imply a testicular tumor. This is probably a rather petty objection, but reflects opinions expressed nearly 20 years ago by Emil Novak.

The designation *arrhenoblastoma* was coined by Meyer for this group of tumors, which were thought to originate in certain male-directed cells persisting in the ovary from fetal life. Although they may lead to masculinizing tendencies, this is not inevitable. Pathologists in the past have been almost uniform in indicating that cellular morphol-

ogy rather than endocrine effect should be the criterion for diagnosis. Today it is almost completely accepted that distinction between certain gonadal stromal tumors is often impossible microscopically without knowledge of any hormone effect, although Teilum might disagree.

The degree of differentiation or dedifferentiation, as stressed by Meyer, is important in the endocrine function of different members of this group, but apparently more factors are involved than this. For example, relatively little is known about the relationship between the gonads and the adrenal cortex, which are embryologically intimately related. It is therefore not surprising that lesions of the ovary and certain ones of the adrenal cortex have similar masculinization potentialities, which may be difficult to distinguish preoperatively.

One great merit of Meyer's work has been his demonstration of the familial relationship existing between tumors of widely different histologic structure. At one end of the scale is the *highly differentiated tumor* originally described by Pick (1905) and designated as *testicular adenoma,* in which the reproduction of the male testicular apparatus in the ovary is quite perfect. At the other extreme is the *highly undifferentiated variety* in which the histologic picture is essentially that of sarcoma, although usually meticulous

523

examination reveals clues to its probable histogenesis.

Between those two groups of differentiated and undifferentiated arrhenoblastoma, all gradations may be encountered, so that Meyer has distinguished an *intermediate group* in which such criteria as tubule formation and the occurrence of interstitial cells are developed to greater or lesser degree.

PATHOLOGY

Gross Characteristics

As encountered at operation, the arrhenoblastoma is generally of moderate size (Fig. 27–1), and may be very small, but in at least a few recorded instances the tumor has weighed over 11 kg. (25 lb.) (Fig. 27–2). It is almost always unilateral (95 per cent). The surface is smooth, and the cut surface is grayish-yellow (Fig. 27–3). The consistency is generally firm, but cystic degeneration is frequent, with focal areas of hemorrhage throughout the yellowish tumor matrix.

Microscopic Characteristics

The microscopic diagnosis of arrhenoblastoma is not always simple, and it presupposes a knowledge of the normal embryology of the testis as well as the ovary. No stereotyped picture can be described. In the *testicular adenoma* variety, the resemblance to seminiferous tubules may be perfect, and

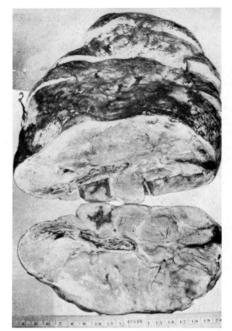

Figure 27–2. Arrhenoblastoma of the ovary. (Courtesy of Dr. R. K. Hancock.)

rete structures may likewise be present (Figs. 27–4 and 27–5).

In the intermediate group, on the other hand, only imperfect attempts (Fig. 27–6) at tubule formation may be seen, or there may be only slender zigzag columns of cells with nuclei arranged transverse to the long axis of the column. *Interstitial cells*, with characteristic lipoid content, may be present (Figs. 27–7 and 27–8). It is probable that their pres-

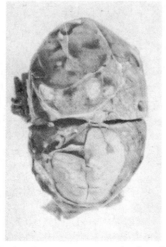

Figure 27–1. Gross appearance of arrhenoblastoma.

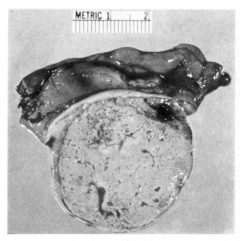

Figure 27–3. Arrhenoblastoma showing characteristic yellowish color with focal hemorrhage and smooth capsule.

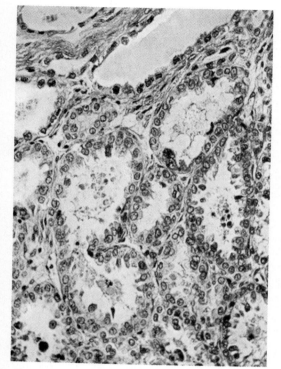

Figure 27–4. Highly differentiated tubular variety of arrhenoblastoma (testicular adenoma), the least common type.

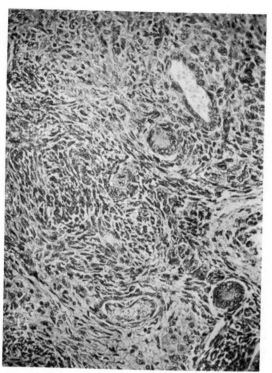

Figure 27–6. Intermediate variety of arrhenoblastoma, with imperfect tubule formation not resembling testicular tubules.

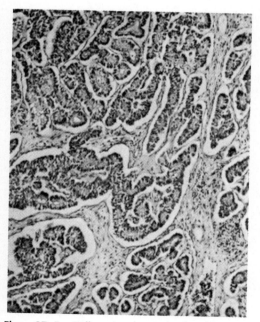

Figure 27–5. Differentiated type of arrhenoblastoma.

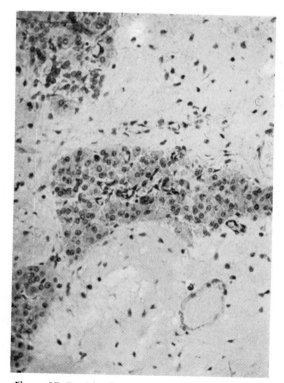

Figure 27–7. Islands of interstitial cells found in same case as shown in Figure 27–6.

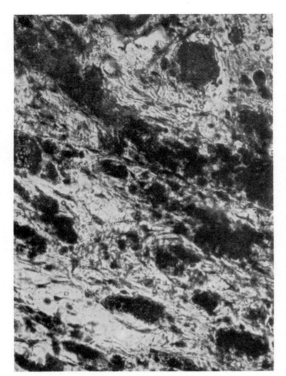

Figure 27–8. Differential fat stain (black) showing richness of lipoid material.

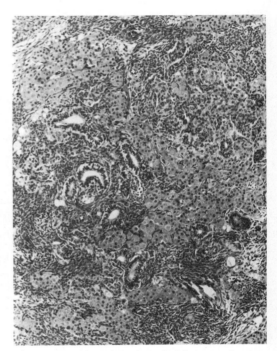

Figure 27–10. Moderately well differentiated arrhenoblastoma with many interstitial cells, a rather uncommon occurrence.

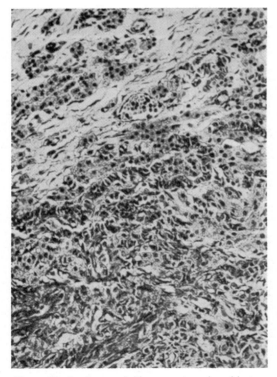

Figure 27–9. Sex-cord–like areas in arrhenoblastoma, with interstitial cells in upper left.

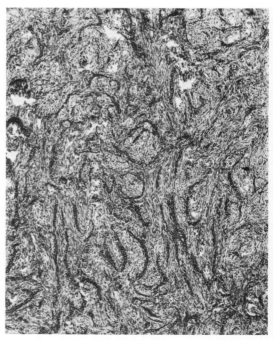

Figure 27–11. Undifferentiated variety of arrhenoblastoma, with cordlike arrangement of cells.

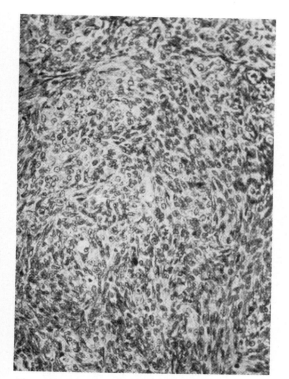

Figure 27–12. Sarcoma-like variety of arrhenoblastoma, although other areas showed a few imperfect tubules.

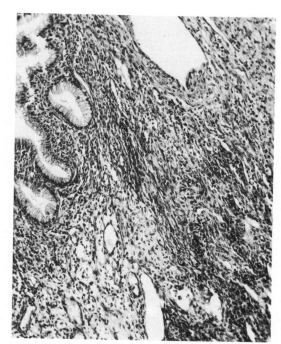

Figure 27–13. Occasional association of arrhenoblastoma with benign cystic teratoma (upper left).

ence alone determines the function or non-function of the tumor. *Reinke crystalloids* are often demonstrable.

Certainly the highly differentiated arrhenoblastoma (testicular adenoma) is less commonly associated with masculinization than is the more undifferentiated tumor. The explanation may lie in the extreme rarity of interstital cells in conjunction with the adenomatous type of arrhenoblastoma, although this occurs on occasion (Figs. 27–9 and 27–10).

Finally, in the very undifferentiated variety, the picture may be that of sarcoma (Figs. 27–11 and 27–12), although associated virilizing interstitial cells seem to explain the frequent functional capability of this group. Moreover, in the majority of cases, very thorough examination, perhaps involving the study of many blocks, reveals the cordlike arrangement of cells, imperfect tubule formation, or lipid-containing cell elements, which indicate the arrhenoblastomatous nature of the tumor. The fact remains, however, that the clinical history is of the greatest value to pathologists in the microscopic examination of these tumors, and they are certainly entitled to the benefit of data. The co-association of arrhenoblastoma with (be-

nign cystic) teratoma, as noted in our review of Ovarian Tumor Registry material, may not be significant (Fig. 27–13), but indicates the association of germ cell and gonadal stromal tumors (in addition to the gonadoblastoma).

CLINICAL CHARACTERISTICS

Arrhenoblastoma is characteristically a tumor of young women, the greatest incidence being in the decade between 20 and

Table 27–1 AGE GROUPS OF PATIENTS WITH ARRHENOBLASTOMA

Age	Number of Patients
Under 20	27
20 to 30	40
30 to 40	18
40 to 50	11
50 to 60	8
60 to 70	7
Total	111

(From Novak, E. R., et al.: Novak's Textbook of Gynecology. 8th Ed. Baltimore, Williams & Wilkins Co., 1970–71.)

30, although it has occurred in a $2\frac{1}{2}$ year old girl as well as a 70 year old woman. Analysis of Ovarian Tumor Registry cases indicates that 75 per cent of such patients were less than 40 years old, and 66 per cent were less than 30 years old. Goldstein and Lamb, and Jensen and co-workers, indicated various fa-

milial tendencies, and the latter also notes associated thyroid abnormalities.

The characteristic clinical history is dependent upon the fact that the tumor, through its endocrine function, first brings about certain phenomena that are probably interpreted as *defeminizing* rather than mas-

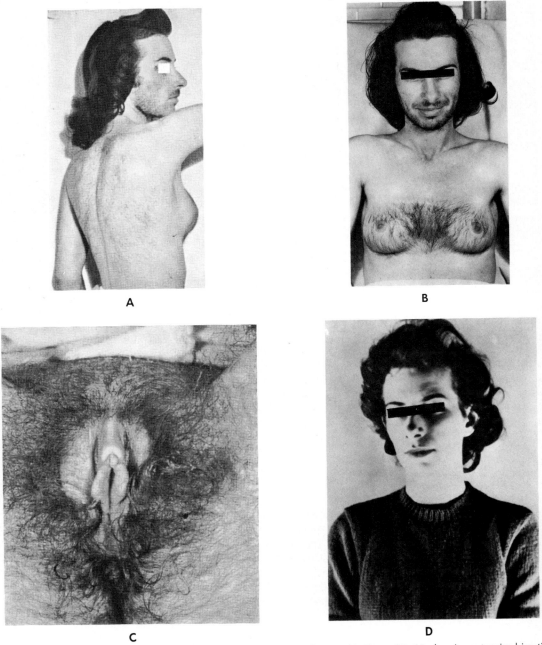

Figure 27–14. *A*, Appearance of patient with the arrhenoblastoma illustrated in Figure 27–15, showing extensive hirsutism with moderate flattening of breasts, which had previously been very large. She had not menstruated for 3 years. *B*, Front view of same patient. *C*, Hypertrophy of clitoris in same patient. *D*, Same patient postoperatively.

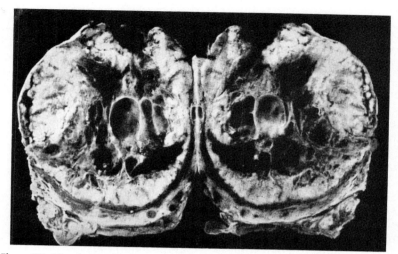

Figure 27–15. Arrhenoblastoma of the ovary found in patient shown in Figure 27–14.

culinizing. This is followed by a secondary phase in which definite *masculinization* manifestations are produced. Hirsutism alone, even with menstrual irregularity, does not imply the presence of an arrhenoblastoma. One must always be mindful of such entities as adrenal pathology and the Stein-Leventhal syndrome in differential diagnosis, although hirsutism may have diverse causes.

The usual sequence can be illustrated by sketching the developments in a single case. The patient, age 25, had an 11 month history of complete amenorrhea after normal menses except with a single normal full term pregnancy 7 years previously. Shortly after cessation of the menstrual function the breasts flattened. Neither the amenorrhea nor the atrophy of the breasts can be considered evidence of masculinization. They represent merely a subtraction from the feminine habitus, and are therefore properly considered defeminizing rather than masculinizing. On the other hand, the subsequent appearance in this patient of facial and body hirsutism, the deepening and roughening of the voice, and the hypertrophy of the clitoris are of positive rather than negative significance, indicating a genuine masculinizing effect.

Finding, on pelvic examination, of a small tumor of the right ovary about the size of a golf ball, left little doubt of the diagnosis, especially in the absence of any evidence of adrenal disease. The tumor proved to be a typical arrhenoblastoma of the intermediate group, and following the operation, men-

struation was reestablished, the breasts again developed, and the other symptoms retrogressed (Figs. 27–14 to 27–16).

Rather characteristically the first menstruation, in most of the recorded cases, has occurred about one month after removal of the tumor. The disappearance of the genuine masculinization phenomena is generally much slower and may be incomplete. Indeed, some enlargement of the phallus and hirsutism have been observed over 20 years

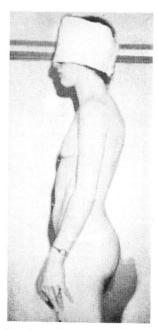

Figure 27–16. Lateral view of another patient with arrhenoblastoma, showing flattening of breasts.

postoperatively, as with the patient noted in Figure 27–14.

It is interesting to note that a considerable number of pregnancies have ensued following removal of an arrhenoblastoma. A rare occurrence is pregnancy complicated by arrhenoblastoma, and one would have to postulate that conception occurred before secretion of enough androgen to inhibit ovulation. In reporting 14 cases of arrhenoblastoma associated with pregnancy, Galle and coauthors note a markedly impaired salvage rate.

Verhoeven and associates have discussed comprehensively the problems of virilization with pregnancy. Whereas the male infant in association with a virilizing tumor is normal, the female may be normal but may exhibit either transient virilism or evidence of pseudohermaphroditism. Only a few cases are on record. Following conservative surgery, however, pregnancy is not uncommon, as noted in the extensive review compiled by Pedowitz and O'Brien.

The case report by Graber and co-workers, which was studied extensively from an endocrinologic standpoint, suggests that determination of the various urinary ketosteroids and corticosteroids is not helpful in pinpointing the diagnosis, although the more recent case studied by Mahesh and associates suggests that on occasion the 17-ketosteroid level may be extremely high. Scully indicates that small unmeasurable amounts of the potently virilizing testosterone may lead to profound masculinization. Other, less virilizing steroids may lead to a markedly elevated 17-ketosteroid level with no androgenic trends. These observations agree with our own.

Malignancy

It is quite difficult to evaluate the degree of malignancy of this tumor group. Most cases have been reported promptly because of their rarity and their biologic interest, so that insufficient time has elapsed to judge their ultimate course. As with other tumors of the functioning group, the degree of malignancy is unquestionably much less than that of the common types of primary ovarian cancer, but much greater than some appear to believe. It is still difficult to express the incidence of recurrence and metastasis with precision, for late recurrence may occur. Our recent survey of Ovarian Tumor Registry

material indicates a nearly 33 per cent 5 year recurrence rate. A review by Ireland and Woodruff suggests a considerably lower incidence; however, they amended the expressed Ovarian Tumor Registry diagnoses by the component members instead of adhering to them, as in our study.

GYNANDROBLASTOMA

A small group of ovarian tumors has been reported in which there has been an apparently paradoxic combination of granulosal or thecal elements together with those which microscopically are typically arrhenoblastoma (Figs. 27–17, 27–18, and 27–19). The first of these cases was reported in 1930 by Meyer, who applied to this tumor type the designation of *gynandroblastoma*. From a clinical standpoint, the masculinizing effect of such tumors appears to have been generally the dominant one, but in some cases such estrogen-induced manifestations as excessive bleeding have also been noted. Judging from Novak's study of eight gynandroblastomas from the Ovarian Tumor Registry, it would appear that androgenic trends

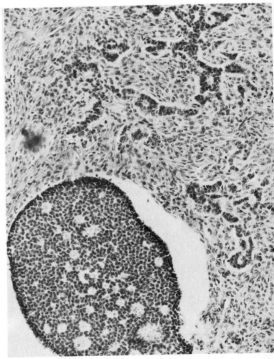

Figure 27–17. Typical granulosal pattern (below) with arrhenoblastoma (above).

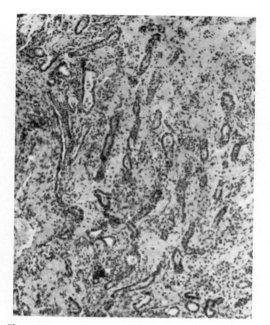

Figure 27–18. Arrhenoblastomatous area in gynandroblastoma. See also Figure 27–19.

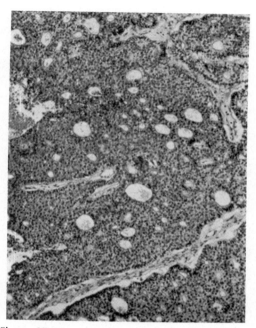

Figure 27–19. Granulosa cell areas in same tumor shown in Figure 27–18.

usually predominate, although not always (Fig. 27–20).

In view of the innumerable variations in the histologic patterns of both granulosa cell tumors and arrhenoblastomas, caution should be exercised in making such a diagnosis as gynandroblastoma unless the two types are clearly and separately demonstrated in the same tumor. In view of the differentiating potency of the gonadal mesenchyme and the biochemical similarity of the estrogenic and androgenic steroids, there seems to be no reason why both feminizing and masculinizing neoplastic tissue should not occasionally coexist, and this has been noted by both Sandberg and Warner and colleagues. We suspect that admixtures of both male and female hormones are produced by many of these gonadal stromal tumors regardless of the histologic appearance, with any clinical effect being the result of a dominance of androgen or estrogen.

ADRENAL TUMORS OF THE OVARY

Tumors of this type are rare and are usually benign; they are not of gonadal stromal origin. It is uniformly accepted that in embryologic life the adrenal gland evolves in close juxtaposition with the ovary, so that it is easy to conceive of aberrant tissue. That lesions of adrenal cell origin may occur in the ovary seems likely, and these may closely resemble the ovarian lutein cell. Whether an actual neoplasm may evolve from such an evanescent structure as a lutein cell poses a question, and it is very unlikely that this is important in the production of virilization. However, certain granulosa or theca cell tumors may undergo complete luteinization; these are prone to be associated with a feminizing or no particular hormonal pattern, but certainly not masculinization.

Histogenesis

Should small clumps of adrenal cells be regarded as nests or adenomas in the sense that the term adenoma is usually employed to designate localized collections of functionally active hormone-secreting cells? Certainly aberrant adrenal tissue is frequently observed along the course of the ovarian or spermatic vessels, although less commonly in the ovary itself (Fig. 27–21). As a rule, these small deposits of adrenal cells are not associated with virilization, and it seems of academic importance whether they are classified as rests or small adenomas. Al-

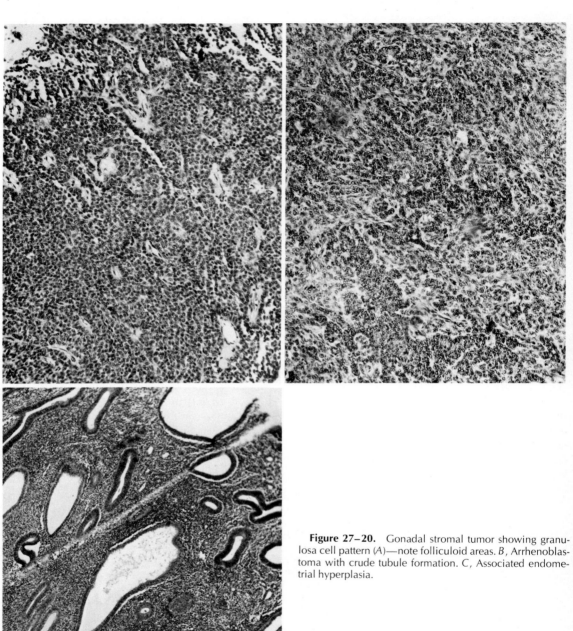

Figure 27–20. Gonadal stromal tumor showing granulosa cell pattern (A)—note folliculoid areas. B, Arrhenoblastoma with crude tubule formation. C, Associated endometrial hyperplasia.

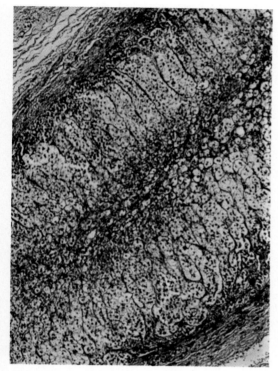

Figure 27–21. Adrenal tissue rest in broad ligament near ovary. There are no sex character changes.

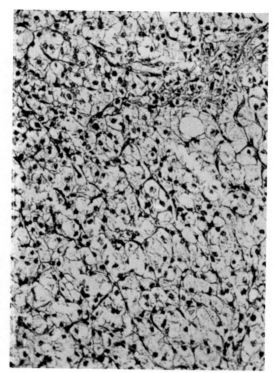

Figure 27–22. Section of adrenal tumor which produced masculinization symptoms identical to those of arrhenoblastoma.

though Norris and Chorlton question the finding of adrenal tissue in the ovary, we have seen several cases in which all different zones of the adrenal have been noted in the ovarian cortex; admittedly these are more common in the mesovarium.

Large ovarian tumors of adrenal origin *may*, of course, produce virilization. It seems plausible to believe that if the parent cell is capable of masculinizing potencies, the mere quantity of these cells may be the determinative factor in manifesting virilism over the typical female pattern (Fig. 27–22). If such an endocrine function is present, clinical characteristics indistinguishable from arrhenoblastoma may be produced. We have recently observed a case of bilateral adrenal tumors associated with profound virilization.

Morphologically similar tumors may be found in which there is no suggestion of hormonal activity. In previous years the terms *hypernephroma* or *hypernephroid* tumor were utilized, as was the ill-defined term *masculinovoblastoma*, originally proposed by Rottino and McGrath. Our tendency is to consider most of these as of adrenal origin or

as clear cell mesonephromas. Histologically, distinction may be impossible but clinical masculinization suggests an adrenal tumor rather than a clear cell mesonephroma.

It seems worthwhile to reevaluate the lipoid tumors of the ovary; indeed, all of the functioning neoplasms need clarification in many respects. Teilum's classification of certain ovarian tumors (as will be discussed shortly) is an effort to overcome this confusion, but seems to us to be of rather dubious value at present.

Hughesdon believes that adrenal and hilus cell tumors are of common ancestry (the ovarian stromal cell), and he utilizes the generic name *lipoid cell tumor* for these neoplasms. Wong and Warner have noted ovarian thecal cells within the substance of the adrenal. Other histologically similar lesions are luteinized granulosa-theca cell tumors, which are thought to be better classified under this particular category. Hughesdon's paper reflects a complete and painstaking study but of only *three* cases. We wonder if even the most thorough study of a very few cases represents the behavior and histogenesis of all cases of any tumor type.

HILUS OR LEYDIG CELL TUMORS

Only a small proportion of virilizing tumors of the ovary arise from the hilus cells which occur predominantly in the ovarian hilus, but may present in the mesovarium or even in the cortical stroma. In cryostat (often serial) sections of the postmenopausal ovary, it is apparent that these cells are found in at least 80 per cent of all climacteric gonads, perhaps as a result of the markedly increased amounts of postmenopausal gonadotropin. Whether these cells originate from the stroma or from nerve cell is uncertain; we believe that a stromal origin seems much more likely.

Although the hilus cell tumor is usually associated with androgenic tendencies, Novak and Mattingly, in a review of 18 cases from the Ovarian Tumor Registry, observed endometrial hyperplasia (a presumed estrogenic effect) in most cases in which the endometrium could be studied, despite clinical virilism. A recent case report by Mohamed and co-workers details a well-studied case of a hilus cell tumor with endometrial carcinoma (the sixth such case in the literature). In an earlier histochemical study (Novak et al.) the hilus cell showed histochemical properties strongly suggesting androgen production, although associated with a clinical status indicating an estrogen stimulus (postmenopausal endometrial hyperplasia or adenocarcinoma). We believe that the postmenopausal hilus cell is an active vector of androgenic steroids with conversion to estrogen at other areas, possibly the uterine end-organ.

These cells are usually distinguishable from adrenal cells in that they are smaller, darker, have a distinct nucleus, and are apt to be arranged in an adenomatous fashion with a connective tissue matrix (Fig. 27–23). Originally described by Berger (1923) and designated as sympathicotrophic cells, they are now believed to be identical to the Leydig cells of the testis. This is suggested by their morphology, and even more by the fact that the cells contain the same Reinke albuminoid crystals that distinguish Leydig cells. The exact nature and function of these Reinke crystalloids remain obscure despite the comprehensive study by Janko and Sandberg (Fig. 27–24).

The review by Boivin and Richart reports 36 cases, although these authors do not include 10 cases (in which the diagnosis was

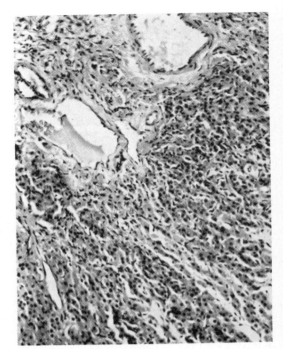

Figure 27–23. Virilizing hilus cell tumor. Contrast with Figure 27–22.

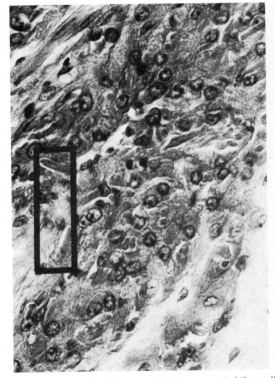

Figure 27–24. Reinke crystalloids apparent in hilus cell tumor. Though pathognomonic, they are not mandatory for diagnosis. (Courtesy of W. F. Peterson, Washington, D.C.)

verified by the Ovarian Tumor Registry) because of lack of individual description. With these cases, Novak and Mattingly were of course totally dependent on outside observation, but their acceptance by such an august body as the Tumor Registry leaves little doubt of their validity. A more recent report by Dunniho and associates notes some 50 cases of recorded hilus cell tumors.

In our own study of 18 cases, Novak and Mattingly observed Reinke crystalloids in less than 50 per cent, but believe that their presence is not mandatory for diagnosis. The tumors were always small (less than 5 cm.), unilateral, and uniformly benign in spite of incomplete surgery. Despite uniform clinical virilism, the endometrium when available for study showed an estrogenic effect, such as hyperplasia or hyperplastic polyps. Plate and Goodwin and co-workers have separately recorded hilus cell tumors with estrogenic manifestations, but more thorough study has put the validity of this diagnosis in doubt. Indeed the Ovarian Tumor Registry opinion was that Plate's case represented a luteinized granulosa-theca tumor, a very legitimate error. Stewart and Woodard report a malignant hilus cell tumor, and the histology and clinical behavior seem irrefutable, despite some observations that the tumor was of the granulosa-theca variety. In the sections observed by us, Reinke crystalloids were plentiful, which strongly suggests a hilus cell origin. Echt and Hadd have discussed the androgen excretion pattern in another malignant metastatic hilus cell tumor.

Scully and Cohen have described hilus cells with Reinke crystals in an adrenal tumor. This, of course, raises considerable speculation of the distribution and exact nature of these cells. Hawkins and Lawrence reported a case of hilus cell hyperplasia, which on chemical analysis showed a marked decrease in estrogen, androgen, and progesterone following surgery. Perhaps the hilus cell is capable of manufacturing diverse types of steroids.

HOMOLOGY OF CERTAIN OVARIAN AND TESTICULAR TUMORS

A provocative approach to the study of this functioning group of tumors has been suggested by Teilum, who believes in the homology of certain tumor groups occurring in the ovary and testis. Although his concept seems fundamentally sound, we believe that it is based too much on extremely uncertain cellular distinction superimposed upon various unproved embryologic data.

Teilum stresses basically two types of tumors. *First* are the endocrine varieties of *androblastoma* that are derived from the primitive mesenchyme, and that reflect the various phases in the embryologic development of testicular elements. These embrace: (a) Certain tumors of a tubular or adenomatous variety (presumed by many to be of granulosa-theca origin) as well as the so-called folliculoma lipidique (the dominant hormone-producing cell type being the Sertoli cell). All of these are considered feminizing; in addition we believe Teilum recognizes the estrogenic tendency of certain granulosa-theca cell tumors evolving from the mesenchyme. (b) Arrhenoblastomas, as recognized by Meyer, in which the virilization is supposedly due to a predominance of Leydig cells, although these are often sparse and difficult to find. (c) Leydig (or hilus cell) tumors which were previously classified as adrenal tumors of the ovary, luteoma, or masculinovoblastoma. Although we agree with Teilum's attempts to delete the so-called luteoma and masculinovoblastoma from our terminology, we do recognize adrenal tumors as an entity.

Second, Teilum notes a group of *germ cell tumors* occurring in male or female. Primary, of course, is the dysgerminoma/seminoma of the female/male. Also included, however, are the tumors considered to be the mesonephromas of Schiller, the endodermal sinus tumor, and the ovarian teratoma. Although we agree with the genesis of teratoma, we do not believe that mesonephromas have a germ cell origin, although we must admit an uncertainty of the exact cell from which mesonephromas are derived. We consider Teilum's studies extremely provocative, but not convincing enough to make this classification of tumors preferable to others. Teilum feels that the morphology of the tumor rather than the endocrine effect should be instrumental in formulating a diagnosis; his concepts of these gonadal lesions are summarized as follows:

Hormonal secretion alone does not contribute a logical basis for classification of gonadal stromal tumors. R. Meyer intended to emphasize the masculinizing properties by using "arrheno-" (Mannlich). The term *androblastoma* is a designation for neoplasms derived from the primitive embryonic mesenchyme of *both testis and ovary,* morphologically reflecting various phases in the development of the male gonad, irrespective of the qualitative hormone-producing properties. The tumors may contain cells comparable to Sertoli and/or Leydig cells. The virilizing properties of Meyer's ovarian arrhenoblastoma depend on the androgenic activity of stromal cells analogous to Leydig cells, whereas testicular and ovarian androblastoma associated with feminization show a predominance of effective estrogen-producing Sertoli cells.

These feminizing androblastomas in either sex are actually estrogen-producing Sertoli cell tumors. The fact that the diffuse androblastoma patterns are morphologically indistinguishable from the patterns of the undifferentiated granulosa, as well as the occurrence of the gynandroblastoma has supported the concept of a common blastemic origin for both androblastoma and tumors of granulosa-theca cell type.

The recognition of embryologic homology of Sertoli cells to granulosa cells and of Leydig cells to theca cells and the occurrence of feminizing granulosa cell tumors of folliculoid type in the testis emphasize a common histogenesis of the series of homologous and identical tumors, both occurring in the testis and ovary. The possibility that the arrhenoblastoma is a masculinizing variant of granulosa cell tumors has been suggested and denied in the past. McKinlay considered the granulosa cell as the parent of the Sertoli cell and proposed designating the entire group granulosa cell tumors; such an interpretation is inaccurate. As emphasized by Warner, "There are two major criticisms: (1) the testicular homologues are ignored, (2) it is unlikely that they are essentially female more than essentially male." The tumor cells in such ovarian neoplasms are chromosomally female regardless of differentiation and proliferation of cell types characteristic of the male gonad, a fact which also applies to the hilus (Leydig) cell of the ovary, which nevertheless are male cells. Neither the view that the term granulosa cell tumor should be restricted to lesions that occur in females who are genetically female nor the postulate that Sertoli cells in the female gonad only occur in cases of testicular feminization is valid.

Warner and co-workers (1960) have provided experimental evidence of the homology and identity of these tumors which, arriving in the testis or the ovary, are derived from the same blastoma. These authors assume there is a considerable lability of gonadal organization during embryonic differentiation, and this can be affected by a variety of experimental procedures.

It is generally believed that the gonadal sex depends on the outcome for dominance between the medullary and cortical components of the primitive bipotential gonads, and that factors determining the differentiation include sex-determining genes on X and Y chromosomes, medullary and cortical inductor substances, and environmental factors. It has been emphasized that the adult ovary has retained in its stromal and epithelial elements a higher degree of pluripotentiality, and suggests that substances arising within certain ovarian tissues may act like embryonic inductors by direct diffusion through the tissues. It is possible that similar mechanisms are involved in the morphogenesis of these tumors, reflecting the bipotential capacity of the gonad.

Exceptions from the blastemic origin are of course hilus cell tumors arising from Leydig cells in the hilus of the ovary, certain well-documented cases of androblastoma originating in the medulla, and rare cases of gynandroblastoma showing a sharp distinction between cortical and medullary elements.

It should be emphasized again that because of the various hormone-producing properties of specific cell types derived from the mesenchymal core of the gonad, the term androblastoma for identical ovarian and testicular tumors reflecting stages in development of the male gonad has a purely morphologic connotation and, in contrast to the term arrhenoblastoma, does not necessarily imply virilization. Androblastomas may therefore exhibit no endocrine effect on the host. Whether male or female, they may be feminizing or virilizing, depending on the type of effective functioning cells. The apparent contradiction that some androblastomas in the testis as well as the ovaries are estrogen-producing is well founded in the studies of estrogenic properties of the testis and ovary, and simply reflects a form of testicular feminization.

In addition, the term androblastoma emphasized the blastemic origin of the tumor. Since the Sertoli cell does not occur in the normal ovary, all ovarian Sertoli cells are blastemic in origin, and therefore produce androblastomas. Sertoli cell tumors of the testis may arise from an undifferentiated blastoma or from Sertoli cells of preexisting tubules.

Certain of these tenets are difficult to accept although the basic concept seems sound.

GONADAL STROMAL TUMORS

In the past we have always stressed our belief that granulosa-theca cell tumors (estrogenic) and arrhenoblastomas (virilizing) were separate entities with a different histogenesis. At the same time it was emphasized that the morphology of the tumor is the prime criterion in diagnosis.

Today, however, we are forced to modify these opinions, not only because of a host of outside observations, but also because of many personal impressions in evaluating ovarian tumors. Well-trained gynecologic pathologists must adopt a defeatist attitude by admitting that there are certain microscopic limitations that the human eye and brain cannot surmount. The distinction between poorly differentiated granulosa-theca lesions and certain arrhenoblastomas is frankly impossible, as is the problem of differentiating various Leydig (hilus) cell tumors from luteinized granulosa-theca or adrenal tumors. We might mention such other problems as distinguishing between the so-called Sertoli cell tumor, certain tubular granulosa-theca lesions, and the folliculoma lipidique. Nor does it follow that a histologically classic feminizing or virilizing tumor has any endocrine effect.

It is of course obvious that evaluation of a few microscopic sections of any large ovarian tumor encompasses only a small segment of the contained pathology; indeed, unless serial sections are routine, it is theoretically possible to overlook certain vital diagnostic features. Although this may occur, review of many similar tumors might be expected to afford an accurate composite, and yield a positive method of anticipating clinical effect from the histologic pattern.

This premise may be valid, but recent studies of the gonadal stromal tumors, both virilizing and feminizing, from the Ovarian Tumor Registry seem to illustrate the futility of correlating the general pattern, component cells, and endocrine effect. Whether the endocrinologically active tumor is tubular, cordlike, or solid, and contains many or no androgenic (interstitial) or estrogenic (granulosa-theca) cells, is often in total disagreement with the clinical effect.

We subscribe to Sandberg's doctrine that endocrine effect should be the index of classifying functionally active tumors, and because he presents persuasive evidence that they all arise from mesenchyme, the generic term of *mesenchymoma* or *gonadal stromal tumor* seems logical. While certain embryologists may disagree on the derivation of the so-called tubules and cords (whether mesenchyme or infolding germinal epithelium), if the coelomic epithelium evolves from mesoderm, does it really matter?

We believe that the ovarian stromal cell is capable of profound differentiating possibilities, into diffuse or cordlike tumors of the granulosa-theca, theca lutein, or Leydig cell type. It can possibly convert into tubular structures such as are present in arrhenoblastomas. Whether this is a capability of the adult stromal cell or results from certain reserve cells, as suggested by Warner and associates, seems academic.

Such a concept permits classification of certain indistinguishable tumors as *mesenchymal* or *gonadal stromal tumors* with qualification by the prefix *inert, masculinizing,* or *feminizing* according to the observed effect, with masculinizing the suggested prefix even if endometrial hyperplasia should coexist with virilism. It must also be recognized that the ovarian stroma with many types of tumors is capable of conversion to a cell that may occasionally secrete an estrogen or an androgen.

MacKinlay's painstaking review of granulosa cell tumors suggests the possible convertiblity of granulosa and theca cells, normally estrogenic, into hilus or luteinized cells capable of androgen secretion. As he states, "granulosa and Sertoli cells have a common histogenesis from the primitive sex cord, and certainly they are indistinguishable." Why then utilize the term Sertoli cell at all, or indeed utilize any designation that is foreign to the ovary? We would rather reemphasize the tremendous differentiating potencies of the gonadal stroma.

If this premise is accepted, it might be feasible to delete such uncertain designations as androblastoma, and even arrhenoblastoma and granulosa-thecoma, from the literature. Admittedly, Teilum has performed a service in portraying homologus ovarian and testicular tumors, yet considerable confusion has arisen from the terms evolved. Let us accept the fact that the stroma with *any* ovarian tumor can exert an endocrine influence, either estrogenic or androgenic, and Morris and Scully aptly refer to them as *tumors with a functioning matrix.* A multitude of ovarian tumors not classically endocrine-secreting in type are hormonally active because of the behavior of the stroma (Brenner, Krukenberg, serous, mucinous [Figs. 27–25 and 27–26], and other tumors), and these have been thoroughly tabulated by Scully and Cohen, Spadoni and co-workers, and others. Seemingly the stroma is stimulated by adjacent tumor implants and con-

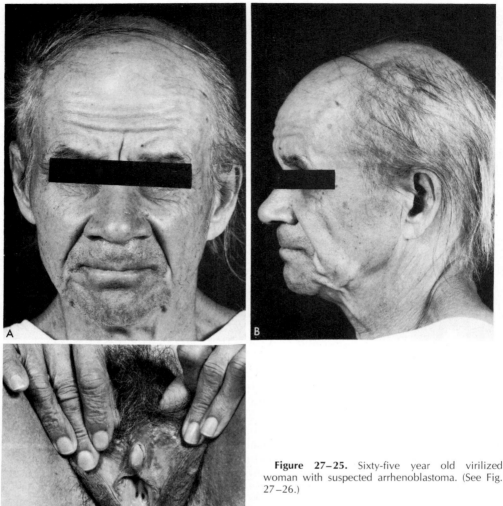

Figure 27–25. Sixty-five year old virilized woman with suspected arrhenoblastoma. (See Fig. 27–26.)

verted into Leydig-like or theca-like cells capable of steroid production.

Many authors, such as Jeffcoate, have commented on the ability of the normal ovary to secrete both estrogens and androgens. Study of many functioning tumors has suggested that some produce a mixture of androgens and estrogens, with one or the other predominating and leading to the clinical effect observed. The close chemical kinship of the virilizing and feminizing hormones with the likelihood of a variable equilibrium makes this possible regardless of the histologic pattern. Perhaps many arrhenoblastomas or granulosa cell tumors are actually gynandroblastomas (Fig. 27–26), with one steroidal effect being dominant.

TREATMENT

Therapy of gonadal stromal tumors is obviously surgery, but because of the low grade malignancy of both the *feminizing* and *masculinizing* neoplasms, the type of operation seems dependent on (1) the age of the patient, and (2) the extent of the disease.

In the youthful patient anxious for subse-

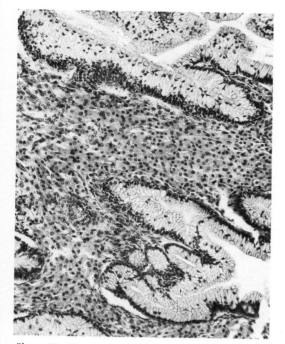

Figure 27–26. Androgenic mucinous tumor with stroma morphologically and histochemically similar to interstitial cells.

quent pregnancy, unilateral salpingo-oophorectomy seems feasible if the lesion appears to be confined to one ovary (capsule intact). In the older patient or when there is extreme disease, complete operation is recommended. Should the tumor show extraovarian extension less than 2 cm. in diameter, the M. D. Anderson Group utilizes irradiation. In the case of advanced disease Schwartz and Smith recommend chemotherapy, but caution that triple drug therapy rather than a single agent is necessary. Actinomycin D, cyclophosphamide, and 5-fluorouracil (5-FU) seemed effective in the feminizing tumors, with vincristine replacing 5-FU with the virilizing neoplasms.

REFERENCES

Berendsen, P. B., Smith, E. B., Abell, M. R., and Jaffe, R. B.: Fine structure of Leydig cells from an arrheoblastoma of the ovary. Am. J. Obstet. Gynecol., *103*: 192, 1969.

Berger, L.: La glande sympathicotrope du hile de l'ovaire; ses homologies avec la glande interstitielle du testicule. Les rapports nerveuses des deux glandes. Arch. Anat., *2*:255, 1923.

Berger, L.: Sur l'existence de glandes sympathicotropes dans l'ovaire et le testicule humains; leur rapports avec la glande interstitielle du testicule. C. R. Acad. Sci., *175*:907, 1922.

Berger, L.: Tumeur des cellules sympathicotropes de l'ovaire avec virilisation. Rev. Canad. Biol., *1*:539, 1942.

Boivin, Y., and Richart, R. M.: Hilus cell tumors of the ovary. Cancer, *18*:231, 1965.

Chan, L. K. C., and Prathrop, K.: Virilization in pregnancy associated with an ovarian mucinous cystadenoma. Am. J. Obstet. Gynecol., *108*:946, 1970.

Dunniho, D. R., Grieme, D. L., and Wolfe, R. J.: Hilus cell tumors of the ovary. Obstet. Gynceol., *27*:703, 1966.

Echt, C. R., and Hadd, H. E.: Androgen excretion patterns in a patient with metastatic hilus cell tumor of the ovary. Am. J. Obstet. Gynecol., *100*:1055, 1968.

Galle, P. C., et al.: Arrhenoblastoma during pregnancy. Obstet. Gynecol., *51*:359, 1978.

Goldstein, D. P., and Lamb, E. J.: Arrhenoblastomas in first cousins. Obstet. Gynecol., *35*:444, 1970.

Goodwin, J. W., Ehrmann, R. L., and Leavitt, T., Jr.: An apparently estrogenic hilum cell tumor of the ovary. Obstet. Gynecol., *19*:467, 1962.

Graber, E. A., O'Rourke, J. J., and Sturman, M.: Arrhenoblastoma of the ovary. Am. J. Obstet. Gynecol., *81*:773, 1961.

Greenblatt, R. B., and Roy, S.: The Hirsute Female. R. G. Greenblatt (Ed.). Springfield, Ill., Charles C Thomas, 1963.

Hawkins, D. F., and Lawrence, D. M.: Virilizing ovarian hilus cell hyperplasia with special reference to hormone excretion. J. Obstet. Gynaecol. Br. Commonw., *72*:285, 1965.

Hughesdon, P. E.: Ovarian lipoid and theca cell tumors; their origins and interpretations. Obstet. Gynecol. Surv., *21*:245, 1966.

Hughesdon, P. E., and Frasier, I. T.: Arrhenoblastoma of ovary. Acta Obstet. Gynecol. Scand., *32*:1, 1953.

Ireland, K., and Woodruff, J. D.: Masculinizing ovarian tumors. Obstet. Gynecol. Surv., *31*:83, 1975.

Janko, A. B., and Sandberg, E. C.: Histochemical evidence for the protein nature of the Reinke crystalloid. Obstet. Gynecol., *35*:493, 1970.

Jeffcoate, S. L., and Pronty, F. T. G.: Steriod synthesis in vitro by a hilar cell tumor. Am. J. Obstet. Gynecol., *101*:684, 1968.

Jeffcoate, T. N. A.: The androgenic ovary, with special reference to the Stein-Leventhal syndrome. Am. J. Obstet. Gynecol., *88*:143, 1964.

Jensen, R. D., et al.: Familial arrhenoblastoma and thyroid adenoma. Obstet. Gynecol. Surv., *29*:646, 1974.

Johnston, J. W., Kernodle, J. R., and Saunders, C. L., Jr.: Arrhenoblastoma of the right ovary. Am. J. Obstet. Gynecol., *78*:800, 1959.

Lees, D. H., and Paine, G. G.: Lipoid masculinizing tumors of the ovary. J. Obstet. Gynaecol. Br. Emp., *65*:710, 1958.

Loubet, R., and Loubet, A.: Le système des cellulaires hilaires de l'ovaire, hyperplasies et tumeurs. Soc. Fránç. Gynécol., *33*:589, 1963.

MacKinlay, C. J.: Male cells in granulosa cell ovarian tumors. J. Obstet. Gynaecol. Br. Emp., *64*:512, 1957.

Mahesh, V. B., McDonough, P. G., and Deleo, C. A.: Endocrine studies in an arrhenoblastoma. Am. J. Obstet. Gynecol., *107*:183, 1970.

Maldman, J. E., et al.: Steroid metabolism in arrhenoblastoma. Obstet. Gynecol., *44*:33, 1974.

Merrill, J. A.: Ovarian hilus cells. Am. J. Obstet. Gynecol., *78*:1258, 1959.

Meyer, R.: Pathology of some special ovarian tumors and their relation to sex characteristics. Am. J. Obstet. Gynecol., 22:697, 1931.

Meyer, R.: Über Adenoma malignum ovarii. Z. Geburtsh. Gynäk., 76:616, 1915.

Meyer, R.: Tubuläre (testikuläre) und solide Formen des Andreioblastoma ovarii. Beitr. Pathol. Anat., 84:485, 1930.

Mohamed, N. C., et al.: Hilus cell tumor and endometrial carcinoma. Obstet. Gynecol., 52:486, 1978.

Morris, J. M., and Scully, R. E.: Endocrine Pathology of the Ovary. St. Louis, C. V. Mosby Company, 1958.

Norris, H. J., and Chorlton, I.: Functioning tumors of the ovary. Clin. Obstet. Gynecol., 17:189, 1974.

Novak, E. R.: Gynandroblastoma of the ovary (review of eight cases from the Ovarian Tumor Registry). Obstet. Gynecol., 30:709, 1967.

Novak, E. R., and Long, J. H.: Arrhenoblastomas of the ovary. A review of the Ovarian Tumor Registry. Am. J. Obstet. Gynecol., 92:1082, 1965.

Novak, E. R., and Mattingly, R. F.: Hilus cell tumors of the ovary (with a review of 18 cases). Obstet. Gynecol., 15:425, 1960.

Novak, E. R., Woodruff, J. D., and Linthicum, J. M.: Evaluation of the unclassified tumors of the Ovarian Tumor Registry. Am. J. Obstet. Gynecol., 87:999, 1963.

Pedowitz, P., and O'Brien, F. B.: Arrhenoblastoma of the ovary. Obstet. Gynecol., 16:62, 1960.

Pick, L.: Über Adenoma der männlichen und weiblichen Keimdrüse. Berl. Klin. Wchn., 42:502, 1905.

Plate, W. P.: Oestrogene Functie van de Tussencellon in de Gonade. Ned. T. Verlosk., 63:83, 1963.

Sachs, B. A.: Leydig (sympathicotropic) cell tumor of ovary: Report of case with virilism, including postmortem findings. J. Clin. Endocrinol., 11:878, 1951.

Sandberg, E. C.: The virilizing ovary. Obstet. Gynecol. Surv., 17:165, 1962.

Schneider, G. T.: "Functioning" ovarian tumors. Am. J. Obstet. Gynecol., 79:921, 1960.

Schwartz, P. E., and Smith, J. P.: Treatment of ovarian stromal tumors. Am. J. Obstet. Gynecol., 125:402, 1976.

Scott, J. S., Lumsden, C. E., and Levell, M. J.: Ovarian endocrine activity in association with hormonally inactive neoplasia. Am. J. Obstet. Gynecol., 97:161, 1967.

Scully, R. E., and Cohen, R. B.: Ganglioneuroma of adrenal medulla containing cells morphologically identical to hilus cells (extra parenchymal Leydig cells). Cancer, 14:421, 1961.

Shippel, S.: The ovarian theca cell. J. Obstet. Gynaecol. Br. Emp., 62:321, 1955.

Sobrinho, L. G., and Kase, N. G.: Adrenal rest cell tumor of the ovary. Obstet. Gynecol., 36:895, 1970.

Spadoni, L. R., Lindberg, M. C., Mottet, N. K., and Herrmann, W. L.: Virilization coexisting with Krukenberg tumor during pregnancy. Am. J. Obstet. Gynecol., 92:981, 1965.

Sternberg, W. H.: Morphology, androgenic function, hyperplasia and tumors of the human ovarian hilus cells. Am. J. Pathol., 25:493, 1949.

Sternberg, W. H., and Roth, L. M.: Ovarian stromal tumors containing Leydig cells. Cancer, 32:940, 1973.

Stewart, R. S., and Woodard, D. E.: Malignant ovarian hilus cell tumor. A.M.A. Arch. Pathol., 73:13, 1962.

Teilum, G.: Special Tumors of the Ovary and Testis. Philadelphia, J. B. Lippincott Co. 1971.

Verhoeven, A. T. M., et al.: Virilization in pregnancy. Obstet. Gynecol. Surv., 28:597, 1973.

Warner, N. E., Friedman, N. B., Bomze, E. J., and Masin, F.: Comparative pathology of experimental and spontaneous androblastomas and gynoblastomas of the gonads. Am. J. Obstet. Gynecol., 79:971, 1960.

Wolff, E., et al.: Virilizing luteoma of pregnancy. Am. J. Med., 54:229, 1973.

Wong, T. W., and Warner, N. E.: Ovarian thecal metaplasia in the adrenal gland. Arch. Pathol., 92:319, 1971.

Younglai, E. V., et al.: Arrhenoblastoma: in vivo and in vitro studies. Am. J. Obstet. Gynecol., 116:401, 1973.

Chapter 28

ECTOPIC PREGNANCY

Types

The term ectopic pregnancy is more inclusive than extrauterine pregnancy. Pregnancy may be definitely ectopic and still not be, strictly speaking, extrauterine, as in interstitial pregnancy, or pregnancy in a rudimentary uterine horn. Ectopic pregnancy is a gestation in which the fertilized ovum implants itself at some site other than the usual one in the endometrium. The term therefore embraces (1) pregnancy in any portion of the tube (*tubal pregnancy*) (Figs. 28–1 and 28–2), including its interstitial portion (*interstitial pregnancy*) (Fig. 28–3); (2) pregnancy in a *rudimentary uterine horn,* even when completely separate from the uterus (Fig. 28–4 A) (Cohn and Goldenberg); (3) *cornual pregnancy* (Fig. 28–4B) (4) *intramural pregnancy* in which the gestation is separate from the uterus and tube and is completely surrounded by myometrium (McGowan) (Fig. 28–5); (5) *ovarian pregnancy;* (6) *abdominal pregnancy,* either primary or secondary; and (7) *cervical pregnancy,* which is rare (Fig. 28–6). In addition to these, occasionally the fertilized egg finds nidation in an endometrial pocket within the wall of a uterus which is the seat of adenomyosis.

Tubal pregnancy is by far the most common form of ectopic gestation, its incidence, according to older references, being one in every 300 cases of pregnancy. This figure varies considerably with the proportion of clinic patients who have a greater incidence of salpingitis and tubal constriction. Actually, a study by Fontanilla and Anderson showed that, in Baltimore, ectopic gestation occurred in 1 of 200 pregnant white women and in 1 of 120 Negro patients, a difference of nearly 100 per cent. Breen's New Jersey study of predominantly black patients notes one ectopic to every 87 deliveries.

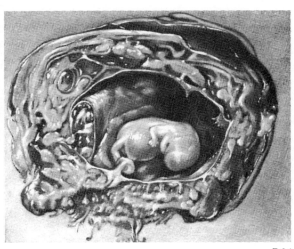

Figure 28–1. Cut surface of tubal pregnancy sac at 2½ months, showing embryo alive at time of operation.

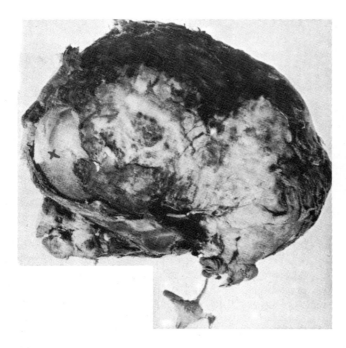

Figure 28–2. Extreme stretching and thinning of tubal wall, with amniotic sac (×) showing through.

Widespread use of the IUD has undoubtedly led to an increased incidence of ectopic pregnancy, since it seems more effective in preventing uterine implantation than tubal or particularly ovarian pregnancy, as noted subsequently. Hallatt records 70 cases in IUD users.

Douglas (1963) states that in Jamaica there is the astounding ratio of one ectopic pregnancy to every 28 live births, presumably because of the high incidence of salpingitis.

Following a tubal gestation, the possibility of a second (repeat) ectopic pregnancy in our clinic appears to be roughly 10 per cent, and this corresponds to the recent reports of Schoen and Nowak, and Hallatt; an intrauterine pregnancy occurs in more than 25 per cent of women in whom the uterus is retained.

Ectopic pregnancy is a potentially hazardous problem. Schneider and associates record 102 deaths in Michigan in a 25 year

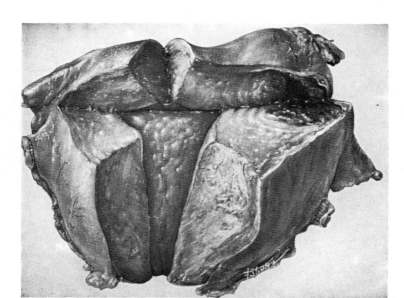

Figure 28–3. Interstitial tubal pregnancy.

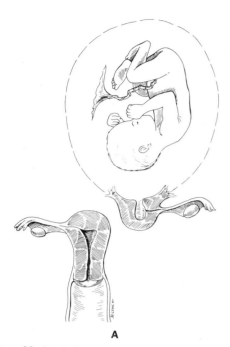

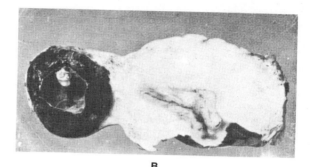

A

B

Figure 28–4. *A*, Pregnancy in an unattached uterine horn. (Courtesy of F. L. Cohn and R. L. Goldenberg: Obstet. Gynecol., *48*:234, 1976.) *B*, Cut surface of uterus and cornual pregnancy. Note the thick decidua still in situ, although evidences of its impending separation are already apparent.

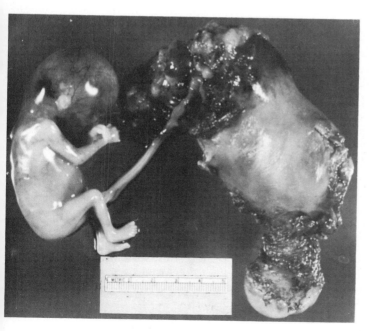

Figure 28–5. Ruptured intramural pregnancy; extrauterine fetus with cord leading to intrauterine placenta. (Courtesy of L. McGowan: J.A.M.A., *192*:637, 1965.)

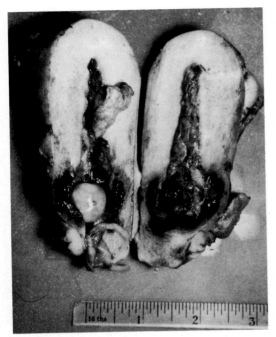

Figure 28–6. Cervical implantation; an ectopic pregnancy with a uterine site of gestation. (Courtesy of Dr. L. Resnick, South Africa.)

period, mostly due to hemorrhage, and they estimate mortality between 2 and 4 per 1000. An even more recent publication by May and associates is in agreement.

ETIOLOGY OF TUBAL PREGNANCY

Although many causes have been suggested for the occurrence of tubal pregnancy, they can all be placed in two chief groups, viz.: (1) factors which delay or prevent the passage of the fertilized egg into the uterine cavity; and (2) factors which increase the receptiveness of the tubal mucosa to the implantation of the fertilized egg.

Factors Which Delay or Prevent Passage of the Fertilized Egg Into the Uterine Cavity

Of this group, undoubtedly the most important is *chronic inflammatory disease.* The role played by inflammatory disease is most apt to be a mechanical one, through narrowing of the lumen, or through the production of blind alleys as a result of agglutination of adjacent tubal folds. The latter change

is especially conspicuous in cases of *follicular salpingitis,* and it is not strange, therefore, that this form of tubal inflammation is considered by many as most frequently involved in tubal implantation. Peritubal inflammation, through the angulation or constriction produced by adhesions, is another possible factor to be considered, and the importance of tubal infection in such anatomic changes has been stressed by Bone and Greene. Nevertheless, antibiotics seem so effective in treating acute salpingitis that normal intrauterine pregnancy frequently follows an adequately treated tubal infection.

Aside from the purely mechanical role of inflammation, one must remember that it may be responsible for marked *impairment of ciliary activity and muscular peristaltic activity,* with resulting retardation of the progress of the egg. Halbrecht notes that, in the few women who become pregnant following *medical treatment for endometrial tuberculosis* (and inevitable salpingitis), there is a high incidence of tubal pregnancy —about two thirds. Concomitant ectopic gestation and active tuberculous salpingitis is uncommon, but Overbeck reports nine cases with no exacerbation of the tuberculosis following unilateral salpingectomy and appropriate chemotherapy.

Greenhill has noted an increasingly common cause of tubal pregnancy, namely previous plastic operation on the tube. Of 405 pregnancies following tuboplastic procedures, ectopic gestation occurred in 15 per cent of the pregnancies. We suspect that (laparoscopic) tubal sterilization may be followed by a certain number of tubal pregnancies; we have witnessed several cases in the few years since this procedure has been in use. Brenner and associates and Sheikh and Yassman have discussed this possibility.

(Congenital) diverticula have been noted by Persaud in nearly 50 per cent of tubal pregnancies, and these may offer lodgment to an egg that has strayed from the tubal lumen proper, as may *accessory ostia* which frequently end blindly. The same statement may be made concerning the relatively rare cases in which the tubal lumen is congenitally duplicated throughout all or part of its course. *Tumors outside the tube,* such as uterine myomas or ovarian cysts, may occasionally cause constriction of the tubal lumen, as may possibly the rare case of *intra-*

tubal polypoid growth, or *tubal endometriosis.*

In a series of studies, Iffy proposes an interesting theory of the cause of ectopic gestation. He suggests that conception may occur late in the cycle so that adequate implantation is not achieved before ensuing menstruation. The menstrual flow propels the fertilized ovum up and into the tube (as in the tubal regurgitation theory of endometriosis). This is an intriguing concept that Iffy has expanded to explain other complications of pregnancy, but it is difficult to accept in toto. The exact time of conception is difficult to assess, and although an implanted ovum may be necessary to inhibit impending menstruation, there may be variations in the time from fertilization to implantation. Nevertheless, Iffy's concept of late implantation warrants consideration.

It appears that partial tubal occlusion resulting from a variety of causes (most frequently inflammatory disease) is the most frequent etiologic factor in the causation of tubal pregnancy, although other factors may play some role.

Factors Increasing Receptiveness of Tubal Mucosa to Fertilized Egg

There seem to be two reasons why the egg does not normally implant itself in the tube, where it is commonly fertilized. One of these is that its burrowing apparatus, *the trophoblast, is not normally developed until after the egg reaches the uterus.* The other seems to be that under normal conditions *the tubal mucosa is not structurally or functionally designed for implanation.* The first reason impresses us as the more cogent, and it would seem that partial retardation of the progress of the fertilized egg is the most important etiologic factor, permitting development of the trophoblast while the egg is still in the tube.

The assumed unreceptiveness of the endosalpinx is based chiefly on the fact that it is not as capable of decidual reaction as is the endometrium, although in some tubes the mucosa at least approximates the endometrium's receptivity to the egg. We are impressed with the fact that pregnancy often occurs in tubes which otherwise seem normal, although it may be difficult to exclude the presence of diverticula on routine sections without serial or radiographic studies.

Finally, the occurrence of definite decidual tubal response in at least some cases of pregnancy, uterine or tubal, is now admitted by practically all authors. For these reasons, we do not think that occasional receptivity of the tubal mucosa can be dismissed in the consideration of the etiology of tubal pregnancy, although the evidence indicates the greater importance of the first group of causes.

NIDATION IN THE TUBE

The fundamental phenomena of implantation in tubal pregnancy are like those of normal uterine gestation, with allowance for the striking deficiency of decidual response of the tubal wall. The villi, through the erosive action of the trophoblast, penetrate the tubal wall, often to the serosa itself. Intra-abdominal bleeding may thus result, and if a large vessel is eroded, such bleeding may be massive. Deportation of trophoblast and villi may be seen similarly to intrauterine pregnancy.

The villi have the same characteristics as in intrauterine pregnancy. When well preserved, they show the two layers of trophoblast, the cytotrophoblast (Langhans layer) and the syncytium, just as in the villi of normal pregnancy. The fastening villi show large masses of trophoblast at their tips, these trophoblastic nodules consisting chiefly of Langhans cells, with streamers of syncytium at the periphery. The trophoblast can, in properly cut sections, be traced by direct continuity far out into the tubal wall, and these invading cells have often been mistaken for decidua (Fig. 28–7).

After the death of the embryo, which usually takes place in the early weeks of pregnancy, the villi undergo degeneration (Fig. 28–8), though many embryologists believe that the trophoblast may remain functionally active, and that it may continue its erosive invasion for a time after the somatic death of the embryo. Studies by Shintani and co-workers indicate adequately that this occurs in some animals. There is also good ground for this belief on the basis of clinical evidence, as tubal perforation frequently occurs a considerable time after the death of the embryo and long after a negative pregnancy test. Perhaps the erosive action of the trophoblast persists after it has lost its capacity to produce gonadotropin. Whatever the

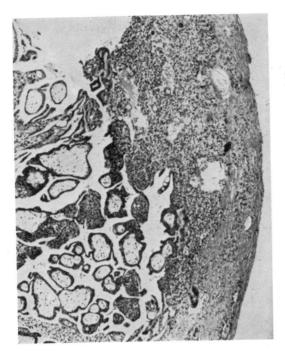

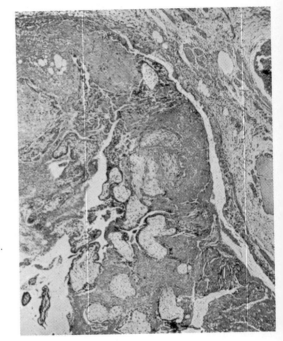

Figure 28–7. Wall of interstitial pregnancy sac in case showing numerous young villi and marked trophoblastic invasion of wall, often mistaken for decidua.

Figure 28–8. Degenerated villi in tubal gestation.

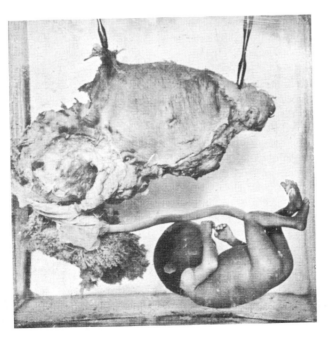

Figure 28–9. Ruptured interstitial pregnancy with fetus.

mechanism, we have seen several such cases weeks after the pregnancy test became negative (Fig. 28–9).

Occurrence of Decidua in the Tubes

Whether genuine decidual tissue may be observed in the tubes has long been controversial. However, opinion on this subject has crystallized, and practically all writers now agree that a true but patchy decidual reaction may occur in the tube with an intra-uterine or a tubal pregnancy. On the other hand, there is general agreement that the decidual cells rarely form a continuous and intact layer, such as one sees in the uterus. The reaction at best is an imperfect one, and in most routine sections cannot be detected (Fig. 28–10).

Much of the confusion on this subject has no doubt been due to incorrect microscopic interpretations. For example, a diagnosis of decidual tissue is frequently made when the connective tissue cells of the tube show only a moderate hypertrophy, or when the edema so often present teases the cells apart, causing them to swell, perhaps giving the tissue a somewhat mosaic appearance (Fig. 28–11). It is difficult, at times, in the known case of tubal pregnancy, to distinguish such decidual-like changes from a genuine transfor-

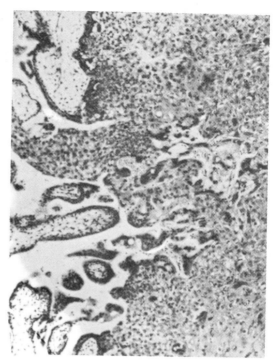

Figure 28–11. Extensive trophoblastic infiltration of tubal wall, showing both syncytium and Langhans cells.

mation. The characteristic decidual changes of the endometrial stroma are the real morphologic criterion in this respect (Fig. 28–12).

In most cases of tubal pregnancy it is rare to observe decidual transformation of the tubal connective tissue. The obvious pitfall in making such a diagnosis is to mistake for decidua the trophoblastic cells which invade the tubal wall extensively. In many cases the trophoblastic nature of the cells is easy to recognize, as when the cells are directly continuous with the trophoblastic villous covering, or when some of the characteristic syncytial giant cells can be seen among them. The syncytial cells can scarcely be mistaken for decidual cells. When the invading cells are of the Langhans type and the continuity with the villous covering is not shown in the particular section under study, the diagnosis is much more difficult.

In other cases, the appearance of the decidual cells is so typical, the existence of definite transition stages from the normal tubal stroma is so clearly demonstrable, and the separateness of the area from the placental site is so evident that the diagnosis of decidual tissue is obvious. When such changes

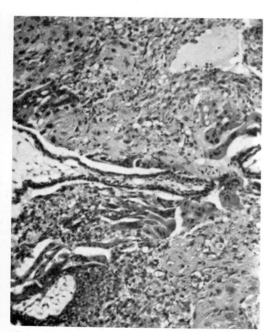

Figure 28–10. Tubal pregnancy, showing both the syncytial and Langhans cells of chorionic villi.

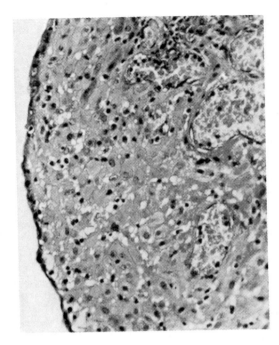

Figure 28–12. High power view of marked decidual change in tubal fold well removed from implantation site.

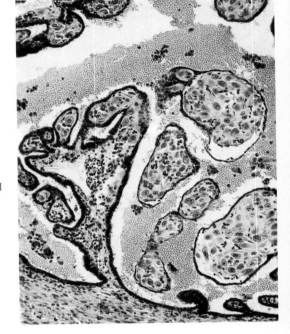

Figure 28–13. Marked decidual reaction within tubal rugae in conjunction with intrauterine pregnancy.

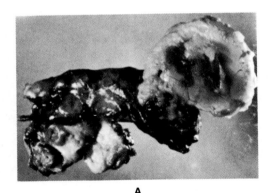

A

B

Figure 28–14. *A*, Tubal abortion protruding out fimbriae. *B*, Opened specimen.

are seen in a distant tissue, as in the opposite tube, the possibility of their being trophoblastic can be eliminated (Fig. 28–13). Never, however, is there in the "pregnant" tube a decidual layer which can be compared in extent and degree to that seen in the uterus with normal pregnancy.

Later Course

The unfavorable environment of the implanted egg is responsible for certain departures from the normal progress of pregnancy. These often develop in the early weeks of pregnancy, and are responsible for the common early death of the ovum. Whereas in the normal uterine implantation area, the egg is embedded in a thick decidua, in the tubal variety this is lacking, so that only a spurious *decidua basalis* and *capsularis* are formed. The former consists of an imperfect layer of decidual cells, and connective tissue and muscle cells which are partially destroyed by the erosive action of the trophoblast, with the production of a necrotic or fibrinoid layer.

TERMINATIONS OF TUBAL PREGNANCY

Tubal Abortion

When the ovum is actually separated from the tube wall, we have to deal with tubal abortion, and in such cases bleeding into the tube (*hematosalpinx*) is likewise an important feature (Fig. 28–14). The ovum may be expelled into the abdominal cavity, and intraperitoneal hemorrhage through the tubal orifice may be profuse. Hematosalpinx is presumptive evidence of tubal pregnancy even in the absence of demonstrated villi, although it is a rare sequel of tumor or infection.

Tubal Rupture

This is a frequent occurrence, producing abdominal bleeding which may be slight but repeated, or profuse and even at times fatal. As already discussed, it is due to the erosive action of the trophoblast upon the tubal tissues and blood vessels. On the other hand, if the bleeding results from perforation along the lower margin of the tube, it is enclosed between the folds of the broad ligament, with the production of a hematoma.

Although tubal rupture may be associated with massive degrees of intraperitoneal hemorrhage, far more often the bleeding is scantier and sporadic; Parker and Parker aptly call it a *chronic ectopic pregnancy*. Repeated episodes of bleeding with spontaneous clot formation may occur so that a large mass may form, mimicking inflammatory disease, endometriosis, or an ovarian tumor. Diagnosis in such cases is difficult.

Secondary Abdominal Pregnancy

In many of the older descriptions, it was stated that if the fertilized ovum is expelled through tubal abortion or perforation, it might occasionally retain its vitality and reimplant itself upon the peritoneum, most often on the tube, broad ligament, or upon adherent portions of the intestine. Such a mechanism for secondary abdominal implantation is incredible, for the embryo succumbs the moment its separation from the tubal wall is complete. The correct explanation of these cases is that the placenta remains attached even though the embryo is extruded through the perforation or the fimbriated orifice. Moreover, the villi begin to grow outward through the rupture point, so that more and more of the placental area, and eventually the entire placenta, may be found outside. This is probably the correct explanation of all secondary abdominal pregnancies, many of which progress to term. Sonography may be of considerable diagnostic value, as noted by Stafford and Ragan.

Broad Ligament (Intraligamentary) Pregnancy

When the tubal rupture takes place at some point along the line of attachment of the mesosalpinx, the embryo may be extruded between the folds of the broad ligament. The placental growth then proceeds more and more into the intraligamentary space, as described with secondary abdominal pregnancy. The placenta may be weaned away entirely from the tube, and in the latter stages is often entirely distinct from it. Broad ligament pregnancy often progresses to late stages of development, and in many instances has continued to full term. Paterson and Grant have provided a recent extensive review of advanced ligamentary pregnancies, many of which progress to viability.

Spontaneous Regression

Not every case of tubal pregnancy comes to operation, for the embryo may succumb and the implantation area undergo gradual retrogression, in the absence of bleeding or other symptoms sufficiently severe to compel medical attention. This is indicated by the occasional finding of old organized and usually hyalinized villi in tubes which otherwise may seem normal, and with no history to justify the suspicion of recent gestation (Fig. 28–15). In cases of this type, however, a careful inquiry may elicit evidence indicating the probable occurrence of tubal gestation many months previously.

Lithopedion Formation or Mummification

A tubal pregnancy may pass unrecognized even when it has advanced to a later stage. In such cases the fetus may be retained for many years, with calcification and lithopedion formation, or mummification. On the other hand, passage of fetal bones may occur via rectum, cul-de-sac, or abdomen, and we can recall instances of all of these.

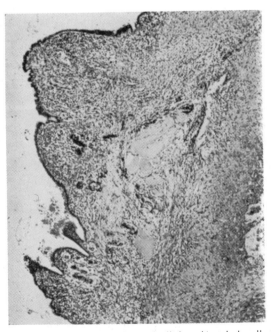

Figure 28–15. Old hyalinized villi found in tubal wall of patient operated upon for an unrelated condition, and representing remains of tubal pregnancy that had occurred long before.

Tubal Hydatidiform Mole or Chorionepithelioma

Although rare, either one of these pathologic entities may follow tubal pregnancy (see Chapter 33).

BEHAVIOR OF UTERINE MUCOSA IN CASES OF TUBAL PREGNANCY

Very soon after fertilization, decidual transformation of the endometrium is noted. There is no sharp dividing line between the histologic picture of premenstrual hypertrophy of the endometrium and that of the young decidua. The former is properly spoken of, from a teleologic standpoint, as a pregravid endometrium. In other words, the endometrium of every woman during reproductive life prepares itself once every month for the reception of an impregnated ovum. If pregnancy does not occur, the preparation in the endometrium is rendered unnecessary and the transformed endometrium, or at least a considerable portion of it, is cast off.

If, on the other hand, the egg is fertilized, it finds a bed already prepared for it in the modified endometrium, which passes by easy stages into frank decidua (Figs. 28–16 and 28–17). The histologic structure of the latter is described in Chapter 7. Suffice it to say that decidual transformation is noted whether pregnancy be intrauterine or extrauterine, but with fetal death, the decidua may gradually be exfoliated, so that if curettage is performed, any type of endometrium may be found, particularly with the chronic ectopic pregnancy; tubal rupture may still occur because of viable invasive trophoblast, despite a negative pregnancy test.

It seems safe to assume, although there is little direct evidence on the point, that in the rare case of tubal pregnancy advancing without interruption to the later months, the uterine decidua exhibits the same features as the decidua vera of intrauterine pregnancy, with perhaps the absence of such thinning and atrophy as is explained by the mechanical pressure of the amniotic contents. Unfortunately, however, the course of the tubal fetus does not run so smoothly as does that of the more happily located uterine embryo. It usually survives only a short time, and its death exerts a profound influence upon the uterine decidua. This is shed, either in one

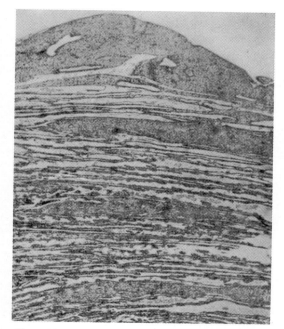

Figure 28–16. Decidua vera in a case of tubal pregnancy in which the embryo was living (2½ months). Note the superficial compacta with its broad fields of decidual cells, and the spongiosa made up largely of very tortuous glands, here shown running parallel to surface, as is often the case. The basalis is not shown.

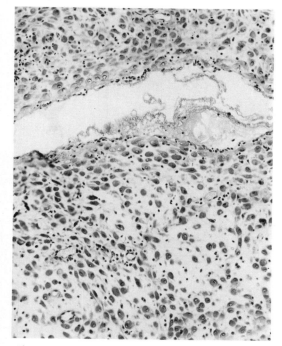

Figure 28–17. Extensive endometrial stromal deciduosis with gland showing almost complete loss of lining epithelium. (Tubal pregnancy of approximately 10 weeks' duration.)

large cast of the uterine cavity or in much smaller particles.

Arias-Stella Reaction (ASR)

In 1957 Arias-Stella noted atypical changes occurring in the endometrium of women with ectopic pregnancy. He believed that this atypicality may be so extreme as to resemble adenocarcinoma and that it may be due to a hormonal effect. Sturgis points out that he described exactly the same findings years before Arias-Stella, and review of his publications confirms this. Novak indicates the difficulty in establishing the diagnosis in borderline cases, especially where there is no knowledge of a coexisting pregnancy. This may account for the wide variation in the Arias-Stella reaction with ectopic gestation (10 to 70 per cent).

Marked cellular atypism and mitotic activity occur with extreme glandular proliferation and striking evidence of progesterone influence on the cells lining the glands. Extensive tufting, budding, and infolding may occur, and the tall pale-staining hypersecretory epithelium (Fig. 28–18 A) itself is suggestive of a markedly adenomatous process. The individual cellular atypia may persist after the hypersecretory pattern has regressed as a result of fetal death, and an alert pathologist may suggest the possibility of a clinically unsuspected ectopic pregnancy (Fig. 28–18 B). It may also occur in ectopic endometrium (endometriosis). We are in full accord with concepts that a prolonged endocrine stimulus might lead to an abnormally profound secretory response to progesterone, although admittedly there are many histologic similarities to certain estrogen-induced atypical hyperplastic endometria. Polyploidy seems usual with the Arias-Stella reaction, unlike the diploidy or occasional aneuploidy observed with endometrial adenocarcinoma (Thrasher and Richart).

In any case, we believe a full-fledged Arias-Stella reaction occurs in only a minority of endometria associated with pregnancy, and we doubt that the incidence is greater than 25 per cent regardless of the site of the pregnancy, despite the study by Lloyd and Fienberg, who indicate a 70 per cent reaction in intra- and extrauterine pregnancy. The frequency varies considerably according to the individual pathologic interpretation; when influenced by the knowledge that a pregnancy has occurred, the pa-

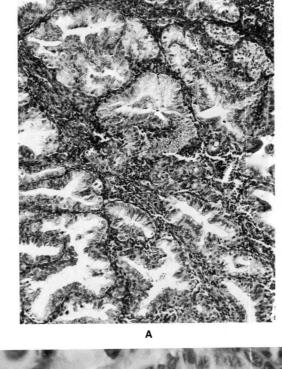

A

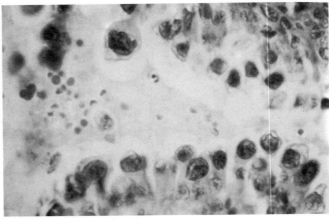

B

Figure 28–18. *A,* Arias-Stella pattern in conjunction with incomplete abortion. Hysterectomy was advised because of presumed adenocarcinoma but refused. Patient is well with two subsequent pregnancies. *B,* High power view of Arias-Stella reaction. Note hyperchromatic nuclear clumping and cellular abnormality. (Courtesy of Dr. E. Friederichs, Milwaukee, Wis.)

thologist can often find areas suggestive of a reaction, but a florid, full-fledged reaction is uncommon. It may occasionally be noted in the endocervix.

Decidual Casts

In any event the patient may note the expulsion of a cast, but in a large proportion of cases, the physician does not have an opportunity to study it. Only too frequently it is not observed or its importance is not appreciated by the patient, and the tissue is not secured for study. The expulsion of uterine casts occurs far more frequently than is commonly believed, but usually intrauterine degenerative changes cause a distintegration of the cast before expulsion. Moreover, the decidua is in many cases shed in small particles, so that no complete uterine cast is expelled by the patient.

The separation and expulsion of the uter-

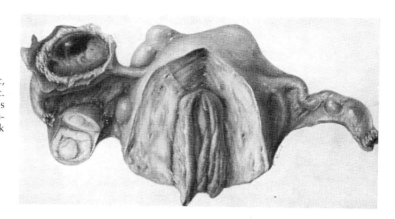

Figure 28–19. Tubal gestation sac, laid open to show embryo in amniotic sac. The large corpus luteum of pregnancy is seen in the ovary of the same side; the interior of the uterus shows the very thick decidua.

ine decidua in cases of tubal pregnancy must at once call to mind the casting off of the corresponding layers in the nonpregnant woman at menstruation, and this may give rise to the so-called *membranous dysmenorrhea*. The compact layer and a portion of the spongy layer are characteristically shed at the menstrual periods, and regeneration of the endometrium proceeds chiefly from the basal layer, which is retained. There is every reason to believe that regeneration after the expulsion of the uterine cast seen with ectopic pregnancy proceeds in essentially the same manner (Fig. 28–19). Decidual casts may be passed in the absence of pregnancy by patients taking contraceptive pills—a presumed hyperreactivity to the exogenous hormones.

Evidence indicates that the life of the uterine decidua is bound up with that of the fertilized ovum. As long as the embryo—uterine or tubal—is alive, the decidua is intact. When the embryo dies, the decidua undergoes the degenerative changes described. However, it must not be assumed that the sequence is always an immediate one, for a number of days may elapse between the death of the embryo and passage of the decidua. In other words, the expulsion of a cast signifies that the embryo has succumbed, but just how long before, one cannot say.

If the uterus is curetted in a case of tubal pregnancy, and the latter proceeds in its development, a new decidual reaction takes place in the uterus. This is exactly what one would expect, and although there is only infrequent opportunity to demonstrate this histologically, it seems generally correct. One such patient had been curetted 10 days before admission to the hospital. The abdominal operation was preceded by another curettage, the curettings showing a definite

decidual reaction. A small living embryo was found in the tube when the abdomen was opened.

Structure of Decidual Casts. Just what thickness of the decidual layer is cast off is difficult to determine, except by a study of the structure of uterine casts or an examination of the uterus after the tissue has been shed. The latter is rarely possible before regeneration has advanced, so that information must come chiefly from the microscopic examination of the casts (Fig. 28–20).

When in a good state of preservation, the casts are observed to consist of the upper or *compact* layer of the decidua with at times a

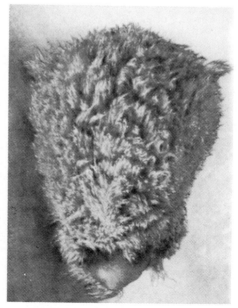

Figure 28–20. Decidual cast thrown off at approximately the sixth week of extrauterine pregnancy. (From Kelly: Operative Gynecology. D. Appleton-Century Co., Publishers.)

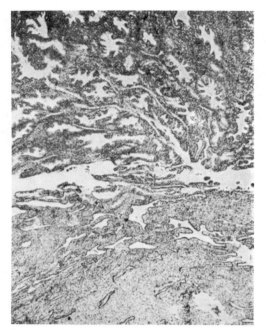

Figure 28–21. Line of separation of decidual cells is evident in this case of tubal pregnancy.

portion of the deeper or *spongy* layer. The surface of a typical cast is covered with a single layer of flattened epithelium. Beneath this is a great field of typical decidual cells, characterized by their mosaic arrangement, polygonal outline, and large, rather pale nuclei (Fig. 28–21). Among these cells are thin-walled venous channels, frequently thrombosed. When decidua without villi are noted, one must always be concerned about the possibility of an ectopic pregnancy. If the decidua is "dirty" (with associated infection and necrosis), one is probably dealing with an abortion, even though villi or trophoblast cannot be demonstrated.

Glands are sparse in the compact layer. They occur usually in the form of slitlike lumina lined by a flat endothelium-like epithelium. In some casts there is a considerable amount of the spongiosa below the compact layer just described. In these are seen many characteristic pregnancy glands. These are, in very young decidua, markedly tortuous, with low and pale-staining epithelium. In the slightly older patient the glands lose some of their tortuosity, possessing large and only slightly irregular lumina lined by flat epithelium. At times, indeed, it is difficult on superficial examination to distinguish them from lymphatic spaces.

VALUE OF DIAGNOSTIC CURETTAGE IN TUBAL PREGNANCY

At times the microscopic examination of uterine curettings is invoked in the diagnosis of tubal pregnancy. Often this is justifiable, as in suspicious cases of uterine bleeding occurring in obese women. It may be impossible to distinguish between the bleeding of a tubal pregnancy which cannot be palpated and that of incomplete early abortion of an intrauterine pregnancy. The occasional diagnostic value of curettage in cases of suspected tubal pregnancy has been noted by many authors, but it should be emphasized that the value is only occasional. Sonography and laparoscopy are much more helpful.

If definite decidual tissue is obtained at curettage, and *if it is not accompanied by chorionic villi*, one is justified in considering the probability of extrauterine pregnancy. This, however, does not invariably prove to be correct, but it might be regarded as a good indication for endoscopic inspection of the pelvic organs (Fig. 28–22).

One must never forget that premenstrual hypertrophy of the nonpregnant endometrium frequently is so pronounced as to completely simulate the appearance of decidua. As a rule, the stromal cells show only a suggestion of the true decidual transformation,

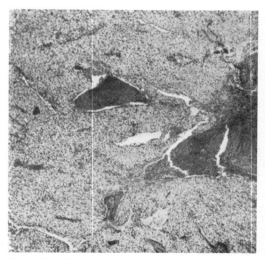

Figure 28–22. A thick cast, comprising the entire compact layer, with also a small portion of the spongiosa. Note the broad field of decidual cells, the thrombosed veins, the infiltrating leukocytes, and the flat epithelium of the few glands that are shown.

and the glandular hypertrophy is also less marked. At times, however, the distinction is not possible unless chorionic tissue is present. The Arias-Stella endometrial response has already been discussed, and has been of some value in the diagnosis of ectopic pregnancy. This may occur in the nonpregnant state as an exaggerated response to progesterone in the premenstrual era, just as a decidual stromal response may be noted.

When curettage is done in cases of tubal pregnancy, it is almost always in cases in which uterine bleeding has been present for a considerable time, i.e., when the embryo has long since died and usually been absorbed, and when the decidua has previously been cast off. Under these conditions microscopic examination commonly yields a normal endometrium with no evidence of the decidual change which was present earlier. The picture is usually that of a postmenstrual or interval type of endometrium (Fig. 28–23). The statement is often made that tubal pregnancy causes uterine decidual change, without proper chronologic qualifications. Hence, one frequently hears surprise expressed if a normal nondecidual endometrium is observed in association with a tubal gestation.

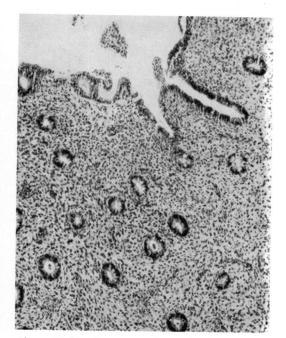

Figure 28–23. Postmenstrual type of endometrium, with no suggestion of decidual change, in case of tubal pregnancy. In other cases, more or less pronounced decidual changes may still be present.

In a large proportion of cases, more particularly in those in which bleeding has been a symptom, little or no information of diagnostic value is to be looked for from the microscopic examination of the uterine scrapings. In a study of certain earlier cases in which the endometrium was available for study, 50 per cent showed a normal postmenstrual or interval type, so that curettage in such cases would have given no help in the diagnosis. In less than 25 per cent there was definite decidual change, so that in these, some help would have been obtained from curettage. In practically all of these, however, curetting would have been contraindicated because there was amenorrhea, with of course the possibility of an intrauterine pregnancy. Lastly, the lutein cyst, so commonly clinically confused with ectopic pregnancy, may produce such a profound progesterone influence that it causes a decidual reaction. Contraceptive pills may on occasion produce not only a decidual appearance but also an Arias-Stella reaction.

SOURCE OF EXTERNAL BLEEDING IN TUBAL PREGNANCY

It has been definitely established that the source of the external bleeding in cases of tubal pregnancy is the endometrium, although in some cases of the interstitial type, the bleeding may have its origin partly from the tubal placental site itself. Although this is true in a minority of cases, the characteristic metrorrhagia of tubal pregnancy is really of endometrial origin, and is at least initiated by the separation of the decidua. The latter, as noted, is caused by the death of the embryo. In other words, as long as the embryo is alive, the decidua is intact and there is no bleeding except perhaps occasional staining.

The most interesting group of cases is that in which there is no uterine bleeding. The clinical diagnosis of such conditions is obviously more difficult than when the characteristic metrorrhagia is present. The amenorrhea in such cases may persist for many months, and is shown at operation to be due to the presence of a living fetus. In the rare case of combined intrauterine and extrauterine pregnancy, a living embryo in the uterus may inhibit bleeding even though the tubal pregnancy has been terminated by rupture.

PREGNANCY TESTS IN TUBAL PREGNANCY

Pregnancy tests are of limited value in that they do not designate the site of pregnancy; positive or negative results depend chiefly upon whether the trophoblast is still functionally active in the production of the chorionic hormone. If the embryo has not succumbed, and probably for some time after embryonic death, the test will be positive. Rasor and Braunstein have indicated the value of the beta-subunit radioimmunoassay in early diagnosis of pregnancy; it will not indicate the site. In many cases, however, degeneration of the villi is eventually followed by cessation of the hormonal function of the trophoblast, so that a negative pregnancy test may be expected. Despite this negative test, rupture of the tube may occur weeks later, and we have seen several such cases.

Indeed, the studies of Douglas and associates suggest that, in addition to chorionic gonadotropin, actual trophoblast is present in the circulation of many pregnant women. Its inability to obtain a foothold and grow probably depends on maternal resistance factors, as is true with trophoblastic disease (Chapter 33).

OVARIAN PREGNANCY

Criteria of Diagnosis

The generally accepted criteria of diagnosis, formulated by Spiegelberg, are: (1) that the tube, including the fimbria ovarica, be intact and the former clearly separate from the ovary; (2) that the gestation sac definitely occupy the normal position of the ovary; (3) that the sac be connected with the uterus by the ovarian ligament; and (4) that unquestionable ovarian tissue be demonstrable in the walls of the sac.

Mechanism of Ovarian Pregnancy

When one recalls that the ovum as it exists in the ovary is incapable of being fertilized until it undergoes certain maturation changes which are completed only during its passage through the tube, it is easy to understand the rarity of ovarian pregnancy. Within recent years, however, there has been rather general acceptance of the view that implantation is not necessarily within the follicle

from which the ovum was discharged, especially now that we know that the secretion of the corpus luteum is essential for implantation. After its discharge, the ovum may be fertilized and then take root in the follicle or corpus luteum (intrafollicular implantation), but these are soon penetrated by the trophoblast, which pushes into the deeper ovarian structure (Fig. 28–24).

However, the most common mechanism seems to be through cortical implantation of the egg. A logical explanation for this might be the frequency with which endometrium is found in the ovary, and the probability, according to many, that this is because of the differentiating potency of the germinal epithelium. The latter might thus afford a favorable anchoring place for the fertilized ovum. There is much difficulty, however, in many cases of ovarian pregnancy in establishing the method of implantation.

Boronow and colleagues, in reporting four cases, thoroughly discuss the possible etiologic factors concerned with the occurrence of ovarian pregnancy. They regard as authentic 62 cases reported (in the English literature) between 1950 and 1963. Studies by Lehfeldt and co-workers and by others suggest that ovarian pregnancy is disproportionately common in women using an IUD. We can only speculate as to whether this may be

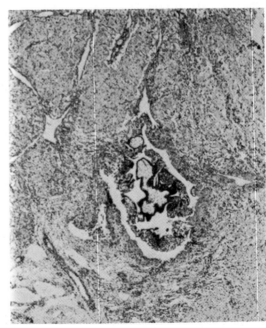

Figure 28–24. Chorionic villi in ovarian pregnancy in which the implantation may have been in the corpus luteum, which can be seen surrounding the villi in this section.

caused by impaired tubal motility so that the fertilized egg is prepared for implantation while still in the tube, or some form of mechanical irritation to the endometrium, as indicated in the recent report by Fernandez and Barbosa. In any case it would appear that the IUD is quite effective in preventing uterine (99 per cent) and tubal (95 per cent) pregnancy, but has little effect in an ovarian location which now constitutes 10 per cent of all ectopic gestations.

One may wonder why ovarian pregnancy is not more common than it is, because many spermatozoa undoubtedly escape from the fimbriated end of the tube. It should be remembered, however, that the ovum, as it exists in the ovary and immediately after its extrusion, is immature and incapable of being fertilized because the extrusion of the second polar body and thus complete maturation is believed to occur in the outer portion of the tube. That ovarian pregnancy does at times occur indicates that maturation must in some cases be completed when the ovum is still in or on the surface of the ovary. Mofid and associates report a full term ovarian gestation.

Course and Termination

The early implantation changes do not differ materially from those of uterine or tubal pregnancy, except for the absence of decidua. Although termination of the pregnancy through early rupture is the usual rule, in a considerable proportion—much higher than with the tubal variety—the pregnancy advances to full term, although the fetus succumbs after a spurious labor if operation is not carried out. Another possible termination, as with tubal pregnancy, is lithopedion formation.

Ovarian Hydatidiform Mole and Chorionepithelioma

This is exceedingly rare, but at least 18 cases are recorded by Marrubini; only one has been noted in our laboratory (Fig. 28–25). The latter is of great interest, because of the typicality of the hydatidiform mole and because of the striking hyperreactio luteinalis which is found throughout the ovary (see Chapter 33). There seems to be no reason why chorionepithelioma might not occur, though there appears to be no authentic report of the primary form of this tumor in the ovary except in association with teratoma (Gerbie et al.).

PRIMARY ABDOMINAL (PERITONEAL) PREGNANCY

Until recently there had been much scepticism as to the possibility of the fertilized egg implanting itself directly on the pelvic peritoneum, outside the genital canal, but the case reported in 1942 by Studdiford seems to establish this possibility beyond question. Moreover, this author has accepted as probably authentic several other

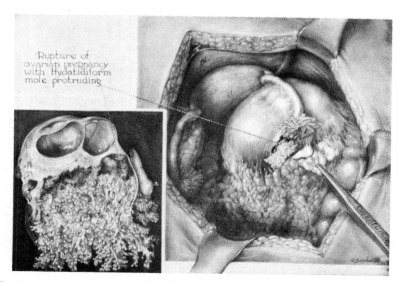

Figure 28–25.   Ovarian pregnancy associated with hydatidiform mole. (Courtesy of Dr. Henry G. Bennett, Oklahoma City.)

cases from the older literature. Stafford and Ragan have provided a more recent review.

Studdiford suggests the following criteria on which proof of this type of pregnancy must rest: (1) that both tubes and ovaries are normal with no evidence of recent pregnancy; (2) the absence of any evidence of a uteroperitoneal fistula; and (3) the presence of a pregnancy related exclusively to the peritoneal surface and young enough to eliminate the possibility of secondary implantation following a primary nidation in the tube.

In any case, it is well known that the corpus luteum is often found on the side opposite the pregnant tube. *External transmigration of an ovum* seems to be a factor in some cases of ectopic pregnancy, and would be highly compatible with primary abdominal pregnancy.

CERVICAL PREGNANCY

Although exceedingly rare, cervical pregnancy is possible. Just as in placenta previa the egg may implant itself in the region of the internal os, so it may, in rare instances, implant on the cervical mucosa (Fig. 28–6). An excellent study of the subject is that of Resnick, who collected a considerable group of cases from the literature. As would be expected, this bizarre type of pregnancy produces profuse bleeding in the early months of pregnancy and necessitates surgical intervention, which may be difficult and serious.

INTERSTITIAL PREGNANCY (FOLLOWING SALPINGECTOMY)

This is a rare occurrence, because primary salpingectomy is not particularly common. However, about 1 per cent of ectopic gestations are located in this area even when there has been previous salpingectomy. For this reason, cornual excision seems a preferable adjunct to salpingectomy. The review by Kirschner and Kimball is highly appropriate.

COMBINED PREGNANCY (INTRA- AND EXTRAUTERINE)

There are now several hundred reported cases of combined pregnancy, one embryo being implanted normally within the uterus,

the other ectopically in the tube. Interesting diagnostic problems may arise with such a combination. For example, rupture of the tubal pregnancy may cause serious intra-abdominal bleeding, with none from the vagina because the integrity of the uterine decidua is maintained by the presence of the living intrauterine embryo. For a discussion of the clinical connotations of combined pregnancy, however, the reader must be referred to textbooks of obstetrics, but Goodno and Sentry have reviewed the diagnostic difficulties. An excellent review is that of Schaefer.

COMBINED PREGNANCY (TUBAL)

Simultaneous pregnancy in both tubes may of course occur, and many such cases have been noted. Less common is unilateral tubal twin pregnancy, only 87 cases having been noted in the review by Storch and Petrie, who emphasize that such twins are usually monozygotic. Forbes and Natale have recorded a triplet pregnancy in one tube (Fig. 28–26).

POSTHYSTERECTOMY ECTOPIC PREGNANCY

Although we have seen a few cases of prolapsed fallopian tubes in which the tubal fimbriae protruded through the vaginal vault

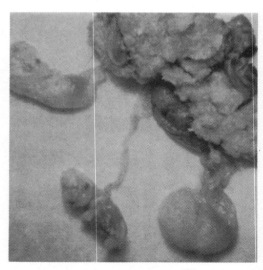

Figure 28–26. Placenta and three fetuses from tubal pregnancy. (Courtesy of Dr. Don Forbes, Springfield, Mass.)

following hysterectomy, our impression is that an ectopic pregnancy is unlikely. The physiology of such a prolapsed tube without an intermediate uterus would seemingly be so impaired that the possibility of pregnancy would be minimal.

Although posthysterectomy tubal pregnancy is rare, the careful clinician cannot absolutely promise the patient that she will not become pregnant following removal of the uterus. Hanes reports 11 cases of pregnancy following abdominal or vaginal hysterectomy. In four instances, the conception probably antedated the operation and was not recognizable at the time of surgery. Perhaps this occurs much more often than realized, with subsequent anemia and pelvic induration being construed as intra-abdominal bleeding incurred by the surgery itself. Often this is self-limited, and does not require operative intervention. Neibyl expands the number of cases to 21.

In other instances, years have elapsed between the hysterectomy and the ectopic gestation so that we have no recourse but to assume that there is some tract whereby the sperm cells can ascend to fertilize an extruded ovum. We might also speculate that passage down the tube by the fertilized egg has been retarded, allowing the trophoblast and villi to undergo sufficient development to permit implantation in the tube or, less commonly, the abdomen.

REFERENCES

Arias-Stella, J., and Gutierrez, J.: Frequencia y significando de las atypias endometriales en el embarazo ectopico. Rev. Lat.-Amer. Anat. Patol., *1*:81, 1957.

Beacham, W. D., Hernquist, W. C., Beacham, D. W., and Webster, H. D.: Abdominal pregnancy at Charity Hospital in New Orleans. Am. J. Obstet. Gynecol., *84*:1257, 1962.

Bernhardt, R. N., Bruns, P. D., and Drose, V. E.: Atypical endometrium associated with ectopic pregnancy (the Arias-Stella reaction). Obstet. Gynecol., *28*:849, 1966.

Bisca, B. F., and Felder, M. E.: Coexistent interstitial and intrauterine pregnancy following homolateral salpingo-oophorectomy. Am. J. Obstet. Gynecol., *79*:263, 1960.

Bone, N. L., and Green, R. R.: Histologic study of uterine tubes with tubal pregnancy: search for evidence of previous infection. Am. J. Obstet. Gynecol., *82*:1166, 1962.

Boronow, R. C., McElin, T. W., West, R. H., and Buckingham, J. C.: Ovarian pregnancy. Am. J. Obstet. Gynecol., *91*:1095, 1965.

Breen, J. L.: A 21 year survey of 654 ectopic pregnancies. Am. J. Obstet. Gynecol., *106*:1004, 1970.

Brenner, P. F., et al.: Ectopic pregnancy following tubal sterilization. Obstet. Gynecol., *49*:323, 1977.

Brody, S., and Stevens, F. L.: Combined intra- and extrauterine pregnancy. Obstet. Gynecol., *21*:129, 1963.

Cavanagh, D.: Primary peritoneal pregnancy. Am. J. Obstet. Gynecol., *76*:523, 1958.

Cohn, F. L., and Goldenberg, R. L.: Term pregnancy in an unattached rudimentary uterine horn. Obstet. Gynecol., *48*:234, 1976.

Demick, P. E., and Cavanagh, D.: Unilateral tubal and intrauterine pregnancy. Am. J. Obstet. Gynecol., *76*:533, 1958.

Douglas, C. P.: Tubal ectopic pregnancy. Br. Med. J., *2*:838, 1963.

Douglas, G. W., Thomas L., Carr, M., Cullen, N. M., and Morris, R.: Trophobast in circulating blood during pregnancy. Am. J. Obstet. Gynecol., *78*:960, 1959.

Fernandez, C. M., and Barbosa, J. J.: Primary ovarian pregnancy and the intrauterine device. Obstet. Gynecol., *47* (Suppl.):9S, 1976.

Fontanilla, J., and Anderson, G. W.: Further studies on racial incidence and mortality of ectopic pregnancy. Am. J. Obstet. Gynecol., *70*:312, 1955.

Forbes, D. A., and Natale, A.: Unilateral tubal triplet pregnancy. Obstet. Gynecol., *31*:360, 1968.

Friedrich, E. G., and Rankin, C. A.: Primary pelvic peritoneal pregnancy. Obstet. Gynecol. *31*:648, 1968.

Gerbie, M. V., et al.: Primary chorioca cenoma of the ovary. Obstet. Gynecol., *46*:720, 1976.

Goodno, J. A., and Sentry, W.: Coexistent interstitial and intrauterine pregnancy. J.A.M.A., *179*:135, 1962.

Grant, A.: Fertility after ectopic pregnancy. Clin. Obstet. Gynecol., *5*:861, 1962.

Greenhill, J. P.: Plastic operation on fallopian tube. Am. J. Obstet. Gynecol., *72*:516, 1956.

Halbrecht, I.: Healed genital tuberculosis: new etiologic factor in ectopic pregnancy. Obstet. Gynecol., *10*:73, 1957.

Hallatt, J. G.: Ectopic pregnancy associated with the intrauterine device: a study of 70 cases. Am. J. Obstet. Gynecol., *125*:754, 1976.

Hallatt, J. G.: Repeat ectopic pregnancy: a study of 123 consecutive cases. Am. J. Obstet. Gynecol., *122*:520, 1975.

Hanes, M. V.: Ectopic pregnancy following total hysterectomy. Obstet. Gynecol., *23*:882, 1964.

Honore, L. H., and Nickerson, K. G.: Combined intrauterine and tubal pregnancy; possible superfetation. Am. J. Obstet. Gynecol., *127*:885, 1977.

Iffy, L.: Time of conception in pathologic gestations. Proc. Roy. Soc. Med., *56*:1098, 1963.

Iffy, L.: Embryologic studies of time of conception in ectopic pregnancy and first-trimester abortion. Obstet. Gynecol., *26*:490, 1965.

Irwin, H. I.: Intraligamentous and abdominal extrauterine pregnancy. Obstet. Gynecol., *16*:360, 1960.

Kirschner, R., and Kimball, H. W.: Interstitial pregnancy following unilateral salpingectomy. J.A.M.A., *175*:146, 1962.

Kleiner, G. J., and Roberts, T. W.: Current factors in the causation of tubal pregnancy. Am. J. Obstet. Gynecol., *99*:21, 1967.

Kornblatt, M. B.: Abdominal pregnancy following a total hysterectomy. Obstet. Gynecol., *32*:488, 1968.

Laiuppa, M. A., and Cavanagh, D.: The endometrium in ectopic pregnancy. Obstet. Gynecol., *21*:155, 1963.

Lathrop, J. C., and Bowles, G. E.: Methotrexate in abdominal pregnancy. Obstet. Gynecol., *32*:81, 1968.

Lehfeldt, H., Tietze, C., and Gorstein, F.: Ovarian pregnancy and the intrauterine device. Am. J. Obstet. Gynecol., *108*:1005, 1970.

Lloyd, H. E. D., and Fienberg, R.: The Arias-Stella reaction. A nonspecific involutional phenomenon in intra- and extrauterine pregnancy. Am. J. Clin. Pathol., *43*:428, 1965.

Maas, D. A., and Slabber, C. F.: Diagnosis and treatment of advanced extra-uterine pregnancy. S. Afr. Med. J., *49*:2007, 1975.

Mall, F. P.: On the fate of the human embryo in tubal pregnancy. Contrib. Embryol. Carnegie Inst. Wash. Publ. No. 221, 1915.

Marrubini, G.: Primary chorionepithelioma of the ovary. Acta Obstet. Gynecol. Scand., *28*:251, 1949.

May, W. J., et al.: Maternal deaths from ectopic pregnancy. Am. J. Obstet. Gynecol., *132*:140, 1978.

McGowan, L.: Intramural pregnancy. J.A.M.A., *192*:637, 1965.

Mofid, M., Rhee, M. W., and Lankerani, M.: Ovarian pregnancy with delivery of a live baby. Obstet. Gynecol., *47*(Suppl.):5S, 1976.

Niebyl, J.: Pregnancy following total hysterectomy. Am. J. Obstet. Gynecol., *119*:512, 1974.

Nokes, J. M., Claiborne, H. A., Thornton, W. N., and Hso, T.: Extrauterine pregnancy associated with tuberculous salpingitis and congenital tuberculosis in the fetus. Obstet. Gynecol., *9*:206, 1957.

Novak, E. R.: The endometrium. Clin. Obstet. Gynecol., *17*:31, 1975.

Overbeck, L.: Tubal pregnancies concurrent with active tuberculous salpingitis. Geburtsh. Frauenheilkd., *24*:700, 1964.

Parker, S. L., and Parker, R. T.: "Chronic" ectopic tubal pregnancy. Am. J. Obstet. Gynecol., *74*:1174, 1957.

Paterson, W. G., and Grant, K. A.: Advanced intraligamentous pregnancy. Obstet. Gynecol. Surv., *30*:715, 1975.

Pent, D., and Loffer, F. D.: The natural history of an hematosalpinx. Obstet. Gynecol., *47*(Suppl.):2S, 1976.

Persaud, V.: Etiology of tubal ectopic pregnancy. Obstet. Gynecol., *36*:257, 1970.

Piven, M. S., Baer, K. A., and Zachary, T. V.: Ovarian pregnancy with intrauterine device. J.A.M.A., *201*:107, 1967.

Rasor, J. L., and Braunstein, G. D.: A rapid modification of the beta-HCG radioimmuno assay. Obstet. Gynecol., *50*:353, 1977.

Resnick, L.: Cervical pregnancy. S. Afr. Med. J., *36*:73, 1962.

Riggs, J. A., Wainer, A. S., Hahn, G. A., and Farell, D. M.: Extrauterine tubal choriocarcinoma. Am. J. Obstet. Gynecol., *88*:637, 1964.

Rimdusit, P., and Kasatri, N.: Primary ovarian pregnancy and the intrauterine contraceptive device. Obstet. Gynecol., *48*:575, 1976.

Schaefer, G.: Extrauterine pregnancy with concomitant term intrauterine pregnancy. Clin. Obstet. Gynecol., *5*:875, 1963.

Schneider, J., et al.: Maternal mortality due to ectopic pregnancy. Obstet. Gynecol., *49*:557, 1977.

Schoen, J. A., and Nowak, R. J.: Repeat ectopic pregnancy: a 16-year clinical survey. Obstet. Gynecol., *45*:542, 1975.

Sheikh, H. H., and Yussman, M. A.: Ectopic pregnancy following laparoscopic tubal ligation. Am. J. Obstet. Gynecol., *125*:569, 1976.

Sherwin, A. S., and Berg, F. P.: Cervical pregnancy. Am. J. Obstet. Gynecol., *79*:259, 1960.

Shintani, S., Glass, L. E., and Page, E. W.: Studies of induced malignant tumors of placental and uterine origin in the rat. 1. Survival of placental tissue following fetectomy. Am. J. Obstet. Gynecol., *95*:542, 1966.

Simpson, J. W., Alford, C. D., and Miller, A. C.: Interstitial pregnancy following homolateral salpingectomy. Am. J. Obstet. Gynecol., *82*:1173, 1961.

Smythe, A. R., II, and Underwood, P. B.: Ectopic pregnancy after postcoital diethylstilbestrol. Am. J. Obstet. Gynecol., *121*:284, 1975.

Spiegelberg, O.: Zur Kasuistik der Ovarialschwangenschaft. Arch. Gynäk., *13*:73, 1878.

Stafford, J. C., and Ragan, W. D.: Abdominal pregnancy. Obstet. Gynecol., *50*:548, 1977.

Stangel, J. J., et al.: Conservative surgical management of the tubal pregnancy. Obstet. Gynecol., *48*:241, 1976.

Storch, M. P., and Petrie, R. H.: Unilateral tubal twin gestation. Am. J. Obstet. Gynecol., *125*:1148, 1976.

Studdiford, W. E.: Primary ovarian pregnancy. Am. J. Obstet. Gynecol., *44*:487, 1942.

Sturgis, S. H.: Arias-Stella phenomenon. Am. J. Obstet. Gynecol., *116*:589, 1973.

Tan, K., and Yeo, O.: Primary ovarian pregnancy. Am. J. Obstet. Gynecol., *100*:240, 1968.

Thrasher, T. V., and Richart, R. M.: Ultrastructure of the Arias-Stella reaction. Am. J. Obstet. Gynecol., *112*:113, 1972.

Vago, T., Rikoven, M., and Reif, A.: Ectopic pregnancy associated with tuberculous salpingitis. Obstet. Gynecol., *16*:360, 1960.

Wagner, D., and Richart, R. M.: Polyploidy in the human endometrium with the Arias-Stella reaction. Arch. Pathol., *85*:475, 1968.

Webster, H. D., Barclay, D. L., and Fischer, C. K.: Ectopic pregnancy: 17 year review. Am. J. Obstet. Gynecol., *92*:23, 1965.

Whittle, M. J.: Cervical pregnancy with local excision. Br. Med. J., *3*:795, 1976.

Chapter 29

PELVIC ENDOMETRIOSIS

Definition and General Characteristics

Pelvic endometriosis refers to the condition in which tissue resembling more or less perfectly the uterine mucous membrane occurs aberrantly in various locations in the pelvic cavity. Although the occurrence of ectopic endometrium in the ovary had been described as far back as 1899, it was not until the classic contribution of Sampson in 1921 that there was any appreciation of the frequency of endometriosis, or of its pathologic and clinical characteristics. Although not so frequent as Sampson's first figures would indicate, it is a very common lesion.

There is a close kinship between *endometriosis* and *adenomyosis* of the uterus, and a frequent clinical association. In the latter the endometrium likewise exhibits aberrant growth, invading the uterine musculature, so that it is often logically spoken of as *endometriosis interna*, in contradistinction to the extrauterine variety, *endometriosis externa*, found at various sites in the pelvis. Although both processes show the common property of misplaced endometrium, in certain other respects, such as the age and fertility of the women involved and the histogenesis, there is a vast difference between the *internal* and *external* varieties of the disease.

Sites

The chief locations in which the aberrant endometrial development may occur are the following: (1) ovaries; (2) uterine ligaments; (3) rectovaginal septum; (4) the pelvic peritoneum, covering the uterus, tubes, rectum, sigmoid, and bladder; (5) umbilicus; (6) laparotomy scars; (7) hernial sacs; (8) appendix;

(9) vagina; (10) vulva; (11) cervix; (12) tubal stumps; (13) lymph nodes.

Although Williams and Pratt find endometriosis in 50 per cent of consecutive laparotomies, it is our personal belief that we are seeing fewer cases of endometriosis than in earlier years. This may be a sequel to the anovulation incurred by the use of contraceptive pills, or it may reflect a tendency of the younger endometriosis-prone woman to visit a more contemporary gynecologist. Although Acosta and co-workers have proposed a clinical classification for endometriosis, it would seem that there are too many variables for this to be satisfactory.

OVARIAN ENDOMETRIOSIS AND ENDOMETRIAL CYSTS OF THE OVARY

Gross Characteristics

In the ovary, endometriosis presents either in the form of small superficial implants of endometrial tissue or in the more important form of endometrial cysts of various sizes (chocolate cysts). The superficial areas of endometriosis usually vary from pinpoint size to perhaps 5 mm. in diameter. They occur most frequently on the convex free border or the lateral surfaces of the ovary. They are, as Sampson has said, of a raspberry color, resembling small areas of fibrinous deposit except for their dark reddish blue and puckered appearance. Even in small areas there is a tendency, as the endometrium grows into the ovary, to the formation of tiny cysts, which soon become hemorrhagic because of the menstrual reaction of the endo-

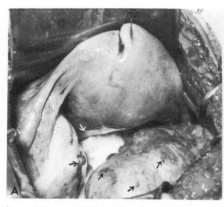
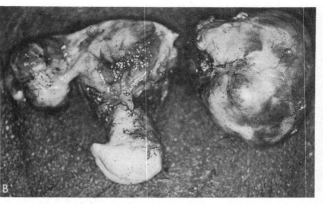

Figure 29–1. *A*, Bilateral endometrial cysts adherent to the posterolateral pelvic walls. Typical implants are evident on surface of ovaries and uterus (arrows). *B*, Posterior aspect of *A* after removal. Note the extensive endometriosis on the posterior surface of uterus and the multiple small implants.

metrium. As they grow larger they penetrate more deeply into the ovary, the content being of dark hemorrhagic character, resembling thick chocolate syrup. However, one may find extensive pelvic endometriosis with no palpatory evidence, for extreme degrees of diffuse punctate disease may occur. Women so afflicted may have severe symptoms without overt evidence of endometriosis and unfortunately may be regarded as chronic complainers.

Even when very small, the cysts show a strong perforative tendency, the contained menstrual blood escaping and causing the ovary to adhere to any contiguous structure,

generally the posterior surface of the broad ligament or the uterus. This perforative tendency is retained as the cyst grows larger, so that characteristically the ovary containing the endometrial cyst, as well as the adjacent tube, is firmly fixed to the broad ligament or uterus (Fig. 29–1). From the standpoint of operating room diagnosis, the important feature is that when such an adherent ovary is dissected from its attachment, there occurs a gush of thick chocolate-colored fluid from the cyst cavity. When this is noted, a presumptive diagnosis of endometrial cyst can be made, even before microscopic examination (Fig. 29–2).

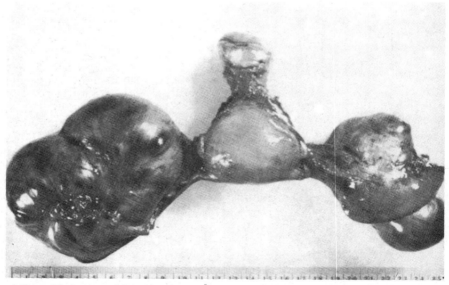

Figure 29–2. Large bilateral endometrial cysts removed without rupture—the exception.

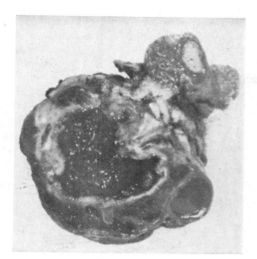

Figure 29–3. Cut surface of endometrial cyst showing dark hemorrhagic inner wall and whitish capsular layer.

When the ovary containing an endometrial cyst is cut into, the cyst characteristically presents as a small round or ovoid cavity whose walls are usually very dark red or brownish red, even after the chocolate-like bloody content has escaped. Surrounding the cyst on cut section one commonly sees a whitish or yellowish capsular layer convoluted. The larger cysts may penetrate deep into the substance of the ovary, the smaller ones being superficial (Fig. 29–3).

The term chocolate cyst, originally applied to these cysts by Sampson, is an expressive one, but it lends itself readily to misapplication if one notices only the chocolate-covered hemorrhagic content. A somewhat similar content may be found in some follicle or lutein hematomas, and the fluid content of a cystadenoma may be chocolate-colored because of hemorrhagic admixture. For this reason, the term *endometrial cyst* is a better one, predicating the existence in the cyst wall of microscopically demonstrable endometrial tissue (Fig. 29–4).

The endometrial type of cyst rarely reaches extreme size, and is rarely larger than a orange or grapefruit. This is explained by the fact that in such cases the early perforative tendency has been lacking, and such cysts are therefore likely to be less adherent, thicker-walled and larger than usual. On the other hand, when perforation does occur in large cysts, it may bring about acute abdominal symptoms resembling either ruptured extrauterine pregnancy or acute appendicitis; Golditch points out that 8 per cent of endometriosis patients present with acute abdominal symptoms, and Pratt and Shamblin reaffirm this observation.

Microscopic Characteristics

In the microscopic diagnosis of ovarian endometriosis one must remember that a wide variation of pictures may occur. The criterion of diagnosis is the observation of endometrial tissue, preferably both glands and stroma. At one extreme, cases are seen in which the endometrium is so typical both histologically and functionally that it cannot

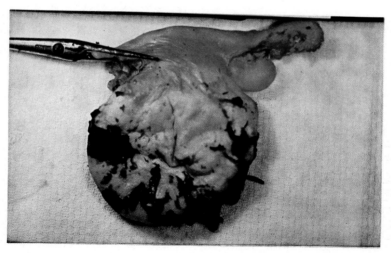

Figure 29–4. Ovary showing superficial endometrial lesion and typical chocolate-colored content having its source partly in an endometrial cyst of other ovary. Note the puckered appearance produced by the superficial lesions.

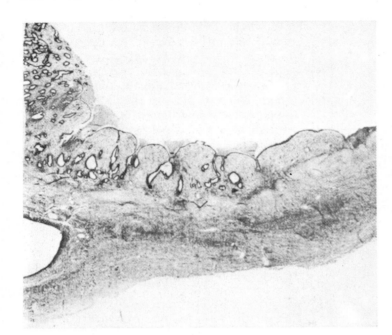

Figure 29–5. Endometrial cyst with lining endometrium identical to that of the uterus.

be distinguished from the normal mucosa of the uterus (Fig. 29–5). At the other extreme are cases in which, as a result of repeated menstrual bleeding and desquamation into a small closed cavity, all trace of the original endometrium may be lost, so that the diagnosis is presumptive rather than absolute. Between these two extremes all gradations are encountered. Germinal inclusion cysts are often mistaken for endometrial glands. Admittedly, the distinction may not always be easy but endometriosis usually shows such other stigmata as stroma, hemorrhage, and pigment-laden macrophages (Fig. 29–6).

There is no difficulty in the diagnosis of cases in which one sees, either on the ovarian surface or in the cyst wall, endometrium with glands, epithelium, and stroma all as clearly defined as in the uterus. The stromal tissue, however, is frequently poorly marked or completely absent, and the glands are often sparse and not well defined. Where the ovary is adherent to the posterior wall of the uterus, adenomyosis may penetrate through the serosal surface to produce the pattern noted in Figure 29–7. In many endometrial cysts, large areas of the wall may have lost the endometrial lining completely, although one often finds remnants in the invagination and indentation so common in the walls of the cyst (Fig. 29–8). During surgery, the surgeon may observe a number of typical endo-

metrial cysts and nodules in which subsequent pathologic examination reveals no vestige of endometrial tissue. Recurrent hemorrhage and pressure atrophy may obliterate all of the microscopic architecture, and it has been reliably estimated that *no specific pathologic diagnosis can be made in about one third of typical endometriosis cases* (Fig. 29–9). Our laboratory policy is to index such lesions as "hemorrhagic" or "sid-

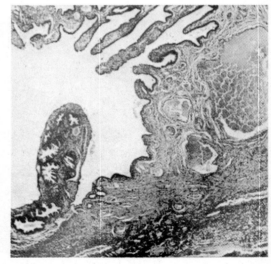

Figure 29–6. Surface endometrial growth on ovary near tubal orifice. Note secretory reaction of glands.

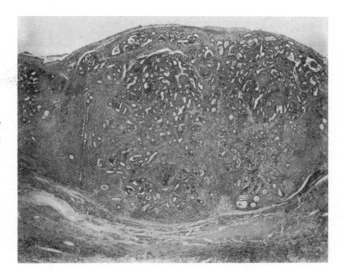

Figure 29–7. Nodule of adenomyosis in wall of large endometrial cyst, adherent to posterior surface of the uterus.

erophagic" cysts (compatible with endometriosis) (Fig. 29–10).

Hughesdon points out that the inside of a chocolate cyst is really the outside of the ovary, with the ovarian cortex identifiable by the primordial follicles. This obviously suggests a surface origin of the endometriosis, and implies a genesis by implantation or metaplasia rather than via the lymphatics which enter in the hilus.

A characteristic feature of the endometrial cyst, though not a constant one, is the presence just beneath the degenerating endometrium, or often in lieu of the latter, of a broad zone rich in large phagocytic cells laden with blood pigment (hemosiderin). These are *endothelial leukocytes* or *pseudoxanthoma cells* (Fig. 29–11). They are large and polyhedral, so that when present in large numbers they may have a superficial resem-

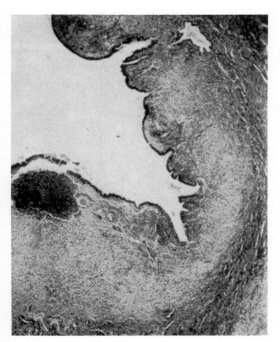

Figure 29–8. Wall of endometrial cyst showing typical epithelium, but sparse stroma and glands.

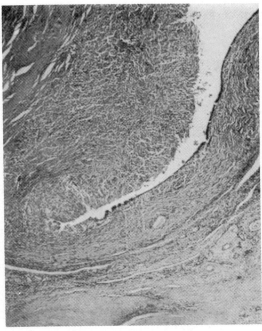

Figure 29–9. Endometrial cyst in which epithelium has been lost over considerable areas. No glands or stroma are to be seen.

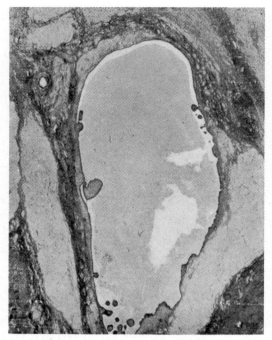

Figure 29–10. Endometrial cyst resembling a miniature uterine cavity and filled with blood.

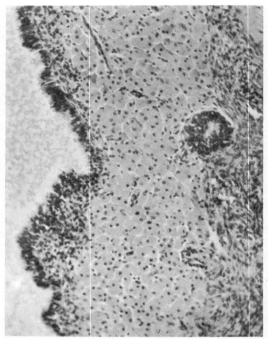

Figure 29–11. High power view of part of cyst shown in Figure 29–10. Note the large pseudoxanthoma cells or endothelial leukocytes.

blance to lutein cells, although there is not the characteristic "festooned" pattern. The presence of such a zone about a hemorrhagic cyst leaves little doubt of its endometrial nature, even when no epithelium or glands can be demonstrated. Surrounding this layer, one often finds a broad zone of hyalinized fibrous tissue, occasionally showing some muscle fibers.

In some cases the endometrium of these cysts exhibits the same functional cyclic response as does uterine mucosa, so that during the premenstrual phase one sees the characteristic predecidual picture, with scalloping and tortuosity of the glands and marked secretory reaction of the gland epithelium (Fig. 29–12). This phase is in turn followed by typical menstrual desquamation. There are, however, many exceptions to this rule, and usually the endometrium is of a purely proliferative type, with no such cyclic response, as has been described by many authors. In these cases the abnormal endometrial tissue in the ovary appears to be immature or unripe, and not capable of the full cyclic response of normal endometrium. In cases of this type one may often see a typical Swiss-cheese hyperplasia pattern.

In the occasional case of endometriosis

complicating pregnancy, either uterine or ectopic, the aberrant endometrium may exhibit a typical decidual response (Fig. 29–13). It should be mentioned that the presence of ectopic decidua does not necessarily imply the presence of pregnancy or, indeed, of endometriosis.

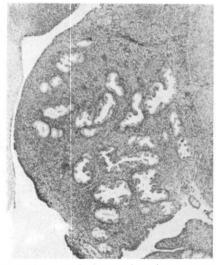

Figure 29–12. Marked premenstrual secretory reaction in lining of endometrial cyst.

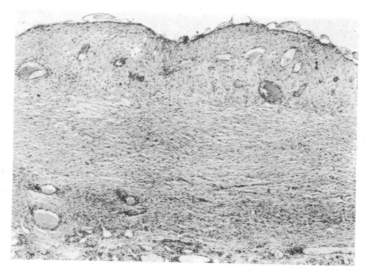

Figure 29–13. Decidual changes in wall of endometrial cyst in pregnancy.

Finally, it should be remembered that in some cases, the aberrant mucous membrane in the ovary represents tubal mucosa rather than an endometriosis, the epithelium being tall and often ciliated, with absence of gland elements and of endometrial stroma, and at times even showing a tendency to the formation of folds like those of the tubal mucosa itself. Cases of this type have been designated *endosalpingiosis* (Sampson) rather than endometriosis. The views held as to their histogenesis are discussed in the section on histogenesis (page 574).

ENDOMETRIOSIS OF UTEROSACRAL LIGAMENTS

An extremely common location for endometriosis is the uterosacral ligaments. Those who advocate Sampson's implantation theory of the origin of endometriosis stress the fact that endometrial particles regurgitating through the fimbriated ends of the tubes, or given off from the perforation of endometrial cysts in the ovary, naturally gravitate toward the cul-de-sac and plant themselves on the uterosacral ligaments. Here they form bluish, somewhat puckered nodules, single or multiple, occasionally tiny, in other cases of considerable size; sometimes involving one ligament, but often both (Fig. 29–14). The nodules are often palpable on rectovaginal examination, and this constitutes the most valuable diagnostic sign. These endometrial lesions swell just before and during menstruation, which explains why, in so many cases of endometriosis, the patient complains of severe dysmenorrhea referred to the rectum or to the lower sacral or coccygeal regions.

Microscopically, these endometrial implants in the uterosacral region show typical endometrial tissue, with usually small cystic cavities filled with dark old menstrual blood. They may at times show a marked fibrotic reaction, with even the formation of muscle tissue. When, as is often the case, they form definite tumor-like nodules, the designation of *endometrioma* may properly be applied.

ENDOMETRIOSIS OF RECTOVAGINAL SEPTUM

An extension of the endometrial lesion just described is brought about when the process extends still deeper, causing endometrial infiltration of the anterior rectal wall, or into the rectovaginal septum. The rectum may thus be solidly welded to the posterior surface of the cervix, and its walls may in extreme cases show such massive infiltration by the endometrial process that it closely simulates malignancy, as noted by Davis and Truehart. The lumen of the bowel may be occluded, with symptoms of obstruction, although the mucosa itself is intact, an important differential.

Formerly it was thought necessary to resect portions of the bowel or perform colostomy as a part of the surgical treatment of these cases of adenomyoma of the septum, although this procedure has been generally

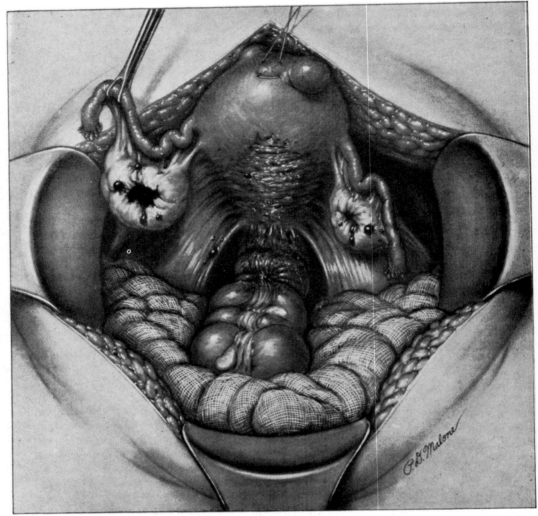

Figure 29–14. Uterosacral, rectovaginal, and ovarian involvement in endometriosis. (From TeLinde: Operative Gynecology. 4th Ed. Philadelphia, J. B. Lippincott Co.)

abandoned since it is apparent that complete removal of ovarian tissue brings about endometrial regression in such lesions, just as it does in the uterus. The infiltration of the endometrium into the septum may bring about a large, firm, nodular enlargement readily palpable through the vagina or the rectum. Rectal bleeding may at times be produced (Fig. 29–15).

The lesion may penetrate through the vaginal wall, producing dark blue, hemorrhagic polyps which cause vaginal bleeding. The endometrial nature of such bluish hemorrhagic nodules or polyps in the vaginal vault should always be suspected, especially if there are other evidences of endometriosis, such as the presence of nodules in the uterosacral area or infiltration of the rectovaginal septum.

A few cases of carcinoma of the rectosigmoid have been noted with pelvic endometriosis. This rare association by no means justifies bowel resection for benign rectosigmoidal endometriosis, unless there is definite microscopic evidence (by frozen section) that malignancy coexists. However, certain young women with extensive endometriosis of the bowel might better be treated by intestinal resection than castration; great individualization seems desirable.

In all cases of such benign lesions the *microscopic diagnosis* is simple, revealing endometrial tissue which, however, may not al-

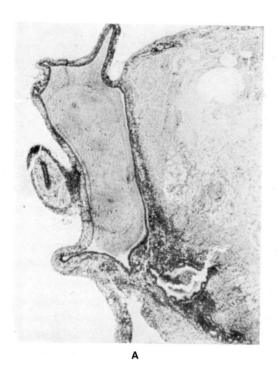

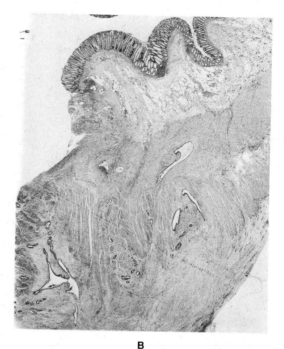

A

B

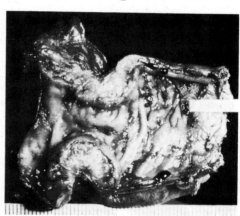

Figure 29–15. *A*, Small endometrial island on surface of sigmoid colon. The section represents the entire dark hemorrhagic lesion; there was no trace of endometriosis in the ovary or elsewhere. *B*, Bowel mucosa at right with endometriosis invading muscularis. *C*, More massive involvement of rectosigmoid with partial obstruction. Note *intact mucosa* with extrinsic lesion. (*C*, Courtesy of Dr. E. Ingalls, Minneapolis, Minn.)

C

ways be entirely typical. The stroma, for example, is often lacking, but the characteristic clinical picture is strongly suggestive of the diagnosis.

ENDOMETRIOSIS OF ROUND LIGAMENTS

Small endometrial islands are frequently found on the round ligaments, as on other parts of the pelvic peritoneum; one may find definite nodules, sometimes of considerable size, and composed not only of endometrium but also of involuntary muscle fibers. The histologic picture is like that seen in adenomyosis of the uterus itself. Either the intraperitoneal or the extraperitoneal portions of the round ligament may be the seat of such tumors. In the latter case they are palpable in the region of the inguinal canal, so that they may give rise to interesting diagnostic problems. Finally, one may at times find ectopic endometrium in the *canal of Nuck* when this is the seat of a hernia or hydrocele. When the content of the latter is hemorrhagic, microscopic examination usually reveals endometrium in the wall of the sac.

ENDOMETRIOSIS OF UMBILICUS

In a considerable group of cases endometrial tissue has been found at the umbilicus. This group is of interest in the discussion of histogenesis because it seems impossible to explain such cases on the basis of Sampson's theory, and some other explanation must be invoked. The most favored is that at the umbilicus one normally finds remnants of the original coelomic epithelium, which is embryologically capable of endometrial differentiation.

On the other hand, Scott believes that various lymphatics connect the peritoneal cavity with the umbilicus. These course along the obliterated umbilical vessels, and Scott has demonstrated their existence by injecting certain dyes or radioactive material into the peritoneal cavity and recovering them in the umbilicus. This communication between peritoneum and navel might explain the rare instance of the so-called *Cullen's sign*—discoloration of the umbilicus in association with hemoperitoneum, most commonly in conjunction with ectopic pregnancy, as well as endometriosis of the umbilicus.

Umbilical endometriosis presents as a small nodule often of bluish hue, and characterized by increased size, with pain and tenderness, at the menstrual periods. External menstrual bleeding has been noted in a number of the reported cases. Histologically the endometrial tissue often occurs in scattered small islands, but in some cases larger areas, with well-defined stroma and perhaps marked hemorrhage, may be noted (Fig. 29–16).

ENDOMETRIOSIS IN LAPAROTOMY SCARS

Still another location of endometriosis which has given rise to much discussion is in laparotomy scars. Here again the chief point of discussion has been about the histogenesis, there being two chief viewpoints. According to one, the endometrial nodules result from implantation of endometrial tissue at the time of operation, although others believe that the doctrine of coelomic metaplasia must be invoked. This subject will be further discussed under the heading *Histogenesis of Endometriosis.*

The endometriosis in this group of cases occurs clinically in the form of small or large

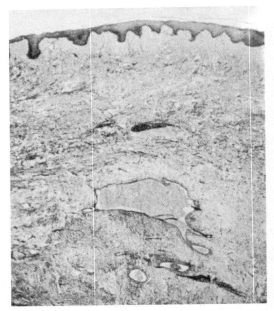

Figure 29–16. Endometriosis of umbilicus in underlying tissue with intact ectoderm.

tender nodules which usually lie deep in the abdominal wall, and are apt to infiltrate the muscle and fascial layers, so that they are fixed and diffuse rather than circumscribed. As with umbilical endometriosis, they swell at the menstrual periods, with increased pain and tenderness, and they may, through penetration of the skin, be associated with external menstrual bleeding. As a matter of fact, Steck and Helwig have commented on cutaneous endometriosis.

Such lesions have been reported after many different types of operation, including those in which the endometrium of the uterus is not invaded. Curiously enough, they rarely occur after cesarean section, in which the uterine cavity is directly opened. On the other hand, they have occurred after simple appendectomy, performed many years previously and before the onset of menstrual function. Figure 29–17 is a good example of the microscopic appearance of such lesions, showing the typical endometrial tissue in a matrix of fibrotic tissue.

OTHER SITES OF ENDOMETRIOSIS

Endometrial islands may occur on any part of the pelvic peritoneum, involving the surface of any pelvic organ, though characteristically they are not found in the abdominal

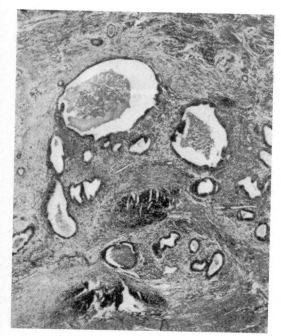

Figure 29–17. Endometriosis of laparotomy scar, following cesarean section 3 years previously.

viscera above the pelvic brim (Fig. 29–18). The *appendix* or the *small intestine* may seem to be exceptions, but probably only because they are often found in the pelvis. The *rectum* or *sigmoid* may be involved, and in

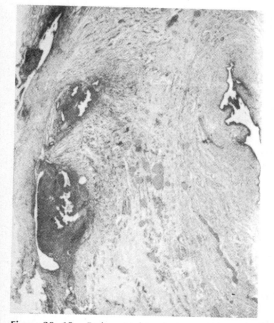

Figure 29–18. Endometrial implants on surface of tube (lumen at right).

such instances the clinician might consider bowel resection rather than castration in the younger woman when there is not too diffuse a disease process, as recommended separately by Ecker et al. and by Gray.

Although in most cases one also finds ovarian endometriosis, this is by no means invariable. A frequent finding is small isolated islands of endometrial tissue, presenting as bluish or bluish-red elevations on the rectum, sigmoid, or posterior surface of the uterus even when there is no suggestion of ovarian involvement. In rather rare cases, endometriosis of the *bladder* may penetrate to the interior of the organ, or there may be periureteral endometriosis with compression and upper tract damage, as noted by Langmade. Endometriosis of the *kidney* has been recorded by Hajdu and Koss, and would seem to represent hematogenous spread of the disease.

Of considerable interest is the recent report in which there was uterine penetration by an IUD with subsequent omental endometriosis (Uohara and Kovara).

Many cases of *cervical* disease have been reported, and care must be taken not to confuse these with an adenocarcinoma. Such cases are often not associated with endometriosis in other locations, although in some instances it seems to be a sequel of downward extension of cul-de-sac endometriosis or adenomyosis; in any case the aberrant tissue was deep and well below the cervical mucosa.

More recently, we have seen additional cases to strengthen our concepts of the occurrence of surface implantation, at least in the lower genital canal. Sufficient cases have accrued in which there is definite evidence of surface endometriosis of the cervix (Fig. 29–19). Many of these patients had previous cervical cauterization, and we must assume that cervical or lower genital tract endometriosis seems to be a frequent sequel to some kind of trauma in tissue over which endometrium is spilled.

Novak and Hoge point out the frequency of lower genital tract endometriosis, especially following some type of trauma (as cervical cauterization). The endometriosis is generally of surface type, and its usual responsiveness to the progestational hormone suggests a mature endometrium, as might be expected if surface endometrium were implanted; in direct contrast is deep cervical endometrium, which is usually an extension

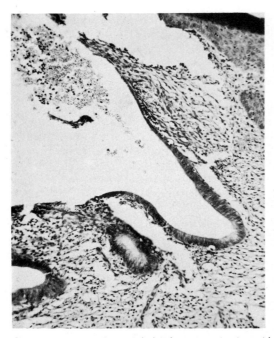

Figure 29–19. Endometrial glands communicating with surface; squamous epithelium is present at upper right.

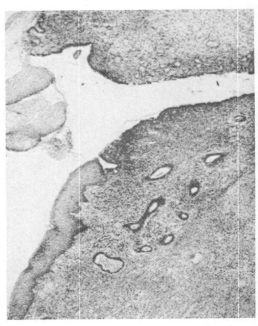

Figure 29–20. Endometriosis of vaginal vault.

of cul-de-sac endometriosis or adenomyosis. This exhibits an almost uniform failure to respond to a biphasic hormone stimulus, and the disparity of humoral response might suggest a different etiology.

Scott, and others have reported other implantation cases. As Scott noted, "it is a wonder that it does not occur more frequently," and he was inclined to attribute this to a varying capability of cast-off endometrium to survive. Decidua is least likely to implant, whereas postmenstrual endometrium is most apt to; in view of the usual tendency to perform cauterization immediately after menstruation, one must wonder at the relative infrequency of cervical endometriosis. Similar cases of typical endometriosis have been observed in the *vulva*, episiotomy scars, site of excised Bartholin gland, and perineum. All of these foci strongly suggest the validity of the implantation theory.

Other observations include posthysterectomy endometriosis of the *vaginal* vault with cyclic bleeding, or pseudomenstruation (Fig. 29–20). Most of the women have had hysterectomy with conservation of an ovary because of pelvic endometriosis, and it is easy to visualize the further spread of such endometriosis through the vaginal vault. This observation does not strengthen the im-

plantation doctrine as much as the few cases in which endometriosis was not present at laparotomy but was found later in the vaginal vault.

Yet, how often does endometriosis follow total hysterectomy, a procedure in which a healing vaginal vault seems to be an ideal nidus for endometrium expressed at any stage of the cycle to implant and flourish? How often is vaginal hysterectomy with repair of cystocele or rectocele followed by vaginal endometriosis despite almost uniform conservation of ovaries? Certainly both are uncommon, and until there is a more frequent sequence, there must be some skepticism of the general applicability of the implanting tendencies of uterine endometrium.

In rare cases endometriosis may arise in *hernial sacs*, which Sampson explains as due to implantation of endometrial particles from the tube or ovary, and others attribute to metaplasia. When the canal of Nuck is thus involved, nodules may occur in the *inguinal region*. Sampson has called attention to the fact that endometriosis is often found arising from the mucosa of tubal stumps that have resulted from amputation of the tubes, presumably as a result of metaplastic changes in the endosalpinx. Finally, there are a number of reported instances of what is apparently unquestionable endometriosis of both the *upper* and *lower extremities* as well as the pleural cavity. One would be inclined to invoke the hematogenous route in the explanation of these bizarre cases, and this will be discussed more fully in the next section.

HISTOGENESIS OF ENDOMETRIOSIS

The question of the histogenesis of endometriosis has been a source of constant discussion since Sampson, in the same paper in which he described this clinical and pathologic entity (1921), advanced a theory of its origin. This was to the effect that the abnormal endometrium in the pelvis arises from the implantation on the ovaries and other pelvic structures of endometrial particles "regurgitated" through the tube as a result of retrograde menstruation. In other words, during menstruation, blood may pass outward from the uterus through the tube into the pelvic cavity, carrying with it endometrium capable of implanting and further developing in the pelvis (Fig. 29–21 A).

In favor of this explanation, Sampson submitted much impressive evidence, such as: (1) the actual demonstration of menstrual regurgitation in at least some cases, especially when the normal exit of the menstrual blood through the cervix was retarded by myoma or retroflexion; (2) the distribution of the pelvic endometrium is about what one would expect if it arose from endometrial particles dropped from the fimbriated ends of the tube; (3) the tubal lumina are usually patent in cases of endometriosis; (4) in animal experiments endometrium has been observed to grow when planted in the peritoneal cavity.

Many objections to the general applicability of Sampson's theory have been raised. Among these are the following: (1) retrograde menstruation, although it may occur, is rarely observed, as contrasted to the great frequency of endometriosis; (2) it is difficult to believe that endometrium cast off in the uterus could enter the small uterine orifice of the tube, travel outward against the current, and still be capable of implanting itself and growing upon the pelvic structures; (3) endometrium shed at menstruation is already degenerated or dead, so that it is not easy to conceive of its taking root in the peri-

toneum; (4) experiments which show that endometrium can grow in the peritoneum have dealt with the normal, healthy endometrium of animals.

Such possibilities have always been conceded by opponents of this theory, the main objection being that the endometrium shed at menstruation is degenerated, nonviable, and incapable of planting itself on the peritoneum. Such were earlier conclusions based on experiments with monkeys, in which menstrual blood was allowed to escape directly into the pelvic cavity through an experimentally created utero-abdominal fistula.

Recent years have witnessed a considerable number of cases in which there was a uterine abnormality, generally a bicornuate uterus with one horn having no cervical egress for menstrual blood. A frequent observation has been hematosalpinx (of retrograde nature) with the advent of pelvic endometriosis. We have seen several such cases, and must admit that they seem to strengthen the argument for the retrograde theory of endometrosis and the probability that desquamated endometrium can implant and grow. Schifrin and associates discuss endometriosis in teen-age girls, and their findings are confirmatory.

A much more elaborate study, however, was made on a considerable group of monkeys by Scott and TeLinde, who devised an ingenious operative procedure whereby the menstrual blood was made to regurgitate into the pelvis, the normal vaginal egress being completely bypassed. In some of these animals endometrial islands were later demonstrated, though usually not for many months, and in one case, three years. Scott and Wharton have treated this aberrant endometrium with various hormones with results similar to those observed in humans.

These highly suggestive observations might be explained on the basis of peritoneal metaplasia as a result of the long continued irritation of the escaped blood, just as Teilum and Madsen explained islands of endometrium on the ovary following the escape of oily solutions through the tubes as a result of salpingography. However, repeated intraperitoneal injection of venous blood has failed to produce endometriosis after more than 5 years' attempts by Wharton and coworkers. Merrill has utilized an endometrium-filled, escape-proof Millipore filter to produce endometriosis in adjacent tissues,

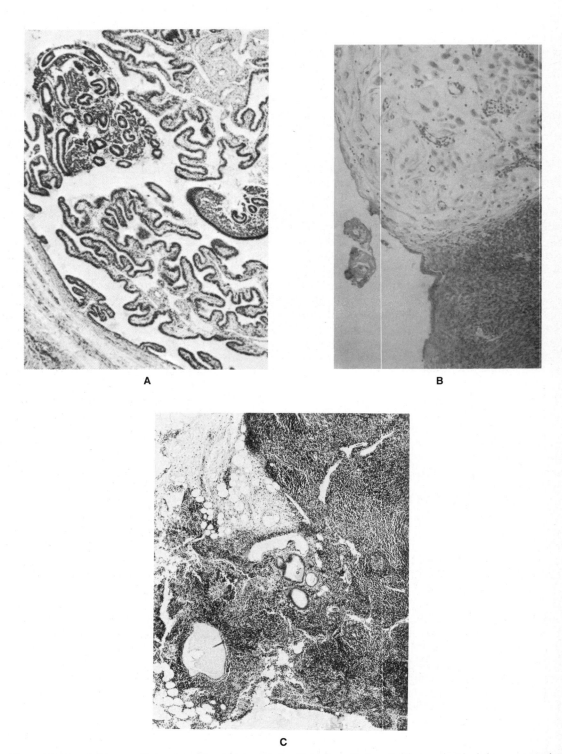

Figure 29–21. *A*, Menstruating endometrium in tube; tubal wall above and below. *B*, Obvious decidual changes on surface of ovary indicative of metaplastic properties. *C*, Endometrial glands in lymph node.

and he suggests an induction principle in the endometrium; however, this must still be regarded as speculative.

Ridley obtained shed endometrium for implantation into the fascia of women selected for future lapatotomy (usually for myoma). One of eight patients did develop typical endometriosis in the implantation area. It may be significant that the one woman developing endometriosis was the sole patient who was not Negro and was under 30.

The majority of those opposed to Sampson's explanation are inclined to favor the view that the aberrant endometrium has its origin from *abnormal differentiation in the coelomic epithelium* from which all the genital mucous membranes arise. The müllerian duct is developed from an invagination of the primitive peritoneum or coelomic epithelium, and from this duct are formed the uterus, tubes, and cervix. The endometrium and endosalpinx both represent only a modified and differentiated coelomic epithelium, whereas the germinal epithelium of the ovary represents the original coelomic epithelium with most of its differentiating potency unused and thus stored. In ovarian endometriosis the germinal epithelium for some reason—perhaps hormonal or inflammatory—differentiates into tissues embryologically capable of forming endometrium, endosalpinx, or endocervix (Fig. 29–21 *B*). The same possibility exists wherever coelomic epithelium or vestiges occur, this including any of the pelvic peritoneal surfaces, the umbilicus, and hernial sacs. The theory, therefore, is a much more inclusive one than that of Sampson.

There are still other theories of endometriosis, such as the concept that the aberrant endometrium arises from desquamated endometrial particles transported by the lymphatics to various locations in the pelvis. Although few believe the lymphatic route is the usual means of endometrial spread and growth, most students are willing to accept this as a possibility (Fig. 29–21 *C*), and the report by Koss of an adenoacanthoma in an obturator node would seem to substantiate this possibility.

Spread of endometrium *by blood* may be unusual but must be considered as the only plausible explanation of the rare cases occurring in arm, leg, etc. There is evidence to suggest an extrapulmonic arterial communication between the abdomen and upper thorax to explain the means whereby endometrium avoids a pulmonary focus more frequently. There are reports, however, of an occasional case involving the pleura, and of a patient who had a lobectomy while pregnant. Instead of a supposed pulmonary tumor, sections showed a massive chunk of decidua (Fig. 29–22). This would be difficult to explain on any other than a hematogenous method of spread. Kovarik and Toll, in tabulating the literature, note 10 cases of thoracic endometriosis, 6 involving the lung parenchyma and 4 the pleura. Labay and Feiner have reported endometrial sarcoma arising from pleural endometriosis.

It now seems fair to state that almost all gynecologists believe that there is more than one method for the origin of endometriosis, and that no one of these theories is satisfactory to explain all cases. The concept of tubal regurgitation with secondary implantation is probably accepted as the usual explanation for most cases of pelvic endometriosis; yet only a few would contend this explains the genesis of all ectopic endometrium. Indeed, the most vociferous proponents of the two commonly invoked theories of histogenesis. Sampson (for the implantation method) and Novak (for the coelomic metaplasia doctrine), were in considerable agreement after many years of hotly contested debate.

ENDOMETRIOSIS AS A SOURCE OF OVARIAN CARCINOMA

In 1925 Sampson described a small group of cases of ovarian cancer in which he believed the malignant ovarian growth had its origin from abnormal endometrium in the ovary. The presence of endometrium side by side with a type of ovarian cancer similar to adenocarcinoma of the uterine endometrium lends much plausibility to Sampson's suggestion, as does the histologic similarity of some ovarian adenocarcinomas and endometrial carcinoma.

Five cases of coexistent ovarian or sequential adenoacanthomas of the ovary and endometrium are reported by Campbell and associates. They consider the tumors as independent rather than metastatic, and imply that a hormonal carcinogenic stimulus to uterine and ectopic ovarian endometrium might be a causative factor. This obviously parallels what may have occurred in Figure 29–23. Gray has also indicated the frequency of neo-

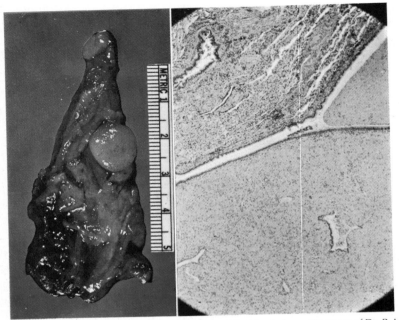

Figure 29–22. Gross and microscopic appearance of decidua in lung. (Courtesy of Dr. R. Lattes.)

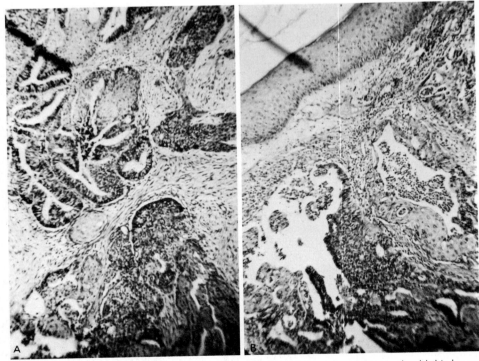

Figure 29–23. *A,* Typical adenoacanthoma of ovary. *B,* Adenoacanthoma of umbilicus—should this be regarded as a solitary metastasis or simultaneous acanthosis of logical sites of endometriosis? We suspect the latter. (Courtesy of Dr. Arthur Hoge, Fort Smith, Ark.)

plasis among multiple areas of the lining germinal epithelium due to an uncertain stimulus.

In our laboratory we have been impressed by the not uncommon finding of tumors of multicentric origin, involving ovary, endosalpinx, endometrium, and endocervix. The most common combination is ovary and endometrium, and where these two organs are involved the salvage is far better than would be expected with any type of metastatic tumor, further implying simultaneous stimulation to malignancy, rather than transtubal or other spread of the disease (Woodruff and Julian).

Even though ovarian carcinoma may arise from ectopic endometrium, it would be difficult to establish in most cases because all traces of the original endometrium are blotted out. However, in a small group of cases such an origin has been established beyond question by demonstration of the adenocarcinoma springing from the ectopic endometrium (Figs. 29–24 to 29–26). Most of these growths have been adenoacanthomas, which supports the endometrial origin of such growths, in view of the frequency of adenoacanthoma in the uterus itself, and the rarity of any acanthomatous tendency in other types of ovarian adenocarcinoma. Although these are generally of low-grade malignancy,

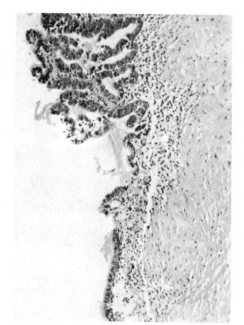

Figure 29–25. Transition zone of benign and malignant growth. (Courtesy of Dr. J. Dan Thompson, Atlanta, Ga.)

Koss reports a small adenoacanthoma with extension to an obturator lymph node. In rare cases there may be extensive spread, but adenoacanthoma is a generally favorable type of adenocarcinoma.

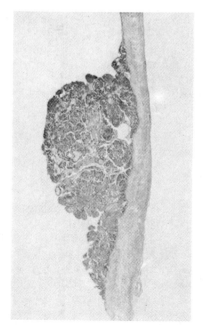

Figure 29–24. Adenoacanthoma arising from benign endometrial cyst of ovary. (Courtesy of Dr. J. Dan Thompson, Atlanta, Ga.)

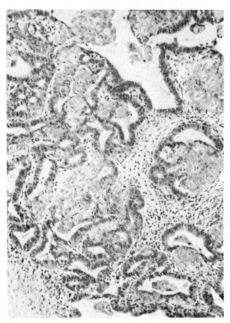

Figure 29–26. Typical adenoacanthoma deeper in tumor. (Courtesy of Dr. J. Dan Thompson, Atlanta, Ga.)

Enough of these cases of adenoacanthomas have been amassed to make some authors state that endometriosis might be regarded as a premalignant disease, which thereby deserves more than expectant therapy. A much more rational approach to the problem is advocated by Thompson, who points out that sarcomatous change in a myoma is such an infrequent complication that it does not influence the method of handling the patient. Why then should the much less common malignancy in endometriosis mandate any sort of radical treatment?

Carcinosarcoma, a rather rare lesion in the ovary, may arise from endometriosis, as has been noted by Azoury and Woodruff, and by Fenn and Abell. Prognosis is extremely poor.

ENDOMETRIOID CARCINOMA OF THE OVARY

Most adenoacanthomas seem to arise from ectopic endometrium even though it may not always be possible to demonstrate transitional phases between the benign and the malignant. On the other hand, adenocarcinomas (without acanthosis) may arise from the ovary or the endometrium, and even the best pathologist cannot name the primary site (Fig. 29–27).

In their study of 20 cases of endometrioid tumors, Long and Taylor list suggested criteria for a possible endometrial origin, although except for acanthosis, their criteria are very difficult to apply. Familarity with the appearance of endometrial carcinoma (Chapter 9) is the only help we can offer.

Schueller and Kirol indicate that the prognosis with endometrioid carcinoma is twice as good as with the more common papillary serous cystadenocarcinoma, and, although their series is small (37 cases), their observations are in complete accord with our own impressions. In a recent FIGO report concerning 469 cases of *combined* endometroid and mesonephric carcinoma Kottmeier notes a 37 per cent 5 year salvage (as compared to 22 per cent for serous tumors). Fathalla suggests that 12 per cent of malignant ovarian tumors arise from endometriosis, a higher incidence than observed in most clinics (Fig. 29–28).

Scully and Barlow have suggested that ovarian mesonephromas arise from pre-existing endometriosis, and they present im-

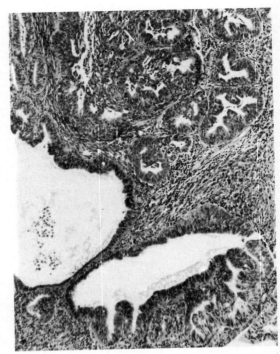

Figure 29–27. Well-differentiated adenocarcinoma (above) probably evolving from endometriosis (below), but such a malignancy can be primarily ovarian without preexisting endometriosis.

pressive photomicrographs showing combination and transition forms between endometrioid carcinomas and mesonephromas. It would seem more likely that the ovarian mesothelium led to both lesions, for serous, mucinous, endometrioid, and mesonephric patterns may be seen in a single tumor, as noted by Kurman and Craig. An extremely interesting case of a clear cell adenocarcinoma arising from retroperitoneal endometriosis has been reported by Brooks and Wheeler. This emphasizes the increased frequency of diverse epithelial lesions that are being recognized today.

CLINICAL CHARACTERISTICS OF ENDOMETRIOSIS

Endometriosis is characteristically a disease of reproductive life, occurring most frequently between 30 and 40 years of age. The *white private patient* is most commonly afflicted, perhaps because she marries and has children later, and might not have the presumably beneficial effect of protracted spells

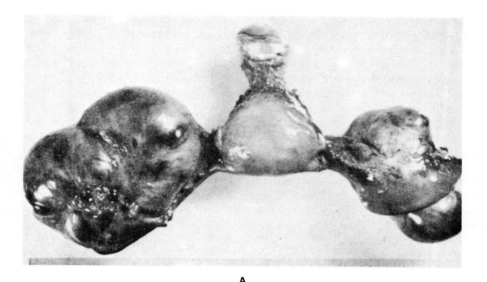

A

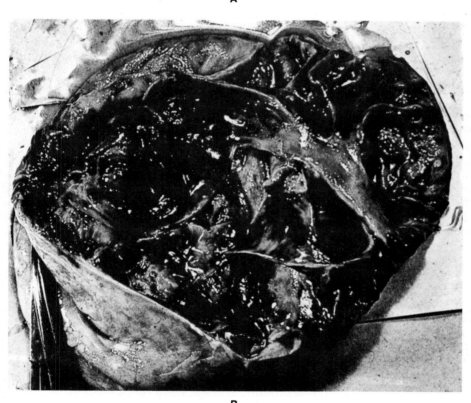

B

Figure 29–28. *A*, Large bilateral endometrial cysts removed without rupture (the exception). *B*, Cut surface of endometrial cyst showing dark hemorrhagic inner wall and whitish capsular layer. Microscopic malignancy was noted.

of amenorrhea. However, anovulation may occur (Soules et al.) and perhaps be responsible for the frequently observed infertility. It should not be inferred that *only* white patients contract endometriosis, for Chatman

has indicated that it is by no means rare in the black race.

A fundamental point in the consideration and the management of pelvic endometriosis is that the aberrant endometrium, like that of the uterus itself, is under the physiologic and trophic control of the ovary. As long as functioning ovarian tissue is present, there is always the theoretical possibility of persistence and extension of the endometriosis, but Kempers and co-workers report frequently active postmenopausal endometriosis, even without hormone therapy. However, there are wide individual variations in the clinical significance of the condition.

At one extreme is a considerable group of cases in which the endometriosis is of greater scientific than clinical significance. Small areas of endometriosis may be accidentally found at operation or on routine laboratory examination in the ovaries or other pelvic organs, with no symptoms referable to such lesions, and with little or no tendency to progress, as observed in the subsequent course of such patients. In the case pictured in Fig. 29–15, for example, there was no other suggestion of endometriosis in the pelvis, the ovaries being entirely normal in appearance. Nor has there been any clinical suspicion of endometriosis for many years since operation. At the other extreme are cases in which the process extends rapidly with widespread involvement of the pelvic structures and the production of severe symptoms, including intestinal obstruction.

Between these two extremes is the largest and clinically most important group, in which, for example, one finds endometrial cysts of one or both ovaries, with or without moderate involvement of the uterosacral ligaments, rectum, or other organs. These are the cases which often require careful judgment on the part of the surgeon. This is not the place for details of surgical treatment, except perhaps to urge conservative treatment when the age of the patient and the desirability of future reproductiveness are important considerations, because in many cases there are no recurrences or, at any rate, they are not serious. An excellent treatise on the medical or surgical treatment of endometrioses has been provided by Ingersoll.

Indeed, Sheets and the Mayo Clinic group believe that hysterectomy alone is frequently curative in patients with symptomatic endometriosis; removal of the uterus may remove the source of viable cells for implantation, and diffuse islands often burn themselves out despite conservation of the ovaries. This occasionally seems apparent to all clinicians, but we have also seen conservation of ovarian tissue attended by activation of residual pelvic endometriosis. There must be considerable variation among individual patients.

Endocrine therapy of many types as advocated by some seems best utilized as a transient means of delaying action prior to surgery. The vogue for oral progestogens, as advocated by Kistner, does not demand discussion in a pathologic text except to note that these can convert aberrant endometrium in many areas into a typical decidual appearance, at the same time producing a prolonged amenorrhea (pseudopregnancy) with marked but often temporary relief of symptoms.

The *symptomatology* simulates chronic pelvic inflammatory disease, except that in many cases severe dysmenorrhea is present and that it is frequently referred to the rectum or sacrococcygeal region. This is explained by the premenstrual and menstrual swelling of the uterosacral endometrial islands often present. This type of involvement is often of much diagnostic aid on pelvic examination. The presence of one or more definite nodules in the uterosacral region, in a case which might otherwise resemble chronic pelvic inflammatory disease, should always make one consider the strong possibility of endometriosis. *Laparoscopy* is frequently of extreme diagnostic value.

ENDOMETRIUM FOLLOWING PROGESTOGEN THERAPY

This pathologic textbook does not propose to explore the treatment of endometriosis, which is often properly surgical in the older parous woman, but sometimes medical in the younger woman. Many authors have pointed out the efficacy of progestational agents in suppressing the symptoms and apparent clinical course of endometriosis. Such drug therapy seems distinctly worthwhile in the symptomatic young female, and women so treated attain considerable amelioration of their symptoms. At the same time, one should be reluctant to utilize medical treatment when there is an adnexal (ovarian) mass despite overwhelming evidence of pelvic endometriosis. The ovarian lesion, although probably an endometrial cyst, could be much more ominous, for endometriosis may coexist with a variety of more lethal tumors. In any case, surgery is usually the

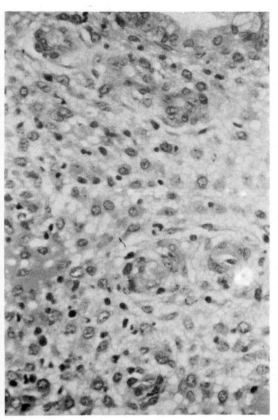

Figure 29–29. Apparent glandular-stromal disparity following Danazol administration.

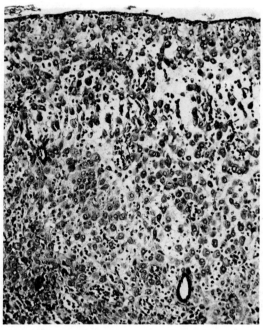

Figure 29–30. Striking features of endometriosis after progestogen therapy are marked decidual reaction in the stroma with profound edema and almost complete glandular exhaustion.

optimal therapy (Andrews and Larson) and is followed by a higher incidence of pregnancy; preoperative progesterone therapy may facilitate surgery when there is extensive disease.

In treating endometriosis by progesterone, the tendency is to produce a pseudopregnancy by gradual increments of the hormone so that an amenorrhea of many months' duration may be obtained. Just as genuine pregnancy may lead to marked remission of symptoms in the patient with endometriosis (if she is fortunate enough to become pregnant), so the pseudopregnancy may lead to similar symptomatic relief, and this form of therapy is being widely utilized today, although it may be replaced by Danazol, an antigonadotropin. This agent has received FDA approval, and is thoroughly discussed in the symposium by Greenblatt. Microscopically, the endometrium in a Danazol-treated patient will reveal glandular exhaustion with a stromal fibrosis rather than the decidual stroma found following progester-

one therapy, although there may be enough stromal edema so that a decidua-like appearance is produced with a glandular-stromal disparity (Fig. 29–29). Obviously, the microscopic appearance is dependent on dosage and its duration—if insufficient, ovulation will not be suppressed.

The pathologist should be familiar with the appearance of an endometrium following prolonged progestogen administration, for breakthrough bleeding, necessitating curettage, may occur. The most striking feature of an endometrium so treated is the profound stromal response with a marked resemblance to the decidua of pregnancy (Fig. 29–30). There is concurrent widespread edema and a loss of the glandular elements (glandular exhaustion). There is considerable variation in the pattern with individual endometria and with the duration of treatment.

Previous chapters have noted the use of progesterone in the treatment of endometrial adenocarcinoma. As might be expected,

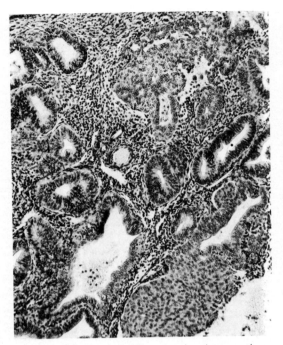

Figure 29–31. Well-differentiated adenoacanthoma. Note apparent transition of glandular epithelium into squamous cells at lower right.

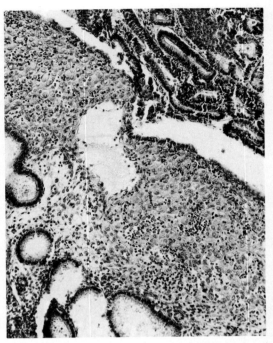

Figure 29–32. Persistent tumor (upper right) despite otherwise good response to large dosages of progesterone.

it is also beneficial in the occasional adenoacanthoma of the ovary, which metastasizes or recurs, although this type of gonadal tumor is usually rather innocuous. In a case reviewed recently, a typical adenoacanthoma recurred one and a half years following surgery. After six months' progesterone therapy, bowel obstruction occurred and laparotomy was performed. Biopsies showed an area of residual tumor (upper right), with the remaining tissue showing a normal glandular pattern and a marked decidual reaction in the tumor matrix. The response was identical to those observed with endometrial cancer (Chapter 9) but are reillustrated here for convenience (Figs. 29–31 and 29–32).

REFERENCES

Acosta, A. A., et al.: A proposed classification of pelvic endometriosis. Obstet. Gynecol., 42:19, 1973.

Allen, E., Peterson, L. F., and Campbell, Z. B.: Clinical and experimental endometriosis. Am. J. Obstet. Gynecol., 68:356, 1954.

Andrews, W. C., and Larsen, G. D.: Endometriosis: treatment with hormonal pseudopregnancy and/or operation. Am. J. Obstet. Gynecol., 118:643, 1974.

Azoury, R. S., and Woodruff, J. D.: Primary ovarian sarcoma. Obstet. Gynecol., 37:920, 1971.

Bachman, E.: Paradoxical metastasis and transpulmonary cancer spread. Am. J. Roentgenol., 72:499, 1954.

Barnes, J.: Endometriosis of the pleura and ovaries. J. Obstet. Gynaecol. Br. Emp., 60:823, 1953.

Barnes, J. J., and Wheeler, J. E.: Malignancy in extragonadal endometriosis. Cancer, 40:3065, 1977.

Boles, R. S., and Hodes, P. J.: Endometriosis of the small and large intestine. Gastroenterology, 34:367, 1958.

Campbell, J. S., Magner, D., and Fournier, P.: Adenoacanthomas of ovary and uterus occurring as coexistent or sequential primary neoplasms. Cancer, 14:817, 1961.

Charles, O.: Endometriosis and hemorrhagic pleural effusion. Obstet. Gynecol., 10:309, 1957.

Chatman, D. L.: Endometriosis in the black woman. Am. J. Obstet. Gynecol., 125:987, 1976.

Davis, C., Jr., and Truehart, T. R.: Surgical management of endometrioma of the colon. Am. J. Obstet. Gynecol., 89:453, 1964.

Dockerty, M. B.: Malignancy complicating endometriosis. Am. J. Obstet. Gynecol., 83:175, 1962.

Dmowski, W. P., and Cohen, M. R.: Treatment of endometriosis with an antiogonadotropin, Danazol. Obstet. Gynecol., 46:147, 1975.

Ecker, J. A., Doane, W. A., and Dickson, D. R.: Endometriosis of the gastrointestinal tract. Am. J. Gastroenterol., 41:405, 1964.

Fathalla, M. F.: Malignant transformation of ovarian endometriosis. J. Obstet. Gynaecol. Br. Commonw., 74:85, 1967.

Fenn, M. E., and Abell, M. R.: Carcinosarcoma of the ovary. Am. J. Obstet. Gynecol., 110:1066, 1971.

Fertano, L. R., Hertz, H., and Carter, H.: Malignant endometriosis. Obstet. Gynecol., 7:32, 1956.

Freidlander, R. L.: The treatment of endometriosis with Danazol. J. Reprod. Med., 10:197, 1973.

Frey, G. H.: Familial occurrence of endometriosis. Am. J. Obstet. Gynecol., 73:418, 1957.

Garcia, C. R., and David, S. S.: Pelvic endometriosis. Am. J. Obstet. Gynecol., 129:740, 1977.

Goldfarb, W. S.: A case of endometriosis in the episiotomy scar. Am. J. Obstet. Gynecol., 66:191, 1953.

Golditch, I. M.: Endometriosis presenting as an acute abdominal emergency. Obstet. Gynecol., 26:780, 1965.

Gray, L. A.: Endometriosis of the bowel. Southern Med. J., 58:815, 1965.

Gray, L. A., and Barnes, M. L.: Relationship of endometriosis to carcinoma of the ovary. Ann. Surg., 163:713, 1966.

Green, T. H., and Meigs, J. V.: Pseudomenstruation from posthysterectomy vaginal vault endometriosis. Obstet. Gynecol., 4:622, 1954.

Greenblatt, R. B. (Ed.): Recent Advances in Endometriosis. Excerpta Medica, March 1975.

Hajdu, S. I., and Koss, L. G.: Endometriosis of the kidney. Am. J. Obstet. Gynecol., 106:314, 1970.

Hartz, P. H.: Occurrence of decidua-like tissue in the lung. Am. J. Clin. Pathol., 26:48, 1956.

Henson, S. W., Jr.: Endometriosis of the rectum simulating carcinoma. J.A.M.A., 187:1026, 1964.

Hughesdon, P. E.: Structure of endometrial cysts of the ovary. J. Obstet. Gynaecol. Br. Emp., 64:481, 1957.

Ingersoll, F. M.: Medical or surgical treatment of endometriosis. Clin. Obstet. Gynecol., 20:849, 1977.

Irani, S., et al.: Pleuroperitoneal endometriosis. Obstet. Gynecol., 47 (Suppl.): 72S, 1976.

Kempers, R. D., Dockerty, M. B., Hunt, A. B., and Symmonds, R. E.: Postmenopausal endometriosis. Surg. Gynecol. Obstet., 111:348, 1960.

Kistner, R. W.: Newer progestins in treatment of endometriosis. Am. J. Obstet. Gynecol., 75:264, 1958.

Koss, L. G.: Miniature adenoacanthoma arising in an endometriotic cyst in an obturator lymph node. Cancer, 16:1369, 1963.

Kottmeier, H. L. (Ed.): Annual Report on the Results (1954–63) of Treatment in Carcinoma of the Uterus, Vagina, and Ovary. Volume 15. Stockholm, Sweden, 1973.

Kovarik, J. L., and Toll, G. D.: Thoracic endometriosis with recurrent spontaneous pneumothorax. J.A.M.A., 196:221, 1966.

Kurman, R. J., and Craig, J. M.: Endometrioid and clear cell carcinoma of the ovary. Cancer, 29:1653, 1972.

Labay, G. R., and Feiner, F.: Malignant pleural endometriosis—endometrial sarcoma arising in pleural and pelvic endometriosis. Am. J. Obstet. Gynecol., 110:478, 1971.

Langmade, C. F.: Pelvic Endometriosis and ureteral obstruction. Am. J. Obstet. Gynecol., 122:463, 1975.

Lauersen, N. H., et al.: Danazol: An antigonadotropic agent in the treatment of pelvic endometriosis. Am. J. Obstet. Gynecol., 123:742, 1975.

Lattes, R., et al.: A clinical and pathological study of endometriosis of the lung. Surg. Gynecol. Obstet., 103:552, 1956.

Leverton, J. C. S.: Uterus didelphys with endometriosis. Obstet. Gynecol., 1:681, 1953.

Long, M. E., and Taylor, H. C.: Endometrioid carcinoma of the ovary. Am. J. Obstet. Gynecol., 90:936, 1964.

McArthur, J. W., and Ulfelder, H.: The effect of pregnancy upon endometriosis. Obstet. Gynecol. Surv., 20:709, 1965.

McCann, T. O., and Myers, R. E.: Endometriosis in the rhesus monkey. Am. J. Obstet. Gynecol., 106:516, 1970.

Meigs, J. V.: An interest in endometriosis and its consequences. Am. J. Obstet. Gynecol., 79:625, 1960.

Merrill, J. A.: Endometrial induction of endometriosis across Millipore filters. Am. J. Obstet. Gynecol., 94:780, 1966.

Mukherjee, T. K., et al.: Ectopic endometrium in omentum. Uterine perforation by Lippes loop. Obstet. Gynecol., 45:105, 1975.

Novak, E. R.: Pathology of endometriosis. Clin. Obstet. Gynecol., 3:413, 1960.

Novak, E. R., and Hoge, A. F.: Endometriosis of the lower genital tract. Obstet. Gynecol., 12:687, 1958.

Nunn, L. L.: Endometrioma of thigh. Northwest Med., 48:474, 1949.

Overton, O. H., Wilson, R. B., and Dockerty, M. B.: Primary endometriosis of the cervix. Am. J. Obstet. Gynecol., 79:768, 1960.

Parsons, L.: Conservative surgical management of external endometriosis. Obstet. Gynecol., 32:576, 1968.

Pratt, J. H., and Shamblin, W. R.: Spontaneous rupture of endometrial cysts of the ovary. Am. J. Obstet. Gynecol., 108:56, 1970.

Ranney, B.: Endometriosis. I. Conservative operations. Am. J. Obstet. Gynecol., 107:743, 1970. II. Emergency operations due to hemopheritoneum. Obstet. Gynecol., 36:437, 1970. III. Complete operations. Am. J. Obstet. Gynecol., 109:1137, 1971. IV. Hereditary tendencies. Obstet. Gynecol., 37:734, 1971.

Ranney, B.: The prevention, inhibition, palliation, and treatment of endometriosis. Am. J. Obstet. Gynecol., 123:778, 1975.

Ridley, J. H.: The histogenesis of endometriosis. Obstet. Gynecol. Surv., 23:1, 1968.

Roddick, J. W., Jr., Conkey, G., and Jacobs, E. J.: The hormonal response of endometriosis in endometriotic implants and its relation to symptomatology. Am. J. Obstet. Gynecol., 79:1173, 1960.

Rodman, M. H., and Jones, C. W.: Catamenial hemoptysis due to bronchial endometriosis. N. Engl. J. Med., 266:805, 1962.

Sampson, J. A.: Perforating hemorrhagic (chocolate) cysts of the ovary, their importance and especially their relation to pelvic adenomas of the endometrial type. Arch. Surg., 3:245, 1921.

Sampson, J. A.: Pathogenesis of postsalpingectomy endometriosis in laparotomy scars. Am. J. Obstet. Gynecol., 50:597, 1946.

Schifrin, B. S. et al.: Teen-age endometriosis. Am. J. Obstet. Gynecol., 116:973, 1973.

Schlicke, C. P.: Endometriosis of thigh. J.A.M.A., 132:445, 1946.

Schueller, H. F., and Kirol, P. M.: Prognosis in endometrial carcinoma of the ovary. Obstet. Gynecol., 27:850, 1966.

Scott, R. B.: Malignant changes in endometriosis. Obstet. Gynecol., 2:283, 1953.

Scott, R. B., and TeLinde, R. W.: External endometriosis. Ann. Surg., 131:697, 1950.

Scott, R. B., and TeLinde, R. W.: Clinical external endometriosis. Obstet. Gynecol., 4:502, 1954.

Scott, R. B., TeLinde, R. W., and Wharton, L. R., Jr.: Further studies on experimental endometriosis. Am. J. Obstet. Gynecol., 66:1052, 1953.

Scott, R. B., and Wharton, L. R., Jr.: Large doses of stilbesterol and endometriosis. Am. J. Obstet. Gynecol., 69:573, 1955.

Scott, R. B., and Wharton, L. R., Jr.: Effect of estrone and progesterone on growth of experimental endometriosis in rhesus monkeys. Am. J. Obstet. Gynecol., 74:852, 1957.

Scott, R. B., and Wharton, L. R., Jr.: The effect of testosterone on experimental endometriosis in rhesus monkeys. Am. J. Obstet. Gynecol., 78:1020, 1959.

Scully, R. E., and Barlow, J. F.: Mesonephroma of the ovary: tumor of müllerian origin related to the endometrioid carcinoma. Cancer, 20:405, 1967.

Sheets, J. L., Symmonds, R. E., and Banner, E. A.: Conservative management of endometriosis. Obstet. Gynecol., 23:625, 1964.

Shmuel, J., Shtamler, B., and Suprun, H.: External endometriosis of the vermiform appendix with acute symptoms. Int. J. Gynaecol. Obstet., 8:38, 1970.

Sotrel, G., and Dmowski, W. P.: Endometriosis and its management. Obstet. Gynecol. Dig., June 1976, p. 26.

Soules, M. R., et al.: Endometriosis and anovulation: a coexisting problem in the infertile female. Am. J. Obstet. Gynecol., 125:412, 1976.

Spangler, D. B., Jones, G. S., and Jones, H. W.: Infertility due to endometriosis. Am. J. Obstet. Gynecol., 109:850, 1971.

Steck, W. D., and Helwig, E. B.: Cutaneous endometriosis. J.A.M.A., 191:101, 1965.

Tate, G. T.: Acute obstruction of the large bowel due to endometriosis. Br. J. Surg., 50:771, 1963.

Teilum, G., and Madsen, V.: Endometriosis ovarii et peritonei caused by histerosalpingography. J. Obstet. Gynaecol. Br. Emp., 57:10, 1950.

TeLinde, R. W., and Scott, R. B.: Experimental endometriosis. Am. J. Obstet. Gynecol., 60:1147, 1950.

Thompson, J. D.: Primary ovarian adeno-acanthoma. Obstet. Gynecol., 9:403, 1957.

Uohara, J. K., and Kovara, T. Y.: Endometriosis of the appendix. Am. J. Obstet. Gynecol., 121:423, 1975.

Weed, J. C., and Holland, J. B.: Endometriosis and infertility. Fertil. Steril., 28:135, 1977.

Wentz, A. C., et al.: Progestational activity of Danazol in the human female subject. Am. J. Obstet. Gynecol., 126:378, 1976.

Williams, T. J., and Pratt, J. H.: Endometriosis in 1000 consecutive celiotomies. Am. J. Obstet. Gynecol., 129:245, 1977.

Williams, J. F., Williams, J. B., and Harper, J. W.: Thoracic endometriosis. Am. J. Obstet. Gynecol., 84:1512, 1962.

Woodruff, J. D., and Julian, C. G.: Multiple malignancies in upper genital tract. Am. J. Obstet. Gynecol., 103:810, 1969.

Wynn, T. E.: Endometriosis of the sigmoid colon. Arch. Pathol., 92:24, 1971.

Zeidman, I., and Buss, J.: Transpulmonary passage of tumor cells. Cancer Res., 12:731, 1952.

Chapter 30

FERTILIZATION, IMPLANTATION, AND PLACENTATION

CARL J. PAUERSTEIN

FERTILIZATION

The human chromosomal complement consists of 22 pairs of autosomes and one pair of sex chromosomes. In contrast the male and female gametes contain only 22 autosomes (one member of each pair) and a single sex chromosome. This reduction to the haploid complement is accomplished by meiotic division.

Primary spermatocytes contain the full diploid chromosomal complement. During spermatogenesis, the primary spermatocyte divides by mitosis into two secondary spermatocytes, (each with diploid number of chromosomes), and each of these divides by meiosis into two spermatids. These meiotic divisions assure that the spermatozoa, the end products of spermatogenesis, have the haploid chromosome number.

In the female the primordial germ cells divide freely by mitotic division while migrating to the gonad from the hind gut. Upon reaching the surface of the genital ridge, the germ cells, now designated oogonia, continue mitotic division. At completion of mitotic proliferation, the oogonia enter meiotic prophase and differentiate into oocytes. Upon encapsulation in the primordial follicle, cell replication ceases in prophase of the first meiotic division. Meiotic prophase with subsequent maturation ordinarily does not resume until the particular ovum is destined to be released from the follicle. The first meiotic division is completed as oocyte maturation continues. Maturation includes disappearance of the nuclear membrane, extrusion of the first polar body, and alignment of chromosomes at metaphase of the second meiotic division. In most mammals, maturation is completed within the follicle prior to ovulation. Thus, the ovum, at its encounter with the fertilizing spermatozoan, is in metaphase of the second meiotic division.

Before fertilization can occur the sperm undergoes maturational changes in the male reproductive tract during epididymal transit, and biophysical changes in the female reproductive tract—e.g., *capacitation* and the *acrosomal reaction.*

Capacitation, the acquisition of the ability to penetrate the zona pellucida, has not been described in humans. Thus, we are dependent upon observations made in other species. The phenomenon of capacitation was first described in 1951 in rabbits and rats. Since those early experiments many investigators have found that freshly ejaculated or epididymal sperm are unable to fertilize ova in vitro while capacitated ones can immediately penetrate ova. Originally it was felt that a sojourn in the female reproductive tract was mandatory for capacitation. However, it is now known that in some species capacitation can be achieved in vitro without exposure to female genital tract fluids. An important step in capacitation lies in the removal of *stabilizing* or *inhibitory* material from the sperm surface (Austin, 1975). Chang's findings regarding reversal of capacitation by exposure to seminal plasma (decapacitation) and regaining of capacitation (recapacitation) by reexposure to the female tract (Chang, 1957) strongly support this view. Capacitation seems to be a necessity for fertilization in many species so far examined, although this has not been completely resolved for the primate.

Fertilization entails the union of the spermatozoon and the ovum with the fusion of the limiting membranes of the two cells so that they become a single cell. The process involves penetration of the spermatozoon into the egg, formation of male and female pronuclei, and union of their chromosomes. Some paternal cytoplasmic elements are also added to the embryo via the tail of the sperm. In penetrating the ovum, the sperm encounters the cumulus oophorus, the zona pellucida, the perivitelline space, and the vitelline membrane.

The cumulus oophorus is composed of granulosa cells embedded in a hyaluronic acid matrix. The densely packed cumulus cells immediately surrounding the ovum are designated the corona radiata. Although considerable species differences may exist, in man spermatozoa enter the ovum while it is still partially enclosed by cumulus.

The zona pellucida, a protein polysaccharide layer formed by the ovum and the granulosa cells during follicular growth, apparently functions to exclude noncapacitated sperm and to limit polyspermy and heterospecific fertilization.

The *zonal block to polyspermic fertilization* is probably a function of vitelline cortical-granules released after penetration of the vitellus by the fertilizing sperm. After passing through the zona pellucida, the head of the first sperm that enters the perivitelline space contracts and fuses with the vitelline membrane. This fusion may be responsible for the penetration of the spermatozoon into the vitellus and for activating the block to polyspermy, so that later arrivals are unable to penetrate the vitellus. The efficiency of the vitelline block to polyspermy varies with species and weakens with increasing maternal age.

Intact ova can generally be penetrated only by sperm of the same species. Rat and hamster ova can be penetrated by mouse sperm only if the zona is removed. Although mouse, rat, and hamster ova are penetrated to some extent by sperm of the rat, hamster, and rat or guinea pig, respectively, no male pronuclei are formed, and the second maturation division does not occur. The zona, therefore, also appears to provide an incomplete barrier to interspecies fertilizations.

Fertilization takes place in the ampulla of the fallopian tube, just above the ampulla-isthmus junction. Physicians dealing with infertility problems and with the development of contraceptive methodology need to know the fertilizing life span of the sperm, and the fertilizable life span of the ovum. The fertilizable life of the mammalian ovum begins with the resumption of the first meiotic division and varies, depending on the species, from 5 to 30 hours following division. Available data suggest that the human ovum is fertilizable for less than 24 hours. The fertile life of sperm within the female genital tract is shorter than the motile life and varies from 12 hours in the mouse, through 30 hours in the rabbit, to 100 hours or more in the bitch, mare, and ferret. The fertile life of sperm in women has not been accurately determined but has been estimated to be about 48 hours. Recently Ahlgren recovered motile sperm from human fallopian tubes 85 hours after coitus. Thus, the fertilizing life span of the human sperm may be longer than previously estimated.

The zygote resides in the ampulla for a variable time after fertilization. In women and subhuman primates, ova remain in the ampulla for about 48 hours after fertilization, and then traverse the isthmus, to enter the uterus 68 to 80 hours after ovulation. Although we have no definitive data on transport of human embryos, fertilized and unfertilized rabbit ova are transported at similar rates. During tubal transport each cell of the embryo undergoes a series of mitotic divisions, forming first the *morula* and then the *blastocyst*. Human embryos apparently enter the uterus in the early blastocyst stage.

Among the zygotes recovered from the human tube and uterus prior to implantation, Hertig and Rock considered four cleavage stages with 5, 8, 9, and 11 to 12 cells to be abnormal, whereas others, comprising 12, 58, and 107 cells, were thought to be normal. In the 58-celled conceptus, the outer and inner cells, as well as the beginning segmentation cavity, are clearly demarcated, and in the 107-celled blastocyst a delicate trophoblast forms the outer wall of the fluid-filled segmentation cavity. The zygote with 107 cells is no larger than that of the earlier cleavage stages. In the human, the free blastocyst period is about four days, and in that time, loss of the zona pellucida occurs, which seems to be prerequisite for implantation. After "hatching," i.e., release from the confines of the zona pellucida, *the expanded blastocyst* is ready for implantation. Implantation in the human is *interstitial* and can be divided into three main stages: (1) muscular, dealing with transport, (2) adhesive, whereby the blastocyst attaches to the surface epithelium, and (3) invasive, wherein the trophoblast penetrates the endometrial wall.

IMPLANTATION

The human uterus simplex is formed from the embryonic right and left paramesonephric ducts by a process first of fusion, and then of recanalization. Thus, the anterior and posterior walls of the uterus are constituted from what was the antimesometrial side of each paramesonephric duct. Human implantation normally occurs on either the anterior or posterior uterine wall, near the fundus. Thus human implantation is designated *antimesometrial*, but it is also *interstitial* because the blastocyst sinks below the endo-

metrial surface. The site of entrance is first covered by fibrin, and then reepithelialized. In the past, various writers have speculated that the endometrial decidual response somehow limits the depth of trophoblastic invasion. However, Ramsey's elegant studies have negated this assumption. In *Macaca mulatta*, implantation is superficial. The entire blastocyst does not sink below the endometrial surface, as in the human. Yet, this species does not develop a generalized decidual reaction, but rather forms an epithelial plaque in the immediate vicinity of the invading trophoblast. The baboon, which exhibits a similar shallow implantation has neither decidual reaction nor plaque. Thus, the decidua clearly does not regulate the depth of invasion.

The human blastocyst probably implants on the sixth day after ovulation. The wall of the blastocyst is composed of a single layer of trophoblast at this time (this stage has not been observed in humans, but we may make certain assumptions by analogy from *Macaca mulatta*). The inner cell mass, from which the embryo will develop, can be distinguished on the inner surface of one pole of the blastocyst. This pole enters the endometrium first. The earliest human implantation

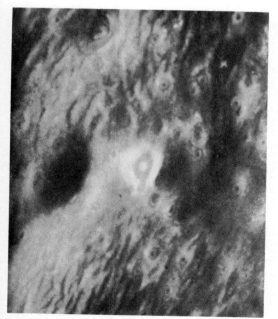

Figure 30–1. The Hertig-Rock egg, 7 to 7½ days old, the youngest as yet described. A surface view, magnified 35 times, of implantation site, showing collapsed blastocyst attached to endometrium. (Courtesy of Drs. A. T. Hertig and J. Rock.)

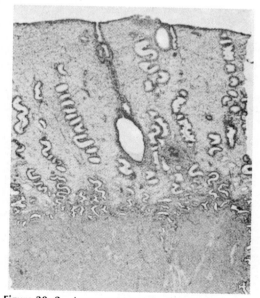

Figure 30–2. Lower power view of implantation site of the Hertig-Rock egg. The endometrium in about the twenty-second day of cycle shows marked physiologic edema. The glands are actively secretory except in their basal part. The superficial portion of the ovum is evident at the top of the picture. (Courtesy of Drs. A. T. Hertig and J. Rock.)

recorded is at about 7½ days postovulation (Figs. 30–1 and 30–2). This implantation measures 0.45 × 0.30 × 1.12 mm. The embryo is well anchored to the endometrium. Later stages demonstrate trophoblastic proliferation, and differentiation of the trophoblast into cytotrophoblast (Langhan's cells) and syncytiotrophoblast. The latter lies between the cytotrophoblast and the maternal tissue. The syncytiotrophoblast is a product of the cytotrophoblast, and is a more highly differentiated tissue, particularly with regard to the production of hormones and enzymes. As development continues, sheets of trophoblast invade the maternal tissues. At the interface of the trophoblast and the maternal tissues, a layer of fibrinoid is deposited. In the human this fibrinoid deposit is called Nitabuch's stria (Fig. 30–3). Similar accumulations of fibrinoid when located at the base of the intervillous space are designated Rohr's stria. Although these layers are sometimes said to be barriers to trophoblastic penetration, in my opinion they are more likely markers of destroyed cells, fetal or maternal or both.

The full decidual response of the endometrium is not elicited until the trophoblast has eroded the superficial uterine epithelium, perhaps in response to histamine or a histamine-like substance present at the site of blastocyst attachment. The process of implantation, although incompletely understood, is know to be under the control of estrogen and progesterone.

Not only does a local rise in pH induce adhesion but in addition the alkalinity that accompanies discharge of bicarbonate from the abembryonic hemisphere of the blastocyst results in dissociation of the cellular uterine epithelium, while the trophoblast remains intact. In the rabbit, Larsen has observed a fusion of the trophoblastic syncytium and the uterine symplasma in the implantation site, with a common cytoplasmic matrix for both maternal and fetal nuclei. Progesterone, which stimulates blastocystic expansion and even spacing of these structures along the rabbit cornu, apparently serves an additional function at the implantation site by augmenting carbonic anhydrase activity and removal of carbon dioxide. The interplay of these various mechanisms has not been fully elucidated in humans.

For several days after implantation, development of decidua occurs in the endometrium, first appearing perivascularly and then spreading throughout the uterus. The stromal cells enlarge and take a round or polygonal shape with a translucent membrane encompassing a round, vesicular nucleus, and abundant, slightly basophilic cytoplasm. The purpose of decidualization is not clear. The critical determinants of optimal nidation are largely unknown. It appears that many factors, such as adequate preparation of the endometrium, good nutrition, normal endocrine support, genetic background, uterine vascularity, freedom from intrinsic disease or anatomic defect, normal immunologic responses, play a role in successful implantation and early placentation.

PLACENTATION

As development continues, columns of trophoblast grow into the endometrium and are called *primary villi*. These columns are separated by spaces called lacunae (Fig. 30–4). The human uterus, as that of all menstruating animals, is equipped with spiral arteries which supply the endometrium. The invading trophoblast, early in implantation, erodes into the endometrial capillaries, and then into the tips of the spiral arteries. Blood thus enters the *lacunar spaces* in the trophoblast, and the lacunae in turn expand and begin to communicate with each other. The

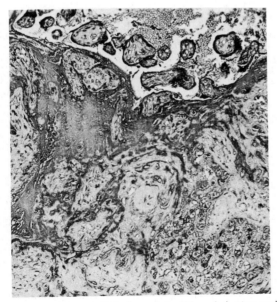

Figure 30–3. Section through junction of chorion and decidua basalis showing a zone of fibrin between the trophoblastic and decidual tissues.

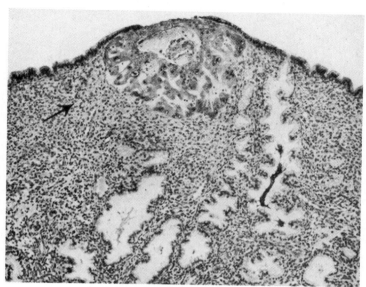

Figure 30–4. A thin section of ovum obtained on twenty-fifth day of cycle, 9½ days or less after conception. Area still exposed to uterine lumen, 0.38 x 0.26 mm. Syncytiotrophoblast, a complex network, fills enlarged implantation site. Within cytotrophoblastic shell are two-layered embryo and amnion-forming cells. Arrow indicates zone of enlarged stromal cells. Photomicrograph × 100. Carnegie Collection No. 8004. (From A. T. Hertig and J. Rock: Contrib. Embryol., *31*:65, 1945.)

lacunar spaces will become the *intervillous space.* The human placenta thus is a *hemochorial* placenta in Grosser's classification, because no maternal tissue intervenes between the mother's blood and the trophoblast.

Certain phenomena involving the invasiveness of trophoblast are of great interest to the reproductive biologist. As noted above, the trophoblast invades the lumina of the maternal arteries early in implantation. Later the intraluminal trophoblast invades the arterial wall and replaces its substance. In addition to the intravascular invasion, individual trophoblastic cells invade the endometrium (termed syncytial endometritis) and the myometrium (syncytial myometritis) (Fig. 30–5). Some of these trophoblastic cells also invade the arterial walls from the outside. Finally, masses of trophoblast may break off in the blood vessels, and be "deported" to remote sites, such as the lung (Fig. 30–6).

Although there is some controversy, primatologists and students of human placentation believe that the mesoderm of the early blastocyst forms a membrane (Heuser's membrane) surrounding a central cavity (Fig. 30–7). This cavity is designated the *primitive yolk sac,* and is the precursor of the definitive yolk sac. The primitive yolk sac is therefore limited by the endodermal plate of the inner cell mass, and by the mesoderm. The cells of the endodermal plate proliferate to form the *definitive yolk sac* suspended

within the primitive yolk sac. The definitive yolk sac becomes surrounded by mesoderm. The *exocelomic cavity* is formed within the mesoderm. As the inner cell mass continues to grow and differentiate, the roof of the definitive yolk sac becomes incorporated into the midgut of the embryo. With further de-

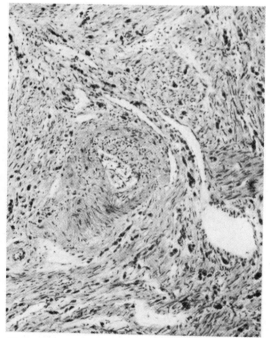

Figure 30–5. Trophoblastic invasion of musculature beneath implantation area. This is a normal process but has at times been wrongly diagnosed as syncytioma or chorioepithelioma.

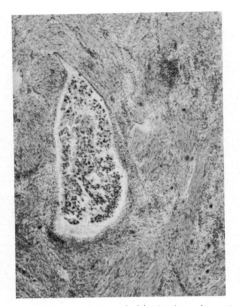

Figure 30–6. Mass of trophoblastic tissue in a uterine vein deep in the muscle. Note also the wandering trophoblastic cells in the muscle (lower right).

velopment the communication narrows, and becomes known as the *vitelline duct*.

The allantois arises as a diverticulum from the hind gut. The human placenta is *chorioallantoic*. Although the allantois itself is rudimentary in humans, all of the vasculature of the villi is derived from the vascularized mesodermal wall of the allantois.

During the third week of embryonic life, mesoderm begins to grow into the columns of trophoblast of the primary villi, to form the *secondary villi*, characterized by a central core of mesoderm, surrounded by a layer of cytotrophoblast, which is in turn surrounded by synctiotrophoblast (Fig. 30–8). At about the same time, the mesodermal cores of the villi begin to be vascularized. Some of these vessels may arise by angiogenesis in situ, but the bulk of the vasculature is the product of the vessels of the allantoic stalk. As the villi grow, and develop finer and finer branches, the blood vessels undergo the same ramifications. Some of the main stem villi grow all

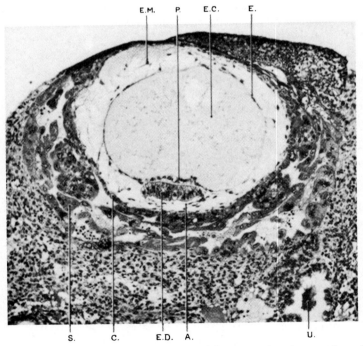

Figure 30–7. Human ovum of previllous stage. Free cells are delaminating from inner surface of trophoblast around its entire circumference, forming amnion adjacent to germ disc. *E.D.*, Embryonic disc; *P.*, primitive endoderm; *A.*, amnion; *E.*, exocoelomic membrane; *E.C.*, primitive yolk sac; *C.*, cytotrophoblast; *S.*, syncytium; *E.M.*, extraembryonic mesoblast; *U.*, uterine gland removed on the twenty-ninth day after the onset of the last menstrual period. Its age is estimated as 12 days. ×120. Carnegie Collection No. 7700. (From A. T. Hertig and J. Rock: Contrib. Embryol., *31*:65, 1945.)

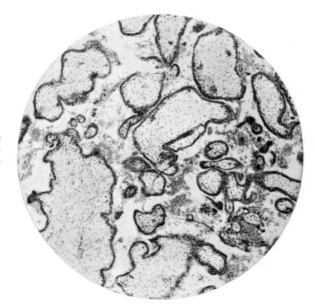

Figure 30–8. Normal chorionic villi, which even with the low power show the two layers of trophoblast found in early pregnancy. Note occasional budding of the syncytium, and also the syncytial or placental giant cells formed by cross section of these buds (upper right).

the way to the decidua and anchor to the decidual plate and to the sides of the placental septa, whereas the majority of villi float freely in the intervillous space. Each main stem villus and its ramifications constitute a *fetal cotyledon*. The villi are thereafter known as *tertiary villi*.

During the early stages of pregnancy, vascularized villi are distributed over the entire surface of the chorionic membrane, and the entire mesodermal lining of the gestational sac is vascularized. Because of a lack of nutrition, the villi disappear from all locations except those underlying the embryonic pole of the sac. The villi in this location form a disc, which will become the definitive placenta. The remainder of the chorion is now called the *chorion laeve* (Fig. 30–9).

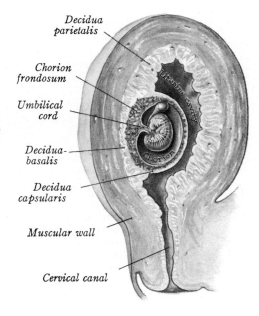

Decidua parietalis

Chorion frondosum

Umbilical cord

Decidua-basalis

Decidua capsularis

Muscular wall

Cervical canal

Figure 30–9. Gravid uterus of slightly over one month, in semi-diagrammatic section to indicate the relations of the embryo to the deciduae. About natural size. (From L. B. Arey: Developmental Anatomy. Philadelphia, W. B. Saunders Co.)

From the maternal side, blood enters the spiral arteries, driven by maternal systemic arterial pressure. The chorionic villi, bathed in this blood, are densely crowded in the intervillous space, except at the placental margin and just below the chorionic plate. Each fetal cotyledon exhibits a central space, which is usually directly above the entrance of each spiral artery. The markedly decreased villous density of the central space is probably due to increased oxygen concentration and mechanical pressure from the pulsatile jets of arterial blood. A pressure gradient exists from the spiral artery through the intervillous space and into the maternal veins distributed beneath the placenta.

The amniotic cavity of the human forms by a coalescence of spaces in the area of the inner cell mass closest to the trophoblast (Fig. 30–10). The resultant cavity is lined by ectoderm, which is surrounded by mesoderm. Thus, the amnion is bilaminar, and avascular. Early in embryogenesis, the amniotic sac is in apposition to the trophoblast over a broad area. Later, the mesoderm connecting the amnion and trophoblast becomes longer and narrower, and attaches to the embryo. The allantoic diverticulum grows into the connecting stalk from the hindgut. The intraamniotic portion of the connecting stalk is called the *body stalk*, and the part outside the amniotic sac is designated the *connecting stalk*. Eventually the blood vessels in the chorionic plate converge at the connecting stalk (now umbilical cord) to form the umbilical arteries and vein, which connect the placental vascular system with that of the fetus.

A spiral artery and a fetal cotyledon make up the functional unit of the placenta. As stressed by Ramsey, the distinction between maternal and fetal cotyledons must be kept clear. The mature placenta is divided by the septa into 15 to 20 maternal cotyledons. Although Ramsey believes that the cores of the septa are of maternal origin, Khudr and associates concluded from quinacrine fluorescence and anti-HCG immunofluorescence that the septal cores are of fetal origin. This view was confirmed by Maidman and coworkers. The margins of the septa are made up of trophoblast, and attached anchoring villi. Two or three fetal cotyledons may be included in a single maternal cotyledon (sometimes called a lobe or lobule). Because there is a one to one correspondence between fetal cotyledons and spiral arteries, two or three of the latter may enter a single maternal cotyledon.

The mature placenta at term measures 15 to 20 cm. in diameter, and is 1.5 to 3 cm. thick. The average weight is 464 g. and the usual ratio of fetal weight to placental weight ranges from 6.4:1 to 7.9:1. The surface area available for fetomaternal exchange at term has been estimated at about 14 sq. m., and the total length of the villous capillary bed at about 56 km. (35 miles).

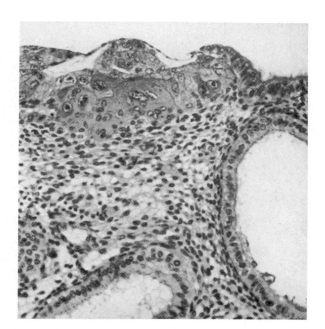

Figure 30–10. High power view of section through middle of ovum and the immediately surrounding endometrium. The bilaminar nature of the germ disc is evident. The early primordium of the amniotic cavity appears as a small cleft between it and the cytotrophoblast. (Courtesy of Drs. A. T. Hertig and J. Rock.)

REFERENCES

Ahlgren, M.: Sperm transport to and survival in the human fallopian tube. Gynecol. Invest., 6:206, 1975.

Arey, L. B.: Developmental Anatomy. 7th Ed. Philadelphia, W. B. Saunders Company, 1974.

Austin, C. R.: Membrane fusion events in fertilization. J. Reprod. Fertil., 44:155, 1975.

Boving, B. G.: Analysis of implantation in the rabbit. In R. M. Wynn (ed.): First Conference on Fetal Homeostasis. New York, New York Academy of Sciences, 1965, p. 138.

Boyd, J. D., and Hamilton, W. J.: The Human Placenta. Cambridge, W. Heffer and Sons, Ltd., 1970, pp. 30–287.

Brewer, J. I.: A normal human ovum in a stage preceding the primitive streak. Am. J. Anat., 61:429, 1937.

Brewer, J. I.: A human embryo in the bilaminar blastodisc stage (the Edwards-Jones-Brewer ovum). Contrib. Embryol., 27:85, 1938.

Brosens, I.: A study of the spiral arteries of the decidua basalis in normotensive and hypertensive pregnancies. J. Obstet. Gynaecol. Br. Commonw., 71:222, 1964.

Chang, M. C.: A detrimental effect of seminal plasma on the fertilizing capacity of sperm. Nature (Lond.), 179:285, 1957.

Cheviakoff, S., et al.: Ovum transport in women. In Harper, M.J.K., et al. (eds.): WHO Symposium—Ovum Transport and Fertility Regulation. Copenhagen, Scriptor, 1976.

Eddy, C. A., Garcia, R. G., Kraemer, D. C., and Pauerstein, C. J.: Detailed time course of ovum transport in the rhesus monkey (Macaca mulatta). Biol. Reprod., 12:363, 1975.

Eddy, C. A., Turner, T. T., Kraemer, D. C. and Pauerstein, C. J.: Pattern and duration of ovum transport in the baboon (Papio anubis). Obstet. Gynecol., 47:658, 1976.

Hertig, A. T., and Rock, J.: On the development of the early human ovum, with special reference to the trophoblast of the previllous stage: A description of 7 normal and 5 pathologic human ova. Am J. Obstet. Gynecol., 47:149, 1944.

Hertig, A. T., and Rock, J.: On a human blastula recovered from uterine cavity 4 days after ovulation (Carnegie No. 8190). Anat. Rec., 94:469, 1946.

Hertig, A. T., and Rock, J.: A series of potentially abortive ova recovered from fertile women prior to the first missed menstrual period. Am. J. Obstet. Gynecol., 58:968, 1949.

Hertig, A. T., Rock, J., Adams, E. C., and Mulligan, W. J.: On the preimplantation stages of the human ovum. Contrib. Embryol., 35:199, 1954.

Keibel, F., and Mall, F. P.: Manual of Human Embryology. Philadelphia, J. B. Lippincott Co., 1910–1912.

Khudr, G., Soma, H., and Benirschke, K.: Trophoblastic origin of the X cell and the placental site giant cell. Am. J. Obstet. Gynecol., 115:530, 1973.

Larsen, J. F.: Electron microscopy of the implantation site of the rabbit. Am. J. Anat., 109:319, 1961.

Maidman, J. E., Thorpe, L. W., Harris, J. A., and Wynn, R. M.: Fetal origin of X-cells in human placental septa and basal plate. Obstet. Gynecol., 41:547, 1973.

Page, E. W., Villee, C. A., and Villee, D. B.: Human Reproduction. Philadelphia, W. B. Saunders Company, 1972.

Pauerstein, C. J.: Physiology. In C. J. Pauerstein: The Fallopian Tube: A Reappraisal. Philadelphia, Lea & Febiger, 1974.

Ramsey, E. M.: The Placenta of Laboratory Animals and Man. Developmental Biology Series. New York, Holt, Rinehart, and Winston, Inc., 1975.

Reynolds, S. R. M.: Formation of fetal cotyledons in the hemochorial placenta. Am. J. Obstet. Gynecol., 94:425, 1966.

Rock, J., and Hertig, A. T.: Some aspects of early human development. Am. J. Obstet. Gynecol., 44:973, 1942.

Rock, J., and Hertig, A. T.: Information regarding time of human ovulation derived from study of 3 unfertilized and 1 fertilized ova. Am. J. Obstet. Gynecol., 47:343, 1944.

Rock, J., and Hertig, A. T.: The human conceptus during the first two weeks of gestation. Am. J. Obstet. Gynecol., 55:6, 1948.

Streeter, G. L.: A human embryo of the presomite period. Contrib. Embryol., 9:389, 1920.

Streeter, G. L.: The "Miller" ovum—the youngest normal human embryo thus far known. Carnegie Contrib. Embryol., 18:31, 1926.

Streeter, G. L.: Developmental horizons in human embryos. Carnegie Inst. Washington, Publ. 541, p. 211; Publ. 557, p. 27, 1945.

Wilkin, P.: In C. A. Villee (ed.): The Placenta and Fetal Membranes. Baltimore, Williams & Wilkins, 1960, pp. 225–233.

Chapter 31

ABNORMALITIES AND DISEASES OF THE PLACENTA AND APPENDAGES (OTHER THAN HYDATIDIFORM MOLE AND CHORIOCARCINOMA)

CARL J. PAUERSTEIN

According to Mossman, the normal mammalian placenta is an apposition or fusion of the fetal membranes to the uterine mucosa for physiologic exchange. The transfer of oxygen and metabolites between the maternal and fetal blood is the critical feature of placental function. Unlike any other organ in the human body, the placenta has a life span of only about nine months; and despite its very temporary function, quantitatively it is the most potent endocrine organ in the body.

In 1909, Grosser called attention to the fact that the proximity of the maternal and fetal circulations is unequally established in the uteri of different mammals during pregnancy. Based on this characterization, he devised a classification of chorioallantoic placentas. His terminology indicated which maternal and fetal tissues were juxtaposed. He implied that the placental barrier is essentially a passive filter and that the transfer of gases between the maternal and fetal blood is inversely proportional to the resistance offered by the tissues that separate the two circulations. Some placentas have six layers of tissue interposed between the fetal and maternal blood (epitheliochorial; the sow); some five (syndesmochorial; the goat); others four (endotheliochorial; the cat); and still others three (hemochorial; the guinea

pig, rabbit, rat, and human). Hemochorial placentas may be either labyrinthine (trophoblast forms lamellae between blood-filled spaces) or villous (trophoblast erosion of maternal vessels with formation of large sinusoids and trabeculae across the blood-filled spaces). The human placenta is of the latter type. Because rapid diffusion occurs across the avascular amniochorion, the chorion laeve has been referred to a paraplacental organ, corresponding to that of certain animals.

Although Grosser's hypothesis of four morphologic types of chorioallantoic placentas has been useful, it has limitations because it attempts to explain all placental exchange on the basis of diffusion and filtration; whereas, in fact, the highly complex membrane participates actively in the facilitation of metabolic transport. Moreover, it is more appropriate to the mature placenta since, at term, association between the respective organisms is more intimate than in earlier development. Pressure differences between the two sides and the surface available for diffusion also influence transfer. Exchanges across the chorion laeve are not taken into account in the Grosser classification. With certain exceptions, substances of a molecular weight under 1000 daltons appear to pass through the placenta by simple diffusion and tend to assume equal concentrations on both sides of the placental barrier. However, recent work demonstrates the need for greater attention to the chemical, histochemical, and cytologic structures of the barrier with respect to the mode of passage of different kinds of substances. The critical determinants of the passage of a given substance are the ionization of the substance, and the charge on the barrier membrane. Placental transport can occur by one of several mechanisms: simple diffusion; active transport; facilitated transport; pinocytosis, and through breaks on the continuity of the barrier membrane. Active transport mechanisms are responsible for most feto-metabolic exchanges.

Placental transfer probably depends as much, if not more, upon the cytologic and cytochemical structures of the placental barrier as upon simple diffusion and filtration. The transport of whole particles of plasma across the placenta may occur through the formation of invaginations in the surface of the syncytium, which close to form fluid-filled vacuoles (*pinocytosis*). The electron microscopic study of the placenta has confirmed the exceedingly complex arrangement of the trophoblast.

Placental Hormones

The placenta produces both steroid and protein hormones. The protein hormones include human somatomammotropin (HCS), human chorionic gonadotropin (HCG), and possibly human thyrotropin (HCT). This last hormone has not been as well characterized as the other two. In addition, there is evidence for the production of luteinizing hormone releasing factor (LRF) and some evidence for the production of thyroid-stimulating hormone releasing factor (TRF) (Siler-Khodr). With the exception of LRF and possibly TRF, and in spite of much controversy in the past (Gey *et al.*, Thiede and Choate, Pierce and Midgley, Dreskin *et al.*, Sciarra *et al.*), all of the protein hormones are now thought to be manufactured in the syncytium.

Wynn and Davies have indicated that only the syncytium contains the subcellular organelles required for synthesis of proteins, particularly abundant endoplasmic reticulum and well developed Golgi complexes. Cytotrophoblasts are ultrastructurally sim-

ple and may play a role primarily restricted to cellular growth and differentiation.

In pregnancy, steroidogenesis is accomplished by a complimentary interplay of enzymes along the maternal, fetal, and placental units. Biosynthesis of estrogen by the human placenta is contingent upon provisions for adequate C19 precursors since this organ has very little, if any, desmolase required to convert C21 steroids to C19 steroids (Ryan). That is, it lacks the C21 side chain cleavage enzymes C16 and C17 hydroxylases and reductases for the A ring. The fetal adrenal cortex has the capability of synthesizing dehydroepiandrosterone where also this compound may be 16α-hydroxylated or sulfurylated. The fetal liver likewise has this 16α-hydroxylating capacity and thus contributes to estrogen synthesis. The maternal adrenal gland may provide up to about one half of these precursors during pregnancy. The placenta has a powerful aromatizing system capable of converting a variety of C19 precursors to estrogen. Estrone and 17β-estradiol are synthesized in the placenta utilizing androstenedione and testosterone as intermediate precursors from the available dehydroepiandrosterone which is transported primarily as a sulfate. The sulfate group is removed in the placenta by active sulfatases. Utilizing similar pathways, estriol is synthesized from 16α-hydroxydehydroepiandrosterone which is transported primarily as a sulfate. The synthesis of estriol in the placenta, which is dependent upon a 16α-hydroxylated neutral precursor from the fetus, accounts for the elevated estriol excretion in the pregnant woman (Siiteri and MacDonald).

Estrogens are produced in presumed excess but the estriol fraction is sulfated and therefore biologically inactive. Moreover, active 15α-hydroxylases and others within the fetal liver result in even less active hydroxylated compounds, apparently offering protection to the fetus against biologically active estrogens. Serial determinations of estrogens (estriol) in maternal serum, urine, or amniotic fluid have become important clinical tests for estimating fetoplacental status. Insults which may give rise to defects in fetal adrenal or liver function may be attended by lowered concentrations of estrogens in these media (Page et al.).

The placenta possesses the 3β-ol-dehydrogenases and $\Delta^{4,5}$ isomerases which the fetus lacks, and has the capacity to convert cholesterol to C^{21}-Δ^4 steroids (Diczfalusy). Progesterone can be synthesized from maternal or fetal acetate or cholesterol precursors. The presence of active 20α-reductases metabolizes progesterone to the weaker compound, 20α-dihydroprogesterone, which can be converted to pregnanediol by both the maternal and fetal livers. This compound, which is excreted in its conjugated form (glucosiduronate), can be measured in maternal urine to serve as a useful guide in estimating placental function independent of the fetal status.

Although a wide variety of adrenocortical steroids appear in high concentrations in the placenta, there is no conclusive evidence that they are produced in that organ. The several-fold increase in the concentration of cortisol and 17-OH corticosteroids in maternal blood is explainable on the basis of enhanced binding capacity (transcortin). The fetal adrenal is capable of synthesizing cortisol from progesterone and de novo from acetate. How much of the total in the maternal blood is contributed by the fetus is unknown; however, production rates of cortisol by the newborn (corrected for size) are equal to that of the adult. Whereas aldosterone production rates are likewise markedly increased in the pregnant woman, this may very well be the result of increased activity of the renin-angiotensin systems.

Placental Immunology

It has been suggested that the trophoblast has an important function in assuring survival of the pregnancy, in which the presence of a fertilized egg implanted upon the endometrium creates the immunologic characteristics of a homograft. According to this hypothesis, trophoblast forms an anatomic and immunologic buffer between the mother and the fetus to prevent rejection of the homograft. In support of this concept, Lanman and co-workers demonstrated that when fertilized rabbit ova are transferred to a recipient's uterus, the pregnancy is unaffected by prior exposure of the foster mother to skin grafts from the parents or reexposure to homografts from these donors at the time of egg transfer or at midpregnancy.

Although many explanations and theories have been offered for the success of the placenta as a homograft, current opinion holds that pericellular sialomucins coating the tro-phoblast are responsible for the immunologic protection of the placenta (Currie et al.).

Gross Characteristics of the Placenta

The human placenta is a discoid organ measuring 15 to 20 cm. in diameter and 1.5 to 3 cm. in thickness. According to Torpin, almost all discoid placentas at term cover one fifth to one fourth of the area of the uterine cavity wall. The placenta, as it is cast off from the uterus after the birth of the fetus, takes the form of a flattened, round, or oval organ. It presents two surfaces and a margin—the surface which was in contact with the decidua basalis designated as the maternal, and that directed toward the cavity of the ovum as the fetal. The placenta proper comprises the chorionic villi with a thin decidual plate on the maternal surface and a chorionic plate on the fetal surface. The maternal surface is divided by depressions of varying depth into a number of irregularly shaped areas, the so-called cotyledons, which vary considerably in number, as many as 20 being observed, corresponding to major maternal vascular units (average about 12). These maternal cotyledons grow in size throughout pregnancy, although less actively in the last month, but the total number remains the same until the end of gestation.

Although the DNA content of the total placenta ceases to increase at about the thirty-fourth gestational week (or after the fetus has attained a weight of about 2500 gm.), indicating a cessation of cellular growth, the RNA content and placental weight continue to increase to term.

It is customary to differentiate between the maternal cotyledon, which is the portion of the placenta lying between placental septa running from decidua to chorion, and the fetal cotyledon, which is the portion of the placenta related to the arborization of a single main stem villus. The appendages include the fetal membranes and the unbilical cord.

The fetal membranes extend from the margins of the placenta, and consist of the amnion, chorion, and a thin layer of decidua.

The amnion, the innermost of the membranes, is a thin, transparent, glistening structure, which, according to Bourne, has five layers (0.02 to 0.5 mm. in thickness), comprising, from within outward, epithelium, basement membrane, the compact layer, the fibroblastic layer, and the spongy layer. The outermost spongy layer has a distensible mucoid structure which allows the amnion to slide along the fixed underlying chorion. The chorion is thicker, vascular, and more opaque than the amnion and contains ghost villi and a scant decidua at its outermost margin. This membrane has four layers consisting, from within outward, of a cellular layer, a reticular layer, a pseudobasement membrane, and trophoblast. The amniochorion offers little resistance to the passage of certain molecules, and this site is important in the diffusion of carbohydrates and possibly other nutrients for the fetus. The prominent fetal veins and the less conspicuous fetal arteries fan out across the fetal surface of the placenta from their point of convergence at the insertion of the umbilical cord.

The weight of the placenta in the early weeks is considerably greater than the weight of the fetus; however, as the end of pregnancy approaches, there is a reversal of this ratio. The term placenta, together with the cord and contiguous membranes, weighs approximately 450 to 500 grams. The fetal-placental weight ratio, according to Adair and Thelander, varies from 6.35:1, to 7.9:1 for full term infants. In such conditions as syphilis and erythroblastosis this ratio may be greatly diminished. In the latter diseases, for instance, the placental weight may exceed 2000 grams. On the other hand, the fetal-placental ratio is occasionally increased to 9 or 10:1; and under such circumstances, fetal growth may be retarded.

The smallest subdivision of the human placenta is a lobule which can be regarded as representing a single "placentome" possessing one fetal cotyledon (Boyd and Hamilton). The larger placental lobes in this interpretation are compound placentomes, and represent fusions containing a number of fetal cotyledons (fetal villous systems) projecting into a single compartment of the intervillous space. According to these authors, the average number of lobes is 22 (extremes of 10 to 38), whereas the corresponding figure for the fetal cotyledons or trunci chorii is considerably greater. The human placenta shares this structure with Old World monkeys and the great apes. At term, the human placenta contains about 40 trunci. According to Boyd and Hamilton, the extremes range between 22 and 76 when

counts are based on radiographs derived from fetal blood vessel dye injections. Crawford's counts range up to 200 villi but about one half of these were tiny fetal cotyledons arising from very small vascular projections from the chorionic plate.

There are complex, multiple factors that limit fetal growth and influence ultimate placental size, such as litter size, implantation site, and blood and nutrient supply. A primary influence of estrogen on placental growth (which in turn affects fetal growth) is suggested by some experimental evidence. According to this hypothesis, estrogens exert an inhibitory effect on cell division in the placenta. At about 34 weeks of pregnancy, cell multiplication ceases, and continued increase in placental size is due only to hypertrophy (Abdul-Karim et al.).

Abnormal Placental Configuration

The ultimate localization of the placenta in the wall of the vesicle and the determination of its size and shape depend upon degeneration of part of the villi that originally cover the entire outer surface of the chorionic vesicle. The villi gradually undergo atrophy and disappear from the portion of the chorionic vesicle poorly nourished by the maternal blood supply. Under normal circumstances the definitive placenta occupies only about one fifth of the surface of the chorionic sac. However, when degeneration proceeds irregularly, the configuration of the placenta may be distorted. The shape and size of the placenta depend upon the number and arrangement of primordial villi at the implantation pole.

One of the most common abnormalities of placental configuration is its division into one or more lobes. If it is divided into two or three lobes, usually attached in the region of cord origination, it is designated as bipartite (bidiscoidal) or tripartite. As many as seven small lobes (placenta septuplex) have been described in rare instances. The lobes are connected by vessels, membranes, and a thinned portion of placenta. If there is a defect in the central thinned portion, the placenta is termed fenestrate. If one or more groups of villi persist apart from the main portion of the placenta, they form accessory or succenturiate lobes, which are connected to the principal portion of the placenta merely by vessels and membranes. When the vascular connections are lacking, the accessory lobe is referred to as placenta spuria.

These variations in gross form are without clinical significance except occasionally in the case of the succenturiate lobe, which is of practical importance for several reasons: (1) The vessels connecting the aberrant lobe with the main portion of the placenta may traverse the region of the internal os, a condition known as vasa praevia. Such vessels frequently rupture in the course of labor and severe hemorrhage may ensue, which may be fatal to the fetus (Fig. 31–1). (2) Unless meticulous inspection of the placenta and membranes is carried out, a succenturiate lobe may be retained in utero after delivery of the main placenta with consequent likelihood of hemorrhage and infection. (3) The succenturiate lobe may be implanted low (placenta praevia) with subsequent premature separation.

Rarely, the entire surface of the ovum is covered by functioning villi, a condition known as placenta membranacea. An incomplete or partial variety of membranacea is referred to as a zonary type. This abnormality may occur when the ovum implants too deeply. In this event, the decidua capsularis is so abundantly vascularized that the chorion in contact with it fails to undergo atrophy. The increase in the surface occupied by the placenta may cause it to extend over the internal os. Hertig and Sheldon, in an analysis of 1000 spontaneous early fetal deaths, found a placental factor in 96 cases, and two of these were instances of placenta membranacea. Finn reported two cases with sufficient constant vaginal bleeding to necessitate cesarean sections at the twenty-sixth and twenty-third weeks, respectively. Bleeding is often seen as early as the second trimester, and the clinical picture is that of central placenta previa.

Another common gross abnormality is the circumvallate placenta, characterized by a thick, round, white opaque ring around the periphery of the placenta. The remainder of the chorionic surface is normal in appearance, but the fetal vessels are limited in their course across the placenta by the ring (Fig. 31–2). The membranes, although attached to the extrachorionic portion of the placenta, can easily be stripped from it. As seen in Figure 31–3, the white ring is made up of a double reflection of membranes and an intervening layer of necrotic and dehydrated villi, chronic fibrous tissue, detached decidua, and fibrin.

The condition may be either complete or partial according to the amount of circumference involved. Usually the extrachorionic portion of the placenta is only 2 to 3 cm. in depth and so of little clinical significance. However, it may be of such magnitude that

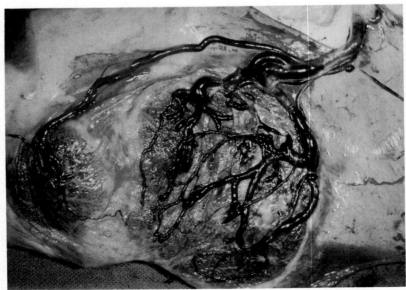

Figure 31–1. Succenturiate lobe showing fetal vessel traversing the membranes between the primary placenta and the aberrant lobe.

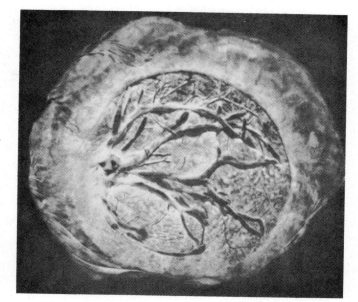

Figure 31–2. Circumvallate placenta. ×½.

the uteroplacental circulation becomes embarrassed, and fetal death, abortion, or premature labor may result.

Hertig reports that about 30 per cent of nontoxic placental separations are due to this

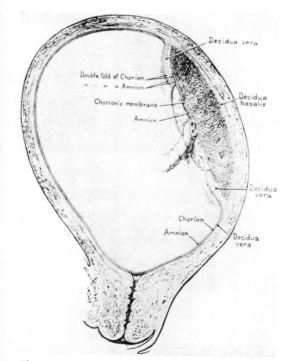

Figure 31–3. Diagram showing circumvallate placenta in situ. Note the relationship of the membranes and decidua over the extrachorionic portion of the placenta. (From Williams.)

anomaly and that it is a common cause of midtrimester abortion. Circumvallate placenta is a relatively common cause of painless antepartal hemorrhage. Scott reports that 18 per cent of 3161 consecutive placentas examined were placentas extrachoriales and 47 per cent of these showed evidence of extrachorial hemorrhage.

The etiology of the condition has been reviewed extensively by Benirschke and Drescoll. It may result from an abnormality of implantation, due apparently to an inability of the implanting ovum to dissolve sufficient decidua; or perhaps, because of the depth of implantation, a smaller portion of the early ovum than usual becomes converted into the chorion frondosum, with the result that the chorionic plate becomes too small and subsequent growth on the part of the villi can take place only by invasion of the surrounding decidua.

Torpin, on the other hand, in rejecting these speculations, indicates that the ring cannot be formed without peripheral decidual hemorrhage. At its origin, the ring lies on the extreme margin of the oversized and immature placenta. He contends that, once begun, the inside diameter of the ring remains constant as the placenta of the true placental site increases in size. The fixed ring is then drawn anterior to the margin as the true placental area increases. In this manner an "early excess area" placenta is gradually reduced to the normal size at term.

Bühler applies the term subchorial closing ring to the zone between the internal and external margins of the placenta. The internal margin corresponds to a line joining the most peripheral points of penetration of the umbilical vessels. The external margin is the boundary between the placenta proper and the chorionic portion of the fetal membranes. There is doubt as to the origin of the ring, whether it is decidual or trophoblastic, but, according to Boyd and Hamilton, these marginal structures (decidua, basal plate, trophoblast, cell islands of the most peripheral placental septa, etc.) must be taken into account in the explanation of placenta circumvallata.

Multiple Pregnancy

The frequency of twins in the United States is about 1 in 90 births but such factors as race, maternal age and therapeutic induction of ovulation influence the rate of multiple gestation. The placenta associated with twin pregnancy may be either single or double. The possible arrangement of membranes is shown in Figure 31–4. According to Boyd and Hamilton the frequency of monozygotic twins varies between 20 and 34 per cent.

Strong and Corney in an excellent review reported that 36.5 per cent of their 200 twins were monozygotic, and of these, 60 per cent were monochorial. Among 25 monozygotic dichorial twins, 13 had fused chorions and 12 had separate chorions. Monozygotic twins exhibit the following types of placental arrangements:

1. Monochorial and diamniotic with one placenta;
2. Monochorial and monoamniotic with one placenta;
3. Fused or separate dichorial and diamniotic with one or two placentas.

According to Benirschke and Kim, the ultimate morphologic type depends upon the stage in which the partitioning of the formative material occurred, i.e., whether it was upon separation of the early blastomeres, duplication of the inner cell mass, duplication of the embryonic rudiment of the germ disc, or incomplete duplication of the germ disc (conjoined twins with a monochorial, monoamniotic placenta). Separation of the early blastomeres (apparently as early as the two-cell stage) gives rise to a dichorial placenta with two chorions, either separate or fused.

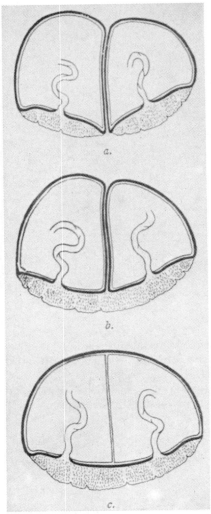

Figure 31–4. Diagram showing relation of placenta and membranes in double- and single-ovum twin pregnancy: a, double-ovum twins; b, double-ovum twins, double membranes, single placenta; c, single-ovum twins, one chorion, two amnions, and one placenta.

All later duplications involving the inner cell mass or germ disc result in monochorial placental types. Duplication after germ disc development gives rise to a monoamniotic type while duplication of the inner cell mass results in a diamniotic placenta.

Thus, placenta and membrane relationships can frequently but not always be relied upon to determine zygosity. That is, all dizygotic twins possess a dichorial diamniotic placenta, but, in some cases, early separation of blastomeres gives rise to the same type. Moreover, among dichorial dizygotic twins, the chorions may be fused in about one half of the cases (Benirschke) and, likewise, placental masses may be fused, perhaps related to the site of implantation of the two blastocysts.

The type of placental arrangement has clinical significance. For example, fetuses with placentas possessing a single amnion (monoamniotic twins) are subjected to substantial risks, as discussed in an excellent review by Benirschke. Knotting of the intertwining cords is responsible for a high perinatal mortality rate in these cases.

Dye injection into the fetal circulation in multiple pregnancy is helpful. A common circulation is indicative of a monochorial arrangement. Benirschke, in his study of 60 consecutive monochorial diamniotic twin placentas, found artery-to-artery communication to be the most common anastomosis and artery-to-vein shunts to be the next most frequent. Vein-to-vein anastomoses, particularly appearing in isolation, were quite uncommon.

The significance of these vascular communications is that variations in blood supply greatly influence fetal welfare. One twin may be plethoric while the other becomes anemic (twin transfusion syndrome). The recipient fetus may develop polycythemia, with cardiomegaly and associated hydramnios, whereas the other becomes anemic, with associated oligohydramnios. In the extreme, the donor fetus becomes exsanguinated and, depending upon degree, there may be anomalous development, fetal death, and abortion. The fetus at birth may be a shapeless mass of tissue (acardius amorphus) or may be retained, macerated, and compressed to form the fetus papyraceus. It has been estimated that perhaps as many as one third of twins with monochorial placentation might be expected to show some features of this syndrome. In dizygotic twinning an infrequent occurrence of vascular anastomosis may give rise to blood chimerism whereby the cells of one twin are liberally admixed with that of the other (Benirschke; Gill). There may be a small area of vascular communication in a fused placenta.

In triplet pregnancies three possibilities of placental arrangement exist. There may be either one large placenta with a single chorion and separate amnions, three entirely separate placentas, or a double placenta with one chorion and two amnions and a complete, separate placenta. The latter is the most common condition. Fusion of amniotic sacs may result in two or more fetuses sharing a single sac (see Boyd and Hamilton for more details). The placentas associated with multiple pregnancy occupy a much larger part of the uterine surface than those associated with single pregnancy. As a result low implantation, placenta previa and premature separation are more common. Postpartum hemorrhage due to atony of the uterus is also a more frequent occurrence.

Aging of the Placenta

Definite morphologic and physiologic modifications take place in the placenta during its limited life span, and the term aging, because it implies change of structure with time, is perhaps an acceptable one to indicate this process. It must be understood, though, that this altered morphology is not a wearing out but in all probability a change that benefits the fetus. Morphologic changes are accompanied by increased rates of some placental functions and decreased rates of others. Undoubtedly they are indications of maturation and should be considered normal.

In the beginning, that portion of the trophoblast to form the placenta depends merely upon which part of the circumference of the ovum implants first and, although this is usually the embryonic pole, it need not necessarily be so. Soon after implantation the trophoblast, taking added nourishment from the uterine mucosa, begins to grow. Growth takes place around the entire periphery of the ovum and proceeds to the point of the formation of primitive villi. However, that area which was first and is now deepest implanted is the best nourished and most rapidly growing. While the remainder atrophies, the chorion frondosum develops into the placenta. The outermost trophoblast cells or syncytiotrophoblasts grow out with great vigor and invade the decidua. There is considerable necrosis of adjacent endometrium and a deposition of fibrinoid material constituting a rather amorphous boundary between trophoblast and maternal cells.

The trophoblast cells perforate small uterine vessels and thus pools of maternal blood are formed. At the same time these rapidly growing trophoblast cells form large cytoplasmic vacuoles which coalesce, and thus intercommunicating lacunae are formed which are rapidly filled with blood from the already ruptured uterine vessels. This whole

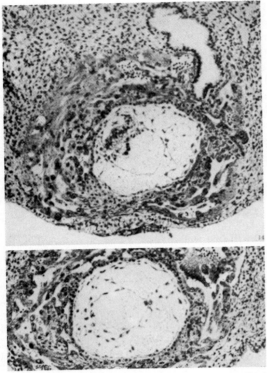

Figure 31–5. Eleven day ovum. × 125. (Courtesy of A. T. Hertig and J. Rock.)

from the cell columns, syncytium, and decidua from the basal plate constitute the floor of the intervillous space. The cell columns are anchored to the decidual plate and arise from the tips of the villi as proliferating cellular trophoblast. At 12 weeks, placental villi are easily recognizable morphologically (Fig. 31–6), although the cytotrophoblast shell has been developing rapidly since the fourth week.

By means of electron microscopy Wislocki and Dempsey have been able to see structures which cannot ordinarily be visualized with the light microscope. Beneath the cytotrophoblastic cells of Langhans, which rest upon a basement membrane, is the fetal connective tissue. All the metabolites that are transferred across the trophoblastic barrier have not only to traverse the syncytium, but also to cross the cytoplasm of the Langhans cells following a complicated route. The syncytial layer is complex, and is provided with cytoplasmic tufts and streamers, or with a brush border, which may be thick and dense, or scanty and irregular. In the areas possessing the so-called brush border the surface of the syncytium of the villi shows filaments (microvilli) of up to 3 μm. in height

process is beautifully seen in Hertig's 11-day ovum (Fig. 31–5). (See Chapter 30 for a more detailed description of these crucial early developments.)

From about the eighteenth day there is a progessive branching of the primordial villi, which continues throughout the first trimester. When seen by light microscopy, the chorionic membrane consists of an inner connective tissue layer and an epithelial layer that differentiates into an inner layer of cuboidal cells with clear cytoplasm and light-staining vesicular nuclei (cytotrophoblast or Langhans cells) and an outer layer of syncytium made up of continuous elongated cells, coarsely granular cytoplasm, and irregularly scattered flat, dark-staining nuclei (syncytiotrophoblast). The connective tissue consists of spindly cells with protoplasmic processes contained within a loose matrix. Branching fibrocytes are separated by a loose matrix of ground substance. The roof of the intervillous spaces is the chorionic plate composed of trophoblast externally and fibrous mesoderm internally. Cytotrophoblast

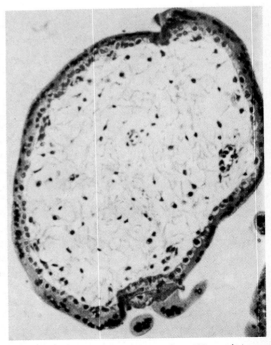

Figure 31–6. Human placenta from 12 weeks' pregnancy. × 50.

and with diameters of 40 to 100 nm. (Fig. 31–7). The cytoplasm of the syncytium has a vesicular structure in which vacuoles, mitochondria, and large osmiophile granules can be identified (Fig. 31–8).

Boyd and Hughes have correlated the presence of many vacuoles beneath the syncytial surface with the presence of microvilli; these authors and others suggest that these areas are regions of absorption, probably of a pinocytotic nature. Dempsey visualizes the syncytium as an ameboid mass of tissue that is continuously flowing and streaming, thereby effecting an active engulfing of plasma into the substance of the syncytium. Placental permeability depends in part upon this selective activity which the placenta appears to exhibit in relation to certain substances. The stroma at this time is made up of loosely knit fibroblasts and a few blood vessels lined with large and immature endothelial cells. Throughout the stroma are many Hofbauer cells, which are merely large mononuclear phagocytes. Their cytoplasm is vacuolated and with proper staining these

vacuoles can be shown to contain fat. Wynn has shown these cells to be of exclusively fetal origin and to be distinct from plasma cells. Some of these cells appear to be degenerative, apparently arising from several different elements in the placental mesenchyme, while others are phagocytic in type.

Mitotic figures are absent in the syncytium, whereas they may be seen readily in the cytotrophoblast. Galton has noted cellular proliferation within the cytotrophoblast followed by coalescence of daughter cells in the syncytium; thus, perhaps, indicating that not only is the syncytium derived from the cytotrophoblast but also that it is an end stage of mitotic division. Nevertheless, the syncytium is complex inasmuch as it contains abundant endoplasmic reticulum, Golgi bodies, mitochondria, secretory droplets, lipid granules, and plasma membranes. Also, the deoxynucleoprotein content is high, as is the ribonucleoprotein, as evidenced by abundant ribosomes and granular endoplasmic reticulum.

Villee and others have pointed out that the

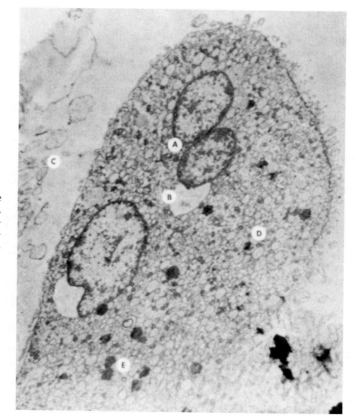

Figure 31–7. Syncytial tag, 9 weeks: *A*, three nuclei that have no intervening cell boundary; *B*, vacuole; *C*, brush border from neighboring syncytium; *D*, syncytium filled with "packages" of ergastoplasm; *E*, mitochondria. (Courtesy of Dr. E. W. Dempsey.)

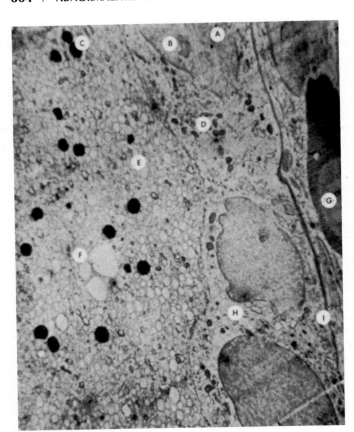

Figure 31–8. Synctium and cytotrophoblast, 9 weeks: *A*, Langhans cells; *B*, nucleolus; *C*, osmiophilic lipid droplets containing steroid hormones; *D*, mitochondria; *E*, profuse spherical structures containing ribonuclear proteins (ergastoplasm); *F*, process of pinocytosis (transfer of plasma); *G*, nucleated fetal red cell; *H*, irregular plasma membrane between cytotrophoblast cells; *I*, fetal capillary wall. (Courtesy of Dr. E. W. Dempsey.)

early placenta has a high concentration of glycogen and that it can secrete glucose. These biochemical observations suggest that the placenta regulates the blood glucose level before the fetal liver is able to do so, but this function declines gradually as gestation proceeds. Thus, the placenta serves as an auxiliary liver in early gestation when glycogen concentration and glucose-6-phosphatase activity in the fetal liver are nil. As this function of the placenta declines, these activities in the fetal liver increase rapidly over the same period. The intervillous space, which is filled at all times with maternal blood, even during uterine contractions, serves as a depot of transfer because at this site there is an active interchange through the chorionic epithelium between fetal and maternal circulations.

At 19 weeks, the villi are smaller and more numerous (Fig. 31–9). The syncytial nuclei have begun to gather together in knots and Langhans cells are less conspicuous. The fetal capillaries are more numerous and the stroma of the villi more closely knit.

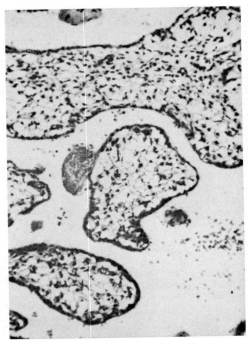

Figure 31–9. Human placenta from 19 weeks' pregnancy. × 100.

By the twenty-eighth week the villi are smaller still (Fig. 31–10). The syncytial layer shows many clear areas with prominent nuclear knots. Despite the formerly held belief that the Langhans cells disappear completely by the sixth or seventh month, Wislocki and Dempsey and others have shown that some persist until full term as flattened cells compressed between the syncytium and the basement membrane upon which the trophoblast rests. These cells retain their ultrastructural simplicity, even to term, possessing abundant free ribosomes but scant ergastoplasm and a few specialized organelles. In certain pathologic conditions of the placenta, such as erythroblastosis and diabetes, these cells become more evident. The collagen-rich stromal connective tissue decreases and one sees relatively fewer Hofbauer cells and fibroblasts. The endothelial cells of the fetal capillaries are more mature, which means that the cells are spaced farther apart and that the nuclei are smaller.

At term, the villi are smaller still and more finely branched (Fig. 31–11). The increase in surface area of approximately 10 sq. m. (Aherne and Dunnill) is associated with decline in the diameter of the villi, trophoblast thinning, and increased villous vascularity.

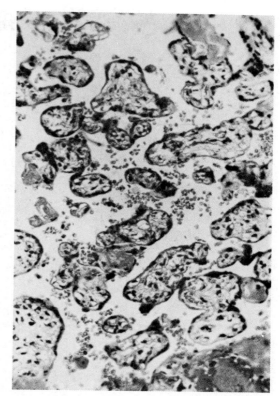

Figure 31–11. Human placenta from 40 weeks' pregnancy. ×100.

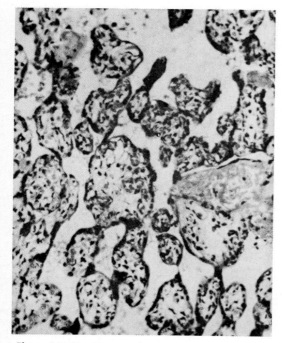

Figure 31–10. Human placenta from 28 weeks' pregnancy. ×100.

The stem villi at term have diameters ranging between 500 μm. and 1500 μm. (Boyd and Hamilton). There is general agreement that only the villus structures in the two thirds of the placenta closest to the decidual plate are important absorptive units of the villous system. Although terminal villi may be found arising abruptly from major stems close to the chorion, it is not likely that these are important structures in metabolic exchange. The syncytium has become a thin acidophilic membrane with the nuclei gathered in knots. The exceptionally thin barrier that separates maternal and fetal blood can be seen in Figure 31–12. Langhans cells are inconspicuous, and the stroma is more than two thirds composed of fetal capillaries, which have become extremely thin-walled. The remainder of the stroma is composed of more or less dense connective tissue. Hofbauer cells are not found in the term placenta (Fig. 31–13). The fetal spiral arteries arise from the major subchorionic vessels and represent the main vascular channels for the primary villus stem.

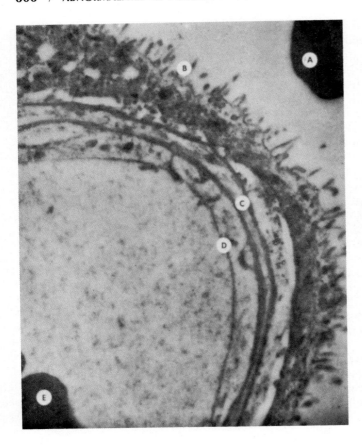

Figure 31–12. Tip of villus, at term: *A*, part of maternal red cell; *B*, brush border of syncytium; *C*, double layer of fetal connective tissue with fibrils between; *D*, endothelium of fetal capillary; *E*, part of fetal red cell. (Courtesy of Dr. E. W. Dempsey.)

It is incorrect to regard syncytial knotting as solely a degenerative process or a response attributable only to local hypoxia. These clustered nuclei are seen in sproutings in the early placenta, and in the mature placenta such formations may be reversible. Although syncytial degeneration does occur under hypoxic insults it is interesting that a concomitant proliferation of cytotrophoblast may occur which might represent an attempt at repair (Page et al.). Regardless of the true nature of these knots it seems clear that they frequently break off and escape the uterus. Although they appear to be trapped and lysed in the maternal lung, it is possible that their excessive release and breakdown may be clinically important in initiating intravascular coagulation under certain circumstances.

Burgos and Rodriguez have noted that the

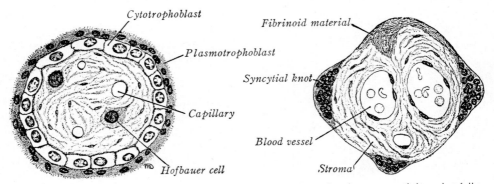

Figure 31–13. Human chorionic villi in transverse section in the early weeks of pregnancy (left) and at full term (right). ×265. (From L. B. Arey: Developmental Anatomy. Philadelphia, W. B. Saunders Co.)

trophoblastic cells of the free chorionic villi at term have two principal zones. The first of these, the alpha zone, is thinner and presents the characteristic ultrastructure of cells specialized in absorption or active transport of substances. Mainly formed by syncytium, they have microvilli, pinosomes, apical canaliculi, phagosomes, lysosomes, and basal infoldings. The second, or beta zone, is thicker and contains numerous nuclei as well as both syncytium and cytotrophoblast. This zone shows a great development of the organelles related to cellular synthesis, i.e., ergastoplasm, ribosomes, polysomes, mitochondria, Golgi bodies, and vesicles.

The primary villus stem vessels have a spiral course. By simultaneous double injections of vinylite the tips of terminal arterioles are seldom found to be separated by more than 1 mm. from the beginning of the connected venules. Two types of capillary complexes occupy this 1 mm. interval: one, a superficial network within terminal villi; the other, a paravascular network providing extra villous shunts from artery to vein, which act as safety valves to prevent overloading of the villous circulation (Ramsey).

Krantz has demonstrated smooth muscle in the chorionic plate extending into the villus stems as far as the precapillary arterioles of the villi. This muscle is probably chemically activated and may play a role in controlling fetal and maternal blood flow by expanding and contracting the villi. Recent descriptions of the presence of nerve trunks and fine fibrils surrounding fetal capillaries as well as possibly ganglia raise doubts, however, that the placenta is free of nerves and that all responses are humoral in type. Reynolds has shown that blood is delivered to the placenta in the umbilical artery at a relatively high pressure and little pressure is lost before the capillary networks are reached. On the venous side, pressure is still high and is maintained by the action of the sphincter between the umbilical vein and the ductus venosus. Pressure in the placental capillaries greatly exceeds the resting pressure in the intervillous space (approximately 10 mm. Hg).

Wislocki and Dempsey have contributed to understanding the aging process of the placenta through histochemical studies. Acid phosphatase accumulates in the trophoblastic syncytium of the human placenta near the end of gestation. It occurs principally in the nuclei of the syncytium and to a lesser extent in the perinuclear cytoplasm. Alkaline phosphatase begins to appear in the syncytium in the first months of pregnancy and increases steadily until term. Thus, these two enzymes characterize the aging placenta. They occur in inverse proportion to cytoplasmic basophilic substance (ribonucleoprotein), which diminishes steadily as the placenta ages. The changes may reflect a disturbance in the placental metabolism of nucleoproteins.

Vesicles within the syncytium communicate with conduits in the endoplasmic reticulum. Substances can be transported or processed in either direction through channels between the intervillous space and fetal capillaries. There are different assigned functions for the smooth and rough endoplasmic reticulum. Presumably the smooth variety is concerned primarily with separation and transport of nonprotein materials while the rough form is involved in synthesis of polypeptides. The assemblage of these compounds and their incorporation into secretory granules occurs in the Golgi apparatus. Cytotrophoblastic cells, which contain large nuclei, prominent nucleoli, and mitochondria, but do not have the complex ultrastructure of the syncytiotrophoblast cells, are almost free of endoplasmic reticulum.

Fat droplets occur in the syncytium throughout gestation, but diminish in size and number by the end of pregnancy. At term, the droplets have almost completely disappeared from the epithelial plates. Glycogen is never present in the syncytium at term. Although it is widely distributed throughout the placenta, glycogen is associated with relative avascularity and is not demonstrable in metabolically active areas. Mitochondria (phospholipids) are abundant in the syncytium early in pregnancy but decline in number as gestation advances. Relatively few are still present in the syncytium at term. Nevertheless, the large mitochondria within the syncytium provide energy sources and may be required for active transfer of vital nutrients. Iron and calcium are demonstrable in considerable quantities in the first half of gestation in the stroma of the chorionic villi, where they are mainly deposited just beneath the trophoblastic epithelium. In the same localities and during the same period, traces of acid and alkaline phosphatases are also encountered.

The reason for these changes is imperfectly understood, but experiments performed during the last several years indicate that this is not merely a wearout process. From the morphologic viewpoint this process should increase the ease of transfer. Not only does the placenta increase in size but the villi become smaller and more numerous, and the fetal blood comes into more and more intimate contact with the maternal blood. These alterations in the villus with advancing pregnancy appear to increase placental permeability, involving not only diffusion but selective transfer as well.

The experiments of Gellhorn and co-workers with radioactive sodium show that the rate of transfer of this ion is increased sixfold per gram of placenta from the twelfth to the fortieth week of pregnancy. Paralleling this increased rate of transfer Wang and Hellman have shown a decrease in oxygen consumption per gram of placenta. Although these two lines of investigation may be taken to indicate that the placenta changes from an organ of active to one of passive filtration and gains in efficiency by so doing, the study of Mandel and associates on nucleocytoplasmic ratios of various aged placentas indicates that they follow a decreasing logarithmic curve similar to that established for age and rate of growth of various other tissues.

These experiments indicate that the process of aging increases the rate of transfer across a barrier. Any terminal sharp decrease in placental permeability as term approaches should be regarded as pathologic.

The placenta also acquires a physiologic capability to maintain fetal homeostasis by reacting to the metabolic needs of the fetus. These regulatory mechanisms of the placenta are only partially understood but they involve the number of functioning capillaries within the placenta and the surface available for transfer. When terminal villi are explanted for organ culture, and the concentration of oxygen in the chamber is reduced from 26 to 6 per cent, morphologic changes occur in syncytiotrophoblast. The nuclei, together with some cytoplasm, cluster at one pole of the villus, leaving only a thin layer of cytoplasm over the basement membrane (Tominaga and Page). The distance from the intervillous space to the nearest fetal capillary is reduced by 25 per cent, thus permitting a comparable increase in the quantity of oxygen transferred per unit of time. The clustering of nuclei and thinning of the syncytial covering are interpreted by these authors to be a slow accommodation of the placenta to chronic hypoxia.

In recent years, "postmature" pregnancies have been regarded with concern by many clinicians. This concern, based originally upon the oxygen studies of Walker, emanates from data which purported to demonstrate a progressive diminution in oxygen content and saturation in the cord blood as pregnancy advances beyond term. The perinatal mortality rate in protracted pregnancies (294 days or more) is several-fold that noted in pregnancies terminated at or near the expected date of confinement.

Clifford describes a typical clinical picture for certain infants associated with intrauterine existence beyond the normal time. He divides the infants into three clinical groups according to the stage of placental dysfunction encountered. The ratio between fetal and placental weights is not usually altered by prolongation of pregnancy; however, a high incidence of gross placental abnormalities has been reported; and, in some instances of severe maternal uterine circulatory impairment (hypertensive cardiovascular disease, toxemia, placental dysfunction syndrome), the placenta is small, meconium-stained, and degenerated.

In a comprehensive review of this subject Clifford reported that the placentas were abnormal in 90 per cent of fetal deaths on or after day 294; 84 per cent showed gross meconium staining; degenerative pathologic changes, with or without hemorrhage, were present in 34 per cent, a low figure because the grossly meconium-stained placentas were not examined microscopically; 15 per cent of the placentas showed extensive infection, also a low figure and for the same reason. This interesting obstetric question must be regarded as unsettled at present, but valuable information could be gained from more detailed studies of the placenta, correlating these findings with gestational age and the clinical picture of the infant.

Degenerative Changes in the Placenta

To understand the significance of the degeneration of any organ, its sources of nutrition must be clear. The placenta derives its nourishment from the maternal circulation; Young, Strachan, Siddall and Hartman, and Stander, as well as more recent workers, have all supported this concept. Any factor that interferes with the maternal blood supply, whether it be placental absorption, thrombosis of maternal vessels, intervillous thrombosis, or encasement of the villi in fibrin, causes death of the affected villi. In the first place, fetal death does not cause placental death, but merely a disuse endarteritis of the villous vessels. Second, the placenta can be present and alive without a fetus, as in pathologic ova, in which only placenta and membranes are present, Type II or III of Mall's Carnegie classification, or Type I of the same classification (hydatid mole). Third, the villi grow prior to the formation of chorionic vessels and during the period before they form a continuous system, as shown in Hertig's paper (1935). Fourth, the results of animal experiments show that the fetus is not necessary for growth or full term delivery of the placenta, because when the fetus is removed in the last months of pregnancy the placenta continues to develop in situ until the usual duration of term, when it is expelled. This was first demonstrated in the mouse by Newton, and later confirmed in the rat by Kirsch, and in the monkey by van Wagenen and Newton.

Placental Infarcts. Deposition of fibrin is the earliest and most frequently noted degenerative change in the placenta.

The deposition of fibrin occurs, according to Webster, as early as the fourth week in the layer of Nitabuch and inconstantly in Rohr's stria at the third month. Nitabuch's layer appears where the invading trophoblast comes in contact with the decidua. It is absent whenever the decidua is defective, and has some clinical importance in cases of placenta accreta. Rohr's stria refers to the inconstant deposition of fibrin at the bottom of the intervillous space and surrounding the fastening villi in this area.

More important than these two layers is the deposition of fibrin beneath the chorion of the fetal surface. This is generally called *subchorionic infarction*, although it is not an infarct. The subchorionic deposition of fibrin is seen in nearly every placenta after the sixth month. It is characterized grossly by flat, creamy white plaques varying from 1 mm. in size to much larger ones occupying the entire chorionic plate (Fig. 31–14). The thickness of the average plaques is 2 to 5 mm., although in this dimension also there is great variation. These plaques are pyramidal in shape and extend downwards with their apices in the intervillous space. The larger plaques frequently show central degeneration with liquefaction. These liquefied areas are sometimes called chorionic cysts, although they bear little resemblance to the true cysts of the chorion. According to Strachan this type of degeneration takes place as early as the fourth month.

Occasionally, fibrin depositions about the intercotyledonary septa result in infarcts with the base at the maternal surface and the apex pointing toward the chorionic plate. Patchy oval infarcts may likewise by seen within the central portions of the placenta. The process results in disappearance of the trophoblast.

Nearly every term placenta shows a yellowish white ring at its edge. This condition, often termed a marginal infarct, may be superficial or it may extend to involve the deeper placental tissues. In late pregnancy, preexisting islands of fibrinoid degeneration

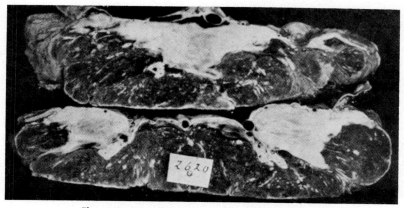

Figure 31–14. Subchorionic fibrin deposition. ×⅓.

of the trophoblast elements in the septa and at the margins fuse to form large pale-staining masses (Fig. 31–15). Areas of glistening, smooth, slightly laminated fibrin, often elongated, although occasionally round, may be located anywhere in the intervillous space. On section there are strands of fibrin between which are sometimes ghosts of red cells.

As the placenta passes into the last half or third of its existence, degenerative lesions may occur which result in fibrinoid degeneration, calcification, and ischemic infarction. Ischemic necrosis of villi may thus result from deposition of fibrin over their surfaces or from sudden coagulation of intervillous blood leading to thrombosis. Similarly, deteriorated syncytium may result in hemovillous degeneration when clotting occurs in the maternal blood in contact with the exposed subepithelial villous tissues. Coagulation of blood in the intervillous space occurs where the circulation is slowest. Vascular lesions of the decidua (abnormalities in the spiral arterioles) resulting in accelerated syncytial degeneration, intervillous thrombosis, and placental infarction are common occurrences in toxemia of pregnancy.

The gathering of syncytial nuclei in small areas on one side of the villus (syncytial knots) which may represent a physiologic

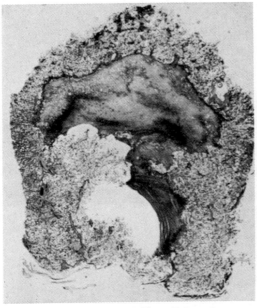

Figure 31–15. Intervillous fibrin. ×3.

contraction of the villus in response to stress is a common feature in beginning syncytial degeneration. Later, the epithelial layer breaks away and the villous stroma undergoes hyalinization. Exposed maternal blood may clot and, as the latter propagates, hemovillous degeneration may involve considerable numbers of villi. The villi in the center of these infarcts are completely hyalinized, whereas those at the periphery are better preserved. The villi enmeshed in the organized fibrin are excluded from their source of nourishment, the maternal circulation.

Only rarely are these placental infarcts massive, or of sufficient degree to produce placental insufficiency and fetal death. Holland arbitrarily attributed fetal death to this cause when the placental-fetal ratio was over 1:10, or when 90 per cent or more of the functioning units of the placenta were destroyed by intervillous fibrin or thrombosis. He reported 17 fetal deaths from this cause; and in 10 fetuses, the placental findings were the only pathologic changes noted.

In our experience, this pathologic finding is considered to be a primary factor responsible for perinatal death in only about one in 500 cases. Gruenwald has noted, however, that the finding of vascular chorionic villi correlates fairly well with the occurrence of fetal malnutrition, and he recommends further extensive investigation of the significance of this placental lesion. One of the basic problems in any of these assessments of the placenta is that histopathologic changes within the tissue are so diverse that no particular area can be called typical or pathognomonic for any underlying etiology.

Intervillous Thrombosis. Grossly, this lesion is characterized by coagulation of blood in the intervillous space (Fig. 31–16). The clot is smooth, firm, and reddish brown. It is laminated, and on microscopic examination shows beginning phagocytosis of red cells. In all probability this lesion is several days old. The trophoblastic endothelial junctions are said to be particularly susceptible to a number of pathologic changes.

Javert and Reiss have pointed out that these junctions are vulnerable to stretching when intracapillary pressure is increased; to spasm, degeneration, and aging; and to rupture of either spontaneous or traumatic origin. Structural damage permits fetal blood cells to enter intervillous spaces where coagulation of the mixture of cells produces the macroscopic intervillous hematomas. Ex-

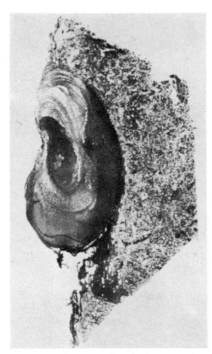

Figure 31–16. Intervillous thrombosis. ×3.

posed connective tissues denuded by the breaking away of syncytium and knots can create the nidus for clotting and propagation to other villous surfaces. Furthermore, the accelerated rate of normal syncytial degeneration in association with toxemia may be one of the predisposing causes since there is hyalinization of both the villi and the decidual vascular walls.

The incidence of intervillous hematomas according to the duration of gestation at delivery of the placenta ranges from 7.7 per cent in the first half of pregnancy to 28.5 per cent in the last half. According to the above authors, when the maternal blood vessels rupture, decidual hemorrhage is produced, which characterizes both premature separation of the placenta and placenta previa but has no relationship to the formation of the intervillous coagulation hematomas.

Bartholomew and co-workers have emphasized the importance of intervillous hematomas and placental infarction as the characteristic lesions of eclamptic toxemia and have attributed their formation to obstruction in the fetal circulation secondary to the vascular changes initiated by the hypercholesteremia of pregnancy. According to Bartholomew, the amount and location of infarction, the degree of vessel obstruction in the

placenta, and the rapidity of autolysis determine whether preeclampsia of mild or severe degree, or abruptio placentae, occurs.

Although degeneration and coagulation of intervillous blood frequently accompany the toxemic process, these lesions of the placenta are not confined to this group of patients. Marais believes that the common denominator of all degenerative lesions appearing in the placenta in association with toxemia is degeneration of decidual spiral arterioles, and his classification of lesions is based on this hypothesis. Williams referred to ischemic degeneration in association with occlusion of spiral arterioles in the decidual plate as "atypical white infarcts."

Ischemic Necrosis of Villi Due to Fibrin Deposition (Figs. 31–15 and 31–17). On gross section the surface of this lesion is firm, dry, roughly granular, and yellowish-white. Microscopically, the granularity of the gross section is seen to represent villi enmeshed in a fibrin matrix. Glycogen accumulates in the stromal connective tissue, followed by an increase in intercellular ground substance and deposition of large amounts of collagen. If this lesion is old enough the chorionic vessels show beginning endarteritis, the end result of which can be a complete obliteration of the chorionic vessels.

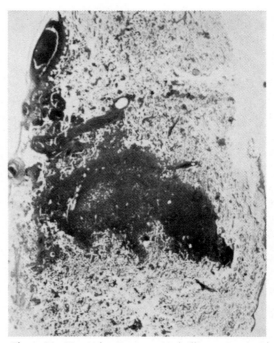

Figure 31–17. Ischemic necrosis of villi associated with intervillous fibrin deposition. ×3.

Ischemic Necrosis of Villi Due to an Interference with the Maternal Circulation (Fig. 31–18). Frequently the areas of hemorrhage or thrombosis in the decidua associated with such necrosis can be demonstrated. The areas of ischemic necrosis are more regular in shape than the preceding type. They are roughly round, sharply demarcated, located near the decidual plate, and on gross section, if recent, they are slightly firmer than the rest of the placenta. The surface is dark red, compact, and finely granular. Microscopically, one sees only tightly compressed villi with very small intervillous spaces. If the lesions are older, the cut surface is yellowish-white, finely granular, dry, and firm. Microscopically, the villi are closely packed and frequently adherent. According to the age of the lesion the endarteritic process in the villous vessels is present to a greater or lesser degree.

Ischemic Necrosis of Villi, Mixed Type (Fig. 31–19). Primary syncytial degeneration and vascular infarcts may appear together and give rise to a variety of mixed lesions in the placenta, which may cause

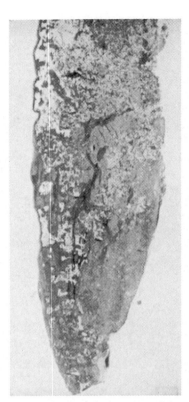

Figure 31–19. Placental degeneration of the combined type. Note that the upper portion of the lesion shows ischemic necrosis of villi associated with intervillous fibrin, whereas the lower portion represents ischemic necrosis due to a more remote interference with the maternal circulation. ×3.

ischemic necrosis of villi throughout its substance and at the margin. Probably all the lesions described are related with respect to underlying etiology, and extensive classifications serve more to confuse than to clarify the subject. Syncytial deterioration seems to be one common feature in all lesions, and vascular changes the other.

PLACENTAL LESIONS IN TOXEMIA OF PREGNANCY

The significance of true degenerative changes, especially those concerned with maternal ischemia and subsequent necrosis of villi, is not clearly understood. That they are in some way related to age of the placenta is evident. Their relationship to the toxemias of pregnancy, and especially those of the more chronic type, is not proved in spite of the interesting theories of Bartholomew. Pathologic lesions found in placentas of tox-

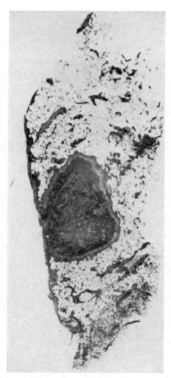

Figure 31–18. Ischemic necrosis of villi associated with disturbance of maternal circulation in the decidual plate. ×3.

emic women are probably secondary changes caused by obstructive lesions in the maternal circulation to the placenta.

Wislocki and Dempsey note changes in the direction of premature aging in the placentas of patients with severe toxemia. The chorionic villi are prematurely aged as judged by their cytologic and histochemical appearance. Aging of the syncytium is characterized by thinning, loss of basophilia, increased affinity for acid dyes, and some deterioration of nuclei, whereas a few of the smallest villi show complete necrosis of both stroma and syncytium.

Ribonucleoproteins (cytoplasmic basophilia) may be prematurely reduced, whereas alkaline and acid phosphatases are often appreciably increased. There may be noticeable changes in the amount and distribution of both calcium and glycogen. The decrease in cytoplasmic basophilia associated with a premature increase in phosphatases suggests a possible disturbance of nucleoprotein metabolism in this disease.

Thickening of the basement membranes of the fetal capillaries and of the trophoblast, a normal observation in placentas after about the thirty-fifth week, may occur sooner and in a more marked degree in toxemia. These findings, first noted by McKay, Hertig, and co-workers, may be the cause of decreased permeability of the fetal capillary membrane and fetal malnourishment, often seen in this complication of pregnancy. More recently, Anderson and McKay described three types of placental changes in toxemia: (1) an apparent increase in the number of cytotrophoblastic cells of the Langhans layer, (2) a thickening of the subtrophoblastic basement membrane of the villus most prominent in regions of intervillous fibrin deposition, and (3) an increase in the number of bulbous microvilli on the surface of the syncytium.

In some cases, a great majority of the villi appear as degenerated structures with only a thin hyalinized non-nucleated surface covering. The degree of this change seems to be directly proportional to the severity of the toxemia. It should be pointed out that in certain placentas that have been subjected to mild ischemia, there may be growth of the cytotrophoblast. These cells may appear in villi in which endarteritis and syncytial degeneration are prominent histologic features.

According to Hellman and co-workers, the chemical and morphologic changes of the placental villi in toxemia could indicate either early aging or chronic ischemia of the placenta or both. If the effect of chronic ischemia of the placenta is one of premature aging, the oxygen uptake or the anaerobic glycolysis, or both, should show an acute decrease in toxemia beyond that evident in the normal placenta. Such a change was not shown in the study of Hellman. Oxygen consumption and anaerobic glycolysis were not significantly altered in cases of severe, acute toxemia including eclampsia.

Abundant evidence suggests that during toxemia placental function is impaired, in regard to the elaboration of enzymes and hormones and in its capacities for transmission. Although, at present, there are no pathognomonic histologic lesions common to all placentas of toxemic women, considerable evidence points to a vascular basis for the diffuse trophoblastic injury and placental dysfunction frequently noted in this disease. In addition, vascular lesions are the basis for intervillous thrombosis and abruptio, lesions of the placenta that occur more frequently in toxemic women.

Calcification

As mentioned before, calcification occurs in areas of degenerating trophoblast. No term placenta is entirely free of it, nor is calcification of clinical significance. It occurs most frequently in the decidual plate but can occur along the main stems of the villi or in the placental septa.

Cysts

True cysts of the placenta probably occur only in the chorionic plate (Fig. 31–20). They have been described in the placenta and in the amnion. In the placenta proper the so-called cysts occur as areas of degeneration and liquefaction in the placental septa or in foci of intervillous fibrin. In the amnion, cysts are probably formed by adherent amniotic folds. Cysts in the chorionic plate reach considerable size, although they are probably rarely of clinical significance. Formerly, small placental cysts were thought to be abscesses because of their grumous contents. They occur frequently near the implantation of the umbilical cord, and are filled with slightly cloudy yellow fluid and occasionally grumous material. They are

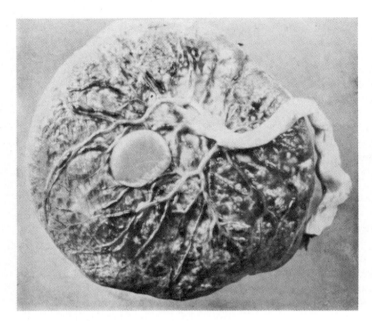

Figure 31–20. Chorionic cysts. $\times \frac{1}{2}$

lined with a single layer of flattened epithelium.

Inflammatory Change in the Placenta

Frequently collections of polymorphonuclear leukocytes are seen in the chorionic plate, not associated with either prolonged labor or febrile puerperia. The cause of this mild inflammation of the chorionic plate is not known, but it may be related to degeneration of underlying trophoblast. Inflammatory reactions in the absence of bacteria are sometimes noted in the chorion when it is exposed to meconium. Similar findings may occur in response to hypertonic saline, or to a long retained dead fetus. Also, inflammatory cells appear in the chorion approximately six hours after rupture of the membranes. The degree of leukocytic infiltration is much more severe in instances of septic abortion, prolonged labor, or premature rupture of the membranes of long duration. The placenta is involved secondarily from infection within the decidua, usually caused by pyogenic bacteria. The chorionic plate becomes loaded with inflammatory cells, and frequently bacteria can be demonstrated. If the infection is severe, the decidual plate, intervillous space, and finally the villi become involved. With maternal bacteremia abscesses of the placenta or its decidual plate are sometimes formed (Fig. 31–21).

In severe cases of intrapartum infection there may be an extension of the deciduitis, chorioamnionitis, and placentitis to involve the umbilical cord (funistis) and the fetus. The latter represent progression of the infection and occur much less commonly than decidual and placental inflammation. General

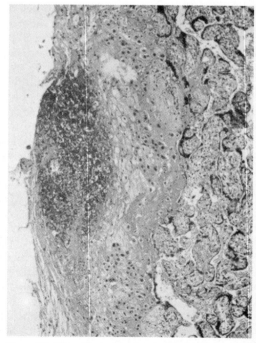

Figure 31–21. Abscess in the decidual plate associated with subacute bacterial endocarditis of the host. $\times 100$.

infection of the fetus may occur when pyogenic bacteria gain access to the chorionic vessels by invading the fetal surface of the placenta or by extension from a placentitis. In advanced cases, the fetus may exhibit evidence of congenital or neonatal pneumonia, otitis, sinusitis, meningitis, enteritis, and general sepsis. Identification of the same bacteria in the lung of the fetus and in the placenta and lower generative tract constitutes strong evidence of ascending infection (Maudsley et al.). Ordinarily, viral infections, which presumably gain access to the fetus via the placenta, do not cause inflammation of cord or chorion (Blanc).

In a study of 2000 consecutive placentas, Mechanic and co-workers found the incidences of chorioamnionitis and umbilical phlebitis to be 13 per cent and 18 per cent, respectively. The incidence of chorioamnionitis rose sharply after prolonged rupture of membranes or prolonged labor of over 12 hours. Their stillbirth rate was 6.3 per cent; there was higher association of chorioamnionitis with prematurity.

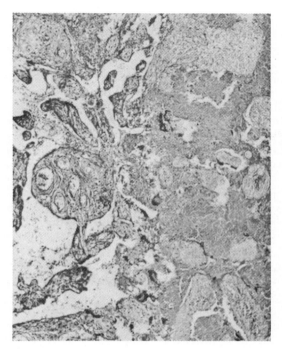

Figure 31–22. Caseous tuberculosis of the placenta. ×100.

SPECIAL DISEASES OF THE PLACENTA

There is no specific disease of the placenta which does not also involve the host, the offspring, or both. There are, however, certain conditions of the mother and fetus which involve the placenta and its appendages to such a degree that they can be called specific diseases of that organ. Tuberculosis, syphilis, and erythroblastosis fall into this category. Although malarial parasites do not produce changes in the structure of the placenta, they may be found in the maternal blood in the intervillous spaces of the placenta in the presence of a maternal infection.

Tuberculosis

The finding of tubercles in the placenta is a rare occurrence. However, the placenta should always be carefully sectioned in every case of suspected active tuberculosis of the host. The observation of tubercles in the placenta should lead one to suspect active disease in the fetus, and this is usually confirmed. Tubercles of the placentas are small, gray, firm areas sometimes showing caseation. Microscopically, there is a whorllike proliferation of endothelial cells (Fig.

31–22). Multinucleated giant cells are present and tubercle bacilli can be demonstrated. It cannot be too strongly emphasized that the search for tubercles and tubercle bacilli can be successful only if many sections of placenta are cut. It is uncommon to discover acute inflammatory lesions in the placenta proper in the absence of infection in the amniotic sac. There have been over 100 reported cases of congenital tuberculosis. About one third of these infants died within the neonatal period (Morison).

Syphilis

Prior to the widespread use of modern chemotherapeutic agents, congenital syphilis was far more common than now. The syphilitic placenta came to be recognized as a pathologic entity and the diagnosis was made with relative ease; however, in reviewing the literature on this subject, and it is ample, there is an evident lack of critique. Not only was there frequent failure to find the spirochete, which is perhaps understandable, but the diagnosis was frequently made on large placentas showing fibrosis of villi and diminution of chorionic vessels, although not the slightest stigma of the disease could be found in either parent or offspring.

The syphilitic placenta was first described by Fränkel and has since been extensively studied. It is described by Williams as being a large, boggy placenta. The maternal surface is pale yellow, with large, greasy, friable cotyledons. The weight of the placenta may be one fourth to one half as much as the fetus.

Microscopic section shows the villi to be large and club-shaped. The stroma is the site of extensive fibrosis with diminution of fetal vessels. Spirochetes can be found rarely in such placentas. This is not surprising, for they are difficult to demonstrate in any tissue and frequently can be differentiated from bits of connective tissue fiber only by the expert. Syphilis elsewhere in the body is a disease affecting smaller arterioles. There is an infiltration of their walls with lymphocytes, resulting in occlusion of the vessels. A chronic and granulomatous degenerative lesion is formed, the end result of which is a gumma. In investigating the question of placental syphilis, such changes should be sought.

The fetus is capable of forming antibodies to treponema antigen by the twentieth gestational week, the time when the spirochete is first able to penetrate the placental barrier. Thus, the traditional concept that intrauterine syphilitic infection was a common cause of abortion is unfounded. Recently Harter and Benirschke described the presence of *Treponema pallidium* in five fetuses and placentas of 10 weeks' gestation. This disproves the accepted theory of the 20 week placental barrier to syphilitic infection. After that period, however, fetal death or congenital syphilis in the newborn is a substantial risk in the untreated case. With rare exceptions, adequate treatment with penicillin, which crosses the placenta freely, will cure the infected fetus.

One of the most significant misconceptions in placental pathology to be clarified in recent years concerns the histologic changes considered diagnostic for fetal syphilis, namely, clubbing of villi, fibrosis, and endarteritis. The similarity of the placentas described by Hellman and Hertig, which were associated with erythroblastosis, in which syphilis was excluded beyond reasonable doubt, leads one to consider the diagnosis with caution. Moreover, it has been shown that the placental changes formerly considered pathognomonic of syphilis may merely represent secondary fibrotic changes in the placenta after fetal death in utero.

When fetal death in utero occurs there may be maceration of the fetus and cord, but death does not necessarily occur concomitantly in the placenta unless it becomes separated. A progressive endarteritic process occurs in the villous vessels. A cuff of fibrous connective tissue appears in the walls of the vessels, thus narrowing and frequently obliterating the lumens. Hyalinization eventually leads to complete obliteration of the vessels and to fibrous overgrowth of the villous stroma. The villi are clubbed and resemble closely the histologic changes of syphilis. These changes, however, are strictly degenerative. It is probable that eventually the fibroblasts can overgrow the entire placenta. This is evidenced in the placental eye transplants and tissue cultures of Gey and associates (Fig. 31–23). Ordinarily, there is much more fibrosis and vascular lesions are more prominent in the placenta of the syphilitic woman than in hydrops fetalis associated with erythroblastosis.

A renewed alertness about the prospects of congenital syphilis and familiarity with its

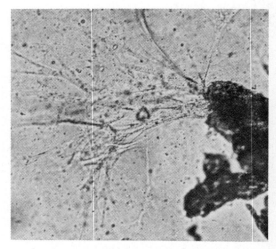

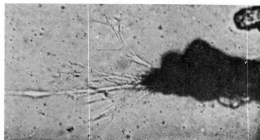

Figure 31–23. Tissue culture of chorionic villus. ×50. Primary explant shows overgrowth of nonepithelial elements.

pathologic features and manifestations are mandatory in the light of rising venereal disease rates. Some authors have reported as much as a sixfold increase in congenital syphilis at their institutions in the past decade (Coblentz et al.). Moreover, increasing numbers of penicillin-resistant strains of spirochetes are being encountered, and at least one fetus and one newborn have been reported recently to be totally refractory to standard therapy (Hardy et al.).

Erythroblastosis

This is a hemolytic disease affecting about 1 per cent of all newborn infants, caused by a particular incompatibility of the fetal and maternal blood. Although the condition has been known since antiquity, and its pathologic manifestations adequately described for some years, it was not until the crucial observation of Levine and Stetson in 1939, that certain mothers may be immunized by the blood of their infants, that the way was paved for an understanding of the pathogenesis of erythroblastosis fetalis. A series of observations during the following three years by Levine, Wiener, and others established that 90 per cent of the mothers of all erythroblastotic children are Rh-negative and their fathers are Rh-positive.

Although a host of factors in the blood are immunologically and genetically important there are at least nine red cell factors representing significant genetically independent antigen systems. These "families" include Rh, ABO, MNS, Kell, Duffy, Kidd, P, Lewis, and Lutheran, as well as a growing list of others, mostly rare, which are as yet unclassified. Practically all blood factors are inherited as mendelian dominants. With the discovery of three specific anti-Rh sera, a constellation of eight Rh types, which fall into two groups of four each, was distinguished; the distinction is related to the presence or absence of the antigen D (Rh_0). For each of the Rh antigens there is an allelomorphic Hr antigen (Fisher-Race designation). The Rh factor is a polysaccharide attached to the red cell of 85 per cent of the U.S. white population and inherited as a mendelian dominant. It is capable of causing antibody formation if injected into people who do not possess it. These people are spoken of as Rh-negative, whereas the former are referred to as Rh-positive.

An Rh-positive man and an Rh-negative woman produce, if the father is homozygous, an Rh-positive infant. Small amounts of the fetal blood may leak through the placental barrier into the mother's blood and produce an antibody in her plasma. Apparently, as little as 0.1 ml. of Rh-positive blood can produce sensitization. Approximately 13 per cent of all marriages between white persons in the United States take place between an Rh-negative woman and an Rh-positive man. Despite this, isoimmunization occurs in only 7 per cent of Rh-negative gravidas, the great majority becoming sensitized by the fourth pregnancy. An even smaller percentage results in fetal damage; the likelihood of fetal involvement will of course depend upon the husband's zygosity with respect to the Rh factor. All offspring of a homozygous Rh-positive male will be Rh-positive; there is a chance of Rh negativity in 50 per cent of the offspring of heterozygous Rh positive males (the former exceed the latter by about 3 to 1). The likelihood of sensitization also depends upon the quantity of fetal red cells reaching the maternal circulation, and possibly upon relative antigenicity of the Rh factor, host responsiveness, and other factors. Extravasations of fetal Rh_0 (D) cells are the most antigenic.

Escape of fetal cells into the maternal circulation during the antepartal period is rare; thus, isoimmunization in the first pregnancy is not a significant potential risk unless there has been an unsuspected abortion or incompatible blood transfusion. On the other hand, a fetomaternal transfusion of more than 50 cu. mm. has been found in at least one fifth of women at delivery (Finn et al.). The greatest risks of transfer of fetal red cells appear to be at the end of a pathologic pregnancy (i.e., placental abruption, placenta previa, toxemia, etc.) and during labor, especially with obstetric intervention and operative manipulations.

The clinical degree of anemia, hyperbilirubinemia, and physical manifestations at birth is variable, and the prognosis differs accordingly. In the mildest form the fetus is only anemic without other stigmas and the outlook is good. A more serious stage is designated icterus gravis in which there is jaundice which deepens progressively. Hepatosplenomegaly and extramedullary erythropoiesis are regularly present. With transfusion in utero if necessary or optimal exchange transfusions in the neonatal period, the prospects of survival are fairly good today. The most serious stage is the hydrops fetalis which rarely responds even to the most expert modern therapeutic regimes. One of the most serious potential postnatal complications is kernicterus, which is characterized by yellowish pigmentation of the basal nuclei, as well as other portions of the infant's brain. Approximately 6 per cent of those who survive the first week of life develop signs of central nervous system damage—particularly premature or hypoxic infants, or those experiencing protractedly high levels of free bilirubin. In management, an effort is exerted to keep bilirubin levels low to minimize this grave risk.

In many cases it is possible to improve the chances of fetal survival by instituting appropriate obstetric measures based on clinical and laboratory estimates of the degree of affectation. Tranfusion in utero and/or timely removal of the fetus from exposure to maternal antibodies may be lifesaving. Fetal status can be judged on the basis of Rh antibody titers (albumin type); indirect Coombs titer —mixing of the patient's serum with Rh-positive cells and testing with antiglobulin; the height of the 450 nm. peak on the spectral absorption curve of amniotic fluids (Liley); and certain hormonal assessments. More refined management has succeeded in reducing the overall perinatal mortality rate to 15 to 20 per cent. The future is promising, not so much because of these improved techniques and therapeutics but because it has been clearly demonstrated that high-potency, anti-D gamma globulin administered to unsensitized Rh-negative mothers within 48 to 72 hours of delivery is nearly totally protective against the formation of Rh antibodies.

That this abnormality of the newborn infant is associated with an enlarged and edematous placenta was recognized by Ballantyne. The fetal-placental ratio is described by Hellman and Hertig as being 3:1 or less. The maternal surface is made up of large, pale, yellow-gray cotyledons that are extremely friable (Fig. 31–24). Although an enlarged hypertrophic edematous placenta is seen most commonly with hydrops fetalis associated with erythroblastosis, the same striking enlargement of the chorionic villi is often encountered in diabetes mellitus and occasionally in cases of cardiac decompensation in the fetus. Microscopic section shows the villi to be enlarged (Figs. 31–25 and 31–26). There is an absence of degenerative changes in the syncytium, with a partial persistence of Langhans' layer. In some instances, a marked rise in the urinary excretion of chorionic gonadotropin warns of advancing severity of the hemolytic process. There are frequently ectopic foci of erythropoiesis present, particularly noticeable in the subchorionic regions. Two types of villous stroma are seen, the edematous and the hyperplastic. There are numerous Hofbauer cells whose cytoplasm contains droplets of fat. The villous vessels are relatively diminished in number. Their endothelium is immature and there are many areas of intra-

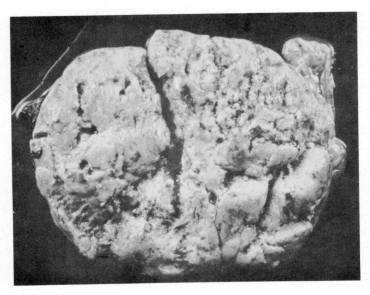

Figure 31–24. Placenta associated with erythroblastosis of the hydrops variety.

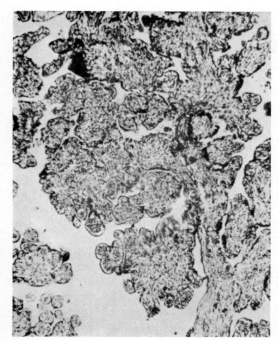

Figure 31–25. Erythroblastotic full term placenta. Note the resemblance to the syphilitic placenta (see page 616). ×45.

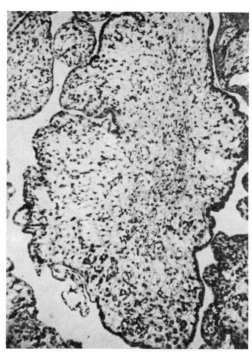

Figure 31–26. Villus of erythroblastotic placenta. Note the hyperplastic and edematous types of stroma and the areas of intracapillary erythropoiesis. ×120.

capillary erythropoiesis. In extreme cases, the placental tissue is so vesicular and friable that it is virtually molar in type. There may be associated polyhydramnios and, with fetal death, development of a maternal toxemia-like syndrome.

The pathologic changes in the placenta of fetuses with less severe forms of the disease are similar to those associated with the hydrops variety, but are present to a much milder degree. The size and gross appearance of the placenta are frequently normal, however, when the fetus is not edematous at birth.

In spite of the seeming pathologic specificity of the lesions included in this syndrome, it now seems probable that they all result from an effort on the part of the fetus to compensate for the anoxia resulting from the tremendous destruction of its red cells. This, if true, would help explain the confusing similarity between the placental changes in erythroblastosis and other pathologic conditions, e.g., syphilis or diabetes.

Approximately 20 to 25 per cent of all pregnancies are heterospecific in the sense that the fetal red blood cells possess an agglutinogen, A or B, not present in the mother,

whereas the maternal serum contains the corresponding agglutinin, which is antagonistic to the fetal blood group. Because the A and B factors are present in tissue cells, Levine and Stetson believe that the specific reaction produced throughout the body by maternal anti-A and anti-B agglutinins may occasionally exert a far more lethal effect on the fetus than the specific reaction of anti-Rh on the fetal blood cells exclusively. Usually, however, the disease is much milder than that associated with the Rh factor. Moreover, only about 5 per cent of those with a major maternal blood group incompatibility, or 1 per cent of all infants, actually develop hemolytic disease. Unlike Rh hemolytic disease, infants of primigravidas are frequently affected and fetuses in subsequent pregnancies will not necessarily be diseased. Although erythroblastosis is generally less severe than Rh factor-provoked disease, it is interesting that affected infants are as susceptible to kernicterus.

In both homospecific and heterospecific pregnancies, the patterns of isoantibodies against A and B remain stationary and only in the postpartal period does a minority of cases of heterospecific pregnancy exhibit a specific immune response to the fetal blood group antigen. Unlike isoimmunization problems involving the Rh factor, there are no adequate methods now available for antenatal diagnosis of ABO hemolytic disease.

It should be noted that a variety of drugs and other agents may induce hemolysis of fetal red cells. All drugs administered to the mother should be evaluated for placental transmission, method of conjugation for excretion, hemolytic effect, ability to bind proteins, and effect on hepatocellular function. Moreover, many biologic compounds, including steroids, sulfonamides, carboxylic acid, and phenols, may compete with bilirubin for conjugation and lead to high levels of the free toxic form in the newborn, regardless of the underlying cause for the hemolysis.

ABNORMALITIES OF IMPLANTATION AND SEPARATION

The placenta is usually implanted on the anterior or posterior surface of the fundus and rarely crosses the lateral midline. Misplacement of the placenta results in a serious prognosis for the infant and frequently in maternal difficulties. From the morphologic viewpoint abnormal implantation inside the uterus does not differ markedly from the normal. Even when the placenta is implanted near the internal os, the formation of decidua and the attachment of the placenta to it is apt to be entirely normal. In low implanted placentas and placenta previas, premature separation frequently takes place at the time of dilatation of the internal os or thinning of the lower uterine segment. This is associated with gross hemorrhage in and on the decidual plate. Microscopically, the decidua is destroyed by hemorrhage and an infiltration of leukocytes. The etiology of low implantations is unknown; however, advanced parity and atrophic changes in the endometrium appear to favor its occurrence.

Tubal, ovarian, and *abdominal pregnancies,* although they are usually incompatible with full term development of the fetus because of an abnormal environment, may show a surprisingly normal chorionic villus development. The details of implantation and decidual response in these ectopic sites have been discussed previously. Suffice it to say that in the great majority of ectopic gestations, death of the embryo takes place in the early weeks of pregnancy because of the unfavorable environment of the implanted ovum. The decidual layer is imperfectly formed or absent, and subjacent necrotic and fibrinoid tissue is formed through erosion of connective tissue and muscle cells by the trophoblast. In advanced ectopic gestations there is a high incidence of developmental anomalies of the fetuses, and the placentas frequently show varying degrees of hydropic degeneration.

Implantation in the tube or ovary is usually terminated with rupture of that organ because of the rapid growth of the products of conception. The subsequent hemorrhage may be violent, for the fetus with its demands on the mother causes a great increase in size of the blood vessels. In abdominal pregnancy the fetus is not confined in any limiting viscus. It may grow to full size but it frequently dies because of failure of delivery at term. It may be resorbed or become calcified, or it may have to be removed surgically because of bleeding into the abdominal cavity. In these cases if the placenta can obtain enough circulation it is usually normal in appearance. It may be implanted on bowel, parietal peritoneum, or any other abdominal viscus. In any event, the absence of decidua makes normal separation of these placentas an impossibility, and as they can only be forcefully torn from their beds they are frequently wisely allowed to remain in situ and be resorbed.

Placenta accreta is not only an abnormality of separation but also one of implantation. Irving and Hertig have reviewed this subject and have pointed out the importance of partial placenta accreta. The etiology seems to be a defect in the decidua resulting from scarring of the endometrium. The placenta becomes implanted on areas partially or completely lacking normal endometrium. This is well shown in Figure 31–27. Muscle fibers lie directly beneath the villi and are drawn up into the placental septa. They can be well demonstrated by the use of special stains. The primary histologic features of placenta accreta can be summarized, as outlined by Millar and others: (1) defective decidua, (2) dense fusion of Rohr's and Nitabuch's fibrin layers, and (3) hyalinization of the uterine muscle. In rare instances the chorionic villi have not only made contact with but have also actually penetrated the uterine muscle. This condition is referred to as *placenta increta.*

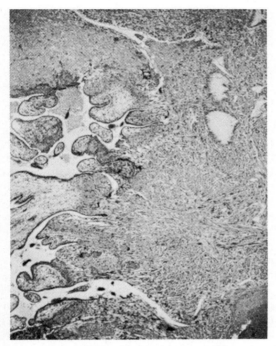

Figure 31–27. Placenta accreta. × 100.

Placenta percreta is a condition in which the chorionic villi have penetrated the whole thickness of the uterine wall and reached its serosal covering, sometimes rupturing into the peritoneal cavity. Old scars with or without inflammation can frequently be seen in the uterine wall in the region of trophoblastic penetration. The cause of such scarring is not known. However, it can probably be caused by chronic infection, and mechanical factors, such as curettage, may play an etiologic role.

Several cases of simultaneous placenta previa and placenta accreta have been reported. More recent reports give rise to the suspicion that this association is more commonly encountered than was suspected heretofore. In more than 70,000 deliveries at the Johns Hopkins Hospital not a single case of complete accreta has been observed; according to Eastman, placenta increta and percreta are even rarer occurrences. Focal areas of placenta accreta are seen more commonly.

Abruptio Placentae

Normally, separation of the placenta occurs through the spongy layer of the decidua, after the delivery of the fetus. With the fetus no longer present, contraction of the uterus tears off the placenta through the large vascular spaces of the spongiosa—just as a postage stamp is torn off through the perforations—since this is the weakest layer of the decidua. Little bleeding accompanies this process because the contracted uterus effectively tamponades the arteries supplying this area; however, a small hematoma forms between the separating placenta and the remaining decidua and its propagation undoubtedly accelerates the cleavage. If separation of the placenta occurs, even to a minor degree, prior to delivery of the infant, the vessels cannot be constricted by the contracting uterus, and bleeding usually eventuates. The placenta may become completely separated from the uterine wall while the membranes remain adherent and, in other circumstances, the blood may gain access to the amniotic sac through rupture of the membranes.

The thin-walled arteries and veins of the decidua basalis are easily torn or ruptured, especially if they are diseased, and the consequent extravasation of blood produces a retroplacental hematoma. All degrees of placental separation may occur, from an area of only a few millimeters in diameter to the entire placenta, with all gradations of clinical signs and symptoms. The classic signs and symptoms are pain, shock, and uterine rigidity, often in association with fetal distress or death, and in the severe forms accompanied by shock, hypofibrinogenemia, and acute renal failure. There may be the remote problem of hypopituitarism among survivors.

A majority of the cases of moderate or marked antepartum hemorrhage are due to some form of premature separation. The reported incidence of this complication is about 1 in 150 deliveries or less, depending upon the diagnostic criteria employed. Spotting or minimal loss of blood per vaginum is more likely to be due to lesions of the lower generative tract, but proper steps must be taken in all such cases to exclude placental complications, even though up to one half of all cases of antepartal bleeding are not assignable to a placental cause.

When the placenta is partially or totally disrupted from the uterine wall prior to delivery of the fetus, it is followed by bleeding from maternal vascular sinuses; and if the tear extends to the margin of the placenta, vaginal bleeding is noted. If the separation is central and does not extend to the margin, a hematoma develops between the placenta and uterine wall and the villi in this area become compressed. In the earliest stages hemorrhage into the decidua basalis, resulting from pathologic small uterine vessels or from vascular damage within the placenta itself, causes a splitting of the decidua, hematoma formation, and ultimate separation, compression, and loss of function within adjacent placental tissue. Usually, there is progression of the hemorrhage and an expanding area of separation which eventually disrupts the placenta at its margin. In some instances, blood gains access to the amniotic cavity after rupturing the membranes or, occasionally, external bleeding is prevented when the membranes remain opposed to the uterine wall even though the placenta may totally disrupt. The wall of the uterus, especially in the lateral portions, may become infiltrated by blood. The uterus assumes a deep purple color, and is described as a Couvelaire uterus (about 5 per cent or less of all cases of abruptio placentae). Hemorrhage is present between muscle bundles, in perivascular tissue, and in the subserosa (Fig. 31–28). The decidual spiral arterioles may show acute atheromatous processes with accumulation of foamy macrophages and fibrinoid degeneration of the intima encroaching upon the lumen. Degeneration and

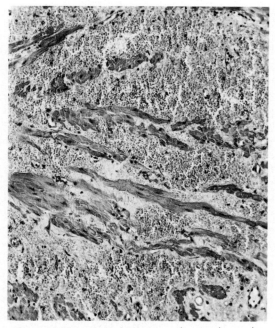

Figure 31–28. Couvelaire uterus showing hemorrhage between muscle bundles.

thrombosis of spiral arterioles in the decidua may be conditioned by previous hypertension and toxemia. Marais has demonstrated a wide range of degenerative vascular lesions in the decidua (sclerosis, necrosis, formation of aneurysms) which lead to rupture or occlusion of the vessels.

The frequency with which abruptio placentae is preceded by hypertension has been reported as being 25 to 60 per cent, depending upon the severity of toxemia. However, this association is significant to this degree with respect only to the most advanced cases of abruption. Previously, certain degenerative lesions involving the intima of the small uterine arteries were incriminated, but now such changes are considered to be merely variations or extensions from the norm. The basic etiology is obscure and such postulations of the cause as shortness of the umbilical cord, compression of the inferior vena cava, folic acid deficiency, and others, remain unproved. It is true nonetheless that direct trauma to the uterus and sudden decompression of the uterus are infrequent but well documented causes of placental abruption. Parity rather than increasing maternal age seems to be an associated factor, although both age and hypertensive disorders increase with parity.

The most important identified cause of fetal death in utero is abruptio placentae. Fetal loss varies with the degree of placental disruption and the presence of associated toxemia. Sexton and co-workers report that the fetal mortality is as high as 66 per cent in cases of abruptio placentae associated with severe grades of toxemia, although the range for all cases is nearer 30 to 60 per cent (Golditch and Boyce).

Marginal Sinus Rupture (Figs. 31–29 and 31–30). Separation of the placenta at its margin should be classified as one form of partial abruptio, not as a separate entity. Roughly one half of all abruptions may fall into this category. Special significance was formerly attached to this condition because of Spanner's theory of placenta circulation which routed all venous flow to the placental margin where the blood drained into a channel called the marginal sinus. More recently, Ramsey and others have dispelled this theory by demonstrating venous drainage through the central portion of the placenta.

Based upon serial and cineradioangiographic visualization of maternal circulation in the primate hemochorial placenta, Ramsey

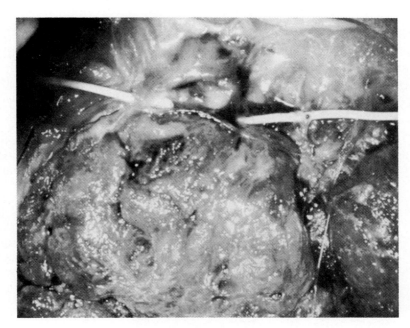

Figure 31–29. Ruptured marginal sinus; superficial clot removed.

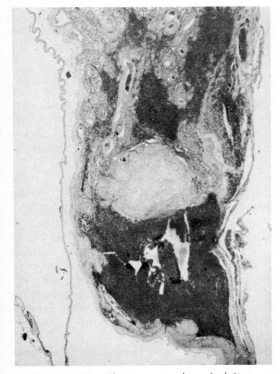

Figure 31–30. Clot in a ruptured marginal sinus.

and co-workers have demonstrated that both arterial entrances and venous exits are distributed over the entire base of the placenta. The head of maternal pressure drives the entering arterial blood high up toward the chorionic plate before lateral dispersion occurs. After bathing the chorionic villi, the blood drains through venous orifices in the basal plate and enters the maternal placental veins. Although the arterial flow has been referred to as localized spurts (Borell's "jets"), Ramsey indicates that there is continuous flow of varying velocities from the arteries.

According to Reynolds, the entire cotyledonary structure and fetal placental vascular bed are under a distending pressure from the back-pressure within it, resulting in a gentle erectile action of all placental tissues. The arterial blood pressure in cotyledonary arteries at term is estimated to be 50 to 60 mm. Hg. Each cotyledon is a terminal arterial glomus from which blood filters slowly through the surrounding fetal villi into the intervillous space proper. The cotyledonary venous pressure is estimated to be about 15 mm. Hg.

The flow rate of the blood in the intervillous space is influenced by uterine activity and pressure as well as the status of the arteriolar walls. Martin and coworkers have shown that arterial blood spurts may appear or disappear independent of myometrial activity or significant change in maternal blood pressure, thus implicating vasomotor tone as a factor in regulating blood flow. Not all endometrial spiral arterioles are continuously patent nor do they all necessarily spurt blood into the intervillous space simultaneously

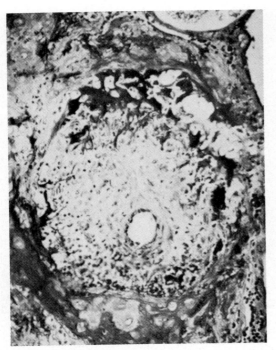

Figure 31–31. Endarteritis of spiral vessel associated with premature separation. ×100.

(Fig. 31–31). Moreover, strict countercurrent is precluded by the random distribution of villi. The force of the spurts is dissipated by the compact villi and provides time for diffusion and metabolic exchange. Apparently, between 20 and 30 spiral arterioles may open into the intervillous space and, as the blood emanating from these orifices slows, small lakes of about 5 mm. in diameter are created about half way toward the chorionic plate. According to Ramsey, injected dye is delayed in making its appearance in the veins of the uterine wall during a strong contraction and intervillous space pressure may be decreased to the point at which blood cannot be expressed against the prevailing myometrial pressure.

Confirmatory evidence for this physiologic explanation, formulated and championed by Ramsey, is provided by several studies. Rates of disappearance of radioactive material from the choriodecidual space, reported by Browne and Veall, suggest that each local region has its own venous drainage system. Moreover, the recordings of intrauterine pressures by Caldeyro-Barcia have established absolute values indicating that the head of maternal pressure is 60 to 70 mm. Hg greater than that prevailing in the intervillous space, whereas the latter exceeds the 8 mm. of venous pelvic pressure by several millimeters during myometrial diastole. With myometrial contractions, pressures are observed up to 80 mm. Hg and concomitant rises are observed in intra-amniotic and intervillous space pressures.

Thus, it appears that too much emphasis has been placed upon marginal drainage of the placenta and the constancy and importance of the marginal sinus as a specific entity. However, from a clinical viewpoint, hemorrhage from the margin of the placenta may be of sufficient severity to cause appreciable separation of the decidual plate in a medial direction. On the other hand, the hemorrhage may be relatively slight and of short duration.

NEW GROWTHS

New growths of the placenta are few, consisting primarily of one benign tumor (the chorioangioma); one potentially malignant tumor (hydatidiform mole); and one malignant tumor (choriocarcinoma). Hydatidiform mole and choriocarcinoma are discussed elsewhere (Chapter 32). Although any tumor with hematogenous spread can theoretically metastasize to the placenta, such occurrences are exceedingly rare. Of the 17 cases of this type reported to date, one third were malignant melanomas (Rothman et al.).

Chorioangioma

Although hemangiomas (chorioangiomas) are the most common benign tumors of the placenta, they occur in only about 1 per cent of the specimens studied, according to recent reports (Benirschke, 1 in 100; Wentworth, 1 in 77 placentas examined). The tumors are round, firm, reddish purple, somewhat lobulated in appearance, and easily shelled out of the depths of the placenta (Fig. 31–32). Usually they are subchorial in location and situated paracentrally with respect to the cord insertion. Characteristically they are encapsulated. They are rubbery and vary considerably in size, although some may be 5 cm. or more in diameter. Fibrous trabeculae can be seen extending across the surface, creating lobules of various sizes which bleed freely on pressure. The trophoblast layer around the tumor is intact, or partially so, and in some cases there is

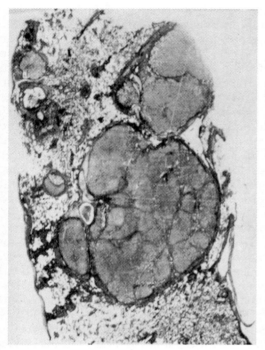

Figure 31–32. Hemangioma (chorioangioma). ×3.

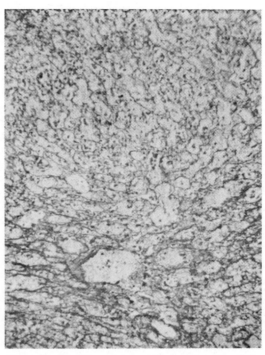

Figure 31–33. Hemangioma (chorioangioma). ×150.

marked proliferation, fibrinoid deposition, and calcification. Frequently these tumors are mistaken for areas of intervillous thrombosis.

Microscopically, the tumors show a well differentiated capillary pattern of benign endothelium supported by a loose network of fibrous tissue and chorionic stromal cells which form spaces containing fetal blood (Fig. 31–33). There may be intervillous thrombi or white fibrin infarcts in nearby areas of the placenta. Because of the abnormal overgrowth of blood vessels and chorionic tissue, these tumors are more properly designated as chorioangiomas. Williams described several types of hemangioma, based on the ratio of vascularity to connective tissue. Tumors in which the capillary-like blood vessels are particularly evident may be designated as angiomyxomas. This variety of tumor may extend into the umbilical cord and frequently contains varying amounts of myxomatous tissue similar to that in the normal cord. Rarely, such tumors may occur only in the cord.

These tumors may be a rare cause of placental insufficiency, especially when they are large, and may be associated with hydramnios, fetal anomalies, premature birth,

fetal microangiopathic hemolytic anemia, thrombocytopenia, and chromosomal disorders (Froehlich et al.).

ABNORMALITIES OF THE AMNION

Disorders of Squamous Epithelium

One of the commonest conditions has been known by several nondescriptive names, such as *amniotic plaques* or *amniotic caruncles*. Small white or dull gray plaques appear on the fetal surface of the amnions in nearly 70 per cent of placentas. They are most frequently located near the insertion of the umbilical cord. The plaques are usually 1 to 2 mm. in diameter with irregular contours. They are raised and their surface is rough and granular. When they are scraped off the surface of the amnion, a slightly rough and whitened area remains.

Microscopic study of these lesions reveals all stages of development from a mere piling up of the usual single layer of columnar epithelium to true metaplasia. In the most completely developed form there are layers of true stratified squamous epithelium with

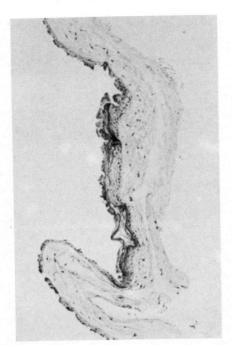

Figure 31–34. Squamous metaplasia of the amnion. ×100.

keratinization (Fig. 31–34). Occasionally, these areas undergo a degenerative change and are seen as small nodules of amorphous, hyaline material in which only shadows of epithelial cells remain. Squamous metaplasia of the amnion is perhaps only of academic interest. Its etiology is unknown, but its occurrence illustrates the totipotential character of the amniotic epithelium. Amniotic folds may fuse occasionally with resultant accumulation of fluid to form small cysts which are lined by typical columnar or cuboidal epithelium. Rarely, a condition known as amnion nodosum appears on the surface of the amnion in cases complicated by a complete lack of amniotic fluid or with oligohydramnios. The presence together of amnion nodosum, oligohydramnios, and renal aplasia is designated "Potter's syndrome." It is uncertain whether the condition arises primarily from the amnion or results from the incorporation of fetal ectodermal derivatives (Bartman and Driscoll).

Amniotic Defects and Bands

On rare occasions the amnion is incomplete and does not cover all the chorionic surface so that part or all of the fetus is extra-amniotic. Occasionally also, amniochorionic mesoblastic fibrous strings and amniotic bands occur and, according to Torpin, these may be associated with constricting fetal malformations or fetal death. If at any time during pregnancy the amnion ruptures while the chorion remains intact in a raw, denuded state, fibrous strings as well as the free floating amnion may become entangled with fetal extremities, particularly fingers and toes, with resulting digital amputations. Rarely, according to Torpin, the umbilical cord or fetal neck may become entwined with these bands and fetal death or abortion may result.

The majority of such cases reveal no histologic evidence that they are inflammatory. Recently, 24 patients with amniotic band syndrome were examined and several different deformities and amputations were found (Ossipoff and Hall). The only etiologic factors found were trauma during pregnancy and discontinuance of oral contraceptives within one month of conception.

Disorders of Amniotic Fluid

The amount of amniotic fluid varies in late pregnancy from about 400 to 1500 ml., according to Elliott and Inman. About 1000 ml. at term is considered normal, and 2000 ml. or more is considered excessive (this occurs in fewer than 1 in 100 deliveries). About one third of the water is exhanged each hour; however, the mechanisms of exchange for different elements are independent of one another (Hutchinson et al.). On the basis of these studies, it has been determined that the net amount of water transferred from fetus to amniotic fluid in hydramnios is much greater than in normal pregnancy, which leads to the clinical observation that fetal anomalies predispose to excess fluid accumulation in the amniotic sac. Failure of normal fetal water interchange may likewise be responsible for placental hypertrophy, which accounts for the increased placental weights observed in hydramnios. The amniotic fluid is both slightly alkaline and hypotonic, and during the latter half of pregnancy a considerable amount of particulate matter is present. At this time, a principal pathway for removal of the fluid is fetal swallowing, about 450 ml. per day according to Pritchard, whereas the chief pathway for its replacement is fetal urination. It has been observed that in the absence of swallowing, as in esophageal atresia, excess fluid accumulates (hydramnios or polyhydramnios), whereas oligohydramnios (too little fluid) develops in the presence of renal agenesis or complete urethral obstruction in the fetus. Too little fluid is also encountered in some cases of placental insufficiency, particularly in association with chronic vascular disease. Hydramnios is common in multiple pregnancy, severe erythroblastosis, maternal diabetes, and in the presence of fetal anomalies. The composition of the fluid in hydramnios is ordinarily the same as in normal conditions.

ABNORMALITIES OF THE UMBILICAL CORD

Normal Structure

The umbilical cord normally contains two arteries and a vein. These are surrounded by a clear gelatinous substance known as Wharton's jelly. The entire mass is covered by the amnion except that where it approaches the fetus an epithelial covering is substituted. Apparently the purpose served by Wharton's jelly is protection, for Browne has demonstrated experimentally that the vessels are protected from undue torsion and compression by the gelatinous consistency of this coat.

In the opinion of Reynold's, however, this jelly-like substance may play an important role in the propulsion of blood through the umbilical vessels. In the living condition, Wharton's jelly is stretched taut around the blood vessels as a thin band of connective tissue which exerts a force tending to make the blood vessels collapse. The vessels do not collapse, however, because there is resistance to the outflow of blood, which is under the control of a sphincter situated at the origin of the ductus venosus at the umbilical recess. Thus, in the normal state, the arteries are smaller in diameter than the vein but all three are greatly distended. The distention prevents easy obliteration of the vessels and facilitates flow of blood by reducing the friction loss of energy against the vessel walls. Finally, after delivery, Wharton's jelly, through its high water content, may

serve the additional function of facilitating desiccation and the dropping off of the cord. Marked water retention of the cord may occur in association with a macerated fetus or one that is edematous.

When an artery of the human umbilical cord is fixed in the normally distended state, transverse intimal folds forming crescentic bands are noted across part of the lumen. These folds are commonly referred to as the "folds of Hoboken." At present they have no known function.

Gross Abnormalities

The umbilical cord shows great variation in length and diameter. The average length is 55 cm. For purposes of classification, umbilical cords over 70 cm. and under 30 cm. in length are described as abnormal. It is questionable whether such classification serves any practical purpose.

Frequently abnormally long cords become entangled with the fetus and may be so compressed as to cause anoxia. However, the same twining of the funis about the neck of the infant is seen when the length of the cord is normal or even unduly short. Moreover, unusually long cords are said to predispose to prolapse and compression of vessels; however, in most cases of prolapse, the umbilical cord is of normal length.

Some authors claim that short umbilical cords may give rise to dystocia, with subsequent inversion of the uterus of separation of the placenta, but in the experience of most obstetricians such accidents are exceedingly rare. Varices of the umbilical vessels are common, and are known as *false knots*. These too, are clinically insignificant.

Abnormalities of Insertion

The relation of the attachment of the umbilical cord to the surface of the placenta is determined at implantation by the postion of the inner cell mass in relation to the uterine wall. In about three quarters of placentas the umbilical cord is inserted eccentrically. It is inserted at the margin of the placenta in 7 per cent, giving rise to the so-called *battledore placenta*. When the cord is implanted on the membranes away from the margin of the placenta, the insertion is termed *velamentous*. The incidence of this is much higher in mul-

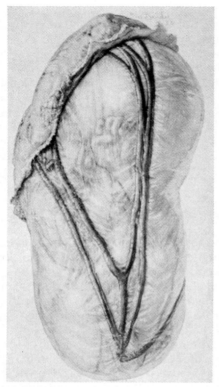

Figure 31–35. Vasa praevia with breech presentation. ×⅓. (From Williams.)

tiple pregnancy. When a velamentous insertion is of such magnitude that the chorionic vessels traverse the entire surface of the membrane and the vessels cross the internal os, the condition is known as *vasa praevia* (Fig. 31–35).

It is conceivable that an abnormal position of the inner cell mass at the time of implantation could give rise to these anomalies. Clinically, only the marginal and velamentous insertions are significant. Rupture of the chorionic vessels during labor is frequently associated with these abnormalities. It is difficult to distinguish fetal bleeding from the bleeding of premature separation, but demonstration of nucleated red cells or fetal hemoglobin is diagnostic. Rupture of fetal vessels frequently causes profound anoxia of the newborn infant.

Knots of the Cord

True knots of the funis are common and may be extremely complicated. Occasionally they become so taut that fetal anoxia occurs; but fortunately the cord vessels are rarely drawn tight enough to seriously embarrass the circulation.

According to Spellacy and co-workers, the incidence of true knotting is 1.1 per cent and the associated perinatal loss is 6.1 per cent. Loops of cords about the fetal neck are rarely a cause of fetal death, although, in monoamniotic twining, cord entanglements are common and much of the fetal risk involved is related to this problem.

Absent Umbilical Artery

The absence of one artery is noted in about 1 per cent of all umbilical cords and up to 6 per cent of the cords of at least one twin. The perinatal mortality rate is elevated and, according to Benirschke, 20 to 40 per cent of all infants with one umbilical artery have associated congenital anomalies. Esophageal atresia and imperforate anus with or without fistula are the most common defects. The birth weight is likely to be lower than normal. Abnormalities are not confined to any single organ of the fetus.

Torsion of the Cord

Undue twisting of the cord, especially in the portion near the fetus at which Wharton's jelly is less abundant, probably can cause fetal anoxia (Fig. 31–36). In the case illustrated, death of the fetus occurred about a week before delivery and was preceded by a period of violent fetal movements. Serial section of the twisted portion of the cord showed complete obliteration of the vessels. However, as has frequently been pointed out, it can never be definitely proved that twisting of the cord does not take place after death of the fetus. Undoubtedly, extreme degrees of torsion occur only after fetal death. The turgor in the umbilical cord of a viable fetus whose vascular dynamics are normal is sufficiently great to minimize greatly any risks of torsion and prolapse.

Hematomas of the Cord

Rarely hematomas of the umbilical cord lead to fetal anoxia from partial or complete compression of one or more of the umbilical vessels. The incidence of this condition is 1 case in 5505 deliveries, with an immediate fetal mortality of 47 per cent.

The hematomas are usually located near the umbilicus and most often arise from rup-

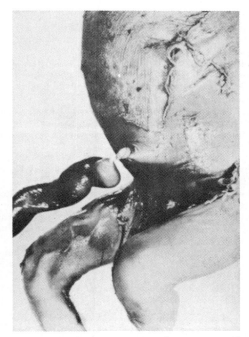

Figure 31–36. Torsion of the umbilical cord. $\times \frac{1}{3}$.

ture of the wall of the umbilical vein. The hematomas vary greatly in size, the diameter ranging from 1 to 5 cm. or more. Mechanical forces probably play an important etiologic role, but there is no truly adequate explanation for the occurrence of hematomas. Before delivery, the only clinical evidence of the presence of a hematoma of the cord is fetal distress or, rarely, vaginal bleeding. Rupture of the cord vessel occasionally occurs and results in fetal exsanguination (Benirschke and Driscoll).

Neoplasms of the Cord

Neoplastic tumors of the umbilical cord may take the form of myxomas, myxosarcomas, dermoids, and teratomas, although they are extremely rare. The most common tumor is the angiomyxoma described previously for the placenta. Cysts may form in the umbilical cord from remnants of the umbilical stalk or allantois, or much more frequently from liquefaction of the myxomatous tissue of the cord; but they probably do not jeopardize fetal circulation. The great edematous change in the umbilical cord frequently seen in association with certain macerated fetuses is effect rather than cause. Although varices of the cord are not neoplasms, they may rarely rupture as the result

of undue stress and thus may be clinically significant to the extent that this accident can result in fetal death.

Inflammation

Dominguez and co-workers found leukocytic infiltration in the umbilical cord in about one quarter of all single births, although not all such findings are indicative of true inflammation. The Wharton's jelly and the adventitia of the funic vessels become infiltrated with inflammatory cells when the cord begins to be macerated after death of the fetus or in cases of severe intrapartum infection. Bacteria may occasionally enter the fetal circulation directly from the wall of the uterus. Bacteria may enter fetal vessels traversing the cord or membranes without going first to the maternal circulation. The low frequency of such infections of the fetus, however, makes this hazard more theoretical than real. Leukocytic infiltrations of the cord occur occasionally without demonstrable cause, and have been mistaken for manifestations of syphilis. Scrapings from the intima of the vessels may be subjected to darkfield examination to rule out the presence of *Treponema pallidum*.

REFERENCES

Abdul-Karim, R. W., Nesbitt, R. E. L., Jr., Drucker, M. H., and Rizk, P. T.: The regulatory effect of estrogens on fetal growth. 1. Placental and fetal body weights. Am. J. Obstet. Gynecol., *109*:656, 1971.

Ackermann: Der weisse Infarct der Placenta. Virchows Arch. Pathol. Anat., *96*:439, 1884.

Adair, F. L., and Thelander, H.: A study of the weight and dimensions of the human placenta in its relation to the weight of the newborn infant. Am. J. Obstet. Gynecol., *10*:172, 1925.

Aherne, W., and Dunnill, M. S.: Morphometry of the human placenta. Br. Med. Bull., *22*:1, 1966.

Anderson, W. R., and McKay, D. G.: Electron microscope study of the trophoblast in normal and toxemic placentas. Am. J. Obstet. Gynecol., *95*:1134, 1966.

Ballantyne, J. W.: The Disease and Deformities of the Foetus. Edinburgh, Oliver and Boyd, 1892, 1895.

Barry, F. E., McCoy, C. P., and Callahan, W. P., Jr.: Hemangioma of umbilical cord. Am. J. Obstet. Gynecol., *62*:675, 1951.

Bartholomew, R. A.: Pathology of the placenta, with special reference to infarcts and their relation to toxemia of pregnancy. J.A.M.A., *111*:2276, 1938.

Bartholomew, R. A., and Kracke, R. R.: The probable role of the hypercholesteremia of pregnancy in producing vascular changes in the placenta, predisposing to placental infarction and eclampsia. Am. J. Obstet. Gynecol., *31*:549, 1936.

Bartman, J., and Driscoll, S. G.: Amnion nodosum and

hypoplastic cystic kidneys. Obstet. Gynecol., 32:700, 1968.

Benirschke, K.: Origin and clinical significance of twinning. Clin. Obstet. Gynecol., 15:220, 1972.

Benirschke, K.: Chimerism and mosaicism—two different entities. In R. Wynn (ed.): Obstetrics and Gynecology Annual. New York, Appleton-Century-Crofts, 1974.

Benirschke, K., and Drescoll, S. G.: The Pathology of the Human Placenta. New York, Springer Verlag, 1967.

Benirschke, K., and Kim, C. K.: Multiple pregnancy. N. Engl. J. Med., 288:1276, 1329, 1973.

Blanc, W. A.: Pathways of fetal and early neonatal infection: viral placentitis, bacterial and fungal chorioamnionitis: J. Pediat., 59:473, 1961.

Borell, U., Fernström, I., and Westman, A.: Arteriographic study of the placental circulation. Geburtsh. u. Frauenheilk, 18:1, 1958.

Bourne, G. L.: The Human Amnion and Chorion. Chicago, Year Book Medical Publishers, 1962.

Bourne, G. L., and Benirschke, K.: Absent umbilical artery. Arch. Dis. Child., 35:534, 1960.

Boyd, J D., and Hamilton, W. J.: The Human Placenta, Cambridge, W. Heffer & Sons, 1970, pp. 114–189; 313–334.

Boyd, J. D., and Hughes, A. F. W.: Observations on human chorionic villi using the electron microscope. J. Anat., 88:356, 1954.

Browne, F. J.: Abnormalities of the umbilical cord which may cause fetal death. J. Obstet. Gynaecol. Br. Emp., 32:17, 1925.

Browne, J. C. M., and Veall, N.: The maternal placental blood flow in normotensive and hypertensive women. J. Obstet. Gynaecol. Brit. Emp., 60:141, 1953.

Bühler, F. R.: Randbildungen der menschlichen placenta. Acta Anat. 59:47, 1964.

Burgos, M. H., and Rodriguez, E. M.: Specialized zones in the trophoblast of the human term placenta. Am. J. Obstet. Gynecol., 96:342, 1966.

Caldeyro-Barcia, R.: In Physiology of Prematurity. J. T. Lanman (Ed.): Transactions of the First Conference. New York, Josiah Macy, Jr., Foundation, 1957.

Caldeyro-Barcia, R.: Oxytocin and contractility of the pregnant human uterus. In The Uterus. Transactions of New York Academy of Sciences, 1958.

Chacko, A. W., and Reynolds, S. R. M.: Embryonic development in the human of the sphincter of the ductus venosus. Anat. Rec., 115:151, 1953.

Clemenz, E.: Kritische und historische Untersuchungen üben die weiten Nekrösen der Placenta. Z. Geburtsch: Gynäk., 84:758, 1922.

Clifford, S. H.: Postmaturity, with placental dysfunction. J. Pediat., 44:1, 1954.

Coblentz, D. R., Cimini, R., Mikity, V. G., and Rosen, R.: Roentgenographic diagnosis of congenital syphilis in the newborn. J.A.M.A., 212:1061, 1970.

Crawford, J. M.: Vascular anatomy of the human placenta. Am. J. Obstet. Gynecol., 84:1543, 1962.

Currie, G. A., Van Doorninck, W., and Bagshawe, K. D.: Effect of neuraminidase on the immunogenicity of early mouse trophoblast. Nature (Lond.), 219:191, 1968.

Curtius, F.: Nachgeburtsbefünde bei Zwillingen und Ähnlichkeitsdiagnose. Arch. Gynäk, 140:361–366, 1930.

Dempsey, E. W.: Discussion. Gestation. Transactions of the First Conference. New York, Josiah Macy, Jr., Foundation, 1955, p. 38.

Dempsey, E. W., Wislocki, G. B., and Amoroso, E. C.: Electron microscopy of pig's placenta, with especial reference to the cell-membranes of the endometrium and chorion. Am. J. Anat., 96:65, 1955.

Diczfalusy, E.: Endocrine functions of the human fetoplacental unit. Fed. Proc., 23:791, 1964.

Dominguez, R., Segal, A. J., and O'Sullivan, J. A.: Leukocytic infiltration of the umbilical cord. Manifestation of fetal hypoxia due to reduction of blood flow in the cord. J.A.M.A., 173:346, 1960.

Dreskin, R. B., Spicer, S. S., and Greene, W. B.: Ultrastructural localization of chorionic gonadotropin in human term placenta. J. Histochem. Cytochem., 18:862, 1970.

Eastman, N. J., and Hellman, L. M.: Williams Obstetrics, 13th ed. New York, Appleton-Century-Crofts, 1966, p. 949.

Eden, T. W.: A study of the human placenta, physiological and pathological. J. Pathol. Bact., 4:265, 1897.

Enders, A. C.: A comparative study of the fine structure of the trophoblast in several hemochorial placentas. Am. J. Anat., 116:29, 1965.

Elliott, P. M., and Inman, W. H.: Volume of liquor amnii in normal and abnormal pregnancy. Lancet, 2:835, 1961.

Finn, J. L.: Placenta membranacea. Obstet. Gynecol., 3:438, 1954.

Finn, R., Clarke, C. A., Donohoe, W. T. A., McConnell, R. B., Sheppard, P. M., Lehane, D., and Kulke, W.: Experimental studies on the prevention of Rh haemolytic disease. Br. Med. J., 1:1486, 1961.

Fränkel, E.: Über placentär Syphilis. Arch. Gynäk., 5:1, 1873.

Freedman, W. L., and MacMahon, F. J.: Placental metastasis. Review of the literature and report of a case of metastatic melanoma. Obstet. Gynec., 16:550, 1960.

Froehlich, L. A., Fujikura, T., and Fisher, P.: Choriangiomas and their clinical implications. Obstet. Gynecol. 37:51, 1971.

Galton, M.: DNA content of placental nuclei. J. Cell Biol., 13:183, 1962.

Gellhorn, A., Flexner, L. B., and Hellman, L. M.: The transfer of sodium across the human placenta. Am. J. Obstet. Gynecol., 46:668, 1943.

Gey, G. O., Seegar, G. E., and Hellman, L. M.: The production of a gonadotropic substance (prolan) by placental cells in tissue culture. Science, 88:306, 1938.

Gill, T. J.: Chimerism in humans. Transplant. Proc., 9:1423, 1977.

Golditch, I. M., and Boyce, N. E.: Management of abruptio placentae. J.A.M.A., 212:288, 1970.

Grosser, O.: Vergleichende Anatomie und Entwicklungsgeschichte der Eihäute und der Placenta mit besonderer Berücksichtigung des Menschen. Vienna, W. Braumüller, 1909.

Gruenwald, P.: The Placenta. Baltimore, University Park Press, 1975.

Hardy, J. B., Hardy, P. H., Oppenheimer, E. H., Ryan, S. J., Jr., and Sheff, R. N.: Failure of penicillin in a newborn with congenital syphilis. J.A.M.A., 212:1345, 1970.

Harter, C. A., and Benirschke, K.: Fetal syphilis in the first trimester. Am. J. Obstet. Gynecol., 124:705, 1976.

Hellman, L. M., Harris, B. A., and Andrews, M. C.: Studies of the metabolism of the human placenta, II. Oxygen consumption and anaerobic glycolysis in relation to aging and severe toxemia. Bull. Johns Hopkins Hosp., 87:203, 1950.

Hellman, L. M., and Hertig, A. T.: Pathological changes in the placenta associated with erythroblastosis of the fetus. Am. J. Pathol., 14:111, 1938.

Hertig, A. T.: Personal communication; angiogenesis in

the early human chorion. Contrib. Embryol., No. 146, 1935.

Hertig, A. T.: Pathological aspects. In The Placenta and Fetal membranes. Baltimore, Williams & Wilkins, 1960, pp. 109–124.

Hertig, A. T., and Rock, J.: Two human ova of the previllous stage. Contrib. Embryol., 184:127, 1941.

Hertig, A. T., and Sheldon, W. H.: Minimal criteria required to prove prima facie case of traumatic abortion or miscarriage. Ann. Surg., 117:596, 1943.

Holland, E.: Reports on public health and medical subjects (report on the causation of foetal death). London Ministry of Health, No. 7, 1922.

Hutchinson, D. L., et al.: The role of the fetus in the water exchange of the amniotic fluid of normal and hydroamniotic patients. J. Clin. Invest., 38:971, 1959.

Irving, F. C., and Hertig, A. T.: A study of placenta accreta. Surg. Gynec. Obstet., 64:178, 1937.

Javert, C. T., and Reiss, C.: The origin and significance of macroscopic intervillous coagulation hematomas (red infarcts) of the human placenta. Surg. Gynecol. Obstet., 94:257, 1952.

Kirsch, R. E.: Study on control of length of gestation in the rat with notes on maintenance and termination of gestation. Am. J. Physiol., 112:68, 1938.

Krantz, K.: Personal communication.

Lanman, J. T., Dinerstein, J., and Fikrig, S.: Homograft immunity in pregnancy: Lack of harm to fetus from sensitization of mother. Ann. N. Y. Acad. Sci., 99:706, 1962.

Levine, P., and Stetson, R. E.: Unusual case of intragroup agglutination. J.A.M.A., 113:126, 1939.

Liley, A. W.: Liquor amnii in the management of pregnancy complicated by rhesus sensitization. Am. J. Obstet. Gynecol., 82:1359, 1961.

Liley, A. W.: Intrauterine transfusion of foetus in haemolytic disease. Br. Med., J., 2:1107, 1963.

Mandel, H. S., Graff, S., and Graff, H.: Placental senescence and the onset of labor. Am. J. Obstet. Gynecol., 50:471, 1945.

Marais, W. D.: Human decidual spiral arterial studies. Part V. Pathogenetic patterns of intraplacental lesions. J. Obstet. Gynaecol. Br. Commonw., 69:944, 1962.

Martin, C. B., et al.: Intermittent functioning of the uteroplacental arteries. Am. J. Obstet. Gynecol., 90:819, 1964.

Maudsley, R. F., Brix, G. A., and Hinton, N. A.: Placental inflammation and infection: a prospective bacteriologic and histologic study. Am. J. Obstet. Gynecol., 95:648, 1966.

McKay, D. G., Hertig, A. T., Adams, E. C., and Richardson, M. V.: Histochemical observations on the human placenta. Obstet. Gynecol., 21:1, 1958.

Mechanic, K., Nasab, A. R. H., and Borazjani, G. R.: Bacterial infection of the fetus and placenta 1. Pathologic examination of 2000 cases in Iran. Int. J. Gynecol. Obstet., 8:304, 1970.

Millar, W. G.: A clinical and pathological study of placenta accreta. J. Obstet. Gynaecol. Br. Emp., 66:353, 1959.

Morison, J. E.: Foetal and Neonatal Pathology. Washington, D.C., Butterworths, 1963, pp. 512–513.

Mossman, H. W.: The rabbit placenta and the problem of placental transmission. Am. J. Anat., 37:433, 1926.

Mossman, H. W.: Comparative morphogenesis of the fetal membranes and accessory uterine structures. Contrib. Embryol., 26:129, 1937.

Nesbitt, R. E. L., Jr.: Prolongation of pregnancy: a review. Obstet. Gynecol. Surv, 10:311, 1955.

Nesbitt, R. E. L., Jr.: Postmature pregnancy: a clinical and pathologic appraisal. Obstet. Gynecol., 8:157, 1956.

Nesbitt, R. E. L., Jr.: Perinatal Loss in Modern Obstetrics. Philadelphia, F. A. Davis Co., 1957, pp. 91–146.

Nesbitt, R. E. L., Jr., and Anderson, G. W.: The Pathologic Aspects of Fetal Death in Utero, Pregnancy Wastage. E. T. Engle (Ed.). Springfield, Ill., Charles C Thomas, 1953, pp. 89–123.

Nesbitt, R. E. L., Jr., and Anderson, G. W.: Perinatal mortality: clinical and pathologic aspects. Obstet. Gynecol., 8:50, 1956.

Newton, W. H.: Hormones and the placenta. Physiol. Rev., 18:419, 1938.

Ossipoff, V., and Hall, B. D.: Etiologic factors in the anmiotic band syndrome: a study of 24 patients. Birth Defects, 13:117, 1977.

Paddock, R.: Recent observations on certain pathological conditions of the amnion. Am. J. Obstet. Gynecol., 8:546, 1924.

Page, E. W.: The Hypertensive Disorders of Pregnancy. Springfield, Ill., Charles C Thomas, American Lecture Series, 1953.

Page, E. W., Villee, C. A., and Villee, D. B.: Human Reproduction. 2nd Ed. Philadelphia, W. B. Saunders Company, 1976.

Pierce, G. B., Jr., and Midgley, A. R., Jr.: The origin and function of human syncytiotrophoblastic giant cells. Am. J. Pathol., 43:153, 1963.

Pritchard, J. A.: Deglutition by normal and anencephalic fetuses. Obstet. Gynecol., 25:289, 1965.

Race, R. R.: "Incomplete" antibody in the human serum. Nature, 153:771, 1944.

Ramsey, E. M.: Maternal and foetal circulation of the placenta. Irish J. Med. Sci., 140:151, 1971.

Ramsey, E. M.: Vascular adaptations of the uterus to pregnancy. In The Uterus. Transactions of New York Academy of Sciences, 1958.

Ramsey, E. M.: The placental circulation. In The Placenta and Fetal Membranes. C. A. Villee (Ed.). Baltimore, Williams & Wilkins, 1960, pp. 36–62.

Ramsey, E. M., Corner, G. W., Jr., and Donner, M. W.: Serial and cineradioangiographic visualization of maternal circulation in the primate (hemochorial) placenta. Am. J. Obstet. Gynecol., 86:213, 1963.

Reid, D. E., Ryan, K. J., and Benirschke, K.: Principles and Management of Human Reproduction. Philadelphia, W. B. Saunders Co., 1972.

Reynolds, S. R. M.: The proportion of Wharton's jelly in the umbilical cord in relation to distention of the umbilical arteries and veins with observations on the folds of Hoboken. Anat. Rec., 113:365, 1952.

Reynolds, S. R. M.: Hemodynamic characteristics of the fetal circulation. Amer. J. Obstet. Gynec., 68:69, 1954.

Reynolds, S. R. M.: Formation of fetal cotyledons in the hemochorial placenta. Am. J. Obstet. Gynecol., 94:425, 1966.

Romney, S. L., and Reid, D. E.: Observations on the fetal aspects of placental circulation. Am. J. Obstet. Gynecol., 61:83, 1951.

Rooth, G., and Sjövall, A.: Acid-base status of amniotic fluid during delivery. Lancet, 2:371, 1966.

Rothman, L. A., Cohen, C. J., and Astarloa, J.: Placental and fetal involvement by maternal malignancy. Am. J. Obstet. Gynecol., 116:1023, 1973.

Sciarra, J. J., Kaplan, S. L., and Grumbach, M. M.: Localization of anti-human growth hormone serum within the human placenta: Evidence for a human chorionic growth hormone—prolactin. Nature (Lond.), 199:1005, 1963.

Scott, J. S.: Placenta extrachorialis (placenta marginata and placenta circumvallata): A factor in ante-partum hemorrhage. J. Obstet. Gynaecol. Br. Emp., 67:904, 1960.

Sexton, L. I., et al.: Premature separation of the normally implanted placenta: a clinicopathological study of 476 cases. Am. J. Obstet. Gynecol., 53:13, 1950.

Shute, E.: Observations on aetiology of abruptio placentae and its response to vitamine E therapy. J. Obstet. Gynaecol. Br. Emp., 44:121, 1937.

Siddall, R. S., and Hartman, F. W.: Infarcts of the placenta. Am. J. Obstet. Gynecol., 12:683, 1926.

Siiteri, P. K., and MacDonald, P. C.: The utilization of circulating dehydro-iso-androsterone sulfate for estrogen synthesis during human pregnancy. Steroids, 2:713, 1963.

Siiteri, P. K., and MacDonald, P. C.: The biogenesis of urinary estriol during human pregnancy (abstract). Clin. Res., 12:44, 1964.

Siler-Khodr, T. M., and Khodr, G. S.: Content of luteinizing hormone–releasing factor in the human placenta. Am. J. Obstet. Gynecol., 130:216, 1978.

Simpson, J. Y.: Pathological observations on diseases of the placenta. Edinburgh Med. Surg. J., 265:45, 1836.

Smith, G. V., and Kennard, J. H.: Progestin and estrin of 19 placentas from normal and toxemic cases. Proc. Soc. Exp. Biol., 36:508, 1937.

Spanner, R.: Mütterlicher und Kindlicher Kreislauf der menschlichen Placenta und Seine Strombahnen. Z. Anat. Entwickl.-Gesch., 105:163, 1935. (Trans. Harris, B. A., Jr., Am. J. Obstet. Gynecol., 71:350, 1956.

Spellacy, W. N., Gravem, H., and Fisch, R. O.: The umbilical cord complications of true knots, nuchal coils and cords around the body. Am. J. Obstet. Gynecol., 94:1136, 1966.

Stander, H. J.: In Williams' Obstetrics. N. J. Eastman and L. M. Hellman (Ed.). D. Appleton-Century-Crofts, New York, 1936.

Strachan, G. I.: The development and structure of the human placenta. J. Obstet. Gynaecol. Br. Emp., 30:611, 1923.

Strong, S. J., and Corney, G.: The Placenta in Twin Pregnancy. Oxford, Pergamon Press, 1967.

Thiede, H. A., and Choate, J. W.: Chorionic gonadotrophin localization in the human placenta by immunofluorescent staining. II. Demonstration of HCG in the trophoblast and amnion epithelium of immature and mature placentas. Obstet. Gynecol., 22:433, 1964.

Thomson, V. M.: Amnion nodosum. J. Obstet. Gynaecol. Br. Emp., 67:611, 1960.

Tominaga, T., and Page, E. W.: Accommodation of the human placenta to hypoxia. Am. J. Obstet. Gynecol., 94:679, 1966.

Torpin, R.: The human placenta; its shape, form, origin, and development. Springfield, Ill., Charles C Thomas, 1969.

van Wagenen, C., and Jenkins, R. H.: An experimental examination of factors causing ureteral dilatation of pregnancy. J. Urol., 42:1010, 1939.

van Wagenen, G., and Newton, W.H.: Pregnancy in the monkey after removal of the fetus. Surg. Gynecol. Obstet., 77:539, 1943.

Villee, C. A.: Biochemical differentiation of human fetal tissues with age. Prematurity, congenital malformation, and birth injury. Proceedings of a conference, sponsored by Association for the Aid of Crippled Children. New York, John B. Watkins Co., 1953, p. 78.

Villee, C. A.: Regulation of blood glucose in human fetus. J. Appl. Physiol., 5:437, 1953.

Villee, C. A.: The metabolism of human placenta in vitro. J. Biol. Chem., 205:113, 1953.

Villee, C. A.: Biochemical aspects. In The Placenta and Fetal Membranes. Baltimore, Williams & Wilkins, 1960, pp. 100–108.

Walker, J.: Fetal anoxia. J. Obstet. Gynaecol. Br. Emp., 61:162, 1954.

Wang, H. W., and Hellman, L. M.: Studies in the metabolism of the human placenta. Bull. Johns Hopkins Hosp., 73:31, 1943.

Webster, C. J.: Human Placentation. Chicago, W. T. Keener & Co., 1901.

Wentworth, P.: The incidence and significance of haemangioma of the placenta. J. Obstet. Gynaecol. Br. Commonw., 72:81, 1965.

Wiener, A. S.: A new test (blocking tests) for Rh sensitization. Proc. Soc. Exp. Biol., 56:173, 1944.

Williams, J. W.: Obstetrics. New York, Appleton-Century-Crofts, 1931.

Wislocki, G. B., and Bennett, H. O.: Histology and cystology of human and monkey placentae with special reference to the trophoblast. Am. J. Anat., 73:335, 1943.

Wislocki, G. B., and Dempsey, E. W.: Histochemical age-changes in normal and pathological placental villi (hydatidiform mole, eclampsia). Endocrinology 38:90, 1946.

Wislocki, G. B., and Dempsey, E. W.: Electron microscopy of the human placenta. Anat. Rec., 123:133, 1965.

Wynn, R. M.: Origin, cytochemistry and ultrastructure of the Hofbauer cells. Obstet. Gynec., 25:425, 1965.

Wynn, R. M.: Cytotrophoblastic specializations: an ultrastructural study of the human placenta. Am. J. Obstet. Gynecol., 114:339, 1972.

Wynn, R. M., and Davies, J.: Comparative electron microscopy of the hemochorial villous placenta. Am. J. Obstet. Gynecol., 91:533, 1965.

Young, J.: The aetiology of eclampsia and albuminuria and their relation to accidental hemorrhage. J. Obstet. Gynaecol. Br. Emp., 26:1, 1914.

Chapter 32

PATHOLOGY OF ABORTION (IN UTERUS, PLACENTA, APPENDAGES, AND OVOFETUS)

CARL J. PAUERSTEIN

Definition

The term "abortion" designates a pregnancy that has terminated prior to the period of fetal viability. This period is arbitrarily set at 20 completed weeks of gestation. The fetus at this stage of pregnancy weighs approximately 500 gm. and its crown to rump length is about 18 cm.

Incidence

Precise information concerning the incidence of fetal deaths prior to the twentieth gestational week is not available. A relatively wide range has been reported, but about 10 per cent may be taken as the mean probability that a pregnancy will end in spontaneous abortion. These calculations are based by necessity upon clinically recognizable abortions. Pregnancy wastage in the first month is quite high but the rate in this preclinical phase is unknown. The peak incidence of abortion occurs during the eighth to twelfth weeks, the average date of expulsion being 10.2 weeks of menstrual age, according to Hertig. It is clear, however, that many early cases go unrecognized. The symptoms of pregnancy may escape notice, or the patient may attribute her problem to a transient menstrual abnormality. More recent studies suggest that 15 per cent may be a more accurate figure.

On the basis of studies of ova obtained from fertile patients, Hertig has indicated a theoretical abortion rate of 29 per cent, once the first menstrual period is missed. This figure is in keeping with the fate of potential embryos estimated from random groups of domestic animals. Casida has shown that in these animals the estimated percentage of actual embryos dying varies from about 30 to 60 per cent. Only one third of the ova in animals that produce litters reach a stage of development that coincides with a clinically recognizable pregnancy. The remaining two thirds of all ovulated ova fail to become fertilized or to undergo segmentation or implantation. The defective ova that produce clinically evident pregnancies but die before term may be analogous to the 10 per cent of human pregnancies that end in clinical abortion.

Etiology

Defective ova have been demonstrated in all species of animals. Abnormalities of embryonic development inconsistent with life are present in the human in about one half of all early abortions (Hertig and Sheldon). The reported incidence of gross chromosomal defects in abortuses is quite high, varying from 22 to 60 per cent in various series. Many aborted fetuses have XO set chromatin ab-

633

normalities and, since they are chromatin negative, the assumption has been that male fetuses are aborted more frequently than female fetuses. Nevertheless, according to Lauritzen, the male to female ratio was found to be 0.96 in a cytogenetic study of 288 abortuses. The incidence of defective development of the ovum in spontaneous abortions decreases progressively after the first four to six weeks of gestation.

Evidence has accrued to indicate that both intrinsic and environmental factors are responsible for abortion. It is customary to classify abortions into two major groups: those believed to be due to ovular or fetal factors and those due to maternal factors. Although the classification has some merit for recording purposes, it is too crude to convey precise information concerning the etiology of abortion. A complete analysis of all causative factors involved is impossible.

Which comes first in the early pathology of implantation, the death of the egg from lethal and sublethal genes originating in the germ cells or the pathologic environment of the uterus? This may be a moot question in the individual case. In some instances the primary cause of the embryonic defect may be clear, but in the majority the attempt to separate genetic factors and those of the environment is futile and ignores the interaction of the two.

Warburton and Fraser have emphasized that the interaction of the fetal genotype and its environment decides the course of development. The fetus' environment, its mother's uterus, is determined by another heredity-environmental complex, namely, the interaction of the mother's genetic makeup and her environment. Abnormal fetal development may be caused by a defect in any one of the components of this system.

It is now apparent that many of the genetically based malformations and embryonal deaths noted in Drosophila in the early 1900's by Bridges and others have clinical counterparts in human reproduction. Defective germ plasm resulting in the development of a rudimentary embryo has been noted in one vesicle of double-ovum twins, whereas the other contained a normal embryo. This finding seems to incriminate a genetic fault because both ova were implanted upon the same decidua. Boué and co-workers found chromosomal anomalies consisting of polyploidy (30 per cent), autosomal trisomy (50 per cent), and monosomy X (20 per cent) in nearly 60 per cent of cases of spontaneous abortion.

Most recent studies indicate that the incidence of such abnormalities is high (Carr, Lauritzen, Kajii et al.). The incidence of chromosomal errors has been related to gestational age. Spontaneous abortions in the first 6 weeks have the highest incidences of cytogenetic aberrations (70 per cent). When the first 10 weeks are included, the incidence falls to 50 per cent, and when all abortions (0 to 20 weeks) are included the incidence will be 20 per cent. The variation in chromosomal errors found in different series probably originates from differences in gestational ages of the abortuses studied.

Aberrations of the maternal environment may bring about defective embryonic development and antenatal death at any early stage of pregnancy, depending upon the degree and duration of insult. The factors that affect intrauterine environment are only partially understood, but it is apparent that growth and development of the embryo may be seriously affected by local conditions in the uterus or by factors removed from the ovum itself. Moreover, a variety of insults, such as radiation, viruses, and chemicals, may affect both the embryo and the intrauterine environment, and may lead either to abortion or to anomalous development of the fetus. Trauma and psychogenic factors have perhaps been overemphasized in the etiology of abortion.

The two viruses definitely known to produce fetal anomalies are those of rubella and cytomegalic inclusion disease, while many others, notably those of hepatitis, herpes simplex, variola, chickenpox, and mumps, may infect the embryo or fetus and cause abortion, fetal death, or neonatal disease. Other infections, notably certain protozoa, spirochetes, and bacteria, which disseminate by the bloodstream, can result in transplacental infection and fetal jeopardy. For example, *Listeria monocytogenes* can occur in utero, causing fetal infection early in pregnancy, or, apparently, in repeated pregnancies, resulting in abortion.

The tendency for abortion to occur more often in certain women than in others indicates that at least some of the causes are recurrent. This tendency may be due to persistent factors in the mother's environment or, possibly, to the aftermath of the initial insult. At present there is no clear evidence to suggest which of the genetic mechanisms may be a cause of repeated abortion. Moreover, there does not appear to be any sound evidence that relates semen quality to habitual abortion, although it seems clear that occasionally sperm capable of fertilization can be responsible for the production of defects in embryogenesis.

It has become increasingly apparent that faulty environment may be a factor common to a spectrum of fetal wastage, including early and late fetal death, premature birth, and malformations. Recurring factors which are inimical to fetal welfare are responsible for disproportionate perinatal wastage in certain segments of the population. The following interrelated factors seem to be particularly important in contributing to pregnancy inefficiency:

1. Very young or advanced maternal age;
2. Previous perinatal losses;
3. Poor socioeconomic status;
4. Prolonged conception-effort time;
5. Impaired maternal health (hypertension, diabetes, infections, syphilis, chronic debilitation);
6. Anatomic defects of generative tract (myoma, adenomyosis, congenital uterine anomalies, incompetent cervical os);
7. Adnexal or pelvic pathology (tumor or infection);
8. Blood incompatibilities between mother and fetus;
9. Psychogenic factors;
10. Endocrine imbalance;
11. Out-of-wedlock pregnancies.

ENDOCRINE FACTORS

Endocrine dysfunction is one of the best documented etiologic factors common to patients who have experienced repeated abortions; however, despite this fact, such insults rarely can be incriminated as causal in the isolated case. Many of these patients exhibit evidence of a fundamental endocrine imbalance over a period of years, often taking the form of long periods of infertility or disturbances of menstruation. The reproductive problem may be looked upon merely as one clinical expression of a basic derangement of reproductive physiology. A properly prepared progestational endometrium, which furnishes proper nutritive conditions for nidation and retention of the ovum, is dependent upon proper ovarian function and a uterus capable of responding to the steroids elaborated by the ovary. When this preparation is defective, the ovular bed collapses, and death or pathologic development of the conceptus is a probable eventuality.

The relationship between the endometrium, chorion, and formation of the decidua is crucial in determining the type of placenta that develops. A well developed placenta produces and secretes adequate amounts of estrogen and progesterone. These steroids not only keep the decidua alive but also maintain the metabolic processes that are essential for fetal growth. There is a synergism between the secretion of chorionic gonadotropin by the trophoblast and the secretion of progesterone and estrogen by the ovary. A vicious cycle may ensue, however, when ovarian function is poor, because the trophoblast may fail to develop properly if the endometrium is not supported adequately. The defective trophoblast, in turn, fails to secrete adequate quantities of chorionic gonadotropin. Consequently, the poorly stimulated corpus luteum may not elaborate enough steroids to prevent further deterioration of the decidua.

Proper hormonal support of the endometrium during implantation and placentation is important to satisfactory fetal growth and development. Although the process of implantation is complex and varies greatly from one species to another, experimentation seems to indicate that a subcritical dose of progesterone administered at the time of implantation in certain castrated animals (rabbit, rat) may result in maldevelopment of the placenta. The progestational support of the endometrium may be sufficient to permit implantation but inadequate to promote placental growth or to sustain the embryo beyond a certain stage of development.

The close correlation between the endocrine pattern and the pathologic type of abortus is amply documented by the studies of Braunstein and co-workers, who studied 256 women in the first 100 days of gestation. In this report, the authors were able to document low gonadotropin production in 57 per cent of pregnancies that terminated in spontaneous abortion, 100 per cent of ectopic pregnancies, and 60 per cent of multiple pregnancies. Thus, a low production of chorionic gonadotropin indicates a poor prognosis for the pregnancy and presumably indicates a defective trophoblast. Similarly, a persistently low excretion of placental steroids portends poorly for the pregnancy and

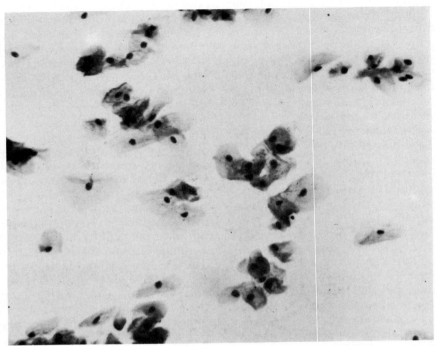

Figure 32–1. Normal vaginal smear of pregnancy showing predominance of precornified cells.

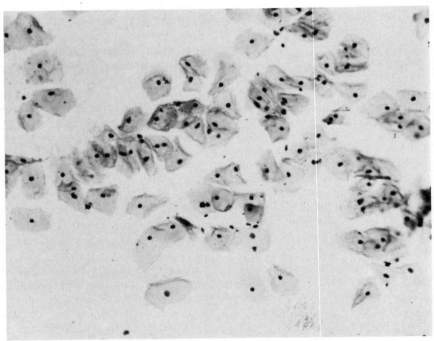

Figure 32–2. Abnormal vaginal smear of pregnancy showing predominance of cornified, superficial cells (high karyopyknotic index).

may connote a primary trophoblastic defect (Nesbitt et al.). At this late stage the vaginal smear, which mirrors the degree of progestational domination, usually reveals a high proportion of karyopyknotic, eosinophilic superficial cells (Figs. 32–1 and 32–2).

It is not possible to incriminate progesterone deficiency as the primary factor in abortion because the deficiency may be either cause or effect.

It is possible to make certain inferences about the patient's endocrine status by taking note of the pathologic types of previous abortuses. This information may be a helpful guide in selecting the appropriate work-up for these patients. If the patient has aborted well-formed fetuses, the likelihood of this fundamental defect is much less. If an endocrinopathy exists, it is likely to be mild. The presence of abnormal staining reactions, vascular thrombosis, and infiltration of erythrocytes and leukocytes in the stroma of the decidua obtained by biopsy in patients who were bleeding during the first 4 months of pregnancy enabled Rutherford to differentiate between patients with and without blighted ova. It should be noted that McCombs and Craig have demonstrated that decidual hemorrhage is common even in normal early pregnancies.

In cases of late abortion it is advisable to search for other etiologic factors, such as medical diseases, anatomic defects (congenital anomalies of the uterine corpus, i.e., double or bicornuate uterus, septate or subseptate uterus, etc.), uterine or pelvic pathology, and cervical incompetence.

PROGESTATIONAL PHASE ENDOMETRIUM

Current interest in preconceptional work-up and therapy to detect and prevent a faulty nidation environment deserves special comment. The uterus is the target organ in these investigations, and, because the endometrium reflects the function of the hypothalamus-pituitary-ovarian system, attention is properly directed to the end organ response. The primary objective in these assessments is to select from a group of patients with repeated abortions those whose progestational endometrial responses are definitely and consistently underdeveloped (Hughes et al.,

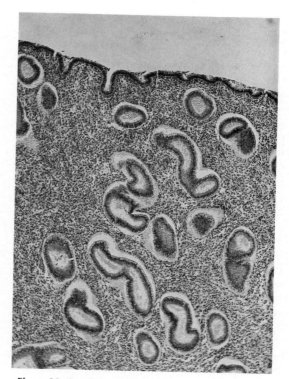

Figure 32–3. Premenstrual endometrium showing inadequate and underdeveloped secretory responses.

Noyes) (Fig. 32–3). Tissue is obtained by uterine curettage or by biopsies taken from the endometrium at about the middle of the progestational phase when secretory development is optimal. The most developed areas of the endometrium should be dated on the basis of standardized, histologic criteria and compared with menstrual dates and the basal body temperature curve. These evaluations should be made through several cycles to assure an accurate diagnosis, particularly if substitution therapy is contemplated. Defective luteal function can also be identified by demonstrating abnormal steroidogenesis, or a decreased luteal span, or both. The normal luteal phase is characterized by a biphasic basal body temperature, in which the temperature rise is sustained for more than 12 days. The following biochemical criteria of normalcy have been cited: (1) The estrogen rise bears the proper temporal relationship to the LH peak; (2) the LH peak occurs at least 13 days prior to the onset of menses; (3) an initial rise in plasma 17-hydroxyprogesterone levels occurs coincident with the LH rise; (4) a second rise in plasma 17-hydroxyprogesterone occurs later, coincident with the rise in plasma progesterone; (5) plasma progesterone begins to rise at the LH peak, and reaches a maximum six to eight days after the LH peak; (6) estrogen secretion attains appropriate levels.

The reader is referred to Chapter 8 for a summary discussion of cyclic and pregnancy changes in the endometrium. Suffice it to say here that in the midprogestational phase maximal secretion is observed in the glandular lumina. During active secretion the stroma is edematous, mitosis is absent, and the spiral arterioles are prominent.

Although there is widespread use of progesterone therapy to avert abortion in cases of suspected progestational deficiency or as a prophylactic measure, reported results are conflicting and difficult to evaluate. Certainly, once bleeding, persistent brown vaginal discharge, or cramps develop, the outlook is exceedingly poor, and seems to be uninfluenced by such therapy. It should be noted that these events are rarely causal and usually become clinically apparent several weeks following death of the embryo.

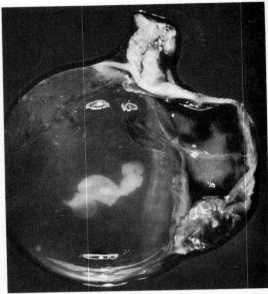

Figure 32–4. Abortus, Carnegie type V. The cephalic pole of the embryo is easily recognizable.

MECHANISM OF ABORTION

Regardless of the primary cause, the precipitating cause of abortion is the regressive decidual change, necrosis and hemorrhage, and separation of the placenta. In most instances the pathologic changes are secondary to fetal death, which occurs an average of 6 weeks before the abortus is expelled.

There is a progressive deterioration of placental function following death of the fetus, and a reduction in steroid production, which thus fails to maintain the integrity of the decidua. The uterus becomes increasingly irritable and eventually labor is initiated, which results in the expulsion of the products of conception.

In the early months of gestation the uterine attachments are somewhat tenuous and, in the course of labor, the fetal sac and the decidua are usually extruded intact. The expelled conceptus is likely to present as an opaque, fluid-filled sac with a thickened area representing the placenta over part of the surface (Fig. 32–4). In some instances, a decidual cast of the uterus is attached or the ovum may be encapsulated by a layer of clotted blood and intermixed villi (blood or carneous mole). When the ovum is nodular in

appearance because of the presence of subchorial hematomas of varying size, the specimen is referred to as a tuberous mole. The villi may be thick and distended with fluid and there may be some constriction of the base of the saclike branches where they arise from their villous stems. The embryo may be absent, represented by a small amorphous mass, macerated, compressed, or even mummified, depending upon the length of time the conceptus is retained after death of the embryo as well as other factors.

At a somewhat later date and until about the fourteenth gestational week, portions of the villous structure may be torn from the uterine wall and expelled in the course of labor, but some chorionic tissue usually remains adherent. The pathologic specimen is incomplete but fragmented, and may be obtained in full only through uterine curettage. After this stage of pregnancy, a normal third stage mechanism of labor is possible, however, and it is not unusual for the complete placenta and membranes to be expelled shortly after delivery of the fetus. In these cases of late abortion, the placental detachment may occur initially in the center of the placenta, with the development of a retroplacental hematoma or at the periphery of the placenta, much like noted in more advanced pregnancy.

PATHOLOGIC CHARACTERISTICS OF THE OVOFETUS

A careful, systematic examination of the ovofetus should be carried out in all cases with a view toward proper classification of the pathologic observations. Mall and Meyer, Hertig and co-workers, and Javert have devised classifications for pathologic ova. The basic classification of Mall and Meyer (Carnegie Classification), as modified by Hertig, has met the test of time, although certain minor alterations may seem desirable to meet the requirements of a particular institution. The basic classification may be summarized as follows:

Group I. Villi Only. The specimen contains only chorionic villi, whether normal or abnormal. This group includes true hydatidiform moles without even traces of chorionic membrane.

Group II. Villi and Chorion Only. There is no derivation of the inner cell mass and the amnion is absent.

Group III. Villi, Chorion, and Amnion Only. There is no evidence of an embryo. If the sac has been ruptured, one should exclude the possibility that an embryo was formed by making certain that a torn stump of umbilical cord is not present. Rupture of the sac makes it difficult occasionally to distinguish between this category and the preceding one characterized by an absence of the amnion. It is advisable, therefore, to designate a subgroup indicating the state of the sac (intact or ruptured).

Group IV. Chorion and Amnion Containing a Nodular Embryo. The embryonic mass consists merely of a disorganized group of cells. Care should be taken not to confuse a macerated stump of umbilical cord for a nodular embryo.

Group V. Chorion and Amnion Containing a Cylindric Embryo. One pole of the embryo is recognizable, usually the head end (Fig. 32–4.)

Group VI. Chorion and Amnion Containing a Stunted Embryo. The embryonic form is easily recognizable, but it is stunted when a comparison is made of its size and the gestational age (Fig. 32–5). One or more portions of the embryo may be atrophic, deformed, or degenerated (Fig. 32–6).

Group VII. Chorion and Amnion Containing a Macerated Embryo. In some classifications this group is eliminated, because the fetuses are anatomically normal and their

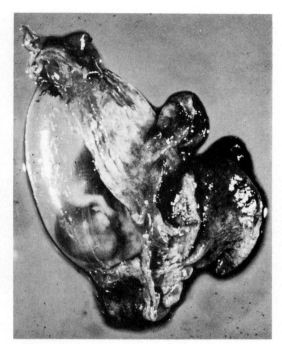

Figure 32–5. Abortus, Carnegie type VI. The embryonic form is easily recognized, but it is stunted when a comparison is made of its size and the gestational age.

growth pattern until death is commensurate with the gestational age (Fig. 32–7). They may possess localized anomalies, such as deformed limb buds or neuroskeletal defects, but these are not necessarily incompatible with full term development of the fetus. The presence or absence of such localized defects and their types, as well as the state of tissue preservation, should be listed in one or more subgroups of this major category. Macerated fetuses showing major developmental defects should not be assigned to this category but placed in their appropriate group as outlined. Nearly one half of all the fetuses subjected to study show maceration in some degree. Most of these are actually missed abortions, although this is not always apparent clinically.

CLASSIFICATION OF INCOMPLETE SPECIMENS

The vast majority of early pathologic ova available for complete study fall into Groups II, III, and IV. However, a large proportion of the pathologic material derived from spontaneous abortions is incomplete and is

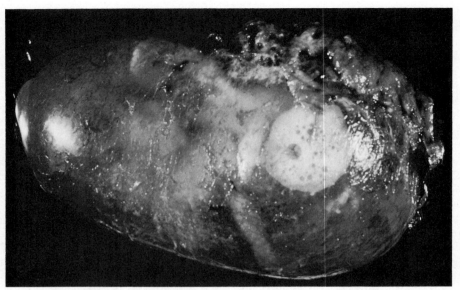

Figure 32–6. Abortus, Carnegie type VI. The caudal portion of the embryo is degenerated.

recovered by uterine curettage (Fig. 32–8). The fragments of placental villi and decidual tissue from these incomplete abortions are not classifiable according to one of the major categories. A separate group may be devised to include these specimens ("decidua without villi" or "villi only") or this material may be included as a subcategory in Group I of the basic classification, to distinguish it from a true mole.

Certain curettings show only old hemorrhagic, necrotic, inflamed tissue without villi, which is hardly discernible as decidua (Figs. 32–9 and 32–10). In some cases of this

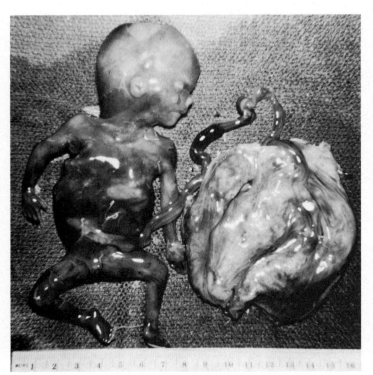

Figure 32–7. Abortus, Carnegie type VII. Formed fetus commensurate in size with gestational age.

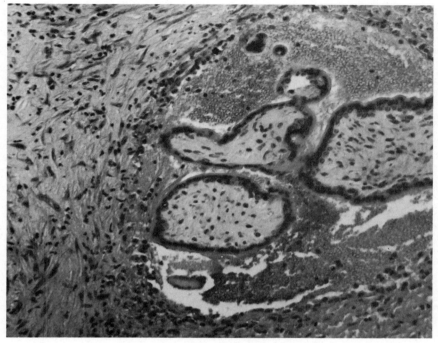

Figure 32–8. Uterine curettings showing decidua and chorionic villi in spontaneous abortion.

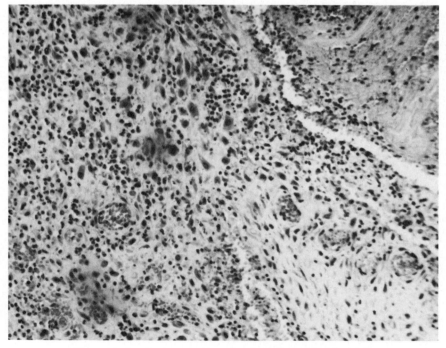

Figure 32–9. Uterine curettings showing inflamed decidual tissue.

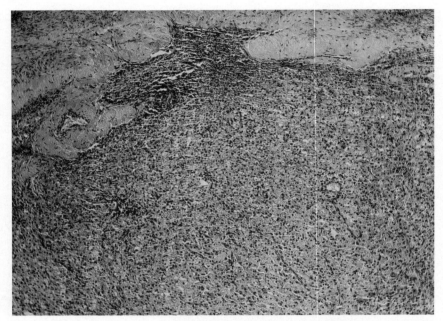

Figure 32–10. Uterine curettings showing necrotic, markedly infected decidua without villi.

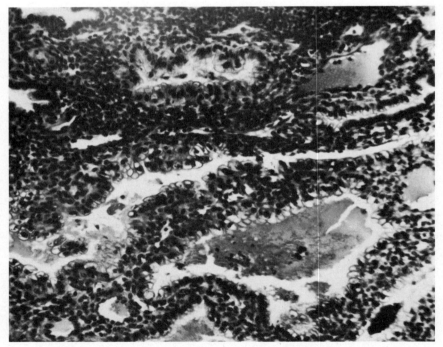

Figure 32–11. Endometrial glands showing Arias-Stella phenomena.

type the diagnosis of pregnancy is presumptive. Many of these cases are septic abortions with necrosis, liquefaction, and suppuration of the retained secundines. A careful medical history and assessment of the patient's clinical course may help to establish the correct diagnosis.

In 1954, Arias-Stella described atypical, focal, adenomatous changes in the endometrium arising as a result of the presence of chorionic tissue in the body. It was possible to demonstrate these changes in both intrauterine and extrauterine pregnancy and also in cases of hydatidiform mole and choriocarcinoma. The endometrial glands present a mixed and atypical pattern characterized by proliferative as well as secretory gland types, intraluminal budding, atypical cell changes, nuclear hypertrophy and hyperchromasia, cellular reduplication, mitoses, and syncytial masses of vacuolated cells (Fig. 32–11). These histologic changes are of diagnostic value only when positive, because the endometrium may not show these characteristics when the chorionic tissue, wherever located, is dead or markedly degenerated.

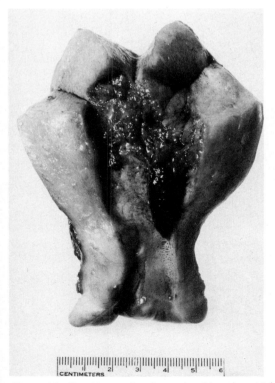

Figure 32–12. Uterus showing polypoid endometrial hyperplasia.

Certain patients may experience profuse uterine bleeding following a period of amenorrhea. These patients, who may be considered pregnant at the time of curettage, often show well-developed endometrial hyperplasia. In some instances this pathologic finding is a consequence of exogenous estrogen therapy. Javert refers to these cases as pseudo- or phantom abortions. If an endometrial polyp is present in association with the hyperplastic endometrium, the problem of differential diagnosis may be even more confusing (Fig. 32–12). Rarely, tuberculous endometritis may be encountered under similar clinical circumstances or in association with abortion.

CLASSIFICATION OF SPECIMENS IN SPECIAL CLINICAL GROUPS

For the sake of complete recording, it is desirable to extend the rather broad classification of abortuses to include, whenever possible, any specific medical, anatomic, or endocrinologic condition which might account for death of the fetus and its ultimate expulsion from the uterus. When specific information is lacking, however, it is far better to indicate this fact than to hypothesize that the ovum is defective or to incriminate some vague lethal gene as the causative factor.

In multiple pregnancy, comparisons of each fetus are made according to the standard classification. The pathology of twin fetuses and placentas is essentially the same as that observed in single gestation, although the incidence of significant pathologic changes appears to be increased in the former (Fig. 32–13).

In twin gestation there may be a gradually increasing area of the communicating portion of the placenta which is monopolized by one embryo, so that the blood supply providing nourishment to the twin is compromised. In extreme cases, the compromised twin may be represented by a shapeless mass, *acardius amorphus*. However, it seems possible that this condition comes from an original failure of parts to form, and not from secondary atrophy.

When one fetus reaches an advanced state of maceration because of long retention in the uterus, it may become compressed between the uterine wall and the membranes of the living twin. Under such circum-

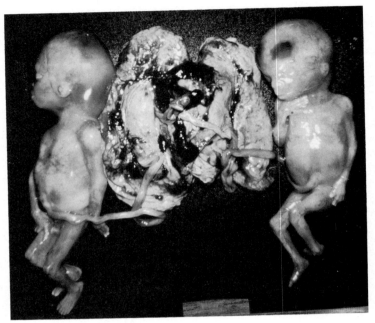

Figure 32–13. Twin abortuses. Carnegie type VII.

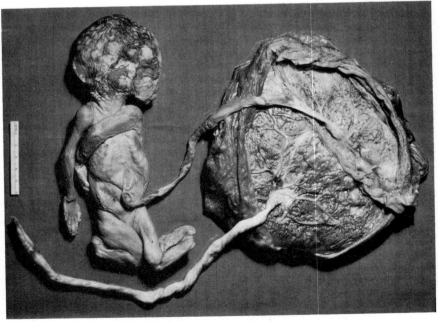

Figure 32–14. Fetus papyraceus.

stances, the tissues of the dead fetus become dehydrated, flattened, and partially mummified, a condition known as *fetus papyraceus* (Fig. 32–14).

CHANGES IN THE DECIDUA AND UTEROPLACENTAL AREA

Many specimens are derived from missed abortions and may be expelled from the uterus in a state of advanced deterioration. Necrosis, hemorrhage, and thrombosis throughout the decidual plate are common pathologic changes noted in these cases. Among patients whose clinical courses are septic, there may be marked inflammatory changes. The pathologic specimen is usually fragmented material passed spontaneously or recovered by curettage of the uterus. In almost all instances there is hemorrhage, thrombosis, necrosis, and inflammation, in some degree. Leukocytic infiltration may be prominent only in areas of tissue destruction, or there may be diffuse inflammation with focal abscesses throughout the decidual plate. The bacteria most commonly encountered are coli-aerogenes and anaerobic streptococci, whereas hemolytic streptococci, staphylococci, and clostridia are seen less frequently.

In some cases of abortion, a distinct retroplacental hematoma is present. This lesion is characterized by an adherent, organized blood clot which is discolored, laminated, and surrounded by decidual necrosis and pigmented phagocytes. These gross and histologic observations in spontaneous abortion are also noted in placental abruptions at later stages of pregnancy. Placenta previa may be encountered in abortion material, although this problem is primarily seen in the late second and third trimesters. In the abortion period, the specimen may show evidence of molding by the cervical canal, in addition to an organized blood clot at the lower margin of the placenta.

Discrete endometrial polyps may be found occasionally in curettage specimens. The histologic findings in these specimens include hemorrhage, necrosis, inflammation, and hyaline degeneration. Young, as well as Hertig and Rock, and Javert have reported cases in which an early human ovum and implantation site were lodged in a structure resembling a polyp.

It seems clear that certain alterations of the placental structure may have their origin in an ill-prepared and poorly sustained decidua which leads to faulty placentation. An implantation defect or poor decidual response may lead to a persistence of functioning villi over the surface of the ovum that are evident at term (placenta membranacea). Under similar circumstances, there may be a conversion of a smaller than normal portion of the ovum into the chorion frondosum. The resulting chorionic plate is due to repetitive peripheral hemorrhages that lead to the formation of circumvallation. Circumvallate placenta is the most common pathologic condition in second trimester abortion. These defects, in the extreme, may lead to serious complications in the course of pregnancy and to fetal death.

CHANGES IN THE PLACENTA

The placenta undergoes progressive deterioration following death of the fetus, but it is remarkable that this organ may remain fairly well preserved, even though the fetus may be absent or markedly macerated. Placental observations noted in abortion specimens are similar to those encountered in pregnancies that proceed beyond the period of fetal viability, although the stage of pregnancy influences greatly the frequency of their occurrence.

The placentas of late abortuses may exhibit abnormalities of attachment, separation, and form and, very rarely, benign tumors are present (see Chapter 33). Likewise, these specimens may show the specific lesions of tuberculosis and hemolytic disease or there may be nonspecific degenerations in association with maternal diabetes, hypertensive disorders, and chronic wasting diseases of the mother. In endemic areas, malarial parasites are commonly found in the vascular spaces of the placenta. Likewise, *Brucella abortus, Listeria monocytogenes, Toxoplasma,* and other organisms implicated in abortion are demonstrable in the aborted tissues on occasion.

A common histologic feature of placentas recovered from spontaneous abortions is fibrinoid degeneration of chorionic villi. This lesion may be patchy or diffuse and may be found in association with syncytial degeneration, endarteritis, fibrosis, and clubbing of the terminal villi (Fig. 32–15). Intervillous thrombosis and infarction of the pla-

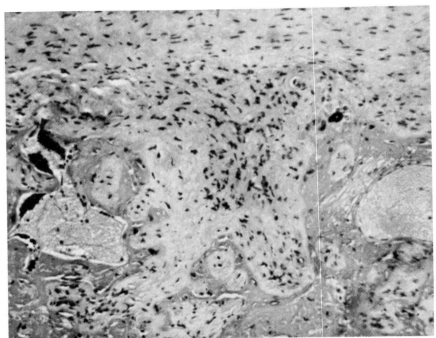

Figure 32–15. Fibrinoid degeneration of chorionic villi showing fibrosis, clubbing, endarteritis, and disappearance of trophoblast.

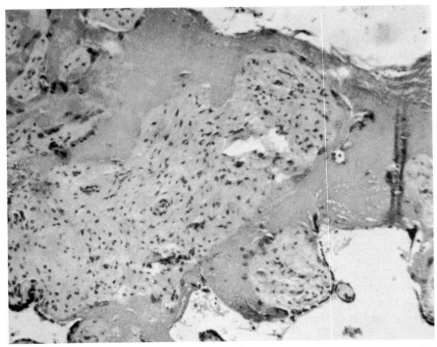

Figure 32–16. Intervillous thrombosis with fibrosis and ischemic necrosis of chorionic villi.

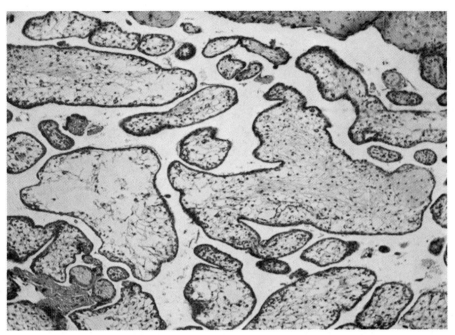

Figure 32–17. Chorionic villi showing hydropic degeneration.

centa in the involved areas are seen less commonly (Fig. 32–16). Large infarcts may seriously interfere with metabolic exchange within the placenta and ultimately lead to the death of the fetus.

Careful study of the villous structures reveals areas of hydropic degeneration in some degree in a relatively high percentage of aborted specimens (Fig. 32–17). Hertig observed degenerative changes of this type in 63 per cent of abnormal ova. When this histologic change is diffuse, one may occasionally have difficulty in distinguishing it from true hydatidiform mole. The significant finding in the latter condition is proliferation of the trophoblast rather than changes in the villous stroma. When attention is directed to this histologic feature, one can usually distinguish between the two lesions without difficulty (see Chapter 33).

Hydropic degeneration of villi, with either an empty sac or a degenerated embryo, and evidence of recent hemorrhage, necrosis, and inflammation of the decidua, are often found in combination. The incidence of significant changes in the placenta is highest among pathologic ovofetuses and least when the fetus is normal.

Hertig and Sheldon found abnormalities of the placenta in association with normal embryos in 9.6 per cent of 1000 abortuses subjected to careful histologic study. The most common derangements were circumvallate placenta (4.5 per cent), hypoplasia (2.0 per cent), and Breus's mole (1.9 per cent). Patients who had anatomically normal ova constituted 26.6 per cent of the entire series. In a study of placentas of abnormal karyotypes, Honoré and co-workers found that the most common pathologic lesion is that of depressed growth activity and dysmorphogenesis. Many of these changes are degenerative in type, however, and should not be implicated as causative factors in abortion.

CHANGES IN THE PLACENTAL APPENDAGES

Degenerative changes and inflammation are common findings in fetal membranes. The specific lesions are amnionitis and chorionitis and, in some cases, focal abscesses in the subchorionic regions (Fig. 32–18). Many of these patients will have experienced premature rupture of the membranes, instrumental interference, and a septic clinical course, although these antecedents are not invariably present. Fre-

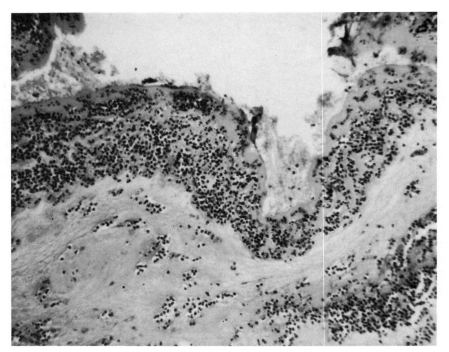

Figure 32–18. Acute chorioamnionitis.

quently, the mother's clinical course is benign and the membranes remain intact until the time of abortion.

An important feature of the pathologic examination of the abortion specimen is careful, systematic examination of the umbilical cord. The incidence of abnormal conditions of the umbilical cord among aborted specimens is high, although most of these are minor deviations from the norm and seem to be of little consequence. Javert has demonstrated that many so-called normal but macerated fetuses are associated with cord complications. He emphasizes that certain primary cord lesions may cause secondary anoxia and, finally, death in utero.

In addition to the common finding of degeneration, the umbilical cord may show a variety of pathologic conditions, either congenital or acquired. The most common congenital lesions are absence or rudimentary development of the cord, coarctation, absence of one artery, and other types of vascular anomalies. Rarely, one may discover a cyst, midgut herniations into the cord, or other evidence of faulty development of the abdominal stalk. Acquired conditions include mechanical problems of torsion, knotting, rupture of vessels with hematoma for-

mation, prolapse, and looping. Marked edema of the cord may be present, but this is usually found in association with a vascular obstruction secondary to looping or torsion. The latter complications appear to be found most commonly in cords of excessive length, although this is not a constant relationship.

Necrosis, hemorrhage, edema, and inflammation are common findings in the cord of abortion specimens. Acute or chronic inflammatory cells may be aggregated about the vascular structures or distributed diffusely throughout Wharton's jelly (Fig. 32–19). Inflammation may be of primary importance or secondary to any one of the previously noted pathologic conditions. Usually, this lesion of the cord is found in association with amnionitis, chorionitis, and deciduitis, or, less frequently, with inflammation of the fetal tissues.

HABITUAL ABORTION

It was formerly believed that when a patient had three or more consecutive abortions (habitual abortion), the prognosis for a subsequent pregnancy without appropriate therapy was so poor that one was justified in postulating a recurring etiologic factor.

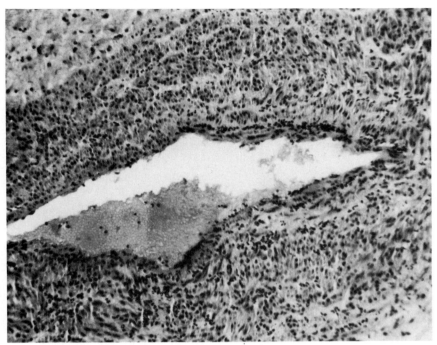

Figure 32–19. Acute inflammation of funis showing inflammatory cells aggregated about the umbilical vein.

Bishop gives the incidence of habitual abortion as 0.41 per cent of all pregnancies, and remarkably similar figures have been quoted by Hertig and by Javert. However, the ominous predictions of Malpas and of Eastman, according to which the risk of abortion increases progressively after each loss, appear to be exaggerated. The chance of repetition following a first abortion is about doubled, but thereafter, despite subsequent losses, the risks remain surprisingly constant—approximately 25 per cent. Cure rates of the order of 75 to 80 per cent reported for a host of therapeutic approaches must therefore be viewed with temperance.

Although abnormal sperm morphology has been incriminated as a rare cause of such repetitive losses, the majority are due to faulty environment. Aside from the endocrinologic aspects of the problem, medical diseases, anomalous conditions of the generative tract, pelvic pathology, and mechanical factors of the cervix have been implicated as occasional etiologic factors. A chromosomal etiology has been advanced by many authors. Khodr found that 6 per cent of the parents in cases of habitual abortion harbor a cytogenetic aberration.

Hardly germane to this chapter is a discus-

sion of the incompetent cervix in which an extremely lax internal os, often due to lacerations, infection, and scarring from previous trauma, may give rise to increased uterine contractility causing expulsion of the products of conception, usually in the second trimester. The latter specimens show no distinctive pathology, although the overall incidence of pathologic findings among second trimester aborters seems to be less than that observed in the specimens representing first trimester losses.

Pathologic ovofetuses occurring in habitual aborters were found in 27.4 per cent of 51 cases studied by Javert and in 36 per cent of 100 cases reported by Wall and Hertig. Lesions of the placenta were found in 31 per cent and 5 per cent, respectively, in these two studies. In Javert's study, the chief lesion of the placental membranes was infection. Javert reported a lower incidence of pathologic changes in the ovofetus, placenta, and cord in habitual abortion than in spontaneous abortion material taken as a whole. But in either group, the frequency of these lesions was substantially greater than that noted among patients whose pregnancies had been terminated by therapeutic abortion.

REFERENCES

Arias-Stella, J.: Atypical endometrial changes associated with the presence of chorionic tissue. Arch. Pathol., 58:112, 1954.

Bishop, P. M. F.: Studies in clinical endocrinology. "Habitual abortion"; its incidence and treatment with progesterone and vitamin E. Guy's Hosp. Rep., 87:362, 1937.

Boué, J., Boué, A., and Lazar, P.: Retrospective and prospective epidemiological studies of 1500 karyotyped spontaneous human abortions. Teratology, 12:11, 1975.

Braunstein, G. D., et al.: First trimester chorionic gonadotropin measurements as an aid in the diagnosis of early pregnancy disorders. Am. J. Obstet. Gynecol., 131:25, 1978.

Bridges, C. B.: Non-disjunction of the sex chromosomes of drosophila. J. Exp. Zool., 15:587, 1913.

Carr, D. H.: Chromosomes and abortion. In: Advances in Human Genetics, 2:201, 1971.

Casida, L. E.: Pregnancy Wastage. Springfield, Ill., Charles C. Thomas, 1953, p. 27.

Hertig, A. T.: Human Trophoblast. Springfield, Ill., Charles C Thomas, 1968.

Hertig, A. T., and Rock, J. A.: Series of potentially abortive ova. Am. J. Obstet. Gynecol., 58:968, 1949.

Hertig, A. T., and Sheldon, W. H.: Analysis of 1000 spontaneous abortions. Ann. Surg., 117:596, 1943.

His, W.: Anatomie Menschlicher Embryonen. Leipzig, F. C. W. Vogel, 1880, p. 39.

Honoré, L. H., Dill, F. J., and Poland, B. J.: Placental morphology in spontaneous human abortuses with normal and abnormal karyotypes. Teratology, 14:151, 1976.

Hughes, E. C., Lloyd, C. W., Van Ness, A. W., and Ellis, W. T.: The role of the endometrium in implantation and fetal growth. In Pregnancy Wastage. Springfield, Ill., Charles C Thomas, 1953, p. 51.

Javert, C. T.: Spontaneous and Habitual Abortion. New York, McGraw-Hill Book Co., The Blakiston Division, 1957, p. 104.

Kajii, T., Ohama, K., Nükawa, N., Ferrier, A., and Avirachan, S.: Banding analysis of chromosomal karyotypes in spontaneous abortion. Am. J. Hum. Genet., 25:539, 1973.

Khodr, G.: Cytogenetics of habitual abortion. Obstet. Gynecol. Surv., 29:299, 1974.

Lauritzen, J. G.: Aetiology of spontaneous abortion. Acta Obstet. Gynecol. Scand., Suppl. 52, 1976.

Mall, F. P., and Meyer, A. W.: Studies on abortions: survey of pathologic ova in Carnegie embryological collection. Contrib. Embryol., 12:56, 1921.

McCombs, H. L., and Craig, J. M.: Decidual necrosis in normal pregnancy. Obstet. Gynecol., 24:436, 1964.

Nesbitt, R. E. L., Jr.: Perinatal Loss in Modern Obstetrics. Philadelphia, F. A. Davis Co., 1957, pp. 29–55.

Nesbitt, R. E. L., Jr., Aubry, R. H., Goldberg, E. M., and Jacobs, R. D.: Correlated hormone excretion patterns and cytohormone variations in normal and complicated pregnancies. Am. J. Obstet. Gynecol., 93:702, 1965.

Novak, E. R., and Jones, G. S.: Novak's Textbook of Gynecology. 7th Ed. Baltimore, Williams & Wilkins, 1961.

Noyes, R. W.: The underdeveloped secretory endometrium. Am. J. Obstet. Gynecol., 77:929, 1959.

Rutherford, R. N.: The significance of bleeding in early pregnancy as evidenced by decidual biopsy. Surg. Gynecol. Obstet., 74:1139, 1942.

Velardo, J. T.: The Endocrinology of Reproduction. New York, Oxford University Press, 1958, pp. 111–125.

Wall, R. L., and Hertig, A. T.: Habitual abortion: a pathologic analysis of 100 cases. Am. J. Obstet. Gynecol., 56:1127, 1948.

Warburton, D., and Fraser, F. C.: Genetic aspects of abortion. Clin. Obstet. Gynecol., 2:22, 1959.

Young, J.: The uterine mucosa in menstruation and pregnancy: the action of the chorionic cells and the function of the decidua. Proc. Roy. Soc. Med., 4:291, 1910.

Chapter 33

HYDATIDIFORM MOLE AND CHORIOCARCINOMA (TRD)

Incidence

Trophoblastic disease (TRD), an inclusive term for hydatidiform mole and choriocarcinoma (chorionepithelioma), represents an unusually complex pathologic problem, as will become apparent in this chapter. In addition, there is little opportunity to study TRD in animals, as will be noted.

Hydatidiform mole is a relatively uncommon disease, which occurs in the United States in approximately 1 in every 2000 to 2500 pregnancies. For unknown reasons certain areas of the Far East, such as the Philippine Islands, as well as our own geographic neighbors (Mexico, for instance), have a 10 times greater incidence—up to an amazing 1 in 82 pregnancies in Taiwan. Most of the patients are of the extremely poverty-stricken group wherein an inadequate diet is standard. Protein deficiency is frequently cited as a factor in the development of trophoblastic disease, and seems a more likely cause than a rice diet. The excellent review by Reynolds suggests a submarginal absorption of folic acid and histadine at a time when this is mandatory for adequate fetal angiogenesis. Frequent gastrointestinal malabsorption (as with tropical sprue, vitamin deficiency, etc.), or the overcooking of such borderline protein foods as beans and rice might well serve as contributory factors.

Fox and Tow find definite differences between ethnic groups. A low chorionic gonadotropin (HCG) level at 7 to 17 weeks is predominant in Chinese women, who have a high incidence of mole and whose socioeconomic status is also exceedingly low, in contrast to various ethnic groups in India and Pakistan. Other groups react differently.

The interest in these disease of the trophoblast—*hydatidiform mole* and *choriocarcinoma*—has in recent years been heightened because of increased knowledge of the biologic properties they possess, and their importance in diagnosis and prognosis. Recently this measurable endocrine response to abnormal trophoblastic tissue has become more important than pathologic criteria in the vital decision as to the type and extent of treatment in certain patients; determination of HCG (human chorionic gonadotropin) is indicative of functioning trophoblast in areas where biopsy diagnosis is difficult or impossible.

Despite increasing knowledge of the disease and ability to adequately suppress certain trophoblastic lesions, there remain many uncertain features. That choriocarcinoma is frequently preceded by mole is certain; that mole only rarely progresses to choriocarcinoma is likewise true. In the report from Sweden by Ringertz, only 3.5 per cent of 654 cases of mole progressed to invasive mole or choriocarcinoma. The exact percentages may be difficult to stipulate because of continued inability to comprehend many facets of benign hydatidiform mole and its malignant counterpart, choriocarcinoma or chorionepithelioma. Although they are both diseases of the trophoblast, they may have different modes of origin, although choriocarcinoma is often an apparent sequel to mole.

There is still much to learn concerning these abnormalities of pregnancy. In proportion to their infrequency, more mistakes of diagnosis are probably made in this field than in almost any other encountered in the average pathology laboratory. In addition, the clinical pattern does not always follow the given rules for its histologic type.

Pseudomalignant Properties of Normal Trophoblast

Before discussing the lesions to which this chapter is devoted, it may be well to recall that normal trophoblast exhibits some of the attributes ordinarily associated with malignancy. The very implantation of the fertilized ovum in the endometrium is due to the *invasive* properties of the trophoblast, whereas the maintenance of its early nutrition is dependent upon the maternal blood set free by the destructive penetration of the maternal blood vessels by the advancing trophoblast. In addition, a species of physiologic *metastasis* of trophoblast is seen in the deportation to the lungs of such tissue.

As early as 1893 this *deportation of villi* was described by Schmorl, and his work has been amply confirmed by other authors. A study by Attwood and Park suggests that trophoblast is found in the lungs of nearly half (43.6 per cent) of all pregnant women, although villi are uncommon.

On the other hand, one must remember that the reaction of the maternal organism to trophoblast is very different from that with malignant tumors. The invasion of the uterine wall by trophoblast is restricted, being held within normal limits by a *local* defensive mechanism probably residing in the decidua, although its exact nature remains obscure. In addition to this local defensive factor, it is clear that there must by one of *systemic* nature, probably in the nature of an antigen-antibody reaction.

More recent studies by Douthwaite and Urbach suggest that trophoblast has a *sialomucin* coating and that, despite antigenic incompatibility, this tends to prevent detection by immunologically competent cells. While it is apparent that there are profound immunologic factors in the failure to reject trophoblast, the precise mechanisms remain uncertain, although the possibilities are discussed by Billingham and by Bagshawe.

Adcock and co-workers suggest that HCG may represent a trophoblastic cell surface antigen which blocks rejection of the trophoblast by maternal lymphocytes, and

that lymphocyte response is important in the prognosis of TRD. Various studies by Siiteri and associates indicate that the high level of progesterone in early gestation may be immunosuppressive. Bagshawe was unable to correlate the clinical course with the HLA antigen of the patient, her husband, or antecedent child. The recent review by Fuller and co-workers stresses the many uncertainties in the immunologic mechanisms involved in TRD, but obviously such are operative. Certain blood groups (type A) seem more likely to contract such malignant disease as choriocarcinoma, but this is uncertain, as is regression of TRD after paternal skin grafts.

How else can one explain the spontaneous lysis of the trophoblast which migrates to the lung in normal pregnancy? How, other than by the assumption of local and systemic defensive factors, can we explain the disappearance of the trophoblastic residua left in the uterine wall after full term pregnancy or miscarriage, or the frequent disappearance, without later sequelae, of the often fairly massive trophoblastic residua left deep in the uterine wall after the evacuation of a hydatidiform mole?

An additional problem in the comprehension of trophoblastic disease is its extreme rarity in the usual laboratory animal. Lindsey and colleagues record a case of a bona fide choriocarcinoma which developed spontaneously in a rhesus monkey—the only known example in a nonhuman primate. Ramsey and co-workers caution against the common tendency to make comparisons between humans and animals and point out various dissimilarities in monkeys, baboons, and humans.

On the other hand, Shintani and associates have induced choriocarcinoma (as well as other types of uterine malignancy) by removing the fetus from a pregnant rat and instilling benzanthracene into the fetal sac. Other, similar early studies are reviewed by Shintani and co-workers.

HYDATIDIFORM MOLE

There is still a difference of opinion as to whether hydatidiform mole is to be considered a degenerative or a neoplastic lesion. Hertig and Mansell believe that mole is a degenerative process, though capable of neoplastic change (i.e., choriocarcinoma), and the direct causation of the hydatid process is seemingly an agenesis of the fetal cardiovascular structure in conjunction with a functioning maternal apparatus and intact trophoblast. Indeed, mole should be considered merely as a form of missed abortion, although this viewpoint is difficult to reconcile with the occasional occurrence of a viable fetus in conjunction with mole (when there is a single placenta). A few cases of intrauterine pregnancy (with normal placenta) coexisting with hydatidiform mole have been reported (Jones and Lauerson). Baggish hypothesizes that mole might arise by endoreduplication of the second polar body. This might explain the twin pregnancy (mole and fetus) and the frequency of chromatin-positive moles (Fig. 33–1 B). Perhaps there is more than one method of genesis.

Carr has suggested that hydropic changes are especially common following discontinuance of oral contraceptives. Hydatid change or mole may be related to a chromosomal anomaly, generally triploidy, and a hormone imbalance. Evaluation of chromosomes in TRD may present considerable technical difficulties.

Microscopic Characteristics

The pathologic changes that characterize hydatidiform mole are trophoblastic proliferation, hydropic degeneration of the villous stroma, and scantiness of blood vessels (Fig. 33–2).

Until the epoch-making studies of Marchand (1895), the stromal degenerative changes were looked upon as of cardinal importance, but there have been many who stressed the vascular as well as the stromal changes. Many years ago Meyer, on the basis of extensive studies at the Carnegie Institute of Embryology, urged this viewpoint, stating that "a villus with a normal stroma and normal vascularization never was found to have undergone true hydatidiform degeneration, but one with a normally active epithelium—both Langhans layer and syncytium—often was truly hydatidiform" (Fig. 33–3). Most investigators believe that early hydatidiform degeneration, commonly unrecognized because unaccompanied by trophoblastic changes, explains many early abortions for which there is no other apparent cause.

Trophoblast. Although it is possible that earlier and as yet unrecognized phases will be demonstrated in the future, the prevailing viewpoint has been that the most important factor in hydatidiform mole is the trophoblastic proliferation, involving both the Langhans layer and the syncytium (Fig. 33–4).

Electron microscopy suggests that the syncytiotrophoblast is derived from the cytotrophoblast (Langhans layer), and various apparent intermediate transition cells have been demonstrated. Garancis and co-workers confirm this, as well as provide important information about the mucoprotein lining of the trophoblast.

Moderate and localized proliferation of these layers is seen even in normal pregnancy, but in mole it is much more marked. Yet in many sections of benign hydatidiform mole one is struck by the complete, or almost complete, absence of trophoblastic activity. Usually, however, this is because such sections come from villi that have undergone degenerative changes as a result of growing away from their blood supply in the uterine wall. The hydatidiform vesicles that are expelled from the uterus, for example, commonly exhibit this absence of trophoblastic activity, as do many of the vesicles that are evacuated from the uterine cavity at operation. The same mole, however, may show a very different picture in the villi still attached to the uterine wall, for here trophoblastic proliferation is often so marked that it may lead to the suspicion of malignancy (Fig. 33–5). Epithelial proliferation is characteristically much less conspicuous in hydatidiform moles developing at an early stage of pregnancy.

It is because of these variations in the degree of trophoblastic overgrowth of evacuated or expelled molar tissue, as contrasted with the histologic picture of the same mole in situ in the uterine wall, that there is great hazard in utilizing the microscopic picture of the former in attempts at appraising the benign or malignant nature of the lesion, as Hertig and Sheldon have suggested. On the basis of the degree of trophoblastic proliferation and the presence or absence of evidences of what they designate as anaplastic change, which is unquestionably difficult to establish with lesions of the trophoblast, they attempted to distinguish six groups, as follows: benign, probable benign, possible benign, possible malignant, probable malignant, and malignant. It is difficult to believe that such delicate nuances of differentiation could be of practical value,

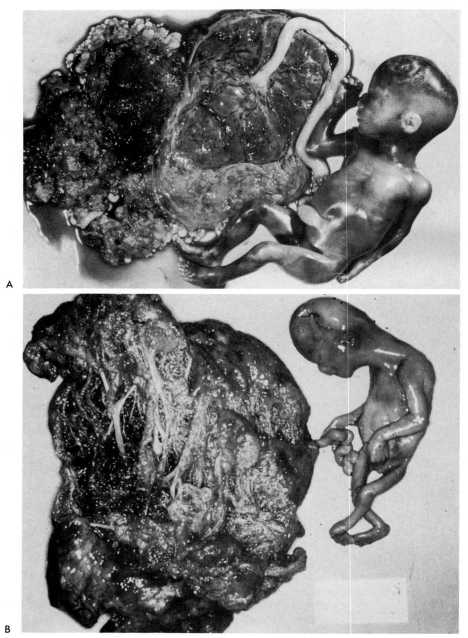

Figure 33–1. *A,* Six month fetus in association with hydatidiform mole. (Courtesy of Dr. N. A. Beischer, Melbourne, Australia) *B,* Similar fetus (Courtesy of Drs. C. M. Cabaniss and J. F. Clark, Washington, D. C.) *C,* Endoreduplication of second polar body with possible sequelae. (Courtesy of Dr. M. S. Baggish, Hartford, Conn.)

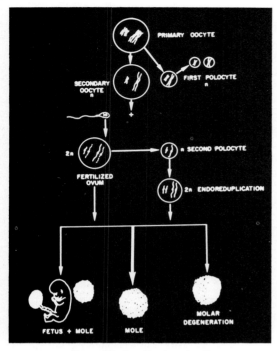

Figure 33–1. Continued. C

especially as most pathologists have only infrequent opportunity to examine molar tissues. Indeed, in a more recent publication, Hertig and Mansell have modified their *pathologic* classification into apparently benign, potentially malignant, and apparently malignant hydatidiform moles. *Clinically* there is an increased tendency to speak of TRD as *nonmetastatic* or *metastatic*.

It is easy to distinguish the Langhans cells from syncytium in the trophoblastic overgrowth. The former appear as well-differentiated cells, usually of cuboidal or polyhedral shape, with large, round, heavily stained nuclei. The syncytium, on the other hand, appears in the form of sheets of fenestrated amorphous masses with a disproportionately big nucleus and scant cytoplasm; on occasion only a large, dark nucleus is evident (Fig. 33–6).

The two elements, in other words, are practically identical to the two layers of the normal trophoblast; while there is some difference of opinion, it is generally accepted at this writing that the cytotrophoblast actively produces HCG, which is merely stored in the syncytium. In the syncytium are found numerous large and intensely stained nuclear masses. The budding tendency of the

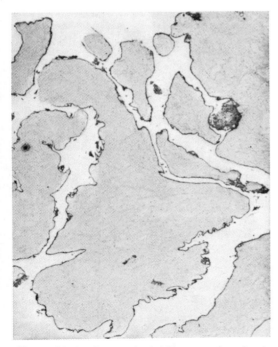

Figure 33–2. Benign hydatidiform mole, showing marked hydropic degeneration of stroma, no blood vessels, and no trophoblastic proliferation, probably because it has grown away from its blood supply.

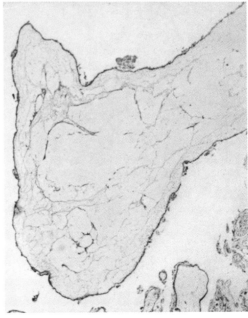

Figure 33–3. Giant villus of benign mole, with central cystic degeneration.

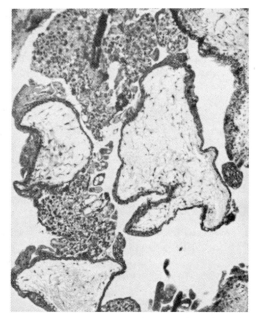

Figure 33–4. Benign hydatidiform mole with moderate trophoblastic proliferation.

syncytium produces on section the characteristic syncytial giant cells found in the vicinity of the villi, and often containing one or many central nuclei. Vacuolization is common with all trophoblast, and must not be mistaken for villi, which are generally larger and have a cellular lining.

Stroma. The stroma shows marked edema and myxomatous degeneration, with scant nuclei and with an absence of blood vessels. The remains of the stroma are often compressed into a thin zone flattened out against the wall of the villus, with a large central cavity filled with clear fluid. This waterlogging of the villus often makes it of gigantic size, transforming the villi into the large or small grapelike vesicles that characterize the mole macroscopically.

Summary of Characteristics of Benign Mole. The frankly benign hydatidiform mole, therefore, is characterized microscopically by a well-preserved villous pattern, by edema and degeneration of the stroma, scantiness of blood vessels, a considerable degree of trophoblastic activity, no tendency to penetrate into the stroma, and no destructive invasion of the uterine tissues such as characterizes the malignant prototype. It may, however, invade the blood channels (Fig. 33–7), as does the normal trophoblast. A positive chromatin pattern is almost uniform (Baggish et al.); the chromosomal pattern seems most uncertain, for there is con-

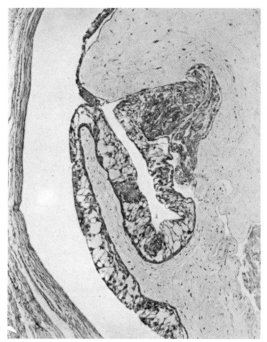

Figure 33–5. Large hydatidiform villus, with marked trophoblastic overgrowth and vacuolization.

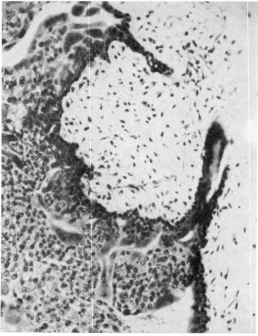

Figure 33–6. Marked proliferative overgrowth of trophoblast in (ovarian) hydatidiform mole.

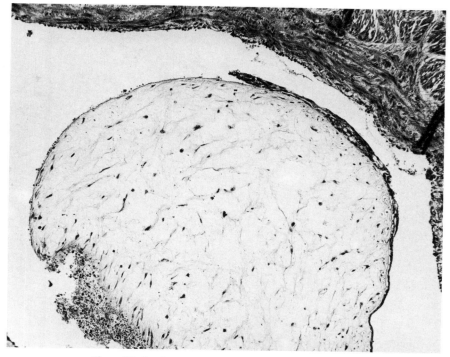

Figure 33–7. Innocuous appearing villus in uterine vein.

siderable divergence of opinion despite Carr's impression that triploidy is usual.

A frequent question involves differentiation between the placenta with hydatid degeneration and mole. The answer is more difficult, but when the process is diffuse, with associated trophoblastic proliferation, a mole is likely (Park). Szulman and Surti believe that mole (without fetus) exhibits a diploid pattern; hydatid degeneration is characterized by triploidy.

INVASIVE HYDATIDIFORM MOLE

(CHORIOADENOMA DESTRUENS)

Unfortunately, the criteria are not sharply defined in all cases. For example, the trophoblastic proliferation may be very pronounced and may invade the uterine muscle to a considerable distance, even though the villous pattern may be well retained (Fig. 33–8). A moderate number of mitoses may be seen. Various deviations from a frankly benign clinical course may be observed.

It is not strange, therefore, that an interme-

diate group has received separate classification under such designations as *malignant* or *invasive mole*, or *chorioadenoma destruens*. The latter term was applied by Ewing to this group, though it seems an ill-advised one. The term chorioadenoma was applied because of a supposed analogy of the chorionic villi with glands, but the comparison is not a good one. They are more nearly analogous, it seems, to the villi of the small intestine, both functionally and anatomically. A better term, therefore, for the destructive type of mole seems to be the older one of invasive mole, but the term chorioadenoma destruens appears to have established itself, in spite of its inappropriateness.

These cases are characterized by a pronounced tendency to invade the uterine and pelvic blood vessels, though distant metastases are rare. Indeed, in a report of 20 cases, Wilson and co-workers note 8 instances of pulmonary metastasis. In their study, as well as in others, actual histologic proof by lung biopsy was available on occasion. Thus it is obvious that metastasis may occur with these seemingly benign tumors, and on occasion with minimal histologic proliferative tendencies. Certainly, however, this is much

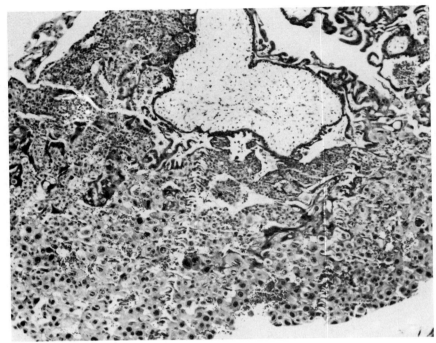

Figure 33–8. Section of chorioadenoma destruens, classified on basis of enormous trophoblastic proliferation and evidence of local invasion.

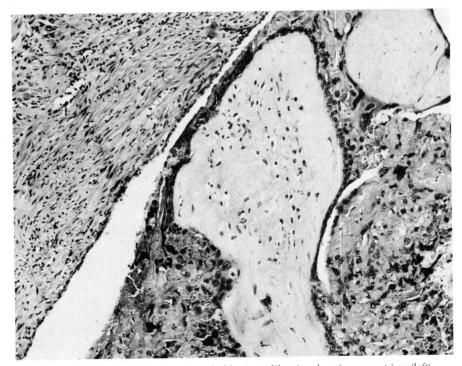

Figure 33–9. Villus with marked trophoblastic proliferation deep in myometrium (left).

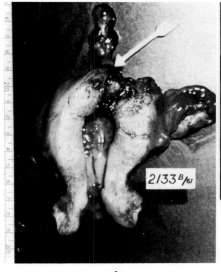

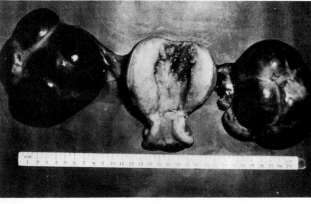

B

Figure 33–10. *A*, Early invasive mole with perforation dome of fundus. *B*, Bilateral theca lutein cysts with invasive mole (though may be associated with other forms of trophoblastic disease). (Courtesy of Dr. M. S. Baggish, Hartford, Conn.)

A

less frequent than with choriocarcinoma and, despite the pseudometastatic phenomenon, all cases were alive and well for 4 years or longer without definitive treatment, illustrating the ability of the uncertain systemic defense mechanism to neutralize the aberrant pulmonary trophoblast associated with invasive mole (Fig. 33–9).

Even perfectly benign moles may penetrate the blood channels of the uterus very deeply, so that in this respect the difference is a quantitative one. They show no such tendency to bulky trophoblastic invasion of the uterine muscle, with destruction of the latter, as characterizes invasive mole. Yet the vascular invasiveness, with the formation of metastatic nodules in the uterine wall and perhaps the penetration of the latter, brings about a condition which may run a clinically malignant course, with death from massive hemoperitoneum or vaginal bleeding (Fig. 33–10). They should, however, be regarded as generally benign, despite a mortality of 5 to 10 per cent.

Figure 33–11. Locally invasive mole (chorioadenoma destruens) with infiltration of myometrium. No metastases and patient well 5 years after hysterectomy.

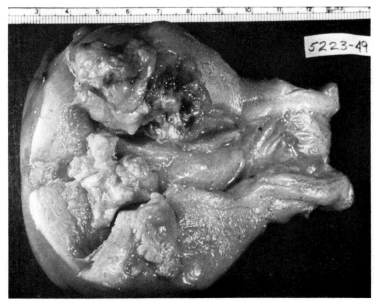

To sum up, therefore, the clinical criterion of the malignant mole is *local invasiveness with rare distant metastasis*. The pathologic criteria are (1) *abnormal penetration* into the uterine, parauterine, and adjoining vaginal tissue of moles which histologically may be similar to those of frankly benign type (Figs. 33–11 and 33–12); and (2) *excessive degrees of trophoblastic proliferation*, obviously a vaguer and more individual interpretation. When only undue penetration without excessive trophoblastic overgrowth is seen, the logical explanation, it seems, is an inadequacy of the local defensive mechanism against trophoblastic invasion. On the other hand, the presumed systemic defense mechanism has the capability of eliminating any hematogenous trophoblastic spread, although it apparently occurs on occasion.

As a general rule, the more complex and threatening the microscopic pattern, the greater the chances for subsequent malignant degeneration. On the other hand, we have seen malignant degeneration, metastatic phenomena, and death with even histologically benign disease. One simply cannot formulate specific rules for the behavior of trophoblast, although it is highly probable that there are varying degrees of cancer potentiality in moles, especially of the so-called chorioadenoma destruens group (Fig. 33–13). It is not always possible to determine these by the histologic appearance of

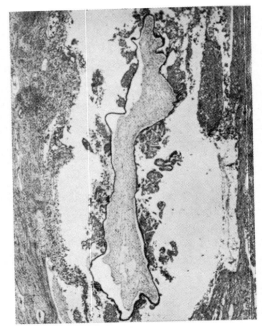

Figure 33–13. Chorioadenoma destruens of penetrative type. Histologically entirely benign, but patient died of deep penetration and intra-abdominal hemorrhage.

evacuated molar material. A persistently elevated or increasing HCG level is probably of more value to the clinician in evaluating persistent trophoblast that may or may not be acquiring malignant propensities (Fig. 33–14).

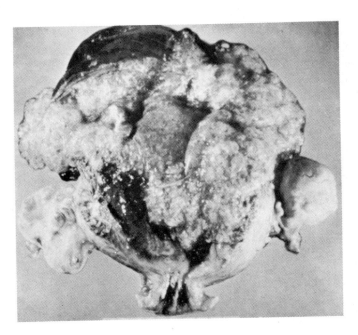

Figure 33–12. Another case of chorioadenoma destruens with marked local extension. (Courtesy of Dr. Paul Hodgkinson.)

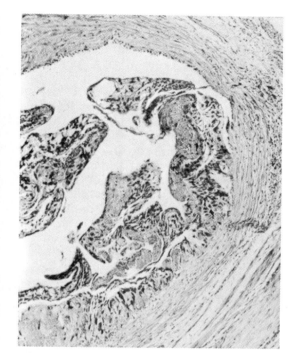

Figure 33–14. Large trophoblastic mass in uterine sinus. HCG was strongly postive 2 months after evacuation of a mole, probably because of the presence of such trophoblastic islands, which are often inaccessible to the curette. The lesion was clinically benign, as the patient remained well for 5 years after operation.

CHORIOCARCINOMA

The term choriocarcinoma seems to have generally replaced the older term chorionepithelioma, but actually these words may be used interchangeably. The chief distinguishing feature of genuine choriocarcinoma is invasion of the uterine wall by trophoblastic cells, with destruction of the uterine tissues, accompanied by necrosis and hemorrhage (Fig. 33–15). Chorionic villi are absent because the trophoblast grows in such extensive columns and masses as to completely obliterate the original villous pattern. Numerous blocks of curettings fail to show any trace of villi, though it must be repeated that their presence does not negate a diagnosis of subendometrial choriocarcinoma, for adequate representative tissue is not always passed vaginally or removed by the curette.

It is appropriate to note that choriocarcinoma is a tumor not of the uterus but of the embryonic chorion, the uterus being only secondarily involved through the local invasion of the tumor. It may be looked upon as a carcinoma arising from the villous epithelium or trophoblast much as an epidermoid

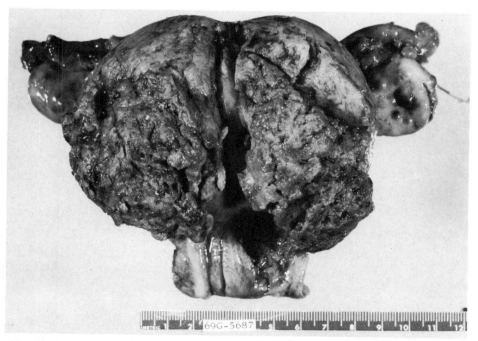

Figure 33–15. Choriocarcinoma with extensive involvement of the uterine wall though with no metastases (the exception).

carcinoma, for example, arises from the squamous epithelium of the cervix.

Microscopic Characteristics

The characteristic histologic picture of choriocarcinoma is that of columns or alveoli of trophoblastic cells, often separated by spaces filled with clotted blood, and pushing into the muscle tissue, the irregular line of advance being marked by destruction of the muscle. Hemorrhage and necrosis are constant features, to the extent that they may make identification of tumor cells difficult (Figs. 33–16 and 33–17).

Both layers of the trophoblastic epithelium participate in the malignant process, though there may be a predominance of either. It was once believed that growths showing a great predominance of syncytial elements are less malignant than those in which the Langhans elements predominate (Fig. 33–18), but this seems totally unpredictable. Although it is emphasized by most investigators that the trophoblast in choriocarcinoma shows definite and marked anaplastic activity, it should be remembered that evidences of anaplasia in the tropho-

blast are not always so clearly defined as in most other tissues. Hyperchromatism, with numerous large, heavily stained and perhaps multiple nuclei, is frequently seen (Figs. 33–19 A and 33–20), but may be found also in the benign hydatidiform mole, or even in normal trophoblast. Disparity in the nuclei and cytoplasm of the Langhans cells is more readily recognizable than in the syncytium, but is of little diagnostic aid. Cell changes are of less importance in diagnosis than the growth pattern of the tumor, for trophoblast itself is undifferentiated and active in its appearance. An Arias-Stella reaction may concur with TRD (Fig. 33–19 B).

Disappearance of Uterine Tumor

It must always be borne in mind that the invaded organ is by nature endowed with the capacity of resisting the encroachment of trophoblast. This resistance is not ordinarily sufficient to hold in check the invasiveness of malignant trophoblast, but in at least a small proportion it is. A considerable group of cases is recorded in which the uterus has completely thrown off the choriocarcinoma, the genuinely malignant nature of the origi-

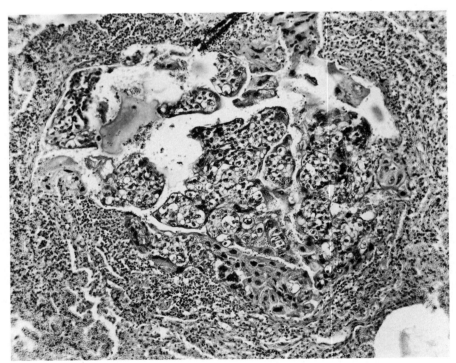

Figure 33–16. Typical picture of choriocarcinoma showing both syncytial and Langhans elements with extensive muscle necrosis.

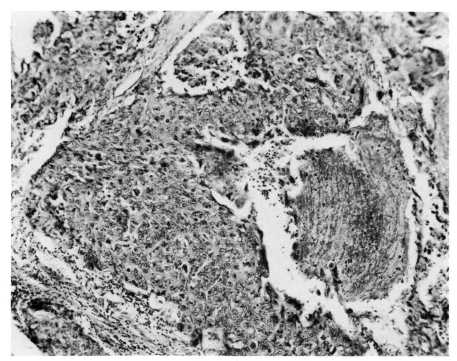

Figure 33–17. Extensive coagulation of invaded myometrium (right) with partial obliteration of tumor architecture due to necrosis and hemorrhage.

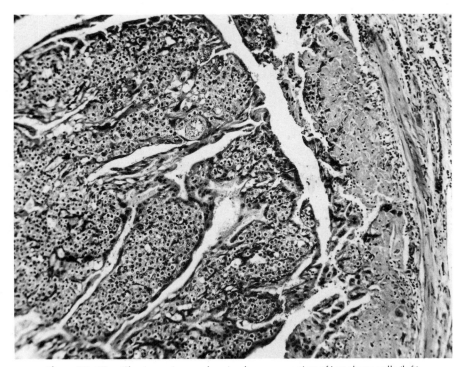

Figure 33–18. Choriocarcinoma showing large proportion of Langhans cells (left).

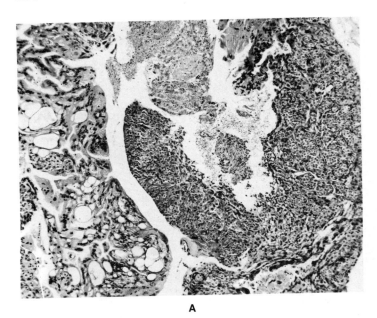

A

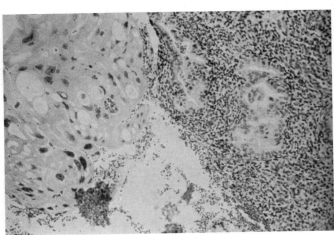

B

Figure 33–19. *A,* Chorionepithelioma-tous tissue obtained at curettage. Note extensive vacuolization which must not be mistaken for villi. *B,* Arias-Stella reaction (right) associated with choriocarcinoma (*A*).

nal uterine growth being verified because the patient has died from extensive extrauterine metastases. Such a case was reported by Novak and Koff, who collected other, similar instances from the literature. This has been well substantiated by Acosta-Sison, by Arias and Bertoli, and by other recent authors who have enumerated a number of cases with appropriate references. In addition, study of autopsy material from fatal cases of choriocarcinoma has presented an apparently retrogressive picture in some of the metastatic foci, especially in the lung. This must always be reckoned with, and it probably explains some of the vagaries of this disease.

The histologic picture presented in frank

choriocarcinoma is distinctive, and few mistakes are made in the diagnosis. Although false negatives (so to speak) should be rare, the false positives have created confusion in the evaluation of cases. *The diagnosis of choriocarcinoma has in innumerable instances been made in cases of benign mole, syncytial endometritis, and even entirely normal pregnancy.*

The presence of large masses of trophoblastic cells of both types but in varying proportion, often with mitoses and other anaplastic manifestations, which are more easily demonstrable in the Langhans cells than in the syncytium, the necrosis and hemorrhage, and *the almost invariable absence of villi*—all these compose a pattern difficult to mis-

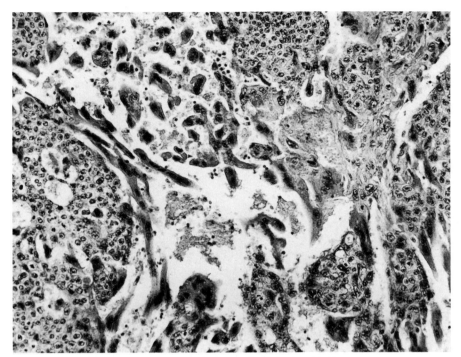

Figure 33–20. Another example of chorioepithelioma.

take, and quite different from the benign choriomas already described. One should abstain from a diagnosis of choriocarcinoma in the presence of well-formed villi, regardless of the amount of trophoblastic overgrowth.

Only once (Fig. 33–21) did definite villi occur in a choriocarcinoma (whose malignancy had been established beyond all doubt by extensive metastasis and death) in the long experience of Emil Novak. There is no doubt that in an occasional case villi may persist in isolated areas of transition from the normal or hydatidiform villi from which such tumors have their origin, but the occurrence must be rare. The exceptions are the cases of early choriocarcinoma, as noted in the next section.

Most cases show a varying combination of Langhans and syncytial elements, and it would not seem that the predominance of one or the other cell type is a determining factor in the ultimate prognosis of the case. It likewise seems impossible to correlate the proportion and amount of cyto- and syncytiotrophoblast with the level of the chorionic gonadotropin. Today, it is generally accepted that the cytotrophoblast is the more likely source of this hormone, and a high titre

is the rule, if *adequate* study of the serum is performed for HCG, despite reports of negative results in urinary assays with choriocarcinoma.

Early Choriocarcinoma

An exception to the usual form of malignant chorionic disease is exemplified by two initial cases reported by Brewer and Gerbie, of metastatic choriocarcinoma with a term pregnancy; villi were present in the very early placental lesion. These occurred in patients with a nonmolar pregnancy who had small lesions located in a grossly normal placenta, with a living fetus. Despite hysterectomy, death ensued because of metastatic choriocarcinoma. Van der Werf and associates have recently tabulated 17 cases of metastatic choriocarcinoma with pregnancy. Most patients presented with a vulvar or vaginal lesion with an advanced pregnancy. Serial sections of the placenta at delivery were necessary to establish the diagnosis.

In such cases chorionic villi may be present, as is a vascular supply, but the usual necrosis and hemorrhage found with most choriomas are absent. No villi are found in the metastatic lesions, perhaps because it is

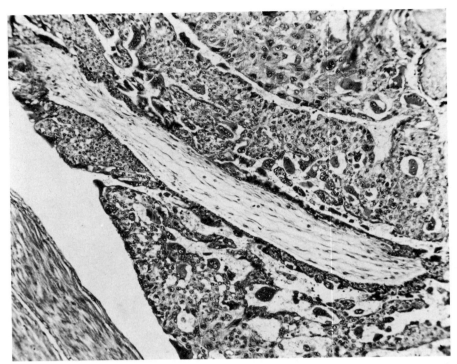

Figure 33–21. True choriocarcinoma with fatal pulmonary metastasis, uniformly accepted by Chorionepithelioma Registry. Note, however, well developed villus.

the proliferating trophoblast rather than the placental villus that is prone to erode into a vascular sinus. As the disease progresses there is invasion of the villous stroma by trophoblast and ultimate loss of the villous structure.

That these are exceptions to the usual histologic pattern of choriocarcinoma is apparent, but the cases reported are unusually early lesions; in the vast majority of instances, the criteria as noted seem valid.

SYNCYTIAL ENDOMETRITIS

This term refers to a postpregnancy condition of the uterine wall characterized by trophoblastic, chiefly syncytial, infiltration, with marked inflammatory reaction and perhaps necrosis. Its designation as a tumor is unjustified, as it represents only an unusual persistence of trophoblastic elements at the placental site after full term pregnancy or, more frequently, after abortion (Fig. 33–22).

It must be remembered that even in normal pregnancy the decidua is often infiltrated with trophoblastic cells. There is simi-

lar invasion of the myometrium beneath the implantation area, sometimes extending deep into the uterine wall, so that the term *syncytial (myo) metritis* might be more appropriate (Fig. 33–23). What has been said

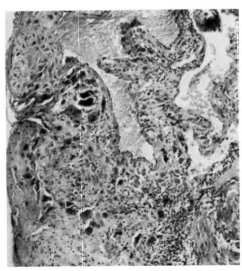

Figure 33–22. Syncytial endometritis in uterus removed by hysterectomy in a woman of 41 years, with large myomas and intrauterine pregnancy.

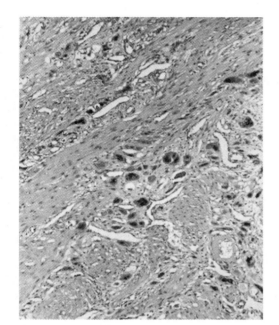

Figure 33–23. Trophoblastic invasion of myometrium, often seen in normal pregnancy and benign mole, and frequently mistaken for chorionepithelioma.

about normal pregnancy applies also to hydatidiform mole, in which such trophoblastic infiltration is sometimes very marked.

Such lesions may readily be mistaken for malignant mole or chorionepitheliomatous invasion, and this is an exceedingly common error for those not familiar with these changes. It is easy to see how the statistics of chorionepithelioma have been vitiated by the inclusion of cases thus wrongly diagnosed.

There are two chief points of difference between the normal trophoblastic invasion of the uterine wall and that seen in choriocarcinoma. In the former the cells infiltrate along the tissue spaces singly, and they produce none of the destructive or lytic effect which the more massive invasion of choriocarcinoma inflicts upon the maternal tissues. Not only do the infiltrating cells stain sharply and clearly, but so does the muscle in which they are scattered.

By contrast, the invasion of the uterine wall in choriocarcinoma is in the form of large columns or masses of trophoblast that destroy the muscle as they advance, so that varying degrees of coagulation necrosis and hemorrhage are seen. Other differences, such as anaplastic changes in the invading trophoblast, especially the Langhans cells, are of lesser importance. Syncytial endome-

tritis is therefore a very common observation on curetting done because of hydatidiform mole or abortion, and it should not be mistaken for evidence of malignancy.

TROPHOBLASTIC PSEUDOTUMOR

This lesion, as described by Kurman and associates, is characterized by extreme degrees of myometrial involvement by rather large clumps of trophoblastic cells without necrosis or destruction of the muscle fibers. Seemingly this represents an extreme degree of syncytial myometritis, but warrants careful observation. The vast majority of patients in this series revealed no evidence of disease for years, suggesting innocuous behavior of this trophoblastic hyperactivity which may persist for months or even years.

DIAGNOSIS OF CHORIOCARCINOMA FROM CURETTINGS

It is unfortunate that some of the characteristics of chorionepithelioma cannot be determined until after removal of the uterus. Indeed, hysterectomy itself is sometimes of no help insofar as a definite diagnosis is concerned, for as noted on page 663, cases have been reported in which the choriocarcinomatous lesion seemed to have completely disappeared from the uterus even though the patient was dying of autopsy-proved pulmonic chorionepithelioma. One must assume that there has been a belated resurgence of the local defense mechanism which obliterated all uterine evidence of the disease, although a breakdown of the general systemic process has permitted metastasis and death. It has also been suggested that trophoblast disseminated to the lung, as may occur during normal pregnancy, becomes malignant.

In many cases, however, the problem of accurate pathologic diagnosis arises, generally on the basis of tissue removed from the uterus by the curette. The decision as to malignancy may be difficult or impossible, and yet there are certain cases in which the diagnosis can be made with reasonable assurance. In other words, a positive diagnosis is conclusive but a negative finding does not exclude the possibility of malignant degeneration, especially if there is a rising HCG level.

When the microscope reveals large amounts of trophoblastic tissue without villi, and with anaplastic activity in the trophoblast, there is little doubt as to malignancy. When, on the other hand, one finds well-preserved villi, one should certainly hesitate in the diagnosis of choriocarcinoma, though it cannot be excluded. One must be careful not to mistake the extensive vacuolization seen with all trophoblastic disorders for chorionic villi. The presence of even considerable trophoblastic proliferation is entirely compatible with a benign mole, as already mentioned, and the presence or absence of such attributes as vascular or myometrial invasion cannot usually be determined from the curettings, so that diagnosis in such cases is obviously difficult and hazardous, since in a considerable proportion of cases chorionepithelioma develops beneath the surface within the uterine wall, so that curettage may yield little or no trophoblastic tissue.

GROSS CHARACTERISTICS OF HYDATIDIFORM MOLE AND CHORIOCARCINOMA

Hydatidiform mole may be either partial or, far more frequently, complete. In the latter, the entire villous structure is involved, with no trace of the embryo. In the former, only a very limited number of villi are affected. In such cases a small cluster of hydatidiform villi is found at some point in an otherwise normal placenta, and as noted earlier, it may be difficult to distinguish between hydatid degeneration and a frank mole.

In the mole the embryo succumbs at an early stage because of the completeness of the villous disease, and the mole presents the characteristic appearance of a mass of grapelike vesicles which fill the uterine cavity. If the mole has advanced to a fairly late stage, the evacuated vesicular mass may be of enormous bulk. The hydropic villi are of various sizes, depending on the degree of

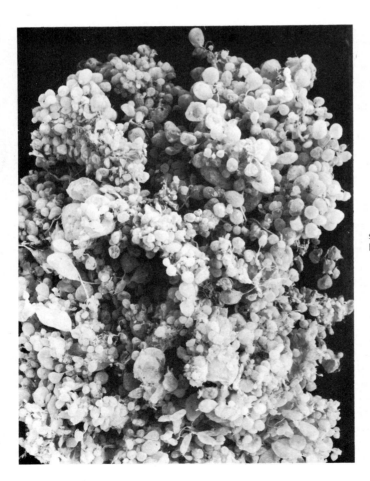

Figure 33–24. Extensive hydatidiform mole showing vesicles of varying size. (Courtesy of Dr. Jan Smalbraak, Bloemendaal, Holland.)

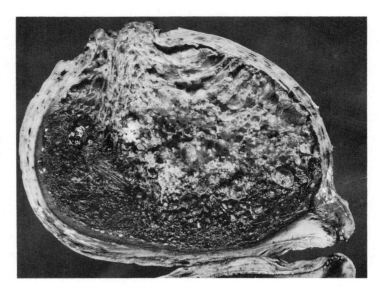

Figure 33–25. Hemisected uterus with typical mole. (Courtesy of Dr. J. Smalbraak.)

edema and the presence or absence of degenerative changes. Some of the villi, therefore, are like large ripe grapes, others like small withered ones, all held tightly by stems of connective tissue, which may be very frail. When still attached to the uterine wall, the vesicles may lie deep in the latter, and, even in the benign mole, tiny clusters may be seen far out in the uterine structures (Figs. 33–24 to 33–27).

Choriocarcinoma most frequently presents as a somewhat circumscribed, raised nodular tumor of dark reddish, hemorrhagic appearance and of grumous consistency, in-

volving some portion of the uterine fundus (Fig. 33–28). Less often it is rather diffuse and only slightly raised above the surface, and in rare cases it may be distinctly polypoid. The hemorrhagic tendency in such tumors makes them often resemble old hematomas. It is important, however, to remember that the tumor frequently develops in the uterine wall beneath the surface, which may be quite intact. This is one of the reasons why diagnostic curettage may be misleading. As the disease advances, the surface may show necrosis and ulceration, whereas in the other direction, the lesion

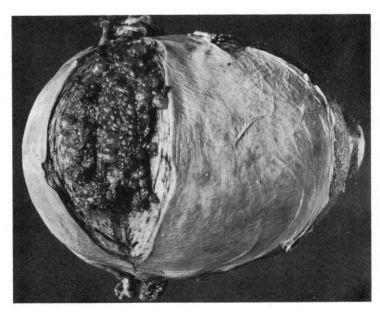

Figure 33–26. Mole protruding from incised uterus. (Courtesy of Dr. J. Smalbraak.)

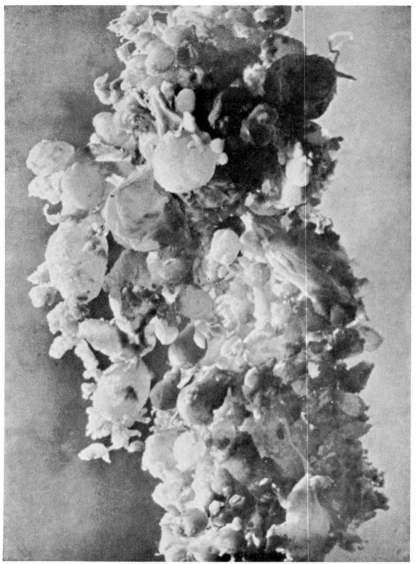

Figure 33–27. Detail of the grapelike gross pattern of hydatidiform mole. (Courtesy of Dr. Lyman W. Mason, Denver, Colo.)

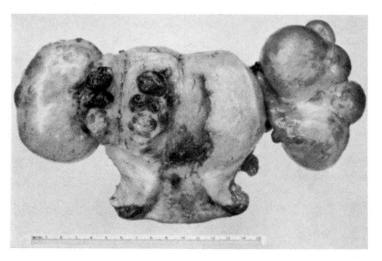

Figure 33–28. Choriocarcinoma associated with bilateral lutein cysts. (Courtesy of Dr. Clayton Beecham, Sunbury, Pa.)

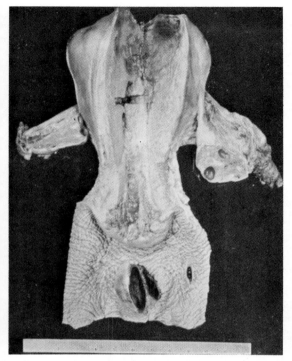

Figure 33–29. Choriocarcinoma of uterus with vaginal metastasis. (Autopsy specimen.) (Courtesy of Dr. Karl H. Wilson, Rochester, N. Y.)

may penetrate the uterine wall or vagina (Figs. 33–29 and 33–30), and infiltrate the parametrium and broad ligaments. When, as is so commonly the case, the disease follows hydatidiform mole, masses of vesicular tissue may still be present at various parts of the uterine wall, especially in the earlier stages of the disease.

CHIEF CLINICAL FEATURES

Mole has been reported in a 12 year old girl (Bobrow and Friedman) and in a postmenopausal woman (Dockerty et al.), but predominantly young adult women are afflicted. There is considerable variation in statistics of the incidence of hydatidiform mole, but a good average in the United States would probably be about 1 in every 2500 pregnancies. Its chief symptom is the appearance of uterine bleeding, usually at some time between the third and fifth months of pregnancy, often with enlargement of the uterus beyond the size to be expected from the presumed duration of the pregnancy. The symptoms are noted in Table 33–1. The spontaneous expulsion of

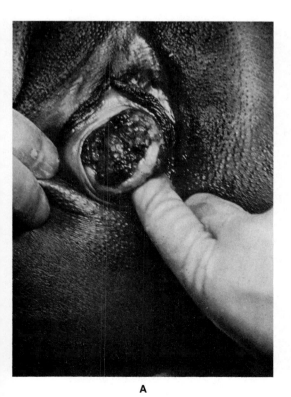

A

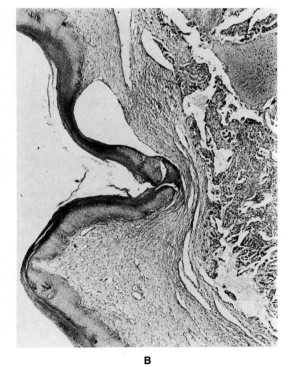

B

Figure 33–30. *A,* Gross appearance of choriocarcinoma with vaginal metastasis. *B,* Microscopic appearance of choriocarcinoma metastatic to vaginal wall.

Table 33–1 CLINICAL SIGNS OF MOLAR PREGNANCY IN 189 PATIENTS

Sign	Incidence	
Vaginal bleeding	189	(100%)
Uterine enlargement	102	(54%)
Toxemia	42	(22%)
Hyperemesis	48	(28%)
Hyperthyroidism	19	(10%)
Trophoblastic emboli	4	(2%)

(Courtesy of Dr. D. P. Goldstein, Boston, Mass.)

vesicular tissue often occurs, and of course makes the diagnosis complete. The absence of fetal heart sound and fetal movements, as well as the failure to palpate the fetal parts when these signs are normally present, are all of great diagnostic aid. Indispensable aids at present are the quantitative biologic tests of pregnancy, which will be discussed later. Increased usage of sonography and arteriography has been extremely helpful (Figs. 33–31 and 33–32) and seems less innocuous than intrauterine dye injection.

An infrequent but potentially serious complication of mole is thyrotoxicosis caused by pituitary stimulation of the thyroid gland. A thyroid storm with cardiac failure may ensue, as noted in the recent review by Hershman and Higgins. Management of molar pregnancy is well discussed in ACOG Technical Bulletin 33, August, 1975.

The proportion of cases of hydatidiform mole that become malignant is estimated variously at from 1 to as much as 10 per cent.

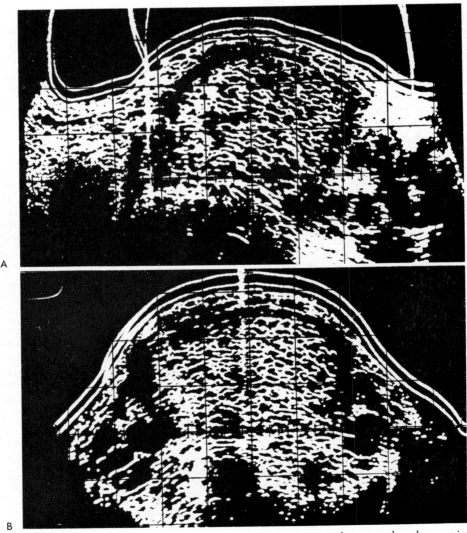

Figure 33–31. *A,* Right marker is at pubis; *left,* umbilicus. Note characteristic honeycomb molar mass in center. Each grid 3 cm. *B,* Transverse view. Note absence of fetal sac. Diffuse echoes with "snowstorm effect" (high sensitivity settings).

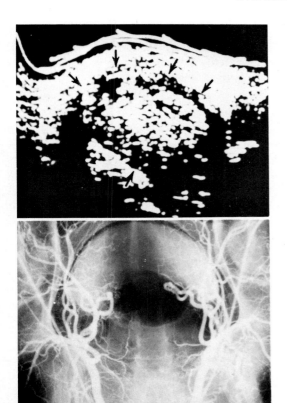

Figure 33–32. A, Uniform "snowstorm" of internal echoes corresponds to grape-like macrostructure of hydatidiform mole. Ventral line at left indicates umbilicus; arrows outline uterine margins. B, Arteriogram of above case. (Courtesy of Dr. J. C. Birnholz, Boston, Mass.)

Although personal experience inclines us to the lower figure, we concur with the opinions of many Far Eastern gynecologists who see many more cases of trophoblastic disease than the usual American clinician, and who are unanimous in their impression that the older woman with a hydatidiform mole has a much greater chance of malignant degeneration. In addition, many cases of presumed postmolar malignancy in reality represent only incompletely removed moles, which are benign despite considerable trophoblastic proliferation and a sustained or rising HCG level. In any case, malignant degeneration is so rare that it should not mandate *routine* drug therapy if there are opportunities for adequate HCG determinations.

Delfs is highly opposed to a single course, which might incur drug resistance should there be subsequent recurrence. Goldstein has likewise revised his original views and recommends therapy only when patients cannot or will not be followed.

Chorionepithelioma, as has already been stated, is an exceedingly rare disease, far more so than hydatidiform mole. While malignant degeneration of mole is rare, most choriocarcinomas are preceded by mole, and repeated studies indicate that choriocarcinoma is preceded by mole in 50 per cent, abortion in 30 per cent, and normal pregnancy in about 20 per cent of all cases. In an occasional case there is no personal knowledge or suggestive history of an antecedent pregnancy; seemingly a first pregnancy may on occasion "go bad" and eventuate in a malignancy termed "de novo" by Beischer and "ab initio" by Acosta-Sison.

Choriocarcinoma may develop during pregnancy, or there may be a latent period, sometimes very long, between the parturition or miscarriage and the development of the chorionepithelioma. When, as in a number of reported cases, this latent period comprises many years, one must always consider the possibility that an unsuspected abortion has intervened. However, we have seen a choriocarcinoma evolve nearly 4 years after a normal pregnancy, at which time tubal ligation was carried out because of hypertension and Lathrop and co-workers have reported a similar occurrence.

The most frequent though not always the first symptom of chorionepithelioma is the appearance or the continuance of bleeding after the evacuation of a vesicular mole, or during or after full term pregnancy, or after miscarriage. As has already been stated, there may be no evidence of the malignancy for a long time after any of the previously mentioned events. Moreover, the first indication of the disease may be the appearance of metastasis in one organ or another, especially in the vagina or vulva, but often in distant organs, such as the lung, brain, or liver. With extension of the uterine disease, bleeding becomes increasingly profuse, with the development of anemia, sepsis, and cachexia, terminating in death.

On the other hand, there are occasional cases such as that reported by Paranjothy and Samuel in which a patient with choriocarcinoma, treated by hysterectomy alone, developed a recurrence 12 years later. The reader must be cautioned, for their report states that "an occasional villus was noted," which makes the diagnosis questionable.

EXTENSION AND METASTASIS IN CHORIOCARCINOMA

Although many of the pathologic characteristics of chorionepithelioma suggest a carcinoma arising from the chorionic epithelium, its propagation more closely resembles sarcoma than carcinoma. Its predominant mode of extension is via the vascular route although the lymphatics may also be infiltrated. The broad ligament structures as well as the tube and ovary are also frequently involved. More characteristic, however, are the metastases which occur through retrograde transport of tumor emboli to the vagina and, less frequently, to the vulva. Vaginal metastasis or extension (Fig. 33–30) may occur in nearly 50 per cent of cases, the vaginal lesion presenting as a dark, reddish or bluish raised nodule which may resemble an angioma or an old hematoma. Indeed, excision of such a nodule, with subsequent microscopic examination, may be the first clue to the existence of chorionepithelioma; metastatic phenomena frequently are the first sign.

Metastasis to the lung is extremely frequent with chorionepithelioma (Figs. 33–33 and 33–34), and is probably the main cause of the patient's ultimate demise. Spiegel had commented on endoarterial choriocarcinoma of the lung, a condition in which there is sufficient blockage of the pulmonary circuit to lead to right ventricular dilatation, hypertrophy, and cardiac embarrassment. He reports 10 cases in addition to his own. Although the pulmonary spread of chorionepithelioma is common, it is not peculiar to the malignant type of trophoblastic disease, for a number of authors report this occurrence even with such benign processes as simple hydatidiform mole, although in most cases of the latter, there are no sequelae because of the suppressive action of the defense mechanism.

Cerebral metastasis is likewise a rather frequent eventuality with choriocarcinoma, as noted by Gurwitt and co-workers and by Jones (nearly 10 per cent). Tedeschi and Toy have commented on this paradoxic type of trophoblastic dissemination, and have found that the human apparently has a vastly different pulmonary capillary bed from the rabbit, which has an almost insurmountable barrier to the dissemination of chorionic elements. However, in the human it seems that destruction and invasion of lung tissue may open pathways for the tumor to completely bypass the capillary bed and enter into large arterial channels with subsequent dissemination to the brain. It appears that this is more likely than some type of extrapulmonary shunt. Cerebral spread may represent the primary symptom of the disease and is a

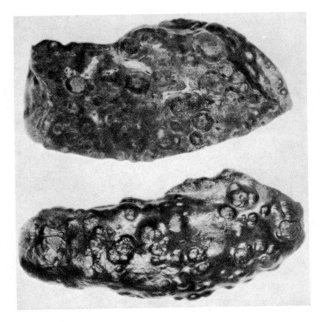

Figure 33–33. Pulmonary metastasis in case shown in Figure 33–28.

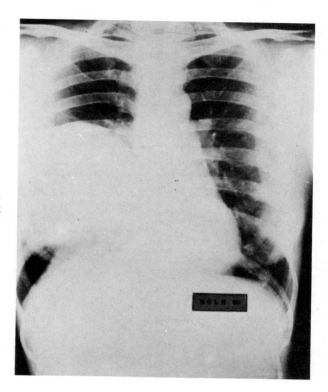

Figure 33–34. Massive pulmonary metastasis with postmolar choriocarcinoma which regressed following treatment with methotrexate. (Courtesy of Dr. M. S. Baggish, Hartford, Conn.)

serious complication, requiring irradiation therapy to the brain as well as chemotherapy. A recent patient at our clinic presented with cranial symptoms two years after passage of a mole, but with an intervening normal pregnancy.

Many other organs may be involved by metastatic phenomenon, such as the liver, kidneys, and indeed every possible site. Mercer and Buckell, with their respective co-workers, have found choriocarcinoma in both mother and fetus, either by direct extension or via the hematogenous route; other cases of maternal and fetal tumor have been noted, with some salvage since the advent of chemotherapy.

MALIGNANCY OF CHORIOCARCINOMA

This particular type of tumor is properly looked upon as one of the most highly malignant of all pelvic neoplasms, although the use of the newer chemotherapeutic drugs, as discussed subsequently, has drastically curtailed the formerly almost universal mortality. In any case, accurate assessment of the degree of malignancy of TRD has always been confused by reports of many supposed cures in cases in which the diagnosis is obviously incorrect.

In the prechemotherapeutic era surgical treatment of choriocarcinoma produced less than a 20 per cent 5 year salvage. A more modern and realistic approach to treated patients with trophoblastic disease is included under the section on Treatment of this particular disease.

In spite of the high degree of malignancy of these tumors, there is apparently general agreement that in a small proportion, less than 10 per cent *spontaneous regression and cure* is noted not only in the primary tumor but also in metastases (in the prechemotherapeutic era). A considerable group of cases has been reported in which the primary tumor completely disappeared, with death from the metastases.

Other cases have been recorded in which, after incomplete operation, or even without operation, the disease disappeared spontaneously, even though vaginal or other metastases appeared. The probable explanation seems to lie in some unknown factor of general body resistance to the inroads of the disease. That such an immune response to trophoblastic growth must be present in at least a limited degree seems to be indicated by the spontaneous regression of the trophoblastic islands found in the lungs of many pregnant women. Whatever the cause, *regression* of any type of trophoblastic disease seems to occur spontaneously on occasion; all of these cases occurred in the prechemotherapeutic days.

VAGARIES OF BENIGN MOLES

While attempting to correlate the pathologic pattern with the biologic behavior of trophoblastic tumors, it must be appreciated that on occasion one may find a complete disparity between the histologic appearance, biologic behavior, and the outcome of the case. For example, we are acquainted with at least two cases in this community of perfectly benign moles which have metastasized to lung, liver, skeleton, etc. with a fatal outcome, although autopsy continued to confirm the benign molar pattern of the metastatic disease. Hsu and co-workers and many other authors have commented on these histologically benign but clinically malignant cases, which fortunately are rare. That even benign hydatidiform mole may be associated with pulmonary deposition of trophoblast is being increasingly appreciated; in most instances, however, the presumed "systemic defense mechanism" seemingly is adequate to cope with and cause regression of this aberrant trophoblast.

On the other hand, we have seen cases in which a benign mole was evacuated, but later bioassays showed a persistently high level of HCG despite repeatedly normal curettings and x-ray of the chest, and even hysterectomy showed no evidence of trophoblastic disease. On occasion the level persisted for years, with even an intervening normal pregnancy before the appearance of clinical evidence of a rapidly advancing and fatal choriocarcinoma. How else can one explain such phenomena other than by postulating benign extrauterine trophoblastic elements held temporarily in check by a maternal defense mechanism that finally became attenuated and was overcome?

Today, however, the situation is vastly changed from that of 10 years ago. Persistent HCG more than two months after evacuation of a mole would almost certainly be treated empirically with one of the newer chemotherapeutic drugs, as will be mentioned in the section on Treatment. Indeed, the recent usage of new chemotherapeutic drugs has completely changed concepts of the treatment of trophoblastic disease. Hysterectomy is becoming an unusual feature of the therapeutic program, except in the case of elderly women with hydatidiform mole, or those few patients who are placed on some form of chemotherapy but show a constantly high or rising titre, or in cases where there is vaginal or intra-abdominal hemorrhage.

In view of the extremely good results in many patients treated by drugs, there seems to be relatively little indication for such procedures as lobectomy, laminectomy, and other extensive extrapelvic surgery for removal of metastatic foci, as was advocated previously. As a rule, metastasizing choriocarcinoma spreads diffusely in sarcoma-like fashion, and there seems slight justification for surgically excising one or two extrauterine sources of tumor, when almost certainly others are also present. Similarly, such forms of medical treatment as hormones, nitrogen mustard, and different methods of radiotherapy must be regarded as extremely unusual and indicated only if there is no chemotherapeutic response.

ECTOPIC CHORIOCARCINOMA

The fact that choriocarcinoma may at times occur in teratomatous tumors, especially of the testis, seems to explain the rare occurrence of undoubted chorionepithelioma in extrauterine situations, like the lungs or ovaries, even when there is no trace of tumor in the uterus. Although this theoretical possibility cannot be excluded in some cases, it is certainly not the correct explanation in all cases of extragenital choriocarcinoma.

In a case of our own, it was possible to establish by curettings, taken several months before the patient's death from a chorionepitheliomatous tumor of the brain, that the disease had originally existed in the uterus, though not a trace of the uterine lesion could be found at autopsy. In such cases it is possible that the curette may remove a localized uterine tumor which has already metastasized. It seems more likely that certain unknown factors of local resistance have eradicated all intrauterine disease, but only after the trophoblast has undergone general dissemination. From a clinical standpoint, there are few cases in which previous pregnancy can be excluded.

Even when choriocarcinoma does not occur in the trophoblast of the implantation, one must remember that it may arise in the trophoblastic villi transported to the lungs or elsewhere, though such an explanation is obviously difficult to prove. In view of the occasional occurrence of chorionepithelioma in teratomas of the testis, one might invoke such an explanation for an ovarian lesion. The tumor is, however, exceedingly rare in the ovary. Response to chemotherapy by the trophoblastic tumors of germ cell origin in the gonad is inferior to that of uterine lesions. Benjamin and Ronat discuss this problem.

A report of eight cases of ovarian choriocarcinoma by Gerbie and associates notes four deaths but four remissions following triple drug therapy. This represents a marked improvement, since extrauterine TRD seemingly did not respond to a single drug.

TUBAL AND OVARIAN HYDATIDIFORM MOLE AND CHORIOCARCINOMA

There seems no reason why hydatidiform mole and chorionepithelioma should not develop from the trophoblast of tubal or ovarian pregnancies, and a small group of such cases has been reported (Fig. 33–35), as recorded by Riggs. One must recall that focal hydatid degeneration may occur with tubal gestation. Ovarian hydatidiform mole is exceedingly rare, as would be expected from the rarity of ovarian pregnancy, but an interesting specimen was observed in our laboratory (although not reported) by Dr. Henry Bennett. Chorionepithelioma of the tube in conjunction with a viable intrauterine pregnancy has been reported by Crisp.

OVARIAN CHANGES ASSOCIATED WITH HYDATIDIFORM MOLE AND CHORIOCARCINOMA

The characteristic multiple lutein cysts of the ovary so often found in association with these conditions have been recognized for many years (Fig. 33–36), but they have assumed much greater interest in recent years because of growing knowledge of the endocrinology of pregnancy. The *incidence* is variable, although sonograms suggest these

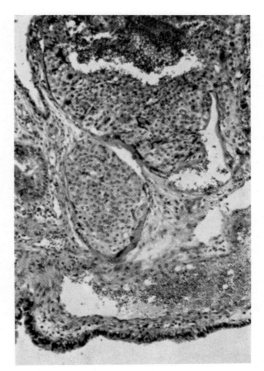

Figure 33–35. Choriocarcinoma of tube following tubal pregnancy. Endosalpinx below; choriocarcinoma with predominant cytotrophoblast above.

occur in over 50 per cent of women with TRD. Such cysts may occur with normal pregnancy or nontrophoblastic complications of pregnancy; Girouard and co-workers enumerate 17 cases.

The presence of these characteristic ovarian changes cannot always be determined by palpation alone. As will be emphasized later, very characteristic hyperreactio luteinalis may occur with ovaries which are of normal size or only slightly enlarged. Termination of pregnancy by hysterectomy (and frequent concomitant oophorectomy) reveals various lutein changes in many grossly normal ovaries.

Such changes may be discoverable only on histologic examination, and this is only occasionally possible because laparotomy in not always indicated in hydatidiform mole, by far the more frequent of the two causative lesions. However, the character and degree of ovarian change probably differ according to the stage of the intrauterine lesion, and, to add to the confusion, this relation does not appear to be chronologically parallel. Thus, the ovaries may become cystic even after evacuation of the uterine contents, although this is unusual.

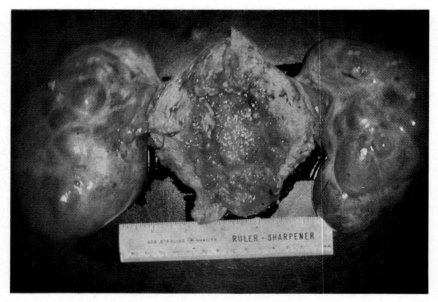

Figure 33–36. Large cystic (theca lutein) ovaries which occur almost exclusively with hydatidiform mole and choriocarcinoma (as in this figure).

Gross Characteristics of the Multiple Lutein Cysts

In the most striking cases, the ovarian cysts may reach enormous size and may give rise to troublesome pressure symptoms. Occasionally they are described as the size of a man's head, whereas in other cases the ovaries may show little or no gross enlargement, although characteristic microscopic changes may be present. All gradations between the extremes mentioned may be noted.

When the ovaries are large and polycystic, there is a tendency to preserve the original ovoid ovarian contour, but the surface is apt to be more or less lobulated. The individual cysts are of varying size, with thin walls, whereas the ovarian stroma is commonly edematous. The walls of the cyst are smooth and usually of a yellowish tinge. The contained fluid is most often clear and of amber tinge, but in some locules is either blood-tinged or definitely bloody.

In cases in which the ovarian response is less pronounced, the gross changes are inconspicuous, and the ovaries may show little or no enlargement. The corpus luteum of pregnancy may be detectable on the surface, but is often revealed only on section of the ovary. Some degree of lutein change is almost always seen, and the cysts may show the characteristics already described for the larger, genuinely polycystic ovaries.

Course of the Ovarian Lesions

There can be little doubt that spontaneous retrogression and disappearance of the ovarian lesion is the rule within a few months after removal of the hydatidiform mole or chorionepithelioma. Mention has already been made that some authors have noted the ovarian enlargement only after evacuation of the mole; that is only temporary, and is ordinarily followed by spontaneous disappearance. It is only in the occasional case, when the tumors give rise to troublesome pressure symptoms, incarceration, or torsion of the pedicle, that their removal may be indicated.

Microscopic Characteristics

During normal pregnancy there is noted in the ovaries an increase in the process of atresia folliculi. Moreover, in the later stages there is often seen a striking hypertrophy of the theca interna cells, which assume an alveolar arrangement, and often invade the stroma in large irregular masses (Figs. 33–37 to 33–39).

Certainly these theca lutein cells are not morphologically comparable to the granulosa lutein cells of the corpus luteum. They resemble much more closely the so-called paralutein cells seen in many corpora lutea, which is not surprising when one considers that their histogenesis is identical to that of the latter.

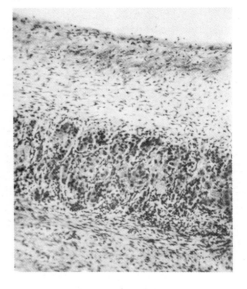

Figure 36–37. Wall of one of multiple lutein cysts with hydatidiform mole, the lutein cells being obviously of thecal origin. The granulosa is seen below.

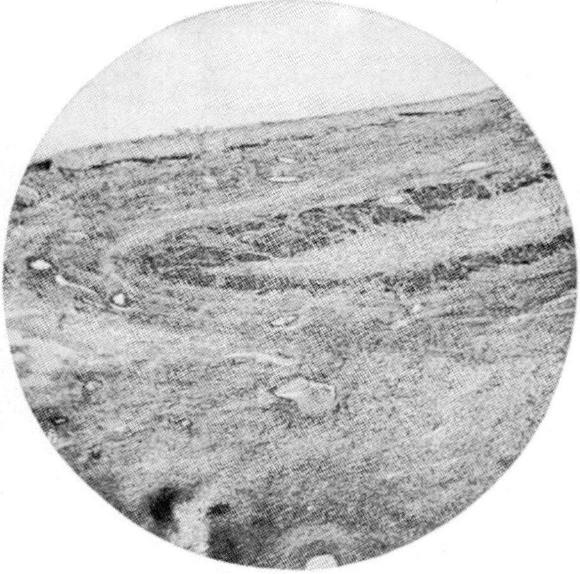

Figure 33–38. Theca lutein cells in wall of old atretic follicle (the dark-staining cells). This patient had a multiple lutein cyst with a hydatidiform mole.

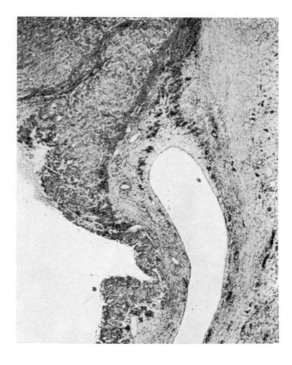

Figure 33–39. Theca lutein cells adjoining a corpus luteum (upper left) in a case of ovarian hydatidiform mole.

The microscopic picture of the ovarian lesions associated with hydatidiform mole or chorionepithelioma is varied, not only in different cases but often in different parts of the same ovary. The degree and the stage of the condition are probably chiefly responsible for the individual differences observed. The earlier studies would indicate that the lutein cells observed in the walls of the cysts are of thecal origin. In other words, not only is there an exaggeration of the process of atresia, with the production of many large follicle cysts, but the theca interna cells and ovarian stroma undergo a striking lutein transformation (Fig. 33–40).

Cause and Significance of Ovarian Changes

Although many formerly believed that these ovarian changes were actually the cause of the hydatidiform disease, there can now be no question that the reverse is the case. In other words, just as the normal trophoblast produces certain characteristic ovarian changes, so the exaggerated trophoblastic overgrowth of hydatidiform mole brings about an abnormal and excessive ovarian response. Morrow and associates indicate a high incidence of persistent TRD with theca lutein cysts greater than 5 cm.

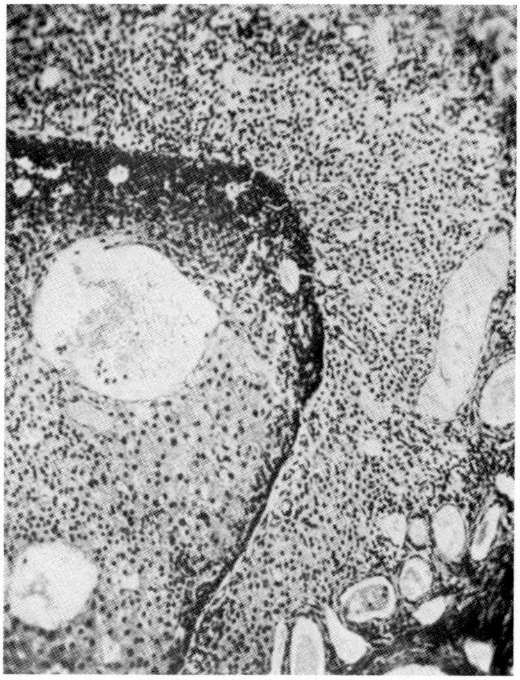

The chorionic gonadotropic hormone produced by the trophoblast naturally suggests itself as the responsible agent, but the answer is probably not as simple as this. It is now well established that the normal human ovary, unlike that of some laboratory animals, is not always influenced by the administration of the chorionic hormone found in the urine of pregnant women, although certain abnormal ovaries (Stein-Leventhal) literally "balloon up" after gonadotropic stimulation. The characteristic changes found in the ovaries of patients with hydatidiform mole resemble those which have been produced experimentally by the anterior pituitary sex hormones themselves. It thus seems that in some way, perhaps through the operation of an "activator" principle, the abnormally excessive production of the chorionic hormone evokes an exaggerated anterior pituitary sex hormone production, with hyperreactio luteinalis in the ovary as a result. One should note, however, that enlarged cystic ovaries, with a mole and an elevated HCG, which revert to normal following evacuation of the mole, may not increase in size with the advent of choriocarcinoma and a recurrent increased HCG levels.

Figure 33–40. Luteinization of both granulosa and theca with hydatidiform mole.

BIOLOGIC TESTS IN HYDATIDIFORM MOLE AND CHORIOCARCINOMA

Pregnancy tests are based upon the fact that normal living trophoblast produces a gonadotropic hormone, which penetrates the maternal blood and urine, so that injection of the latter into a mouse or rabbit produces characteristic changes in the animal's ovaries. With hydatidiform mole and chorioepithelioma, an excessive amount of trophoblast is present, and inordinately high levels of hormone are produced. Various dilutions may be injected into laboratory animals to obtain a quantitative level of the HCG.

In recent years, however, various immunologic methods of determining pregnancy have been developed, and have proved to be of considerable accuracy. Many immunologic methods of quantifying urinary chorionic gonadotropin have been devised, although there is some question of their accuracy with lower values of HCG. It is becoming increasingly apparent to most gynecologists that determination of the HCG is at least as important in deciding on the mode of therapy for the patient as any tissue removed for pathologic examination or evaluation of the clinical course of a woman harboring a hydatidiform mole (Elston and Bagshawe). Perhaps this should be extended to women with postpartum or postabortal bleeding despite a negative curettage. We are aware of one recent case of choriocarcinoma which arose postabortally, and the absence of a report on HCG levels was of importance in subsequent medicolegal problems. However, routine HCG study would probably not be feasible.

Nevertheless, it should be appreciated that bioassays do have definite limitations. For example, even in normal pregnancy there is at 8 to 10 weeks (about one month after the first expected but missed menstruation) a sudden high peak of chorionic hormones, so that the urinary titer may show larger amounts than one occasionally finds in hy-

datidiform mole or choriocarcinoma (Fig. 33–41). Although there have been many reports that pregnancy tests may be negative in cases which subsequently are revealed to definitely be moles or choriocarcinoma, our own experience is that, if bioassay is performed on serum, the results are dependable. TRD is also characterized by low estrogen, progesterone, and placental lactogen levels (Goldstein). These seem of secondary importance to the elevated HCG level.

On occasion a high titre may persist for months after the expulsion or evacuation of perfectly benign moles. The patient who has harbored a hydatidiform mole should be followed with determinations of the HCG level, with the firm admonition to avoid pregnancy, for this contingency obviously influences subsequent bioassays.

Although there have been more recent articles, the most authoritative one was published many years ago by Delfs. In studying 90 patients with hydatidiform mole, she

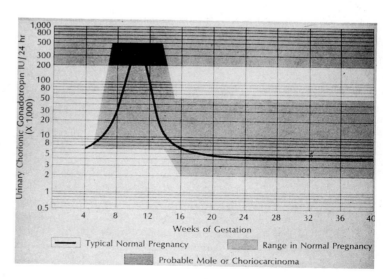

Figure 33–41.

found that of the 81 who had evacuation of the mole, 73 (90 per cent) retained their uteri and remained well. The HCG level reverted to negative within two months after delivery of the mole in more than 75 per cent of the cases, with almost 15 per cent more becoming negative later. Of the 10 per cent treated by hysterectomy because of a persistently high titre, all were found to have either an invasive mole or a choriocarcinoma. Her conclusion was that assay of HCG levels was the most important single factor in determining the patient's condition, in indicating treatment, and in formulating prognosis of trophoblastic disease.

This observation, made long before the advent of chemotherapy, is of even greater importance today. Its main value lies perhaps not so much in early diagnosis of hydatidiform mole, for multiple pregnancy and other abnormalities of pregnancy are difficult to distinguish by their HCG level. Following termination of a pregnancy, evacuation of a mole, or persistence of the titre if hysterectomy should be performed, a sustained high level of HCG becomes an increasingly ominous factor. Delfs, like many others, indicates that persistence of the HCG 60 *days* after evacuation of molar material is an extremely important determinative point, after which therapeutic measures should be considered.

It would seem preferable to obtain both bioassays and immunoassays which reflect different activities: hormonal action (bioassay) and antigen-antibody reaction (immunoassay). The two tests should parallel one another as do temperature and pulse in a temperature chart as noted by Lau, but he points out that when this no longer occurs, and the plotted lines cross or diverge, there is potential trouble. Schreiber and associates imply that urinary assays are more reliable than serum.

In recent years it has been noted that HCG and LH have a different and measurable *beta-subunit*, although the alpha-subunit is similar. Thus, it is possible to know that any detectable gonadotropin is chorionic in origin, and if radioimmunoassays are utilized, any hormonal activity can be detected in the milliunit stage. Consequently, appropriate (chemo)therapy may be initiated at an early stage in the event of an incipient recurrence (Jones, Goldstein). Schreiber warns that very low levels of HCG may not be detected even by beta-subunit determimation.

Certain cancers that originate outside the genital tract may be associated with an elevated HCG, possibly because of conversion of tumor to trophoblastic cells. This might suggest HCG studies in any patient with cancer, irrespective of the primary site, and Rutanen and Seppola have reviewed this problem. As noted earlier, HCG may represent a trophoblastic cell surface antigen that blocks trophoblastic rejection by maternal trophoblast in normal pregnancy and TRD. CEA evaluation would also seem appropriate in this disease with such profound immunologic implications.

TREATMENT OF TROPHOBLASTIC DISEASE

Earlier editions of this text emphasized the importance of repeated bioassays of HCG following removal or expulsion of any molar tissue. Curettage was often utilized, especially when the titre remained high, and, when this persisted longer than 8 to 10 weeks after evacuation of the uterine contents, hysterectomy was considered the proper treatment, although various less serious entities, such as residual mole or syncytial endometritis, were far more frequent operative findings than choriocarcinoma.

Today plans of treating trophoblastic disease have become completely revolutionized because of the outstanding studies of certain workers, notably Hertz and his associates (generally Ross, Lewis, and Lipsett), who have utilized a chemotherapeutic approach to the treatment of trophoblastic disease by use of the drug *methotrexate* (MTX), and various others in case of drug resistance to this (as indicated by a persistently elevated HCG level.) MTX was used initially to produce abortion but was found to be too toxic.

In previous years methotrexate was considered in purely an adjuvant role to surgery, i.e., when hysterectomy revealed choriocarcinoma and the level of HCG remained high with or without demonstrable evidence of residual or recurrent trophoblastic evidence of residual or recurrent trophoblastic disease. The encouraging results stimulated Hertz and his co-workers to a trial of *primary chemotherapy without surgery*. The astoundingly successful salvage has prompted optimism that there may be an adequate chemotherapeutic approach to at least certain types of genital malignancy.

Table 33–2 RESULTS OF CHEMOTHERAPY IN 111 PATIENTS WITH METASTATIC TROPHOBLASTIC DISEASE*

Treatment	Choriocarcinoma		Mole, Destruens and Others		Total		
	Cases	Remissions	Cases	Remissions	Cases	Remissions	Per cent
MTX initially	58	29	29	16	87	45	51%
Actino after MTX	17	10	6	2	23	12	52%
Actino initially	7	3	6	4	13	7	54%
MTX after Actino	5	2	2	2	7	4	57%
Other†	–	–	–	–	35	4	9%
			Total		111	72	64%

*10/1/63.
†Vincaleukoblastine; combination therapy; 6-mercaptopurine; Cytoxan; HN_2; DON.

(Courtesy of R. Hertz, National Institute of Health, Bethesda, Md.)

Although there have been many publications by these authors, the most significant concerns 111 women with metastatic trophoblastic disease, of whom 75 were presumed to have choriocarcinoma, whereas the others had some other form. With methotrexate, and occasionally such other agents as Vincaleukoblastine and actinomycin D, an outstanding remission rate of 64 per cent was produced, although not necessarily 5 years (Table 33–2). Of 75 patients with choriocarcinoma the remission rate was noted to be 60 per cent; of 36 patients with mole and chorioadenoma destruens it was found to be 75 per cent (Table 33–3). More recent studies by Ross and co-workers, Lewis and associates and Hammond and Parker indicate a 75 per cent remission rate for metastatic trophoblastic disease, and over 90 per cent when the disease is localized. Jones prefers to divide his cases into four very logical categories, as noted in Table 33–4. Group I yielded a nearly 100 per cent salvage without any chemotherapy. The salvage in Group II approached 90 per cent with sequential methotrexate and actinomycin D, while Group III dropped to 70 to 80 per cent despite combination therapy even with rather toxic actinomycin D, methotrexate, and either chlorambucil, cytoxan, or 6-mercaptopurine. The Group IV patients necessitate combined chemotherapy and irradiation and showed a 50 per cent salvage. This is a markedly improved result, since in earlier years there were few survivors with metastatic liver or brain disease. The dosage and therapeutic schedule are adequately documented in Jones' treatise (1975b).

This represents much better figures than the compilation by Brewer and co-workers of women treated by surgery alone, for in 122 patients who had hysterectomy alone, the 5 year salvage was 41 per cent when there were no metastases, but only 19 per cent in metastatic disease. Indeed, primary chemotherapy alone gives better results than when combined with surgery, and this has prompted Hertz to speculate about the danger of tumor emboli being disseminated by the manipulation of surgery.

A later study by Brewer and associates of 28 cases reaffirms the preferential role of

Table 33–3 COMPLETE REMISSION FOLLOWING CHEMOTHERAPY IN 111 CASES WITH METASTASES

Histology	Cases	Remissions	Per Cent Remissions
Choriocarcinoma	75	45	60
Mole, destruens and other	36	27	75
Total	111	72	64

(Courtesy of R. Hertz, National Institute of Health, Bethesda, Md.)

Table 33–4

A. THERAPEUTIC CLASSIFICATION OF GESTATIONAL TROPHOBLASTIC DISEASE BASED ON PROGNOSIS

Group	Metastases	Titer >100,000 (IU/24 hr) or Duration (4 mo)	Liver or Brain Involved	Prognosis
I	–	±	–	Excellent
II	+	–	–	Good
III	+	+	–	Fair
IV	+	±	+	Poor

B. CHEMOTHERAPY AND RESPONSE OF GESTATIONAL TROPHOBLASTIC DISEASE BASED ON THERAPEUTIC GROUP

Group	Therapy	Per Cent Remission
I	Single-agent chemotherapy	100
II	Single-agent chemotherapy	80–90
III	Combination chemotherapy	70–80
IV	Combination chemotherapy, Brain or liver irradiation or both	50

chemotherapy, although pointing out, as do other authors, that hysterectomy may occasionally be necessary if there is failure of response or extreme toxicity to the different drugs. Indeed, many believe that chemotherapy alone should be reserved for the youthful patient desiring further pregnancy, and that combined chemotherapy and surgery should be the usual method of treatment. Such authors as Acosta-Sison and others indicate that hysterectomy is sometimes indicated, although acknowledging the tremendously beneficial results of chemotherapy. Occasionally massive bleeding necessitates hysterectomy; preoperative drug therapy is preferable.

Admittedly it is beneficial for the young patient to retain her uterus, and yet be assured a considerable chance of cure for what has previously been considered to be one of the most lethal forms of cancers. From the standpoint of the pathologist, it is frustrating because, without hysterectomy, it is usually impossible to know what is being treated (except an elevated level of HCG), and a recent article by Bagshawe reaches similar conclusions. Curettage alone is rarely diagnostic and, indeed, hysterectomy is not always informative (as in those cases in which

no uterine tumor is present, although it probably arose in this organ, and was obliterated by the previously mentioned defense mechanism). Many cases of presumed metastatic trophoblastic disease are probably treated only because of a persistent HCG and vague x-ray shadows (not biopsy-confirmed) which may be due to many more innocuous causes than choriocarcinoma. Indeed, we think it is remarkable that the diagnosis of choriocarcinoma has been made with presumed assurance in so many cases without hysterectomy.

In addition, MTX is a toxic drug, and must be administered cautiously because of such severe side-effects as dermatitis, alopecia, bone marrow depression, renal or hepatic complications, stomatitis, and actual ulceration of the gastrointestinal tract. Deaths from this form of therapy were not uncommon initially, but as familiarity with these drugs has increased, morbidity and mortality have decreased; nevertheless it seems that such a toxic agent should be utilized for treating only a serious disease like choriocarcinoma. Goldstein advocates associated citrovorum factor to minimize toxicity and makes a persuasive case for routine chemotherapy of all cases of trophoblastic disease by indicating a markedly decreased incidence of complications in treated cases (Table 33–5), but, as noted earlier, he has since amended his views. Chemically, methotrexate is 4-amino-N^{10}-methyl pteroylglutamic acid, a folic acid antagonist which may be given orally or intravenously in dosages varying according to the body weight, but generally up to 25 mg. per day. A five-day course with a week's resting stage is followed by repeated dosages, meanwhile measuring the level of the HCG (Fig. 33–42). Failure of response after sev-

Table 33–5 OVERALL RESULTS OF PROPHYLACTIC CHEMOTHERAPY

Results	Number of Patients	
	Untreated*	Treated
Normal involution	93	67
Persistent disease		
Nonmetastatic	18 (16%)†	6 (8%)
Metastatic	5 (4%)	0
TOTALS	116	73

*Follow-up begun within 2 weeks after evacuation.
†HCG level elevated 8 weeks after evacuation.

(Courtesy of Dr. D. P. Goldstein, Boston, Mass.)

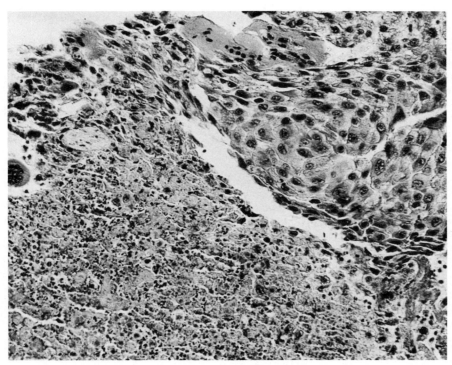

Figure 33–42. Viable choriocarcinoma (upper right) with beginning necrosis and obliteration of tumor after two 5-day courses of methotrexate (premature laparotomy because of suspected uterine perforation).

eral courses might suggest trial of the less toxic actinomycin D, but again if there is no decrease in the bioassay result, hysterectomy deserves strong consideration. Advanced cases and those with brain or liver involvement may necessitate combination drug therapy, although this is extremely toxic (Jones).

Retention of the uterus permits further pregnancy, and Van Thiele and colleagues record 88 pregnancies in 50 women following chemotherapy, generally methotrexate. There were no cases of subsequent trophoblastic disease, but a disproportionately higher incidence of placenta accreta was noted. It is speculated that this may result from a maternal or placental defect in the immunologic regulation of placental trophoblastic invasion. Walden and Bagshawe suggest that patients who develop TRD have a poor obstetric record.

A negative bioassay for one year is considered a prerequisite for further attempts at pregnancy; during the year contraception should be practiced; Kistner has indicated that oral contraceptives do not affect the level of HCG. The offspring of methotrexate-treated mothers are normal; indeed, one of the more interesting case reports is that of Freedman and co-workers concerning a woman who previously had an invasive mole and was observed to have a rising titre of HCG. She was treated vigorously for three months with methotrexate before it was observed that she had an intrauterine pregnancy at which time chemotherapy was discontinued. Normal delivery of a term twin pregnancy subsequently occurred, despite the presumably toxic effects of chemotherapy.

Hertz and associates state that when extrauterine trophoblast is present, the histopathologic pattern is of only academic importance, and is not a factor as a prognostic index. It seems to us that true metastatic phenomena occur only with true choriocarcinoma, excluding such entities as deportation of villi and certain rare instances in which specific tumor types simply fail to follow the usually accepted behavioral pattern.

Of particular interest is their statistically valid observation that a lesion of *short duration* (less than four months) and a *low titre* of HCG (less than 1 million mouse units or 100,000 I.U.) seemingly affords a *much more favorable prognosis*. On the basis of these criteria (along with the presence or absence of metastases), most studies are divided into good and poor risk categories. Only a few moles progress to choriocarcinoma, and Husel has reported six consecutive moles without progression of the disease. Yet, many if not most choriocarcinomas are preceded by mole, and it might be preferable to think of mole as potentially but not inevitably malignant.

The contributions by Hertz and associates are monumental, and we heartily applaud their outstanding work in at least partially subjugating one of the most lethal types of malignancy so often afflicting young women. At the same time, it is difficult to quote their statistics because of the constantly increasing number of patients with a sometimes uncertain pathologic diagnosis, who have had diverse treatment. Probably, some of the patients would have experienced spontaneous remission. Indeed, space limitations have compelled us to delete from this edition certain references (found in earlier editions) of many cases of malignant trophoblastic disease that were seemingly cured spontaneously or by surgery, nitrogen mustard, irradiation, and other agents.

REFERENCES

Acosta-Sison, H.: Apparent metastatic chorionepithelioma (without trace of primary disease in the uterus). Obstet. Gynecol., 10:165, 1957.

Acosta-Sison, H.: Changing attitudes in management of hydatidiform mole (196 cases). Am. J. Obstet. Gynecol., 88:634, 1964.

Adcock, E. W., et al.: Human chorionic gonadotropin: its possible role in maternal lymphocyte suppression. Science, 181:845, 1973.

Arias, R. E., and Bertoli, F.: Metastatic choriocarcinoma without primary lesion. Obstet. Gynecol., 13:737, 1959.

Attwood, H. D., and Park, W. W.: Embolism to the lungs by trophoblast. J. Obstet. Gynaecol. Br. Commonw., 68:611, 1961.

Baggish, M. S.: Gestational trophoblastic neoplasia. Clin. Obstet. Gynecol., 17:259, 1974.

Baggish, M. S., et al.: Sex chromatin pattern in hydatidiform mole. Am. J. Obstet. Gynecol., 102:362, 1968.

Bagshawe, K. D.: Choriocarcinoma. London, Edward Arnold (Publishers) Ltd., 1969.

Bagshawe, K. D.: Risk and prognostic factors in trophoblastic neoplasia. Cancer, 38:1373, 1976.

Barr, F. G., and Oktay, A.: Primary hydatidiform mole of ovary. Am. J. Obstet. Gynecol., 79:1088, 1960.

Behrman, S. J.: Rhesus and squirrel monkey placental specific antigens. Am. J. Obstet. Gynecol., 118:616, 1974.

Beischer, N. A.: Significance of chromatin pattern in cases of hydatidiform mole with associated fetus. Aust. New Zeal. J. Obstet. Gynaecol., 6:127, 1966.

Benjamin, F., and Ronat, E.: Primary gestational choriocarcinoma of the ovary, Am. J. Obstet. Gynecol., 131:343, 1978.

Billingham, W. D.: Transplantation immunity and the placenta. J. Obstet. Gynaecol. Br. Commonw., 74:834, 1967.

Birnholz, J., and Barnes, A. B.: Early diagnosis of hydatidiform mole by ultra sound imaging. J.A.M.A., 225:1359, 1973.

Bobrow, M. L., and Friedman, S.: Hydatidiform mole in 12-year-old girl. Am. J. Obstet. Gynecol., 73:448, 1957.

Brandes, J., and Peretz, A.: Recurrent hydatidiform mole. Obstet. Gynecol., 25:398, 1965.

Brandes, J., Grunstein, S., and Peretz., A.: Suction evacuation of the uterine cavity in hydatidiform mole. Obstet. Gynecol., 28:689, 1966.

Brewer, J. I., et al.: Hydatidiform mole. . J. Obstet. Gynecol., 101:557, 1968.

Brewer, J. I., and Gerbie, A. B.: Early development of choriocarcinoma. Obstet. Gynecol., 94:692, 1966.

Brewer, J. I., Rhinehart, J. J., and Dunbar, R. W.: Choriocarcinoma: report of five or more years survival from Albert Mathieu Chorionepithelioma Registry. Am. J. Obstet. Gynecol., 81:574, 1961.

Brinck-Johnson, T., Solc, J., and Galton, V. A.: Urinary excretion of estrogens in women with hydatidiform mole and choriocarcinoma. Obstet. Gynecol., 36:671, 1970.

Buckell, E. W. C., and Owen, T. K.: Chorionepithelioma in mother and infant. J. Obstet. Gynaecol. Br. Emp., 61:329, 1954.

Canlas, B. D.: Benign lesions of aberrant trophoblast in the lung. Obstet. Gynecol., 20:602, 1962.

Carr, D. H.: Cytogenetics and the pathology of hydatidiform degeneration. Obstet. Gynecol., 33:333, 1969.

Clark, P. B., Gusdon, J. P., Jr., and Burt, R. L.: Hydatidiform mole. Obstet. Gynecol., 35:597, 1970.

Curry, S. L., et al.: Hydatidiform mole: diagnosis, management, and long-term followup of 347 patients. Obstet. Gynecol., 45:1, 1975.

Crisp, W. E.: Choriocarcinoma of the fallopian tube coincident with viable pregnancy. Am. J. Obstet. Gynecol., 71:442, 1956.

Delfs, E.: Quantitative chorionic gonadotrophin. Obstet. Gynecol., 91:1, 1957.

Delfs, E.: Hydatidiform mole. Obstet. Gynecol., 45:295, 1975.

Dimmette, J. E.: Studies of human pregnancy. I. Immunoglobulins attached to the trophoblast. Obstet. Gynecol., 47:730, 1976.

Dockerty, C. M., et al.: Choriocarcinoma in postmenopausal women. Am J. Obstet Gynecol., 132:700, 1978.

Douthwaite, R. M., and Urbach, G. I.: In vitro antigenicity of trophoblast. Am. J. Obstet. Gynecol., 109:1023, 1971.

Driscoll, S. G.: Choriocarcinoma: an "incidental finding" within a term placenta. Obstet. Gynecol., 21:96, 1962.

Elston, C. W., and Bagshawe, K. D.: The diagnosis of trophoblastic tumors from uterine curettings. J. Clin. Pathol., 25:111, 1972.

Fox, F. J., and Tow, W. S. H.: Comparative immunological chorionic gonadotrophin levels in normal pregnant Chinese, Indian/Pakistani, Malay and Swedish women. Obstet. Gynecol., 27:795, 1966.

Freedman, H. L., Magagnini, A., and Glass, M.: Pregnancies following chemically treated choriocarcinoma. Am. J. Obstet. Gynecol., 83:1637, 1962.

Fuller, A. F., Jr., et al.: Immunity, trophoblast, and trophoblastic neoplasia. Clin. Obstet. Gynecol., 20:681, 1977.

Garancis, J. C., Pattillo, R. A., Hussa, R. O., et al.: Electronic microscopic and biochemical patterns of the normal and malignant trophoblast. Am. J. Obstet. Gynecol., 108:1257, 1970.

Gerbie, M. J., et al.: Primary ovarian carcinoma. Obstet. Gynecol., 46:720, 1973.

Girouard, D. P., Barclay, D. L., and Collins, C. G.: Hyperreactio-luteinalis: Review of literature and report of two cases. Obstet. Gynecol., 23:513, 1964.

Goldstein, D. P.: Five years' experience with the prevention of trophoblastic tumors by the prophylactic use of chemotherapy in patients with molar pregnancy. Clin. Obstet. Gynecol., 13:945, 1970.

Goldstein, D. P.: The chemotherapy of gestational trophoblastic disease. J.A.M.A., 220:209, 1972.

Goldstein, D. P.: Endocrine assay in chorionic tumors. Clin. Obstet. Gynecol., 18:41, 1975.

Gurwitt, L. J., et al.: Cerebral metastatic choroiocarcinoma: a postpartum cause of "Stroke." Obstet. Gynecol., 45:583, 1975.

Hammond, C. B., and Parker, R. T.: Diagnosis and treatment of trophoblastic disease. Obstet. Gynecol., 35:132, 1970.

Hammond, C. B., et al.: Treatment of metastatic trophoblastic disease: good and poor prognosis. Am. J. Obstet. Gynecol., 115:451, 1973.

Henderson, S. R., and Lund, C. J.: Severe preeclampsia, disseminated intravascular coagulopathy, and hydatidiform mole complicating a 20-week pregnancy with fetus. Obstet. Gynecol., 377:22, 1971.

Hershman, J. M., and Higgins, H. P.: Hydatidiform mole; a cause of clinical hyperthyroidism. N. Engl. J. Med., 284:573, 1971.

Hertig, A. T.: The placenta: some new knowledge about an old organ. Obstet. Gynec., 20:859, 1962.

Hertig, A. T.: Human trophoblast: normal and abnormal. Am. J. Clin. Pathol., 47:249, 1967.

Hertig, A. T., and Mansell, H.: Atlas of Tumor Pathology. Section IX, Fascicle 33. Armed Forces Institute of Pathology, Washington, D.C., 1956.

Hertig, A. T., and Sheldon, W. H.: Hydatidiform mole: a pathological-clinical correlation of 200 cases. Am. J. Obstet. Gynecol., 53:1, 1957.

Hertz, R.: Eight years' experience with the chemotherapy of choriocarcinoma and related trophoblastic tumors in women. In Choriocarcinoma. J. F. Holland and M. M. Hreshchyshyn (Eds.). New York, Springer-Verlag, 1966, 1967.

Hertz, R., Ross, G. T., and Lipsett, M. B.: Chemotherapy in women with trophoblastic disease: choriocarcinoma, chorioadenoma destruens, and complicated hydatidiform mole. Ann. N.Y. Acad. Sci., 114: (Art. 2) 881, 1964.

Holland, J. F., and Hreshchyshyn, M. M. (Eds.): Choriocarcinoma. New York, Springer-Verlag, 1967.

Hsu, C., Huang, L., and Chen, T.: Metastases in benign hydatidiform mole and chorioadenoma destruens. Am. J. Obstet. Gynecol., 84:1412, 1962.

Hsu, C. T., et al.: Some aspects of trophoblastic diseases peculiar to Taiwan. Am. J. Obstet. Gynecol., 24:1918, 1964.

Husel, D. H.: Six recurrent hydatidiform moles. Am. J. Obstet. Gynecol., 93:287, 1965.

Hutchison, J. R., Peterson, E. P., and Zimmerman, E. A.: Coexisting metastatic choriocarcinoma and normal pregnancy. Obstet. Gynecol., 31:331, 1968.

Jones, W. B.: Treatment of chorionic tumors. Clin. Obstet. Gynecol., 18:247, 1975.

Jones, W. B., and Lauersen, N. H.: Hydatidiform mole with coexistent fetus. Am. J. Obstet. Gynecol., 122:267, 1975.

Jones, W. B., and Lewis, J. L.: Treatment of gestational trophoblastic disease. Am. J. Obstet. Gynecol., 120:14, 1974.

Kistner, R. W.: Gynecology. Chicago, Year Book Medical Publishers, Inc., 1964.

Koren, Z., Behrman, S. J., and Paine, P. J.: Antigenicity of trophoblastic cells indicated by fluorescein technique. Am. J. Obstet. Gynecol., 104:50, 1969.

Kurman, R. J., et al.: Trophoblastic pseudotumor of the uterus: An exaggerated form of "syncytial endometritis" simulating a malignant tumor. Cancer, 38:1214, 1976.

Lathrop, J. C., et al.: Choriocarcinoma following tubal ligation. Obstet. Gynecol., 51:477, 1978.

Lau, L.: Personal communication.

Levin, D. C., et al.: Complementary role of sonography and arteriography in management of uterine choriocarcinoma. Am. J. Roentgenol. Radium Ther. Nucl. Med., 125:462, 1975.

Lewis, J. L., Jr.: Chemotherapy for metastatic gestational trophoblastic neoplasms. Clin. Obstet. Gynec., 10:330, 1967.

Lewis, J. L., Jr.: High risk pregnancy: hydatidiform mole and choriocarcinoma. J. Reprod. Med., 7:33, 1971.

Lindsey, J. R., Wharton, L. R., Jr., Wharton, J. D., and Baker, H. J.: Intrauterine choriocarcinoma in a rhesus monkey. Pathol. Vet., 6:378, 1969.

Llewellyn-Jones, D.: Trophoblastic tumors (geographical variation). J. Obstet. Gynaecol. Br. Commonw., 72:242, 1965.

Marchand, F.: Über die sogenannte decidualen Geschwülste im Anschluss an normale Geburt, Blasenmole und Extrauterinschwangerschaft. Mschr. Geburtsh. Gynäk., 1:419, 1895.

Marrubini, G.: Primary chorionepithelioma of the ovary. Acta Obstet. Gynecol. Scand., 28:251, 1949.

Mercer. R. D., Lemmert, A. C., Anderson, R., and Hazard, J. B.: Choriocarcinoma in mother and infant. J.A.M.A., 166:482, 1958.

Moore, J. H.: Hydatidiform mole in 53 year old patient. Am. J. Obstet. Gynecol., 69:205, 1955.

Nelson, J. H., Jr., et al.: The effect of trophoblast in immune state of women. Am. J. Obstet. Gynecol., 117:689, 1973.

Novak, E.: Pathological aspects of mole and choriocarcinoma. Am. J. Obstet. Gynecol., 59:1355, 1950.

Novak, E., and Koff, A. K.: Chorioepithelioma. With especial reference to disappearance of the primary uterine tumor. Am. J. Obstet. Gynecol., 20:153, 1930.

Novak, E., and Seah, C. S.: Choriocarcinoma of the uterus. Am. J. Obstet. Gynecol., 67:933, 1954.

Novak, E., and Seah, C. S.: Benign lesions in chorionepithelioma registry. Am. J. Obstet. Gynecol., 68:376, 1954.

Osathanondh, R., et al.: Actinomycin D as the primary agent for gestational trophoblastic disease. Cancer, 36:863, 1975.

Paranjothy, D., and Samuel, I: A rare case of choriocarcinoma recurring 12 years after hysterectomy. Am. J. Obstet. Gynecol., 110:410, 1971.

Park, W. W.: Experimental trophoblastic embolism in the lungs. J. Pathol. Bacteriol., 25:257, 1958.

Patillo, R. A., et al.: In vitro identification of the trophoblastic stem cell of the human villous placenta. Am. J. Obstet. Gynecol., 100:582, 1968.

Posner, A. C., Kushner, J. I., and Posner, L. B.: Repeated hydatidiform mole. Obstet. Gynecol., 5:761, 1955.

Ramsey, E. M., et al.: Interreactions of trophoblast and maternal tissues in three closely related primate species. Am. J. Obstet. Gynecol., 124:647, 1976.

Reynolds, S. R.: Hydatidiform mole: a vascular congenital anomaly. Obstet. Gynecol., 47:244, 1976.

Riggs, J. A., et al.: Extrauterine tubal choricarcinoma. Am. J. Obstet Gynecol., 88:637, 1964.

Ringertz, N.: Hydatidiform mole, invasive mole, and choriocarcinoma in Sweden, 1958–1965. Acta Obstet. Gynecol. Scand., 49:195, 1970.

Robinson, E., Shulman, J., Ben-Hur, N., Zuckerman, H., and Neuman, Z.: Immunological studies and behaviour of husband and foreign homografts in patients with chorionepithelioma. Lancet, 1:300, 1963.

Ross, G. T.: Congenital anomalies among children born of mothers receiving chemotherapy for gestational trophoblastic neoplasms. Cancer, 37(Suppl.) 1043, 1976.

Ross, G. T., Goldstein, D. P., Hertz, R., et al.: Sequential use of methotrexate and actinomycin D in the treatment of metastatic choriocarcinoma and related trophoblastic disease. Am. J. Obstet. Gynecol., 93:223, 1965.

Rutanen, E. M., and Seppola, A.: The HCG beta-subunit in nontrophoblastic gynecological tumors. Cancer, 41:692, 1978.

Schmorl, G.: Pathologisch-anatomische Untersuchungen uber Puerperal-eklampsie. Leipzig, Vogel, 1893.

Schreiber, J. R., et al.: Limitation of the specific serum radioimmunoassay for human chorionic gonadotropin in the management of trophoblastic neoplasms. Am. J. Obstet. Gynecol., 125:705, 1976.

Shintani, S., Glass, L. E., and Page, E. W.: Studies of induced malignant tumors of placental and uterine origin in the rat. II. Induced tumors and their pathogenesis with special reference to choriocarcinoma. Am. J. Obstet. Gynecol., 95:550, 1966.

Spellacy, W. N., Meeker, H. C., and McKelvey, J. L.: Three successful pregnancies in a patient treated for choriocarcinoma with methotrexate. Obstet. Gynecol., 25:607, 1965.

Szulman, A. E., and Surti, Y.: The syndromes of hydatitorm mole. I. Cytogenetic and morphological considerations. Am. J. Obstet. Gynecol., 131:65, 1978.

Szulman, A. E., and Surti, Y.: Evolution of complete and partial mole. Am. J. Obstet. Gynecol., 132:20, 1978.

Tedeschi, L. G., and Toy, B. L.: Experimental transpulmonary migration of trophoblast. Obstet. Gynecol., 21:55, 1962.

Van der Werf, A. J. M., et al.: Metastatic choriocarcinoma as a complication of pregnancy. Obstet. Gynecol., 35:78, 1970.

Van Thiel, D. H., Ross, G. T., and Lipsett, M. B.: Pregnancies after chemotherapy of trophoblastic neoplasms. Science, 169:132, 1970.

Van Thiel, D. H., et al.: Partial placenta accreta in pregnancies following chemotherapy for gestational trophoblastic neoplasms. Am. J. Obstet. Gynecol., 112:54, 1972.

Walden, P. A., and Bagshawe, K. D.: Reproductive performance of women successfully treated for gestational trophoblastic tumors. Am. J. Obstet. Gynecol., 125:1108, 1976.

Wei, P., and Ouyang, P. Trophoblastic disease in Taiwan. Am. J. Obstet. Gynecol.., 85:844, 1963.

Wilson, R. B., Hunter, J. S., and Dockerty, M. B.: Chorioadenoma destruens. Am. J. Obstet. Gynecol., 81:546, 1961.

Wu, F. Y.: Recurrent hydatidiform mole. A case report of nine consecutive molar pregnancies. Obstet. Gynecol., 41:200, 1973.

Wynn, R. M., and Davies, J.: Ultrastructure of transplanted choriocarcinoma and its endocrine implications. Am. J. Obstet. Gynecol., 88:618, 1964.

Wynn, R. M., and Harris, J. A.: Ultrastructure of trophoblast and endometrium in invasive hydatidiform mole (chorioadenoma destruens). Am. J. Obstet. Gynecol., 99:1125, 1967.

Yenen, E., Dinvana, S., and Barbano, C.: Ectopic choriocarcinoma. Obstet. Gynecol., 30:556, 1967.

Chapter 34

GYNECOLOGIC AND OBSTETRIC CLINICAL CYTOPATHOLOGY

JOHN K. FROST, M.D.

Many aspects of health and disease are reflected accurately in both *tissue* and *cellular* patterns. Clinical cytopathology brings about *detection* and *diagnosis* of many diseases at stages earlier than ever before possible. It first indicates the need for further essential *diagnostic* procedures, and then evaluates their accuracy. Likewise, through its use, proper *treatment* is indicated and then evaluated for efficacy. Further, and perhaps of even greater significance, it builds an understanding of the basic biologic processes with which we are dealing in both health and disease.

Clinical cytopathology was first successfully introduced by Papanicolaou and Traut in 1943. Since that time, after extensive use and proof of reliability, it has become an integral part of quality medical practice. It detects *cancer* and other diseases early, identifies numerous infections (Fig. 34–1 *C*) where other methods fail, offers further understanding of *endocrine* status (Fig. 34–1*A*) and *chromosomal* makeup, and is useful in assessing a patient's *prognosis* and response to therapy.

Its *clinical* simplicity places cytopathologic consultation at the fingertips of every practicing physician regardless of specialty, training, or experience. On the other hand, the *microscopic* examination is long and meticulous and its interpretations and recommendations for utilization by clinicians require the knowledge and wisdom of a physician skilled in clinical cytopathology, Cytotechnologists play a key role in extending the cytopathologist's skills to more clinicians and their patients.

To guide securely and not mislead, both clinician and consulting cytopathologist must have a clear and accurate picture of each other's problems and perspective. Striving for a complete understanding of the patient, intercommunication of history and physical examination, as well as microscopic finding are essential to accurate diagnoses, recommendations, and clinical action.

Clinical cytopathology is a form of tissue examination using *microbiopsies*—cellular specimens. It is more inclusive in area coverage than is classic biopsy, however, and is far less disturbing to the biologic behavior of the lesion.

When the specimen is inadequate, the accuracy of any examination is doubtful. The degree to which it is satisfactory must be evaluated and related from the pathologist to the clinician, and heeded by the latter for proper patient care.

NORMAL SQUAMOUS CELL MORPHOLOGY

Nonmalignant cells usually have predictable morphology (Fig. 34–1 *A,B*). Variations in the level of biologic activity, degenerative or inflammatory changes, and preneoplastic

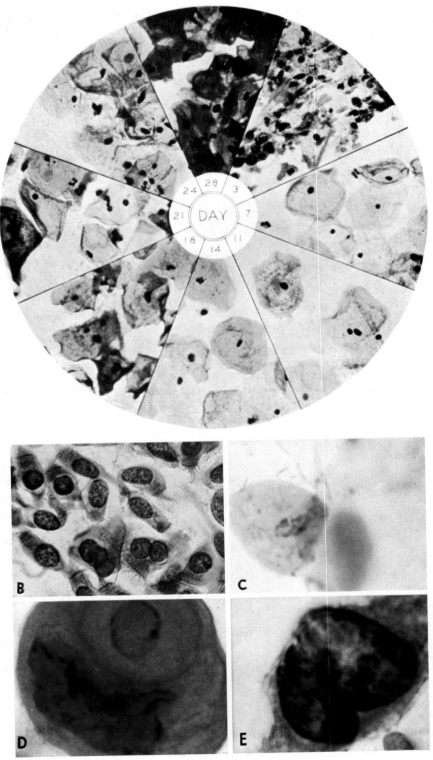

Figure 34–1. *A, The menstrual cycle.* Vaginal pool cellular spreads taken at three to four day intervals in a normal 28 day cycle. Menstruation commenced on the twenty-ninth day. Age 21. At ovulation (day 14) the Maturation Index is $\overrightarrow{0/40/60}$, the cells lie singly and flat, and the background is "clean." Before menstruation (day 28) the Maturation Index is $\overline{0/70/30}$, cells are clumped and curled, and the background is "dirty." Note endometrial cells and erythrocytes on day 3. Papanicolaou stain. ×70.

Legend continued on the following page

development can produce morphologic changes in nonmalignant cells which can be extremely confusing to the unwary in differentiating from malignancy.

Whereas columnar cells line the fallopian tubes, endometrium, and endocervix (Fig. 34–1 B), the greatest number of epithelial cells encountered in vaginal specimens is shed from the noncornified, stratified squamous epithelium covering the vaginal vault and the portio vaginalis of the cervix (Fig. 34–1 A; Fig. 34–2).

Squamous epithelium is so named because its most mature cells lie flattened, scale-like (squamous) upon the surface (Fig. 34-2 A). Thus, mature squamous cells orient *parallel* to the basement membrane, whereas mature columnar cells orient *perpendicular* to it.

Cells exfoliated from this squamous epithelium generally have round or oval *nuclei* with a reticular chromatin pattern. In each cell the nucleus is centrally placed in a symmetric cytoplasm (Fig. 34–2 B,C). As the cell matures the nucleus changes, with its fine reticular pattern gradually becoming slightly more coarse and granular, suddenly becoming pyknotic (karyopyknosis), and eventually breaking up and disappearing (karyorrhexis and karyolysis).

With maturation, the *cytoplasm* first loses its green staining qualities and then its blue, finally becoming yellow or red (Fig. 34–1 A). Concurrently, it loses its elasticity and assumes, with maturity, the hard qualities of keratin and its precursors. Thus, the least mature cell becomes round when exfoliated and appears small and thick. The older cells flatten in the tissue and, upon exfoliation, retain their extreme thinness (Fig. 34–2 C), appearing as large, wafer-thin polygon-shaped cells.

Germinal Cell

The true basal cell, or germinal cell, lies upon the basement membrane as the so-called stratum columnum (Fig. 34–2 A). It is normally *not* exfoliated, even with rigorous scraping of the epithelium. When there is erosion or ulceration of the epithelium down to the basement membrane, this germinal cell is too degenerated from the trauma or inflammation to be of diagnostic value, or even to be separately identified.

Parabasal Cell

In older, discarded nomenclature, this cell has also been called the prickle cell, basal cell, pavement cell, malpighian cell and even intermediate cell. Its most distinguishing feature is the thickness of its rounded *cytoplasm* from nucleus to cellular border (Fig. 34–2 A,B). The less mature the cell is, the more elastic and rubbery is the cytoplasm, which, when released into the vaginal fluid, assumes more of a spherical shape. The upper, more mature parabasal cells spread more upon a glass slide, but not to the wafer-thin thickness of the cytoplasm of the squame (intermediate or superficial cell).

Figure 34–1. *Continued*

  B, Ciliated columnar cells. These endocervical cells have prominent acidophilic cilia and terminal plates. Note the abundant cytoplasm at the luminal end of the cell, and scant tail of cytoplasm at the end which rests upon the basement membrane. The round or oval nuclei have a uniform granular chromatin pattern. Multinucleation is frequent. ×520.

  C, Trichomonas vaginalis lying on the edge of the red cytoplasm of a superficial cell covering the right half of the field. Whereas the cytoplasm of this organism is green, it can take the color of any cytoplasm. Within the organism are red granules, placed in three orderly longitudinal rows. The nucleus is a definite structure, but it is small and pale. Flagella are not visible usually, but when present diverge from the cytoplasm near the nucleus. Papanicolaou stain. ×1378.

  D, Malignant pearl shed from squamous cell carcinoma. The cellular borders of both cells are sharp and extremely well defined. The cytoplasm of the small cell is divided between a foamy perinuclear endoplasm in which the nucleus resides and the hyaline ectoplasmic rim. Within this rim of ectoplasm, hyaline rings can barely be discerned. Note the malignant criteria of the large nucleus. The cytoplasm of both cells has a hyaline glassy quality and is extremely orangophilic, both suggestive of keratinization. The small cell lying on the large cell cytoplasm in a stratifying manner gives first an impression of "cannibalism" or phagocytosis. By focusing up and down, however, it is easily resolved into a typical pearl formation of stratifying squamous differentiating cells. ×1378.

  E, Malignant criteria in the nucleus. There is massive chromatin clumping free within the nucleus and plastered against the inner border of the nuclear membrane. The chromatinic rim is minimally irregular in shape but massively irregular in thickness, being extremely thin in the right and upper left and massively thick in other areas. To the right of center is an angular jagged nucleolus. In the center is an area of abnormal parachromatin clearing. The cytoplasmic border is indistinct. Papanicolaou stain. ×1378.

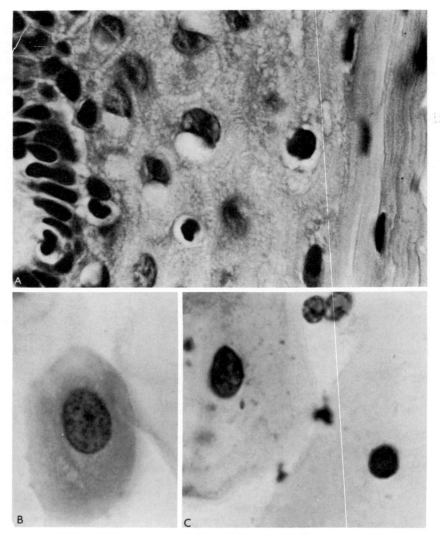

Figure 34–2. Noncornified stratified squamous epithelium of the vaginal vault. *A*, Tissue section, from left to right: basement membrane; germinal (basal) cell layer; parabasal (prickle) cell layer; intermediate cell layer; superficial cell layer. × 1100. *B*, Exfoliated parabasal cell in vaginal smear. The cytoplasm is rounded and is *thick* from nucleus to cellular border, as compared with the bit of adjacent intermediate cell cytoplasm in the upper right corner. The centrally placed nucleus is vesicular, with a reticular chromatin pattern. ×1500. *C*, Exfoliated squames (intermediate cell, *left*, and superficial cell) in vaginal smear. Cytoplasm of both is uniformly *wafer-thin* from nucleus to cellular border, with keratinizing granules in the left. The intermediate cell has an oval vesicular nucleus, which has retained a definite chromatin pattern with beginning prekaryopyknotic blurring. The superficial cell has a small, dark pyknotic nucleus with complete loss of chromatin pattern. × 1500.

The thickness can accurately be determined by moving the plane of focus of the microscope up and down through the cell.

The centrally placed vesicular *nucleus* is round or oval. The nuclear membrane is regular and smooth, while the chromatinic rim against the membrane is delicate and uniformly thin. The chromatin pattern is regular and consists mainly of thin strands in reticular mesh. The sex chromocenter is easily identified (Fig. 34–3) with other occasional small chromocenters and rare, inconspicuous nucleoli present. At times the nucleus is pyknotic, but it is still recognizable as a parabasal cell if the cytoplasm is thick.

Normal parabasal cells are not to be confused with the moderately mature and immature dyskaryotic cells shed from metaplasia or dysplasia (see Fig. 34–32). The latter have larger nuclei of dyskaryotic type with an abnormal chromatin pattern and a higher than normal nucleo-cytoplasmic ratio.

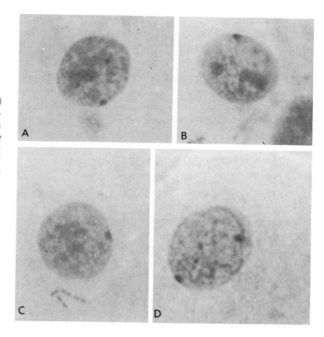

Figure 34–3. Four interphase (resting, metabolic) nuclei of epithelial cells. ×2000. An X chromatin (female sex chromocenter, Barr body) lies against each nuclear envelope. It appears as an oval (*A, D*), a triangle (*B*), a rectangle (*C*), or combination, averaging about 1.0 μm. in diameter, and is found at any point around the nuclear rim. To be diagnostic, it must meld with the chromatinic rim, which is shaped by the invisible nuclear membrane. *A, B,* and *C* are from buccal smears; *D* is from a vaginal-pancervical Fast smear.

In fully mature and intact epithelium, parabasal cells lie between the germinal cells and the overlying squamified intermediate cells (Fig. 34–2 *A*) and do not normally exfoliate (Fig. 34–1 *A*). When parabasal cells appear in naturally exfoliated cellular material, however, they are lying *upon* the surface of the epithelium at the time of their exfoliation (Fig. 34–2 *B*). This occurs in inflammation (see Figs. 34–42; 34–53) or in states in which there are low or altered maturation factors (i.e., estrogens, progestogens, corticoids) (see Figs. 34–9; 34–11).

Intermediate Cell

This cell type previously was called the precornified cell. The most distinguishing features of the intermediate cell (Fig. 34–2 *A,C*) are its *thin* wafer-like (a true "squame") cytoplasm and its *vesicular* (not pyknotic) nucleus.

The *cytoplasm* of the cells abruptly becomes squamous (platelike) as the cells mature from the parabasal (Fig. 34–2 *B*) to the intermediate type. This sudden thinning is uniform from nucleus to cytoplasmic rim (Fig. 34–2 *C*). Because of this great cytoplasmic attenuation, the cell appears larger; actually its volume has not increased. It is usually blue or green (Fig. 34–1 *A*) but can be acidophilic, especially in inflammation or as a result of drying artifacts.

The *nucleus* remains vesicular and retains its round or oval shape. Although the reticular chromatin pattern may become somewhat coarse, with prominent chromocenters, it definitely retains the open meshwork pattern of an actively metabolic intermitotic nucleus and clearly displays the female sex chromocenter if it is present (Fig. 34–3). Nucleoli are usually absent, but may be small and inconspicuous.

In fully mature epithelium, intermediate cells lie between the parabasal cells and the overlying superficial cells (Fig. 34–2 *A*). When they appear in naturally exfoliated material (Fig. 34–2 *C*), however, they actually were lying upon the surface of the epithelium at the time of exfoliation, indicating that the epithelium had reached only that level of maturation (see Figs. 34–7; 34–10).

Superficial Cell

Previously incorrectly called the cornified cell, the superficial cell lies above the intermediate cell and upon the surface of the fully matured noncornified stratified squamous epithelium (Fig. 34–1 *A,C*). Its most distinguishing features are a *thin* wafer-like cytoplasm and a *pyknotic* (not vesicular) nucleus.

The cytoplasm is uniformly thin from nuclear to cell border (Fig. 34–2 *C*), like the intermediate cell. Although it is usually acidophilic (Fig. 34–1 A,C), the superficial cell cytoplasm may be blue-green. Too many artifacts (i.e., fixation, drying, inflammation) cause cytoplasm to stain acidophilic so that this cytoplasmic tinctorial reaction cannot be relied upon for differentiating the cell type. True cornification does not normally occur in the vaginal mucous membrane. When it does appear, as in hyperkeratosis, the nucleus is usually lost, granules appear in the cytoplasm and it becomes extremely orangophilic and glassy (hyalinized).

Pyknosis of the nucleus is the most reliable feature differentiating a superficial cell from an intermediate cell. The chromatin pattern of the pyknotic nucleus disappears into a hyperchromatic structureless mass (Fig. 34–1 C), while its size shrinks to less than 6μm.

Anucleate Superficial Cell

This cell is not present in the normal non-cornified stratified squamous epithelium of the female genital tract. When found in gynecologic material, it represents contamination by the introitus or an epithelial abnormality with hyperkeratosis or leukoplakia. In these states it lies on the surface of the epithelium above the normal, nucleated superficial cells.

The cytoplasm retains a wafer-thin squamous character but the nucleus is lost, at times with a central nuclear "ghost" occurring as a round, clear area in the cytoplasm (see Fig. 34–14). The cytoplasm may retain nuclear fragments or contain keratinizing granules of dark amorphous keratohyalin or acidophilic hyalinized keratin.

X Chromatin

In the normal female and in other individuals with a pair of XX sex chromosomes, a conspicuous peripheral chromocenter is identifiable in the metabolic (intermitotic, resting) nucleus of exfoliated squamous cells (Fig. 34–3). This heterochromatic chromatin mass measures approximately 1μm. in diameter (0.7 to 1.4μm.), and appears as a thickening of the nuclear chromatinic rim, projecting inward. It occurs at any random point upon the nuclear membrane so that when it does not lie on the lateral margin of a nucleus it cannot be positively identified.

As identified in this strict manner, the X chromatin (sex chromocenter, Barr body) can be recognized in 20 to 60 per cent of well-preserved normal female nuclei, and in virtually *no* normal XY males. To be *diagnostic*, the X chromatin must be a part of the nuclear chromatinic rim, blending indistinguishably therewith under oil immersion magnification in a well-preserved cell. Deviation from these strict criteria leads to false identifications.

Using these strict criteria, one does not find a like body in normal male nuclei. With only high dry objective magnification, however, more deeply placed chromocenters in cells of both sexes may appear to involve the nuclear chromatinic rim and lead to false identification as a female chromocenter if oil immersion is not utilized. Since early degeneration can cause chromatin condensation and peripheral aggregation onto the nuclear envelope, mimicking the sex chromocenter, only well-preserved vesicular nuclei with sharp chromatin patterns should be evaluated. Occasionally, even when an apparently normal XX chromosome pair is present, the Barr body may appear abnormally large or small, or even paired. Rarely, a very large or very small Barr body may indicate an abnormally large or small X sex chromosome, which only cytogenetic study can confirm.

Truly double (not paired) Barr bodies appear when XXX sex chromosomes are present (see Fig. 34–15). Triple and quadruple Barr bodies are found in the presence of XXXX and XXXXX sex chromosomes in mosaic individuals.

The number of X chromatin bodies observed *plus* one, corresponds to the least number of X sex chromosomes present in that cell.

Multiple Barr bodies are at times present in dyskaryotic cells shed from dysplasia, because of hyperploidy, and from in situ and invasive squamous cell carcinoma. The buccal smear is preferred for evaluating the presence of X chromatin (Fig. 34-57). A vaginal smear can be used, but it introduces the confusion of many more artifacts, and frequently in the presence of inflammation there is poorer nuclear preservation. A good nuclear stain should be utilized. Although numerous stains are available, a permanent aceto-orcein stain is excellent for routine diagnostic work.

CYTOHORMONAL EVALUATION

The vaginal epithelium is extremely sensitive to the constant interplay of many humoral agents. It reacts in characteristic patterns to estrogens, progestogens, other hormones and other agents. The ways in which the vaginal epithelium can react are limited, but they can occur singly or in complex patterns. They include maturation of the epithelium, retention or exfoliation of individual cells, formation of glycogen, and secretion of mucus. These in turn affect the bacterial flora, the pH of the vaginal fluid, and the inflammatory elements.

Progestogens cause squamous cells to curl (naviculate), to stick together in agglutinated clumps, and to exfoliate at the intermediate cell level of maturation (Day 28, Fig. 34–1 A). Estrogens cause them to lie flat and singly, and to exfoliate at the superficial cell level (Day 14, Fig. 34–1 A). Most clinically desirable information can be obtained from well-made and accurately interpreted *vaginal pool spreads* prepared in the routine manner for cancer detection. Additional tests more specific for glycogen, mucus, bacteria, pH, or occult blood are available to supply a bit more hormonal information, but are usually unnecessary.

Reactions of cells to their complex endocrine milieu is the basis of cytohormonal evaluation. This evaluation is thus dependent upon *types* of hormonally active compounds present, their dose *levels* of activity, and the patient's ability for tissue *response*. The last is dependent upon the patient's thyroid status, previous injury to the tissue (e.g., radiation), and differences in response inherited by tissues of the end organ.

Although all living tissues respond to their endocrine-enzymatic milieu, some change their morphologic state with greater sensitivity. These reflect acutely the delicate hormonal balance present throughout the body at a given time. The vaginal epithelium is a mirror for the systemic interplay of clinically important substances. It is extremely sensitive to the sexually active compounds (estrogens, progestogens, and androgens) and in varying degrees to others (corticoids, thyroxins, vitamins, tetracyclines, digitoxins, etc.). The buccal mucosa, the external skin, and the urinary tract epithelium show similar responses, which are much weaker and less dependable.

None is as sensitive an indicator as the epithelium of the vaginal vault in quality, quantity, and rapidity of response. The vaginal epithelium at both ends—that which is near the introitus and that covering the fornices and the ectocervix—is less sensitive endocrinologically and much less reliable than the vaginal epithelium lining the middle portions of the vaginal tube.

The *lateral vaginal wall,* approximately opposite the tip of the cervix, is the most hormonally sensitive and accurate area for obtaining a cellular specimen. Scrapings of this region and material from this region in the vaginal pool are two most valuable specimens for indicating hormonal activity. Because of the ease of obtaining *vaginal pool* material and because it is a part of most routine cytologic preparations (e.g., Fast smear, see Fig. 34–56), it is the most widely used hormonal specimen (Fig. 34–56). When using vaginal pool material, however, one must be very careful to evaluate only material from the vaginal wall and not material coming from the cervix. With experience and care, this important distinction can be made consistently.

In *children* and the *aged,* great care must be exercised so that the specimen is obtained from the vaginal vault only. Contamination from touching the labia, vestibule, or the ungloved examiner's finger gives false cytohormonal evaluations. A reliable cytohormonal specimen is obtained from a child by using a nonabsorbent cotton swab, moistened with saline or serum, and introduced *through* a nasal speculum, a pediatric vaginal speculum, an otic speculum, or a drinking straw.

The use of Rakoff's rapid stain allows immediate recognition of overt abnormalities and prompt institution of therapy. This is a temporary preparation, however, and a permanent specimen also should be taken for more thorough inspection of important fine details as well as for future reference. Thus, the routine diagnostic cellular specimen for cancer detection, if it contains vaginal pool material, also allows a complete evaluation of endocrine changes to compare with previous and subsequent preparations. Scrapings or aspirations from the cervix do *not* yield accurate endocrine evaluation, and should not be used for cytohormonal evaluation.

Cellular Morphology Response

The most dependable and valuable information of the endocrine status is gained from cellular morphology, both in the relationships of one cell to another and their individual state of cellular maturation. The former includes mainly their sticky behavior with clumping *vs.* the tendency to remain separate as individual cells; and a cytoplasmic naviculation and enfolding upon itself *vs.* the tendency to lie flat. These relationships are extremely difficult to evaluate objectively and to communicate to others.

The most objective indicator of endocrine status is the stage of maturation which the cells of the vaginal epithelium attain at their time of exfoliation—the Maturation Index or M.I. Obviously, natural exfoliation is of basic importance to hormonal evaluation. Lateral vaginal wall scraping should be gentle and uniform from examination to examination. Vaginal pool material, obtained by either physician or patient, is generally uniform and yields accurate, reproducible, and clinically useful information, if not contaminated from cervicitis.

The endocrine-enzymatic milieu in which the squamous cells are bathed has the greatest influence upon the length of time these cells remain attached as part of the epithelium and upon the stage of maturation to which they develop. Compounds reach the cells with effectiveness either systemically from vessels below the basement membrane or topically from the vaginal lumen above the epithelial surface to produce cellular effects characteristic of the substance.

Indices and Values

A few clinically useful cellular indices have developed through general use, which express the stage of maturation attained by the cells of the squamous epithelium at their time of exfoliation. They yield the most objective and reproducible cytologic evaluation of endocrine status.

The Karyopyknotic Index (K.I.) is the percentage of squames (intermediate and superficial cells) having nuclear pyknosis. The percentage of squames showing cytoplasmic acidophilia is termed the Cornification Index (C.I.) or Eosinophilic Index (E.I.). Both of these exclude, however, the important parabasal-type cell exfoliation.

The Maturation Index (M.I.) gives a more completed cytohormonal picture, including parabasal cell evaluation, and is useful in more clinical situations. More complicated methods of expression are in use, but they appear to offer little more clinical assistance than those mentioned.

The Maturation Value (M.V.) assigns weights to each cell type (i.e., parabasal = 0.0; intermediate = 0.5; superficial = 1.0), providing a single value from the M.I., which is more easily fed into computers. Thus, an M.I. of $\overline{0/100/0}$, characteristic of intermediate cell estratrophy, is represented by an M.V. of 50; however, so is an M.I. of $\overline{33/34/33}$, which is found in severe inflammation and has nothing to do with estratrophy. More accurate and reproducible information regarding epithelial maturation is conveyed by use of the complete Maturation Index.

Maturation Index (M.I.)

There is a delicately changing ratio in the level of cellular maturation attained by the squamous cells at their time of exfoliation which is directly related to hormonal interplay and the endocrine status. It is determined by performing, in vaginal pool or lateral vaginal wall material, a randomized differential wall count of three major cell types shed from the stratified squamous epithelium listing percentages with the less mature cell on the left and the most mature on the right, viz.: parabasal cells, intermediate cells, and superficial cells (Fig. 35–2). Thus $\overline{0/75/25}$ represents the Maturation Index of a patient exfoliating no parabasal cells, 75 per cent intermediate cells, and 25 per cent superficial cells; furthermore, it reflects their ratio on the surface of the intact vaginal epithelium at their time of exfoliation. A shift of the Maturation Index to the left (i.e., $\overleftarrow{30/70/0}$) denotes the release of less mature cells, whereas a shift to the right ($\overrightarrow{0/30/70}$) indicates a greater degree of cellular maturation before exfoliation (Fig. 34–1).

The three cell types are identified first by their *cytoplasmic thickness*. If the cytoplasm is thick, the cell is parabasal; if it is wafer-thin, the cell is a squame of either intermediate or superficial type (Fig. 34–2). In the latter group, the *nuclear status* is the indicator which separates the intermediate from the superficial cell type. If the cell has a plump and vesicular nucleus with an intact chromatin pattern, it is an intermediate cell. If the nucleus is pyknotic, shrunken below 6μm., hyperchromatic, and lacks a chromatin pattern, the cell is a superficial cell.

The most accurate and reproducible differentiation between intermediate and superficial cells is thus made on nuclear pyknosis alone. There is fairly good, but unpredictable, correlation between cytoplasmic color of intermediate and superficial cells (Cornification Index) and the degree of nuclear maturation (Karyopyknotic Index). Cytoplasmic color is frequently misleading because of drying, fixation, inflammation and other unpredictable artifacts, and it is disregarded for the determination of the Maturation Index. It gives a rapid, but rough, impression of the level of cellular maturation utilizing Papanicolaou, Shorr, or Rakoff stain. For objective accuracy, however, the three individual cell types are evaluated with strict adherence to cellular morphology (i.e., cytoplasmic maturation, *thick vs. thin;* nuclear maturation, *metabolic vs. pyknotic).*

The pyknotic nucleus of the superficial cell shines with a peculiar reddish gleam when examined with the phase contrast microscope. When the routine Papanicolaou stain is used, a sharp distinction is obvious on properly fixed material (Fig. 34–2). In unsatisfactory nuclear stains and in cellular preparations dried before fixation or incorrectly fixed, a sharp differentiation may be difficult regardless of the visualizing technique.

One must be very careful *not* to include metaplastic or dysplastic cells in the Maturation Index. Such cells, as from endocervical dysplasia, may contaminate the vaginal pool material, but they are recognized by their large abnormal nuclei (see Fig. 34–32). These dyskaryotic cells must be excluded from the Maturation Index. This is, therefore, another important reason why the cervical component is to be *identified* and *not used* in cytohormonal evaluation. One *identifies* the cervical component by recognizing its dyskaryotic cells, its endocervical cells, and the thick inflammatory mucus characteristic of coexisting chronic cervicitis, and *does not use it* for cytohormonal evaluation.

Under a low power lens the vaginal wall material areas of the slide that are free of cervical contamination are determined. These areas are then used for cytohormonal evaluation by picking a random aliquot for evaluation. This is accomplished by counting *only* the *first* two squamous epithelial cells encountered in each *randomly* selected field of the pure vaginal wall material, until 100 or 200 squamous cells have been evaluated.

Anucleate superficial cells are sometimes encountered under abnormal conditions. When they occur in patchy distribution, they are usually shed from areas of hyperkeratotic leukoplakia or from contamination from the introitus. When equally distributed throughout the vaginal material, however, they re-sult from extremely high levels of estrogen or increased tissue sensitivities to the hormone (excessive therapy, tumors of the ovaries and endometrium, etc.) (see Fig. 34-14). This is a usual occurrence in the rhesus monkey at menarche, but occasionally is also a physiologic finding at human menarche.

Under certain conditions parabasal cells have acidophilic cytoplasm which, uncommonly, may be truly keratinized. At times their nuclei may be pyknotic; at other times, they are large and pale. Such abnormal parabasal cells can be found in severe teleatrophy, in inflammation, in an androgenic effect, and in some patients with mammary carcinoma. Their true parabasal cell identity is evident from the *thickness* of the cytoplasm and the absence of the thin squamification of superficial cells.

Artificial Vagina

Grafts from the thigh and other parts of the body to form artificial vaginas may show a slight degree of endocrine response after becoming well established and adapted to the situation. It has been shown that they are even capable of some *sexual secretory activity* characteristic of the normal vaginal wall. The cytohormonal pattern is not normal, however, as the cells tend to retain some true cornification, with extreme shifts of the Maturation Index to the right and exfoliation of anucleate superficial cells.

CYTOHORMONAL PATTERNS: NORMAL

Certain normal cytohormonal patterns and their physiologic variations must be understood as a baseline before attempting to interpret abnormalities. For better comprehension and clinical correlation, the normal female life span is considered in five periods: *childhood, perimenarchal, reproductive, perimenopausal,* and *postmenopausal* (Fig. 34–4). Three of these, the childhood, reproductive, and postmenopausal periods, are well defined clinically by the objective occurrences of *birth, menarche, menopause,* and *death.* The other two, the perimenarchal and the perimenopausal periods, overlap the former at menarche and menopause. Even though clinical definition of the beginning and cessation of menses may appear to be fairly sharp in most individ-

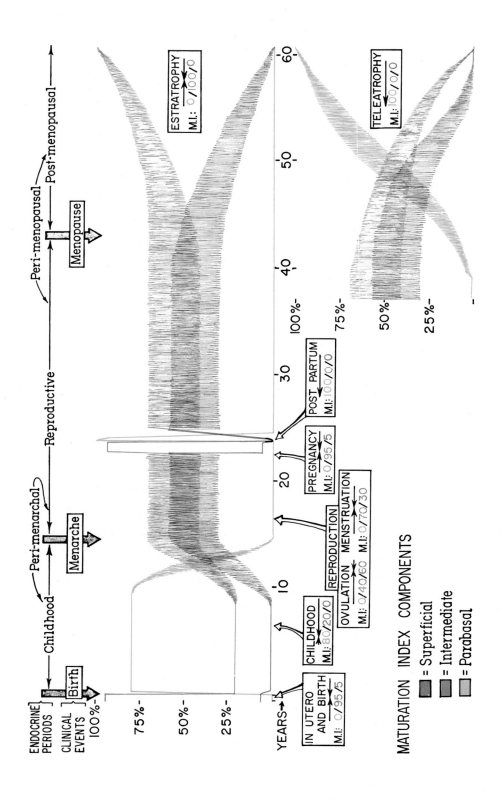

Figure 34–4. A woman's cytohormonal lifetime—a schematic representation of the Maturation Index (M.I.). The endocrine periods of the female —*childhood, perimenarchal, reproductive, perimenopausal,* and *postmenopausal*—and the three major clinical events—*birth, menarche,* and *menopause*—are represented with their coinciding Maturation Indices. This represents the fluctuations of the percentages on the surface of the vaginal epithelium of the three stages of epithelial cell maturation (parabasal cell, intermediate cell, superficial cell), which occur under the influence of various hormones.

Estrogens produce superficial cell maturation (M.I. to the right, toward $\overline{0/0/100}$). A moderate degree of this effect is noted at ovulation (M.I.:.c. $\overline{0/40/60}$).

Progestogens and *cortisone* cause intermediate cell maturation (M.I. to the midzone, toward $\overrightarrow{0/100/0}$). A moderate degree of this effect is noted at menstruation (M.I.:.c. $\overline{0/70/30}$), with extreme effects at both birth and pregnancy (M.I.:.c. $\overline{0/95/5}$) and the postmenopausal intermediate cell maturation (M.I.: $\overline{0/100/0}$).

Lack of all maturing factors, or repression of their effects, causes no maturation beyond parabasal cells at the time of exfoliation (M.I. to the left, toward $\overline{100/0/0}$). A moderate degree of this effect is noted during childhood (M.I.:.c. $\overline{80/20/0}$), whereas an extreme degree occurs during the post-partum period and in postmenopausal parabasal maturation (M.I.: $\overline{100/0/0}$).

Childhood is relatively constant and predictable with a lack of superficial cells. The *reproductive* period is fairly constant from cycle to cycle in a given individual. Atrophy in the *postmenopausal* period is of two main types: intermediate cell maturation (M.I.: $\overrightarrow{0/100/0}$) with complete lack of estrogenic effect (estratrophy), and parabasal cell maturation (M.I.: $\overline{100/0/0}$) with complete lack of effect of all maturing substances (teleatrophy). In contrast, the *perimenarchal* and the *perimenopausal* periods are extremely difficult to predict without cell specimen because of the wide range of normal possibilities serving as an unpredictable baseline.

After conception the Maturation Index takes a wide swing and is locked in place during pregnancy by massive hormone levels (M.I.: $\overleftarrow{0/95/5}$). At term the Maturation Index abruptly swings to the surprising atrophic pattern of post partum. It then gradually returns to normal reproductive levels unless the patient nurses.

For an intelligent cytohormonal evaluation it is thus essential to know all pertinent information about the patient, including age, date of cell specimen, last menstrual period, previous menstrual period, drug therapy, radiotherapy, surgery.

uals, these two periods (perimenarchal and perimenopausal) are exceptionally unpredictable without cytohormonal evaluation because they are times of great endocrine turbulence, with extreme individual variation.

Normal Cytohormonal Patterns of Basic Stimulating Agents

Estrogens

All layers of the squamous epithelium become thickened and proliferated under the influence of this family of hormones, most markedly in the intermediate and superficial cells. Estrogens cause the cells to mature to superficial cells before exfoliation, with the resultant shift of the Maturation Index to the right. Thus, a patient with only parabasal cell maturation (M.I.: $\overleftarrow{100/0/0}$) (see Fig. 34–11), given increasing doses of estrogens, either systemically or vaginally, undergoes a progressive shift of the Maturation Index to the right. Because the degree of shift is proportional to the amount of estrogens administered, a moderate dose produces a partial shift to the right (M.I.: $\overrightarrow{0/50/50}$) whereas an extremely large dose can produce a complete shift to the right (M.I.: $\overrightarrow{0/0/100}$). When estrogenic effect is so extreme (see Fig. 34–14), many of the superficial cells become anucleate.

With the maturation to superficial cells in response to estrogen therapy, clinical and cytologic inflammation caused by teleatrophy disappears (see Fig. 34–11). Degeneration is strikingly reduced and the cellular smear appears "clean," with cells tending to be distributed singly and without curling.

Progestogens

The squamous epithelium of the vaginal vault is also proliferative under the influence of this group of hormones; however, maturation progresses only through the intermediate cell stage, at which time exfoliation occurs. Thus the predominant cell on the surface and in the vaginal smear is the intermediate cell. The Maturation Index shifts toward the midzone and, if the effective level is sufficiently high, reaches $\overrightarrow{0/100/0}\overleftarrow{}$.

When the epithelium has been properly "primed" with estrogens, administration of progestogens causes the edges of the cells' cytoplasm to curl upward, giving a boatlike (navicular) shape peculiar to this hormone's action. The cells appear sticky and clump together in masses (Figs. 34–1 A, 34–5 B and 34–7). At times cytolysis occurs. The background of the cellular spread is "messy" with mucus, neutrophils, and cellular debris.

Superficial cells are not produced by action of progesterone alone. In the absence of irritations, estrogen are needed to mature the epithelium past the intermediate cell stage.

Cortisone

Drugs having the clinical effect of cortisone produce a cellular proliferation which is partially similar to that of progesterone in that the cells mature to the intermediate cell type on the surface of the epithelium before exfoliation, and the Maturation Index approaches $\overrightarrow{0/100/0}\overleftarrow{}$, according to the effective dosage. Contrary to the effect of progestogens, however, the cells do not tend to curl or stick but lie flat and singly in a pattern of intermediate cell maturation, with the cellular spread appearing strikingly "clean" and mucus usually scanty or absent (see Fig. 34–10).

Androgens

This group of hormones does not truly oppose proliferation of the epithelium, contrary to common presumption. In fact, proliferation of different types is the rule under the influence of androgens. Although the cells on the surface usually mature mainly to parabasal cells, they can mature to any of the three cell types. At times all three cell types are present on the epithelial surface, under androgen effect, depending mainly upon the "priming" of the epithelium beforehand. Thus, one can find parabasal cells lying on the surface beside superficial cells and intermediate cells, making the Maturation Index a "spread" pattern approaching $\overleftarrow{33/34/33}\overrightarrow{}$ and mimicking the effect of inflammation. In some patients a preponderance of intermediate cells or parabasal cells is present, approaching either $\overrightarrow{0/100/0}\overleftarrow{}$ or $\overleftarrow{100/0/0}$ Maturation Index. The trend for the index to "spread" under the effect of androgens remains even in these patients, however, and they can produce a few superficial cells.

Androgens do not produce only simple atrophy. That they may be contributing to a given "spread" pattern is suggested by the finding of abnormally small orangophilic superficial cells (wafer-thin polygonal cytoplasm with karyopyknosis) and small *cornified* parabasal cells (thick orangophilic cytoplasm with karyopyknosis). These can be produced also in keratinizing atypical metaplasia, another reason why it is essential that the cervical component and the vaginal wall component *each* be recognized in a vaginal pool specimen, and that only the latter be evaluated cytohormonally; or, preferably, that a pure lateral vaginal wall scraping be obtained to determine definitely the presence of three cell types, so rare in the absence of inflammation. At times mucus is profuse in the background of an androgen pattern.

These cellular findings, however, can also be observed with inflammation. Because an androgenic pattern may appear inflammatory and obscuring, these two conditions can be difficult to discriminate. Furthermore, the pattern resultant from androgens is very dependent on preexisting and coexisting endocrine influences. Thus, while an observed pattern may be very suggestive of the hormone, androgens unfortunately do not produce a diagnostic pattern.

Miscellaneous Substances

Various other compounds can affect the sensitive vaginal epithelium. Digitalis and some broad spectrum antibiotics (e.g., tetracyclines) produce maturation of the epithelium to intermediate cells before exfoliation ($\overrightarrow{0/100/0}$), without causing navicularization and other changes associated with progesterone. Long-term digitalis therapy may also cause a shift of the Maturation Index to the right, mimicking estrogens. However, both the midzone shift and the shift to the right with digitalis are mild and easily obscured by other hormones.

Conversely, the *absence* or severe reduction of some substances may change the cellular response. Severe avitaminosis A causes a shift of the Maturation Index to the right, whereas virtual athyroidism and panhypopituitarism shift the Maturation Index to the left.

Different substances acting together, in succession or simultaneously, produce *compounding* effects which may simply be additive or may qualitatively change the response to each of the others. For example, the effect of progesterone upon an unstimulated atrophic vaginal epithelium differs markedly from that produced by the same hormone upon one primed with estrogen.

Inflammatory Effect

In addition to bringing forth the leukocytes and other inflammatory elements, inflammation alters the level of maturation attained by the cells on the surface of squamous epithelium. Specifically, all three cell types can be found on the surface of the epithelium at the same time and exfoliate, as in the androgenic pattern. The tendency is for the cell types that were in the minority before inflammation to increase at the expense of the cell types that were in the majority (e.g., $\overrightarrow{0/95/5}$ to $\overleftarrow{30/40/30}$). If severe enough, it can shift any pattern to a complete spread ($\overleftrightarrow{33/34/33}$). The degree of spread of the Maturation Index, is roughly proportional to the severity of the inflammation and dependent upon its etiology. However, the effects of inflammation cannot be predicted closely enough to extrapolate in order to obtain the true underlying hormonal pattern, so that it is necessary to clear the inflammation and repeat the cytohormonal evaluation.

Severe inflammation may even mature the surface cell past the nucleated superficial cell type, exfoliating anucleated superficial cells into the vaginal pool. In vaginitis it is distributed *generally* throughout the material. When the severe irritation is restricted to an extremely small area of the epithelium (e.g., chronic inflammation from the irritation of a retained pessary, a localized dermatosis), these extreme cellular artifacts exfoliating into otherwise healthy vaginal secretions may appear paradoxic. Since they are *patchy* and well separated from the healthy secretions, their true nature can be suspected.

In addition to the alteration of cellular maturation, severe inflammation also obscures and destroys cells. In all events, a cytohormonal evaluation should *not* be attempted in the presence of marked inflammation or false and misleading information will be obtained. The one and *only* exception to this rule is parabasal teleatrophy ($\overleftarrow{100/0/0}$) which can be accurately diagnosed even in presence of severe inflammation.

Otherwise, an inflammatory cell specimen is unsatisfactory for cytohormonal evaluation. If vaginitis *is* present, any effective way of reducing the inflammation which does not employ agents altering the epithelial maturation makes it possible for the true hormonal pattern to be evaluated. If there is *no* vaginitis, but cervicitis is present contaminating the vaginal pool and obscuring the cytologic pattern, a lateral vaginal wall scrape yields a satisfactory specimen.

Normal Cytohormonal Pattern of the Endocrine Periods

Childhood Period

The normal cellular pattern of childhood is one of the most dependable and constant basic patterns. Except for the very beginning (neonatal) and end (perimenarchal) of the period, the *superficial cell* is *absent* (Fig. 34–4). Its presence may signal an improper sample (e.g., contamination by introitus, inflammation), an estrogen source (e.g., ingestion), or an abnormality (e.g., ovarian tumor).

At birth the vaginal epithelium of the female infant is thick and lush in response to circulating maternal hormones, including massive progestogens, estrogens, and adre-

nocortical compounds (Fig. 34–5). The cells on the surface consist mainly of intermediate cells so that the Maturation Index is $\overline{0/95/5}$, which is characteristic of birth as well as of pregnancy (Fig. 34–7).

Within the first few weeks following birth, however, there is a mass exfoliation of the lush intermediate cell layers. The epithelium becomes thin and atrophic, so characteristic of childhood, with the cells maturing only to the parabasal cell or intermediate cell type before exfoliation. Reflecting this change, the Maturation Index markedly shifts to the left (from $\overline{0/95/5}$ to about $\overline{100/0/0}$, $\overline{70/30/0}$)—but with *no* superficial cells.

Throughout the rest of childhood until perimenarche, the normal level of maturation which the surface cell attains is the parabasal type cell or the intermediate cell, but with *no* superficial cells. The presence of the latter bears great clinical significance. If there is no inflammation or irritation and no contamination of the vaginal smear with vulvar or introitus cells, the superficial cell is normally absent until the onset of the peri-

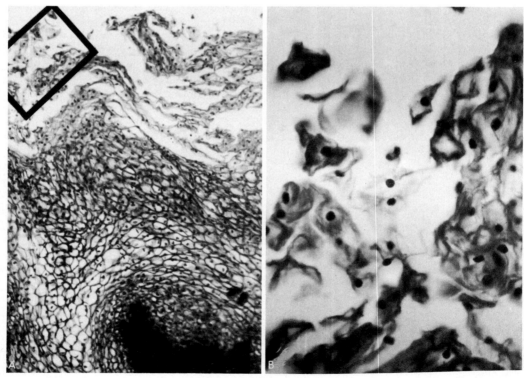

Figure 34–5. Vaginal epithelium, six-month human fetus, hematoxylin-eosin. *A,* The epithelium is lush, composed mainly of intermediate cells. A few layers of parabasal cells are present in the depths of the epithelium, but intermediate cells make up most of its thickness and lie on its surface. ×40. *B,* The surface of the same epithelium is exfoliating intermediate cells almost exclusively (M.I.: 0/95/5) with curling of their edges (*naviculation*). ×160. (See Fig. 34–7 for identical pattern in Fast smear.)

menarchal period. Abnormal estrogenic effect is signaled by the *unexplained* presence of the superficial cell.

Perimenarchal Period

There is great individual variation in the age of onset of the perimenarchal period. Usually beginning around the age of 6 or 8 years, there is a gradual increase in notable sex steroid activity until the reproductive level is reached at menarche, about the age of fourteen (Fig. 34–4). With this gradual increase the vaginal epithelium becomes thicker and more proliferative, with an increasing percentage of the surface cells maturing to the intermediate cell and superficial cell types before exfoliation. Thus, the vaginal cellular spread mirrors the increase of sex hormone production during this perimenarchal period with an increasing shift of the Maturation Index to the right, until the typical cytohormonal pattern of the reproductive age is present at menarche.

Great variation can be encountered in this perimenarchal period because it is a continuing transition from childhood atrophy (M.I.: $\overleftarrow{100/0/0}$ to $\overrightarrow{0/100/0}$) to the lush epithelium of the reproductive period (M.I. about $\overrightarrow{0/30/70}$, $\overrightarrow{0/70/30}$). Although age is the major factor in evaluating endocrine status during this period, individual variations are many. Even after the appearance of menses there is still adjustment for many persons. Some have not yet reached a full reproductive Maturation Index at menarche, whereas others exceed normalcy for a period of time with an extreme shift to the right of the Maturation Index at midcycle. Eventually they settle into their pattern of the reproductive period.

Reproductive Period

Normally the endocrine milieu shows great cyclic fluctuation from menarche to menopause. Following the initial period of endocrine adjustment in the establishment of menses (perimenarche) and extending into the disruption of endocrine interplay (perimenopause) (Fig. 34–4), the hormonal pattern varies widely within each lunar cycle. Each cycle, however, is mirrored in repetition with a given individual. Normally their constancy is broken only by childbearing. The characteristic patterns of the reproductive period are the *menstrual cycle, pregnancy,* and the *postpartum* period.

Menstrual Cycle. The cells on the surface of the vaginal epithelium during the menstrual cycle, and thus in the cellular spread, are both intermediate and superficial cells. Their percentages vary from 30 per cent to 70 per cent in response mainly to estrogen and progestogen levels (Fig. 34–1 A and 34–4).

At *ovulation* the level of estrogen is the highest without opposition (Fig. 34–6). This produces a moderate shift to the right in the Maturation Index (c. $\overrightarrow{0/40/60}$, $\overrightarrow{0/40/70}$). When ovulation occurs, the level of circulating estrogens drops rapidly but promptly rises again with the development of the corpus luteum. During this secretory phase, however, the estrogens are accompanied by progestogens (Fig. 34–6). Just before menstruation this progestogen opposition is at its highest, producing a moderate shift of the Maturation Index toward the midzone (c. $\overleftarrow{0/70/30}$). This is the *biphasic pattern of ovulation* (Fig. 34–1).

During *menstruation* the levels of both estrogens and progestogens drop sharply, but soon the estrogens alone again rise from the developing new follicle during the proliferative phase. This shifts the Maturation Index back to the right until the ovulatory pattern (M.I.: c. $\overrightarrow{0/40/60}$, $\overrightarrow{0/30/70}$) is again reached, and held until ovulation occurs, approximately two weeks before the next menses.

Normally the parabasal cell does not exfoliate during the reproductive period, except for the postpartum period and the later (perimenopausal) years of the reproductive period (Figs. 34–1 A and 34–4). In some patients the parabasal cell may not exfoliate at any time, even during the perimenopausal and postmenopausal periods, if intermediate maturation ($\overleftarrow{0/100/0}$) rather than parabasal maturation ($\overleftarrow{100/0/0}$) develops.

Only limited endocrine information can be obtained from the evaluation of a *single* vaginal cellular spread. Hormonal variations are tremendous during the menstrual cycle. Furthermore, there are many possible combinations of factors which can produce similar cytohormonal patterns when they are viewed statically as a single examination. This is analogous to evaluating a single basal body temperature versus a series.

Thus, to yield valuable dynamic endocrine information, a complete cytohormonal evaluation may at times depend upon *multiple daily* vaginal specimens. It is best that these be vaginal pool aspiration smears, easily prepared by the patient who, at the same time, records her basal body temperature,

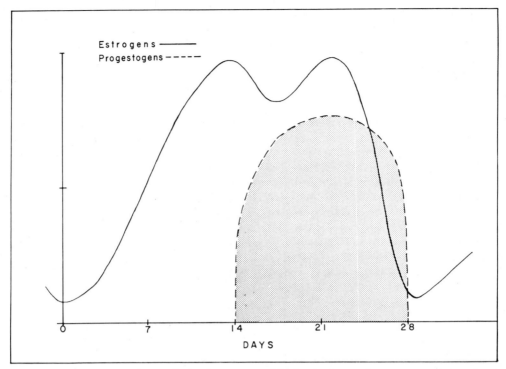

Figure 34–6. The menstrual cycle. An idealized composite of the levels of systemic estrogens and progestogens during the menstrual cycle of a woman in her reproductive period. Their interplay is a prime factor in determining the level of maturation of the vaginal epithelium, of the Maturation Index of the exfoliated cells and of the overall cytohormonal pattern (compare with Fig. 34–1A).

menstrual information, etc. These data may be invaluable for determining time in cycle, ovulation, anovulation, and other endocrinopathies.

Pregnancy. The cytohormonal pattern of normal pregnancy is characteristic and constant. Its time of appearance and degree may vary from patient to patient.

With conception, the normal luteal phase proceeds much as in the nonpregnant menstrual cycle, with a moderate shift of the Maturation Index toward the midzone (Figs. 34–1 A, 34–4, and 34–6). However, when the pattern reaches the menstrual Maturation Index (c. $\overleftrightarrow{0/70/30}$) it does not reverse toward the ovulatory pattern, as in a normal menstrual cycle (Fig. 34–1 A) but continues its midzone shift until, usually within a few weeks, it reaches the pattern that is so characteristic of pregnancy—an extreme *midzone* shift of the Maturation Index to $\overrightarrow{0/95/5}$ (Figs. 34–4 and 34–7). This is maintained throughout normal gestation.

The massive levels of estrogens, progestogens (Fig. 34–8), and cortical steroids strongly maintain this midzone pattern in normal pregnancy. Because of this massive hormonal milieu, the Maturation Index is "locked into" this characteristic midzone pattern ($\overrightarrow{0/95/5}$), and is not altered by the same small therapeutic dosages of hormones that alter the index in a nonpregnant patient. Thus, Wied has shown that, in patients with perimenopausal amenorrhea entering into a pattern of intermediate cell maturation, which might be confused with that of pregnancy (see Fig. 34–10), cellular examinations made before and after administration of small dosages of estrogens given systemically reveal the true condition: the pregnant perimenopausal patient shows no Maturation Index shift; the *non*pregnant perimenopausal patient, however, shows the characteristic estrogenic shift of the Maturation Index to the right.

Vaginitis has a *direct* effect upon the vaginal epithelium. Even with the massive hormonal levels of pregnancy, the epithelium is altered if inflammation is sufficient. The characteristic inflammatory spread pattern of the Maturation Index results (from $\overrightarrow{0/95/5}$ to c. $\overleftrightarrow{33/34/33}$).

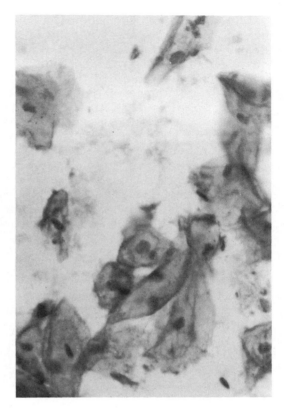

Figure 34–7. Pregnancy pattern. Fast smear of a 23 year old female, seventh month of gestation. The midzone shift of the Maturation Index (0/95/5) is typical of pregnancy and of progestogen/estrogen therapy. It is also found during fetal life (Fig. 34–5) and at birth. There is curling of the intermediate cells into navicular forms. They clump and adhere to each other. There is some cytolysis with bare nuclei resulting. ×160.

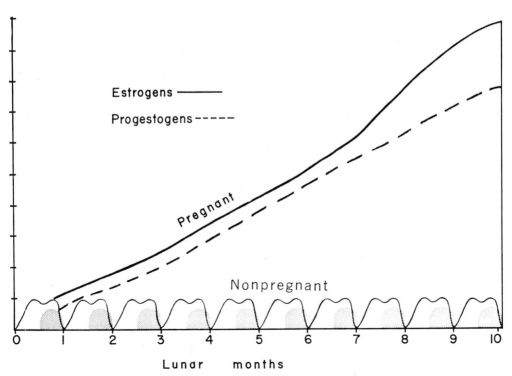

Estrogens ———

Progestogens – – – –

Pregnant

Nonpregnant

Lunar   months

Figure 34–8. Pregnancy. An idealized composite of the systemic estrogens and progestogens of a hypothetical patient, superimposed upon the pattern expected if she were not pregnant.

In the absence of inflammation, it is significant to find appreciable variance in the pregnancy Maturation Index of $\overrightarrow{0/95/5}$, either to the right or to the left. For such an alteration to occur in a pattern normally held by massive levels of hormones, the endocrine derangement must be great. Abortions having an endocrine basis can be heralded by a bizarre Maturation Index, either to the right, to the left, or spread. A threatened abortion with an endocrine basis is usually accompanied by a Maturation Index shift to the right; however, it may be spread or, strongly suggesting death of the fetus, shifted to the left, similar to the postpartum cytohormonal pattern (Fig. 34–9).

Postpartum Period. Around the time of delivery another mammoth hormonal change takes place, which is mirrored in the Maturation Index. Just before delivery the Maturation Index may shift briefly to the right, but then plunges to the left after delivery, toward a teleatrophic pattern characteristic of the postpartum period (Figs. 34–4 and 34–9). It is striking indeed for a normal woman in her reproductive years to develop an apparent cytohormonal atrophy of the parabasal cell type (M.I.: $\overleftarrow{100/0/0}$), and this can be clinically misleading if adequate history is not forthcoming.

This postpartum parabasal cell maturation pattern and its duration vary among individuals depending upon various factors, including whether the woman breast-feeds or receives hormones for suppression of lactation. It gradually returns to the normal cytohormonal pattern of the menstrual cycle.

Pundel observed the brief prepartum shift to the right in a large number of patients, which indicated impending delivery. He also noted a brief prepartum shift to the left in a few cases, associated with postmaturity. In the latter he reports successful rescue of the infants. Not all workers have been able to confirm these observations.

The sex of the fetus does not significantly alter the cytohormonal pattern of the mother. The normal hormonal levels which establish the pregnancy pattern are so massive, relative to the minor alteration which any fetal production might produce, that a change is not recognizable in the cytohormonal pattern.

Perimenopausal Period

For a varying number of years around the clinical menopause there are gradually progressive alterations to the orderly cyclic endocrine patterns of the reproductive period, both prior to and after the actual cessation of menses. These are mirrored in the vaginal epithelium and in its cytohormonal pattern (Fig. 34–4). This alteration commences insidiously in the last years of the reproductive period and continues for varying numbers of years after the clinical menopause, with cyclic hormonal variations decreasing in intensity and frequency. Just as onset is gradual and variable, the cessation of cycles is also insidious and without overt clinical manifestations, but it is detectable with cytohormonal evaluation.

Cytohormonally women fall into two fairly well-defined categories: those who, in their postmenopausal period, are to develop *estratrophy*, intermediate cell maturation (M.I.: $\overrightarrow{0/100/0}$) with lack of observable estrogenic effect (Fig. 34–10), and those who are to develop *teleatrophy*, parabasal cell maturation (M.I.: $\overleftarrow{100/0/0}$) with no evidence of

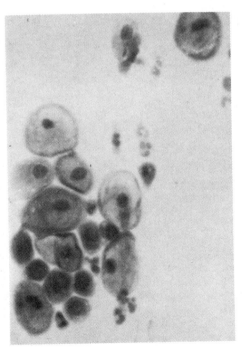

Figure 34–9. *Postpartum lactational pattern.* This is a parabasal cell maturation pattern (M.I.: $\overleftarrow{100/0/0}$) consisting mainly of parabasal cells whose cytoplasm frequently contains golden-brown material. It occurs abruptly at the end of gestation and is a marked change from the lush intermediate cell exfoliation of pregnancy (Fig. 34–7). It lasts for a varying length of time, eventually shifting to the right into the cytohormonal pattern of the menstrual cycle. Fast smear, 25 year old patient, six weeks post partum. ×160.

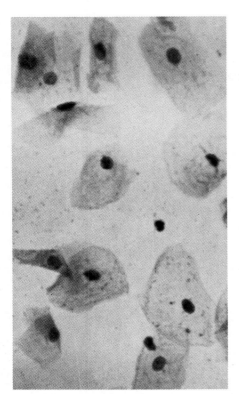

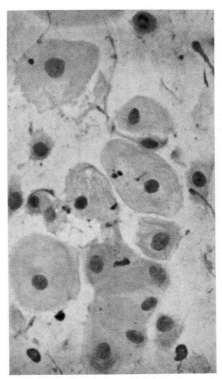

Figure 34–10. *Intermediate cell maturation pattern—* Maturation Index: $\overrightarrow{0/100/0}$. There is a complete lack of observable estrogenic effect (*estratrophy*). The cellular spread contains only intermediate cells (thin, wafer cytoplasm with vesicular nuclei). They typically lie singly and flat, as under cortisone therapy, and do not clump or curl as with pregnancy (Fig. 34–7) and progesterone therapy, which also exhibit an M.I. midzone shift. There is no evidence of estrogenic stimulation (no superficial cells), but in its place are other maturing elements, apparently mainly corticoids, which give abundant proliferation of the epithelium and mature its cells to the intermediate cell stage before exfoliation. This type of epithelium, which is *not* easily infected, is to be distinguished from the thin, atrophic epithelium of parabasal cell maturation (Fig. 34–11) which is frequently inflamed. This Fast smear is of a 55 year old female, 5 years postmenopausal. ×100.

Figure 34–11. *Parabasal cell maturation pattern—* Maturation Index: $\overleftarrow{100/0/0}$. Complete atrophy (*teleatrophy*). There is no evidence of an epithelial maturing factor, as this cellular spread contains only parabasal cells (thick cytoplasm). The thin atrophic epithelium from which these cells are shed shows no effect of maturing hormones; however, it is usually very sensitive to their administration unless this pattern is the result of injury (e.g., postirradiation). This type of epithelium is easily infected, producing senile atrophic vaginitis. This Fast smear is of a 66 year old female, 22 years postmenopausal. ×160.

vaginal epithelial maturation (Fig. 34–11). These two patterns are strikingly and significantly different, both morphologically and clinically. Both were referred to in the older literature as atrophy, which of course is most confusing clinically. Because these are two distinct endocrine situations, care must be taken to separate and identify them clearly.

With the development of *estratrophy* (complete lack of observable estrogenic effect) in the perimenopausal period, an increasing number of *intermediate cells* exfoliate at the expense of superficial cells

without production of parabasal cells (Fig. 34–4), producing the pattern of cortisone effect (Fig. 34–10). This results in a gradual shift toward the midzone until complete intermediate maturation (M.I.: $\overrightarrow{0/100/0}$) is reached, sometimes years after actual cessation of menses. The vaginal epithelium in estratrophy is *not* thin and atrophic but is more lush and resistant to infection than in teleatrophy. Senile atrophic vaginitis is *not* found in this group of patients. If inflammation is present in estratrophy, an etiologic agent should be sought (i.e., *Trichomonas*, fungus, bacteria, virus).

With the development of *teleatrophy* (complete lack of effect of all maturing substances—a hormonal "vacuum" pattern) in the perimenopausal period, there is a gradual increase in exfoliation of *parabasal cells*.

This is usually first at the expense of the superficial cells, and later of the intermediate cells (Fig. 34–4). When complete teleatrophy appears, with parabasal cell maturation and a complete shift of the Maturation Index to the left ($\overrightarrow{100/0/0}$) (Fig. 34–11), vaginal atrophy is clinically present and there is an extremely low resistance to trauma and infection. Senile vaginitis, or atrophic vaginitis, is found frequently in this group of patients.

When a patient is castrated during her reproductive period, the resulting epithelial maturation yields a cytohormonal pattern of intermediate cell maturation, not parabasal cell maturation. Adrenocortical function plays a larger role in vaginal epithelial maturation than is generally appreciated, accounting in great part for the Maturation Index midzone shift of intermediate cell maturation. It is not clear why all patients do not follow the same pattern at the menopause, but unquestionably many factors are at work. There is great individual variation in vaginal epithelial sensitivity and response, in hypophyseal response to feedback, in production of adrenocorticoids and sex steroids, and in cortisone utilization in response to infection and stress.

Thus, there is *no* typical cytohormonal pattern at the time of the last menses, the range of normalcy being extremely wide. Some pass through the menopause with a "young" pattern, whereas others are more atrophic. A cytohormonal evaluation, however, detects these differences and gives good clinical insight as to that particular patient's endocrinologic milieu.

The established pattern appears to be mainly one of default (withdrawal of maturing substances) rather than of strong endocrine control. It is thus very labile and sensitive to small dosages of hormones or to inflammation. The previously discussed differentiation between a perimenopausal pregnancy and a missed menstrual period with intermediate maturation (p. 704) exploits the weak endocrine control over the latter pattern.

Thus, there is a very broad "normal limit" to consider when evaluating patients of the perimenopausal period for endocrine abnormalities. Further, this perimenopausal period is greatly variable in length, and the exact "normal" course to be taken by a given patient is unpredictable. However, when it is clinically of crucial importance to know whether estrogen effect on tissues is present or not, a careful cytohormonal evaluation can be the only source of this vital information.

Postmenopausal Period

As the endocrinologically stormy and unpredictable perimenopausal period passes into the relatively quiescent postmenopausal period (Fig. 34–4), either of the two major patterns (intermediate or parabasal cell maturation), or variations thereof, is assumed. Cyclic fluctuations continue for varying periods, becoming less and less intense.

Estratrophy of intermediate cell maturation (M.I.: $\overrightarrow{0/100/0}\overleftarrow{}$) (Fig. 34–10) is usually asymptomatic because the epithelium is thick, proliferative, and protective (p. 707).

Teleatrophy of parabasal cell maturation (M.I.: $\overrightarrow{100/0/0}$) (Fig. 34–11) is virtually a pattern of an endocrine "vacuum" (p. 707). It is associated with a thin atrophic epithelium which frequently becomes inflamed and infected, producing senile atrophic vaginitis. At times in these individuals, bizarre changes in parabasal cells result from irritation and regeneration, which can produce marked dyskaryosis, morphologically very difficult to differentiate from neoplasia. When this occurs, small amounts of estrogens, administered either orally or vaginally, mature this sensitive epithelium sufficiently for the problem in diagnosis to be dissipated. If no neoplastic process is present, the parabasal maturation pattern gives way to a normal estrogenic pattern. Abnormal cellular changes of epithelial injury and healing may take weeks or months to disappear. However, if cancer is present, the true identity of the neoplastic cells can be determined as the inflammatory process subsides. While this must never replace adequate tissue studies, such estrogen trial can at times provide valuable clinical information otherwise unobtainable, and detect latent, hidden cancer.

One *reliable abnormal finding* in this postmenopausal period is the unexplained presence of appreciable numbers of superficial cells (more than about 10 per cent) in the absence of estrogen administration and inflammation. Superficial cells are present in infection, chronic irritation (procidentia, pessary, etc.), leukoplakia, vaginal dermatoses, certain tumors (endometrial, tubal, ovarian, mammary, adrenal), endocrinopathies, and, of course, contamination of the vaginal cellular specimen with cells from the introitus or vulva.

CYTOHORMONAL PATTERNS: ABNORMAL

Before attempts are made to detect abnormalities or to determine their nature, the normal baseline expected for that given patient must first be clearly determined. One must consider the date of the specimen, last menstrual period (LMP), previous menstrual period, possible hormonal therapy, surgical or radiologic endocrine change, or the effects of various artifacts (e.g., inflammation) which might alter the basic pattern. When all this information has been analyzed in relation to the five normal endocrine periods, one can then proceed to determine variations from this expected "normal" and evaluate their significance.

Neoplasms Producing Hormones

Hormone-producing tumors cause a shift of the Maturation Index that is characteristic of the hormone secreted. The quality of the shift and its degree depend upon the clinical effectiveness of the particular compound being produced, upon the amount reaching the vagina, and upon the responsiveness of the vaginal epithelium.

Estrogen-Producing Tumors

The *estrogens* produced by ovarian granulosa cell tumors are usually potent and, if produced in sufficient quantities, shift the Maturation Index clearly to the right (toward $\overrightarrow{0/0/100}$). On the other hand, estrogens from the adrenal cortex are usually weaker clinically and less physiologic in their activity, and produce estrogenic effects proportionally.

Progestogen-Producing Tumors

Progesterone produced by luteinizing tumors of the ovary varies in potency. If secretion and potency are sufficient, there is a recognizable midzone shift of the Maturation Index (toward $\overrightarrow{0/100/0}$). The cells fold (naviculation), and stick together if sufficient estrogen is also present in the system, even to the point of exactly mimicking pregnancy.

Miscellaneous Hormone-Producing Tumors

Other mesenchymal tumors of the ovary produce mixtures of the steroids, including androgens. The vaginal epithelium, and thus the cytohormonal pattern, reflects the result of these influences. Some virilizing ovarian tumors (arrhenoblastoma, hilus cell tumor) produce *androgens*, whereas others produce mixtures. Some adrenal cortical hyperplasias and tumors also produce mixtures of androgens, estrogens, progestogens, and corticoids with the resultant cytohormonal pattern reflecting the complex hormonal status. Hormones produced by pituitary tumors act upon their specific end organs (e.g., ovary; adrenal) and if the latter produce hormones, these act upon the vaginal epithelium in a manner characteristic of the end organ's hormone (e.g., estrogen; cortisone).

Thus, when pertinent conditions are known and properly understood, the Maturation Index of the vaginal cellular specimen reflects the cytohormonal pattern characteristic of a single hormone, or of the compounding effects of multiple agents on the cytohormonal pattern if two or more are biologically active and present in sufficient quantities.

Neoplasms Without Obvious Hormonal Production

Cystic and solid tumors of the *ovary* (fibroma, cystadenoma, adenocarcinoma, papillary cystadenocarcinoma, etc.) usually are *not* associated with complete atrophy or parabasal cell atrophy, regardless of age. This is also true of hyperplasia and adenocarcinoma of the endometrium, as well as metastatic tumors to the ovary (i.e., stomach, colon). In spite of the lack of known hormonal secretion of these tumors, the Maturation Index frequently is shifted to the right. At times this shift is out of the range of normalcy so that an abnormal hormonal pattern can be identified (Fig. 34–12).

This abnormal cytohormonal pattern may be the only indication of disease, particularly in ovarian, tubal, and endometrial adenocarcinoma (Fig. 34–4B). In vaginal pool material it can account for an additional 15 per cent detection of endometrial carcinoma in the absence of neoplastic cells, and an additional 35 per cent detection of ovarian cancer. This may represent an abnormal hormonal level or an abnormal tissue sensitivity to normal levels of hormones. In metastases to the ovary, the surrounding ovarian stroma is usually hyperplastic, with the cytoplasm laden with steroids appearing to reflect tumor irritation.

A few postmenopausal patients exhibiting this abnormal superficial cell response (M.I.

to the right) appear to be in good health after a thorough examination. With close follow-up, however, some do develop disease and others will reveal a history of successful treatment of one of these lesions. About one quarter of patients with this slight abnormal Maturation Index shift to the right appear to harbor *no* disease, and a marginal inflammation may becloud the significance (Fig. 34–12).

This slight abnormal MI shift to the right for the age and history given, therefore, is not an absolute diagnostic finding; but it may be the *only* indication of disease, and lead to detection of an asymptomatic lesion after careful work-up.

The areas to consider as possibly harbor-ing lesions are the endometrium (hyperplasia, adenocarcinoma), ovary (follicle cyst, cystadenoma, adenocarcinoma, metastatic tumor, hormone-producing tumor), fallopian tube (adenocarcinoma), breast (fibroadenoma, adenocarcinoma) pituitary and adrenal cortex (hyperplasia, adenoma, adenocarcinoma).

Anovulation

Anovulation is clearly demonstrated by daily vaginal smears. There is *no* monthly change of the Maturation Index, which occurs with normal ovulation, from the proliferative pattern (c. $\overline{0/40/60}$) to the secretory pattern (c. $\overrightarrow{0/70/30}$) and back again (Figs. 34–1A

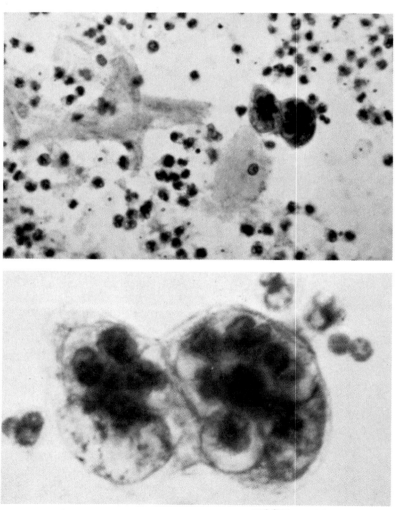

Figure 34–12. A Fast smear of a 71 year old woman. Maturation Index is $\overrightarrow{0/71/29}$, which is abnormal for this age; it is shifted to the right in spite of inflammation (not spread). The patient had a serous cystadenocarcinoma of the ovary. These two malignant cells traveled down the tube and uterus into the vaginal pool. Their hyperdistended secretory vacuoles are packed with well-preserved neutrophils, which are actively phagocytosing the cytoplasm of the cell. ×480 and ×2000.

and 34–4). Thus, in the presence of anovulation, the M.I. is constant during the monthly cycle, and there is no biphasic shift of ovulation (Fig. 34–1). Some persons demonstrate a high level of estrogenic effect (M.I.: c. $\overline{0/20/80}$), some indicate a low estrogenic effect (M.I.: c. $\overline{0/80/20}$), and others fall between the two.

The actual *value* of a given Maturation Index is, therefore, not of great significance in anovulation. The key finding is the *lack of change* in the Maturation Index at the time of expected ovulation, e.g., 14 days *before* menses.

A *single* cytologic examination, therefore, not only assists little in this determination but may give wrong information to the clinician, as patterns can be mimicked. *Two* cytologic evaluations can be helpful if the two samples happen to be taken just at the correct time (i.e., if the first one is obtained just before the estimated ovulation, and the second one two weeks later just before menstruation). Ovulation is implied if the characteristic Maturation Index shift occurs, with a sufficient change in cellular configuration (e.g., curling, clumping) to indicate progesterone effect (Fig. 34–3 A). But the possibility that the two smears are *not* taken at the correct time is too great for reliance, on only two samples.

Daily vaginal smears are by far the most accurate. Vaginal pool aspiration smears can easily be obtained daily by the patient herself (p. 777) *twice a week*, every three to four days (Fig. 34–1A). They indicate ovulation, or its absence, and provide information for detecting the type of endocrinopathy present. The dates of menses and daily basal body temperatures should be supplied for most complete evaluation and clinical value.

Persisting follicular cysts are found in a high estrogenic pattern with a Maturation Index shift to the right, at times extreme, without evidence of ovulatory shift. Although the Stein-Leventhal syndrome occurs in no characteristic cytohormonal pattern (maintaining either a moderate shift to the right, to the midzone, or a spread, its significant finding is constancy *without* ovulatory shift.

Primary Amenorrhea

The evaluation of women of reproductive age who have never menstruated should include cytohormonal pattern, presence of ovulation, and chromosomal sex (p. 694). Such patients will be considered in four clinical categories:

Normal Hormonal Pattern with "Positive Chromatin"

This is found in anatomic variants with XX sex chromosome constitution (e.g., congenital atresias, absence of portions of the generative system other than ovaries) or otherwise normal females with systemic disease or endocrinopathies insufficient to place the hormonal pattern outside the normal range. In the former, a normal ovulatory shift in the cytohormonal pattern (M.I.) is present if there are normally functioning ovaries. In the latter the shift is usually absent or abnormal. Very few or very small sex chromatin bodies may indicate mosaicism, translocation, or other genetic abnormalities whose exact nature can be determined only by thorough cytogenetic studies.

Abnormal Hormonal Pattern with "Positive Chromatin"

These individuals have a normal XX sex chromosomal constitution and significant endocrinopathy. First rule out artifacts (hormonal therapy, inflammation, cervical or vulvar contamination of the specimen) and then consider diseases such as dysfunctions of the ovary (agenesis, hypofunction, primary or metastatic tumor), pituitary (dwarfism, Simmonds' disease, tumors), thyroid (marked hypothyroidism, cretinism), adrenal (hyperplasia, tumor), endometrium (hyperplasia, tumor), breast (hyperplasia, tumor), and chromosomes (Down's syndrome, somatic trisomy). An XXX individual has "double positive" chromatin.

Ovulation is usually absent, but if present it may provide key evidence of the site of abnormalities. Intermediate maturation (M.I.: $\overline{0/100/0}$) indicates lack of ovarian function. Parabasal maturation (M.I.: $\overline{100/0/0}$), or a pattern approaching this, is found in pituitary or adrenal dysfunction or in extreme hypothyroidism. One must also consider the rare case of extreme hypospadias in Klinefelter's syndrome with vaginal formation (usually in mosaic pattern), and of a mosaic Turner's syndrome (e.g., XX/XO).

Normal Hormonal Pattern with "Negative Chromatin"

This may be present in testicular feminization with an XY sex chromosomal constitution (feminizing male pseudohermaphroditism). The cytohormonal pattern may be well within normal limits (Fig. 34–13), but when estrogen production or tissue sensitivity is extreme, the Maturation Index may shift excessively to the right, past normal, and at times even with exfoliation of anucleate superficial cells (Fig. 34–14). There is no cyclic cytohormonal shift, thus indicating anovulation.

Abnormal Hormonal Pattern with "Negative Chromatin"

This is found in the usual Turner's syndrome (XO) and in masculinizing male pseudohermaphroditism (XY). In patients with Turner's syndrome, intermediate cell maturation or parabasal cell maturation is present, depending upon the age of the patient. Masculinizing male pseudohermaphrodites

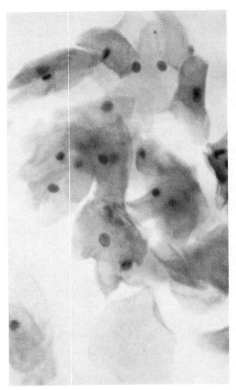

Figure 34–14. Testicular feminization with abnormal cytohormonal pattern (extreme estrogenic response). Fast smear, 17 year old sister of patient of Figure 34–13. The nuclei of these cells also contained no Barr bodies (chromatin negative). This cytohormonal pattern, however, shows a more extreme estrogen response, with numerous anucleate superficial cells (below center) (M.I.: $\overrightarrow{0/32/68}$). Eighteen of the 68 superficial cells were anucleate. She also was a normally developed girl who had never menstruated. Laparotomy revealed testicular feminization. ×160.

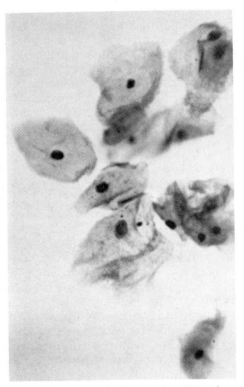

Figure 34–13. Testicular feminization (XY) with normal cytohormonal pattern. Fast smear, 20 year old woman. The nuclei of these cells contained no Barr bodies (chromatin negative) and the cytohormonal pattern revealed good estrogen production (M.I.: $\overrightarrow{0/62/38}$). This well developed, normally feminine appearing girl had good breast development and normal external genitalia. She had never menstruated. Laparotomy revealed testicular feminization. ×160.

may have an androgenic cytohormonal pattern, or may approach intermediate cell or parabasal cell maturation depending on their age. Ovulation and its cytohormonal shift are absent.

Secondary Amenorrhea and Oligomenorrhea

Cytohormonal Pattern Within Normal Range

In anovulation one considers the possibility of systemic illnesses, emotional disturbances, or endocrinopathies of borderline severity. To detect the extremely long menstrual period encountered with many irregular or scanty menses, the presence or absence of ovulation should be determined from menses to menses, which may total more than the usual 30 daily smears. The cytohormonal pattern does not fluctuate in Stein-Leventhal syndrome, nor in persistent follicle cysts with anovulation. Rarely in Sheehan's syndrome with partial pituitary function, there may be a cytohormonal pattern falling within normal range. This is also true in most thyroid disorders, except for extreme deprivation where the Maturation Index shifts to the left.

The ovulatory pattern is normal in simple physical blockage of the genital tract and in endometrial sclerosis (Ascherman's disease).

Abnormal Cytohormonal Pattern

Secondary amenorrhea or oligomenorrhea with abnormal cytohormonal patterns indicates a more severe systemic illness, endocrinopathy, or emotional disturbance. After carefully excluding local inflammation and other artifacts, four major cytohormonal patterns should be sought, either in pure form or combined, viz.: shift of the Maturation Index to the *right*, to the *midzone*, or to the *left*, or a *spread*.

A *right shift* of the Maturation Index (superficial cell maturation, approaching $\overrightarrow{0/0/100}$, Fig. 34–14) indicates *great* estrogenic effect, and may be found in persisting follicular cysts, certain ovarian and adrenal tumors and cytogenetic abnormalities. There may be a less marked shift to the right in some instances of endometrial hyperplasia and adenocarcinomas, in endometriosis, in myomata, and in mammary disease. Estrogen therapy in its many and frequently occult forms of administration must be carefully ruled out.

A *midzone shift* of the Maturation Index (approaching intermediate cell maturation $\overrightarrow{0/100/0}\overleftarrow{}$, Fig. 34–10) indicates a *lack* of estrogenic effect *with* the continued presence of nonestrogenic maturing stimulation to the epithelium (i.e., cortisone) which causes maturation of the intermediate cell layer. This is most frequently found in ovarian failure with adequate adrenocortical function remaining. Oophorectomy, either surgical or following irradiation, during the childbearing age is a prime example in this category, because it removes ovarian estrogen and progestogen production while leaving the adrenocortical function intact. During the

reproductive years the latter normally is overwhelmingly productive of cortisone-type compounds, producing intermediate cell maturation (M.I.: $\overrightarrow{0/100/0}\overleftarrow{}$). Sheehan's syndrome results from pituitary hypofunction with a selective lack of gonadotropins, producing the midzone pattern (M.I.: $\overrightarrow{0/100/0}\overleftarrow{}$) of ovarian ablation and continuing adrenocortical function. When pituitary injury in Sheehan's syndrome is severe, with widespread trophic effects, a spread cytohormonal pattern or even parabasal cell maturation is produced. Pituitary hypofunction of other types (tumors, Simmonds' disease, anorexia nervosa, radiation ablation) may be partial and nonselective with a spread Maturation Index pattern simulating inflammation, or if panhypopituitarism is severe, there may be a complete shift to parabasal cell maturation (M.I.: $\overleftarrow{100/0/0}$). Other menstrual disorders associated with a Maturation Index midzone shift include those caused by functioning ovarian mesenchymal tumors producing progestogens, functional adrenocortical tumors, and certain drugs. *The most frequent cause of secondary amenorrhea with an approximate intermediate cell maturation pattern* ($\overrightarrow{0/95/5}\overleftarrow{}$) *(Fig. 34–7) is pregnancy.*

A *left shift* of the Maturation Index (approaching parabasal cell maturation: $\overleftarrow{100/0/0}$, Fig. 34–11), associated with secondary amenorrhea or oligomenorrhea, indicates that the vaginal epithelium is not maturing. Usually the maturing stimuli are absent or below effective levels, but at times the vaginal epithelium is nonresponsive. Normal vaginal epithelium capable of full maturation may be deprived of specific maturing substances (i.e., estrogens, progestogens, corticoids). In this way parabasal cell maturation occurs in extreme panhypopituitarism of severe Simmonds' disease, anorexia nervosa, and occasional Sheehan's syndrome with massive pituitary ablation. On the other hand, abnormal vaginal epithelium is incapable of reacting to maturing substances in the normal manner (i.e., following extensive irradiation), or when elements basic to cellular metabolism are absent (thyroid deprivation in cretins) and results in parabasal cell maturation.

The most frequent cause of secondary amenorrhea with an approximate parabasal cell maturation (Fig. 34–9) is the postpartum state or lactation.

A *spread* pattern of the Maturation Index (approaching $\overleftrightarrow{33/34/33}$) usually results from inflammation, which must be carefully ruled out and, if present, cleared with properly indicated therapy. Agents effecting vaginal maturation must not be used (e.g., estrogen cream, tetracyclines). Cervical material may show a spread pattern from minor atypias or metaplasia, so that only *lateral vaginal wall scraping* specimens should be evaluated. If after all of this a spread pattern truly is present, androgenic effect (p. 700) may be suspected and the cause searched for (i.e., adrenal tumor, mammary carcinoma, pituitary dysfunction, hilus cell tumor, therapy, or self-administration). Some geriatric vitamin preparations contain androgen-estrogen combinations, which is to be suspected when a spread pattern is found in an elderly patient who appears to be in good health.

Abnormal Hormonal Patterns With Lesions of the Breast

The most frequent mammary lesion of youth, which is at times associated with a Maturation Index shift to the right, is adenofibroma. Chronic cystic mastitis, usually with a normal pattern, can also be associated with a Maturation Index shift to the right or a spread pattern.

Mammary adenocarcinoma takes virtually any pattern, at times extremely abnormal. The Maturation Index may be shifted to the right or to the left. It may even spread, which suggests an androgenic effect (p. 700) or one similar to the postpartum lactational effect (Fig. 34–9).

Cytohormonal Aids in Management of Advanced Breast Carcinoma

Metastatic adenocarcinoma frequently responds dramatically to drastic changes in the existing hormonal milieu. Cytohormonal evaluation of the predominant or the lacking hormone can assist in making the proper choice of therapy to effectively alter the endocrine milieu and effect remission.

Cytohormonal evaluation qualitates and roughly quantitates remaining endocrine activity to indicate estrogenic effect, androgenic effect, or parabasal cell maturation of a "hormonal vacuum" (p. 707). If there is a parabasal cell maturation pattern, estrogen therapy most frequently gives the best clinical response. When there is evidence of extremely good estrogenic activity, androgenic therapy and/or estrogenic ablative therapy give the best therapeutic response.

Monitoring of clinical therapy is aided by follow-up cytohormonal evaluations. When the desired or expected cytohormonal effect is not obtained after a hormone is administered or a procedure is performed to drastically alter the endocrine milieu, a poor clinical response can be expected. Thus, when androgen therapy or estrogen ablation fails to reduce the percentage of superficial cells, a poor clinical response results. Furthermore, after a desirable clinical remission has been obtained, an impending clinical relapse can be preceded by three or four months of an undesirable change in the cytohormonal pattern.

Abnormal Cytohormonal Patterns of Childhood

The normal cytohormonal pattern of childhood (p. 702) has *no* superficial cells (Fig. 34–4). It is so characteristic and predictable, as being between parabasal cell or intermediate cell maturation, that abnormalities are obvious and significant.

Adrenogenital syndrome with adrenocortical hyperplasia has a pattern that varies according to the amounts of estrogens, progestogens, and androgens being produced by the cortex. Because the effect of the androgens usually predominates, the corresponding androgenic Maturation Index spread pattern *without* inflammation (p. 700) is a frequent cytohormonal finding.

Because superficial cells are normally absent during childhood, before perimenarche commences, a Maturation Index shift to the right is distinctly abnormal and indicates the presence of estrogens. Ovarian granulosa cell tumors and feminizing mesenchymal tumors produce significant Maturation Index shifts to the right, as does estrogen therapy for childhood atrophic vaginitis.

Oral estrogens (e.g., mother's birth control pills; grandmother's geriatric vitamins with steroids) and contamination by introitus material from an improperly taken cellular specimen must be carefully ruled out as sources of abnormal superficial cells. A proper childhood cellular specimen (p. 777) is of utmost importance.

Sex Determination: Genetic and Endocrine Bases

Cytologic determination of sex gives invaluable clinical assistance when clinical determination is not straightforward. Moreover, even when the sex appears to be clinically obvious, rare situations of discrepancy exist. In cases of ambiguous genitalia, the true somatic sex should be established in *infancy* so that psychologic difficulties are avoided in rearing the child.

Barr and his co-workers demonstrated a characteristic arrangement of interphase nuclear chromatin in the epithelial cells of the human female that is distinctly and diagnostically different from that in the male. It has subsequently been shown to be the case in almost all cells of the body, but is most accurately present in the epithelial cells of the skin. Present also in skin biopsies, the nuclear chromatin difference can be determined most easily in exfoliated cells (Fig. 34–3). This makes it possible to determine easily the male or female chromosomal make-up without skin or gonadal biopsies, by using simple, painless, properly taken smears of the buccal mucosa lining the cheek pouch (see Fig. 34–57).

Cytogenetic Basis for the Determination of Sex

The genetic basis for the determination of sex is established with the fertilization of an ovum. In addition to the 44 autosomes, a pair of X sex chromosomes is characteristic of normal females (XX). An X and a Y sex chromosome are present in each diploid cell of normal males (XY). This make-up can be altered by abnormal division (nondisjunction) for that individual at subsequent mitoses, and for his offspring at meioses.

At times abnormal numbers of chromosomes are present, either autosomes or sex chromosomes. This is usually the result of nondisjunction, a condition in which the chromosomes fail to separate in the normal manner during cell division, and are distributed abnormally or unequally among the daughter cells. If nondisjunction occurs during the meiotic production of the ova or spermatozoa, the individual resulting from subsequent fertilization has an abnormal genetic endowment which is uniform throughout the body (e.g., XXX). On the other hand, if nondisjunction occurs in a zygote at a mitosis subsequent to fertilization, a *mosaic* pattern is formed in which cells of the individual vary in genetic makeup (e.g., XX becomes XO/XXX). These may be uniformly distributed in mosaic pattern throughout the body or, apparently, may be in localized areas or organs.

The Mitotic Nucleus. At metaphase, the chromosomes are contracted into their characteristic forms. Chromosomal endowment is determined by incubating peripheral blood, preparing "squash" or "dry" preparations, and then microscopically analyzing the individual chromosomes of a dividing cell in metaphase. Previously it was believed that humans had 48 chromosomes. Analyzing the metaphase plates produced by these more exacting techniques has revealed that humans *normally* have 46 chromosomes, of which 44 are autosomes and two are sex chromosomes (XX or XY). By newer banding techniques, in addition to distinctions based on arm length and centromeric position, each individual chromosome can be definitely identified and the origin of abnormal chromosomes (i.e., breaks, translocations, rings) determined.

The Interphase Nucleus. Chromosomes are in the euchromatic state in the enterphase (resting, metabolic) nucleus, appearing threadlike and not individually recognizable. However, when a pair of X sex chromosomes is present in the nucleus, at least one is euchromatic while the other may be heterochromatic. This small bit of heterochromatic chromatin, when it is definitely identified (Fig. 34–2), is referred to as *X chromatin* (female sex chromocenter, Barr body).

X chromatin *identification for clinical use* must be based upon *strict criteria in well-preserved* nuclei (p. 694). It is best identified with the light microscope by using a good nuclear stain such as a permanent aceto-orcein fast green or, less desirably, the hematoxylin stain used in routine diagnostic work. It can also be recognized in fluorescent microscopy using quinacrine stains for Y chromatin identification. When this 1 μm. heterochromatic chromatin mass is present on the lateral equatorial rim of the nucleus as viewed through the microscope, it appears to *merge* with the nuclear membrane (Fig. 34–3). If a chromatin mass can be optically separated from the nuclear membrane when examined using oil immersion (100×) resolution, it should *not* be identified as X chromatin for clinical diagnostic purposes.

An X chromatin definitely identified indicates the presence of two X sex chromosomes. It is felt best that such a nucleus be referred to as being "X chromatin-positive" rather than "female" to decrease any psychologic burden which the latter might bring forth clinically in intersex problems.

In the normal female, X chromatin can be so identified in about 20 to 60 per cent of the well-preserved (immediately wet-fixed, not air-dried) nuclei. Extremely low counts (e.g., 5 per cent) are found in some mosaics (e.g., XO/XX). If repeated, carefully taken buccal smears (Fig. 34–57) that are immediately wet-fixed (not allowed to dry) still reveal this low count, blood karyotyping is necessary to determine the sex chromosome constitution.

The recognition of two X chromatin masses establishes the presence of three X sex chromosomes (XXX) (Fig. 34–15). In the presence of four X sex chromosomes (XXXX), there are three sex chromocenters. In a person with a mosaic cellular pattern, the number of Barr bodies per cell varies according to the mosaic pattern. Rarely, ex-

tremely large X chromatin is encountered. This can occur with translocation onto an X chromosome or with a giant X chromosome.

In the absence of a Barr body, the "X chromatin-negative" nucleus indicates the lack of paired X sex chromosomes. This usually identifies the normal male state (XY), but is also the pattern when one X sex chromosome and no other X or Y sex chromosome is present (XO). There have been no OY or OO individuals reported. These combinations represent lethal variants, as an X sex chromosome appears to be needed for viability.

Thus, the number of X chromatin bodies in an interphase nucleus *plus one* gives the minimum number of X sex chromosomes in that cell.

Many of the characteristics we associate with masculinity and femininity evidently having determining factors residing on the autosomes. The major determinants of sex,

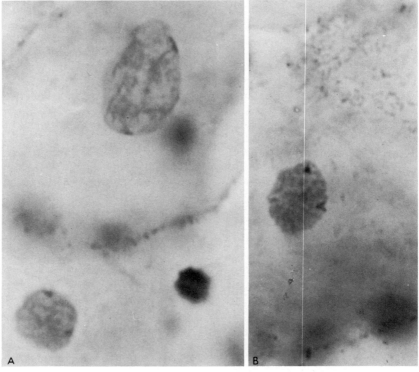

Figure 34–15. Two X chromatin bodies in a "super female" (XXX). Buccal smear. Aceto-orcein Fast green permanent stain. ×2000. *A,* Each nucleus of these two intermediate cells has two diagnostic X chromatins (sex chromocenters, Barr bodies) widely separated on the nuclear membrane. They merge imperceptibly with the chromatinic rim in all four cases. Two Barr bodies in one "double positive" nucleus indicates three X sex chromosomes, such as this (XXX) "super female" and the rare Klinefelter's configuration (XXXY). *B,* The same patient. These are probably two sex chromocenters in the same nucleus; however, the upper chromocenter does not blend in with the membrane in profile, as it is on a superior or an inferior surface of the membrane, so it is *not* diagnostic. The diagnostic Barr body on the right, merging imperceptibly with the chromatinic rim, is a forked single body.

however, appear to reside on the two sex chromosomes.

In newborn females it appears that the X chromatin may not be formed well enough to be morphologically identifiable. An "X chromatin-positive" pattern recognized at birth is dependable evidence of a chromosomal make-up of XX. An "X chromatin-negative" pattern at birth, however, is better redetermined carefully (see Fig. 34–57) during the second or third month of life before submitting a clinical judgment to be sure of sex chromatin absence.

Endocrine Basis for the Determination of Sex

The development of genitalia in utero is dependent upon a distinct hormonal milieu. In the absence of functional gonads, the external genitalia of a fetus develop along normal female lines regardless of its sex chromosomal constitution. The presence of testicular tissue, or the administration of androgenic hormones to the mother of a female fetus during the first trimester, influences fetal development along male lines. The latter (i.e., artificial progestogens with androgenic effect) constitutes a major cause of newborn intersex or female pseudohermaphroditism.

Cytohormonal evaluation can assist in the understanding of sex abnormalities in the newborn. Furthermore, the causes for changes or abnormal development in secondary sex characteristics and external genitalia *after* birth are better understood if the basic cytogenetic and cytohormonal make-up are determined by buccal and vaginal smears.

SEXUAL NORMALCY AND ANOMALOUS SEX SYNDROMES.

Sexual identity is usually clinically clear-cut. Those syndromes and abnormal changes that are complex can be better defined by evaluating the *clinical, cytogenetic,* and *hormonal* relationships that prevail.

The Normal Female (XX)

The genetic endowment of the normal female is 46 chromosomes—44 autosomes and two X sex chromosomes. One of the latter is

heterochromatic and appears as the X chromatin (Barr body) in the interphase nucleus (chromatin-positive) (Fig. 34–3). The genitalia and secondary sex characteristics are those of a normal female and the cytohormonal pattern is the one expected for the age (Fig. 34–4). Failure of normal development (e.g., the presence of vestigial müllerian elements) and endocrinopathies account for most of the clinical problems encountered in this group.

The Normal Male (XY)

The chromosome number of a normal male is also 46 per diploid cell—44 autosomes, one X sex chromosome, and one Y sex chromosome. No X chromatin (Barr body) is present in the interphase nucleus (chromatin-negative). The genitalia and secondary sex characteristics are those of a normal male, unless developmental or endocrine abnormalities complicate the picture.

Gonadal Agenesis (Turner's Syndrome)

About three fourths of the individuals with this condition have 45 chromosomes—44 autosomes and only one sex chromosome, an X sex chromosome (XO). Thus, there is no Barr body in the interphase nucleus (chromatin-negative) and it appears identical to the normal male nucleus.

Individuals with clinical Turner's syndrome occasionally have apparently normal XX or XY chromosome constitutions, but they usually have XO or mosaic chromosomal patterns (e.g., XO/XX, XO/XY). Unlike the XO and XO/XY Turner's syndrome, the nuclei of the XO/XX individuals are chromatin-positive and look like the nuclei of a normal female, but in these patients there is a smaller percentage of chromatin-positive nuclei.

The patients have "streak gonads" and are infertile. Their abnormal cytohormonal pattern is usually that of intermediate maturation (M.I.: $\overline{0/100/0}$), but there is a progressive shift to the left of the Maturation Index, with increasing parabasal cell exfoliation from the third decade on.

The two constant findings are the lack of estrogenic effect (Fig. 34–10) and the lack of the biphasic pattern of ovulation. The former is in marked and diagnostic contradistinction to patients with testicular feminization who, although they likewise are chromatin-negative and have anovulation, have definite estrogenic effects (Figs. 34–13 and 34–14). If estrogen has been given, for breast development or other reason, there will of course be an estrogenic effect.

Testicular Dysgenesis (Klinefelter's Syndrome)

Most individuals having the clinical syndrome first described by Klinefelter, have a 47 chromosome constitution with two X sex chromosomes and one Y sex chromosome (XXY). Because they have two X sex chromosomes, they are chromatin-positive with a single Barr body in the interphase nucleus, identical to the normal female nucleus (Fig. 34–3).

Some persons with Klinefelter's syndrome bear genetic constitutions different from XXY. These patients usually have sex chromosome mosaicism, with some cells having 48 chromosomes, such as XXYY (one X chromatin appearing as a normal female nucleus, Fig. 34–3), or XXXY (two Barr bodies appearing as a "super female" nuclear pattern, Fig. 34–15). Patients with 49 chromosomes (XXXXY) and three Barr bodies per interphase nucleus have been described as clinically having Klinefelter's syndrome, as have some rare persons with 50 or 51 chromosomes, with five X sex chromosomes and one or two Y sex chromosomes in a mosaic polysomy.

Klinefelter's syndrome may thus occur in persons having at least one Y sex chromosome *and* two or more X sex chromosomes.

The "Super Female"

For many years geneticists have known of the existence of "super females" (XXX) in lower forms of life. In humans, these individuals possess 47 chromosomes—22 apparently intact autosome pairs and three X sex chromosomes. Their interphase nuclei have two Barr bodies and are thus X chromatin-double positive (Fig. 34–15). A rare patient with 48 or more chromosomes may be encountered in mosaicism, who will thus have four or more X sex chromosomes (XXXX) and three or more X chromatin bodies in the interphase nuclei of their buccal smears.

Most "super females" encountered have been mentally deficient. Some, however, have been of normal intelligence and, occa-

sionally, even above average. Menses and childbearing have been encountered, although primary amenorrhea and infertility are the rule.

Female Hermaphroditism and Intersex

These individuals have an apparently normal female genetic constitution (XX) as ascertained by current cytogenetic techniques, and a chromatin-positive buccal smear; however, their external genitalia are either male or ambiguous (intersex). Such may result in a female fetus of a mother receiving androgenic hormones, or progestational hormones with androgenic effect.

Masculinization of previously normal female external genitalia, frequently with accompanying male secondary sex characteristics, occurs in patients with adrenogenital syndrome (adrenocortical hyperplasia), in patients with masculinizing tumors (e.g., arrhenoblastoma), and in patients with endocrinopathies (e.g., Cushing's syndrome).

If the abnormal hormone is active at the time of examination, the cytohormonal pattern of these individuals will be adrogenic. However, if the abnormal hormone only acted *previously* (i.e., *in utero*), and is absent at the time of examination, the cytohormonal pattern will be normal female for that age.

Male Hermaphroditism and Intersex

These individuals have an apparently normal male genetic constitution (XY), with 44 autosomes and a chromatin-negative buccal smear; however, their external genitalia are female or ambiguous (intersex). Most of these patients have *male body* types. When estrogens are being produced in the body, male pseudohermaphrodites have extremely *female body* types. Such is the case with testicular feminization, in which the genetic constitution appears to be that of a normal male yet the testicles produce estrogen. Extremely well developed feminine secondary sex characteristics and a marked estrogenic effect in the vaginal smear (Figs. 34–13 and 34–14) are a striking contrast to the male X chromatin-negative pattern of the interphase nucleus.

With the relatively simple methods for cytogenetic determination—the buccal smear for X chromatin identification and the peripheral blood "squash" or "dry" metaphase examination—developments in cytogenetics have been extremely rapid. With this progress, many of our fundamental concepts in physiologic and biochemical genetics are being altered and, thus, also our approaches to clinical problems.

NORMAL CELL MORPHOLOGY

NORMAL SQUAMOUS CELLS

The stratified squamous epithelium, which is present in the female reproductive tract (Fig. 34–2) *noncornified* from the squamocolumnar junction of the uterine cervix to the introitus. It then becomes cornified as it continues onto the external surface of the body.

As the cells of stratified squamous epithelium mature, they orient *parallel* to the *basement membrane*. The most mature cells thus become *squames* (Latin, scales), whereas the less mature cells retain their rounded immature cytoplasm (Fig. 34–2). Cells shed from the epithelial surface are currently categorized into three main types according to their degree of maturity: *parabasal, intermediate,* and *superficial* cells.

Detailed morphology of these *normal* squamous cells has been presented (p. 689). Discussion of abnormally active (dyskaryotic), degenerative, and malignant squamous cells follows.

NORMAL COLUMNAR CELS

Columnar epithelium is present in the female reproductive tract proximal to the squamocolumnar junction of the cervix uteri. Mature columnar cells orient in tissue *perpendicular* to the *basement membrane,* in contradistinction to the parallel orientation of mature stratified squamous cells.

Columnar epithelium ranges in thickness from extremely thin single cell epithelium to extremely thick pseudostratified columnar epithelium, depending upon its functions of defense, secretion, absorption, transportation, reaction to injury, etc. The cells on the luminal surface of thick pseudostratified columnar epithelium remain attached to the *basement membrane* by thin tails of cytoplasm. Interspersed between are the subcolumnar, subcylindrical, parabasal, or reserve cells, with the germinal cells lying upon the basement membrane.

Individual Columnar Cell Morphology

When viewed in profile (Fig. 34–1 *B*) the exfoliated columnar cell has a symmetry about its long axis, and typically appears as an elongated cylinder or cone. The nucleus rests near the basal end of the axis with scanty cytoplasm, usually in the form of a thin tail, extending past it. The opposite luminal end of the cell has abundant cytoplasm and is wide and blunt (Fig. 34–16), frequently with cilia (Fig. 34–1 *B*). This nucleocytoplasmic orientation at times becomes important for identification of cell type.

The *nucleus* is characteristically vesicular and may vary markedly in size, but retains a round or oval shape. The chromatin pattern is uniformly dispersed and tends to be finely granular (Fig. 34–16), differing from the reticular meshwork of squamous cell nuclei (Fig. 34–3). Nucleoli are frequently prominent and multiple, yet are rounded and smooth. Multinucleation is common (Fig. 34–17), especially in irritation, but the chromatin pattern is uniform from nucleus to nucleus within the same multinucleated cell.

The *cytoplasm* is usually abundant. It is characteristically foamy and finely vacuolated (Fig. 34–17), at times containing multiple vacuoles of secretion or even single

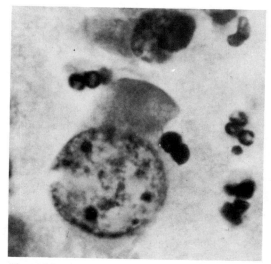

Figure 34–16. Columnar cells. The lower is a ciliated cell which has lost its cilia with only the terminal plate visible at the upper blunt end. The chromatin pattern is uniformly granular. (The large nucleus was so large that in the process of preparation it ruptured, with apparent clear areas which are artifactual.) Three uniform round nucleoli are prominent. Note the immense nuclear size variance; the lower nucleus occupies about six times the area of the upper ciliated cell nucleus. ×1435.

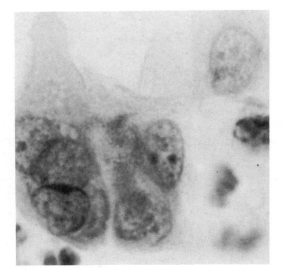

Figure 34–17. "Reactive" columnar cells. The luminal end of these endocervical cells is at the upper left of the field. Note the features of dyskaryosis and proplasia with the multiple nuclei per cell and the regular, finely granular chromatin pattern with occasional prominent but rounded nucleoli. Mature columnar dyskaryotic cells. ×1455.

frankly secretory vacuoles (Fig. 34–18). By the character of their cytoplasmic differentiation for function, one recognizes a *nonsecretory* or serous columnar cell, a mucus *secretory* cell, and a *ciliated* cell.

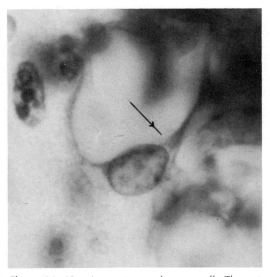

Figure 34–18. A secretory columnar cell. The cytoplasmic tail of this endocervical cell has been drawn up by a huge vacuole. The cytoplasm at the nucleovacuolar angle (arrow) is decreased, indicating a hyperdistended vacuole. Very frequently intact neutrophils lie within such hyperdistended vacuoles of secretion. ×1455.

The so-called *nonsecretory* or serous columnar cell has a uniform, slightly foamy, and usually basophilic cytoplasm (Fig. 34–17). Frequently, fine acidophilic granules are found scattered throughout the cytoplasm. The foamy nature of the cytoplasm and the acidophilic serous granules frequently indicate that these cells are indeed secretory, but the absence of large, frankly secretory vacuoles has characterized these as nonsecretory.

A mucus *secretory* columnar cell may also have multiple cytoplastic vacuoles. However, the secretory vacuole is frequently single and, when large, pushes the nucleus farther into the tail of the cell (Fig. 34–18). At times it is huge with "pouching out" of its hyperdistended vacuole, with loss of cytoplasm at the nucleovacuolar angle, with extreme thinning of the cytoplasm about the nucleus, and with "demilune" compression of the nucleus. Such hyperdistended secretory vacuoles are noted in chronic inflammations (e.g., cervicitis), abnormal hormonal states (endometrial hyperplasia), and neoplasias (adenocarcinomas) (see Figs. 34–45 and 34–46). This large single vacuole is a helpful characteristic to determine secretion (Fig. 34–18) *vs.* degeneration (see Fig. 34–23 *B*) *vs.* phagocytosis (Fig. 34–21 *A*).

A *ciliated* columnar cell has a prominent refractile terminal plate across the broad luminal end of the cytoplasm, from which numerous delicate cilia project perpendicularly (Fig. 34–1 *B*). Both cilia and terminal plates are the same color, usually lavender or red. The cilia are usually the first part of the cell to disappear when it undergoes degeneration, leaving a prominent terminal plate on a conspicuously square-ended cell as the only evidence of ciliation (Figs. 34–1 *B*; 34–16). Endocervical cells, endometrial cells, and cells from the fallopian tubes are frequently ciliated.

Multicellular Tissue Fragments Composed of Columnar Cells

Sheets. Columnar cells in a sheet and viewed on end (*en face*) have a pavement pattern reminiscent of squamous cells, with the nuclei lying symmetrically in the center of the cytoplasm. The cytoplasmic borders, however, abut rather than overlap as do squames, and are sharp and distinct. They are uniformly hexagonal, giving a characteristic honeycomb appearance to the sheets

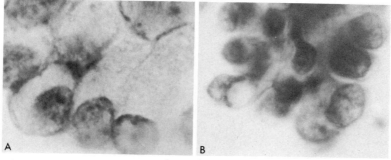

Figure 34–19. Columnar cells in tissue fragments: endocervical *vs.* endometrial. ×1435. *A,* Endocervical cells in a sheet. They have abundant cytoplasm which abuts with resulting *prominent* intercellular borders. There is honey-combing in the upper left field where the cells are viewed *en face.* The cells around the edge of the sheet in the lower field are viewed in profile and thus recognizable as columnar cells. The nuclei are uniformly vesicular with a regular chromatin pattern. *B,* Endometrial cells shed in a tissue fragment. Vaginal pool material. The cytoplasm is very scanty, with *indistinct* cellular borders. The nuclei are more irregular in shape than are the endocervical cells and chromatin tends to be more clumped, but the chromatin pattern is uniform from nucleus to nucleus within this tissue fragment. There is a single secretory vacuole in the cell on the left. As with all clumps, the cells can best be studied about the edge.

(Fig. 34–19 *A*). Around the edge of such a sheet one usually finds cells lying upon their sides, where they can be studied in profile and identified as columnar cells.

Acini, Polyps, Ducts, and Stalks. When a whole gland is shed, the acinus and the duct can be recognized. Because the lumen of an acinus and a duct lies on the *inside* of the tissue fragment, the cells are oriented toward the center with the basement membrane around the outside.

When a villus or papillary frond is shed, the stalk and polypoid tip can be recognized. Interglandular septi are also shed in villus formation with attached stalk, as are actual polyps and micropolyps. In contradistinction to the acinus, the lumen of a polyp and its stalk are at the *outer* margin of the tissue fragment. The cells are thus oriented with their luminal ends facing to the outside, with the basement membrane and stromal tissues in the center of the polyp.

At times it is not possible to definitely identify whether a structure is an acinus or a polyp, and the question becomes academic. What is frequently of the utmost importance, however, is to be certain that it *is* either an organized glandular or a polypoid structure, rather than merely a tissue fragment or aggregate of cells, and thus recognize its columnar cell differentiation.

The fact that a tissue fragment is an acinus or a polyp, rather than simply a fragment of disorganized tissue, can usually be determined definitely by moving the microscope plane of focus up and down through the structure. As the plane of focus must be thin,

the highest power lens is used. In this way, the top level is a sheet of *en face* columnar cells viewed on end with a honeycomb appearance. Moving the plane of focus down, the midplane ring of cells is identified. (At this level of focus one frequently can locate the basement membrane and the luminal portions of the cells, determining, by their orientation, whether one is viewing a glandular or a villous formation.) As the plane of focus is moved downward to the level of the slide, the lower sheet of cells forming the structure appears as a second honeycomb (*en face*) of columnar cells viewed on end. This structural organization is absent in disorganized tissue fragments or aggregates of single cells.

The most frequent cell type to be shed in these acinar or polypoid formations is the endometrial cell at menses. This configuration is also found in endometrial hyperplasias and in adenocarcinomas involving the female genital tract. With polypoid or glandular hyperplasia of the endocervix, the endocervical cells also are shed in such configurations, usually with much more cytoplasm and more vesicular nuclei (Fig. 34–19).

Endocervical Cells

Columnar cells from the endocervix frequently exfoliate in sheets or clumps when a scraping method is used to obtain them. Cytoplasmic molding is prominent, but nuclear molding by adjacent cells is minimal. Intercellular cytoplasmic membranes are con-

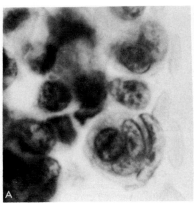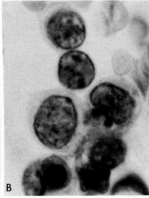

Figure 34-20. Endometrial columnar epithelial cells. ×1435. *A,* The edge of a tissue fragment showing marked nuclear variation in chromatin pattern. Chromatin clumps are rounded, without sharp points. Nuclear molding is moderate. *B,* The cytoplasm is scanty with some nuclear size variation. The chromatin pattern is regular, with a sex chromocenter in midfield.

spicuous and when viewed on end (*en face*) the sheets appear as a honeycomb with round, centrally placed, uniform nuclei (Fig. 34–19 *A*). The cytoplasm of endocervical cells is abundant, with nonsecretory (serous) and secretory (vacuolated) cells intermingled. Hyperdistended secretory vacuoles (Fig. 34–18) appear in chronic cervicitis. At times these huge vacuoles are packed with well-preserved neutrophils, which have entered the cells and are phagocytosing vacuolar material. Ciliated endocervical cells are also encountered from the endocervix (Fig. 34–1 *B*), and at times their detached ciliary tufts (DCT) are encountered.

Endocervical cell nuclei are frequently very bizarre when they are proplastic; this is most often seen in reaction to injury (Fig. 34–17) and in regeneration. They are usually round or oval with a uniformly granular chromatin pattern. Their size can increase five to seven times, especially when there is marked irritation (Fig. 34–16). Under these conditions, multiple nuclei are frequent (Fig. 34–17). They are uniform in shape and

in chromatin pattern *within* each cell, however, even though their size may vary. The nucleoli are frequently multiple, prominent, and gigantic in such reactive cells; but they are characteristically rounded and lack the sharp, pointed irregularity of malignant nucleoli. Hyperchromasia is very disturbing at these times, but the chromatin pattern is rounded and may show smudgy degeneration of varying degrees. When hyperactivity is severe, these proplastic nuclei fall within the designation of Papanicolaou's *dyskaryosis* (pp. 737–743) with varying degrees of cytoplasmic columnar maturation.

Endometrial Cells

Although columnar cells from the endometrium may exfoliate in sheets (*en face*), they are usually shed in disorganized tissue fragments (Fig. 34–19 *B*) or glandular formations of acini or villi. Single endometrial cells (Fig. 34–20 *B*) at times strongly resemble single small histiocytes (Fig. 34–21 *A*)

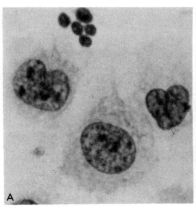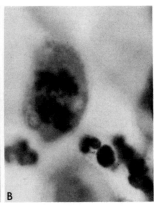

Figure 34-21. Histiocytes. ×1435. *A,* Small histiocytes with typically foamy cytoplasm and eccentric nuclei. The chromatin pattern is uniform with rounding of chromatin clumps. The nuclei are round, oval, kidney-bean, and horseshoe shaped just "ticking" or "bouncing off" the cell membrane on the left. *B,* Small histiocyte in mitosis. Cell division is much more frequently seen in histiocytes than in single malignant cells in naturally exfoliated material.

and it may be impossible to discriminate between some of them morphologically.

The appearance of endometrial cells differs markedly when obtained from *vaginal* or *endometrial* cavity (i.e., by aspiration, brush, irrigation, helix). This is due to two major influences. Endometrial material in the vaginal pool is degenerated from its passage through the uterine canal and is shed only at menses, while material from the endometrial cavity is well preserved and can be obtained at any time in the cycle.

Vagino-Cervical Material. Moderate crowding and molding are frequently found among the endometrial cells. Their cytoplasm is scantier than that of endocervical cells, and intercellular borders are much less distinct (Fig. 34–19). Cytoplasmic vacuolation is present in varying degrees, but it usually appears in the form of single clear vacuoles. At times extreme hyperdistended secretory vacuolation is associated with endometrial hyperplasia and chronic endometritis.

The nuclei are usually rounded, oval, or indented due to wrinkling. They are smaller and less regular than those of endocervical cells. Although they tend to be moderately hyperchromatic with some chromatin irregularity, the borders of the chromatin aggregates are not acutely angular or sharply jagged (Fig. 34–20). At times the nuclei mold about adjacent ones dramatically. The chromatin pattern frequently has the hazy, smudgy appearance of degeneration (Fig. 34–19A). Nuclear size varies less than in endocervical cells, but occasionally increases four to five times.

It is normal to find well-preserved "exhausted" endometrial cells in the vaginal pool material the first few days of the menstrual cycle, with scanty cytoplasm and frequently in acinar or villous formation. As the menstrual period progresses they appear more and more degenerated, at times with alarming nuclear features (i.e., hyperchromasia, folding chromatin clumping) but also those more characteristic of degeneration (i.e., rounded, blurred chromatin). Because of this and of the all too frequent absence of clear-cut criteria in adenocarcinoma, it is safer to repeat the examination at midcycle or during the late luteal phase (e.g., last week of period) for careful reevaluation, or to directly sample the endometrial cavity (e.g., brush; D & C).

Endometrial Cavity Material. Endometrial columnar cells obtained directly from the endometrial cavity (i.e., aspiration, brushing, irrigation helix), are better preserved than the vaginal pool material. They also appear different, according to the time in the menstrual cycle.

At *menstruation* the endometrial cells appear exhausted, with scantycytoplasm. They are usually better preserved when obtained directly from the endometrial cavity than their counterparts appearing in vagino-cervical material.

During the *proliferative* follicular) phase, endometrial cells are proplastic, closely mimicking serous endocervical cells. The cytoplasm is tall, columnar, clear, and abundant. The nucleus is vesicular and large with a uniform chromatin pattern composed of prominent granules with small chromocenters.

During the *secretory* (luteal) phase following ovulation, the abundant cytoplasm is filled with numerous foamy vacuoles. The nucleus becomes smaller and the chromatin pattern is less uniform, with abundant parachromatin and more prominent chromocenters. Nucleoli may be prominent. Toward the end of the secretory phase, the amount of cytoplasm decreases, approaching the low cuboidal type of exhausted endometrium obtained routinely in the menstruum of vagino-cervical material.·

MACROPHAGES

Macrophages, or histiocytes, usually occur singly (Fig. 34–21). When they do clump together they appear as aggregates of individual cells secondarily coming together, rather than cells which primarily grew together in tissue. The clumped histiocytes have small openings or "windows" remaining between the cytoplasmic walls of the rounded cells. This helps to distinguish them from true tissue fragments whose cells primarily grew together and whose nuclei mold around adjacent nuclei (Fig. 34–20 A). Of additional help is the appearance of the outer border of a histiocytic aggregate which seems to be haphazard and does not have the smooth epithelial luminal border which a fragment of epithelial tissue displays. These three points help to distinguish histiocytes, no matter how bizarre, from true tissue fragments of benign cells (i.e., endometrial) or of cancer.

The *cytoplasm* characteristically is foamy

(Fig. 34–21 A) or has multiple vacuoles, with or without debris. The nucleus is round or oval in the resting state with a uniform reticular and granular pattern. It is characteristically eccentric, at times barely touching or "ticking" the cell membrane at one point as if "bouncing off" of it (Fig. 34–21 A).

When a histiocyte becomes "active" in response to phagocytic stimuli, the nucleus becomes proplastic and changes in four morphologic areas, which may appear alarming. The nuclear *shape* becomes irregular—it may be round, oval, flattened on the side near the cytocentrum, indented on that side (kidney-bean shaped), enfolded (Fig. 34–21 A), bilobulated or very rough and irregular on its side nearest the cytocentrum or *hof*. This is in diagnostic contrast to cancer cell nuclear irregularities away from the cytocentrum, or *anti-hof* (see Fig. 34–46 B). The *chromatin pattern* becomes dark and uneven with clumping, cleared parachromatin (conspicuous nuclear sap), prominent nucleoli, and an unevenly thickened chromatinic rim. These chromatin clumps and nucleoli are usually rounded and fuzzy, in contradistinction to the extremely sharp borders and angles of chromatin clumps in well-preserved malignant cells. *Mitoses* are frequent in histiocytic activity (Fig. 34–21 B). Although mitoses are found in freshly broken off true fragments of regenerating tissues and cancer, it is a relatively rare occurrence in such cells shed singly into such nonphysiologic and necrotic material; however, in this degenerated material, histiocytes frequently divide in response to their "call to duty" and their need for more scavengers. *Multinucleation* is a characteristic of histiocytes, resulting in either a binucleated *large* histiocyte or a multinucleated *giant cell* histiocyte (Fig. 34–22). The multiple nuclei within such a cell are identical to each other morphologically in many critical features. In gynecologic material, these multinucleated giant histiocytes are found *most* frequently with *Trichomonas*, but tuberculosis and foreign bodies (i.e., fat, pessary, IUD) are to be considered.

There is another type of multinucleated giant "cell" encountered in vaginal material. This represents a mass of degenerated fuzzy histiocytes sticking together in a conglomeration or pseudosyncytium, which is frequently incomplete, with the holes and cracks of degenerated "windows" to identify the individuality of the cells making up the mass. In contradistinction to the nuclear uniformity within a true multinucleated giant cell, the nuclei of this pseudosyncytial cell can vary strikingly in size, shape, and chromatin pattern. On the other hand, nonuniformity of nuclei in multinucleated *malignant* cells is a good malignant criterion (Fig. 34–38), contrasting with the nuclear uniformity in benign multinucleation (Figs. 34–17 and 34–22), and not to be diagnostically confused with the nonuniformity of nuclei in these *benign* cells coming together in a *pseudosyncytium* of degeneration.

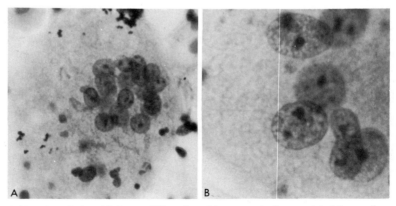

Figure 34–22. Multinucleated giant histiocyte. When found in gynecologic material, this usually means that there is a *Trichomonas* infection; however, foreign bodies and other agents can also be responsible. A, The nuclei are mirror images of each other. They are usually found aggregated together in the centrum, periphery, or in horseshoe fashion. Note nuclear debris of partially digested leukocytes in the abundant, foamy cytoplasm. ×665. B, The nuclear chromatin and nucleolar pattern are uniform in these identical sister nuclei. Note the typically foamy histiocyte cytoplasm. ×2000.

DEGENERATION AND REGENERATION

Degeneration

Retrogressive changes of degeneration in cells and tissues are frequently associated with bizarre retroplastic morphologic changes, which can either *mimic* or *mask* malignancy for the unwary. On the one hand, when their true nature has not been recognized they have been responsible for false diagnoses of cancer; conversely, the appearance of cancer cells can be so changed by degeneration that their morphologic criteria of malignancy, and thus their true neoplastic nature, are unrecognizable.

Causes of degeneration are many, including infection, inflammation, presence of blood, drying *before* fixation, inadequate fixation, cell aging, and death.

Morphologic changes produced by degeneration likewise are many but, for the most part, they are nonspecific. Cytoplasmic *tinctorial* reaction is altered, usually toward the acidophilic (yellow, orange, red), and frequently is mistaken for keratinization. At times this acidophilic change occurs in the improperly fixed center of a cellular clump so that the line of tinctorial change passes through cells, resulting in biphasic acido-basophilic cytoplasm in the same cell. This is in contrast to keratinizing acido-philia, which involves the entire cytoplasm of a

cell. This false acidophilia is present throughout the whole slide when many alcohols other than ethyl (e.g., isopropyl, methyl) are utilized either in fixation or in the staining process. A prominent cytoplasmic *perinuclear halo* develops after long-standing cellular irritation (Figs. 34–23 B, 34–24 B, and 34–25A).

Swelling is frequent in both cytoplasm and nucleus (Fig. 34–23A) with decreased staining intensity proportional to the imbibition of water. As both nucleus and cytoplasm swell, a normal nucleo-cytoplasmic ratio is usually maintained. *Cytoplasmic vacuolation* due to degeneration is multiple (Figs. 34–23 B, 34–24, 34–25) and distributed uniformly throughout the cytoplasm, with neither the nuclear distortion or dislodgment which is produced by secretory vacuoles.

With *rupture* of the cell membrane, there can be complete disappearance of the cytoplasm into the background (Fig. 34–23 C). Because the resulting *bare nucleus* is an obvious sign of a degenerated cell and frequently contains markedly bizarre changes, it should *not* be used as the basis for a *diagnosis* of malignancy lest diagnostic importance be placed upon false criteria due to degenerative changes. When the appearance of such a bare nucleus is sufficiently alarming, it certainly can raise one's *index of suspicion*, and lead to the examination of more, and better preserved, material.

With *nuclear* degeneration, the chromatin

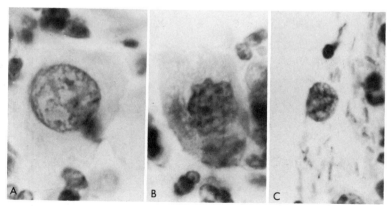

Figure 34–23. Cellular degeneration. *A*, Both nucleus and cytoplasm have imbibed water and are swollen, even though the nucleo-cytoplasmic ratio remains normal. Compare with neutrophils for size. ×1435. *B*, The central nucleus has not been displaced, in spite of multiple vacuoles of degeneration scattered throughout the cytoplasm. There is a beginning perinuclear halo to the left of, and above, the nucleus. The nucleus is degenerating with *wrinkling* of the nuclear membrane, chromatin beading along the left portion of the nuclear envelope, and beginning chromatin smudging. ×1435. *C*, Cytolysis has occurred with rupture and dissolution of the cytoplasm, leaving a *bare nucleus* with minimal chromatin clumping of degeneration. These truly bare nuclei frequently have artifacts of degeneration (i.e., hyperchromasia, clumping, clearing) and thus should not be the basis for a *diagnosis* for malignancy. ×1435.

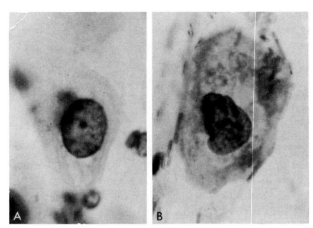

Figure 34–24. Chromatin degenerative clumping and smudging. ×1500. *A,* Chromatin *beading* is beginning at the lower right of the nuclear rim. It is more advanced along the left border, with moderate smudging and beginning chromatin laking. *B,* Beading and smudging along inner surface of left nuclear border. At the left border of both nuclei, note the sharply defined outer surface of the thickened chromatinic rim in contrast to its blurred inner surface and blurring of the other chromatin/parachromatin interfaces. Chromatin clumps are rounded. Small cytoplasmic vacuoles (in both *A* and *B*) are uniformly dispersed within the cytoplasm without displacing the nucleus. There is a partial perinuclear clearing in B.

blurs and either lakes with loss of pattern or condenses into hyperchromatic clumps. Chromatin tends to marginate peripherally and bead along the inside of the chromatinic rim (Figs. 34–23 *B* and 34–24). An important characteristic for recognizing degenerative chromatolysis is the chromatin blurring which occurs at the chromatin/parachromatin interfaces throughout the nucleus. This results in the lack of sharp "cookie cutter" borders on the chromatin clumps and the

inner surface of the chromatinic rim. Although the *outside* border of the chromatinic rim remains sharply defined due to the presence of the invisibly thin true nuclear membrane, the *inside* border blurs, as do the rest of the chromatin/parachromatin interfaces throughout the nucleus (Fig. 34–24). This comparison of the inner and outer borders of the nuclear membrane serves as a most sensitive indicator of early nuclear degeneration. Fortunately, this is in contrast to the

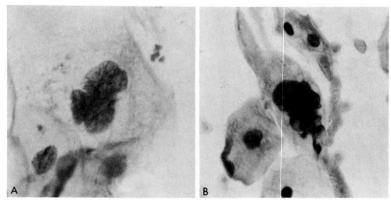

Figure 34–25. Cellular degeneration: benign cell *vs.* malignant cell. Vaginal pool material. Both patients had *Trichomonas* infection with severe cellular degeneration. ×665. *A,* Bizarre changes in a nonmalignant epithelial cell with nuclear gigantism and hyperchromasia. Compare the relatively normal intermediate cell at the lower left. The chromatin pattern of the huge nucleus, under careful scrutiny, is not sharp but has the haziness of degeneration and beginning laking. There is a prominent perinuclear halo with degenerative wrinkling of the nuclear membrane from shrinkage. The degeneration in this dyskaryotic cell makes it appear more worrisome than the minor atypia from which it came. *B,* Degenerative changes in this cell, shed from squamous cell carcinoma, mask the sharp malignant characteristics of the nucleus and make the cell appear less than diagnostic. Haziness of chromatin clumps makes malignant criteria equivocal. The cytoplasm is moderately abundant, with numerous vacuoles of cell degeneration.

sharp, freshly punched-out "cookie cutter" appearance of well-preserved malignant cells (Fig. 34–37).

Degenerating nuclei usually appear either swollen and pale (Fig. 34–32 A) or shrunken and hyperchromatic (Fig. 34–2 C). Both the former (bland) and the latter (pyknotic) nuclei eventually lose their chromatinic pattern and become uniformly laked, fragment, and dissolve. Thus, degenerated nuclei that are large are usually pale; those that are small usually are dark. At times, however, a degenerated nucleus appears paradoxically both swollen *and* hyperchromatic. This occurs when the large nucleus of a dyskaryotic cells undergoes degeneration (Fig. 34–25 A). When this is found, its smudgy degenerative character can bear a striking superficial resemblance to a degenerating malignant cell (Fig. 34–25 B).

At times neutrophils invade the cellular border and lie well preserved within the degenerating cytoplasm of the cell (Fig. 34–12). This appears naively to be phagocytosis by the epithelial cell of the neutrophils; it actually is phagocytosis by the neutrophils of the epithelial cell contents. This is evident by the excellent state of preservation of nearly every neutrophil in the epithelial cells (Figs. 34–45 and 34–46) in contrast to the varying stages of degenerative neutrophils when they are found within phagocytosing histiocytes (Fig. 34–22 A).

Regeneration

Proplastic changes can be very severe in regenerating tissues that are in the healing phases of inflammations, ulcerations, biopsy sites, etc. The *nuclei* are large and may be multiple. The chromatin pattern is granular, but the moderate-sized granules are uniformly dispersed and rounded (Fig. 34–26 C) rather than unevenly distributed and angular, as with cancer (Fig. 34–37). The nuclear membrane is wavy, evidencing increased activity, and the chromatinic rim is of uniform thickness. From cell to cell, however, the rim can vary from extremely thin and pale to thick and hyperchromatic. Nucleoli may be multiple and very prominent, especially in regenerating columnar cells, but they are rounded and not angular as they are when they aid in the diagnosis of malignancy.

Chromatin of regeneration has distinct borders, which are not blurred unless also degenerated. Because of the frequent accompaniment of marked inflammation and degeneration, however, the chromatin of regenerative cells may appear smudged and blurred with cytoplasmic perinuclear halos and vacuolation overlaid upon the features of regeneration.

The cytoplasm is usually of normal amount but is sometimes scanty. It frequently shows very little of its typical specialized functions (e.g., secretory vacuolization), which may be atypical (i.e., hyperdistended secretory vacuoles) (Fig. 34–18). Because of the greater nuclear size, the nucleo-cytoplasmic ratio is frequently increased.

NONSPECIFIC INFLAMMATION, CHRONIC IRRITATION, AND SENILE VAGINITIS

Inflammatory response is brought forth by many conditions and stimuli, including irritation, infection, radiation, trauma, endocrine states, vitamin deficienies, and neoplasia. When severe enough, the resulting cellular distortion and degeneration can *mask* the presence of underlying disease, including malignancy. Further, it is impossible to accurately evaluate hormonal status in the presence of significant inflammation.

A heavy leukocytic infiltrate (Fig. 34–26), hemorrhage, and necrotic debris can cause distortion and degeneration of diagnostic elements and obscure them. The cytohormonal pattern is disrupted with spread of the Maturation Index (approaching $\overleftrightarrow{33/34/33}$), so that cytohormonal evaluation is rendered useless (p. 701). Neoplasia can be hidden by an inflammatory reaction, or rendered unidentifiable; conversely, normal cells can be so severely altered that a false diagnosis may be made by the unwary (Fig. 34–25).

Chronic Trauma

Prolapse, prolonged use of a pessary, foreign bodies, or other sources of chronic irritation can cause an obscuring degenerative inflammation and a Maturation Index shift to the right or spread. Anucleated superficial cells are exfoliated from such leukoplakic areas of hyperkeratosis. Although this renders cytohormonal evaluation worthless, the finding of anucleate superficial cells alerts one to the lesion. Some foreign bodies, such as imbedded sutures or iodinated fat used to

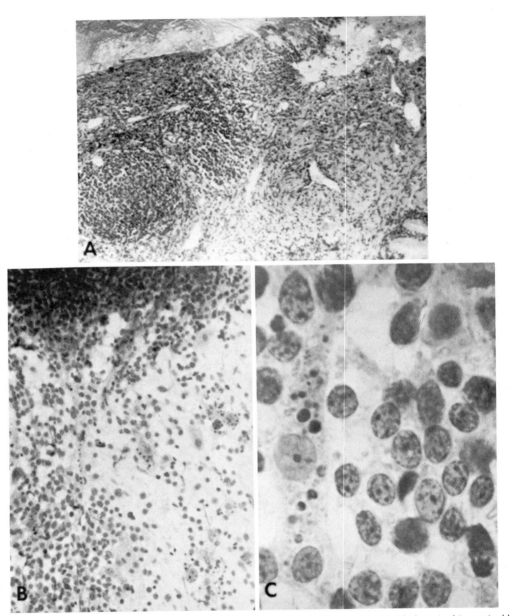

Figure 34–26. Lymphocytic follicular formation in chronic cervicitis. *A,* The overlying epithelium in this cervical biopsy has ulcerated, allowing the underlying follicular elements to exfoliate. Hematoxylin-eosin stain. ×120. *B,* Cervical cellular spread. Cellular elements streaming from the follicle at top of photo are composed almost entirely of young lymphocytes with blood vessels (upper midfield), erythrocytes, and large reticulum cells scattered throughout. ×120. *C,* Cervical cellular spread. Lymphocytic elements on the right are proplastic with a mitosis in lower field. A large phagocytic reticulum cell is on the left and contains cytoplasmic debris. ×1200.

determine tubal pregnancy, can bring forth multinucleated giant histiocytes (Fig. 35–22) with granulomatous chronic inflammatory reaction.

Senile Vaginitis

In the senile vagina with parabasal cell maturation, the vaginal epithelium is thin and completely atrophic (Fig. 34–11). The cells lying on the surface have matured only to the parabasal level by the time they are exfoliated (M.I.: $\overline{100/0/0}$). This teleatrophic epithelium is extremely susceptible to inflammation or nonspecific infection (senile vaginitis) as well as monilial or *Trichomonas* infection.

In contradistinction, intermediate cell

maturation (Fig. 34–10) is not associated with senile vaginitis. When there is vaginitis in the presence of intermediate cell maturation, specific etiologic agents should be sought and identified.

Parabasal cells can be so distorted by irritation, degeneration, and regeneration accompanying teleatrophy that they appear bizarre with cellular changes of dyskaryosis (Fig. 34–32). There is increased nuclear size, nuclear hyperchromasia, chromatin clumping, increased nucleo-cytoplasmic ratio, and grotesque configurations of the cytoplasm (atypical functional differentiation). Artifactually, many features of these reactive parabasal cells are similar to those found in some cells shed from carcioma in situ and from invasive squamous cell carcinoma. Conversely, such inflammatory reaction may distort cancer cells and obscure their recognition or diagnosis.

In senile vaginitis, estrogens, either alone or with antibiotics, bring both clinical relief and clearing of the cytologic picture, usually in about two weeks. Severe epithelial atypias based upon the senile vaginitis may require many more weeks to entirely disappear, but prompt clearing of the vaginitis allows the epithelial lesion to stand out in better preservation, for proper identification. In this way an underlying lesion can be detected and properly diagnosed, or its absence clearly determined.

Postirradiation Changes

Following large doses of radiation to the area of the vaginal epithelium, such as therapy for carcinoma of the cervix, the tissues are severely injured. After such therapy, epithelial cells usually do not mature past the parabasal cell type, and the Maturation Index approaches $\frac{}{100/0/0}$. There may be marked inflammation.

This teleatrophy differs from that of senile vaginitis in that moderate doses of oral estrogen do not affect the cytohormonal pattern, necessitating local estrogen therapy.

Metabolic Disorders

In cases of severe *hypothyroidism*, the teleatrophic epithelium (M.I.: $\frac{}{100/0/0}$) is susceptible to infection. Likewise, the teleatrophic epithelium of *childhood* is very susceptible to general infection. Patients with severe, uncontrolled *diabetes* frequently have fungus and bacterial infection, and any basic inflammatory lesion present is liable to be more severe than in a nondiabetic individual.

INFECTIONS

Outpouring of leukocytes and cellular destruction, which are so prominent in the inflammatory and irritative patterns, are also present in infection. In addition, specific etiologic agents (e.g., *Trichomonas*, bacteria) or hallmarks of their presence (e.g., inclusion bodies, ciliocytophthoria) can frequently be identified. Recognition and identification of these permit a more intelligent approach to prognosis and therapy.

In many infections, the acute phases are vaginal. When they become chronic they are frequently restricted to the periurethral glands, the vulvovaginal glands, or the endocervical glands and canal.

Most infections are mixed. One agent may initiate the process, or develop into the major cause of the inflammation, but usually many agents are involved in any given case. In spite of some very efficacious "shotgun" therapy which might be available for certain situations, it is advantageous to identify specific agents, such as *Trichomonas* and *Candida,* in order to direct specific therapy, which otherwise might not be included in a general broad spectrum approach.

Recognition of teleatrophy (parabasal cell atrophy) of the aged woman or child, a state which is so prone to mixed or nonspecific infections, may allow for the production of a lush and highly resistant epithelium simply by the administration of vaginal estrogens without antibiotic therapy. It is important also to recognize the predilection to infection in the pregnant state, and to provide local vaginal and cervical therapy when indicated.

VIRUSES

Many viruses have been isolated from the female genital tract. Whereas some bring about specific infections, others are associated clinically with nonspecific inflammation or complicate other lesions.

Herpes simplex virus type II (herpes genitalis) is associated with specific intranuclear inclusion bodies in gynecologic smears (Fig. 34–27 A) and vesicular-ulcerated lesions of the female genital tract (e.g., cervix, vagina, introitus). The cells are typical and usually

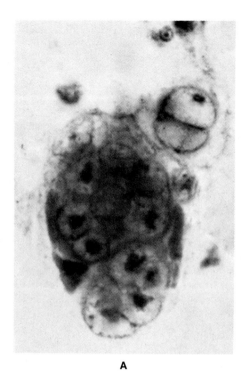
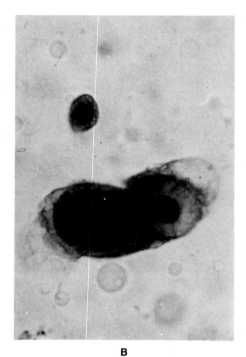

A **B**

Figure 34–27 Viral intranuclear inclusions in epithelial cells. ×1200. *A,* Epithelial changes associated with herpes simplex virus, type II, infection. Fast smear of an 18 year old patient, six weeks post partum. These multiple large nuclei are closely packed and tightly molded within the scant but chromatophilic cytoplasm. The *irregular* intranuclear bodies are mixed eosinophilic and basophilic and have a large clear halo between them and the nuclear membrane. Degenerated chromatin has both mixed with the inclusion bodies and also marginated, smudging the internal border of the nuclear envelopes. Note the neutrophils in the upper background for size comparison. *B,* Cytomegalic inclusion disease. Salivary gland virus changes in renal tubular epithelial cells exfoliated into the urine of a 1 month old female child. Again the nuclei are very large, but each contains a massive, *round* intranuclear body. It is mixed acidophilic and basophilic, and has a large clear halo between it and the degenerated chromatinic rim at the nuclear membrane. The chromatin is mixed with the inclusion, has marginated to the nuclear border, and extends as trans-halo bridges between the inclusion and the chromatinic rim. It is smudgy and degenerated. Cytoplasm is scant. Papanicolaou stain. Millipore (SM) filter membrane preparation.

diagnostic. In contrast to the multiple, huge, degenerated nuclei, the cytoplasm is scanty but very chromatophilic. The nuclei are extremely crowded and mold into each other, suggesting the configuration of seeds in a pomegranate or stones in a gallbladder. They have been mistaken for syncytial trophoblast cells, but rather than the good proplastic nuclear pattern of placental cells, their nuclei have bland, "washed-out," slate gray degenerated chromatin and characteristic prominent single intranuclear inclusions with the scanty, wispy cytoplasm. The nuclear membrane is thickened by degenerated chromatin plastered to its inner surface. There is a large cleared area or halo, surrounding a moderate sized, irregular intranuclear inclusion body. The latter is *acidophilic*, but has varying amounts of hematoxylinophilic smudged chromatin

inseparably mixed with it. Severe dysplasia is at times associated with herpes infection of the cervix, especially in the early, stimulative phases of the infection, with shedding of severely dyskaryotic cells.

Salivary gland virus infection in a pregnant woman produces in the fetus a congenital infection which may result in *cytomegalic inclusion disease* in the newborn. Degenerated renal tubular epithelial cells, containing typical intranuclear inclusion bodies, exfoliate into the child's urine (Fig. 34–27 *B*) but rarely into the mother's, even though virus can be cultivated therefrom. When the cellular changes are typical a clinical diagnosis can be made. The cell is enlarged but, because of the extremely large nucleus, the cytoplasm appears somewhat scanty. The texture of the cytoplasm is coarse and moderately chromatophilic. Although intracytoplasmic inclusions can occur, they are not diagnostic as are the intranuclear changes. The nuclear envelope is ballooned, as with herpes, with degenerating strands of chromatin adhering to the internal surface, but the inclusion body is round, and the nuclei are single. As with herpes, the inclusion body is acidophilic, with an admixture of hematoxylinophilic degenerated chromatin.

Chickenpox and other viral infections can be associated with inclusion bodies. Some (e.g., parainfluenza) produce changes of ciliocytophthoria in the ciliated columnar endocervical cells.

The epithelium overlying chronic infection of the genital tract (i.e., virus, granuloma inguinale, lymphopathia venereum, tuberculosis) is frequently very proplastic, form-

ing *pseudo-epitheliomatous hyperplasia,* which exfoliates dyskaryotic cells (Fig. 34–32). Donovan bodies containing the organism *Donovania granulomatis* can be identified in Wright stained smears from the active lesion of granuloma inguinale. The type of dyskaryotic cells shed from the overlying hyperplastic epithelium reflects the extent of atypicality in the epithelium. When carcinoma develops in this chronically hyperplastic epithelium, carefully taken scrapings of the lesion can detect it in its early developing stages (Fig. 34–28). If the disease extends into the vaginal vault, routine Fast vaginopancervical or vaginal smears are valuable; however, if the vulva is involved, multiple direct smears of the lesion are necessary to obtain sufficient cellular evidence.

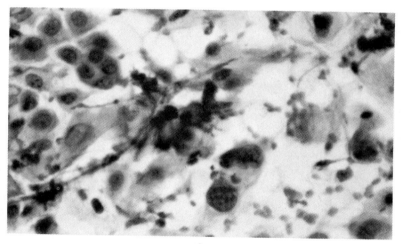

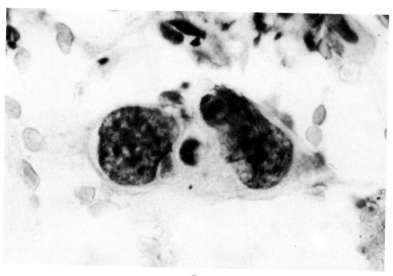

Figure 34–28. *Squamous cell carcinoma developing in granuloma inguinale.* Direct cellular scraping. Papanicolaou stain. *A,* In the upper left and lower right of the field, there are numerous dyskaryotic cells (see Fig. 34–32) shed from the atypical epithelium termed pseudo-epitheliomatous hyperplasia. In the lower center are two large hyperchromatic malignant cells shed from squamous cell carcinoma. ×480. *B,* These cells shed from carcinoma have massive chromatin clumping and hyperchromasia with nuclear irregularity and increased nucleo-cytoplasmic ratio. Fifty-seven year old patient. Donovan bodies demonstrated 5 years earlier. Biopsy revealed squamous cell carcinoma. ×1200.

A

B

BACTERIA

Acute bacterial infections (e.g., Neisseria, streptococci, staphylococci, hemophilus, and pneumococci) are associated with exudation of neutrophils and serum. Blood may be present. Marked cellular destruction is present with obscuring of evidence for both cytohormonal evaluation and cancer detection or diagnosis. *Haemophilus vaginalis* organisms residing on top of squames give a peculiar mosaic pattern referred to by Gardner as the "clue" cell. These organisms must not be confused, however, with tiny bubbles of air that may be trapped on top of squames from momentary drying during cover-slipping.

Tuberculosis produces a chronic granulomatous inflammation with histiocytic activity. The Langhans giant cell, so typical of tuberculosis in tissue, is *not* indicative of this infection in cellular smears; instead, whereas it may rarely be found in gynecologic cellular preparations in tuberculosis, this multinucleated giant cell histiocyte is most frequently found in *Trichomonas* infection. Tubercles involving the cervix are at times associated with a severe metaplasia or epithelial atypia from which dyskaryotic cells are shed.

Actinomycetes is found in gynecologic smears of users of an intrauterine contraceptive device (Fig. 34–29 A,B). Most examined by immunofluorescent techniques (Gupta) have been identified as *A. israelii*. In addition to local endometrial infection about the device, infection has extended into the tubes, with resultant abscess, and into the bloodstream, with metastic foci of infection occurring throughout the body. Penicillin does not affect the infection, but removal of the intrauterine device causes the bacteria to disappear promptly from gynecologic smears. Such infection has also been associated with the use of a vaginal pessary in the postmenopausal period.

Chlamydia trachomatis, one of two species of the genus *Chlamydia*, is the causative agent of a number of human diseases, including lymphogranuloma venereum, salpingitis, trachoma, inclusion conjunctivitis, and possibly interstitial pneumonia of the newborn. Previously called "TRIC agents" (TRachoma–Inclusion Conjunctivitis), they are now believed to be bacteria and, because of confusion with "trich" for *Trichomonas*, the term "TRIC agent" is now in disuse in favor of "chlamydia". While there are serotypic and growth differences between the agent causing lymphogranuloma venereum and that responsible for trachoma and inclusion conjunctivitis, their morphology and cytologic identification in epithelial cells are identical (Fig. 34–29 C). The *initial* body is noninfective but actively metabolic in the cell. Microcolonies of it appear on Papanicolaou stain as multiple small eosinophilic granules just at the limits of the light microscope, surrounded by a poorly defined circular area of cytoplasmic clearing. This condenses into the *intermediate* body (Fig. 34–29 C) which further develops into the infectious stage, the *elementary* body.

FUNGI

Candida albicans, or *Monilia*, is the most frequent fungus encountered in vulvovaginitis. It is easily diagnosed by taking a bit of a "cotton patch" from a vaginal lesion and preparing a crush preparation on a slide with NaOH. It can be found and tentatively identified as a fungus consistent with *Candida* in routine vaginal smears taken for cancer detection. *Candida*, as in its form in tissue, presents as long septate hyphae (long bodies) and budding round yeast (round bodies) producing a tentatively identifiable characteristic morphology (Fig. 34–29 D). Because other fungi are found at times, which have the same morphology (i.e., *Torulopsis glabrata*), it is tentatively identified as a "fungus consistent with *Candida*" and definite identification should be made on the basis of cultural characteristics. Contaminating pollens and other plant bodies can closely mimic morphologic characteristics of fungi.

PROTOZOA

Trichomonas vaginalis is capable of producing either an infestation or an infection. When it infests, it is found without inflammation clinically or cytologically and evidently involves the luminal surface, producing no, or minimal, disease in the epithelium and in the underlying tissue.

On the other hand, it can produce either acute or chronic infection. This is characterized by a prominent vascular and inflammatory phenomenon of the epithelium and subepithelial tissues. With severe infection and

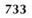

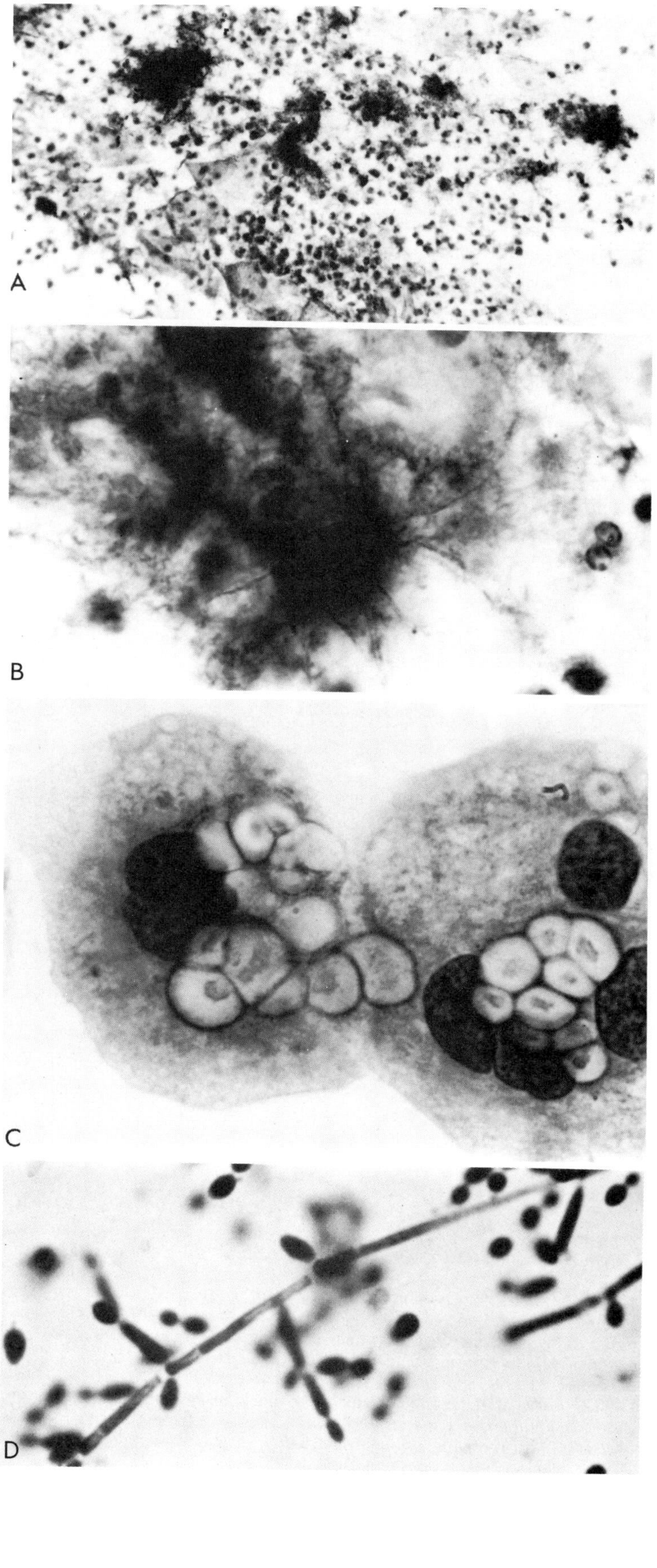

Figure 34–29. *A, B,* Actinomycetes infection in an IUD user; *C,* Chlamydial infection; *D, Candida albicans* (Monilia). *A,* A heavy leukocytic and necrotic inflammation within which, on low power, numerous irregular hematoxylinophilic masses are prominent. *B,* High magnification identifies the branching, delicate rods of the bacteria surrounded by amorphous or granular material, with neutrophils in close association at the periphery. Immunofluorescence identified *A. israelii.* (Courtesy of P. K. Gupta.) *C,* Chlamydial infection in squamous epithelial cells. In midfield, and scattered throughout the cytoplasm, are numerous *initial* bodies, consisting of microcolonies of small eosinophilic bacteria surrounded by indistinctly cleared cytoplasm. The multiple prominently cleared areas with a single centrally condensed particle and thickened membrane are the *intermediate* bodies. There is one *elementary* body, the infectious stage, above the nucleus of the cell on the left. The large and reactive nuclei are moderately dyskaryotic. (Courtesy of P. K. Gupta.) *D, Candida albicans* (Monilia). Long, thin, septate hyphae (long bodies) and small oval budding yeast (round bodies) are morphologically characteristic of Candida. Absolute identification is based upon cultural characteristics. Papanicolaou stain. *A,* × 220; *B, C, D,* × 1400.

host response, there can be invasion of the host cells with epithelial injury, destruction, regeneration, and dysplasia associated with severe inflammatory outpouring.

The severity of the disease from this organism is much greater during certain hormonal states—i.e., pregnancy, late luteal phase, and menstruation. It can be found at virtually any vaginal pH, but it is more florid around pH 6 and pH 7. Pathogenicity varies (a) according to the strain of the organism, (b) between different hosts, and (c) in the given individual according to her state of resistance. As the vaginal pH changes or as other factors become hostile to the organism it retreats to the glands, the urethra, or the endocervix. This results in an outpouring of both acute and chronic elements, serum, and blood into the cellular specimen. Multinucleated giant cell histiocytes are frequently brought forth in the cell spread.

Clinical manifestations are found in two major phases: the *florid* and the *latent*. During the *florid* phase of vaginitis, the patient is troubled and symptomatic. Although a hanging drop examination usually reveals the organism, cytologic examination of the frothy white exudate of the acute phase yields preserved and diagnostic trichomonads (Fig. 34–30), but at times with great difficulty. Cellular destruction can be great, but bizarre epithelial nuclear changes are usually not prominent in this phase.

During the *latent* phase of *Trichomonas* infection, the patient is usually asymptomatic and one has difficulty in finding the organism in the hanging drop examination of vaginal fluid. In addition, routine pelvic examination reveals a healthy vagina and, usually, a perfectly normal appearing cervix or one showing only slight chronic cervicitis. The organism retreats into the endocervix

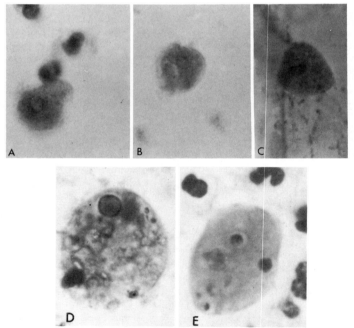

Figure 34–30. *A, B, C, Trichomonas vaginalis; D, E, Entamoeba. A, B, C,* In the routine Papanicolaou preparation and stain, trichomonads are usually poorly preserved so that a meticulous search is required to find *diagnostic* organisms. They are about the size of a small histiocyte (note neutrophils in *A* for comparison of size), and are round, oval, or pear-shaped. The cytoplasmic stain of their bodies is not to be confused with the nuclear stain of a bare epithelial cell nucleus. There must be a definite nucleus, but it should be small, pale, and single. When a florid vaginitis is not present, they are best found in cervical scrapings from their latent sites. *D, Entamoeba histolytica* of cervix. The nucleus (at 12 o'clock position) has a prominent chromatinic rim and centrally placed karyosome. Numerous erythrocytes are present in the cytoplasm. (Courtesy of P. K. Gupta.) *E, Entamoeba,* probably *gingivalis.* Numerous amebae were present in this Fast smear of an asymptomatic user of an IUD. The nucleus (at 9 o'clock position) is pale but is typical of Entamoeba, with a centrally placed karyosome. The numerous hematoxylinophilic bodies of neutrophil nuclear debris in the cytoplasm strengthen the identification of this as most probably *E. gingivalis. Actinomycetes* was also present, and both disappeared promptly upon removal of the IUD. Papanicolaou stain. ×1400.

and urethra, and can be readily identified in cellular spreads of cervical material. The resulting chronic endocervicitis may be inconspicuous or obvious on inspection of the external os but when there is outpouring of serum, blood, necrotic debris, mucus, and inflammatory cells, this greatly obscures the exfoliated cellular pattern.

It is in this latent phase that the organism is most frequently associated with the *serious* epithelial lesions of the endocervix. This should be regarded in two aspects. First, the heavy inflammatory reaction both obscures diagnostic cells and alters their morphologic characteristics, so that the nature of the underlying epithelium may not be definitely identified. Thus, malignant cells may lose their diagnostic criteria, whereas benign cells cause alarm and even false identification of cancer (Fig. 34–31).

Second, continuing injury and regeneration are associated with epithelial atypias, at times of grave concern. Great care must be taken with cytologic interpretation in the presence of severe *Trichomonas* infection with obscuring and cellular destruction. However, when cytologically diagnostic cancer is present, based upon careful evaluation, the mere presence or absence of trichomonads makes no difference in the cytologic assessment.

The presence of alarming cells, which are not diagnostic of cancer, bears the same indications for biopsy when *Trichomonas* is present as it does in the absence of the organism. If cytologic evidence is diagnostic only of a dysplastic lesion and if no cancer is found on satisfactory and adequate tissue examination, intensive therapy should be directed at this chronic endocervical infec-

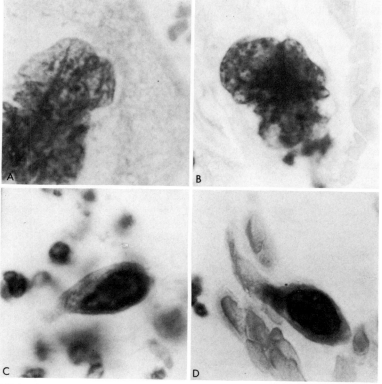

Figure 34–31. Cellular degeneration associated with trichomoniasis in benign (*A* and *C*) and malignant (*B* and *D*) cells. Benign cells can be made so bizarre as to appear neoplastic, whereas malignant cells can lose their unequivocal diagnostic criteria. Papanicolaou stain. ×1435. *A*, Nuclear size increase and hyperchromasia in a *benign* cell with chromatin smudging and perinuclear halo. There is abundant cytoplasm. *B*, A large malignant nucleus with degenerative chromatin smudging and hyperchromasia. The diagnostic value of the nuclear irregularities is greatly diminished; there is loss of sharp detail from degenerative smudging. *C*, Intense nuclear hyperchromasia in this benign cell with scant cytoplasm. The extreme peripheral smudging and central laking of chromatin indicate degenerative changes. *D*, Degenerative smudging in a malignant "tadpole" nucleus. The malignant chromatin clumps are so smudged that their criteria are not conclusive and could be mimicked by a benign process.

tion. Clearing this allows better interpretation of the basic cellular change, with the verification of the malignant or benign character of any existing lesion. Such procedure is often necessary before accurate identification of the most serious lesion can be made either cytologically or histologically (Fig. 34–31).

For a *diagnostic* identification of *T. vaginalis* (Fig. 34–30), one must be careful to rule out a bare epithelial cell nucleus, distorted neutrophil, histiocyte, parabasal cell with a small nucleus, cytoplasmic fragment, or mucus blob—all of these can closely mimic a trichomonad in certain circumstances. Flagella, undulating membrane, axostyle, and fine internal cytoplasmic structures are rarely identified in a routine cytologic smear.

Three morphologic charcteristics are most important as a *minimum* for a positive identification of the organism: the organism must be composed of *cytoplasm* (tinctorially and morphologically) (Fig. 34–1 *C*) which cannot be either a vague mucous accumulation or a bare nucleus; this must contain a *single small, pale nucleus* which is neither dark nor pyknotic; the overall *size* of this rounded organism falls between that of a neutrophil (Fig. 34–30) and a parabasal cell.

Strains of *T. vaginalis* vary greatly in their pathogenicity. In addition, the pathogenicity of a single strain appears to vary markedly from patient to patient. In the same patient, furthermore, the infection waxes and wanes according to various host factors. The reaction of the organism and its destruction of cellular pattern is more severe in the late secretory phase of the menstrual cycle, during menstruation, and during pregnancy.

Entamoeba infections of the female genital tract occur in two distinct types. In geographic areas of the world where intestinal amebiasis is hyperendemic, *E. histolytica* produces major gynecologic disease, including severe granulomatous ulcerations of the cervix, vagina, and vulva, which can be misinterpreted clinically as carcinoma (Fig. 35–30 *D*). In contradistinction to this severe infection, there has recently been described by de Moraes-Ruehsen and co-workers an asymptomatic infection by an *Entamoeba*. Not only does it appear to lack the clinical pathogenicity of *E. histolytica* but, as these authors thoroughly describe, its cellular morphology more closely resembles *E. gingivalis* (Fig. 35–30 *E*). It is found associated with *Actinomycetes* infection in users of an intrauterine contraceptive device and, although susceptible to metronidazole, it disappears without therapy following removal of the device.

HELMINTHS

Ova and larvae of pinworms and other helminths found in the vaginal pool material usually either are picked up on the specimen from the labia or are contaminants from the feces and urine. Occasionally they are associated with genital disease. *Enterobius, Strongyloides*, and *Schistosomas* have been encountered in cytologic material in severe gynecologic disease. Ova must not be confused with pollen or plant cells, which also contaminate and may appear morphologically similar.

THE "SHADES OF GRAY" LESIONS— ABNORMALITIES OF EPITHELIAL DEVELOPMENT, CELLULAR ORIENTATION, AND NUCLEAR AND CYTOPLASMIC RELATIONSHIPS

Female genital tract epithelium undergoes morphologic alterations ranging from normalcy (euplasia) through atypical lesions (e.g., degeneration, repair, stimulation, chronic irritation, intraepithelial neoplasia) to the changes of carcinoma (malignant neoplasia). The atypical lesions, or "shades of gray," are *not* static entities but are transition states in constantly changing processes. They are classified by various terms, such as anaplasia, dysplasia, hyperplasia, metaplasia, atypia, hyperactivity; but their nomenclature is of secondary importance. What is of utmost importance is the recognition of their biologic nature and their proper handling clincally.

There are only a few basic patterns in which epithelium is capable of reacting to the many and varied stimuli it receives. Furthermore, more than one process usually operates at the same time (i.e., injury, degeneration, inflammation, reparation, regeneration, endocrine alterations, neoplasia), which beclouds both cytologic and histologic pictures.

Serial cellular samples, correlated whenever possible with selected tissue biopsies, yield valuable insight into the true biologic nature of the resulting complex lesion. Cellular samples allow repeated examination of maximal surface area (which is larger than the surface area of a biopsy specimen), without disturbance of the lesion. As experience with careful evaluations of cytologic-histologic correlations increases, it becomes obvious that exfoliated cells are not only an accurate mirror for the diagnosis of many morphologic features of the parent epithelium but also aid immensely in understanding their biologic processes.

The Lesion and its Cellular Exfoliation

When a lesion of the epithelium is composed only of mature cells (either squamous or columnar) with normal euplastic nuclei, it exfoliates only that type of cell. Thus, normal mature cells are shed from areas of simple eversion, mature epidermidalization, simple metaplasia, atrophic leukoplakia, and similar lesions. A diagnostic hallmark of simple mature metaplasia, as opposed to normal squamous epithelium, is the *small* amount of cytoplasm of some of the mature squamous cells shed.

As cellular atypia occurs within the epithelium, prompt evidence of it appears in the exfoliated cellular material as dyskaryosis. Even when histologic examination appears to confine abnormal changes to the lower epithelial layers, sufficient cellular alteration usually persists in enough cells as they mature and move to the surface to be detected in exfoliated material. The removal of superficial debris and hyperkeratinized layers may be necessary to procure a specimen containing diagnostic cells from ulcerative, necrotic, or hyperkeratotic lesions.

Dyskaryosis

Atypical cellular activity in tissue is reflected in the exfoliated cell as abnormal nuclear changes (*dyskaryosis*), alteration in cytoplasmic maturation (i.e., *dyskeratosis*, immaturity), or both.

Dyskaryosis is *not* a *clinical* diagnosis. It is *not* synonymous with dysplasia, nor is it a new term, being well established in pathology. Papanicolaou, however, reapplied it specifically to exfoliated cells to characterize a group of cellular abnormalities involving mainly the nucleus, and called them *dyskaryotic* cells (Fig. 34–32).

The Dyskaryotic Cell. The round or oval nucleus of the dyskaryotic cell is hyperchromatic. It is large and the nuclear envelope is wavy or undulated (Fig. 34–32)—not wrinkled or shrunken) (see Figs. 34–23*B*, 34–25 *A*). The parachromatin is cleared and the chromatin is minimally to coarsely granular, depending upon the degree of increased activity, but they are evenly distributed throughout the nucleus. Nucleoli are usually

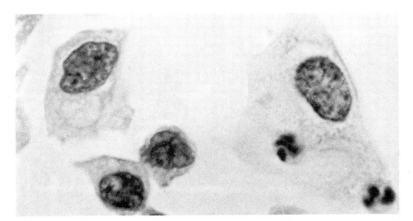

Figure 34–32. Dyskaryotic cells. These abnormal nuclei contain many of the criteria encountered in cancer, but each cell as a whole is not diagnostic of malignancy. These dyskaryotic nuclei are of varying degrees of atypicality, and are located in cytoplasm which exhibits significantly varying degrees of atypicality of maturation and of immaturity. Note the wavy nuclear membrane in the upper left, the uniformly thickened chromatinic rim, the coarse chromatin granules, and the abnormally cleared parachromatin which is uniformly dispersed throughout the hyperchromatic chromatin. Nucleoli, so prominent in dyskaryosis with columnar maturation (Fig. 34–17), are absent in these cells of squamous maturation. Cytoplasm of the two lower cells is scanty and nonsquamified (immature dyskaryotic cells). The cytoplasm of the cell in the upper left is more abundant but is still nonsquamified (moderately mature dyskaryotic cell). The cytoplasm of the cell at the upper right is abundant and squamified (mature squamous dyskaryotic cell). A mature columnar dyskaryotic cell is not shown (see Figs. 34–16, 34–17 and 34–33C.) Papanicolaou stain. ×1200.

not conspicuous in squamous cells, but are very prominent in columnar cells (Figs. 35–16, 35–17, 35–33), urothelial cells, and those of mesodermal origin (i.e., mesothelial cells, muscle, connective tissue). Smudged hyperchromasia or pallid cellular swelling indicates degeneration, which may be found, *with* dyskaryosis but must be distinguished *from* it. Changes in the *cytoplasm* of the dyskaryotic cell, which is of diagnostic help, involve mainly impairment of its ability to mature normally. Hypermaturity produces extreme keratinization or *dyskeratosis;* conversely, *immaturity* brings inability to either squamify or produce columnar forms, and a decrease in the amount of cytoplasm both absolute and relative to the nucleus (increased nucleo-cytoplasmic ratio) (Fig. 34–32).

In gynecologic sites, immaturity of the cytoplasm is more frequent than hypermaturity. Based upon this ability for cytoplasmic maturation, the dyskaryotic cells are considered to be *immature, moderately mature,* or *mature* (squamous or columnar) (Figs. 34–16, 34–17, and 34–32).

Papanicolaou noted the association of dyskaryotic cells with the shades of gray lesions, as well as with the early and late neoplastic lesions of the cervix. He associated the less mature dyskaryotic cells with lesions of greater atypia. In an attempt to classify the dyskaryotic cells, he equated the apparent maturation of the surrounding cytoplasm with the cytoplasm of the most closely identifiable normal cell, and thus subdivided them into the endocervical dyskaryotic cell, the superficial dyskaryotic cell, the intermediate dyskaryotic cell, and the parabasal (deep) dyskaryotic cell. This nomenclature is easily confused with the normal cell types, and has regrettably created the *misconception* that is a classification based on the cell of origin rather than on morphologic similarity. A superficial dyskaryotic cell, for instance, does not usually originate from a normal superficial cell; on the contrary, it is usually the result of maturation of the cytoplasm of another *less* mature dyskaryotic cell rather than the formation of a dyskaryotic cell from a normal cell of like maturity.

This is not a minor academic point. The processes of dyskaryosis which bear the most *serious* connotation are *not* those with only *surface* atypia, wherein a mature cell becomes less mature; neither are they proc-

esses of degeneration, wherein a nucleus undergoes retrogressive changes. It has been shown in animal studies of carcinogenesis that these cells develop as abnormal cells early in their beginning and, in fact, most are daugther cells of abnormal cells.

Another important concept is that the cells of a dyskaryotic series are abnormal and should *not* be included in any evaluation of normal cells (e.g., Maturation Index, Cornification Index).

The complete significance of the dyskaryotic cell is far from settled, and many prefer to avoid the term because it is poorly understood. At least it can be concluded that the changes referred to as dyskaryosis do *not* always mean cancer, but are also associated with benign progressive changes (e.g., stimulation, regeneration, healing) as well as with premalignant and frankly malignant lesions.

Degrees of Cellular Dyskaryosis. As epithelial lesions become more atypical or dysplastic, the cells exfoliated from the surface tend to show: (a) more severe nuclear dyskaryotic changes (e.g., increased hyperchromasia, chromatin granule size, parachromatin clearing, nuclear membrane undulation) and (b) decreased cytoplasmic maturation (e.g., less stratification, less columnar maturation, lesser amount of cytoplasm).

Using the three major categories of dyskaryotic cells, illustrated in Figure 34–32, one can objectively express the degree of atypicality present in the epithelial lesion. Thus, from evaluation of the degree of severity of nuclear change (Fig. 34–32) and of the percentages of *immature* dyskaryotic cells to *moderately mature* dyskaryotic cells to *mature* dyskaryotic cells (an index of dyskaryosis, D.I.) a more objective evaluation of the degree of cellular and tissue abnormalities can be obtained (Figs. 34–33 to 34–36).

With metaplasia of columnar epithelium to squamous epithelium, the matured cell on the surface does not have columnar orientation (perpendicular to the basement membrane) but matures to a squamous orientation (parallel to the basement membrane). If the resulting squamous epithelium is mature, normal squamous cells are exfoliated; these cells, however, tend to have small squamous cytoplasm. If there is minor atypicality of the epithelium, mature squamous dyskaryotic cells are shed (Fig. 34–34).

As the stratified squamous epithelium becomes more atypical and dysplastic, the cy-

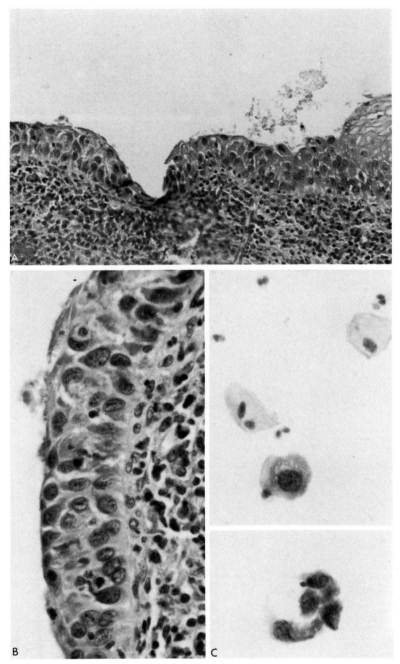

Figure 34–33. Atypical lesion with columnar surface maturation. *A,* Normal noncornified stratified squamous epithelium (right) sharply changes to atypical epithelium. Hematoxylin-eosin stain. ×120. *B,* Both surface and subcolumnar reserve cells are extremely hyperplastic and active (dyskaryotic), with frequent mitoses. Surface maturation is mainly columnar (perpendicular to basement membrane) with occasional squamous maturation (parallel to basement membrane). Hematoxylin-eosin stain. ×400. *C,* Fast smear of same patient. Two normal intermediate cells and neutrophils in the upper field compare with the five abnormal dyskaryotic cells below. Note abnormal nuclear size, chromatin, and granularity. Compare nuclear patterns with *B.* Two mature columnar dyskaryotic cells (below) are in profile and two reserve cells are *en face.* One moderately mature dyskaryotic cell (center) represents the predominant cell in the specimen. (D.I.: 15/65/20.) Papanicolaou stain. ×400. Thirty-eight year old pregnant woman with *Trichomonas vaginalis* infection.

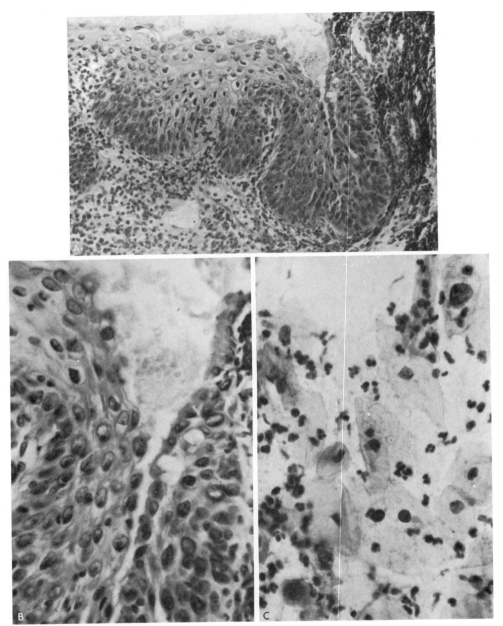

Figure 34–34. Slightly atypical lesion with squamous surface maturation. *A,* Simple columnar endocervical epithelium (right) gives way to stratified squamous epithelium. Hematoxylin-eosin stain. ×120. *B,* Degenerating simple columnar cells are retained on the surface of atypical squamous epithelium for a short distance (right). Nuclei appear very active (dyskaryotic) throughout all layers, even where the cells surface as squames (left). Hematoxylin-eosin stain. ×400. *C,* Fast smear of the same patient. A mature squamous dyskaryotic cell (upper right) and an immature dyskaryotic cell (lower left) have typical abnormal nuclear patterns when compared with the surrounding normal cells. (D.I.: 6/44/50.) Papanicolaou stain. ×400. Thirty-two year old pregnant woman with *Trichomonas vaginalis* infection.

toplasm of the surface cell shows less maturation and is more crowded (less cytoplasm) (Fig. 34–35). This is reflected in the cellular spread as a progressing immaturity of the exfoliated dyskaryotic cell, with the *nuclear* pattern becoming more coarsely granular and hyperchromatic, the *cytoplasm* demonstrating less ability to squamify and becoming less abundant, and the index of dyskaryosis (D.I.) shifting to the left.

When the atypicality of the lesion is extreme, and yet the surface cell matures suffi-

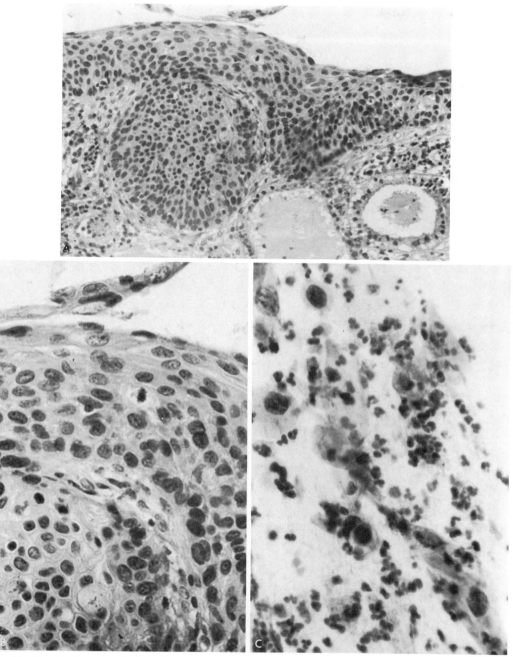

Figure 34–35. Moderately atypical lesion with squamous surface maturation. *A,* There is gland involvement with replacement of columnar cells with metaplastic epithelium. Hematoxylin-eosin stain. ×120. *B,* Throughout all layers, the dyskaryotic nuclei are large and hyperchromatic, and have granular chromatin and frequent mitoses with moderate crowding. Surface cells mature by flattening parallel to basement membrane (squamous maturation). Hematoxylin-eosin stain. ×400. *C,* Fast smear of the same patient. Numerous dyskaryotic cells are shown: mature squamous (lower right), moderately mature (left center), and immature (top, left of center). There are others obscured by this dense inflammatory material. (D.I.: 34/38/28). Papanicolaou stain. ×400. Twenty-two year old pregnant woman with *Trichomonas vaginalis* infection.

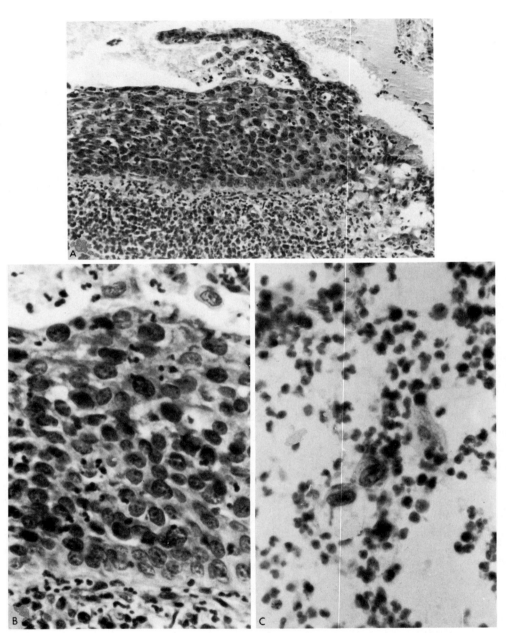

Figure 34–36. Markedly atypical lesion with minimal squamous surface maturation. *A*, This borderline lesion retains a row of normal, simple columnar cells overhanging its margin. Nearly the entire thickness is composed of very hyperactive cells of parabasal maturation with minimal stratification on the surface (left) where retained columnar epithelium had not covered. The stratum germinativum retains orientation. Hematoxylin-eosin stain. ×120. *B*, There is extreme crowding of very large dyskaryotic nuclei. The chromatin is granular and hyperchromatic. There is minimal orientation of the stratum germinativum and minimal stratification on the surface. Note neutrophils and edema throughout all layers. Hematoxylin-eosin stain. ×400. *C*, Fast smear of same patient. Two immature dyskaryotic cells are partially obscured by intense inflammatory background (midfield). Compare these with cells in *B* (D.I.: 48/44/8.) Papanicolaou stain. ×400. Thirty-two year old pregnant woman with *Trichomonas vaginalis* infection.

ciently to be flattened in tissue, then, in the cellular spread, its extremely scanty cytoplasm demonstrates like ability to squamify, even though it may be very slight (Fig. 34–36).

These are extremely valuable hallmarks of cellular dysfunction. When properly fitted into the overall pattern of the cellular spread and pertinent clinical data, they provide valuable information regarding the *biologic behavior* of tissues and the *identification of lesions*.

THE CANCER CELL: CRITERIA OF MALIGNANCY

No *one* morphologic feature characterizes a cancer cell. Usually, cancer cells are abnormal in appearance and a certain number of them show morphologic aberrations sufficient to allow them to be unequivocally recognized as malignant. The appearance of others, however, falls well within normal limits or the limits of nonmalignant abnormality.

From the point of view of diagnosis, it is fortunate that most cancer cells contain certain morphologic changes which, although they occasionally are found in nonmalignant states, are found frequently enough in malignancy to bear diagnostic significance. These are the *criteria of malignancy*. When occurring together in recognized patterns, these cellular changes have been found to be most useful as criteria for recognizing malignant cells in given types of exfoliated material and under defined conditions.

It is to be understood that there is *no absolute* criterion for diagnosing a malignant lesion. That is to say there is no cytologic change which, by itself, unequivocally indicates malignant change; nor is there a cytologic change which, when absent, indicates benignancy. The pattern of multiple criteria indicates the nature of the process being studied, and in this way establishes the diagnosis.

The most valuable criteria of malignancy are found only rarely in bizarre nonmalignant states. In formulating one's own malignant criteria one must be careful not to include certain cellular findings only because they happen to be present in a cell which is known to be malignant. Careful discrimination and a conservative approach reduce to a minimum the possibility of a false interpretation.

One should strive for a *cytologic* diagnosis of malignancy which has the reliability of a *tissue* diagnosis. Therefore, one must strive to recognize the conditions under which an impression might be termed unequivocal, in both cytopathology and histopathology.

Because cellular pathology is a proved and reliable method for diagnosis and clinical assistance in therapy, it must not be approached as a "game" between clinician and pathologist. For the utmost in patient care, the cytopathologist who arrives at his impression from studies of cellular material must be made aware of all information available and of every pertinent fact in the case. As with tissue studies, therefore, and to an even greater degree, cellular evidence is of the greatest clinical value when the type of material, condition of the patient, and condition of the specimen preparation are known.

To arrive at a diagnosis, however, one must have certain objective findings to be observed and weighed in the light of experience and knowledge. For the diagnosis of cancer in cytopathology, these are the criteria. Many of them undoubtedly are artifacts of the method utilized for obtaining and processing the specimen; however, as long as the artifacts are constant, well controlled, and reproducible, they are dependable. Therefore, it is important to note that these discussions are based mainly upon materials *immediately* fixed in 95 per cent *ethyl* alcohol, and stained with a good hematoxylin and counter staining method, preferably the brilliantly multichromatic and transparent one proposed by Papanicolaou.

Thus, one determines the presence or absence of malignancy by evaluating all available evidence, both clinical and pathologic; but especially by evaluating those morphologic changes termed *malignant criteria* and by fitting them into a pattern of recognition.

It is important that only *well-preserved* cells be evaluated in determining criteria for diagnosing malignancy (see section on Degeneration and Inflammation). Disregard for this is probably the greatest single cause of false cancer diagnoses and of missed cancer cases.

The most important criteria fall within three major areas: *irregularity* (e.g., nuclear shape, chromatin pattern), *sharp angularity* (e.g., chromatin clumps, nucleoli, nuclear membrane), and *extremes* (e.g., nucleo-cytoplasmic ratio, thickness of chromatinic rim). Malignant criteria are found in the many disruptions of the normal biologic regularity found in normal cellular components, or normal characteristics being carried to extremes. Only a few criteria involve the cytoplasm; most are present in changes of the *nucleus,* of its *relationship* to the cytoplasm, and of the relationship of *one cell to another.*

THE NUCLEUS

Nuclear *sizes* usually are abnormal. At times extremely small nuclei are formed (Fig. 34–37 A), but most malignant nuclei are larger than their normal counterparts, occasionally reaching huge proportions.

Malignant nuclei have no characteristic or predictable *shape,* unless it is irregularity. Frequently, they are very uniform (Fig. 34–37 B) but at times assist diagnosis by showing extreme sharpness and angularity (Fig. 34–37 C) and by being irregular from one cell to the next (Fig. 34–37 D).

Nuclear *chromasia* is actually hematoxylinophilia, and is imparted mainly by the chromatin and the chromatinic rim. Parachromatin (nuclear sap with finely distributed euchromatin) is very faintly hematoxylinophilic. The nucleoli are acidophilic, frequently with nucleolar associated chromatin. *Hyperchromasia* of the nucleus is usual in malignancy, but by no means is it the rule. In fact, in the same bit of tissue, one cell can be hyperchromatic and its adjacent sibling can have less chromasia than normally expected (Figs. 34–37 D and 34–38). *Irregular chromasia* is frequently found in most malignant cells, with irregular hyperchromatic areas separating large cleared areas of parachromatin (Fig. 34–37 E).

Frequently disregarded is the fact that de-

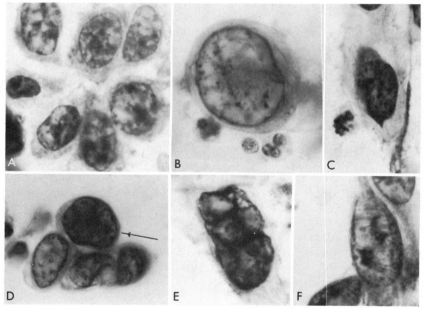

Figure 34–37. General criteria of malignancy. ×1200. *A,* Undifferentiated cells of cancer with scant cytoplasm and indistinct borders. There is only moderate nuclear size variation except for the extremely small malignant cell in left midfield. Note irregular chromatin patterns with large abnormally cleared areas of parachromatin, and chromatin clumps with sharp points and angles. The nuclear chromatinic rims vary abruptly in thickness. *B,* A large cell from cancer (note neutrophil in lower field) with a high nucleo-cytoplasmic ratio. Although the nuclear pattern is pale, it is not degenerated. There are large abnormally cleared areas of parachromatin and chromatin spindles. The cytoplasmic border is sharp. *C,* The nuclear outline is irregular with a sharp pointed angle protruding. Karyopyknosis is beginning. *D,* There is massive chromatin clumping, which is sharp and well preserved. Inside the nucleus at the arrow is a sharply angled nucleolus. Cytoplasm is very scanty with poor cellular borders and crowding of the cells within this tissue fragment. *E,* There is marked hyperchromasia with chromatin clumping and sharply delineated abnormally cleared areas of nuclear sap. Two large and prominent nucleoli are present, which, however, are perfectly round and offer no malignant diagnostic assistance. *F,* There are sharp and pointed nucleoli and chromatin clumps in the large nucleus, with abnormal clearing of parachromatin. The cytoplasm is markedly attenuated over the sides of the nucleus, being drawn tightly around it before tailing off at both ends. Note especially the close nucleo-cytoplasmic association, or hugging, around the upper pole of the nucleus. Papanicolaou stain.

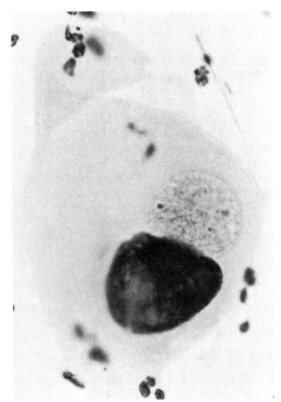

Figure 34–38. Multinucleated squamous cell carcinoma cell. The two daughter nuclei represented are of minimally different size and shape; significantly, however, they vary markedly in chromatin pattern and in chromasia. The nucleus in right center is pale and uniformly granular; however, the nucleus below it is extremely hyperchromatic, with a large aggregation of chromatin to one side of the nucleus and clearing below and to left, with beginning karyopyknosis. The cytoplasm was brilliantly orangophilic and hyaline, with faint refractile rings in the cytoplasm, noted faintly here lying below and to the right of the nuclei. Papanicolaou stain. ×1200.

generation accounts for much hyperchromasia of all cells, benign and malignant. For hyperchromasia to be of valuable diagnostic assistance, therefore, a *well-preserved* chromatin pattern must be retained, no matter how irregular it might be, so that it can be differentiated from the hyperchromasia of nuclear degeneration (Fig. 34–31, C,D, vs. 34–37). To be of reliable diagnostic significance, the chromatin aggregates must have well-preserved, sharply defined borders, as if cut out by a cookie cutter. The smudging of the borders of chromatin clumps and the inner border of the chromatinic rim due to degeneration, is in clear contrast to the sharp "cookie cutter" appearance of well-preserved malignant aggregates. This is an

important concept and, merely because malignant cells are also vulnerable to degeneration with consequent morphologic changes (Fig. 34-31 *D*), one should not lower diagnostic criteria to include smudging.

Very *sharp points* and *acute angles* characterize well-preserved malignant clumping (Fig. 34–37 *C,D,F*). Jagged, sharp, spindly chromatin spears are frequently formed. It is here that good preservation with lack of degeneration is of such basic importance because these are among the most valuable criteria.

Thus, *chromatin pattern* bears the most important diagnostic significance. The uniform chromatin pattern of the normal nucleus is altered into one of marked irregularity, with the chromatic substance clumping into dense hyperchromatic masses, sweeping the nuclear sap clear of its pale-staining hematoxylinophilic material, and leaving behind large, *abnormally cleared* areas of parachromatin (Fig. 34–1 *E* and Fig. 34–37 *E*).

Nuclear membrane irregularities of certain types can be of diagnostic value. The contour of the nuclear envelope frequently consists of sharp and unpredictable foldings and irregularities (Fig. 34–37 *C, E*). This is to be clearly distinguished from the degenerative wrinkling of decreased activity (Figs. 34–24 and 34–31) and the undulation or waviness of increased activity (Fig. 34–32). These are in clear contrast to the sharp irregularities of malignancy whose occurrence is unpredictable by known physiologic reasons.

Nuclear membrane irregularities are very significant, however, in two respects: extreme pointedness and sharpness (Fig. 34–37 *C*) and marked variation in the thickness of the chromatinic rim against the membrane, ranging from areas which are thinner than normally expected (absence of chromatinic rim) to vast thicknesses within the same cell (chromatin aggregates plastered onto the inner surface of the membrane) (Figs. 34–1 *E* and 34–37 *A,C,E,F*).

In degenerative changes and cell multiplication ("active" histiocytes, regeneration, etc.), nuclear patterns may have what appears to be similar chromatin aggregation; but on critical evaluation the aggregates are rounded and there frequently is smudging of the chromatin-parachromatin interfaces (Fig. 34–31 *C*). Chromatinic rim thicknesses and accumulated masses that are sharply punched out in a well-preserved "cookie cutter" manner are of major diagnostic significance, favoring malignancy.

Nucleolar configurations offer valuable malignant criteria in two areas of consideration. One is for there to be great *variation in numbers* of nucleoli present in daughter nuclei of the same cell, or in nuclei of cells in the same tissue fragment. The other is for the outline of *large* nucleoli to be *irregular* and *sharp*, with jagged points and extreme angularity (Figs. 34–1 *E* and 34–45). Merely enlarged nucleoli should be viewed with caution if their contour is rounded and lacks sharp angularity as this may indicate only increased activity. Thus, nucleolar gigantism and multiplicity are of weak diagnostic significance (34–37 *E*), and are liable to be misleading. They all too frequently are found in biologic variants in nonmalignant cells undergoing secretion, regeneration, etc. (Figs. 34–16, 34–17, and 34–22).

Multinucleation is a helpful criterion of increased activity, not of malignancy. It is frequently present in nonmalignant cell variants but these are usually uniform in shape, chromatin pattern, nucleolar pattern, and size (Figs. 34–1 *B*, *34*–17, and 34–22). Malignant nuclei can also appear uniform, and the resulting multiple nuclei may not have sufficient variation to serve as a helpful criterion. When size variation is present, it can be of some value (Fig. 34–39 *A*), but the greatest help is when the daughter nuclei within the same cell differ markedly in chromatin pattern and in numbers of nucleoli per nucleus. Multinucleation offers a good opportunity to observe the nuclear criteria mentioned previously and to observe how irregularly and differently each criterion is portrayed from one daughter nucleus to the next (Fig. 34–38).

Mitotic activity, a valuable criterion of malignancy in tissue *section*, loses most of its significance in *exfoliated* material and is frequently misleading. This is mainly because epithelial cells exfoliating into the secretion of the genital tract are in a foreign medium, which is not conducive to their growth and proliferation. Thus, in contrast to body cavity fluids, only a few mitoses are observed in material naturally exfoliated into gynecologic tract secretions, even in wildly growing tumors; but mitoses may be present if the material has just been removed by scraping or aspiration. On the other hand, histiocytes tend to proliferate in such nonphysiologic material, as if in response to a need for in-

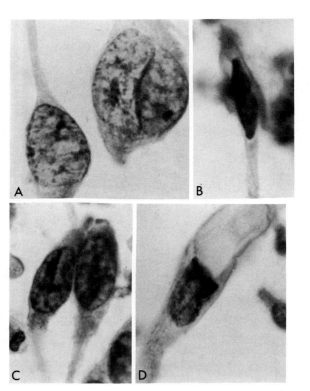

Figure 34–39. Malignant tadpole cells shed from squamous cell carcinoma. ×1200. *A*, Large oval or round nuclei at one end of cell with thin cytoplasmic tails streaming upward. The cell on the right has a tendency to send a second tail downward. Nuclei appear to be malignant and are characteristic of invasive carcinoma with irregular, pointed, sharp chromatin clumping. Small areas of abnormally cleared parachromatin can be noted in the nucleus near midfield. Multinucleation is present but without chromatin pattern variation, which is so helpful when it exists. Extreme cytoplasmic thinning with hugging of the nuclei is significant. *B*, Thin cell with two sharp, pointed nuclei showing the smudging, peripheral clumping, and other degenerative changes of karyopyknosis so characteristic of squamous cell maturation. *C*, Sharp cytoplasmic border with well preserved malignant nuclear criteria consisting of chromatin clumping with abnormally cleared areas of parachromatin. The nuclear membranes have small irregularities of shape, and the chromatinic rims have moderate differences in thickness within each nucleus. *D*, The nuclear border is wrinkled with degenerative smudging of beginning karyopyknosis so common in tadpole and spindle cells. Note the linear markings of the fibrillary apparatus along the tails in *B*, *C*, and *D*.

creased numbers of phagocytes to cope with inflammation and necrotic debris. Abnormal mitoses are more significant indicators of malignancy. Thus, in gynecologic material, normal mitoses should first make one suspicious of histiocytes (Fig. 34–21 *B*).

THE CYTOPLASM

The *amount* of cytoplasm around a malignant nucleus tends to be less than that expected around a normal nucleus of the same size; thus, the nucleo-cytoplasmic ratio (N/C) is greater than for normal cells (Figs. 34–1 *E* and 34–37). This high N/C ratio is a valuable criterion when the nucleus is large, but it is virtually of no value in small cells the size of a lymphocyte.

The cytoplasm must be *present* and intact for other criteria to be of diagnostic importance. A truly bare nucleus represents a portion of a degenerated cell. Degenerative changes in nonmalignant cells dangerously mimic malignant criteria and account for many reported false positives. At times oil immersion may be necessary to resolve the presence or absence of a thin shell of cytoplasm.

A high nucleo-cytoplasmic ratio results from either scanty cytoplasm, nuclear gigantism, or both. Many times the amount of cytoplasm is normal or more than normal, but because of the huge nuclear size the nucleo-cytoplasmic ratio is increased. Because increased nucleo-cytoplasmic ratio is a normal finding in the small blood elements (e.g., leukocytes), it has its greatest value as a malignant criterion in moderate and large sized cells.

RELATIONSHIP OF NUCLEUS TO CYTOPLASM

A peculiar *attenuation* or a *hugging* of the cytoplasm around the nucleus is at times striking in malignant cells (Figs. 34–37 *F*, 34–39 *A*, and 34–41). The attenuation can be extreme, with only scanty cytoplasm between nuclear membrane and cytoplasmic membrane. Artifactual production of this relationship by cellular degeneration or by distortion in the process of smearing must be carefully ruled out. Furthermore, the examiner must be sure he or she is not dealing with a distorted normal columnar cell (Fig. 34–1 *B* and 34–16) in which the attenuation of the cytoplasm about the nucleus is usually of only moderate severity. In addition to the scantiness of cytoplasm, there is at times a peculiar relationship between the two membranes so that they may remain a uniform, constant distance apart for a long way. At times the nucleus is "pushed" uniformly close to the cytoplasmic rim for a long distance and for no apparent reason, abundant cytoplasm being present in the rest of the cell. The cytoplasm maintains its cell membrane a uniform distance from the nuclear membrane over an appreciable distance of the nucleus, then spreads out and displays its ample volume.

TISSUE FRAGMENTS: RELATIONSHIPS OF ONE CELL TO ANOTHER

The *irregularity* and *variability* of the previously discussed criteria of malignancy can be more accurately evaluated and closely compared from sibling cell to sibling cell, within a fragment of tissue. Of significance is the great variability in chromatin pattern, nucleolar number and pattern, multinucleation, and nuclear size and shape. *Nuclear molding* by adjacent nuclei is evidence that the cells grew together as tissue (Fig. 34–43); however, nuclear molding by only soft cytoplasm of an adjacent cell without secretion, favors malignancy. Molding of the cytoplasm bears no significance with regard to malignancy. Cellular *crowding* indicates scanty cytoplasm or high N/C ratio. and accentuates its variations in amounts from cell to cell.

The formation of *tissue structures* foreign to the area of examination is significant and at times is a valuable criterion. Thus, the finding of acini and polyps in abdominal fluid obtained at paracentesis is distinctly abnormal.

By evaluating these malignant criteria, one first determines the presence or absence of *cancer*—mainly by *nuclear* characteristics. Then, if cancer is present, one proceeds to determine the type of neoplasm into which it is differentiating by evaluating *functional differentiating* characteristics—mainly by *cytoplasmic* features.

CANCER DIFFERENTIATION— CELLULAR CHARACTERISTICS OF FUNCTIONAL DIFFERENTIATION

Functional differentiation characteristics are *not* malignant criteria. They are cellular characteristics indicating differentiation into a particular cell type (type-specific modulation). Differentiation of any neoplastic cell is an attempt at differentiation toward the normal cell of that cell type. Roughly, the more differentiation there is in tissue, the more differentiating characteristics there are in exfoliated cells.

Although most criteria of malignancy are in the nucleus, most differentiating characteristics are in the *cytoplasm*. First, the cell must be identified as malignant by the foregoing patterns of malignant criteria, mainly nuclear. Second, the differentiation characteristics are evaluated to determine or to detect cells differentiating toward a certain *type* of malignancy (e.g., establish a malignant cell, determine squamous differentiation, thus infer squamous cell carcinoma). The reverse should never be done (e.g., it is wrong and very dangerous to use the fact that cells are tadpole-shaped to diagnose malignancy—many benign lesions shed tadpole cells).

In cells, as well as in intact tissue, differentiation frequently is not complete; also maturation may not be advanced. Thus, cellular differentiation characteristics may be only suggestive and not diagnostic of a specific cell type produced, and unless one is cautious may even give false information. When the evidence of differentiation is conclusive, it can be diagnostic; when not conclusive, differentiation should not be attempted.

SQUAMOUS CELL CARCINOMA

Invasive Squamous Cell Carcinoma

The Individual Cell. Squamous cell carcinoma tends to shed cells *singly*. Most of their characteristics of differentiation are in the cytoplasm.

The Nucleus. During its process of maturation from an intermediate cell to a superficial cell, the normal squamous cell nucleus undergoes karyopyknosis (Fig. 34–2). This same change occurs in maturing squamous cell carcinoma (Fig. 34–39 *B,C*). By its very nature this characteristic ruins nuclear criteria of malignancy as it progresses in severity (Fig. 34–40). At times nuclear pyknosis in multinucleated squamous carcinoma cells does not progress at the same rate in the different nuclei of the same cell (Fig. 34–38). With karyopyknosis, therefore, criteria are obscured, frequently reducing diagnostic significance. Extremely large nuclear size and sharp nuclear membrane configuration may still remain as criteria (Fig. 34–37 *C*), even after karyopyknosis has ruined all others. This nuclear degeneration of senescence cannot be distinguished from other forms of degeneration (Figs. 34–31 *C, D*).

The Cytoplasm: Keratinizing Tendencies.

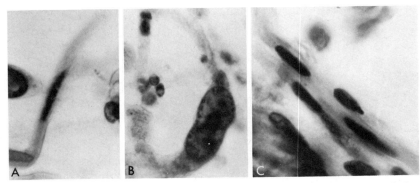

Figure 35–40. Malignant spindle cells shed from squamous cell carcinoma. ×1200. *A,* The extremely thin, pointed nucleus lies midway in an extremely thin, pointed cytoplasm. Little chromatin pattern remains in this pyknotic nucleus. Note that where it is in focus, the cytoplasmic border is sharp and distinct. *B,* The chromatin pattern is retained in this malignant spindle cell nucleus with irregular chromatin clumping and abnormal clearing. *C,* Palisading of malignant spindle cells is frequent. Some of these nuclei retain remnants of chromatin patterns so essential to diagnosis of malignancy, whereas others are completely karyopyknotic and are *not* diagnostic of cancer. Tadpole cells (Fig. 34–39) are frequently associated with spindles.

The cytoplasmic *border* of a normal squamous cell is sharp and crisp (Fig. 34–2 *B,C*). This differentiating characteristic is associated with the process of cytoplasmic keratinization and is present in maturing squamous carcinoma cells as a sharp, distinct, prominent cellular border (Figs. 34–1 *D*, 34–39 *B*, *D*, 34–40, and 34–41). The whole cytoplasm changes in *color* toward acidophilia, eventually becoming a vivid "Halloween" orange and appearing glassy (*hyaline*), both in normalcy (Fig. 34–1 *A*) and in malignancy (Fig. 34–1 *D*). Artifactual acidophilia occurs in degeneration and in many artifactual situations, including drying before fixation, use of improper fixatives (methyl alcohol, isopropyl alcohol, etc.) and pH change (middle of cell clumps). A hyaline cytoplasm that is brilliantly orange or red, however, is highly suggestive of keratinization in the absence of artifactual explanations (Fig. 34–1 *D*).

Under certain states of stress, such as infection and trauma, the cytoplasm of nonmalignant cells atypically keratinizes. The outer portion of the cytoplasm appears to gel in this process of keratinization. A prominent optical interface occurs between the gelled *ectoplasm* (outer hyalinized shell) and the *endoplasm* (inner amorphous cytoplasm) resulting in a sharp ecto-endoplasmic border (Fig. 34–42). This same keratinizing process occurs in malignant cells of squamous cell carcinoma (Figs. 34–1 *D*, 34–41, and 34–43). When the ecto-endoplasmic border is carried into the cytoplasmic tail of elongated squamous cells, either benign (Fig. 34–42) or malignant (Figs. 34–39 *D* and 34–41), a spiral of Herxheimer, or fibrillary apparatus, is formed. Frequently this extends into a bulbous end of the tail and expands into a large endoplasm "waiting for a nucleus," with a thin rim of ectoplasm around it (Fig. 34–41). The nucleus is always within the amorphous endoplasm in which, in tissue culture, it is seen to turn and maneuver actively during its metabolic activities.

Hyalinization of the ectoplasm produces a peculiar glassy appearance in that portion of the cytoplasm—like the colored glass of a church window (Fig. 34–1 *D*). This hyaline quality is not related to the color because the cytoplasm can take any hue, but refers only to its highly refractile appearance.

Refractile *rings* appear in this hyaline outer cytoplasm (Figs. 34–1 *D*, 34–38, and 34–41). These are best appreciated by focus-

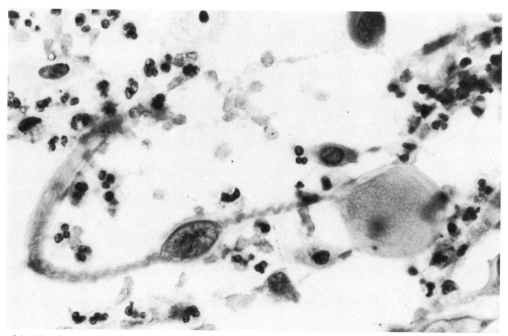

Figure 34–41. Fast smear of cervical squamous cell carcinoma in 55 year old woman, 12 years postmenopausal. Note the clear hyaline ectoplasm enclosing the amorphous endoplasm extending throughout most of the cell. The ecto-endoplasmic border is carried into both cytoplasmic tails as Herxheimer spirals. One tail ends in a large bulbous formation with a copious endoplasm. There is ringing in the ectoplasm. ×160.

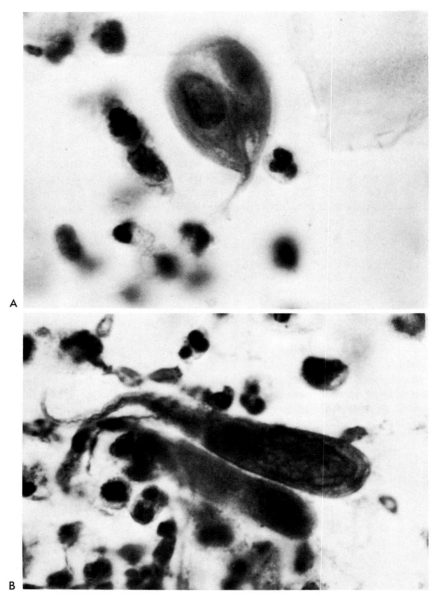

Figure 34–42. Tadpole and Herxheimer spiral formation. Three *benign* tadpole cells resulting from distortion of normal parabasal cells in severe inflammation. Note that the nuclei are not at the head end as in malignant tadpole cells (Fig. 34–39) but are near the cytocentrum. The nucleus in the lower cell is out of focal plane. The nuclear pattern of the cell in *A* is large and finely granular with dyskaryotic characteristics. In all cells there is a sharp cytoplasmic border, a well-formed ectoplasm with hyaline ringing, a sharp ecto-endoplasmic border, and an amorphous endoplasm in which the nuclei lie. The ecto-endoplasmic borders are thrown into numerous linear folds, which extend down the ctyoplasmic tail as a Herxheimer spiral. The same *cytoplasmic* characteristics are found in malignant tadpole cells (Figs. 34–39 and 34–41), but can be identified as malignant, by *nuclear* criteria, whereas these are obviously benign. ×1200.

ing the fine adjustment of the microscope up and down through the cell. They appear to represent interfaces of progressive shells, or rims, laid down by successive gelations during keratinization.

Irregular *keratinizing clumps* at times appear in the cytoplasm of squamous carci-noma cells. They can be strikingly irregular and mammoth. Active *thinning* of the cytoplasm, as the normal squamous cell matures from a parabasal to an intermediate cell, produces a uniformly wafer-thin cell (Fig. 34–2 *B,C*). Likewise, the cytoplasm of malignant squamous cells thins either *uniformly* as a

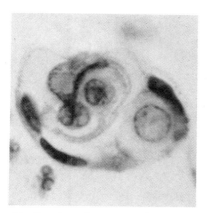

Figure 34–43. A malignant "pearl" shed from squamous cell carcinoma. Three karyopyknotic malignant cells, with extremely thinned squamous cytoplasm, form the floor of this pearl. Their nuclei are extremely thinned and are markedly molded in the one upper right cell and are encircling in the two lower left cells. The three cells in the upper left of center could be interpreted as demonstrating "cannibalism," but this is obviously not true phagocytosis as two cells are lying on the largest cell in a "cup and saucer" arrangement, with the cells in a truly stratified fashion. The small round cell on the right has hyaline cytoplasm with concentric rings in the ectoplasm and a sharp cytoplasmic border. The larger nuclei of this cellular group are *primarily* malignant by their criteria and this is *secondarily* a pearl by its stratified and concentric configurations. Benign pearls can take this same overall intercellular configuration, but in that case their nuclear characteristics indicate benignancy. ×665.

squamous plate, at times arranged in layers much as in mature stratified squamous epithelium (malignant pearl, Fig. 34–43), or in an elongated *bizarre* tail-like manner. The latter occurs frequently, but is best developed in the tadpole and spindle cells (Figs. 34–39, 34–40, and 34–41).

Tissue Fragments. Normal squamous epithelium *stratifies,* so that thin squames lie on top of each other. When this occurs in epithelial crevices and the contents of this plug are exfoliated, it appears as a benign pearl. This same tendency to exfoliate rounded stratified structures of multiple squames as pearly bodies is carried over into the malignant cell trying to differentiate toward squamous cell carcinoma. These *malignant pearls* (Fig. 34–43) are composed of cancer cells by malignant criteria patterns, primarily; then recognized as squamous cells in a pearl formation, secondarily.

When only two cells are involved in this stratified structure, they frequently appear as one cell within another. The first impulse is to call it "cannibalism" (Figs. 34–1 *D* and 34–43), but by fine focusing of the micro-

scope up and down, one observes the layering and stratification of the upper cell lying within a pit on the lower cell's upper surface —as a baseball lies in a catcher's mitt, or like a cup lying on a saucer. At times an inner cell is simply ringed by an outer cell, giving an onionskin appearance.

There are other forms of "cannibalism" which involve *any* malignant cell and are thus not to be confused with these differentiation characteristics found in squamous cell carcinoma. In undifferentiated or anaplastic cancer, one malignant cell can phagocytose another; but this does *not* represent one cell lying on top of another one in the squamous cell differentiation features of *thinning* and *stratification* found in a *pearl.* Likewise, when an "active" histiocyte engulfs a malignant cell, their close association makes it easy to erroneously tag the histiocyte as a malignant cell. At times *columnar* cells tightly curve around each other to form a pseudopearl, which can be differentiated from a true pearl of *squamous* epithelium by careful microscopic discernment of cellular orientation.

The Cell as a Whole. Certain of these differentiation characteristics are found together frequently enough to be recognized as a cellular pattern. These are conveniently loosely grouped as "cell types" of squamous cell carcinoma differentiation.

The Malignant Tadpole Cell. This unilaterally elongated cell has its nucleus at the "head end," with a cytoplasmic tail streaming out (Fig. 34–39 *A,C*). This is distinctly different from a benign columnar cell which, although it may at times be extremely elongated and appear as a tadpole, has its normal appearing nucleus near the tail (Fig. 34–1 *B*). Also not to be confused with the *malignant* tadpole cell are the many bizarre shapes which squamous cells can take under certain degenerative conditions (i.e., inflammation, irradiation) in which the nucleus appears benign and is not placed in the characteristic "head end" (Fig. 34–42).

The key, therefore, is the *nucleus,* which must have sufficient criteria to be diagnostic of cancer before the diagnosis of squamous cell carcinoma can be made. It tends to be round and frequently lies within an amorphous endoplasm surrounded by a hyalinized ectoplasm. The ectoplasm frequently extends down the tail, with the remaining thin endoplasmic tail appearing as a fiber (Fig. 34–39) and at times ending in a bulbous knob (Fig. 34–41). The amount of cytoplasm is usually abundant in these cells, giving a normal nucleo-cytoplasmic ratio.

The Malignant Spindle Cell. Papanicolaou called this cell type a "fiber" cell, but, because of its confusion with the fibrocyte, it is better to use the term spindle cell. The *nucleus* has malignant criteria (Fig. 34–40 B) which are frequently partially or completely obliterated by karyopyknosis (Fig. 34–40 A, C). Usually the nucleus is elongated and at times extremely thinned and pointed at both ends (Fig. 34–40 A) matching cytoplasmic configuration.

The *cytoplasmic* rim is usually thinned and extremely molded as it extends past the nucleus (Figs. 34–37 F and 34–40 B). At times it has ecto-endoplasmic differentiation (Fig. 34–41). The total amount of cytoplasm is abundant, yielding a fairly normal nucleo-cytoplasmic ratio.

Benign spindle cells have nuclei falling within normal limits, which are usually rounded and do not have cytoplasmic thinning around them. They frequently occur from normal intermediate or superficial cells, folded upon themselves and lying on their side. At other times, benign "active" spindle cells may occur in degenerative or irritative situations.

IN SITU SQUAMOUS CELL CARCINOMA

Nuclei of cells shed from in situ carcinoma have many features of nuclei of the severely dyskaryotic cell (Fig. 34–32). They tend to be more hyperchromatic, however (Fig. 34–44), with coarser chromatin granules, clearer parachromatin, and more undulated and prominent chromatinic rims. They are disarmingly round and symmetric (i.e., as if benign), with a uniform distribution of the chromatin granules throughout the parachromatin, uniformly thick chromatinic rims, and a central location in the cytoplasm. Nucleoli are virtually absent or inconspicuous.

The *cytoplasm* also holds a morphologic key to discriminating "classical" or "conservative" in situ carcinoma from severe dysplasias. In the conservatively diagnosed in situ carcinoma, without maturation of the surface cells, the cytoplasm of the diagnostic exfoliated cell is extremely scanty (Fig. 34–44). It appears as a thin rim, giving the cell an extremely high nucleo-cytoplasmic ratio. To

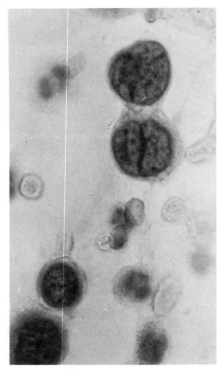

Figure 34–44. Characteristic cell type shed from classical in situ carcinoma. The cells are single, round, and symmetrical with an extremely high nucleo-cytoplasmic ratio. The chromatin pattern is moderately coarsely granular but is uniformly distributed. The chromatinic rims are uniform in thickness, but are wavy or undulated. These nuclei have the characteristics of those found in severe dyskaryosis (compare with Fig. 34–32), but are more extreme. The cytoplasm shows no maturation and is extremely scanty in a markedly thin and attentuated rim. These cells differ from the immature dyskaryotic cell in the extremely scanty amount of cytoplasm present, the increased hyperchromasia, and the more violent undulations of the nuclear membrane (compare with Figs. 34–33 to 35–36).

be diagnostic, there should be no evidence of degeneration or possible artifactual loss of cytoplasm and one must make certain one is not dealing with an active immature subcolumnar or reserve cell of endocervical epithelium.

There is virtually no evidence of maturation or functional differentiation in the scanty cytoplasm of in situ carcinoma (Fig. 34–44) except, at times, a sharply distinct cellular border. It may infrequently contain suggestive concentric rings, or even an ecto-endoplasmic border; however, if these are prominent, or if there is hyalinization or tendencies to elongate and form a cytoplasmic tail (Fig. 34–3 A), microinvasion or frank invasion is to be suspected. Also, invasion is to be expected if nucleoli are present and prominent, if large irregular and sharply angular chromatin masses appear (Fig. 34–37), and if large areas of parachromatin become abnormally cleared, with disruption of the regular chromatin pattern, which is so characteristic of in situ carcinoma (Fig. 34–44).

The *total cell* from in situ carcinoma is round and symmetric. It tends to be found singly or, at times, lying in very loose tissue fragments with poor intercellular borders in a so-called syncytial or, more properly, pseudosyncytial arrangement.

THE SPECTRUM: INVASIVE SQUAMOUS CELL CARCINOMA, MICROINVASIVE CARCINOMA, IN SITU CARCINOMA, AND SHADES OF GRAY LESIONS

Developing cancer and other shades of gray lesions (pp. 736–743) shed cells with distinctive morphologic features (Figs. 34–33, 34–34, 34–35, and 34–36). *In situ* carcinoma sheds cells with additional morphologic alterations, which have come to be recognized as characteristic of the altered biologic behavior of this preinvasive neoplasm. As in situ carcinoma further alters its biologic behavior and begins to invade its host, *microinvasion* is reflected in its exfoliated cells by the appearance of additional key structural changes (e.g., appearance of nucleoli, chromatin clumping, bizarre parachromatin clearing, nuclear irregularity and asymmetry, cellular elongation, atypical functional differentiation). As invasion advances, structural changes continue to evolve in the individual cell, both in tissue and after exfoliation, until it displays the full-blown picture of classical *invasive* squamous cell carcinoma. The morphology of these cells bespeaks the macabre biologic behavior of the parent neoplasm from which they exfoliate.

One *cannot rule out* invasion by exfoliated cells without recourse to *adequate* tissue examination; however, at times adequate cytology *can* rule it *in* when initial tissue studies miss it. One should determine the most severe lesion demonstrated in the cellular material, and then carefully adjudge whether or not that lesion is represented in the biopsy. Inadequate tissue can miss the most severe part of a lesion; thus, a small invasive lesion in the endocervical canal

will be missed in tissue taken only from a neighboring coexisting in situ lesion. Most cervical lesions of this spectrum are multiphasic. Tissue specimens usually sample the areas of highest clinical suspicion, missing inconspicuous ones of more grave biologic potential. Adequate cellular examinations cover the total surface in question.

When in situ carcinoma is present, many dyskaryotic cells (Fig. 34–32) are usually shed from the lesion along with the more characteristic in situ cells (Fig. 34–44). These dyskaryotic cells are shed from both the various shades of gray lesions (e.g., atypical metaplasia, reserve cell hyperplasia, basal cell hyperactivity, spinal cell hyperactivity, dysplasia) which are adjacent to the carcinoma, and from the multiplicity of cell types present in the in situ lesion itself.

In summary, therefore, dyskaryotic cells (Fig. 34–32) are shed from the shades of gray lesions, from in situ carcinoma, and from invasive cancer. In situ cells (Fig. 34–44) are shed from in situ carcinoma and invasive squamous cell carcinoma. Squamous carcinoma cells with bizarre chromatin configurations and nucleoli (Fig. 34–37), extreme asymmetry (Fig. 34–39), aberrant keratinization (Fig. 34–3 *D*), and abnormal thinning (Fig. 34–41) and stratification (Fig. 34–43) are shed from invasive squamous cell carcinoma.

ADENOCARCINOMA

The Individual Cell

Adenocarcinoma tends to shed cells in *tissue fragments* especially the more undifferentiated lesions. The well differentiated or "early" lesions shed a higher percentage of single cells. The cells are basically of the large pleomorphic, undifferentiated type with varying degrees of differentiating characteristics toward glandular and secretory activities.

The Nucleus. Nuclei of adenocarcinoma tend to be vesicular (Fig. 34–45). Karyopyknosis occurs rarely and is a degenerative phenomenon, rather than a feature of functional differentiation as with squamous cell carcinoma. Criteria of malignancy are usually excellent, with some of the sharpest chromatin clumping, jagged nucleoli, and abnormally cleared areas. Occasionally, however, adenocarcinoma nuclei are com-

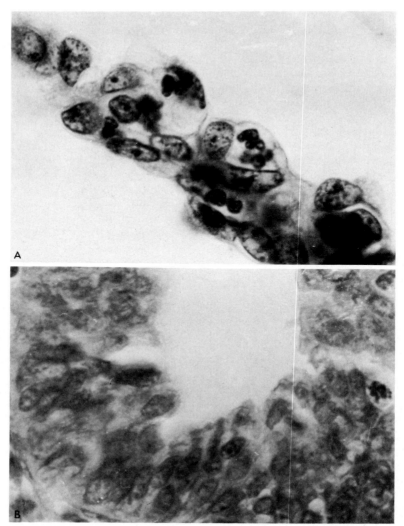

Figure 34–45. Adenocarcinoma of the endometrium. Eighty year old patient with a distinctly abnormal cytohormonal pattern (M.I.: 0/77/23). ×1200. *A,* Cells present in a Fast smear. Note extremely good malignant criteria in the nuclei. A large irregular, triangular clump of chromatin (right lower center) lies within an abnormally large cleared area with irregular thickening of the chromatinic rim. The secretory vacuoles are hyperdistended with thin cytoplasmic walls and markedly thinned semilunar nuclei (upper center). Many neutrophils have invaded and are phagocytosing the cytoplasmic contents. The neutrophils are extremely healthy and well preserved in contrast to degenerated ones in a macrophage. *B,* Tissue obtained at curettage. This malignant gland is lined by cells having many malignant criteria and mitoses.

pletely bland with a powdery gray "ground-glass" chromatin.

The Cytoplasm. Cellular borders are usually indistinct and hazy (Fig. 34–45). *Secretory vacuoles,* frequently present within the cytoplasm, tend to be single in contradistinction to the multiple vacuolation of degeneration or phagocytosis. At times the vacuoles are distended with "pouching out" and loss of the cytoplasm at the nucleo-vacuolar cytoplasmic angle (Figs. 34–45 and 34–46). The cytoplasm is frequently atten-

tuated over the vacuole and is also extremely thinned around the nucleus. Frequently there is molding of the nucleus from the secretory vacuole. In secretion of both normal and cancer cells, it is common to find many neutrophils packed with cytoplasm or secretory vacuoles. The neutrophils have invaded the larger epithelial cell and are phagocytosing its secretory contents; they are not being phagocytosed by the larger cell. Because the neutrophils are the phagocytes, they are well preserved and appear healthy (Fig. 34–45A)

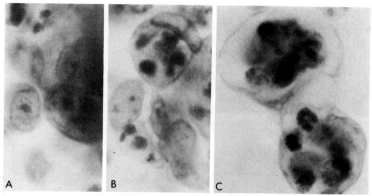

Figure 34–46. Adenocarcinoma cells. ×1435. *A,* The chromatin clumping is angular with nuclear clearing. The cytoplasm is scant and the borders are indistinct. These are undifferentiated type cells. *B,* The "ground-glass" nuclei are large and bland (left and lower) with only occasional chromatin clumping. Cytoplasm is extremely thinned about the nucleus of the upper cell, which has one large hypersecretory type vacuole filled with well preserved neutrophils, which are phagocytosing, *not* being phagocytosed. Note the loss of cytoplasm at the nucleo-vacuolar cytoplasmic angle on the right and the extreme attenuation around the vacuole and nucleus. *C,* Hypersecretory vacuoles filled with well preserved phagocytosing neutrophils. The extremely pale nucleus on the right is molded by the vacuole.

rather than degenerated as they would if they were being phagotosed and digested by the larger cell (Fig. 34–22 *A*).

Cell Groups

Frequently malignant *acini, tubules, villi,* and *polyps* are shed (Fig. 34–47). As with their benign counterparts, they are recognized by focusing up and down through the structure. Thus, the lining malignant cells resting upon the slide surface are identified as a sheet lying *en face;* they are then followed up from the sides of the sheet covering the outer surface of a polyp, or the inner surface of an acinus, with a continuous epithelial luminal border on the lining cells (Fig. 34–47). Moving up to the highest plane of focus, they are then seen to fall back together into the form of a covering sheet (*en face*). Crowding, irregular nuclear and cytoplasmic distribution, and nuclear criteria of malignancy differentiate the malignant from the benign counterpart.

ADENOCARCINOMA TYPES SUGGESTING SITES

Usually adenocarcinoma has no specific cytologic features identifying the site from which it arises. At times, however, there are some characteristics which typify the site of origin, and suggest it as the primary locus.

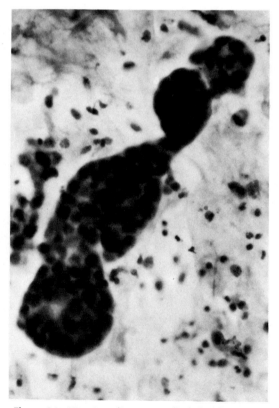

Figure 34–47. A malignant papillary frond shed from papillary cystadenocarcinoma of the ovary. Note the regular epithelial lumen border about the outside of this tissue fragment. The lower portion has the inferior plane of cells in focus (*en face*) whereas the central portion of the frond has the middle plane in focus demonstrating the luminal border on the outer side of the single cells lining the lumen. This 60 year old woman had a slightly high estrogenic pattern for her age (M.I. $\overrightarrow{12/74/14}$). ×400.

Endocervical Adenocarcinoma. The cytoplasm of adenocarcinoma rising from the cervix tends to be abundant and textured (Fig. 34–52), frequently with a blue-lavender tint. At times this is in striking contrast to the scanty clear cytoplasm of endometrial adenocarcinoma cells (Figs. 34–45 and 34–46). The nuclei of endocervical adenocarcinoma cells are frequently larger and more vesicular than the clumped, condensed, and irregular nuclei of those of endometrial origin. The terminal bars holding well-differentiated endocervical adenocarcinoma cells together at the lumen remain intact as the more basal areas of the cells separate. This forms peculiar rosette formations with prominent epithelial luminal borders.

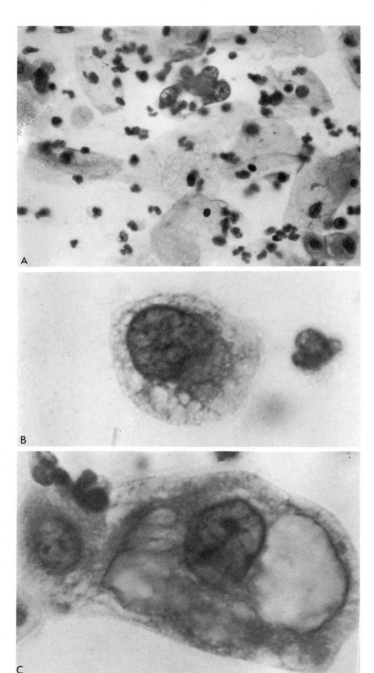

Figure 34–48. Early endometrial adenocarcinoma detected cytologically on a Fast smear from a 58 year old female. *A,* The Maturation Index ($\overrightarrow{0/62/38}$) is shifted moderately to the right for the age and the slight inflammation. A small tissue fragment is present in the upper center, with large hyperdistended single secretory-type vacuoles containing neutrophils. In addition to this individual cell secretion, the tissue fragment is forming a bizarre acinus, the lumen of which contains dark and inspissated secretions. ×480. *B,* Abundant cytoplasm which contains numerous vacuoles of secretion and has a textured, foamy appearance. The nucleus lying near the center has many malignant criteria with chromatin clumping and nuclear membrane irregularities at both the cytocentrum and, significantly, away from it (near the 10 o'clock position in the nucleus). Although this resembles an active histiocyte, it is a tumor cell shed from the cancer. ×1920. *C,* A single adenocarcinoma cell resembling a histiocyte. The abundant cytoplasm is foamy and textured without phagocytic debris. The cytoplasmic border is well defined. There is a lighter stained rim on the outer portion of the cytoplasm. Small significant nuclear irregularities are present in many sites about the nucleus (5, 9, 12 o'clock positions), not only near the cytocentrum, as with histiocytes (see Fig. 34–21A). ×1920.

"Early" Endometrial Adenocarcinoma.
Cells shed from an extremely small, well-differentiated or early carcinoma of the endometrium at times appear distinctly different from those of the full-blown advanced lesions. They may occur singly with abundant and symmetric or slightly eccentric cytoplasm, closely resembling histiocytes (Fig. 34–48 *B,C*). At times the outer portion of the cytoplasm appears as a cleared rim (Fig. 34–48 *C*), not suggesting keratinization but appearing as a biphasic cytoplasm. The cells closely resemble active histiocytes or other benign cells, but if they have sufficiently abundant criteria within their nuclei they may be diagnostically unequivocal cancer cells.

Of extreme significance, in the early lesions as well as in the late lesions, may be a borderline abnormal cytohormonal pattern with a Maturation Index shifted slightly to the right for the patient's age and history (Fig. 34–48 *A*). In 15 per cent of patients with endometrial adenocarcinoma, this occurrence of abnormal numbers of superficial cells presents as the *only* abnormality leading to a cytologic detection.

Ovarian Adenocarcinoma. Nucleoli are frequently very prominent, mainly in size but also in number. Howdon points out the occurrence of a prominent, clear perinucleolar halo about a cherry-red nucleolus in ovarian adenocarcinoma, which is seen significantly more frequently than in other primary sites. The secretory vacuoles in the cytoplasm tend to be extremely large, thin-walled, and hyperdistended. They seek the surface of the tissue fragments, where they characteristically project outward, resembling pox vesicles or bubble gum. They are frequently shed in papillary frond formations (Fig. 34–47) and at times psammoma bodies are present within exfoliated tissue fragments (Fig. 34–49).

ADENOACANTHOMA, MUCO-EPIDERMOID CARCINOMA, AND OTHER CARCINOMAS OF MIXED PATTERNS

At times both squamous cell carcinoma and adenocarcinoma characteristics are found in exfoliated cells. One must be very cautious in interpreting these cells, to be sure that *both* cell types have sufficient criteria showing them to be unequivocally shed from cancer, before diagnosing a biphasic carcinoma.

Frequently shades of gray squamous lesions are present in the cervices of patients having adenocarcinoma. Thus, severely dyskaryotic cells with degrees of cytoplasmic squamous maturation can be enthusiastically mistaken for squamous carcinoma elements in a patient with known adenocarcinoma. Conversely, squamous carcinoma cells are able to degenerate and form cytoplasmic vacuoles. Although these are usually multiple and are not hyperdistended, as with typical secretory vacuoles, they can be improperly categorized as adenocarcinoma. Also, mature columnar dyskaryotic cells from reparative endocervical epithelium shedding along with a coexisting cervical squamous carcinoma may lead to a false impression of an adenocarcinoma element. It is therefore essential that *each* cell by which one is attempting to determine differentiation characteristics is diagnosed as a cancer cell on the basis of its own characteristics. When this condition is completely satisfied, such biphasic tumors can occasionally be identified cytologically.

SMALL-CELL ANAPLASTIC CARCINOMA

Most of the lesions shedding cells of this type represent poorly differentiated squamous cell carcinoma. Wentz and Reagan refer to this type as "nonkeratinizing small-cell carcinoma" and have found that the prognosis is the gravest of their three types of squamous cell carcinomas of the cervix. This is frequently the cell type that recurs following irradiation therapy (Fig. 34–54).

At times small-cell undifferentiated cancer cells are shed from a poorly differentiated adenocarcinoma of the endometrium. They tend to have an eccentric nucleus in a bit more cytoplasm than those from poorly differentiated squamous cell carcinoma, and the nucleus is frequently indented near the cytocentrum.

The Individual Cell

The cells from small-cell undifferentiated squamous cell carcinoma of the cervix are uniformly small. They are slightly larger than small histiocytes and have no differen-

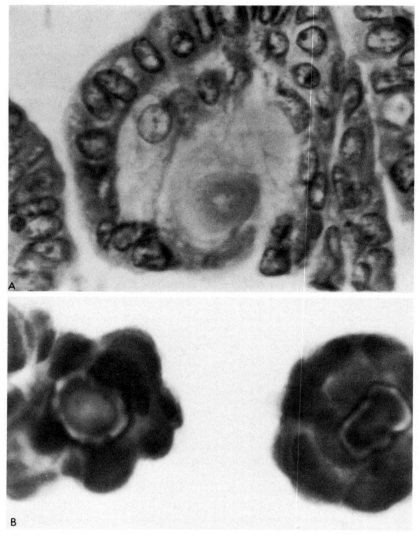

Figure 34–49. Psammoma bodies in adenocarcinoma of the ovary. ×1200. *A,* A papillary frond of a serous cystadeno-carcinoma of the ovary, containing a psammoma body in lower center. *B,* Peritoneal fluid of the same patient containing a psammoma body within each of two cellular groups. The peritoneal fluid was extremely bloody and, as this was the first paracentesis, the cells had been in this degenerating fluid long enough to lose their fine nuclear detail; however, their general nuclear outline supplies evidence of severe molding.

tiation. Some tumors are composed entirely of this small-cell undifferentiated type. Other tumors show areas of differentiation of varying degrees.

The Nucleus. The nucleus is basically round or oval, but has severe molding from the adjacent cells (Fig. 34–54). Although chromatin clumps may not be outstandingly prominent, they are sharp and pointed in their angularity.

The Cytoplasm. The cytoplasm is very scanty and usually wispy; however, for an unequivocal diagnosis it must be present and represent well-preserved cells. At times oil immersion is necessary to determine the presence of intact cytoplasm, or to identify the truly bare nucleus of a degenerating cell. The nuclei tend to be centrally placed in the scanty cytoplasm, in contrast to an eccentric indented nucleus in small cell adenocarcinoma.

LARGE-CELL UNDIFFERENTIATED CARCINOMA

Some totally undifferentiated tumors are composed entirely of this cell type. Adenocarcinoma and most sarcomas shed mainly this type of cell, but they may also shed varying numbers of cells which are sufficiently differentiated to form a basis for tumor differentiation. Large undifferentiated cells also are shed from squamous cell carcinoma, so that one should search carefully for cytoplasmic evidence of differentiation and, lacking this, one is forced to refer to it as the large-cell undifferentiated type of tumor.

The Individual Cell

These cells are extremely pleomorphic, having some of the largest as well as some of the smallest cells encountered in tumors. This is in sharp contrast to the monotonous pattern of small-cell undifferentiated cancer.

The Nucleus. The nucleus is usually vesicular and very irregular (Fig. 34–37 A,D,E) and contains some of the best criteria of malignancy. Large, jagged, angular chromatin clumps are prominent, with abnormally cleared areas and frequently irregular nucleoli. Multinucleation commonly occurs.

The Cytoplasm. The cytoplasm usually has indistinct cellular borders and characteristically varies in amount from scanty to abundant. Pleomorphism is frequently great, with one cell from the same tumor having an extremely high nucleo-cytoplasmic ratio whereas the adjacent one has more than the normal amount of cytoplasm.

If there is the least bit of cellular keratinization, distinct borders or nuclear pyknosis, one suspects a large-cell, nonkeratinizing, squamous cell carcinoma of Wentz and Reagan. Extremely indistinct cellular borders and bubbly cytoplasm should make one suspect adenocarcinoma. Indistinct and wispy cellular borders with a tendency to cytoplasmic elongation should make one suspect sarcoma.

SARCOMAS

Sarcoma cells tend to shed in tissue clumps. Basically they are the "large-cell undifferentiated" type, but the differentiating characteristics of their cytoplasm frequently identify their attempt to mature toward an adult mesodermal cell type.

Characteristically, the *cytoplasmic* border of sarcoma cells is extremely indistinct and fuzzy. When the cytoplasm is elongated, one must consider fiber-forming cells (fibrosarcoma), smooth muscle cells (leiomyosar-

coma) (Fig. 34–50 A,B) and striated muscle cells (rhabdomyosarcoma) (Fig. 34–50 C). The finding of longitudinal fibrillae within the elongated cytoplasm strengthens the possibility of their being muscle fibrils, but the possibility that they might represent folding or Herxheimer's spirals (Fig. 34–42) must be ruled out. The latter are found in cells having sharp cytoplasmic borders, whereas the former are found with extremely indistinct cytoplasmic borders (Fig. 34–50). Of distinct diagnostic value, of course, is the finding of periodic thickenings on the cytoplasmic myofibrillae to give the cross-striated appearance of a voluntary muscle cell, which identifies rhabdomyosarcoma (Fig. 34–50 C).

The *nuclei* may give a hint at times as to cell type. Nuclei of fibrosarcoma, neurofibrosarcoma, and leiomyosarcoma tend to be elongated (Fig. 34–40 A,B), whereas nuclei from rhabdomyosarcoma tend to be more oval and irregular (Fig. 34–50 C). Elongated neurofibrosarcoma cell nuclei at times have undulated, accordioned nuclear membranes.

Rounded cells with vacuoles of the *storage* type, having thick vacuole walls rather than the extremely attenuated ones of secretion, should make one consider liposarcoma. The formation of cartilage or bone should be considered, but these features are so easily mimicked by squamous carcinoma cells, by bizarre endocervical cells, or by mature dyskaryotic cells that they offer little assistance in recognizing differentiation. Malignant melanoma and pigmented basal cell carcinomas have cytoplasmic granules of melanin, unless the tumor is amelanotic. The former may also have extremely prominent, large nucleoli.

LESIONS OF THE CERVIX UTERI

Cervical lesions represent adequately many of the concepts basic to consideration of diseases of the whole female reproductive system. Discussed in detail at this point, these concepts are to be carried over forcefully in the succeeding sections dealing with specific areas of the genital tract.

Epithelial Changes

Under a variety of influences, the covering epithelium of the genital tract undergoes ex-

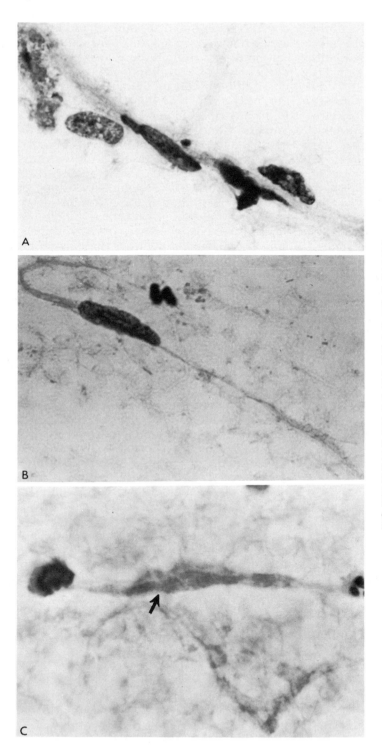

Figure 34–50. Gynecologic cellular specimen with elongated sarcoma cells shed from mixed mesodermal sarcoma. *A, B,* Leiomyosarcoma cells, *C,* Rhabdomyosarcoma cell. *A, B,* The nuclei are elongated and contain malignant criteria. The elongated and extremely attenuated cytoplasm has a wispy and indistinct cytoplasmic border. Running longitudinally within the cytoplasm are thin myofibrils. In *B* the fibrils can be seen fanning out and terminating at either end of the cell. There are no cross striations. *C,* The nucleus is rounded, irregular, and hyperchromatic. The attenuated and elongated cytoplasm contains numerous thin myofibrillae with uniformly periodic constrictions oriented transversely on neighboring fibers to give numerous cross striations throughout the cytoplasm (arrow). Note neutrophil on right for size. (Cellular specimen for *C* courtesy of Drs. John F. Sheehan, Thomas R. Simon and James W. Reagan, 1960 Seminar, College of American Pathologists–Am. Soc. of Clinical Pathologists–American Society of Cytology.) Papanicolaou stain, ×1200.

tensive morphologic alterations. These range from normal epithelium (squamous and columnar euplasia) to that of carcinoma (malignant neoplasia). The questionable lesions lying between—the shades of gray lesions—are classified variously as anaplasia, dysplasia, hyperplasia, metaplasia, atypia, hyperactivity, etc. They are not static entities, but represent stages in constantly changing processes. Their nomenclature is actually immaterial; what is important is that they be recognized, their biologic potential determined, and the condition properly treated.

More than one process is usually operating upon the epithelium at the same time (i.e., injury, inflammation, degeneration, regeneration, endocrine alterations, neoplasia), beclouding both cytologic and histologic pictures. In reaction to many and varying stimuli, however, the epithelium is capable of only a *few* basic patterns of response.

Examinations of *serial* cellular samples yield valuable insight into the nature of the complex lesions resulting from a mixture of these basic patterns, especially if cell studies are correlated with occasional selected surgical biopsies. This allows repeated cellular tissue examination of maximal surface area, relative to the small surface area of a surgical biopsy specimen, with minimal disturbance of the lesion. In this way, the lesion is left intact and viable in the host, rather than altered or even removed completely by biopsy.

Cytologic-Histologic Correlation

Correlation between the exfoliated *cells* and the intact *lesion* approaches absolute when adequate cellular specimens are available for examination. When histologic examination indicates cellular alterations on the surface of the epithelium, the process is reflected in exfoliated cells. Even when the abnormal changes originate in the lower epithelial layers, sufficient cellular alterations persist in enough cells as they mature and move to the surface so that the true lesion usually can be detected and accurately evaluated in exfoliated material. Removal of superficial debris and keratin layers may be necessary in ulcerative, necrotic, or hyperkeratinized lesions in order to produce a specimen containing diagnostic cells. Some lesions exfoliate cells readily, whereas others require surface scraping or aspiration. For this reason the method of procurement is of basic importance and must receive careful, *individual* consideration for each specimen (see pp. 776–778).

When an epithelial lesion is composed only of *mature* elements (squamous or columnar), only mature cells are exfoliated. Normal mature cells are shed from areas of simple eversion, mature epidermidalization, simple metaplasia, atrophic leukoplakia, and

similar processes (Fig. 34–34). As cellular *atypia* increases within the epithelial lesion (anaplasia, dysplasia, hyperplasia, etc.), prompt evidence of this change appears in the exfoliated cell material (e.g., dyskaryosis, dyskeratosis) (Figs. 34–35 and 34–36).

When epithelial lesions become more atypically active or dysplastic, their exfoliated cells tend to increase in nuclear hyperchromasia and chromatin granule size, and to decrease in cytoplasmic maturation. Thus, the ratio of the immature dyskaryotic cell to the moderately mature dyskaryotic cell to the mature (squamous or columnar) dyskaryotic cell indicates the degree of abnormality (see Figs. 34–34 to 34–36). These hallmarks of cellular dysfunction, when properly fitted into the overall pattern of a cellular spread and pertinent clinical data, provide valuable information regarding identification of the lesion and its biologic behavior.

Anatomic Consideration of the Cervix Uteri

The squamocolumnar junction between the noncornified stratified squamous epithelium on the portio vaginalis and the columnar epithelium in the endocervix usually is present *near* the external os. At times the endocervical columnar epithelium extends onto the portio vaginalis (ectropion, etc.) bringing a portion of the squamocolumnar junction into view, while in vaginal adenosis it extends for great and varying distances onto the vaginal fornices and down the vaginal tube. Frequently areas of columnar epithelium within the endocervical canal or within the extent of vaginal adenosis become, through metaplasia, tongues or islands of stratified squamous epithelium, especially in the presence of persistent and chronic cervicitis. In this way the squamocolumnar junction exists high up the endocervical canal, frequently many centimeters above the external os or out onto the vaginal wall.

The *early* lesions of the cervix are associated with this squamocolumnar junction. These are best visualized and sampled under careful colposcopy, as most are confined to the distal 2 cm. of the canal; but there are still some that remain hidden from the view of the examiner.

An *adequate* endocervical scraping must be obtained from as *high* up the endocervical canal as the cervical spatula or swab allows in order to examine this important squamo-columnar junctional area. Over twenty years ago, greatest interest was in the portio vaginalis, which is visible and easy to biopsy. It is now clear, however, that the first 2 cm. up the endocervical canal from the external os is the most critical zone, which must be carefully examined cytologically for lesions. This zone, hidden from the clinician's view but easily accessible to proper cellular examination, harbors the *early* squamous cell carcinomas and their associated shades of gray lesions.

Histologic studies taken in this region to confirm cellular findings, must have *intact* and *adequate* epithelium of the endocervical canal upon which to base a confirming diagnosis and to evaluate the biologic potential of the lesion. Great care must be taken that the overlying epithelium is not removed by the preoperative preparation (Fig. 34–51) or by a preceding dilatation and curettage, that there is no abrasion of the specimens through improper handling during trimming, and that there is no improper orienta-tion of the blocks of tissue with respect to the microtome knife. Such histologic studies are not made to examine the underlying stroma, but are for examination of the *epithelium*, essential to the diagnosis and understanding of early carcinomas and shades of gray lesions.

Chronic Cervicitis

Epithelial changes present in chronic inflammation of the cervix run a wide gamut of reactions. Frequently the lesions are mixed and their exfoliated cells reflect the variety. In simple endocervical *glandular hyperplasia* with proliferation, arborization, or pocketing-off (nabothian cyst formation) of the epithelium and its supporting stroma, mature columnar cells are shed. At times individual cells are proliferative or reactive (Figs. 34–16 and 34–17) and contain hyperdistended secretory vacuoles (Fig. 34–18). The papillary tufts and acinar clefts of this polypoid cervicitis are shed as micropolyps or acini.

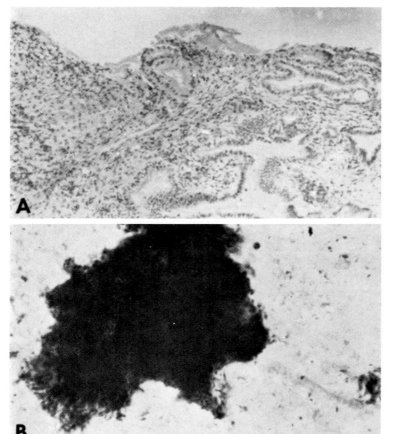

Figure 34–51. *A,* An *unsatisfactory* endocervical biopsy following the introduction of an antiseptic (alcohol) cotton pledget placed gently in the canal to reduce bacterial contamination before the biopsy procedure. The lumen is above. The underlying endocervical glands and stroma are intact; however, the overlying epithelium for which the biopsy was obtained is entirely missing. Impression: biopsy, *unsatisfactory for epithelial examination. B,* Same patient. The cotton pledget was rinsed in saline which was then passed through a Millipore SM cellulose membrane filter. This large sheet is representative of the fragments of epithelial atypia and dysplasia which had been removed. These elements should have been intact on the biopsy for a satisfactory diagnosis of an epithelial lesion. ×30.

As the columnar epithelium repeatedly reacts to injury with repair, both its surface and reserve cells become more hyperplastic and "reactive." *Reserve cell hyperplasia* sheds two types of dyskaryotic cells (Fig. 34–33), one with mature columnar cytoplasm (surface cells) and one with markedly less mature cytoplasm (reserve cell). As the columnar epithelium undergoes *metaplasia*, with the surface cell losing its columnar orientation (perpendicular to the basement membrane) and assuming a squamous orientation (parallel to the basement membrane), mature squamous dyskaryotic cells are shed (Fig. 34–34).

As this metaplastic epithelium becomes more atypical and *dysplastic,* the cells become less mature and more crowded (Fig. 34–35). This is reflected in the cellular spread as a progressive cytoplasmic immaturity of the exfoliated dyskaryotic cell (Fig. 34–32) with the nuclear pattern becoming more coarsely granular and hyperchromatic. As the cytoplasm becomes less abundant and demonstrates less ability to squamify, the index of the dyskaryotic cells shifts to the left. As atypicality becomes more *severe* but the surface cell of the epithelial lesion matures sufficiently to flatten parallel to the basement membrane, the exfoliated cell demonstrates similar restricted ability for its scanty cytoplasm to squamify (Fig. 34–36). These *shades of gray* lesions are common in the cervix, but are also present in the vagina and vulva.

When no maturation is present in the tissue from basement membrane to lumen, and there are complete loss of surface cell stratification, and extreme crowding, classic carcinoma in situ is recognizable. The exfoliated cell becomes extremely dyskaryotic, with scanty and completely nonsquamified immature cytoplasm (Fig. 34–44).

The Gamut of Epithelial Lesions

When in situ carcinoma is present in the cervix uteri, it is usually accompanied by areas of these questionable shades of gray lesions. Likewise, when invasive cancer is present, areas of in situ carcinoma as well as areas of the questionable shades of gray lesions accompany it. Therefore, both cytologic and histologic impressions are based upon recognition of the *most severe* lesion represented. Furthermore, they do *not* preclude the presence, in the patient, of a more serious lesion, which may be absent in the examined specimen.

Because the early lesions of the cervix are small and patchy within the endocervical canal, inadequately sectioned cones and biopsies may miss a lesion. Thus, if repeat cellular spreads continue to demonstrate the presence of a lesion, careful clinical examination (i.e., colposcopy) with well taken tissue and cell studies, and thorough sectioning of existing paraffin blocks will assist in establishing the most serious diagnosis of its site.

In Situ Carcinoma of the Cervix

As the shades of gray spectrum morphologically runs almost imperceptibly into carcinoma in situ, so the biologic behavior of the cells also becomes nearly imperceptibly different. Biologically the cells must differ to be consistent with our basic concepts of autonomous irreversibility. Consistent morphologic separation of these lesions is necessary, correlating their biologic behavior and potential for reversibility or irreversibility and autonomous growth to eventual death of the patient.

One of the most valuable morphologic features correlated with this biologic behavior is the apparent loss of ability of the in situ carcinoma cell to mature in an orderly manner throughout all layers of the epithelium. Thus, in tissues one sees extreme crowding, loss of stratification, and loss of polarity. These phenomena are reflected in the exfoliated material as extremely scanty cytoplasm (high nucleo-cytoplasmic ratio) and loss of maturity (squamification or columnarization) in the individual cells (Figs. 34–32 and 34–44).

Cells from *in situ carcinoma* and the associated *shades of gray* lesions, have varying degrees of the peculiar nucleus described by Papanicolaou as "dyskaryotic" (Figs. 34–32 and 34–44). On the other hand, cells shed from an *invasive squamous carcinoma* take on additional characteristically distinct nuclear features of malignant criteria (Figs. 34–1 D,E and 34–37 to 34–39).

The cellular population of in situ carcinoma tends to be round or oval (Fig. 34–44). Nucleoli are absent or, occasionally, extremely inconspicuous. The scanty cytoplasm is placed symmetrically about the nucleus and is clear, only rarely showing evidence of maturation (keratinization, hyalinization. The cell border is usually distinct, but at times is difficult to discern, with the cells blending together in a false syncytial arrangement.

Departure from this uniform pattern of in situ carcinoma with tendencies toward that of invasive squamous carcinoma strongly indicates the presence of invasion. If sampling of the lesion is adequate, the degree of these tendencies closely reflects the degree of invasion, whether microinvasion, early invasion, or classic invasive disease. Multiple and adequate histologic sectioning of tissue is then required to rule out invasion or to determine its extent. It should be pointed out again, however, that if only cells from dysplasia are present in a patient's smear, it does *not* rule out in situ carcinoma; further, if only cells from dysplasia and in situ carcinoma are present this does *not* rule out the presence of invasive cancer. Small areas are easily missed in obtaining cellular samples, as in tissue samples, and the more severe lesion may not be represented in the cellular population available for examination.

Experience has shown, however, that with adequate cellular samples there is over 80 per cent correlation. Thus, the most advanced lesion represented on the cellular spread will be the most advanced lesion histologically demonstrable. Accuracy of this correlation is directly proportional to the *adequacy* and *interpretation* of both *cellular* and *tissue* samples. The clinical preparation of an adequate and satisfactory specimen is thus of fundamental importance. With proper material (see The Clinical Specimen, pp. 776–778) and interpretation, detection of these early endocervical lesions is well over 95 per cent.

Invasive Squamous Cell Carcinoma of the Cervix

The cellular population of invasive squamous cell carcinoma is characteristically different from that of in situ carcinoma or of the questionable shades of gray lesions. When invasive squamous cell carcinoma is present, the cells that are shed have the sharp, irregular, jagged criteria of malignancy (Figs. 34–1 *D*, 5*E*, and 34–39).

In their *nuclei*, the chromatin is in massive, angular, and irregular clumps. It is abnormally distributed leaving large cleared areas of nuclear sap. Further, there is marked clumping of the chromatinic rim upon the inner surface of an irregular nuclear membrane. This jagged chromatin clumping (Fig. 34–37) is distinctly different from the granular chromatin configurations of the dyskaryotic cell nucleus (Fig. 34–32) and the in situ carcinoma cell nucleus (Fig. 34–44). Further, the nuclei of invasive squamous cell carcinoma lose their round uniformity and become elongated or bizarre in outline.

Strikingly, the *cytoplasm* of cells shed from invasive squamous cell carcinoma show more squamous maturation than that of in situ carcinoma cells. Bizarre and asymmetric shapes are formed (tadpole, spindle) (Figs. 34–39, 34–40, and 34–41), and there is extreme thinning of the cytoplasm. Stratification of the cells, a tendency for squamous epithelium in its maturation process, is reflected as pearls (Fig. 34–1 *D* and 34–43). Keratinization of the cytoplasm is reflected as hyalinization, extreme orangophilia (Fig. 34–1 *D*), the formation of ecto-endoplasm, and the formation of ectoplasmic rings. (See Differentiation Characteristics, pp. 748–753.)

When most of the cells shed from invasive squamous cell carcinoma have abundant asymmetric cytoplasm showing extreme maturation, Wentz and Reagan's classification refers to this as large-cell keratinizing carcinoma. When the cell type has more uniform, symmetric, and abundant cytoplasm with only minimal attempts at squamous cell maturation, this is referred to as large-cell nonkeratinizing carcinoma. When the cytoplasm is scanty and wispy with no squamous cell maturation, and yet the nuclear criteria are those of invasive carcinoma (Fig. 34–54) rather than in situ carcinoma (Fig. 34–44), this is classified as small-cell nonkeratinizing carcinoma. The last has, by far, the poorest prognosis; of the first two, the second bears somewhat better chances for survival).

Adenocarcinoma of the Endocervix

In addition to having adenocarcinoma features, this lesion frequently exhibits additional features indicating its endocervical cell of origin (see p. 721). It tends to have more abundant cytoplasm (Fig. 34–52) which may appear lavender and textured, and frequently forms good epithelial luminal borders not necessarily associated with acinar or polypoid formation. This cytoplasm is extremely soft and easily destroyed; thus, there is a distinct tendency for these

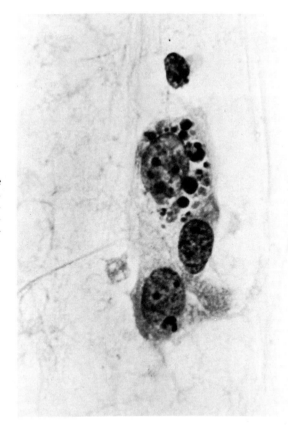

Figure 34–52. Adenocarcinoma of endocervix. Three cells shed from an adenocarcinoma of the endocervix. Note the abundant cytoplasm and large vesicular nuclei. Many neutrophils have invaded the cytoplasm of one cell. ×1200. (Cellular specimen courtesy of Leopold G. Koss, 1961 Seminar, American Society of Cytology.)

cells to appear as degenerated bare nuclei matting together in clusters in striking absence of significant inflammation.

It may be difficult to distinguish cells shed from the very "early" or well-differentiated endocervical adenocarcinomas from the extremely reactive endocervical cells resulting from reparative atypia. Either can have prominent nucleoli, but in the former they can vary significantly in number. Reparative atypias are shed within a background of severe cervicitis; the early neoplasm may have none.

Carcinomas of the cervix having both a squamous cell carcinoma and an adenocarcinoma pattern are not rare, and may shed both cell types. Usually, however, only one cell type is diagnostic of cancer.

Ionizing Irradiation

Ionizing irradiation causes tissue *damage* of a general nature, tissue *changes* of a peculiar host-reaction significance, and dyskaryotic changes of repair and of dysplasia. The damage ranges from changes that are mild and reversible to those that are severe and

irreversible, leading to death of the tissues. It evokes a general inflammatory response with leukocytic and fluid outpouring, which is reflected in the vaginal pool spread as a nonspecific acute inflammation. Graham demonstrated that certain characteristic alterations in the exfoliated nonmalignant cells in patients receiving radiation therapy heralded the body's ability or inability to handle the tumor with eventual survival or death. As a result of ionizing irradiation, cells in exfoliated material show alterations varying with time. They appear more rapidly following radium application and supervoltage irradiation than with conventional x-ray therapy, but all are basically the same.

Cytoplasmic changes are the most significant. Within the first or second week of x-ray therapy small *vacuoles* occur within the cytoplasm (Fig. 34–53). At the same time, *swelling* begins in both the cytoplasm and the nucleus. As they increase in size, both the cytoplasm and the nucleus retain approximately the same amount of chromasia as in the nonirradiated state; therefore, this appears not to be a simple imbibition of water from an injured cell, but to represent actual

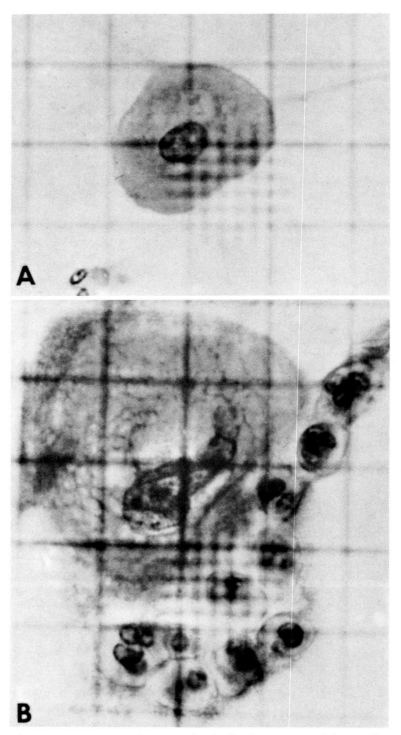

Figure 34–53. Radiation response in nonmalignant parabasal cells of squamous epithelium. *A, B,* Vaginal smears of the same patient treated for squamous cell carcinoma, taken at the same magnification. ×100. *A,* Untreated parabasal cell of normal size and shape. Inconspicuous cytoplasmic vacuolation is present. *B,* Same type of parabasal cell following external irradiation therapy. The cytoplasm and nucleus have both swollen but are not pale. The cytoplasm is vacuolated and there is a small perinuclear halo. The nucleus is distorted, with a fold in the nuclear envelope extending lengthwise in the upper left of the nucleus. There is chromatin clumping within the nucleus and about the membrane. Neutrophils also have swollen. Papanicolaou stain.

increase in cellular protein. Vacuolation and swelling are usually among the first changes to appear during therapy and among the last to disappear after its completion. These cellular changes are frequently present many years after therapy.

Nuclear abnormalities also appear, including folding (Fig. 34–53 B) and wrinkling of the chromatinic rim, multinucleation, hyperchromasia, and chromatin clumping. In the superficial cell, because of karyopyknosis, multinucleation is the only nuclear abnormality which can be detected.

Perinuclear halos appear in approximately the second week. In contradistinction to the perinuclear halos associated with cellular irritation (Figs. 34–23 B, 34–24 B, and 34–25 A), these at times reach gigantic proportions and contain a golden-brown material. In the second or third week, peculiar lavender fibrils appear within the cytoplasm. These disappear completely within a few weeks. Nonspecific inflammation also increases, with accompanying cellular degeneration.

The highest number of cells demonstrate this radiation response usually approximately two weeks following radium application or around the last day of external irradiation therapy.

Recurring Carcinoma of the Cervix

Following radiotherapy, many bizarre cellular changes are present in the normal cells as well as cancer cells (see Ionizing Irradiation). Because of this, elongated degenerated nonmalignant cells can be produced and confused, by the unwary, with malignant tadpole and spindle cells. The nuclei of benign cells following radiation can be very large and at times hyperchromatic, with chromatin irregularity. These changes must be viewed with caution, and critically evaluated as to whether they represent true criteria or are cellular changes from irradiation. It is best to find poorly differentiated or undifferentiated carcinoma cells before an unequivocal cellular diagnosis is made of malignancy present after irradiation therapy, and to be extremely critical of severe postirradiation dyskaryotic changes. Inflammation, infection (particularly *Trichomonas*) and atrophic vaginitis markedly complicate and obscure interpretation. Their removal clinically will greatly help clarify cytologic, as well as histologic, diagnosis. Postirradia-

tion repair can be long and severe, with prominent nucleoli found in markedly reactive cells.

A treacherous cell type which frequently recurs after radiation therapy is the small-cell undifferentiated carcinoma cell. This can appear disarmingly as a moderately small bizarre histiocyte. The nuclear criteria of malignancy indicate its true character as does its high nucleo-cytoplasmic ratio (Fig. 34–54). Further, the nuclei of histiocytes tend to be somewhat eccentric and to just touch, or "tick," the cellular border (Fig. 34–21); the nuclei of recurring small carcinoma cells, however, tend to be centrally placed and to "hug" the cytoplasmic border in extremely close association. The criteria of the nuclei still remain the most potent method of recognizing the true identity of these cells.

When cervical carcinoma recurs in the lumen of the genital tract, it is detected cytologically in a high percentage of cases, provided sufficient and proper cellular specimens are examined. Frequently cellular detection occurs before there is gross evidence of intravaginal recurrence. Extraluminal recurrence does not shed vaginally, of course; but there may be a persisting severe epithelial dysplasia accompanying it, which serves to alert one of its possibility. A continued shift of the Maturation Index to the right with a high Cornification Index, rather than the expected teleatrophic shift following the radiotherapy, has been associated by Wachtel with a high rate of recurrence, both intra- and extravaginally.

Recurrences are usually of the original histologic variety or of the small-cell undifferentiated type. Occasionally in situ carcinoma occurs years after fully treated invasive carcinoma, reactivating the question of recurrence *vs.* second primary. Epithelial damage from radiotherapy may produce a postradiation dysplasia of long standing and persistence, which must be carefully followed to detect a developing neoplasm.

Pregnancy Considerations in Cervical Lesions

Atypical tissue and cellular changes associated with pregnancy do *not* differ basically from those found in the nonpregnant state. There is growing evidence that their *biolo-*

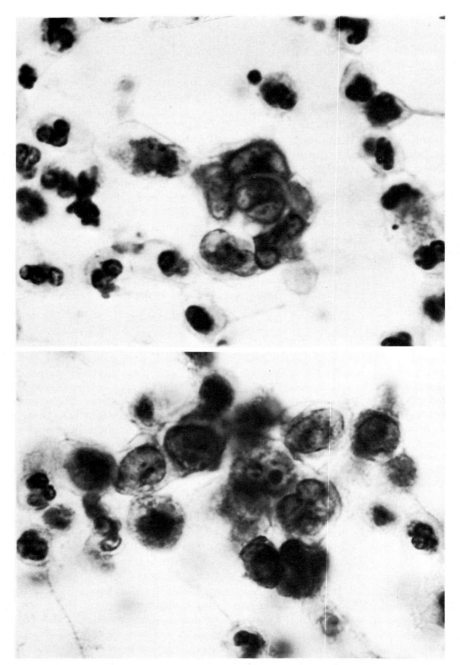

Figure 34–54. Small cell anaplastic carcinoma from postirradiation recurring squamous cell carcinoma. These small undifferentiated cells approximate the size of medium or small histiocytes. Their nuclei tend to be more centrally placed, however, and to "hug" the cell border rather than just touch it at one spot, as do histiocytes. Note good malignant criteria within the nuclei. ×1500.

gic behavior may be accelerated by pregnancy, and their degree of *frequency* as well as *severity* in the younger age group is greater in the pregnant than in the nonpregnant woman. The shades of gray lesions frequently increase in severity during each pregnancy. As a rule, they recede afterwards even though regression is usually incomplete. Thus, in subsequent pregnancies these lesions tend to start at a higher plane of activity than in the preceding gestations. A patient known to have a doubtful lesion in one pregnancy should be carefully studied at each subsequent periodic examination.

The ideal time for a routine cytologic examination of the pregnant patient is the *first* prenatal visit. If peculiar cell changes are noted and a lesion is present which needs clarification, there is still time for the indicated diagnostic procedures and therapy to be carried out. Infection, with cellular degeneration and obscuring, increases as pregnancy progresses, and is frequently severe in postpartum cervical healing. Furthermore, at the six weeks postpartum visit, reparative changes may complicate the cellular interpretations.

Although the average age of pregnant patients is less than the average age of patients having cervical cancer, the incidence of cervical cancer is much greater in the pregnant patient than in the nonpregnant patient of the same age. The age of incidence of cervical carcinoma is lower in the pregnant group. The youngest patient I have seen with invasive cervical carcinoma was a *16 year old pregnant girl, who, in spite of intensive and complete therapy* begun immediately upon cytologic and tissue diagnoses, died 2 years later of her disease.

Of the pregnant patients seen at the Johns Hopkins Hospital both privately and in clinic, 4 per cent have had a sufficient degree of cellular abnormality in their routine cytopathologic examination taken during pregnancy to be investigated further. Carcinoma has been proved in 3.5 per thousand of these pregnant patients, 40 per cent of these lesions being invasive. Increased cancer risk appears to be associated with coitus, especially early in life and with many partners, rather than pregnancy.

Clinical Specimen: Cervical Lesions

Early carcinoma of the cervix is detected in approximately 97 per cent of cases by examining material scraped directly from the squamocolumnar junction within the *endocervical canal* (not only ectocervical) and by endocervical aspiration. When vaginal pool material is examined, the detection of cervical cancer is reduced to 90 per cent, but cytohormonal evaluation becomes possible and detection of endometrial and ovarian neoplasms is increased. For this reason, an adequate *pan*cervical scraping (ectocervical and high endocervical) and vaginal pool specimens are the components of the single slide

Fast smear (Fig. 34–56) used as a routine examination specimen.

LESIONS OF THE VULVA AND VAGINA

Clinical detection of vulvar and vaginal lesions usually follows a thorough pelvic examination and diagnosis is easily confirmed by tissue studies, unless the lesion is small and inconspicuous or is hidden in a fold. Cellular examination is of value in these cases which would otherwise necessitate numerous multiple biopsies (Fig. 34–28).

Leukoplakia

The clinical term leukoplakia or white patch, is a clinical term describing the color of the lesion relative to the color of the epithelium surrounding the area in question. In the cornified squamous epithelium of the *vulva*, in which a keratin layer is normal, leukoplakia is produced by hyperkeratosis. In the noncornified squamous epithelium of the *vagina*, in which keratinization is abnormal, the mere formation of a cornified layer results in leukoplakia. These both exfoliate anucleate superficial cells with keratinized hyaline cytoplasm.

In the delicate columnar epithelium of the *endocervix* and *endometrium*, areas of metaplastic noncornified squamous epithelium offer sufficient contrast to present clinically as leukoplakia. Yet these lesions shed normal nucleated squamous cells from simple metaplasia and, when the leukoplakic areas are atypical in their maturation, they shed abnormal dyskaryotic cells. The quality and degree of nuclear changes present in the exfoliated cell make possible the assessment of the degree of atypical changes of the epithelium. Atypias and dysplasias in leukoplakic lesions, thus are detectable by careful examination of adequate and properly obtained cytologic specimens.

In *vulvar leukoplakia*, information differentiating the atrophic from the hypertrophic forms of Taussig can be obtained from cytologic specimens procured after the anucleate horny layer has been removed. The degree of atypical nuclear change varies from area to area, so that adequate lesion sampling is necessary for assessment. Developing carcinomas are detectable if satisfactory cellular specimens are taken from properly selected areas (Fig. 34–28). Diagnostic cells from these vulvar lesions usually do not exfoliate into the vaginal pool, so that direct scraping of the lesion is usually necessary. At times bizarre, dyskaryotic cells are present in the vaginal pool.

Vaginal leukoplakia, on the other hand, usually exfoliates cells into the vaginal pool in quantities which are sufficient for detection; at times, however, direct smears are necessary to obtain a rich cellular specimen for careful evaluation and diagnosis. Again, the most severe cellular changes observed establish the most serious diagnosis to be made on the specimen; however, they do not rule out the presence of more severe lesions in areas not represented in the cellular samples examined. As in the cervix, the various questionable shades of gray epithelial lesions and the carcinomas frequently occur together.

Lack of cytologic evidence of carcinoma does *not* rule out its presence, any more than do tissue studies—adequacy of sampling is basic. Cytologic studies supplement and complement tissue studies, but do not replace them.

Kraurosis Vulvae

In spite of the severe atrophy of the epithelium and the underlying tissues found in the pure form of kraurosis vulvae, there is exfoliation of relatively normal mature squamous cells. When epithelial hyperactivity or atypicality occurs in kraurosis vulvae, the changes are reflected in the exfoliated cells. As with lesions of the cervix uteri, the degree of this dyskaryotic change is helpful in assessing the lesion's potential biologic behavior. Cytohormonal evaluation of vaginal pool material of patients with kraurosis vulvae usually reveals teleatrophy (Fig. 34–11) with no cellular maturation of the vaginal epithelium past the stage of the immature parabasal cell (M.I.: $\overline{100/0/0}$). Frequently there is inflammation which complicates the picture by obscuring and by cellular degeneration.

Urethral Caruncle

The angiomatous and granulomatous variety of caruncles exfoliate no significant abnormal epithelial cell when the covering epithelium is normal. When the overlying epithelium is reactive, metaplastic, or atypical, as with many papillomatous varieties, the change is reflected in the type and degree of dyskaryosis present in the exfoliated cells. A vaginal pool smear may reveal changes, but a satisfactory cellular scraping may be necessary for proper evaluation.

Papillomas

True epithelial papillomas or developmental tags are covered with, and exfoliate, normal mature squamous cells. Condyloma acuminatum (vulvar, vaginal, cervical), however, sheds mild to moderate dyskaryotic cells, frequently with nonspecific koilocytosis, a perinuclear cytoplasmic clearing of the cytoplasm.

Cancer

Squamous cell carcinoma of the vagina and vulva (Fig. 34–28) is the most frequent lesion. More highly keratinized than most cervical lesions, they otherwise yield the same findings (p. 748), and undergo a similar progression through atypia, in situ, and invasive carcinoma (p. 753).

Of recent years, adenocarcinoma of the vagina has been seen in young women more frequently, which is usually of a clear cell pattern, but frequently mesonephric (Fig. 34–55). It is usually associated with diethylstilbestrol therapy to the mother around 20 years before, during her gestation, but is not restricted thereto. Its cytologic features are basically those of adenocarcinoma (p. 753). At times it presents with a mesonephric pattern, the individual cells having abundant cytoplasm and presenting a hobnailed outer appearance to fragments of tissue exfoliated.

Adenosis vaginae is also more common in these young women a score of years after their mother's stilbestrol treatment. When the lesion is properly scraped, it sheds mature columnar cells resembling endocervical cells of varying degrees of activity from normalcy through atypia, depending upon the activity of the lesion.

Squamous metaplasia occurs frequently in this stilbestrol adenosis. It runs the gamut of atypia found in the cervix, including reported cases of carcinoma (pp. 748–753).

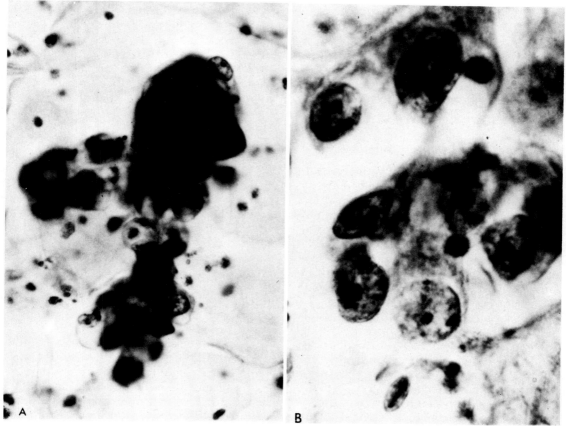

Figure 34–55. Clear cell adenocarcinoma of the vagina. Age 18 years. *A,* The high estrogenic effect in the Maturation Index and clean background are consistent with patient's age. There is a mesonephric hobnail pattern to the cells about the edge of the tumor fragment. ×540. *B,* Nuclear detail of malignancy with abundant clear cytoplasm and secretory activity. Papanicolaou stain. ×1000.

Clinical Specimen: Vulvar and Vaginal Lesions

Depending upon the site of the lesion, either a vaginal pool (p. 777) or a direct scraping (p. 778) is the procedure of choice. A direct scraping of a leukoplakic or condylomatous lesion may be necessary to insure proper cellular representation, due to the highly keratinized surface. Such a specimen is an adjunct to surgical biopsies and compensates for the patchy nature of these biopsies.

LESIONS OF THE ENDOMETRIUM

To properly assess cellular material for lesions of the endometrium, one must evaluate the *general cellular* pattern, the *cytohormonal* pattern, and the pattern of *specific cells* encountered.

The General Cellular Pattern

Bleeding is a frequent occurrence with endometrial lesions. It is fairly well mixed with the cellular specimen, however, not merely in the endocervical portion as with traumatic cervical scrapings. A bloody smear may not be entirely satisfactory and may have to be repeated. Obtaining a cellular specimen should never be postponed, however, merely because the patient is or seems to be menstruating. Many times the bloody smear is the only specimen which will contain diagnostic cells. It is thus well worth the possibility of an occasionally unsatisfactory specimen to obtain smears even during bleeding.

Many *histiocytes* and neutrophils are usually present in neoplastic lesions of the endometrium. Endometritis and pyometra also shed these two cell types in necrotic debris, which may mask an underlying adenocarcinoma.

The Cytohormonal Pattern Relationship

An evaluation of the cytohormonal pattern in the postmenopausal individual is essential to detecting some early preclinical and curable lesions and to a critical understanding and interpretation of many cells resembling endometrial cells. Atypical hyperplasia and early adenocarcinoma of the endometrium are rarely associated with teleatrophy (M.I.: $\frac{}{100/0/0}$) even in the very aged, but show some estrogenic effect.

In postmenopausal women, especially after age 65, superficial cells from the vaginal wall make up less than 10 per cent in the absence of inflammation. Significantly frequently with endometrial hyperplasia and adenocarcinoma, the associated cytohormonal pattern is sufficiently bizarre for the Maturation Index to fall to the right of normal with 10 to 40 per cent superficial cells (Fig. 34–48). If the examiner is aware of its significance, the finding of an abnormal cytohormonal pattern for the age and history of the patient, using vaginal pool material or lateral vaginal wall scraping (*not* cervical scraping), can account for an additional 15 per cent detection of endometrial lesions. It is thus essential that the expected normal variation of the cytohormonal pattern be known for the specific patient under consideration (Fig. 34–4).

The Appearance of Endometrial Cells

Normal endometrial cells shed into the vaginal pool at the time of menstruation appear different from those dislodged directly into the endometrial cavity at varying times in the menstrual cycle and collected by various techniques (aspirate, brush, lavage, helix).

Vaginal Pool Material. The endometrial epithelial cell normally encountered in the vaginal pool material is the "exhausted" and degenerating cell of menstruation. The finding of endometrial-type cells at a time of the cycle other than during the menses and a few days thereafter is abnormal. Degenerated endometrial cells can be present in vaginal material even three or four days after clinical bleeding stops. In the luteal phase of the cycle, however, the presence of endometrial-type cells is distinctly abnormal. Endometrial cells present after the eighth to eleventh day of the period (depending upon age) should be thoroughly investigated.

The cytologic distinction between some degenerated or atypical endometrial cells, "active" histiocytes, distorted endocervical cells, cells from endometrial hyperplasia, and adenocarcinoma cells can be very difficult at times. The use of the term "endometrial-type" cell denotes a group of cells the individuals of which are frequently morphologically separated only with great difficulty. At times this reflects a poor state of preservation, which is due to the long journey down the canal and the bloody fluid in which they sit, as well as a basic difficulty in cytologic and histologic differentiation.

Atypical endometrial cells are shed out of cycle in delayed shedding, endometrial polyps, Arias-Stella reaction, endometrial hyperplasia, and even adenocarcinoma; the lesion present, therefore, should be identified by further study. Some early preclinical adenocarcinoma sheds cells indistinguishable from extremely active histiocytes (Fig. 34–48). *At least* a repeat smear in the late luteal phase should be considered, and preferably also an endometrial cavity sampling (aspiration, brush, lavage, helix), all of which are office procedures. *Dilatation and curettage* should also be considered if clinically or cytologically indicated, and the whole case reevaluated in the light of the new material.

No cytologic procedure should ever keep the physician from performing a dilatation and curettage or other tissue studies if there are clinical indications for them. A negative cytologic report is *not* absolute, but provides additional office-obtained material which frequently provides valuable information.

Endometrial Cavity Material. Endometrial cells in material obtained directly from the endometrial cavity by *aspiration, brush, lavage,* or *helix*) can appear quite different according to the phase of the cycle. In the *proliferative* phase, nuclei are large and hyperchromatic with moderately coarse chromatin granules. The cytoplasm is abundant and frequently the cells resemble sheets of active endocervical cells.

In the *secretory* phase the nuclei become round and seek the tail end of the cell. The luminal end frequently has multiple vacuoles of secretion resembling the picket-fence type of cervical epithelium. In the late secretory and menstrual phases, the cytoplasm becomes extremely scanty and frayed as the cell appears exhausted. Normally, hyperdistended secretory-type vacuoles (Fig. 34–18) are infrequent.

Swiss-cheese hyperplasia sheds sheets of cells resembling those of the proliferative phase. It usually does not shed cells out of cycle into the vaginal pool unless polyps are present.

Adenomatous atypical hyperplasia sheds cells which are markedly proliferative, or proplastic. Cells shed from this lesion into the vaginal pool can be very alarming. At times considerable nuclear hyperchromasia and molding are present, but criteria sufficient for the diagnosis of cancer are lacking. Cytoplasm is moderately abundant and large, hyperdistended, secretory-type single vacuoles are frequently present (Fig. 34–18) at times containing numerous well-preserved phagocytosing neutrophils. Endometrial cells with these single, hyperdistended, secretory-type vacuoles are suggestive of hyperplasia. Although hyperplasia does not show normal secretory activity in tissue examination, this abnormal hyperdistended secretion is not uncommon.

Intrauterine Contraceptive Devices

In the presence of an intrauterine contraceptive device, markedly reactive endometrial cells and tissue fragments can shed, closely mimicking severe hyperplasia or even suggesting adenocarcinoma. A second type of atypical cell shed in the presence of an IUD is small and round with a thin scanty rim of cytoplasm, resembling severe dysplasia of the cervix. With prolonged use of the device, there is an increased incidence of actinomycetes (Fig. 34–29 *A,B*) and entamoeba (Fig. 34–30 *E*) detectable cytologically.

Endometrial Adenocarcinoma

Advanced adenocarcinoma of the endometrium is cytologically typical of adenocarcinoma. First, the cells are cancerous, by virtue of evaluating their malignant criteria; second, they are secretory cells forming acini and polyps. At times they are purely large-cell undifferentiated carcinoma cells (Fig. 34–45). It is not unusual, however, to find hyperdistended secretory-type vacuoles as found in hyperplasia with many well-preserved phagocytosing neutrophils packed within a single vacuole (Figs. 34–45 and 34–46). Frequently the endometrial adenocarcinoma cells are in a poor state of preservation, making the differentiation from normal endometrial cells or cells from hyperplasia extremely difficult.

Endometrial cavity sampling (aspiration, brush, lavage, helix) is extremely valuable in the diagnosis of this lesion, yielding over 95 per cent detection.

The abnormal cytohormonal pattern associated with adenocarcinoma, that of excessive estrogenic stimulation for the age of the patient, is variable but is a most helpful finding in the aged. It is of relatively little value in the woman during the childbearing age because of the normally high estrogenic level at that time in life, or in those women taking estrogens.

Early adenocarcinoma of the endometrium is frequently found with the cytohormonal pattern shifted to the right for the age of the patient (Fig. 34–48 *A*). At times small cellular clumps are shed which show individual cell secretion as well as acinar formation. Although some hyperdistended single vacuole type of secretion occurs, it is more frequent in the early lesions for the vacuolation to be multiple and occur in abundant cytoplasm (Fig. 34–48 *B*). The large and vesicular nuclei are frequently central or minimally eccentric. The abundant cytoplasm is symmetrically arranged about the nuclei and frequently has a sharp cytoplasmic border (Fig. 34–48 *C*). These single cells resemble histiocytes or, at times, immature or moderately mature dyskaryotic cells. A thin rim of cytoplasm about the outer borders of the cell is at times devoid of the "textured" appearance, giving an impression of a different type of cytoplasm. This somewhat resembles the ectoplasm of a hyalinizing squamous cell, from which it must be distinguished. This peculiar cytoplasmic border is not truly glassy nor are there concentric rings or other indications of keratinization.

It is to be remembered that these early lesions of the endometrium are frequently minute and focal. Many sections may be necessary to demonstrate them and, unless great care is taken, they may be entirely missed in routine histologic examination. But these early lesions represent the best chance for cure and, if not detected cytologically, many go undetected until they develop into classic, symptomatic late adenocarcinoma.

Squamous Cell Carcinoma of the Endometrium and Multiphasic Patterns

The rare squamous cell carcinoma of the endometrium sheds cells typical of squamous cell carcinoma (Fig. 34–1 *D*, 34–39, and 34–40). They are not associated with an abnormal cytohormonal pattern, and have no cytologic characteristics differing from the squamous carcinomas primary in the cervix.

Mixtures of squamous and columnar maturation characteristics occur in adenocarcinoma of the uterus with metaplasia, resulting in adenoacanthoma. This adenocarcinoma is usually of a Grade I or II histologically and cytologically. Cytologically, these are basically adenocarcinoma cells with dyskaryotic squamous component cells lacking in sufficient criteria to be unequivocally diagnostic of squamous cell carcinoma. When this cytologic pattern is present, therefore, one should be alerted first for cervical dysplastic lesions associated with adenocarcinoma of the endometrium before establishing a diagnosis of adenoacanthoma on exfoliated cellular material.

When both columnar and squamous cells are unequivocally malignant, the cytologic diagnosis of a tumor of mixed type is possible. The adenocarcinoma component of this type is usually of Grade III or IV.

Miscellaneous Uterine Lesions

At times *endometriosis* and *myomas* are each found in a peculiar cytohormonal pattern, with the Maturation Index shifted to the right of the expected normal for that patient. *No* specific pattern is found with these lesions, however, and most of the cases fall well within normal limits.

Leiomyosarcomas, *rhabdomyosarcomas*, *mixed mesodermal sarcomas*, and *carcinosarcomas* may shed diagnostic cells into the vaginal pool (Fig. 34–50). Necrosis and cellular breakdown are usually severe with sarcomas. As a result, cytologic pick-up and diagnosis are discouraging unless the cervix or vaginal vault is involved to allow for scraping of the surface of the lesion. Cells shed from sarcomas are mainly poorly differentiated. Their nuclear criteria may be excellent, whereas their cytoplasmic borders are usually very indistinct. Rarely, their cell type can be identified by demonstrating fat, myofibrils, cross striations, etc. (Fig. 34–50).

Clinical Specimen; Endometrial Lesions

Cervical scraping yields poor detection of endometrial carcinoma, as opposed to its high rate of detection of cervical carcinoma. For detection of endometrial lesions the vaginal pool specimens are the best available for routine cellular examinations. They contain identifiable cells in 75 per cent of cases (Fig. 34–45) and yield an abnormal cytohormonal pattern in an additional 15 per cent. Endocervical canal aspirations are valuable. The vaginal pool specimen is a component of the single slide Fast vaginal-pancervical combined smear used as a *routine* examination specimen (see Fig. 34–56).

Endometrial aspiration, brush, lavage, or helix yields a higher detection rate of endometrial lesions (over 97 per cent). They are sufficiently more difficult and time consuming and take expertise and experience to reduce the unsatisfactory rate, so that they are not yet accepted at this time as *routine* cancer detection procedures by the average clinician and pathologist. In addition, they require an aspirating cannula, a brush, or other instrument, which must be thoroughly cleansed and sterilized after every use, or which is disposable. This *office* endometrial cavity sampling procedure, however, is economical, convenient for more adequate cell sampling, and has high patient acceptance. Yet it should *not* replace a dilatation and curettage whenever that procedure is indicated clinically. Before its use, intrauterine pregnancy must be excluded.

LESIONS OF THE PLACENTA, TUBES, AND OVARIES

Placenta

While not frequent, trophoblasts can be present in vaginal pool specimens without indicating abnormality, especially during the first trimester. Their presence may indicate a low-lying placenta or a threatened abortion. They can be present with hydatidiform mole, but cytology is of unpredictable assistance in predicting the grade of a mole or the presence of a choriocarcinoma, especially for detecting recurrence. When the latter involves the genital lumen, exfoliated cells can be diagnostic of cancer and, at times, differentiate into malignant syncytial trophoblasts and cytotrophoblasts. Benign syncytial trophoblasts have multiple, large, bland nuclei molding markedly in a moderately abundant cytoplasm. Cells shed from herpes simplex infection (Fig. 34–27A) have been misdiagnosed as synctial trophoblasts; but the former are more degenerated, and the latter have more cytoplasm and lack inclusions.

The presence of decidual cells may be suspected, but is difficult to diagnose with certainty. Their centrally placed nuclei closely resemble moderately mature dyskaryotic cells, but their chromatin pattern is usually bland and their cellular borders indistinct.

Fallopian Tubes

The infrequent adenocarcinoma of the tubes sheds diagnostic cells into the endometrial cavity and the vaginal pool. This lesion is usually not associated with teleatrophy, and may even have an abnormal Maturation Index shifted to the right in women past the menopause. Unexplained adenocarcinoma cells in vaginal or cervical material with an abnormal cytohormonal pattern should stimulate consideration of this lesion. These cells can be present in endometrial cavity office preparations (e.g., aspiration, brush, lavage, helix).

Ovaries

There are four major areas in the cytopathologic consideration of ovarian lesions: lesions *known to produce hormones*, lesions with which *hormone production is classically not associated*, *specific cells* shed from the ovarian lesion, and cells shed from an associated *hyperplastic endometrium*.

Hormone-producing tumors of the ovary display their presence by the cytohormonal pattern characteristic for the endocrine substances being secreted (pp. 709–710). Thus, the granulosa cell tumor shifts the Maturation Index to the right (toward $\overline{0/0/100}$), the degree of shift depending upon the amount and biologic activity of the produced circulating estrogens and upon the age of the patient, with cells lying flat and singly. Luteinized

mesenchymal tumors producing progesterone or cortisone shift the Maturation Index toward the midzone (toward $\overrightarrow{0/100/0}\overleftarrow{}$), with cell curling and sticking. If estrogens are also secreted, the cytohormonal pattern is mixed between the two types, and may even mimic pregnancy if estrogen and progesterone are in correct proportion. Hilus cell tumors and arrhenoblastomas show the Maturation Index pattern of androgens if the level and potency of the hormones are sufficient. Unless malignant and metastatic, these hormone-producing tumors of the ovary do *not* shed diagnostic cells into the vaginal pool, the abnormal cytohormonal pattern being all that is present.

Where *hormone production is classically not associated*, certain lesions of the ovary are still found in cytohormonal patterns *other than* teleatrophy (M.I.: $\overline{100/0/0}$) (Fig. 34–11) regardless of age. About one half of the solid and cystic adenomas, adenocarcinomas, and metastatic tumors to the ovary are associated with a Maturation Index shifted to the right sufficiently to be abnormal for the age (Figs. 34–12 and 34–47) if no hormonal therapy or inflammation is present to interfere with it. There is evidence that the ovarian stromal hyperplasia, frequently associated with such nonfunctional ovarian tumors, may be a factor in this abnormal pattern, or that there may be increased end-organ sensitivity.

Specific cells shed from ovarian tumors into the endometrial and vaginal pool materials can at times identify the lesion of origin (Fig. 34–12). These are mainly papillary adenocarcinomas of the ovary of both the cystic and solid varieties. The identification of papillary fronds (Fig. 34–47) or of psammoma bodies (Fig. 34–49) is very suggestive of ovarian origin. In addition, single hyperdistended secretory-type vacuoles at times "pouch out" of the tissue fragments; these are frequently filled with neutrophils (Fig. 34–12). The nuclei of ovarian adenocarcinoma cells often contain extremely prominent rounded nucleoli with wide and striking perinucleolar halos. Although psammoma bodies (Fig. 34–49) are highly suggestive of this ovarian lesion, it must be remembered that they are also shed from other lesions including adenocarcinomas of the endometrium and tubes, mesotheliomas, and breast carcinomas. Cells can exfoliate from the tumors into the peritoneal cavity and, finding the lumen of the tubes, travel down to appear in the vaginal pool. However, most of these patients with ovarian cancer cells in the vaginal material do have metastases to the tubes, body of the endometrium, or vagina.

When *endometrial hyperplasia* is associated with ovarian tumors, endometrial cells may shed into the vaginal pool which are atypical, shed out of cycle (i.e., after the tenth day), or postmenopausal. The hope of *early* detection of ovarian lesions appears to rest mainly on finding an abnormal cytohormonal pattern or finding endometrial type cells which are either out of cycle or atypical in appearance on routine vaginal-type specimens, or the acceptance of endometric cavity sampling (aspiration, brush, lavage, helix) as a routine office procedure.

Aspiration of the cul-de-sac is a sensitive method for detecting ovarian lesions, especially asymptomatic latent or recurring tumors. It is not suitable for a routine detection procedure, however.

THE CLINICAL SPECIMEN

Identify the slide with the patient's name to prevent mix-up, by using a lead pencil on a frosted-end slide or a diamond-point pencil on a plain slide.

Fix the material *immediately.* It should never be allowed to dry, even on the exploring instrument (spatula, pipette) or at the edges of the smear before immersing in fixative.

Spread *quickly* and *evenly* a sufficient quantity of material, eliminating thick clumps and blank areas. Pipettes and scrapers tend to spread unevenly unless used very carefully. A cellular spreader rapidly produces a uniform film with all but inspissated material (see Fig. 34–56 *E*). Another good method is the use of the gloved fifth finger (rubber glove or finger cot) wiped free from talc. Two rapid motions along the slide lengthwise result in a uniform smear.

However made, the uniform smear must be fixed immediately. It may be made over an open-mouth jar of fixative so that it can *immediately* be dropped therein (Fig. 34–56 *E,F*). Thus, the specimen is transformed from a thick, well protected, mucoid drop into a fixing, thin, even smear in a fraction of a second.

Fixative recommended is 95 per cent ethyl alcohol. Half ether and half alcohol is very

flammable as well as volatile. Alcohols other than ethyl (isopropyl, methyl) too frequently give cellular preparations inferior to those fixed in ethanol, especially in markedly inflammatory and obscuring specimens which so frequently are present with carcinoma. Ethyl alcohol fixative can be reused over and over, if filtered after every use. Malignant cells can drop off from one slide when placed in fixative and be transferred to another; therefore, specimens from only *one* patient should be placed in the same bottle of fixative. If more than one slide is taken on a given patient, a paper clip placed over the name end of alternate slides holds the cellular spreads apart. The specimen is fixed for at least one-half hour or, preferably, overnight.

Satisfactory variants on this fixative are available. Two to 10 per cent Carbowax gives some physical protection to cells that are air-dried *after* fixation for transport. Dispensed in individual disposable packets, dropper bottles, and aerosol cans, a satisfactory fixative is available for nearly every situation. The two primary factors are still essential: a *proper* fixative, applied *immediately.*

For *transporting* to the laboratory, the slides can be left in the bottle of fixative or can be removed *after* adequate fixation (one half hour, preferably overnight) and then transported in a proper slide holder. Glycerin or other materials are *not* needed. A dried smear remains well preserved indefinitely, if dried *after* proper fixation with *no* drying allowed *before* its immediate fixation.

The Fast Smear (Single Slide, Combined Vaginal-Pancervical) for Routine Specimen Preparation

For *routine* use, this Fast smear (Fig. 34–56) offers a high rate of general gynecologic cancer detection; it is fast and simple to prepare clinically, is rapid and economical to process, and affords an even, abundant cellular spread of both *pan*cervical (e.g., *endo*cervical, *ecto*cervical, and cervical os) and vaginal pool material to be microscopically examined. It offers the same high rate of detection of fundal adenocarcinoma as does the vaginal smear (approximately 90 per cent), and has as high a detection rate as a good pancervical scraping (over 97 per cent) in early squamous cell carcinoma of the cervix.

The *Fast smear* has vaginal pool material

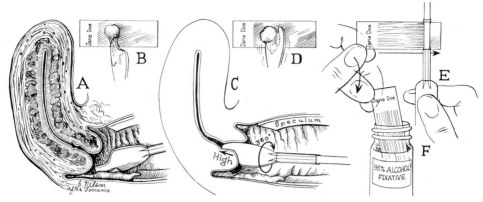

Figure 34–56. Fast combined vaginal-pancervical smear. Identify slide with patient's name. *A,* Posterior vaginal pool mucus is placed upon slide, *B,* without smearing. *C,* Scrape entire cervical os 360 degrees with properly shaped cervical spatula (obtaining a good, high endocervical component) and quickly mix, *D,* with the drop of vaginal mucus on the slide. *E,* Spread with a plastic cell spreader or make two rapid wipes with the gloved fifth finger (not shown) and, *F, immediately* drop into fixative. Specimen from only *one* patient per bottle.

and a pancervical scraping sample mixed on one slide. The *vaginal pool* component provides an accurate hormonal evaluation, a judgment of radiation response, determination of sex, and a high rate of detection of lesions of the endometrium, salpinx, and ovaries. The *pancervical component* gives a high rate of detection of carcinoma of the cervix and its associated lesions. Mixing the pancervical scraping with the vaginal pool material allows the mucus of the latter to protect the pancervical material when it is spread on a slide before fixation. Preservation of material from inflamed cervices, therefore, is better than with a simple cervical scrape smear.

The Fast Smear Technique (Fig. 34–56). (1) Obtain mucus from posterior vaginal pool with spatula and place it as a thick drop upon one side of slide. Do *not* smear. (2) Obtain a pancervical specimen by scraping the endocervical canal, external os, and ectocervix with cervical end of spatula, scraping as *high* as can be reached and completely around the canal (360°). (3) Mix on the slide all of this *pan*cervical scraping material with the vaginal pool drop. (4) Hold slide over *open* bottle of fixative, smear drop with plastic cellular spreader or make two lengthwise *light* strokes of gloved fifth finger (glove or cot). *Immediately* place in fixative.

One should carefully choose the cervical scraper to be of proper configuration for that particular cervix, with the longest thin endocervical tip it will take. Plastic yields a better sample than wood, if its surface has been treated to make it hydrophilic. Cotton-tipped applicators absorb water, producing cell distortion with retention by the cotton and loss to the sample.

Vaginal Pool Smear

Adult. This is excellent for hormonal pattern, radiation response, and fundal cancer detection. It is less valuable than the Fast smear or cervical scraping for detecting early cancer of the cervix. Vaginal pool material from the posterior fornix is obtained by pipette aspiration or spatula and dropped upon the glass slide (previously described Step 1), smeared with a plastic cellular spreader or with the gloved fifth finger and *immediately* dropped into fixative (Step 4). If prepared by the patient for serial cytohormonal evaluations, the pipette can be used to smear the specimen.

Child. This material must *not* be contaminated with cells from the introitus, perineum, or examiner's fingers, because the cytohormonal pattern will be altered. A nasal speculum is introduced into the introitus, or a protective tubing, such as a drinking straw, is used. A nonabsorbent cotton swab (not touched or made with bare fingers) is dipped in physiologic solution or serum, and the excess is expressed. The cotton swab is introduced through the nasal speculum (without touching the introitus) or in its protective tubing, into the posterior fornix, moved laterally gently, and withdrawn. Holding a glass slide over an open bottle of fixative, roll the swab on the slide and *immediately* drop it into the fixative.

Pancervical Scraping Smear

This is excellent for detection of early carcinoma of the cervix but is of very little value in endometrial carcinoma. Cervical scraping material tends to be bloody and to dry very rapidly on the spatula and slide surface. Thus it often gives less satisfactory nuclear preservation than the Fast combined smear. Material from the endocervical canal, external os, and ectocervix is obtained (Fig. 34–56 C, E, F), quickly spread upon a glass slide, and *immediately* placed into fixative.

A moistened, nonabsorbent cotton swab may be used in place of the spatula for an endocervical swab smear. The number of significant cells obtained is decidedly less, however, and their preservation is less satisfactory due to drying from the cotton.

Endocervical Aspiration Smear

Debris and mucus at the site of the external os are gently removed. A plastic or glass pipette with an aspirating bulb attached is gently introduced a few millimeters into the external os. All material present is aspirated. It is withdrawn and all material is blown upon a glass slide, *quickly* spread with a second slide, and both slides are *immediately* immersed in 95 per cent ethyl alcohol.

Endometrial Aspiration Smear

The presence of endometrial *infection* and *pregnancy* must be ruled out. The ectocervix is gently cleansed. A sterile endometrial aspiratory cannula with syringe attached is introduced through the external os and the internal os, into the endometrial cavity where it is halted by the cervical stop provided. The endometrial cavity is then thoroughly aspirated and the cannula is withdrawn. The material is blown upon a glass slide, spread with a second slide, and both are *immediately* immersed in 95 per cent ethyl alcohol.

VCE Smear

VCE designates material from the *v*agina, ecto*c*ervix, and *e*ndocervix. Two wooden spatulas and one moistened nonabsorbent cotton swab are arranged in the examiner's hand, fanwise. The first scrapes the lateral vaginal wall or obtains vaginal pool material, the second scrapes the ectocervix, and the third is gently inserted into the endocervical canal. They are then rapidly smeared in the same succession upon a clean glass slide, side by side—vaginal portion nearest the label, the ectocervical portion next, and the endocervical portion at the end of the slide. The slide is then immersed in fixative.

Owing to even momentary drying before smearing and fixation, cell preservation frequently is not optimal. This technique can give valuable information at times, however, by more closely localizing the site of inflammation and other disease processes.

Vulvar and Vaginal Smears

The best specimens are obtained after the growing margins of the lesions are well soaked with physiologic saline and the necrotic and keratinized debris is removed and discarded. A wooden tongue blade or spatula, or a cotton swab dipped in egg albumin or serum, is then used to abrade the growing margins of the lesion. Collect the cell specimen, spread it onto a slide held over an *open* bottle of fixative, and *immediately* drop it in for fixation.

Buccal Scraping Smears

Clinically, this is the simplest yet most reliable method for determining true chromosomal (somatic) sex. The mouth is opened and the angle drawn laterally with the little finger of the hand holding a clean slide (Fig. 34–57). This reveals the buccal pouch. Gently but firmly a tongue blade is drawn forward a number of times along the upper buccal pouch, *above* and *avoiding* the white dentate line, so that a white milky material is obtained which is rich in cells. While the slide is held over a bottle of fixative, this milky material is quickly spread upon the glass slide and *immediately* dropped into fixative. Spray and dropper fixatives are available commercially which dry rapidly upon the cells giving good preservation. Ninety-five per cent ethyl alcohol is preferred.

CYTOPATHOLOGIC REPORTS AND THEIR INTERPRETATIONS

The disease present and those suspected should be stated in a cytopathology report in

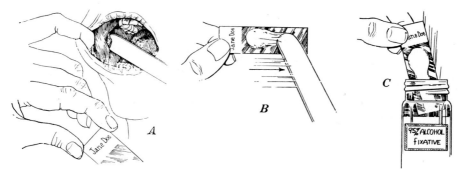

Figure 34–57. Buccal smear. *A,* Draw angle of mouth and cheek laterally, exposing the buccal mucosa of the cheek pouch. Draw a tongue blade forward firmly along the buccal mucosa *above* the white dentate line, being careful to *avoid* the latter, and collect the milky cellular fluid. *B,* Quickly smear onto a glass slide and *C,* immediately drop into fixative.

the same manner and with the same completeness as in a surgical pathology report. It is a consultative report. As such, it represents a liaison of physician to physician. Every effort must be made between pathologist and clinician to make understanding complete and liaison thorough. A shorthand or categorical jargon for snap reports leads to misinterpretation and mishandling of critical patients.

Methods vary widely according to the physician reporting. It is essential that the particular method utilized be thoroughly understood by the clinician. As with most of medicine, not everything in exfoliative cytopathology is as definite as black or white. When shades of gray do exist in disease interpretation, and therefore in clinical handling, the situation must be thoroughly understood and discussed by clinician and pathologist with full understanding of what the significance is for the *given* patient.

Most cases are *negative*, being completely without evidence of cancer. Others contain unequivocal malignant cells, shed from *cancer* and clearly indicating the need for surgical tissue studies.

Between these two extremes in the diagnostic spectrum, there are always *other* cases that are neither clearly free of evidence of cancer nor unequivocally malignant. These cases are inconclusive or equivocal, and their significance is doubtful, but they clearly indicate the necessity for further study of the patient. It is clear, therefore, that regardless of the type of reporting system utilized, complete understanding of the significance of cellular findings must be arrived at between pathologist and clinician.

The cellular sample, as in surgical tissue, must be adequate and properly prepared. The consultation requested upon this specimen should be as highly skilled and experienced as is possible to obtain. For a wise and a thorough interpretation, it is mandatory that there be complete understanding of the patient and liaison between the two physicians. This is basic to *all* consultation, and is especially essential to the proper handling of the borderline or questionable lesions. Here, only free and complete exchange of ideas between physicians results in proper diagnosis, therapy, follow-up, and prognosis of the patient.

REFERENCES

Barr, M. L.: Sex chromatin. Science, *130*:1302, 1959.

Bechtold, E., and Reicher, N. B.: The relationship of trichomonas infestations to false diagnoses of squamous carcinoma of the cervix. Cancer, 5:442, 1952.

Berry, A.: Multispecies schistosomal infections of the female genital tract detected in cytology smears. Acta Cytol., *20*:361, 1976.

Bibbo, M., Ali, I., Al-Naqeeb, M., Baccarini, I., Climaco, L. A., Gill, W., Sonex, M., and Wied, G. L.: Cytologic findings in female and male offspring of DES treated mothers. Acta Cytol., *19*:568, 1975.

Bonte, J., Decoster, J. M., and Ide, P.: Vaginal cytologic evaluation as a practical link between hormone blood levels and tumor hormone dependency in exclusive medroxyprogesterone treatment of recurrent or metastatic endometrial adenocarcinoma. Acta Cytol., *21*:218, 1977.

Brewer, J. L., and Guderian, A. M.: Diagnosis of tubal cancer by vaginal cytology. Obstet. Gynecol., 8:664, 1956.

Christ, M. L., and Haja, J.: Cytologic changes associated with vaginal pessary use, with special reference to the presence of Actinomyces. Acta Cytol., *22*:146, 1978.

Christopherson, W. M., and Scott, M. A.: Trends in mortality from uterine cancer in relation to mass screening. Acta Cytol., 21:115, 1977.

Davis, H. J.: Population screening for cancer of the cervix with irrigation smears. Am. J. Obstet. Gynecol., 96:605, 1966.

deBorges, R.: Findings of microfilarial larval stages in gynecologic smears. Acta Cytol., 15:476, 1971.

deMoraes-Ruehsen, M., McNeill, R. E., Frost, J. K., Gupta, P. K., Diamond, L. S., and Honigberg, B. M.: A *gingivalis*-like *Entamoeba* in the genital tract of IUD users. Acta Cytol., 23 (in press).

Fidler, H. K., Boyes, D. A., Auersperg, N., and Lock, D. R.: The cytology program in British Columbia. I. An evaluation of the effectiveness of cytology in the diagnosis of cancer and its application to the detection of carcinoma of the cervix. Can. Med. Assoc. J., 86:779, 1962.

Fluhmann, C. F.: Carcinoma in situ and the transitional zone of the cervix uteri. Obstet. Gynecol., 16:424, 1960.

Fox, H.: Estrogenic activity of the serous cystadenoma of the ovary. Cancer, 18:1041, 1965.

Fraenkel., L., and Papanicolaou, G. N.: Growth desquamation and involution of the vaginal epithelium of fetuses and children with a consideration of the related hormonal factors. Am. J. Anat., 62:427, 1938.

Frost, J. K.: The Cell in Health and Disease. Baltimore: Williams & Wilkins Co., 1969.

Frost, J. K.: *Trichomonas vaginalis* and cervical epithelial changes. Ann. N.Y. Acad. Sci., 97:792, 1962.

Frost, J. K.: Cytologic evaluation of endocrine status and somatic sex. *In* Novak, E. R., Jones, G. S., and Jones, H. W.: Novak's Textbook of Gynecology. 8th ed. Baltimore, Williams & Wilkins Co., 1970.

Frost, J. K.: Gynecologic clinical cytopathology. *In* Novak, E. R., Jones, G. S., and Jones, H. W.: Novak's Textbook of Gynecology. 9th ed. Baltimore, Williams & Wilkins Co., 1975.

Frost, J. K.: Concepts Basic to General Cytopathology. 5th ed. Baltimore, Johns Hopkins Press, 1972.

Frost, J. K.: Cytology of benign conditions. Clin. Obstet. Gynecol., 4:1075, 1961.

Galvin, G. A., Jones, H. W., and TeLinde, R. W.: The significance of basal cell hyperactivity in cervical biopsies. Am. J. Obstet. Gynecol., 70:808, 1955.

Geirsson, G., Woodworth, F. R., Patten, S. F., Jr., and Bonfiglio, T. A.: Epithelial repair and regeneration in the uterine cervix. I. An analysis of the cells. Acta Cytol., 21:371, 1977.

Graham, R. M., Schueller, E. F., and Graham, J. B.: Detection of ovarian cancer at an early stage. Obstet. Gynecol., 26:151, 1965.

Gupta, P. K., Hollander, D. H., and Frost, J. K.: Actinomycetes in cervico-vaginal smears: an association with IUD usage. Acta Cytol., 20:295, 1976.

Hollander, D. H., and Gupta, P. K.: Detached ciliary tufts in cervico-vaginal smears (DCT). Acta Cytol., 18:367, 1974.

Honigberg, B. M.: Comparative pathogenicity of *Trichomonas vaginalis* and *Trichomonas gallinae* to mice. I. Gross pathology, quantitative evaluation, and some factors affecting pathogenicity. J. Parasitol., 47:545, 1961.

Honigberg, B. M., Livingstone, M. F., and Frost, J. K.: Pathogenicity of fresh isolates of *Trichomonas vaginalis*: The mouse assay *vs.* clinical and pathological findings. Acta Cytol., 10:353, 1966.

Howdon, W. M., Howdon, A. K., Frost, J. K., and Woodruff, J. D.: Cyto- and histopathologic correlation in

mixed mesenchymal tumors of the uterus. Am. J. Obstet. Gynecol., 89:670, 1964.

Hypes, R. A., and Ladewig, P. P.: Leukocytic clusters on epithelial cells in cervico-vaginal smears: a presumptive test for Trichomonas infection. Am. J. Clin. Pathol., 26:94, 1956.

Johnston, W. W., Goldston, W. R., and Montgomery, M. S.: Clinicopathologic studies in feminizing tumors of the ovary. III. The role of genital cytology. Acta Cytol., 15:334, 1971.

Jones, H. W., and Wilkins, L.: The genital anomaly associated with prenatal exposure to progestogens. Fertil. Steril., 11:148, 1960.

Kashgarian, M., Erickson, C. C., Dunn, J. E., and Sprunt, D. H.: A survey of public awareness of uterine cytology in Memphis-Shelby county. Acta Cytol., 10:10, 1966.

Kean, B. H., and Day, E.: *Trichomonas vaginalis* infection. An evaluation of three diagnostic techniques with data on incidence. Am. J. Obstet. Gynecol., 68:1510, 1954.

Klaus, H.: Quantitative criteria of folate deficiency in cervicovaginal cytograms, with report of a new parameter. Acta Cytol., 15:50, 1971.

Koss, L. G.: Diagnostic Cytology and Its Histopathologic Bases. 3rd ed. Philadelphia, J. B. Lippincott Company, 1979.

Koss, L. G., and Wolinska, W. H.: *Trichomonas vaginalis* cervicitis and its relationship to cervical cancer. Cancer, 12:1171, 1959.

Lencioni, L. J.: Comparative and statistical study of vaginal and urinary sediment smears. J. Clin. Endocrinol., 13:263, 1953.

Lichtfus, C. J. P.: Vaginal cytology at the end of pregnancy. Acta Cytol., 3:247, 1959.

Luff, R. D., Gupta, P. K., Spence, M. R., and Frost, J. K.: Pelvic actinomycosis and the intrauterine contraceptive device. A ctyo-histomorphologic study. Am. J. Clin. Pathol., 69:5B1, 1978.

MacGregor, J. E., Fraser, M. E., and Mann, E. M. F.: Improved prognosis for cervical cancers due to comprehensive screening. Acta Cytol., 16:14, 1972.

Marsh, M.: Original site of cervical carcinoma. Obstet. Gynecol., 7:444, 1956.

Masukawa, T.: Vaginal smears in women past 40 years of age, with emphasis on their remaining hormonal activity. Obstet. Gynecol., 16:407, 1960.

Masukawa, T., Lewison, E. F., and Frost, J. K.: The cytologic examination of breast secretions. Acta. Cytol., 10:261, 1966.

McKay, D. G., Terjanian, B., Boschyanchinda, D., Younge, P. A., and Hertig, A. T.: Clinical and pathological significance of anaplasia (atypical hyperplasia) of the cervix uteri. Obstet. Gynecol., 13:2, 1959.

McNeil, R. E., and deMoraes-Ruehsen, M.: Ameba trophozoites in cervico-vaginal smear of a patient using an intrauterine device—a case report. Acta Cytol., 22:91, 1978.

Meisels, A., Fortin, R., and Roy, M.: Condylomatous lesions of the cervix. II. Cytologic, colposcopic and histopathologic study. Acta Cytol., 21:379, 1978.

Ng, A. B. P., Reagan, J. W., and Lindner, E. A.: The cellular manifestations of microinvasive squamous cell carcinoma of the uterine cervix. Acta Cytol., 16:5, 1972.

Nytlicek, O.: Vaginal cytology postpartum and during the lactation period. Acta Cytol., 3:271, 1959.

Oriel, J. D., Johnson, A. L., Barlow, D., Thomas, B. J., Nayyar, K., and Reeve, P.: Infection of the uterine cervix with *Chlamydia trachomatis* J. Infect. Dis., *137*:443, 1978.

Papanicolaou, G. N.: Existence of a postmenopause sexual rhythm in women as indicated by the study of vaginal smear. Anat. Rec. (Supp.), *55*:71, 1933.

Papanicolaou, G. N.: Cytology. Harvard Univ. Press, Cambridge, Mass., 1954.

Papanicolaou, G. N., and Traut, H. F.: Diagnosis of Uterine Cancer by the Vaginal Smear. Commonwealth Fund, New York, 1943.

Patten, S. F., Jr.: Diagnostic Cytology of the Uterine Cervix. 2nd Ed. Basel, S. Karger AG, 1978.

Pryzbora, L. A., and Plutowa, A.: Histological topography of carcinoma in situ of the cervix uteri. Cancer, *12*:263, 1959.

Purold, E., and Savia, E.: Cytology of gynecologic condyloma acuminatum. Acta Cytol., *21*:26, 1977.

Rakoff, A. E., Paschkis, K. E., and Cantarow, A.: Clinical Endocrinology. 3rd Ed. New York: Paul B. Hoeber, 1967.

Reagan, J. W., and Ng, A. B. P.: The Cells of Uterine Adenocarcinoma. 2nd Ed. Basel, S. Karger AG, 1973.

Reagan, J. W., and Patten, S. F., Jr.: Dysplasia: A basic reaction to injury in the uterine cervix. Ann. N.Y. Acad. Sci., *97*:662, 1962.

Richart, R. M., and Vaillant, H. W.: Influence of cell collection technique upon cytological diagnosis. Cancer, *18*:1474, 1965.

Riley, G. M., Dontas, E., and Grill, B.: Use of serial vaginal smears in detecting time of ovulation. Fertil. Steril., *6*:86, 1955.

Rubin, D. K., and Frost, J. K.: The cytologic detection of ovarian cancer. Acta Cytol., *7*:191, 1963.

Schacter, J.: Chlamydia infections. New England Jour. Med. *298*:426, 490, 540, 1978.

Schenck, S. B., and Mackles, A.: Primary carcinoma of fallopian tubes with positive smears. Am. J. Obstet. Gynecol., *81*:782, 1961.

Shrago, S. S.: The Arias-Stella reaction. A case report of a cytologic presentation. Acta Cytol., *21*:310, 1977.

Stern, E., and Neeley, P. M.: Carcinoma and dysplasia of the cervix. A comparison of rates for new and returning populations. Acta Cytol., *7*:357, 1963.

Traut, H. F., and Papanicolaou, G. N.: Vaginal smear changes in endometrial hyperplasia and in cervical keratosis. Anat. Rec., *82*:428, 1942.

Varga, A., and Browell, B.: Vital inclusion bodies in vaginal smears. Obstet. Gynecol., *16*:441, 1960.

Van Niekerk, W. A.: Cervical cytological abnormalities caused by folic acid deficiency. Acta Cytol., *10*:67, 1966.

von Haam, E.: Some observations in the field of exfoliative cytology. Am. J. Clin. Pathol., *24*:652, 1954.

Wachtel, E.: A simple cytological test for cancer cure. Br. Med. J., *1*:20, 1958.

Wentz, W. B., and Reagan, J. W.: Survival in cervical cancer with respect to cell type. Cancer, *12*:384, 1959.

Wied, G. L.: Importance of the site from which vaginal cytologic smears are taken. Am. J. Clin. Pathol., *25*:742, 1955.

Wied, G. L., Boschann, H.-W., Ferin, J., Frost, J. K., Lukasch, F., Meisels, A., Montalvo-Ruiz, L., Terzano, G., Teter, J., and Wachtel, E.: Symposium on hormonal cytology. Acta Cytol., *12*:87, 1968.

Wood, S., Jr., Halyoke, E. D., and Yardley, J. H.: Mechanisms of metastasis production from blood borne cancer cells. Can. Cancer Conf., Vol. 4, 1961.

World Health Organization: The early detection of cancer. WHO Chronicle, *20*:322, 1966.

INDEX

Page numbers in *italics* indicate illustrations; page numbers followed by "t" indicate tables.

783